VASCULAR INVOLVEMENT IN DIABETES

Clinical, Experimental and Beyond

Editor:

Dan CHEŢA

Assistant Editors:

Bogdan Balaş
Dănuţ Cimponeriu
Cristian Panaite
Radu Şerban Vasilescu

VASCULAR INVOLVEMENT IN DIABETES

Clinical, Experimental and Beyond

Edited by **DAN CHEŢA**

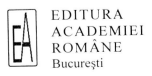

EDITURA
ACADEMIEI
ROMÂNE
Bucureşti

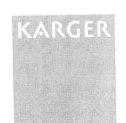

Basel · Freiburg · Paris
London · New York
Bangalore · Bangkok · Singapore
Tokyo · Sydney

A C.I.P. Catalogue record for this book is available from the Library of Congress.

ISBN: 973-27-1120-5

ISBN: 3-8055-7962-4

Published by Editura Academiei Române and S. Karger AG

EDITURA ACADEMIEI ROMÂNE

(THE PUBLISHING HOUSE OF THE ROMANIAN ACADEMY)

Calea 13 Septembrie nr. 13, sector 5

050711, Bucureşti, România

Tel.: +40(0)21 / 411 90 08; Fax. +40(0)21 / 410 39 83

e-mail: edacad@ear.ro

www.ear.ro

S. KARGER AG

P.O. Box

4009 Basel, Switzerland

Tel.: +41(0)61 / 306 11 11; Fax. +41(0)61 / 306 12 34

e-mail: karger@karger.ch

www.karger.com

In all countries, except for Romania and the Republic of Moldavia, sold and distributed by S. Karger AG,
P.O. Box, 4009 Basel, Switzerland

In Romania and the Republic of Moldavia, sold and distributed by Editura Academiei Române
P.O. Box 5–42, 050711, Bucureşti, România

Printed on acid-free paper

Editorial Assistants: OLGA DUMITRU, MONICA STANCIU, DOINA ARGEŞANU, CRISTIANA CHIRIAC

Technical editors: MARIA-MAGDALENA JINDICEANU, LUIZA DOBRIN, RĂZVAN-DAN CURELEŢ

Cover: GIGI GAVRILĂ

Printed in Romania

MOTTO:

If the writer is so cautious that he never writes anything that cannot be criticized, he will never write anything that can be read. If you want to help other people you have got to make up your mind to write things that some men will condemn.

Thomas Merton
(Seeds of contemplation, 1949)

MOTTO:

Diabetes is a state of premature cardiovascular death, which is associated with chronic hyperglycaemia and may also be associated with blindness and renal failure.

Miles Fisher
(Re-definition of diabetes, Dublin 1996)

CONTENTS

VIII

PREFACE

At the beginning of the twentieth century atherosclerotic vascular disease, particularly coronary artery disease, was considered to be an uncommon condition and its pathogenesis was not understood. By the late nineteen fifties it had grown to epidemic proportions in the developed world and it had become clear that hypertension, cigarette smoking and hyperlipidemia were important predisposing factors. In the sixties, diabetes mellitus emerged as an additional important risk factor. Since then we have learned that diabetes and atherosclerosis are closely intertwined in at least four ways. First, patients with type 2 diabetes have an increased likelihood of traditional risk factors for atherosclerosis, such as hypertension and hyperlipidemia. Second, even when these are taken into account, the presence of diabetes confers substantial excess risk for the development of accelerated vascular disease. Third, diabetes mellitus increases markedly the risk of adverse clinical outcomes. For example, when adjusted for age and gender, diabetics with acute coronary syndromes have twice the mortality of non-diabetics. Fourthly, the prevalence of diabetes has been increasing rapidly and at alarming proportions in both the developed and developing regions of the world, especially during the past two decades.

The convergence of these four factors are making a "perfect storm." The growing pandemic of type 2 diabetes (and the closely related Metabolic Syndrome) is responsible for increasing death and disability from atherosclerotic vascular disease, thereby making such disease the most frequent cause of death worldwide, for the first time in human history.

We must now declare war on diabetes mellitus, which has become our mortal enemy. How are we going to win this war? Surely not with a single magic bullet, whether it is changes in lifestyle, a drug, gene or device. Professor Cheţa's excellent book, *Vascular Involvement in Diabetes*, sets out a logical battle plan. First, it helps us to understand the terrain on which this war must be fought. The opening chapter does this by clearly spelling out the enormity of the problem and the demographic forces at play. The book then helps us to understand the enemy by describing the fundamental mechanisms responsible for vascular involvement in diabetes, at multiple levels – genetic, molecular, tissue, organ and organismal. The second half of the book helps us to look the enemy squarely in the eye by providing a detailed description of the varied clinical aspects of the problem. Finally, as in any other war, weapons must be judiciously deployed and the last portion of the book carefully lays out the currently available therapeutic and preventive measures for diabetes.

While diabetes is a stubborn enemy, we are beginning to win a few skirmishes. For example, recent trials have shown that lifestyle changes, angiotensin converting enzyme inhibitors, angiotensin II receptor blockers, biguanides and fibrates each reduce the likelihood of the development of diabetes in individuals at high risk. HMGCoA reductase inhibitors clearly reduce the incidence of adverse outcomes in patients with established diabetes, even those with normal lipid values, while thiazolidinediones may slow the progression of atherosclerotic vascular disease in diabetics. Thus, there are grounds for cautious optimism that ultimately this war can be won.

Professor Cheţa, the field marshal of this war, should be congratulated on selecting the correct topics and authors, and for his skillful editing of their contributions, making this book far more useful than a simple compilation of fine chapters. Special thanks should also be extended to the authors, all distinguished investigators or clinicians. Although the contributors include experts from Belgium, France, Germany, the United Kingdom and the United States, the largest number of contributors, the Editor in Chief and the Assistant Editors are all from Romania. The talents of scientists and clinicians of this nation, as displayed in this book, are impressive and it is reassuring that they are fully engaged in this great struggle.

Vascular Involvement in Diabetes will be enormously useful to both cardiovascular specialists and diabetologists who must care for the growing number of patients with these disorders. It will be equally useful to those who are training to deliver this care. Surely the time has come for cardiologists to learn more about diabetes and for diabetologists to learn more cardiology. Perhaps it is now appropriate to establish a new specialty: "Diabetocardiology", whose practitioners will become the front line troops in this war.

EUGENE BRAUNWALD, M.D.

Boston, MA

EDITORIAL NOTE

The present book, though consistent, is not a treatise. It was not in our intention to exhaust the field of cardiovascular complications in diabetes mellitus, as evidence stands currently. We did intend to bring forward as many data, concepts and current guidelines so that our readers could, on the one hand, benefit from 'up-to-date' information but remain, on the other hand, with the wish to consider them in depths.

We invited distinguished specialists from Romania, the United States, the United Kingdom, France, Belgium, Germany; for the kindheartedness of their response, we remain much obliged to them.

Authors were encouraged to freely shape their ideas (within the general frame of the suggested editorial model). It is due to this reason that the readers who are to cover the whole material may find redundant some topics in etiopathogeny or therapeutics. On the contrary, the readers who are interested only in a couple of chapters or in a particular topic are to find a relatively thorough, comprehensive exposition of the target topic. The chapters' flow aimed to be as familiar as possible, from basic research to current clinical aspects and therapeutic approaches. Professor E. Braunwald's promise to write the preface for this book represented a strong challenge for the hard dedication of both authors and editors.

D.C.

ALPHABETICAL LIST OF AUTHORS

Eduard APETREI, MD, PhD, FESC
Professor, Institute of Cardiovascular Diseases
"Prof.dr.C.C.Iliescu", Bucharest, Romania
258 Fundeni Way, Bucharest 2, Romania
Tel.: +40-21-2402224
Fax: +40-21-2402224
E-mail: apetrei@fx.ro

Pompilia Petruța APOSTOL, PhD Student
Research assistant, Institute of Genetics, University
of Bucharest
1–3 Portocalilor Street, Bucharest, Romania
Tel.: +40-21-2248846
Fax: +40-21-2248846
E-mail: apostol_pompilia@yahoo.com

Katalin BABEȘ, MD, PhD
Assistant Professor, University of Oradea,
31 Piața Independenței, 3700 Oradea, Romania
E-mail: piszekati@yahoo.co.uk

Petru Aurel BABEȘ, MD, PhD
Professor, University of Oradea,
31 Piața Independenței, 3700, Oradea, Romania

Karim BAKRI, MB BS
Renal Unit, Guy's Hospital, London, UK

Rashed BAKRI, MB BS
Renal Unit, Guy's Hospital, London, UK

Cornelia BALA, MD
Diabetes Center and Clinic
2–4 Clinicilor Street, Cluj Napoca, Romania
Tel.: +40-264-599578
Fax: +40-264-594455
E-mail: diabet@insin.hearticj.ro

Bogdan BALAȘ, MD
Medical Resident, "C.I. Parhon" Institute of Endocrinology
36 Bd. Aviatorilor, 011863, Bucharest, Romania
E-mail: bbalas74@yahoo.com

Monica Mariana BĂLUȚĂ, MD
Assistant Professor of Medicine,
St. Pantelimon University Emergency Hospital
Department of Internal Medicine and Cardiology
340 Pantelimon Street, Bucharest 2, Romania
Tel.: +40212552049
Cell: 0722605745

Gheorghe S. BĂCANU, MD, PhD
Professor, Diabetes Clinic, County Hospital, "Victor
Babeș" University of Medicine and Pharmacy,
Timișoara, Romania
156 Bd. Liviu Rebreanu, 300723 Timișoara, Romania

Șerban BĂLĂNESCU, MD, FESC
Lecturer, Cardiology and Internal Medicine Dept.
"Carol Davila" University of Medicine and Pharmacy
Floreasca Emergency Hospital
8 Calea Floreasca, Bucharest 1, Romania
Tel.: +40-21-2300053
Fax: +40-21-2300053

Stuart J. BRINK, MD
Associate Clinical Professor of Pediatrics, Tufts
University School of Medicine, Boston, MA, USA
Senior Endocrinologist, New England Diabetes and
Endocrinology Center (NEDEC)
40 Second Avenue, Suite #170, Waltham MA 02451-
1136 USA
Tel.: 781 890 3610
Fax: 781 890 3612
E-mail: stubrink@aol.com

Ioana Maria BRUCKNER, MD, PhD
Associate Professor – Diabetes, Nutrition and Metabolic
Diseases "N. Malaxa" Hospital,
12 Vergului Street,
Bucharest, Romania
E-mail: diabmalaxa@yahoo.com

Ion Victor BRUCKNER, MD, PhD
Professor of Internal Medicine and Cardiology,
Colțea Hospital
1-3 I.C. Brătianu Street, Bucharest, Romania
E-mail: bruckner@fx.ro

Benone CÂRSTOCEA, MD, PhD
Professor, Head of the Ophthalmology Clinic
The Emergency Central Clinical Army Hospital
134 Calea Plevnei, Bucharest 1, Romania

Anca CERGHIZAN, MD
Diabetes Center and Clinic
2-4 Clinicilor Street, Cluj Napoca, Romania
Tel.: +40-264-599578
Fax: +40-264-594455
E-mail: diabet@insin.hearticj.ro

Dan Mircea CHEȚA, MD, PhD
Professor, 2nd Clinic of Diabetes, Nutrition
and Metabolic Diseases
"N. Paulescu" Institute, Bucharest, Romania
5 Ion Movilă Street, 020475 Bucharest 2, Romania
Tel.: +40212108499, extn.: 113
Fax: +40212111575
E-mail: fpas@fx.ro

Dănuț Gheorghe CIMPONERIU, PhD Student
Research assistant, Institute of Genetics,
University of Bucharest
1–3 Portocalilor Street, Bucharest, Romania
Tel.: +40-21-2248846
Fax: +40-21-2248846
E-mail: dancimponeriu@yahoo.com

**Ruxandra CIOBANU-JURCUȚ,
MD, PhD student,**
Junior Lecturer, Institute of Cardiovascular Diseases
"Prof.dr.C.C.Iliescu", Bucharest, Romania
258, Fundeni Way, Bucharest, 2, Romania
Tel.: +40-21-2402224
Fax: +40-21-2402224
E-mail: rciobanu@fx.ro

Anca Ileana COMAN, MD
"N.Paulescu" Institute of Diabetes, Nutrition
and Metabolic Diseases
5-7 I. Movilă Street, 020475 Bucharest 2, Romania

Ioan Mircea COMAN, MD, PhD, FESC
Lecturer, "Carol Davila" University of Medicine
and Pharmacy
Head of Department,
"C.C. Iliescu" Institute of Cardiovascular Diseases
258 Fundeni Way, Bucharest 2, Romania
E-mail: iocoman@pcnet.ro

Adrian COVIC, MD, PhD
Associate Professor for Internal Medicine and Nephrology
Director of the Dialysis and Renal Transplantation
Center
Nephrology Clinic, Parhon University Hospital
50 Carol 1st Blvd., Iași 6600, Romania
Tel.: +40-232-210940
Fax: +40-232-210940
e-mail: acovic@xnet.ro

Dana DABELEA, MD, PhD
Assistant Professor, Department of Preventive Medicine
and Biometrics
School of Medicine, University of Colorado Health
Sciences Center
4200 East Ninth Ave Box C245
Denver, CO 80262, USA

Tel.: 303-315-1433
Fax: 303-315-101
E-mail: Dana.Dabelea@uchsc.edu

Françoise DESBIEZ, MD
Praticien Hospitalier, Service de Diabétologie
CHU BP 69 63003 CLERMONT-Fd France
Tel.: (33) 4 73 751 533
Fax: (33) 4 73 751 532
E-mail: fdesbiez@chu-clermontferrand.fr

Laura DIACONU, MD
Diabetes Clinic, County Hospital Timişoara, Romania
156 Bd. Liviu Rebreanu, 300723, Timişoara, Romania

Harry DORCHY, MD, PhD
Professor of Pediatrics and of Diabetology,
Free University of Brussels
Head, Diabetology Clinic,
University Children's Hospital Queen Fabiola
Avenue JJ Crocq, 15
B-1020 Bruxelles, Belgium
Tel.: (32)-2-4773175
Fax: (32)-2-4773156
E-mail: hdorchy@ulb.ac.be

Maria DOROBANȚU, MD, PhD, FESC
Head, Cardiology and Internal Medicine Dept.
"Carol Davila" University of Medicine and Pharmacy
Floreasca Emergency Hospital
8 Calea Floreasca, Bucharest 1, Romania
Tel.: +40-21-2300053
Fax: +40-21-2300053

Dinu DRAGOMIR, MD, PhD
Cardiologist,
"Prof. Dr. Dimitrie Gerota" Emergency Hospital
50 Ferdinand Bvd, Bucharest, Romania

Luiza Otilia GAFENCU, MD, PhD
The Emergency Central Clinical Army Hospital
134 Calea Plevnei, Bucharest 1, Romania
E-mail: otilia_g@k.ro

Laurence GALANTI, MD, PhD
Cliniques UCL Mont-Godinne Laboratory
Avenue Therasse, 1
B-5530 Yvoir, Belgium
Tel.: 00 32 81 42 3200
Fax: 00 32 81 42 3204
E-mail: galanti@mexp.ucl.ac.be

Elena GANEA, MD, PhD
Research Scientist, First Degree
Head of the "Posttranslational modifications of proteins"
group

Institute of Biochemistry, Romanian Academy
296, Splaiul Independentei Street, Bucharest, 060031, Romania
Tel.: +40 21 2239069
Fax: +40 21 2239068
E-mail: eganea@biochim.ro

Carmen GINGHINĂ, MD, PhD
Professor , Chief of the 3rd Cardiology Department
"Prof. Dr. C.C.Iliescu" Institute of Cardiovascular Diseases,
258 Fundeni Way, Bucharest, Romania

David J.A. GOLDSMITH, MD
Consultant Nephrologist, Renal Unit, Guy's Hospital
London SEI 9RT, United Kingdom
E-mail: david.goldsmith@kcl.ac.uk

Florin GRIGORESCU, MD, PhD
"Chargé de Recherche" at Institut National de la Santé
et de la Recherche Médicale
IURC, Molecular Endocrinology, 641 Ave. Du Doyen
Gaston Giraud
34093 Montpellier Cedex 5, France
Tel.: (+33) 467.41.59.24.
Fax : (+33) 467.54.27.31
E-mail: florin@montp.inserm.fr.

Cristian GUJA, MD, PhD
Registrar, Research Scientist
1st Clinic of Diabetes, Nutrition and Metabolic
Diseases, "N. Paulescu" Institute, Bucharest, Romania
5–7 Ion Movilă Street, 020475 Bucharest 2, Romania
Tel.: +40 21 210 64 60
Fax: +40 21 210 22 95
E-mail: cristi_guja@fx.ro

Adriana Luminița GURGHEAN, MD
Consultant of Cardiology, Colțea Hospital
1–3 Brătianu Street, Bucharest, Romania
E-mail: adryana173@xnet.ro

Paul GUSBETH-TATOMIR, MD
Assistant Professor, Dialysis and Renal Transplantation
Center,
Nephrology Clinic, Parhon University Hospital
50 Carol 1st Blvd., Iași 6600, Romania
Tel.: +40-(0)745-533788
Fax: +40-(0)745-533788
E-mail: paulgusbeth@hotmail.com

Nicolae HÂNCU, MD, PhD
Professor, "Iuliu Hațieganu" University of Medicine
and Pharmacy Cluj-Napoca
Head of the Diabetes Center and Clinic
2–4 Clinicilor Street, Cluj Napoca, Romania
Tel.: +40-264-599578

Fax: +40-264-594455
E-mail: diabet@insin.hearticj.ro

Claude HANET, MD
University of Louvain Medical School
Division of Cardiology
Avenue Hippocrate 10/2881
B-1200 Brussels, Belgium
Tel.: 32-2-7642803
Fax: 32-2-7642811
E-mail: hanet@card.ucl.ac.be

Mihai IONAC, MD, PhD
"Victor Babeş" University of Medicine and Pharmacy
Surgical Clinic 2, County Hospital
156 Liviu Rebreanu Bvd, 300723, Timişoara, Romania
Tel.: +40256-163001
Fax: +40256-165397

Constantin IONESCU-TÎRGOVIŞTE, MD, PhD
Professor, 1st Clinic of Diabetes, Nutrition and
Metabolic Diseases, "Prof. N. Paulescu" Institute,
Bucharest, Romania
5–7 Ion Movilă Street, 020475 Bucharest 2, Romania
Tel.: 0040 21 210 64 60
Fax: 0040 21 210 22 95
E-mail: cit@paulescu.ro

Billy IQBAL, MD
Honorary Research Fellow Cardiology
Clinical Trials and Evaluation Unit
Royal Brompton Hospital
Sydney Street, London, United Kingdom
Tel.: 0044 207 351 8827
E-mail: mi014j3755@blueyonder.co.uk

Paul JENNINGS, MD, B Med Sci BM BS DM FRCP (E), FRCP (L)
Consultant Endocrinologist/ Honorary Senior Lecturer
York Diabetes Centre, York Hospital
Wigginton Road, York, YO31 8HE, United Kingdom
E-mail: paul.e.jennings@York.nhs.uk

Wolfgang KERNER, MD, PhD
Director of Diabetes and Metabolic Diseases Clinic
Karlsburg
Greifswalder Straße 11 A, 17 495
Karlsburg, Germany
E-mail: prof.kerner@drguth.de

Radu LICHIARDOPOL, MD, PhD
Professor, "Carol Davila" University of Medicine and
Pharmacy
"N. Paulescu" Institute of Diabetes, Nutrition and
Metabolic Diseases, Bucharest, Romania
12 J.S. Bach, Bucharest 2, Romania

Umair MALLICK, MD
Senior Honorary Clinical Research Fellow Cardiology
Clinical Trials and Evaluation Unit
Royal Brompton Hospital
Sydney Street, London, United Kingdom
Tel: 0044-7970 683039
Fax: 0044-777 908 0787
E-mail: umairmallick@hotmail.com

Irina MĂRGĂRITESCU, MD
Medical Resident, Clinic of Dermatology
Central Clinical Emergency Military Hospital
88 Mircea Vulcanescu Street, 010816, Bucharest,
Romania
Tel.: 40-21-2222.783
E-mail: irina_margaritescu@yahoo.com

Mirela MARINESCU, MD
Cardiologist, Emergency Clinical Hospital
8 Floreasca Street, Bucharest, Romania

Laurence MARTEL-COUDERC, MD
Assistant-Chef de Clinique, Service de Diabétologie
CHU BP 69 63003 CLERMONT-Fd France
Tel.: (33) 4 73 751 533
Fax: (33) 4 73 751 532
E-mail: lmartel couderc@chu-clermontferrand.fr

Viorel MIHAI, MD
Department of Cardiology,"N. Paulescu" Institute
of Nutrition, Diabetes and Metabolic Diseases
5–7 Ion Movilă Street, 020475 Bucharest 2, Romania

Mihai NECHIFOR, MD, PhD
Professor, Head of the Department of Pharmacology,
"Gr. T. Popa" University of Medicine and Pharmacy,
Iaşi, Romania
16 Universitatii Street, 700115, Iaşi, Romania
Tel.: +40-232-220875;
Fax: +40-232-211820;
E-mail: nechifor@umfiasi.ro

Dana M. NEDELCU, MD, PhD
Head - Department of Clinical Ultrasonography Central
Clinical Military Hospital, Bucharest, Romania
88 Mircea Vulcanescu Street, 010816, Bucharest,
Romania
Tel.: (401) 224-9405/321
Fax: (401) 222-2783
E-mail: dananedelcu@hotmail.com

Ioan NEDELCU, MD, PhD
Professor & Chair,
Clinic of Dermatology
Central Clinical Emergency Military Hospital
88 Mircea Vulcanescu Street, 010816, Bucharest, Romania

Tel.: 40-21-2222.783
E-mail: ioannedelcu@hotmail.com

Laura-Elena NEDELCU
Medical Student, Faculty of Medicine
"Carol Davila" University of Medicine and Pharmacy,
Bucharest
8 Eroilor Street, 050511, Bucharest, Romania
E-mail: laura_ned@yahoo.com

Anca Maria NEGRILĂ, MD
Internal Medicine Specialist, Colţea Hospital,
1-3 I.C. Brătianu Street, Bucharest, Romania

Gabriela NEGRIŞANU, MD, PhD
Associate Professor, Diabetes Clinic, County
Hospital no.1
"Victor Babeş" University of Medicine and Pharmacy,
Timişoara, România
156 Liviu Rebreanu Bd, 300723, Timişoara, Romania

Tudor NICOLAIE, MD, PhD
Associate Professor, Head – 2nd Clinic of Internal
Medicine, Central Clinical Military Hospital, Bucharest,
Romania
88 Mircea Vulcanescu Street, 010816 Bucharest, Romania
Tel.: (401) 212-6571
Fax: (401) 212-6571
E-mail: nicolae28@yahoo.com

Lawrence Chukwudi NWABUDIKE, MBBS,
Specialist in dermatology, Consultant in dermatology
and diabetes foot care
"N. Paulescu" Institute, Bucharest, Romania
5 Ion Movilă Street, Bucharest 2, Romania
Tel.: +40-0744-330492
Fax: +40-212111575
E-mail: chukwudi@fx.ro

Gabriela ORĂŞANU, MD
Postdoctoral Research Fellow in Medicine
Brigham and Women's Hospital, Harvard Medical School
Cardiovascular Division
77 Avenue Louis Pasteur, NRB 742
Boston, MA 02115, USA
Tel.: 617-525-4365
Fax: 617-525-4380
E-mail: gorasanu@rics.bwh.harvard.edu

Cristian PANAITE, MD
2nd Clinic of Diabetes,
Nutrition and Metabolic Diseases,
"N. Paulescu" Institute, Bucharest, Romania
5 Ion Movilă Street, Bucharest 2, Romania
E-mail: cristip73@yahoo.com

Traian PĂTRAȘCU, MD
Senior Consultant Surgeon
Assistant Professor "Prof. I. Juvara" Department of
Surgery, Cantacuzino Hospital,
5–7 Ion Movilă Street, Bucharest 2, Romania

Jorge PLUTZKY, MD
Assistant Professor of Medicine, Harvard Medical School
Director, The Vascular Disease Prevention Program
Brigham and Women's Hospital
Cardiovascular Division
77 Avenue Louis Pasteur, NRB 740
Boston MA 02115, USA
Tel.: 617-525-4360
Fax: 617-525-4366
E-mail: jplutzky@rics.bwh.harvard.edu

Amorin-Remus POPA, MD
Associate Professor, University of Oradea
143 Louis Pasteur Street, 3700 Oradea, Romania

Rodica POP-BUȘUI, MD, PhD
Assistant Professor of Medicine and Physiology
Division of Endocrinology and Metabolism
Department of Medicine, Medical College of Ohio
3120 Glendale, Toledo, OH 43614 USA
Tel.: 419-383-3707
Fax: 419-383-6244
E-mail: rpbusui@mco.edu

Doina POPOV, PhD
Senior Research Scientist,
Head of the Laboratory "Vascular Dysfunction in Diabetes"
Institute of Cellular Biology
and Pathology "N. Simionescu"
8 BP Hasdeu Street, 050568, Bucharest, Romania
Tel.: 40214115240 extn.:17
Fax: 40214111143
E-mail: popov@simionescu.instcellbiopath.ro

Dorel Lucian RADU, MD, PhD
Head of the Laboratory "Cellular Immunology",
National Institute of Research and Development for
Microbiology and Immunology "Cantacuzino"
103 Splaiul Independenței, Bucharest, Romania
Tel: 40214113800 extn.: 190
Fax: 40214115672
E-mail: dorel.radu@cantacuzino.ro

Irina RADU, PhD
Research scientist III, Institute of Genetics, University
of Bucharest
1–3 Portocalilor Street, Bucharest, Romania
Tel.: +40-21-2248846
Fax: +40-21-2248846
Email: irina@botanic.unibuc.ro

Gabriela RADULIAN, MD, PhD
Lecturer, "Carol Davila" University of Medicine and
Pharmacy, Bucharest, Romania
"N. Paulescu" Institute of Diabetes, Nutrition and
Metabolic Diseases
12 I.L. Caragiale Street, Bucharest 2, Romania
E-mail: dearadulian@hotmail.com

Gordon REID, PhD
Professor, Department of Animal Physiology
and Biophysics
Faculty of Biology, University of Bucharest, 91–95
Splaiul Independenței, 76201, Bucharest, Romania
Tel.: +40 21 410 9720Fax. +40 21 411 3933
E-mail gordon@biologie.kappa.ro

Mihaela ROȘU, MD
"Victor Babeș" University of Medicine and Pharmacy
Diabetes Clinic, County Hospital
156 Liviu Rebreanu Bvd, 300723 Timișoara, Romania
Tel.: +40256-163001
Fax: +40256-165397

Ilinca SĂVULESCU-FIEDLER, MD
Specialist Internal Medicine, Assistant Cardiology
Department, "Colțea" Hospital
1–3 I.C.Brătianu Street, Bucharest, Romania
Tel.: +4021 3113581
Fax: +4021 3110181
E-mail: ilinca_savulescu@yahoo.com

Cristian SERAFINCEANU, MD
Department of Nephrology and Dialysis
"N. Paulescu" Institute of Diabetes, Nutrition and
Metabolic Diseases
5–7 Ion Movilă Street, 020475 Bucharest, Romania

Alexandra SIMA, MD
"Victor Babeș" University of Medicine and Pharmacy
Diabetes Clinic, County Hospital
156 Liviu Rebreanu Bvd, 300723, Timișoara, Romania
Tel.: +40256-163001
Fax: +40256-165397

Anca SIMA, PhD
Group leader of the laboratory "Lipoproteins and
atherogenesis"
Institute of Cellular Biology
and Pathology "N. Simionescu"
8 B.P. Hașdeu Street, Bucharest, Romania
Tel.: 40 21 411 08 60
Fax: 40 21 411 11 43
E-mail: simionescum@instcellbiopath.ro

Maya SIMIONESCU, PhD
Director of the Institute of Cellular Biology
and Pathology "N. Simionescu"
8 B.P. Haşdeu Street, Bucharest, Romania
Tel.: 40 21 411 08 60
Fax: 40 21 411 11 43
E-mail: simionescum@instcellbiopath.ro

Andy SMITH, MB BS MRCP
Diabetes Unit, Guy's Hospital,
London, UK

Martin STEVENS, MD
Associate Professor of Medicine
Division of Endocrinology and Metabolism
Department of Medicine, University of Michigan
1150 W. Med Ctr Dr, Ann Arbor, MI 48109, USA
Tel.: 734-647-3409
E-mail: stevensm@umich.edu

Viorel ŞERBAN, MD, PhD
Professor, Head of Diabetes Clinic, County Hospital,
"Victor Babeş" University of Medicine and Pharmacy,
Timişoara, Romania
156 Bd. Liviu Rebreanu, 300723 Timişoara, Romania
Tel.: +40256-163001
Fax: +40256-165397
E-mail: viorelserban@hotmail.ro

Igor TAUVERON, MD, PhD
Professor, Praticien Hospitalier, Service de Diabétologie
CHU and Université d'Auvergne BP 69 63003
CLERMONT-Fd France
Tel.: (33) 4 73 751 529
Fax: (33) 4 73 751 532
E-mail: itauveron@chu-clermontferrand.fr

Philippe THIEBLOT, MD
Professor, Head, Praticien Hospitalier,
Service de Diabétologie
CHU and Université d'Auvergne BP 69 63003
CLERMONT-Fd France
Tel.: (33) 4 73 751 533
Fax: (33) 4 73 751 532
E-mail: pthieblot@chu-clermontferrand.fr

Romulus TIMAR, MD, PhD
Assistant Professor, Diabetes Clinic, County Hospital,
"Victor Babeş" University of Medicine and Pharmacy,
Timişoara, Romania
156 Bd. Liviu Rebreanu, 300723, Timişoara, Romania

Ion VEREANU, MD, PhD
Senior Consultant Surgeon
Professor and Head, "Prof. I. Juvara" Department of
Surgery, Cantacuzino Hospital,
5–7 Ion Movilă Street, Bucharest 2, Romania

Marius Marcian VINTILĂ, MD, PhD
Professor of Medicine and Cardiology
St. Pantelimon University Emergency Hospital
Department of Internal Medicine and Cardiology
340 Pantelimon Street, Bucharest 2, Romania
Tel: 021/2552049
Cell: 0788363757
E-mail: mariusvintila@zappmobile.ro

Vlad Damian VINTILĂ, MD
Assistant Professor of Medicine
University Emergency Hospital
3rd Internal Medicine and Cardiology Department
160 Independenţei Street, Bucharest, Romania
Cell: 0788363758
E-mail: vladvintila@zappmobile.ro

Adrian VLAD, MD
Assistant Professor, Diabetes Clinic, County Hospital,
"Victor Babeş" University of Medicine and Pharmacy,
Timişoara, Romania
156 Liviu Rebreanu Bvd, 300723, Timişoara, Romania
Tel.: +40256-163001
Fax: +40256-165397

Mihaela Victoria VLĂICULESCU, MD
Internal Medicine Specialist
"N. Malaxa" Hospital,
12 Vergului Street, Bucharest, Romania

Eckhard ZANDER, MD, PhD
Diabetes and Metabolic Diseases Clinic Karlsburg
Greifswalder Straße 11 A, 17 495
Karlsburg, Germany
E-mail: dr.zander@drguth.de

Ouliana ZIOUZENKOVA, PhD
Instructor in Medicine
Brigham and Women's Hospital, Harvard Medical School
Cardiovascular Division
77 Avenue Louis Pasteur, NRB 742
Boston, MA 02115, USA
Tel.: 617-525-4365, Fax: 617-525-4380
E-mail: oziouzenkova@rics.bwh.harvard.edu

ACKNOWLEDGEMENTS

This editorial project was encouraged by the Romanian Academy and the Romanian Academy of Medical Sciences.

The editor and part of the authors cooperated within the frame of a joint European programme for scientific research (COST).

Our colleagues Anne-Marie Crăciun and Bogdana Balaş contributed to final checking and verifying of the manuscript.

Other colleagues from "Nicolae Paulescu" Institute of Diabetes, Nutrition and Metabolic Diseases and the Foundation for Healthy Nutrition gave a helping hand in various stages of this project.

Publishing expenses could be covered due to sponsorship generously offered by the following medical and pharmaceutical companies: **Aventis Pharma, GlaxoSmithKline (GSK), CSC Pharmaceuticals, Eli Lilly, Wörwag Pharma, Pfizer, Servier, Merck Sharp & Dohme (MSD)**, by their Romanian Offices.

INTRODUCTION

1

CARDIOVASCULAR COMPLICATIONS OF DIABETES MELLITUS: MAGNITUDE OF THE PROBLEM

Dan CHEŢA, Cristian PANAITE, Bogdan BALAŞ, Gabriela RADULIAN

Cardiovascular involvement in diabetes mellitus has become a major problem that researchers and clinicians have to deal with. Its growing impact on society is not at all surprising if we take into consideration the increase in incidence of both cardiovascular disease and diabetes *per se*.

This introductory chapter reviews the various manifestations of cardiovascular disease in diabetes, supported by strong epidemiologic data. The peculiar features of both macrovascular (coronary artery disease, peripheral artery disease, and cerebrovascular disease) and microvascular (nephropathy, retinopathy) complications were investigated.

The social and financial aspects we studied revealed the true magnitude of the problem. Huge resources are allocated each year for the treatment of diabetes, vascular complications accounting for the most significant proportion.

In Romania, data regarding the diabetes epidemic and its vascular complications are scarce and sometimes contradictory. The most reliable source is EPIDIAB study, briefly reviewed.

In the light of new studies, several principles emerge on how to diminish cardiovascular risk in diabetes. In our opinion, a multifactorial approach to this matter would be the most beneficial. However, practical difficulties in implementing prevention strategies still have to be overcome before succeeding in this ambitious, yet so necessary endeavor.

Cardiovascular involvement in diabetes mellitus has become increasingly important over the last decades. The impact generated both in the medical (clinical and basic research) and in the socioeconomic field, is growing, whether we are considering direct complications or other morbid associations and conditions (Table 1.1). This is not at all surprising if we accept two fundamental aspects of the modern world: the rise in the incidence of cardiovascular disease along with the dramatic increase in the frequency of diabetes *per se*.

Table 1.1

Vascular involvement in diabetes:
main areas of interest

- EPIDEMIOLOGY – alarming figures
- FINANCIAL AND SOCIAL BURDEN
- CAUSES AND MECHANISMS – complicated
- THERAPY – not easy and not complete
- PREVENTION – still not efficient

There are some semantic difficulties related to this subject. Terms that are more general are not very precise, hence their use in literature is not always rigorous. But one cannot say that we are dealing with real contradictions that might become subjects of debates and classifications (Table 1.2).

Table 1.2

Semantic difficulties

GENERAL TERMS
- Cardiovascular Complications of Diabetes
- Macro- and Microvascular Complications
- Vascular Disease in Diabetes
- Diabetic Angiopathy
- Others

MORE SPECIFIC TERMS
- Diabetic Retinopathy
- Diabetic Nephropathy
- Diabetic Foot
- Diabetic Cardiomyopathy
- Diabetic Heart Muscle Disease
- Others

SURVEY
OF THE EPIDEMIOLOGY

Cardiovascular disease accounted for 16.6 million deaths worldwide in 1998 alone: 13 million deaths (29% of all deaths) in low- and middle-income countries and 3.6 million deaths (45% of all deaths) in high-income countries. By 2020, it is estimated that ischemic heart disease will be the largest single cause of morbidity and mortality in the world [1].

On the other hand, according to WHO estimates, approximately 172 million people had diabetes in 2000 (almost a 50% increase in prevalence compared with 1990). Furthermore, the global prevalence of diabetes is predicted to double and reach over 360 million by 2030 [1].

Coronary artery disease (CAD). Large epidemiological studies have shown that the risk of CAD is increased 2-4 fold in diabetic patients, compared to non-diabetic individuals [2, 3].

The incidence and prevalence of CAD in diabetic subjects are influenced by sex, duration of disease, degree of metabolic control, type of diabetes, associated diseases (dyslipidemia, hypertension, etc.) as well as by other factors [4].

Diabetic patients have a high prevalence of sub-clinical cardiovascular disease, which is a strong predictor of subsequent CAD and cardiovascular mortality [3]. Clinical data suggest that diabetic patients may already have developed vascular disease by the time a clinical diagnosis of diabetes is made [5]. The Chennai Urban Population Study (CUPS) evaluated atherosclerotic markers by non-invasive means, and showed evidence of vascular disease by revealing endothelial dysfunction and increased carotid intima-media thickness in diabetic patients with no history of coronary artery disease [6]. Such findings emphasize the clinical relevance of the "ticking clock" hypothesis that suggests that macrovascular disease (CAD for instance) begins in the prediabetic state, whereas microvascular disease (*e.g.*, retinopathy or nephropathy) usually starts with the onset of hyperglycemia [5]. In fact, several studies demonstrated that hyperglycemia, even in the absence of clinically diagnosed diabetes, is associated with an increased cardiovascular risk [7–14].

Diabetes also worsens early and late outcomes in acute coronary syndromes [3].

The relationship between diabetes and coronary artery disease has been thoroughly analyzed in regard of mortality [1, 3, 4, 8–13]. A population-based study conducted in Finland compared cardiovascular mortality in approximately 1,400 non-diabetic subjects and 1,000 diabetic subjects with and without myocardial infarction (MI). The seven-year incidence of cardiovascular death was:

 – 42.0 and 15.4/100 person-years in diabetic patients with and without prior MI;

 – 15.9 and 2.1/100 person-years, respectively in non-diabetic patients.

Thus, the risk of cardiovascular death in diabetic patients without prior MI was comparable to that of non-diabetic patients who had previously experienced an MI [15]. This statement is still debated by some authors who argue that the duration of diabetes was not taken into account, although it is an important risk factor or that the incidence of cardiovascular disease is high long before the clinical diagnosis of diabetes [16].

It is well known that mortality from coronary heart disease has declined substantially in the United States during the past 30 years. The decrease has been attributed to reduction in cardiovascular risk factors and improvement in treatment of heart disease. Unfortunately, these changes appear to have been less favorable or less effective for people with diabetes, particularly for women [17].

These findings led the Adult Treatment Panel III of the National Cholesterol Education Program to establish diabetes as a CAD risk equivalent mandating aggressive antiatherosclerotic treatment [3, 18].

The gender difference in cardiovascular mortality related to diabetes remains a controversial subject. Mukamal *et al.* remark that diabetes is associated with markedly increased mortality after acute myocardial infarction, particularly in women [19]. A recently published study demonstrates that newly diagnosed diabetic women have higher relative risks for death from cardiovascular disease than diabetic men. The authors consider that a more aggressive control of hyperglycemia as well as of other cardiovascular risk factors might be appropriate in women with asymptomatic hyperglycemia [13].

Laing *et al.* analyzed a cohort of 23,000 patients with insulin-treated diabetes. They conclude that the risk of mortality from ischemic heart disease is exceptionally high in young adult women with type 1 diabetes, with rates similar to those in men with type 1 diabetes under the age of 40. These results emphasize the need to identify and treat coronary risk factors in these young patients [20].

Diabetes mellitus is now largely recognized as a coronary heart disease equivalent [5, 13, 15, 18, 20].

Peripheral arterial disease (PAD). Generally, it is recognized that individuals with diabetes have a 2- to 4- fold increase in the rates of PAD [3, 21].

On the other hand, the presence of diabetes leads to changes in the nature of PAD itself. Thus, diabetic patients more commonly have infrapopliteal arterial occlusive disease and vascular calcification than non-diabetic cohorts [22]. The number of amputations among diabetic subjects continues to remain high all over the globe. For example, it is established that diabetes causes most non-traumatic lower extremity amputations in the United States [3, 23].

Cerebrovascular disease. It is estimated that the risk of stroke is increased 150% to 400% for subjects with diabetes mellitus, and worsening glycemic control relates directly to stroke risk [3, 24].

The main causes and peculiarities of stroke in diabetic patients have been the subject of analysis in many clinical studies [4]. Diabetes considerably increases the risk of stroke among younger individuals [25]. It also increases total and stroke-related mortality [3, 26, 27].

Diabetic nephropathy. Overall, 25–50% of diabetic patients develop kidney disease and require dialysis or kidney transplantation [28]. The mortality rate from all causes in diabetic patients with nephropathy is 20 to 40 times higher than that of patients without nephropathy. Diabetic nephropathy is the single most common cause of end-stage renal disease in Western countries; in some countries diabetic patients comprise over one third of all patients entering renal replacement therapy [28, 29].

Significant differences between type 1 and type 2 diabetes exist [30]. About 50% of patients with type 1 diabetes and overt nephropathy develop end-stage renal disease during the next 10 years, and more than 75% develop it during the next 20 years. Patients with type 2 diabetes exhibit a much slower rate of progression from microalbuminuria to renal insufficiency; after 20 years of diabetes, only about 20% of these subjects progress to end-stage renal disease. Nevertheless, patients with type 2 diabetes account for the major part of the overall incidence of end-stage renal disease because of the higher incidence of this type of diabetes [29].

Diabetic retinopathy. The epidemiology of this condition has been widely investigated [29, 31, 32]. It is considered that the most frequent vascular complication of type 1 diabetes is diabetic retinopathy. It represents, together with senile macula degeneration, the major cause of blindness in Western countries. In fact, blindness is about 25 times more common in individuals with diabetes mellitus than in those without this disease [29].

With regard to this vascular complication, significant differences between type 1 and type 2 diabetes are found. Even earlier, it was observed that patients with type 1 diabetes had a greater risk of developing more frequent and more severe ocular complications [33]. About 25% of these individuals have retinopathy after 5 years and 80% after 15 years of disease. Proliferative diabetic retinopathy, the most vision-threatening form of occular disease, is present in more than 25% of patients with type 1 diabetes of more than 15 years duration [34].

The incidence of diabetic retinopathy is different in type 2 diabetes. The pre-diagnosis period of this disease is usually long. Therefore, about 40% of subjects with type 2 diabetes have diabetic retinopathy at the time of diagnosis [29]. About 30% of patients with type 2 diabetes develop proliferative diabetic retinopathy after 15–20 years of diabetes [34]. Considering the epidemiologic dimension, type 2 diabetes accounts for most patients with severe visual loss [29].

The prevalence of diabetic macular edema does not vary as much with the type of diabetes, and is approximately 18–20% [32].

SOCIAL AND ECONOMIC BURDEN

Social impact, along with costs associated with diabetes, are becoming an increasingly pressing matter [35–38]. For example, direct and indirect expenditures attributable to diabetes in the United States in 2002 were estimated at about 132 billion USD. Direct medical expenditures alone totaled 91.9 billion USD: 23.2 billion for diabetes care, 24.6 billion for chronic complications attributable to diabetes and 44.1 billion for excess prevalence of general medical condition. Indirect expenditures resulting from lost workdays, restricted activity days, permanent disability and mortality due to diabetes totaled 39.8 billion USD. When adjusting for differences in age, sex and ethnicity between the population with and without diabetes, individuals with diabetes had medical expenditures that were ~2.4 times higher than expenditures in the absence of diabetes [36].

The CODE-2 study was the first coordinated attempt made to measure the cost of diabetes in Europe and involved more than 7,000 diabetic subjects. According to this study, the total annual cost of diabetes in 1998 was a massive 29 billion EUR, which means 2,515 EUR per patient [37, 38].

Caro *et al.* tried to model the lifetime costs associated with complications of type 2 diabetes. A cohort of 10,000 diabetic patients was simulated using a model based on existing epidemiological data. Macrovascular disease was estimated to be the largest cost component, accounting for 85% of cumulative costs of complications over the first five years. The costs of complications were estimated on average to be 47,240 USD *per* patient over 30 years. The management of macrovascular disease was estimated to be the highest cost component, accounting for 52% of the costs; nephropathy accounted for 21%, neuropathy accounted for 17%, and retinopathy accounted for 10% of the costs of complications. This study concludes that the complications of diabetes mellitus account for substantial costs attributed mainly to the management of macrovascular disease because of its earlier development and greater extent [39].

Expenditures for health care events with a primary diagnosis of uncomplicated diabetes and diabetes-related supplies were estimated to be 23.2 billion USD for 2002 in the United States, which accounts for 25% of all health care attributable expenditures (Table 1.3). At over 44 billion USD (or 48% of total attributable expenditures), general medical conditions comprise the largest component. Together, the seven chronic conditions associated with diabetes account for the remaining 27% of attributable expenditures, with cardiovascular disease being the single largest contributor [36].

The CODE-2 study showed that cardiovascular medication accounted for the greatest proportion of drug expenditures (33%) in diabetic individuals, followed by oral antidiabetic agents (14%). Lipid-lowering agents accounted for a further 9% of drug expenditures. These kinds of figures highlight the substantial burden of hypertension and cardiovascular disease in the diabetic population [37, 38].

Table 1.3

Health care expenditures in the USA attributable to diabetes, by medical condition, 2002 (in millions of dollars). Adapted from [36]

MEDICAL CONDITION	AMOUNT
Diabetes	23,231
Neurological symptoms	2,748
Peripheral vascular disease	1,121
Cardiovascular disease	17,626
Renal complications	1,879
Endocrine/metabolic complications	426
Ophthalmic complications	422
Other complications	318
Diverse medical conditions	44,091
TOTAL	91,861

Another interesting study demonstrated that the average direct medical cost per patient is increased 1.7-fold by the presence of microvascular complications, 2.0-fold by the presence of macrovascular complications and 3.5-fold by the presence of both micro- and macrovascular complications. Additionally, the presence of both micro- and macrovascular complications increases hospitalization costs 5.5-fold [40].

In a study conducted in US during 1999, Nichols and Brown compared medical costs in 16,180 diabetes patients with and without cardiovascular disease and found that single most expensive category of complications was cardiovascular. Much of the added cost resulted from admission to hospital because of cardiovascular events, including myocardial infarction and heart failure [41, 42].

On the other hand, the costs for treatment of diabetic patients with end-stage renal disease have been estimated to be more than 15.6 billion USD, demonstrating once more the enormous impact of this disease for society as a whole, in addition to the implications for the affected individuals [29]. We will add to the above information some data presented at the ADA Congress in New Orleans, LA, June 2003. Costs of medical care for one diabetic patient in the US can be as high as 15,000 USD/year. Costs of dialysis are expected to reach 55,000 USD/year. In the US, there are currently 100,000 patients that underwent renal transplantation; among them, there are 9,500 patients that received both renal and pancreatic transplantation. Renal transplantation associated costs are estimated to be approximately 143,000 USD. Pancreas transplantation alone costs about 148,000 USD whilst combined renal and pancreas transplantation costs up to 195,000 USD [43].

The socioeconomic impact of diabetic retinopathy is also dramatic. About 5,000 new cases of blindness occur each year in the US because of this complication [29]. On the basis of computer-derived projections, it has been estimated that appropriate treatment of type 1 diabetes results in savings of about 101 million USD and 47,374 person-years of sight annually, and savings of 247.9 million USD and 53,986 person-years of sight for type 2 diabetes, at current treatment levels [29, 44].

A study aiming to develop a model to estimate the direct medical costs associated with type 2 diabetes showed that the annual direct medical costs for white men and women with diet-controlled type 2 diabetes, BMI of 30 kg/m^2, and no microvascular, neuropathic or cardiovascular complications were 1,700 USD and 2,100 USD respectively. Treatment with oral-antidiabetic agents, proteinuria, and peripheral vascular disease were associated with moderate 10% to 30% increases in cost. Insulin treatment, dialysis, angina and myocardial infarction were associated with 60% to 90% increases in cost. Mean annual direct medical costs for diabetic patients with acute MI, stroke and amputation were 36,000 USD, 35,000 USD and 52,000 USD, respectively. The authors concluded that insulin treatment and major diabetes complications have a substantial impact on total annual direct medical costs of type 2 diabetes [45].

In Australia, the total cost of diabetes-attributable non-blood glucose-lowering medications increased two-fold over 4 years and was associated with the presence of CHD and its major risk factors, nephropathy, and obesity at baseline. Using forward stepwise multiple linear regression, costs/year was positively and independently associated with baseline systolic blood pressure, coronary heart disease (CHD), total serum cholesterol, serum triglycerides, serum creatinine, BMI, and educational attainment [46].

All these data clearly demonstrate that diabetes mellitus represents, in our days, a serious and expensive disease because of micro- and, above all, macrovascular complications [37].

WHAT ABOUT ROMANIA?

EPIDIAB is a large epidemiological study, which started in 2000 and aimed to analyze newly-diagnosed diabetes mellitus in 14 counties representing one third of the total population. The number of newly-diagnosed persons with diabetes in the first three years was: 15,057 (7.4% type 1 diabetes and 92.1% type 2 diabetes) in 2001; 15,858 (5.4 type 1 diabetes and 89% type 2 diabetes) in 2002 [47].

Among persons with type 2 diabetes, hypertension was present: 45.3% in 2000, 49.9% in 2001 and 48.3% in 2002. The presence of cardiovascular disease was 32%, 31.6% and 27.7%, respectively. The screening for complications revealed the data included in Table 1.4.

The results confirm the epidemic of diabetes and the high prevalence of cardiovascular disease at diagnosis [47].

HOW TO DECREASE THE CARDIOVASCULAR RISK OF DIABETES?

A simple and apparently logical answer to this question might be: by preventing diabetes itself [42, 48]. Reconsideration, extension and reinforcement of primary prevention are essential to the reduction of the burden of diabetes and its complications [49]. Nowadays, there are some interesting ways of prevention for both type 1 and type 2 diabetes. Moreover, some successful studies give us legitimate hopes [50, 51].

However, at this time, primary prevention of diabetes cannot be viewed as a realistic and efficient solution relative to the decrease of cardiovascular risk. Its implementation in clinical practice is still limited and unsafe. On the other hand, primary prevention is no longer of value for individuals already having diabetes.

The most reasonable solution used to diminish cardiovascular risk associated with diabetes seems to be identification and aggressive treatment of

risk factors [48, 52–58]. In order to realize a most efficient strategy, Hupfeld *et al.* prefers to classify the risk factors in two categories: traditional and non-traditional. Recommendations regarding assessment and management of traditional risk factors are basically similar for diabetic and non-diabetic individuals with several important differences. Traditional factors include hypertension, hyperlipidemia, smoking and age. Several non-traditional risk factors also play an important role in the development of cardiovascular disease in diabetes and need to be addressed if full preventive care is to be provided. From this category, we mention hyperglycemia, hyperinsulinemia, central obesity, hypercoagulability, other lipoproteins, homocysteine [55].

During the last decades, many valuable studies demonstrated that reduction in morbidity and mortality from cardiovascular events in diabetic subjects may be obtained using drugs and/or other interventions directed against one or more risk factors [54, 59–61].

The cardiovascular benefits of glucose lowering in both diabetic and non-diabetic dysglycemic people will be evaluated by the ongoing international ORIGIN study (Outcome Reduction with an Initial Glargine Intervention) [62, 63].

Gradually, a new concept seems to emerge: multifactorial approach to the cardiovascular risk factors in diabetes [48]. It is of use to point out at this moment that the recent Standards of Medical Care for Patients with Diabetes Mellitus of the American Diabetes Association respect this concept (Table 1.5). Thus, not only a good glycemic control is of importance, but also identification and aggressive therapy of other risk factors. Target levels for blood pressure and lipids are more stringent than those recommended for the general population [53].

Table 1.4
Screening for complications of diabetes, according to EPIDIAB-study [47]

Year	Dyslipidemia		Retinopathy		Nephropathy		Diabetic foot	
	Tested	Positive	Screened	Positive	Screened	Positive	Screened	Positive
2000	70.9	48.8	74.9	12.4	60.8	7.3	71.5	24.3
2001	65.7	51.7	59.6	15.8	50.4	5.1	53.7	22.5
2002	69	62.6	65.5	9.9	61	4.9	64.3	19.6
Data in table are %								

Table 1.5

Target levels of risk factors in patients with diabetes mellitus (ADA). Adapted from [53]

- Blood pressure below 130/80 mmHg
- Low density lipoprotein cholesterol below 100 mg/dl
- Triglycerides below 150 mg/dl
- High-density lipoprotein cholesterol above 40 mg/dl
- Glycosylated hemoglobin below 7%

The Steno-2 study, published in 2003, showed that a multifactorial strategy could approximately halve the risk of cardiovascular events in patients with type 2 diabetes [54]. The results of this study are undoubtedly both a reason for new hopes and a source of inspiration.

However, the multifactorial approach cannot reach perfection, not even in theory. A comprehensive and precise knowledge of the causes and mechanisms involved in the generation of cardiovascular complications of diabetes is not at reach. Among the most important difficulties are the practical ones:

– the impossibility of complete and regular follow-up of risk factors in the diabetic population;

– lack of compliance to therapeutic schemes (usually long term and complex);

– high costs (in some circumstances);

– the increased probability of cumulating adverse effects when more than one drug is administered;

– National Health Care Systems do not possess the logistics required to deal with an issue of this magnitude.

We can assume that in the future at least some of these difficulties will be overcome by developing new therapeutic and preventive measures to address several risk factors at the same time, without significant adverse effects.

REFERENCES

1. Wild S. Cardiovascular death and diabetes. In: *Highlights of the International Acarbose Symposium,* Sitges, 28 February – 1 March 2003, Bayer AG, 2.
2. Feskens EJ, Kromhout D. Glucose tolerance and the risk of cardiovascular disease: the Zutphen Study. *J Clin Epidemiol,* **45:** 1327–1334, 1992.
3. Beckman JA, Creager MA, Libby P. Diabetes and Atherosclerosis. Epidemiology, Pathophysiology, and Management. *JAMA,* **287:** 2570–2581, 2002.
4. Tuomilehto J, Rastenyte D. Epidemiology of Macrovascular Disease and Hypertension in Diabetes Mellitus. In: Alberti KGMM, Zimmet P, DeFronzo RA, Keen H (eds). *International Textbook of Diabetes Mellitus,* 2nd edition, Wiley, Chichester, 1997, 1559–1583.
5. Deedwania PC. Diabetes and Vascular Disease: Common Links in the Emerging Epidemic of Coronary Artery Disease. *Am J Cardiol,* **91:** 68–71, 2003.
6. Ravikumar R, Depa R, Shanthirani CS, Mohan V. Comparison of carotid intima-media thickness, arterial stiffness and brachial artery flow mediated dilatation in diabetic and non-diabetic subjects (The Chennai Urban Population Study) [CUPS-9]. *Am J Cardiol,* **90:** 702–707, 2002.
7. Wilson PWF, Cupples LA, Cannel WB. Is hyperglycaemia associated with cardiovascular disease? The Framingham Study. *Am Heart J,* **121:** 586–590, 1991.
8. Barrett-Connor EL, Cohn BA, Wingard DL, Edelstein SL. Why is diabetes mellitus a stronger risk factor for fatal ischemic disease in women than in men? The Rancho Bernardo Study. *JAMA,* **265:** 627–631, 1991.
9. Barrett-Connor E, Ferrara A. Isolated post-challenge hyperglycaemia and the risk of fatal cardiovascular disease in older women and men. *Diabetes Care,* **21:** 1236–1239, 1998.
10. DECODE Study Group: Glucose tolerance and mortality: Comparison of WHO and American Diabetes Association diagnostic criteria. *Lancet,* **354:** 617–621, 1999.
11. DECODE Study Group: Glucose tolerance and cardiovascular mortality: Comparison of the fasting and the 2-hour diagnostic criteria. *Arch Intern Med,* **161:** 394–404, 2001.
12. Saydah SH, Miret M, Sung J, Varas C, Gause Brancati FL. Postchallenge hyperglycemia and mortality in a national sample of U.S. adults. *Diabetes Care,* **24:** 1397–1402, 2001.
13. DECODE Study Group. Gender difference in all-cause and cardiovascular mortality related to hyperglycaemia and newly diagnosed diabetes. *Diabetologia,* **46:** 608–617, 2003.
14. Taubert G, Winkelmann BR, Schleiffer T, Marz W, Winkler R, Gok R, Klein B, Schneider S, Boehm BO. Prevalence, predictors, and consequences of unrecongnised diabetes mellitus in 3266 patients scheduled for coronary angiography. *Am Heart J,* **145:** 285–291, 2003.
15. Haffner SN, Lehto S, Ronnemaa T, Pyorala K, Laakso M. Mortality from coronary heart disease in subjects with type 2 diabetes and in non-diabetic subjects with and without prior myocardial infarction. *N Engl J Med,* **339:** 229–234, 1998.

16. Hu FB. The impact of diabetes and prediabetes on risk of cardiovascular disease and mortality. *Drugs Today (Barc)*, **38:** 760–775, 2002.

17. Gu K, Cowie CC, Harris MI. Diabetes and Decline in Heart Disease Mortality in US Adults. *JAMA,* **281:** 1291-1297, 1999.

18. Executive summary of the third report of the National Cholesterol Education Program (NCEP) Expert Panel on Detection, Evaluation, and Treatment of High Blood Cholesterol in Adults (Adult Treatment Panel III). *JAMA,* **285:** 2486–2497, 2001.

19. Mukamal KJ, Nesto RW, Cohen MC, Muller JE, Maclure M, Sherwood JB, Mittleman MA. Impact of Diabetes on Long-Term Survival after Acute Myocardial Infarction. Comparability of risk with prior myocardial infarction. *Diabetes Care,* **24:** 1422–1427, 2001.

20. Laing SP, Swerdlow AJ, Slater SD, Burden AC, Morris A, Waugh NR, Gatling W, Bingley PJ, Patterson CC. Mortality from heart disease in a cohort of 23,000 patients with insulin-treated diabetes. *Diabetologia,* **46:** 760–765, 2003.

21. Howard BV, Magee MF. Macrovascular Complications of Diabetes Mellitus. In: LeRoith D, Taylor SI, Olefsky JM (eds). *Diabetes Mellitus. A Fundamental and Clinical Text,* 2nd edition, Lippincott Williams & Wilkins, Philadelphia, 2000, 957–962.

22. Jude EB, Oyibo SO, Chalmers N, Boulton AJ. Peripheral arterial disease in diabetic and nondiabetic patient. *Diabetes Care,* **24:** 1433–1437, 2001.

23. Diabetes-related amputations of lower extremities in the Medicare population-Minnesota, 1993–1995. *MMWR Morb Mortal Wkly Rep,* **47:** 649–652, 1998.

24. Kuusisto J, Mikkanen L, Pyorala K, Laakso M. Non-insulin-dependent diabetes and its metabolic control are important predictors of stroke in elderly subjects. *Stroke,* **25:** 1157–1164, 1994.

25. Jorgensen H, Nakayama H, Raaschon HO, Olsen TS. Stroke in patients with diabetes: the Copenhagen Stroke Study. *Stroke,* **25:** 1977–1984, 1994.

26. Tuomilehto J, Rastenyte D, Jousilahti P, Sarti C, Vartiainen E. Diabetes mellitus as a risk factor for death from stroke: prospective study of the middle-aged Finnish population. *Stroke,* **27:** 210–215, 1996.

27. Laing SP, Swerdlow AJ, Carpenter LM, Slater SD, Burden AC, Botha JL, Morris AD, Waugh NR, Gatling W, Gale EA, Patterson CC, Qiao Z, Keen H. Mortality form cerebrovascular disease in a cohort of 23,000 patients with insulin-treated diabetes. *Stroke* **34:** 418–421, 2003.

28. Trevisan R, Viberti G. Pathophysiology of Diabetic Nephrophaty. In: LeRoith D, Taylor SI, Olefsky JM (eds). *Diabetes Mellitus. A Fundamental and Clinical Text,* 2nd edition, Lippincott Williams & Wilkins, Philadelphia, 2000, 898–910.

29. Spranger J, Pfeiffer AFH. Diabetc Microvascular Complications. In: Mogensen CE (ed). *Hypertension & Diabetes,* vol 1, Lippincott Williams & Wilkins, London, 2002, 57–67.

30. Bilous RW, Marshall SM. Clinical Aspects of Nephropathy. In: Alberti KGMM, Zimmet P, DeFronzo RA, Keen H (eds). *International Textbook of Diabetes Mellitus,* 2nd edition, Wiley, Chichester, 1997, 1363–1411.

31. Hamman RF. Epidemiology of Microvascular Complications. In: Alberti KGMM, Zimmet P, DeFronzo RA, Keen H (eds). *International Textbook of Diabetes Mellitus,* 2nd edition, Wiley, Chichester, 1997, 1213–1319.

32. Chew EY. Pathophysiology of Diabetic Retinopathy. In: LeRoith D, Taylor SI, Olefsky JM (eds). *Diabetes Mellitus. A Fundamental and Clinical Text,* 2nd edition, Lippincott Williams & Wilkins, Philadelphia, 2000, 890–898.

33. Klein R, Klein BEK, Moss SE. Visual impairment in diabetes. *Ophthalmology,* **91:** 1–9, 1984.

34. Klein R, Klein BEK, Moss SE, Davis MD, DeMets DL. The Wisconsin Epidemiologic Study of Diabetic Retinopathy. II. Prevalence and risk of diabetic retinopathy when age of diagnosis is less than 30 years. *Arch Ophtalmol,* **102:** 520–526, 1984.

35. Massi Benedetti M, Calabrese G, Cesarini A. Diabetic Life Problems: Social Rights. In: Alberti KGMM, Zimmet P, DeFronzo RA, Keen H (eds). *International Textbook of Diabetes Mellitus,* 2nd edition, Wiley, Chichester, 1997, 1755–1760.

36. American Diabetes Association. Economic Costs of Diabetes in the U.S. in 2002. *Diabetes Care,* **26:** 917–932, 2003.

37. Eschwege E. Counting the costs. In: Highlights of the International Acarbose Symposium, Sitges, 28 February – 1 March 2003, Bayer AG, 3.

38. Jönsson B. Revealing the cost of Type II diabetes in Europe. *Diabetologia,* **45:** S5–12, 2002.

39. Caro JJ, Ward AJ, O'Brien JA. Lifetime Costs of Complications Resulting From Type 2 Diabetes in the U.S. *Diabetes Care,* **25:** 476–481, 2002.

40. Williams R, Van Gaal L, Lucioni C. Assessing the impact of complications on the costs of Type II diabetes. *Diabetologia,* **45:** S13–17, 2002.

41. Nichols GA, Brown JB. The impact of cardiovascular disease on medical care costs in subjects with or without type 2 diabetes. *Diabetes Care,* **25:** 482–486, 2002.

42. Safar ME. The Epidemiology and Costs of Hypertension and Type 2 Diabetes. In: Mogensen CE (ed). *Hypertension & Diabetes,* vol. 1, Lippincott Williams & Wilkins, London, 2002, 29–42.

43. Stratta RJ. Quality of Life and Economics in Pancreas Transplantation. In: Symposia. Clinical Pancreas and Islet Transplantation, 63rd Scientific Sessions ADA, June 13–17, 2003, New Orleans, LA, USA.

44. Javitt JC, Aiello LP, Chiang Y, Ferris FL 3rd, Canner JK, Greenfield S. Preventive eye care in people with diabetes is cost-saving to the federal government. Implications for health-care reform. *Diabetes Care,* 17: 909–917, 1994.

45. Brandle M, Zhou H, Smith BRK, Marriott D, Burke R, Tabaei BP, Brown MB, Herman WH. The Direct Medical Costs of Type 2 Diabetes Mellitus. *Diabetes,* **52(Suppl 1):** A10, 2003.

46. Davis WA, Davis TME, Knuiman MW, Hendrie D. Predictors of diabetes-attributable non-blood glucose-lowering medication costs for type 2 diabetes: the Fremantle diabetes study. *Diabetologia,* **46(Suppl 2):** A105, 2003.

47. Hancu N, Albota A, Babes A, Barbonta D, Calinici A, Creteanu G, Ghise G, Graur M, Morosanu M, Mota M, Petrescu I, Stamoran M, Suciu G, Szilagyi I. Quality of care in newly-diagnosed diabetes mellitus: 'EPIDIAB' program-lessons from the first three years. *Diabetologia,* **46(Suppl 2):** A102, 2003.

48. Solomon CG. Reducing Cardiovascular Risk in Type 2 Diabetes. *N Engl J Med,* **348:** 457–459, 2003.

49. Cheta DM. *Preventing Diabetes. Theory, Practice and New Approaches,* Wiley, Chichester, 1999.

50. Diabetes Prevention Program Research Group. Reduction in the incidence of type 2 diabetes with lifestyle intervention or metformin. *N Engl J Med,* **346:** 393–403, 2002.

51. Tuomilehto J, Lindstrom J, Eriksson JG, Valle TT, Hamalainen H, Ilanne-Parikka P, Keinanen-Kiukaanniemi S, Laakso M, Louheranta A, Rastas M, Salminen V, Aunola S, Cepaitis Z, Moltchanov V, Hakumaki M, Mannelin M, Martikkala V, Sundvall J, Uusitupa M, for the Finnish Diabetes Prevention Study Group. Prevention of type 2 diabetes mellitus by changes in lifestyle among subjects with impaired glucose tolerance. *N Engl J Med,* **344:** 1343–1350, 2001.

52. Turner RC, Millns H, Neil HAW, Stratton IM, Manley SE, Matthews DR, Holman RR. Risk factors for coronary artery disease in non-insulin dependent diabetes mellitus: United Kingdom prospective diabetes study (UKPDS: 23). *BMJ,* **316:** 823–828, 1998.

53. American Diabetes Association. Standards of medical care for patients with diabetes mellitus. *Diabetes Care,* **26(Suppl 1):** S33–S50, 2003.

54. Gaede P, Vedel P, Larsen N, Jensen GVH, Parving HH, Pedersen O. Multifactorial Intervention and Cardiovascular Disease in Patients with Type 2 Diabetes. *N Engl J Med,* **348:** 383–393, 2003.

55. Hupfeld CJ, Wong GA. Current Recommendation for Prevention of Cardiovascular Disease in Patients with Diabetes Mellitus. *Prev Cardiol,* **5:** 34–37, 2003.

56. Zimmet P. The burden of type 2 diabetes: are we doing enough? *Diabetes Metab,* **29:** 6S9–18, 2003.

57. Vinik AI, Vinik E. Prevention of the complications of diabetes. *Am J Manag Care,* **9(Suppl2):** S63–80, 2003.

58. Bate KL, Jerums G. Preventing complications of diabetes. *Med J Aust,* **179:** 498–503, 2003.

59. Pyorala K, Pedersen TR, Kjekshus J, Fsergeman O, Olsson AG, Thorgeirsson G. Cholesterol lowering with simvastatin improves prognosis of diabetic patients with coronary heart disease: a subgroup analysis of the Scandinavian Simvastatin Survival Study (4S). *Diabetes Care,* **20:** 614–629, 1997.

60. Heart Outcomes Prevention Evaluation (HOPE) Study Investigators. Effects of ramipril on cardiovascular and microvascular outcomes in people with diabetes mellitus: results of the Hope Study and MICRO-HOPE substudy. *Lancet,* **355:** 253–259, 2000.

61. Heart Protection Study Collaborative Group. MRC/BHF Heart Protection Study of cholesterol lowering with simvastatin in 20,536 high-risk individuals: a randomized placebo-controlled trial. *Lancet,* **360:** 7–22, 2002.

62. Gerstein HC, Capes SE. Dysglycemia: A key cardiovascular risk factor. *Semin Vasc Med,* **2:** 165–174, 2002.

63. Gerstein HC. Targeting Normoglycemia to prevent Cardiovascular Outcomes – New Opportunities. In: *Symposium. Real Life Strategies for Treating to Target A1c Control,* IDF Congress, Paris, August 2003, Abstract Book (Aventis), p. 8.

BASIC RESEARCH

2

ENDOTHELIAL DYSFUNCTION IN DIABETES

Maya SIMIONESCU, Doina POPOV, Anca SIMA

> *"Man may be the captain of his fate,*
> *but he is also the victim of his blood sugar."*
> **W. Oakey**
> *Trans Med Soc Lond **78**:16, 1962*

The vascular endothelium (lining the entire cardiovascular system) by its strategic position exerts active metabolic and regulatory functions that maintain the body homeostasis. Concomitantly, the endothelial cells (EC) are the first to be exposed and affected by the various insults occurring either in the blood or within the tissues. As a function of the nature, duration and intensity of the deleterious factors (hyperglycemia, hypercholesterolemia, inflammation, high blood pressure, etc.) the EC pass gradually through modulation, dysfunction, injury and cell death.

The endothelial dysfunction may be defined as a localized alteration of EC, causing temporarily and, often reversibly, a modified functional state supported by a phenotypic change. Hyperglycemia induces a functional alteration of EC characterized by: increased cell proliferation, augmentation of vascular permeability, diminishment of the anionic sites density of the luminal plasmalemma, enhanced synthesis of basal lamina and extracellular matrix proteins, expression of new adhesion molecules, imbalanced production of vasodilator/vasoconstrictor molecules and of coagulation/fibrinolysis factors, etc.

Recent studies identified the specific markers of EC dysfunction in diabetes: excessive accumulation of advanced glycation end-products (AGE) and of advanced lipoxidation products (ALE), the augmented oxidative stress, expression of new adhesion molecules by the luminal plasmalemma, alteration of the vascular reactivity and impaired nitric oxide (NO) concentration. At the molecular level, three biochemical pathways were reported to trigger the vascular dysfunction induced by high glucose: (1) increased glucose flux through the sorbitol (polyol) pathway, (2) enhanced formation of advanced glycation end-products and (3) activation of protein kinase C.

Another feature of EC dysfunction in diabetic condition is the reduced bioavailability of NO. Among the mechanisms that generate this process are the deficient expression of endothelial NO synthase (eNOS), the lack of its substrate (L-arginine), a reduced activation of NOS due to altered signal transduction pathways, or the increased inactivation of NO (after its synthesis) by the reactive oxygen species. In addition, the enhanced level of endothelins (mainly of endothelin-1) results in a diminished endothelium-dependent relaxation. The sustained shear stress could activate transcription factors that, in turn, regulate the genes responsive for remodeling of the vascular wall, increasing its mechanical stiffness and conducing finally to the impeded vasorelaxation.

All the recent data on EC dysfunction indicate that the vascular endothelium can be considered a therapeutic target. In recent years, the strategies to improve/reverse endothelial dysfunction are focused to amend the high glucose-disturbed mechanisms, addressing specifically to the molecules in affected signal transduction pathways. Thus, inhibitors of glycation, anti-oxidants, NO scavengers, L-arginine supplementation, inhibition of PARP activity, transplantation of pancreatic islets, lipid lowering and inhibition of the renin-angiotensin system are at present the key approaches for restoring the altered endothelial function.

A new family of nuclear receptors, the peroxisome proliferator-activated receptors (PPAR), were reported to regulate the expression of genes controlling both lipid and glucose metabolism (PPAR-α, PPAR-(β)δ, PPAR-γ). Pharmacological and genetic studies have determined that PPAR-α regulates pathways of fatty acid oxidation and PPAR-γ modulates fatty acid synthesis and storage in adipose tissues. At present, the synthetic agonists of PPARs are used in the treatment of metabolic diseases, such as type 2 diabetes and dyslipidemia: glitazones (which are insulin sensitizers) are synthetic high affinity ligands for PPAR-γ, and fibrates (hypolipidemic drugs) are PPAR-α ligands.

In the restoration of the endothelial function, the effectiveness of the treatment may differ according to the cause of the dysfunction or to the vascular bed involved (arteries, arterioles, capillaries, etc.). At present, cohort trials are necessary to conclusively prove whether reversal of endothelial dysfunction offers the clinical advantage of reduced morbidity and mortality.

Abbreviations List

AGEs – advanced glycation end-products
ALE – advanced lipoxidation end-products
BP – blood pressure
CHD – coronary heart disease
D – diabetic hamsters
EC – endothelial cell
eNOS – endothelial nitric oxide synthase
ET-1 – endothelin 1
GBM – glomerular basement membrane
H – hyperlipemic hamsters
HD – simultaneously hyperlipemic and diabetic hamsters
HNE – 4-hydroxynonenal

LDL – low density lipoprotein
LDL-C – low-density lipoprotein cholesterol
MDA – malondialdehyde
MRL – modified and reassembled lipoproteins
NO – nitric oxide
PARP – poly (ADP-ribose) polymerase
PKC – protein kinase C
PPAR – peroxisome proliferator-activated receptors
RAGE – advanced glycation end-products receptor
ROS – reactive oxygen species
SMC – smooth muscle cells
TRAP – total antioxidant radical trapping potential
VEGF – vascular endothelial growth factor

Diabetes mellitus is commonly accompanied by nephropathy, retinopathy, neuropathy and accelerated atherosclerosis (the main cause of morbidity and mortality in this disease). All these complications involve abnormalities of the large and/or small blood vessels that all commence with alterations of the endothelial cell (EC) functions.

Blood capillaries were first observed by Malpighi in 1661, but for a very long time the vascular endothelium was viewed as an inert cellophane barrier between blood and tissues. In 1960, Palade reported the presence of an unusual large number of plasmalemmal vesicles (known also as caveolae) that populate the EC [1], and numerous further studies (using tracer molecules of various dimensions and chemistry) have demonstrated that these vesicles are involved in active transport of macromolecules across the endothelium (for reviews see Simionescu M and Simionescu N, 1991, Simionescu et al., 2002) [2, 3]. Moreover, using plasma molecules, it was demonstrated that albumin [4], low-density lipoproteins [5], and thyroxin [6] are indeed transported by vesicles across the endothelium, employing various mechanisms of transcytosis (fluid phase, adsorptive or receptor mediated transcytosis), a term and concept coined by N. Simionescu [2, 7].

With time, it was revealed that beside the selective transport of plasma molecules, the EC have numerous other vital functions. They are endowed with the ability to synthesize and release pro- and anticoagulant factors, cytokines, adhesion molecules, collagen, elastin, prostacyclin, balanced amounts of vasodilators (such as nitric oxide, NO) and vasoconstrictors (like endothelin), as well as other vasoactive substances (Plate 2.1). NO is a gas that passes easily the cell membranes of EC and smooth muscle cells (SMC) at the level of which increases the cyclic guanosin mono-phosphate concentration and induces relaxation. NO also has antithrombogenic and antiproliferative effects and inhibits leukocyte adhesion to EC (for review, see Lüscher et al., 2001) [8]. The family of endothelins consists of three peptides (ET-1, ET-2, ET-3). ET-1 has vasoconstrictor effects through activation of ET_A receptors (Plate 2.1) coupled to intracellular G proteins in vascular SMC (reviewed in Lüscher et al., 2001) [8].

In physiological conditions, the release and the concentration of these numerous compounds is under thorough control of EC, so as to maintain the steady state condition, i.e. the body homeostasis. Thus, the endothelium, as a whole, may be considered the largest endocrine organ in the body (having an approximate total weight of 1 kg).

Based on its large and vital properties, the endothelial layer (lining the entire cardiovascular system) exerts numerous active metabolic and regulatory functions, such as plasma homeostasis, blood coagulation and fibrinolysis, interaction with circulating cells, presentation of histo-compatibility antigens, regulation of vascular tone and of the blood pressure, etc. [for review see 9].

However, the properties of the endothelium differ along the vascular tree, and even in various zones of the same vessel [10, 11]; subsequently, differences exist in the reactivity and pathology of endothelium in various locations. Thus, atherosclerotic plaques develop in specific zones of the arterial tree (lesion-prone areas) such as coronaries, aortic arch, aortic valves; thrombosis occur in veins and vascular leakage in small venules [12].

In all afflictions EC by their position between the circulating plasma and all other tissues of the body are the first to be exposed and affected by the various insults occurring either in the blood or within the tissues. As a function of the nature, duration and intensity of the deleterious stimuli, the EC may pass gradually through modulation, dysfunction and finally, injury. The initial response of the endothelium to abnormal stimuli is the *modulation* of its constitutive functions; examples are the increased permeability for circulating lipoproteins in hyperlipemia or hyperglycemia, increased production of NO upon stimulation by acetylcholine, or adaptation to the blood flow changes. In time, abnormal stimuli may generate endothelial *dysfunction:* this is the case of hyperglycemia-induced "activation" of EC that expresses an increased number or new adhesion molecules [13] and an imbalance between secreted relaxation and contraction factors, or inflammation in which the increased production of cytokines (IL-1 and TNF alpha) generates abnormal functionality. Excessive adverse influences resulting in physical damage of EC characterize the altered state of *injury,* that may be reversible through a repair process or by the replacement of the denuded endothelial area (local tissue regeneration), or irreversible, leading to cell death [14].

MULTIPLE CONNOTATIONS FOR ENDOTHELIAL CELL DYSFUNCTION

Largely, the endothelial dysfunction may be defined as a localized alteration of EC, causing temporarily and often reversibly a modified functional state supported by a phenotypic change. The altered condition is generating variations of the specific molecules, such as: basal lamina and extracellular matrix components, adhesion molecules, von Willebrand factor, NO, endothelin-1, tissue type plasminogen activator, plasminogen activator inhibitor-1, and relaxing and contracting factors.

Thus, EC dysfunction is characterized by increased cell proliferation, abnormal augmentation in vascular permeability and the gradual change of the EC to a secretory phenotype (Figure 2.1). The latter modification may explain the significant enhanced synthesis of basal lamina and extracellular matrix proteins, of von Willebrand factor and adhesion molecules that occur in early stages of diabetes and atherogenesis.

Another modification commonly occurring in diabetes is the change of the EC luminal membrane anionic sites from the uniform (Figure 2.2a) to the patchy distribution (Figure 2.2b), as revealed by the decoration with cationized ferritin. The gradual diminishment of the anionic sites density parallels the progression of the disease [15, 16]. By contrast, the venous endothelium (of the heart and hind limb) maintains in a diabetic condition the same uniform distribution of the anionic sites of the luminal plasmalemma as in normal EC (Figure 2.2a) [16]. Since in hyperglycemic animals the platelet membrane anionic sites are markedly reduced [17], one can assume that platelet adhesion to the venous endothelium is enhanced, a process which may explain the predisposition for thrombus formation at the level of the veins. In addition, the number of cationic ferritin detectable anionic sites along the vein traject varies, diminishing gradually towards the venular segment, where it resembles the situation described for capillary and arterial endothelium [18, 19].

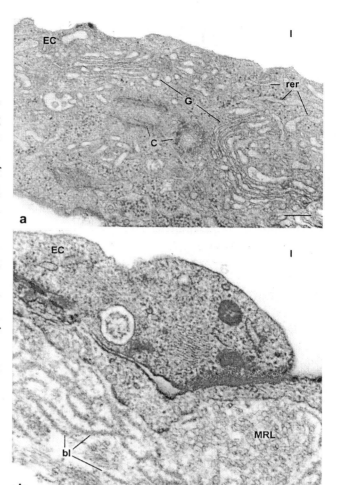

Figure 2.1

Early (2 weeks) ultrastructural changes of the aortic valve endothelial cells (EC) in a hyperlipemic-diabetic hamster:

a – the cell is enriched in numerous copies of biosynthetic organelles such as rough endoplasmic reticulum (rer) and Golgi apparatus (G), centrioles (C); b – as well as in another early modification is the appearance of hyperplasic, multilayered basal lamina (bl), in the meshwork of which numerous modified and reassembled lipoproteins (MRL) are trapped.

l: vascular lumen. Bars: (a): 0.8 μm; (b): 0.6 μm.

Another expression of the endothelial dysfunction is the impairment of NO bioavailability [9, 20]. The factors contributing to the decline in NO are the decreased expression of endothelial NO synthase (eNOS) [21], lack of substrate or cofactors for eNOS [22], a deficient activation of eNOS due to altered cellular signaling [23] and accelerated inactivation of NO by the reactive oxygen species [24].

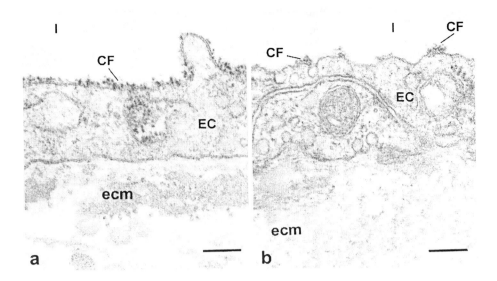

Figure 2.2

Distribution of the anionic sites on the endothelial plasmalemma reacted *in situ* with cationized ferritin (CF). After the vasculature was washed out of blood, CF was perfused for 2 min through the entire vasculature, followed by extensive washing, and the standard protocol for electron microscopy. Note the even distribution of CF-decorated anionic sites on EC of a vein of normal hamsters (a) and the patchy decoration with CF of the EC plasmalemma in a heart capillary of a 15-weeks diabetic hamster (b). l: vascular lumen; EC: endothelial cell; ecm: extracellular matrix. Bars: (a): 0.18 μm; (b): 0.12μm.

As already stated, in physiological conditions the vascular endothelium produces balanced amounts of relaxing and contracting factors, as a result of which the optimal response of the vessel wall to the circulating or locally released agonists occurs. Any deviation from this condition is defined as endothelial dysfunction and specifically, the impairment of vasorelaxation in response to pharmacological and non-pharmacological stimuli, such as acetylcholine, shear stress and cold pressor [25]. Several mechanisms were suggested to be involved in the decreased endothelium-dependent vasodilation: the decreased secretion of vasodilator mediators, the increased production of vasoconstrictors, the increased sensitivity to vasoconstrictors and/or the resistance of the vascular smooth muscle cells to the endothelial vasodilators. In addition, the sustained shear stress could activate transcription factors that, in turn, regulate the genes responsive for remodeling of the vascular wall, increasing its mechanical stiffness and conducting finally to the impeded vasorelaxation [9]. Also, intimal thickening may conduct to decreased vasodilator response to acetylcholine [26].

MARKERS OF ENDOTHELIAL DYSFUNCTION

Plasma circulating markers. Of the circulating markers, the metabolites of NO, namely *nitrites, nitrates* and cyclic GMP (the second messenger of NO) are direct indicators of endothelial dysfunction. Other plasma circulating markers of EC dysfunction are the presence of glycated proteins, peroxidized lipids, the asymmetric dimethylarginine, and the increase in the concentration of endothelin-1, von Willebrand factor, tissue type plasminogen activator, plasminogen activator inhibitor-1. The enhanced number of copies of Weibel Palade bodies expressed particularly by the venous endothelium (Figure 2.3) may account for the reported increase in the circulating von Willebrand factor in diabetic subjects [16, 27, 28, 29]. In type 1 diabetic patients the increased concentration of plasma von Willebrand factor was correlated with increased concentration of circulating C-reactive protein, suggestive of an inflammatory reaction [30].

Increased oxidative stress. Accumulated data indicate an increased level of circulating lipid peroxides, mainly associated with the low-density

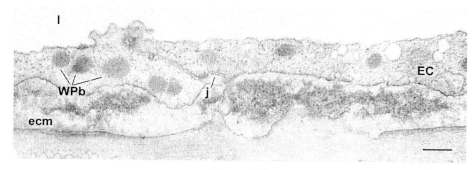

Figure 2.3

The presence of Weibel Palade bodies (WPb) within the endothelium of the saphenous vein
of a diabetic hamster (at 15 weeks after streptozotocin injection).

l: vascular lumen; EC: endothelial cell; ecm: extracellular matrix; j: endothelial junction. Bar: 0.27 μm.

lipoproteins (LDL), both in atherosclerosis and diabetes [31]. In addition, the total level of Cu^{2+} is higher in diabetics than in normal individuals, reaching the highest level in diabetic patients with angiopathy and alterations in lipid metabolism [32]. These data indicate that in the two pathologies there is an increased oxidative stress that, by its deleterious effects on the cells of the vessel wall, may potentiate the atherosclerotic plaque formation.

In diabetes, various sources of free radicals increase the oxidative stress; among these are the non-enzymatic glycosylation of proteins and monosaccharide autoxidation, polyol pathway activity, indirect production of free radicals through cell damage and the reduced antioxidant reserve. In physiological conditions, the free radicals generated in the circulation are efficiently scavenged by various antioxidant systems available in the plasma milieu [33]. These include, apart from different enzymatic-based defenses (*i.e.* superoxide dismutase, catalase), a series of small molecules either lipophilic or hydrophilic, generically known as antioxidants. The lipophilic antioxidants such as tocopherols and carotenoids (mainly associated with plasma lipoprotein particles) contribute together with the hydrophilic molecules like ascorbic acid, to plasma intrinsic antioxidant defense. It has been reported [34] that in diabetic patients, the serum total antioxidant potential is reduced as compared to healthy subjects and the decrease is even higher in diabetic patients with coronary heart disease (Plate 2.2).

Epidemiological trials and experimental studies indicate the potential benefits of both natural and synthetic antioxidants in the development of atherosclerosis (for review see [35]); however, the data are not conclusive yet.

Endothelial cell adhesion molecules. Release or altered expression of endothelial cell adhesion molecules, such as ICAM-1, VECAM-1, E-selectin and P-selectin are other markers indicating the cell dysfunction [9, 13]. Interestingly, the levels of E-selectin and ICAM-1, and the enzymatic activity of serum N-acetyl-β-glucosaminidase were reported as early indicators of vascular changes in diabetic microangiopathy [36].

Vascular reactivity. There are important alterations of the vascular reactivity of the mesenteric resistance arteries of Golden Syrian hamsters rendered hyperlipemics (by a diet supplemented with 3% cholesterol and 15% butter, H group), diabetics (by streptozotocin injection, D group), and simultaneous hyperlipemics-hyperglycemics (by the combination of the two conditions, HD group) [37, 38]. The vascular reactivity of the resistance arteries was measured under isometric conditions by the myograph technique, originally introduced by Mulvany and Halpern (1977) [39]. Compared to the resistance arteries of normal hamsters that relaxed in cumulative doses of acetylcholine (10^{-8}–10^{-4}M) to a maximum of ~ 80 %, the relaxation of the similar vessels in groups H and D was diminished to ~ 64 % and ~ 55 %, respectively; the relaxation of similar arteries in group HD was reduced to ~ 61 % [38].

Several factors were identified to cause the impeded relaxation of the resistance arteries in associated hyperlipemic-hyperglycemic conditions induced in hamsters: a deficit of NO, the thickening of the arterial wall (that presented ~ 10% increase

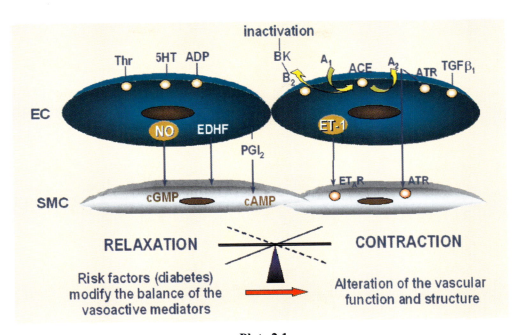

Plate 2.1

Endothelial cells – a source of vasoactive mediators.

The endothelial cells (EC) synthesize and release numerous vasoactive compounds, most of which acting on smooth muscle cell (SMC): vasodilators such as nitric oxide (NO), endothelium-derived hyperpolarizing factor (EDHF) and prostacyclin (PGI_2), and vasoconstrictors like endothelin-1 (ET-1). The surface exposed angiotensin converting enzyme (ACE) simultaneously converts angiotensin-1 (A_1) to the potent vasoconstrictor angiotensin II (A_2) and inactivates bradykinin (BK). (Adapted from Lüscher *et al*. [8]). Thr – thrombin; 5HT – serotonin; ADP – adenosine diphosphate; ATR – Angiotensin receptors; $TGF\beta_1$ – transforming growth factor β_1; ET_AR – endothelin receptor; B_2 – bradykinin receptors.

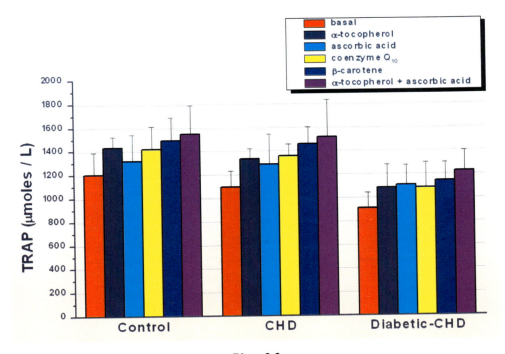

Plate 2.2

Values of the total antioxidant trapping potential (expressed as mean TRAP values) in the sera collected from control subjects, from patients with coronary heart disease (CHD) and from non-insulin diabetic patients with CHD complications.

of the cross sectional area of the intima plus media, ~ 20% diminishment of the lumen area, and ~ 3 fold increase in the wall to lumen ratio), the formation of small calcification centers surrounded by a hyperplasic extracellular matrix within the intima (that induced a rigidity of the arterial wall), and the accumulation of AGE-collagen and pentosidine in the mesenteric vascular bed [38, 40].

As for the contractile response, it was found that simultaneous insult of hyperlipemia-hyperglycemia was associated with the highest contractility of the resistance arteries to $PGF_{2\alpha}$. A reduced effect of cyclooxygenases inhibition, the diminishment of the activity of Ca^{2+} dependent K^+ channels and the enhancement in the protein kinase C were among the mechanisms that explained the augmented contractility to $PGF_{2\alpha}$ [41].

In humans, the endothelial dysfunction can be assessed by the vascular reactivity tests that include assays of the endothelium-dependent vasodilation either by invasive (at the coronary or forearm levels) or by noninvasive techniques (positron emission tomography and ultrasound methods).

To date, endothelial dysfunction is a common "umbrella" not only for the imbalances in EC functions produced by stress, aging, cigarette smoking, drugs or inappropriate nutritional habits, but also for diseased states such as vasospasm, inflammation, leukocytes and platelets adhesion, thrombosis and abnormal vascular proliferation (for review see Vapaatalo and Mervaala, 2001) [9]. It is noteworthy that in diabetes [42], hypertension [43], hypercholesterolemia [44] and coronary heart disease [45], dysfunction of the EC occurs before the development of associated cardiovascular disease and, as such, they may represent an early marker of further vascular complications.

SIGNAL TRANSDUCTION PATHWAYS IN GLUCOSE-INDUCED ENDOTHELIAL DYSFUNCTION

The primary factor that induces endothelial dysfunction in diabetes is the hyperglycemic millieu that flushes the endothelial layer. Three biochemical pathways were reported to trigger the vascular dysfunction induced by high glucose:

(i) increased glucose flux through the sorbitol (polyol) pathway, (ii) enhanced formation of advanced glycation end-products and (iii) activation of protein kinase C (PKC).

(i) The sorbitol pathway comprises two enzymatic steps: reduction of D-glucose to sorbitol by aldose reductase (coupled to oxidation of NADPH to $NADP^+$), and oxidation of sorbitol to fructose by sorbitol dehydrogenase (coupled to reduction of NAD^+ to NADH). In high glucose conditions, the increased free cytosolic NADH / NADPH ratio can be corrected by oral administration of aldose reductase inhibitors [46].

(ii) Advanced glycation end-products (AGEs) result from the reaction of glucose (or other reducing sugars) with the primary amino groups of proteins, lipoproteins, nucleic acids and other molecules. The reversible Shiff bases formed are transformed into Amadori products and then into various irreversible, crosslinked, fluorescent and chemically reactive adducts. Protein modifications by AGEs induce a decrease in solubility and protease resistance, which in tissues conduct to abnormalities of matrix-matrix and matrix-cell interactions [47]. These reactions take place at a slow pace during normal aging and at a faster rate in diabetes. AGEs accumulate on long-lived circulating proteins and affect also the cellular membranes, cytosolic proteins, the components of the basal lamina and of the extracellular matrix. In an original model of diabetes associated with hyperlipemia, it was found that the concentration of AGE-Albumin (AGE-Alb) in circulation paralleled that of blood glucose [18]. In the streptozotocin-induced diabetic rats, AGEs accumulation in endothelial and smooth muscle cells was reported to increase with the duration of diabetes [48]. Circulating lipoproteins (LDL) accumulate in the subendothelium of diabetic hamster and coronary heart disease patients' arteries as modified and reassembled lipoproteins coupled to AGEs [49, 50].

The mechanism that enables the endothelium to take up circulating AGE-proteins involves their recognition by specific AGE-receptor (RAGE), which is a member of the immunoglobulin superfamily of the cell surface molecules [51]. The interaction of RAGE with ligands enhances receptor expression; thus, in diabetic vasculature, expression of RAGE was increased not only in the endothelium, but also in smooth muscle cells and infiltrating mononuclear phagocytes [52]. An unusual feature of RAGE is the ability to engage classes of molecules, rather than individual ligands, propagating cellular perturbations, such as the immune and inflammatory responses (for review see Schmidt *et al.*, 2001) [52]. The progressive accumulation of AGEs in tissues under diabetic conditions suggests that the clearance mechanism fails to function effectively. Accumulation of AGEs and the increase in RAGE expression may explain the role of AGEs in the initiation of macroangiopathy (through RAGE) and the accelerated atherosclerosis associated with diabetes [48].

(iii) The mechanism of glucose-induced protein kinase C activation involves increased production of diacylglycerol, either from agonist-induced phosphatidylinositide hydrolysis or from de novo synthesis from glycolytic intermediates (reviewed in Koya and King, 1998) [53]. Activation of PKC has been linked to changes in permeability of the endothelium, changes in endothelin and prostaglandin production, increases in gene expression and altered responses to the circulating hormones [54].

A potential cascade explaining the multiple effects of high-glucose on the endothelium includes: increase of glucose flux via the sorbitol pathway generating a reductive stress, production of reactive oxygen species (ROS) by the excess cytosolic NADPH, activation of PKC, formation of AGEs and ALEs, interaction of AGEs with RAGE on the endothelium and smooth muscle cells, peroxidation of membrane lipids, calcium influx and endothelium hyperpermeability. To the augmented permeability contributes also the increased concentration of the vascular endothelial growth factor (a proinflammatory and prothrombotic molecule), the mitogen-activated protein kinase (serving as glucose transducers) and of the NO level [55].

ACCUMULATION OF AGEs AND ALEs IN THE DIABETIC VASCULAR WALL

The vascular endothelium is able to remove AGE molecules from the circulation by a receptor-mediated process, which is AGE-specific [56–58]. Experiments performed with AGE-Albumin (AGE-Alb) either radiolabeled or adsorbed to gold particles have revealed that the probe is taken up specifically and saturably by the microvascular endothelial vesicles (caveolae) open to the lumen, after which it is transcytosed and discharged into the subendothelial space. As a general feature, the uptake of circulating AGE-Alb was found increased in diabetic animals (compared to normal) suggestive for an augmented removal of AGE-molecules from the circulation [59]. Competition experiments (performed in the presence of excess unlabelled AGE-Alb) reduced significantly the uptake, indicating the specificity of the process [60]. In hyperglycemic conditions, instead of being removed, the AGE-proteins accumulate in the subendothelial space and induce physico-chemical alterations of low density lipoproteins (LDL) retained within the intima, thus contributing to the altered millieu of the vascular wall and accelerated atherosclerosis, characteristic for diabetes [61].

In addition, the increased risk for atherosclerosis in diabetes may result from the carbonyl production from carbohydrates and the peroxidation of lipids of the lipoproteins accumulated in the vascular wall, leading to the local production of reactive carbonyl species. The latter mediate recruitment of macrophages and chemical modifications of vessels' proteins by advanced lipoxidation end-products (ALE).

The most studied carbonyl intermediates are malondialdehyde (MDA), 4-hydroxynonenal (HNE) and acrolein, which react with cysteine, histidine and lysine residues in proteins, generating characteristic ALEs. Despite their presence in low concentration in proteins, there is growing evidence that protein-bound ALEs and AGEs are mediators of stress responses and tissue damage. MDA-Lys and HNE-Lys have been detected in atherosclerotic plaques of diabetic (D) and simultaneously hyperlipemic and diabetic (HD) hamsters [19], as well as in human plaques [50]. As opposed to normal hamsters, in which only minute quantities of LDL, AGEs and IgG are present in the vessel wall, in D and HD hamsters there is a significant increased concentration of modified LDL and IgG in lesion prone areas [19]. Among other LDL oxidation products, 4-hydroxynonenal can be immunolocalized in the fibrous cap of atherosclerotic plaques, together with AGE-proteins. Concomitantly with the subendothelial accumulation of modified and reassembled lipoproteins (MRL) and alterations of the extracellular matrix, the immunostaining of modified LDL and IgG in the subendothelial space of aortic valves is more prominent. On consecutive cryosections of the aortic arch and valves, deposition of IgG paralleled the accumulation of LDL (revealed with antibody to LDL) and total lipids (stained with Oil Red O). In advanced lesions of the aortic arch, the immunostaining for modified LDL (HNE-adducts, AGEs) and IgG was particularly pronounced in the fibrotic cap and the shoulders of the lesions that appeared strongly labeled. In both D and HD hamsters, AGE-proteins deposits were focally detected at the level of fatty streaks, as well as in advanced lesions. In all types of lesions examined, AGEs were found associated with the extracellular matrix of the vessel intima, in the adventitia, and especially in the macrophage-derived foam cells and some SMC.

In atherosclerotic plaques of patients with diabetes and coronary heart disease modified LDL (Plate 2.3a), lipid peroxidation products as 4-hydroxynonenal (Plate 2.3b) and advanced glycation end-products (Plate 2.3c) were detected. These results indicate that LDL, HNE- and AGE-proteins co-localize in human atheroma; they are present intracellularly (in macrophage-derived foam cells on the shoulder areas and smooth muscle cells of the fibrous cap), as well as extracellularly within the lipid deposits adjacent to the internal elastic lamina [50].

OXIDATIVE STRESS-INDUCED ENDOTHELIAL DYSFUNCTION

The reactive oxygen species (ROS) include free radicals (molecules possessing unpaired electrons) or strong oxidants. Representative for the free radicals are: the superoxide anion ($O_2^{-\cdot}$), hydroxyl radical (HO·), nitric oxide (NO·), and lipid radicals. The strong oxidants that contribute to the oxidative stress are: hydrogen peroxide (H_2O_2), peroxinitrite ($ONOO^-$), and the hypoclorous acid (HOCl). Cellular production of one ROS may lead to the production of several others by radical chain reactions [24].

Several studies advanced various mechanisms by which ROS may induce endothelial dysfunction:

(i) oxidative stress modulates endothelial function by regulating caveolae formation and eNOS expression [62]; (ii) enhancement in glycosylated hemoglobin concentration may result in an increased generation of superoxide anions, that in turn affects the NO levels [63] and (iii) oxidative stress stimulates formation of lipid peroxidation products and of lipid hydroperoxides, that directly injure EC and cause membrane dysfunctions [64].

A large body of evidence suggests that ROS induce accelerated inactivation of NO, that consecutively causes endothelial dysfunction in numerous pathophysiological conditions such as diabetes, hypertension, atherosclerosis or heart failure [65]. There are several explanations for the reduced NO levels in conditions of oxidative stress: inappropriate utilization of arginine for NO synthesis, abnormal eNOS activity due to inadequate cofactors, quenching of NO by AGE-products and increased synthesis of superoxide anion radicals, which destroy NO activity [66]. It has been reported that ROS quench NO and inhibit the synthesis of prostacyclin, conducting to impair antithrombotic and vasodilating properties of the endothelium [67].

In EC, the main enzymatic systems contributing to increased production of ROS are: xanthine oxidase, NADH/NADPH oxidase, and eNOS [24]. Endothelial dysfunction may result from the imbalance of oxidant/antioxidant mechanisms, reduced glutathione and increased oxidized glutathione levels that reflect a depletion of the antioxidant reserve, as reported for patients with chronic renal failure [68].

Another pathway of endothelial dysfunction in diabetes is connected to activation of nuclear enzyme poly (ADP-ribose) polymerase (PARP), subsequent to the oxidant-induced DNA strand breakage; in response to high glucose concentration, an increase in poly (ADP-ribosyl)ation occurs [69, 70]. The latter authors demonstrated that high glucose induces significant PARP-dependent changes in endothelial ATP content and in the pyridine nucleotide levels (NADPH included). Depletion of endothelial NADPH may be directly responsible for the inhibition of eNOS activity (a NADPH-dependent enzyme), conducting to the suppression of endothelium-dependent vasodilation in diabetic vessels.

NO-DEPENDENT ENDOTHELIAL DYSFUNCTION

In diabetic conditions, bioavailability of NO is the result of the equilibrium between its synthesis from L-arginine by eNOS and its inactivation by superoxide anions. The superoxide anions may be generated by the eNOS itself and by the NADH / NADPH oxidase system [71, 72]. Interestingly, the antioxidant superoxide dismutase is advantageously located within the vascular wall, in the compartments where NO may be inactivated by the superoxide anions [73].

In addition to the effects of ROS on NO levels, there is the possibility that endothelial dysfunction results from a diminished endothelial capacity to synthesize and release NO or from an increased inactivation of NO after its synthesis [74]. Another cause of NO-dependent endothelial dysfunction is connected to the loss of eNOS expression, a condition that can be reversed by cerivastatin, which stabilizes eNOS mRNA and upregulates eNOS expression [75].

As already stated, the EC dysfunction is, up to a point, a reversible process. In experimental diabetes, L-arginine (L-arg) administration or syngeneic pancreatic islet transplantation restores endothelial function [40, 76, 77].

L-arginine reverses the impaired relaxation to acetylcholine of the aortic rings of 8-weeks diabetic animals and its action was found to be stereospecific, since D-arginine does not have the same effect. The benefic effect of oral L-arginine administration (~ 600 mg/kg bw/day, for 12 weeks) in simultaneous hyperlipemic-diabetic hamsters was reported [40, 78]. Beside the direct effect on NO synthesis, indirect favorable effects of L-arginine administration were detected on: (i) plasma homeostasis, *i.e.* diminished concentration of circulating glucose and cholesterol, reduced activity of angiotensin converting enzyme and lower osmotic fragility (marker for the oxidative stress) of erythrocytes membrane; (ii) improved endothelium-dependent relaxation of resistance arteries; (iii) decreased thickness of the left ventricular wall, and (iv) restored width of the pericapillary extracellular matrix close to normal dimensions [40].

Recent clinical data showed that asymmetric dimethyl-L-arginine (an endogenous L-arginine agonist) inhibits NO synthesis in hyper-cholesterolemia, thus representing another risk factor for endothelial dysfunction [79].

The favorable effects of transplantation of pancreatic islets are complex and relate to the decreased oxidative stress, enhanced arginine supply and utilization for NO synthesis and improved glycemic control [76].

ENDOTHELIAL DYSFUNCTION GENERATES AN INCREASE IN CIRCULATING VASOCONSTRICTORS

In the pathogenesis of the vascular dysfunction, the balance of mediators released by the endothelium is shifted to angiotensin II and endothelin (ET-1), vasoconstrictor compounds that also enhance the proliferation of smooth muscle cells [67]. ET-1 increases diacylglycerol levels activating PKC, induce ET-1 receptors and stimulate vascular endothelial growth factor (VEGF) synthesis [53, 80]. By interaction with the NO pathway, ET-1 and angiotensin II intervene in the dysfunctional relaxation of the vascular wall [20, 55].

VEGF-MEDIATED VASCULAR DYSFUNCTION IN DIABETES

The elevated levels of growth factors, particularly of VEGF, was reported to be responsible for diabetic vascular dysfunction [55]. Several compounds account for VEGF-mediated vascular dysfunction, such as AGEs, NO, the EC adhesion molecules and the tight junctional proteins, occludin and ZO-1; the latter two proteins were identified as downstream effectors of the VEGF signaling pathway in the retinal circulation [81].

ENDOTHELIAL DYSFUNCTION IN DIABETES-INDUCED ACCELERATED ATHEROSCLEROSIS

Atherosclerosis is common for both type 1 and type 2 diabetes and commonly occurs at an accelerated rate. This complication appears soon after the onset of diabetes, having as end-result myocardial infarction, cerebral stroke or gangrene

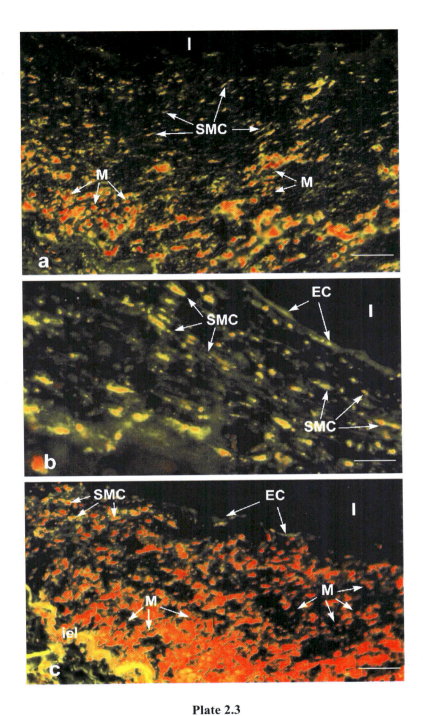

Plate 2.3

Cryosections of human coronary atheroma:

a – immunolocalization of LDL (green fluorescence) in macrophage-derived foam cells (M) and in smooth muscle cells (SMC) in the fibrous cap; b – immunolocalization of 4-hydroxynonenal (green fluorescence) in the fibrous cap and c – immunolocalization of advanced glycation end-products (green fluorescence) in endothelial cells (EC), M and in SMC from the shoulder area. The red fluorescence represents the Oil Red-O staining of the lipid deposits; the yellow color is a result of the superposition of the green and red fluorescence (Nikon Microphot-FXA microscope). l: vascular lumen, iel: internal elastic lamina. Magnifications: × 500 (a); × 1000 (b), × 3000 (c).

of the lower extremities of these patients. The propensity of diabetics for atherosclerosis is due to hyperglycemia, hyperlipidemia, nonenzymatic glycosylation of LDL, the increase in AGE-proteins (in circulation and within the subendothelium); the latter induce chemical modifications of LDL increasing the atherogenicity of the molecule, which is more readily taken up by macrophages to become foam cells [61, 82].

In experimentally induced diabetic (D) and simultaneously hyperlipemic/diabetic (HD) hamsters, ultrastructural data revealed that soon after the induction of the diseases, the large vessels' EC switch to a secretory phenotype and appear as actively dividing cells: the cells are endowed with numerous copies of organelles involved in biosynthesis (rough endoplasmic reticulum and Golgi apparatus) and division (centrioles) (Figure 2.1a). The cells produce an expanded basal lamina and an enlarged subendothelial matrix (Figure 2.1b). Of common occurrence for EC and SMC is the hyperplasia of the extracellular matrix enriched in all components, especially collagen bundles and fibrils. This phenomenon was found to be particularly prominent for microvessels, like the myocardial capillaries, where it impairs the diffusion of gases and the transport of molecules from the plasma to the cardiomyocytes [18]. The enhanced secretion of various proteins and the general change in EC phenotype may represent an adaptation / modulation of EC constitutive functions in response to hyperglycemia and associated dyslipidemia [49].

In large vessels, the proliferation of basal lamina and of the extracellular matrix disrupts the close contact *via* gap (communicating) junctions between EC and SMC, as well as between neighbouring SMC, leading to an altered response of the vessel wall to external stimuli. Within the meshwork of the hyperplasic, reticulated basal lamina, a large accumulation of uni- and multilamellar vesicles (Figure 2.1b) documented to be modified and reassembled lipoproteins (MRL) were found [83]. In MRL rich regions, adherence and diapedesis of blood monocytes within the subendothelium take place. Within the intima, monocytes become activated macrophages that take up MRL and turn into macrophage-derived foam cells embedded within the hyperplasic extracellular matrix. This is the

inception of the atheroma formation, generated by the hyperglycemic conditions.

In acute coronary syndromes, dysfunctional endothelium triggers plaque rupture by promoting the adhesion of circulating leukocytes to EC-expressed adhesion molecules (VCAM-1, ICAM-1, and E-selectin), constriction of the vascular wall, platelet activation and formation of thrombi [84]. Clinical studies have shown a greater incidence of ischemic symptoms in the diabetic than in the control population [85], together with an increased risk of death from ischemic heart disease [86]. Arterial stiffness provides also a link between hyperlipidemia, endothelial dysfunction, hypertension and stroke [87].

ENDOTHELIAL CELL DYSFUNCTION IN DIABETIC MICROANGIOPATHY

The pathogenesis of diabetic microangiopathy is related to hyperglycemia, AGEs, increased synthesis of collagen (especially type IV), decreases in proteoglycans and alteration of biochemical composition of the matrix. A consistent structural modification that occurs in diabetes is the thickening of the basement membrane of capillaries of the kidney glomeruli, myocardium, retina, skin, and muscle leading to altered functionality and characteristic micro-angiopathy of the respective organ.

In experimental diabetes, the changes that occur in the kidney consist, primarily, in the thickening of glomerular capillary basement membrane (GBM) and expansion of the mesangial matrix. Despite the significant hyperplasia of GBM, the capillaries are more leaky than normal, allowing passage of plasma proteins, such as glycated albumin (Figure 2.4 a,b). In addition, in diabetes, GBM exhibits marked irregularities and intercalated nodules, that, together with GBM hyperplasia, may account for the functional changes occurring in the diabetic kidney leading to augmented creatinine levels [38].

The progressive expansion of the mesangial volume is another modification observed in the glomeruli of streptozotocin-diabetic animals, similarly to the human kidney pathology.

The myocardial capillaries in experimental diabetes exhibit structural alterations of the EC and modifications of the perivascular extracellular matrix [18, 19]. The most striking occurrence is the hyperplasia of the extracellular matrix (Figure 2.4 b) that may contribute to the impeded exchange of oxygen and nutrients between the capillaries and the cardiomyocytes. An important feature is the existence of altered, fragmented pericytes surrounding the myocardial capillaries (Figure 2.4b), a process described so far for diabetic retinal capillaries only [18, 49]. About

30% of the myocardial capillaries are compressed and turn into narrowed-lumen vessels.

The retinal capillaries in diabetic animals also display an enlarged pericapillary extracellular matrix, that entraps pericytes in various stages of degradation (Figure 2.5a). As a result of pericyte disappearance and of the pressure exerted by the enlarged matrix (secreted by the EC), the lumen of the retinal capillaries becomes gradually narrowed, a process accelerated by the presence of a

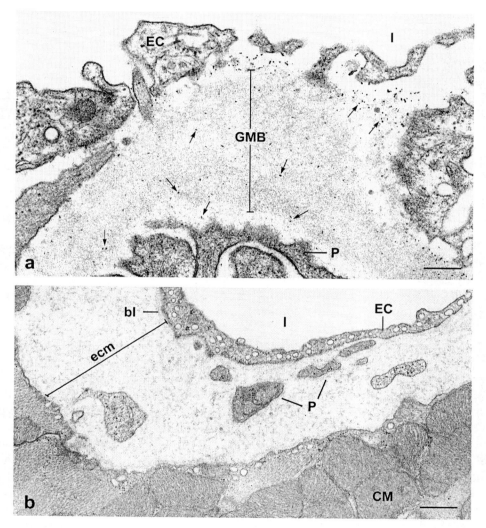

Figure 2.4

Modifications of kidney (a) and myocardial (b) capillaries in 7 weeks diabetic hamsters.

a – segment of a glomerular capillary perfused *in situ* with glycated albumin adsorbed to gold particles (gAlb-Au). Note the significant increase in thickness of the glomerular basement membrane (GBM) and the scattered distribution of gAlb-Au (arrows) throughout the GBM, indicative of disturbances in its selective permeability; b – myocardial capillary exhibiting remnants of a pericyte (P) embedded within a hyperplasic pericapillary extracellular matrix (ecm). l: capillary lumen; EC: endothelial cell; P: podocyte; CM: cardiomyocyte; bl: basal lamina. Bars: (a) 0.20 μm; (b) 0.14 μm.

high concentration of plasma glucose [18]. Interestingly, capillaries of the optical nerve show similar structural modifications with those of the retinal nerve fiber layer of diabetic hamsters (Figure 2.5b). Thus, the secretory phenotype of the endothelium, the collapse of the vascular lumen, the lesions of the renal glomeruli and retina are significant pathogenic elements possibly contributing to the vulnerability of diabetics to neuropathy.

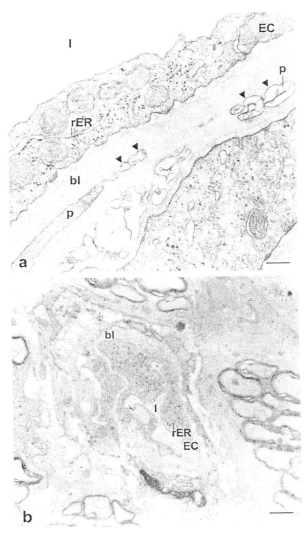

Figure 2.5

Structural changes of the capillaries of the retina (a) and optical nerve (b) in a diabetic hamster.

a – fragment of a retinal capillary endothelial cell (EC) displaying a secretory phenotype, a thick basal lamina (bl) with embedded fragments of disintegrated pericytes (P, arrow heads); b – a collapsed optical nerve capillary (suggestive of impaired blood flow) displays the endothelial cell (EC) with abundant rough endoplasmic reticulum (rer) and disorganized pericapillary extracellular matrix. l: capillary lumen; bl: basal lamina. Bars: (a) 0.19 μm; (b) 0.10 μm.

The alterations of the normal structure of capillaries described in the experimental models of streptozotocin-injected animals, such as mice [59] and hamsters [18, 19, 40], are essentially similar to those encountered in diabetic patients [88]. Moreover, when hyperlipemia is associated with diabetes (in hamsters), the microangiopathic alterations become more severe.

NUTRITION AND ENDOTHELIAL DYSFUNCTION

The correlation between dietary fat and endothelial dysfunction is complex and far from being clarified [89]. Dietary unsaturated fatty acids are easily oxidized and peroxidized and may inhibit endothelial activation [90]. A diet enriched in saturated fat is harmful. We have found that in hamsters, the increase in saturated fat consumption (energetic values: 267.3 and 488.2 kcal % as fat) is associated with: (i) a gradual change in homeostasis, severe hypertriglyceridemia and augmented creatinine levels that relate to disturbances in the renal function, progressing to nodular glomerulosclerosis and nephropathy; (ii) a switch of the aortic endothelium to a secretory phenotype, suggestive of endothelial activation; (iii) severe structural alterations of pancreatic capillaries and acinar β-cells, and kidney glomeruli, and (iv) reduced early insulin secretion in response to glucose [91].

REVERSAL OF ENDOTHELIAL DYSFUNCTION

Notable efforts are ongoing to determine ways that may prevent or stop the progress of complications in diabetes. Tight glucose and blood pressure (BP) control is known to improve to various degrees the vascular status of diabetic patients. Anti-inflammatory drugs and lowering low-density lipoprotein cholesterol (LDL-C) level are also useful. An emerging understanding of the importance of small, dense LDL-C and the anti-inflammatory effects of statins has provided new algorithms for primary prevention of macrovascular disease. Antiplatelet agents have also been shown to be effective in the secondary prevention of cardiovascular events.

In recent years, the strategies to improve/reverse endothelial dysfunction are targeted to amend the high glucose-disturbed mechanisms, addressing specifically to the molecules in affected signal transduction pathways. Thus, inhibitors of glycation, anti-oxidants, NO scavengers, L-arginine supplementation, inhibition of PARP activity, transplantation of pancreatic islets, lipid lowering and inhibition of the renin-angiotensin system are, at present, the key approaches for restoring the altered endothelial function.

Aminoguanidine was the first inhibitor of glycation used [92]; the drug blocks the chain of autocatalytic early glycation by reacting with the reaction intermediates. Once AGE cross-links are formed, the cross-link breakers, such as phenacylthiazolium bromide and ALT 711 reduce AGEs accumulation [93] and restore the vascular reactivity to normal [94].

Among the antioxidants, N-acetylcysteine was reported to abrogate diabetes-induced endothelial dysfunction in rat aorta [95]; in humans, Rosen *et al.* [67] suggest that the antioxidant treatment might be helpful to reduce the cardiac risk in diabetes.

The serum antioxidant potential, measured as total antioxidant radical trapping potential (TRAP), reveals important differences in the mean values recorded for coronary heart disease patients (CHD), with or without diabetic complications [34]. As shown in Plate 2.2, there is a variation in the intrinsic antioxidant values of the serum of diabetic-CHD and CHD patients, compared with healthy subjects. The data obtained demonstrate that the lowest mean TRAP value is in sera from diabetic-CHD patients, it increases in sera from CHD patients and has the highest mean value in sera from normal, healthy subjects. This may be due either to a reduced amount of LDL-associated antioxidants or to the serum hydrophilic antioxidants that cannot balance the circulating free radicals in the sera of diabetic patients; it is also possible that in diabetes, the glycation of proteins and lipoproteins may affect the antioxidant potential. One can safely assume that the low antioxidant status in the plasma of diabetic patients could predispose LDL to oxidative modification, a susceptibility that may be reduced by addition of antioxidants.

The effects of various antioxidants on the intrinsic antioxidant potential of sera were measured *in vitro*, after adding the following antioxidants to the reaction mixture: α-tocopherol, coenzyme Q_{10}, β-carotene (lipid-soluble antioxidants), ascorbic acid (water-soluble antioxidant) or a combination of α-tocopherol with ascorbic acid. In all cases studied, addition of antioxidants increases to various degrees the mean TRAP values of sera. This effect can be explained by the cooperation between exogenous and endogenous antioxidants, resulting in an increased resistance of the antioxidant status to the free radicals. The best results were obtained when a combination of 5 μM ascorbic acid and 3 μM α-tocopherol were employed, which increased serum TRAP value by ~34% for diabetic-CHD patients and ~41% for CHD patients. Also, β-carotene supplementation increased significantly the TRAP values in all analyzed sera (Figure 2.6).

Glycation of proteins can cause inactivation of enzymes and alterations in the structure and function of collagen and membranes, which may play a role in the long-term complications of diabetes [96, 97]. Recent studies in diabetic patients and rats have reported that vitamin E supplementation can reduce the level of blood glycated hemoglobin by inhibiting malondialdehyde formation. Other studies on erythrocytes and endothelial cells have shown that elevated glucose levels can generate oxygen free radicals and cause membrane lipid peroxidation, both processes being reduced by vitamin E supplementation [98, 99, 100].

The imbalance between the production of reactive oxygen species and the antioxidant defense can easily occur *in vivo* [101, 102] and may significantly contribute to the development of diabetes or atherosclerosis. Several drugs and compounds have been shown to have an antioxidant effect on LDL. However, it is not definitely demonstrated that they play a significant role in retarding the atherogenic process.

Taken together, we have data that indicate that: (i) the antioxidant capacity of diabetic-CHD patients sera is significantly lower than that of CHD patients and healthy subjects; (ii) there is a large inter-individual variability among the patients and (to a lesser extent) in healthy subjects, also; (iii) adding antioxidants to sera increases the total antioxidant capacity of serum, but (iv) there is a patients' sera-specific effect of antioxidants.

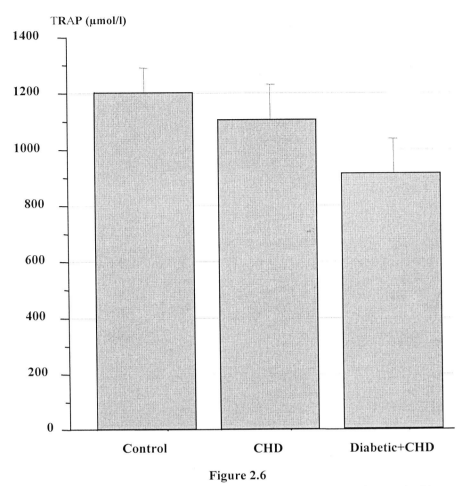

Figure 2.6

Changes in TRAP values induced by the *in vitro* addition of various antioxidants
to the sera collected from coronary heart disease (CHD) patients
and diabetic-CHD patients, as compared to healthy subjects (control).

These data may partially explain the contradictory results of various trials regarding the effects of antioxidants in treatment of atherosclerosis or diabetes and point out to the utility of the individual testing when the antioxidant therapy is to be used. Assessment *via* a simple method of the condition of the patient's serum, as well as measuring the response to specific antioxidants, may be an alternative to random administration of antioxidants. Although clinical trials are important for a general view of the effects of drugs and antioxidants, for their maximal efficiency the individual pathological, dietary and behavioral status should be taken into account. Patient-specific characteristics, such as the presence of hyperlipidemia, hypertension, and diabetes may affect the response to drugs or antioxidant supplementation.

The protective role of L-arginine on endothelial dysfunction [66] is based on the following properties of this molecule: (i) it is the substrate for NO synthesis, (ii) it inhibits lipid peroxidation by scavenging the superoxide anions [103], (iii) it inhibits AGE formation [104], and (iv) by supplementary administration may replenish the diminished arginine stores in diabetic vascular tissue [77]. In simultaneous hyperlipemia-hyperglycemia induced in hamsters, we found that dietary supplementation with L-arginine reversed the dysfunctional condition in myocardial capillaries and in the resistance arteries; thus, the capillaries turned from narrow lumen to largely open structures, the pericapillary matrix was diminished, and the vasodilation of the resistance arteries increased from ~ 62 % in simultaneous hyperlipemic-hyperglycemic hamsters, to ~ 72 % after L-arginine administration for 12 weeks [40]. These data are in good agreement with the clinical reports that indicate that in patients with chronic heart failure, the use of dietary supplementation of L-arginine improves the agonist-mediated endothelium-dependent vasodilation, an effect enhanced when physical exercise was combined with the treatment [105].

The pharmacological inhibition of PARP (by PJ34 given at 10 mg/kg per os) was reported to induce rapid reversal of diabetic endothelial dysfunction [69, 70].

The benefic effects of inhibition of the renin-angiotensin system relies on reduced (angiotensin II-mediated) radical formation and on the increase in NO bioavailability (for review, see Hornig and Drexler, 2001) [106].

The increased incidence of type 2 diabetes is most likely the result of modern life style and the tendency of obesity among the world's population. The treatment of type 2 diabetes has been the focus of pharmaceutical trials, targeting hypertension, obesity and dyslipidemia. Peroxisome proliferator-activated receptors (PPAR) are a group of nuclear receptors that regulate the expression of genes controlling lipid and glucose metabolism [107]. There are three different subtypes: PPAR-α, PPAR-(β)δ, PPAR-γ. PPAR-α is highly expressed in the liver and skeletal muscle, PPAR-γ is expressed in the adipose tissues and PPAR-δ is expressed in most cell types.

Pharmacological and genetic studies have determined that PPAR-α regulates pathways of fatty acid oxidation and PPAR-γ modulates fatty acid synthesis and storage in adipose tissues. Synthetic agonists of PPARs are used in the treatment of metabolic diseases, such as dyslipidemia and type 2 diabetes. The hypolipidemic fibrates are PPAR-α ligands. The antidiabetic glitazones, which are insulin sensitizers, are synthetic high affinity ligands for PPAR-γ. Thiazolidinedione (TZD) PPAR-γ activators, such as rosiglitasone and pioglitasone, have been used for treatment of type 2 diabetes. In obese animal models, TZD and non-TZD glitazones decrease the circulating levels of triglycerides by inducing lipolysis (*via* activation of LPL expression in adipocytes) and clearance of triglyceride-rich lipoproteins. The induction of LPL by PPAR-γ promotes fatty acid delivery. Although, the triglyceride-lowering activity of PPAR-γ activators in animal models is well documented, substantial controversy exists concerning their hypotrigly-ceridemic activity in humans [108].

Is the restoration of endothelial function clinically relevant? It is clear that effectiveness of the treatment may differ according to either the cause of the dysfunction or to the vascular bed explored (large arteries, resistance arterioles) [20]. At present, larger trials are necessary to conclusively prove whether reversal of endothelial dysfunction offers the clinical advantage of reduced morbidity and mortality. However, reversal of endothelial dysfunction is an open and exciting field of investigation, of basic relevance for many diseases and, in particular, for diabetes and atherosclerosis. At present, the scientists are targeting their endeavors to turn-around the condition of the diabetic patient from the "victim of his blood sugar" to the "captain" of his fate.

REFERENCES

1. Palade GE. Blood capillaries of the heart and other organs. *Circulation*, **24**: 368–384, 1961.
2. Simionescu M, Simionescu N. Endothelial transport of macromolecules: Transcytosis and endocytosis. A look from cell biology. *Cell Biol Rev*, **25**: 1–78, 1991.
3. Simionescu M, Gafencu A, Antohe F. Transcytosis of plasma macromolecules in endothelial cells: a cell biological survey. *Microsc Res Tech*, **57**: 269–288, 2002.
4. Simionescu N, Simionescu M. Receptor-mediated transcytosis of albumin: identification of albumin binding proteins in the plasma membrane of capillary endothelium. In Tsuchiya M *et al.* (eds). *Microcirculation-an update*. Excerpta Medica, Amsterdam, 1987, 67–83.
5. Nistor A, Simionescu M. Uptake of low density lipoproteins by the hamster lung. Interactions with capillary endothelium. *Am Rev Resp Dis*, **134**: 1266–1272, 1986.
6. Heltianu C, Dobrila L, Antohe F, Simionescu M. Evidence for thyroxine transport by the lung and heart capillary endothelium. *Microvasc Res*, **37**: 188–203, 1989.
7. Simionescu N. The microvascular endothelium: Segmental differentiations, transcytosis, selective distribution of anionic sites. In: Weissman G, Samuleson B, Paoletti R (eds). *Adv in Inflamm Res*, New York: Raven Press, vol. **1**, 1979, 61–70.

8. Lüscher TF, Spieker LE, Noll G, Cosentino F. Vascular effects of newer cardiovascular drugs: focus on nebivolol and ACE-inhibitors. *J Cardiovasc Pharmacol*, 38 (Suppl 3): S3–S11, 2001.

9. Vapaatalo H, Mervaala E. Clinically important factors influencing endothelial function. *Med Sci Monit*, 7: 1075–1085, 2001.

10. Simionescu N, Simionescu M, Palade GE. Structural basis of permeability in sequential segments of the microvasculature. I. Bipolar microvascular fields. *Microvasc Res*, 15: 1–16, 1978.

11. Simionescu N, Simionescu M, Palade GE. Structural basis . of permeability in sequential segments of the microvasculature. II. Pathways followed by microperoxidase across the endothelium. *Microvasc Res*, 15: 17–33, 1978.

12. Majno G, Palade GE. Studies on inflammation. I. The effect of histamine and serotonin on vascular permeability: an electron microscopic study. *J Biophys Biochem Cytol*, 11: 571–606, 1961.

13. Manduteanu I, Voinea M, Serban G, Simionescu M. High glucose induces enhanced monocyte adhesion to valvular endothelial cells *via* a mechanism involving ICAM-1, VCAM-1 and CD18. *Endothelium*, 6: 315–324, 1999.

14. Simionescu M. Endothelial cell response to normal and abnormal stimuli. Modulation, dysfunction, injury, adaptation, repair, death. In: Simionescu N, Simionescu M (eds). *Endothelial cell dysfunctions*. Plenum Press, New York, 1992, 3–10.

15. Raz I, Havivi Y, Yarom R. Reduced negative surface change on arterial endothelium of diabetic rats. *Diabetologia*, 31: 618–620, 1988.

16. Mompeo B, Popov D, Sima A, Constantinescu E, Simionescu M. Diabetes induced structural changes of venous and arterial endothelium and smooth muscle cells. *J Submicrosc Cytol Pathol*, 30: 475–484, 1998.

17. Lupu C, Manduteanu I, Calb M, Ionescu M, Simionescu N, Simionescu M. Some major plasmalemma proteins of human diabetic platelets are involved in the enhanced platelet adhesion to cultured valvular endothelial cells. *Platelets*, 4: 70–84, 1993.

18. Simionescu M, Popov D, Sima A, Hasu M, Costache G, Faitar S, Vulpanovici A, Stancu C, Stern D, Simionescu N. Pathobiochemistry of combined diabetes and atherosclerosis studied on a novel animal model: the hyperlipemic hyperglycemic hamster. *Am J Pathol*, 148: 997–1014, 1996.

19. Sima A, Popov D, Starodub O, Stancu C, Cristea C, Stern D, Simionescu M. Pathobiology of the heart in experimental diabetes: immunolocalization of LDL, IgG and AGE-proteins in diabetic and/or hyperlipidemic hamster. *Lab Invest*, 77: 3–15, 1997.

20. Taddei S, Virdis A, Ghiadoni L, *et al.* Effects of antihypertensive drugs on endotheial dysfunction. *Drugs*, 62: 265–284, 2002.

21. Wilcox JN, Subramanian RR, Sundell CL, Tracey WR, Pollock JS, Harrison DG, Mardsen PA. Expression of multiple isoforms of nitric oxide synthase in normal and atherosclerotic vessels. *Arterioscler Thromb Vasc Biol*, 17: 2479–2488, 1997.

22. Pou S, Pou WS, Bredt DS, Snyder SH, Rosen GM. Generation of superoxide by purified brain nitric oxide synthase. *J Biol Chem*, 267: 24173–24176, 1992.

23. Shimokawa H, Flavahan NA, Vanhoutte PM. Loss of endothelial pertussis toxin-sensitive G protein function in atherosclerotic porcine coronary arteries. *Circulation*, 83: 652–660, 1991.

24. Cai H, Harrison DG. Endothelial dysfunction in cardiovascular diseases. The role of oxidant stress. *Circ Res*, 87: 840–844, 2000.

25. Hermann J, Lerman A. The endothelium: dysfunction and beyond. *J Nuclear Cardiology*, 8: 197–206, 2001.

26. Asai K, Kudej RK, Shen Y-T, *et al.* Peripheral vascular endothelial dysfunction and apoptosis in old monkeys. *Arterioscler Thromb Vasc Biol*, 20: 1493–1499, 2000.

27. Porta M, La Selva M, Molinatti PA. von Willebrand factor and endothelial abnormalities in diabetic microangiopathy. *Diab Care*, 14: 167–171, 1991.

28. Blann A. von Willebrand factor and the endothelium in vascular disease. *Br J Biomed Sci*, 50: 125–134, 1993.

29. Blann A, McCollum CN. von Willebrand factor, endothelial cell damage and atherosclerosis. *Eur J Vasc Surg*, 8: 10–15, 1994.

30. Schalkwijk CG, Poland DCW, van Dijk W, *et al.* Plasma concentration of C- reactive protein is increased in type I diabetic patients without clinical macroangiopathy and correlates with markers of endothelial dysfunction: evidence for chronic inflammation. *Diabetologia*, 43: 351–357, 1999.

31. Oberley LW. Free radicals and diabetes. *Free Rad Biol Med*, 5: 113–124, 1988.

32. Mateo MC, Bustamante JB, Cantalapiedra MA. Serum, zinc, copper and insulin in diabetes mellitus. *J. Biomed*, 29: 56–58, 1978.

33. Stocker R, Frei B. Endogenous antioxidant defences in human blood plasma. In: Sies H (ed). *Oxidative stress: oxidants and antioxidants*. Academic Press, San Diego, 1991, 213–243.

34. Niculescu L, Stancu C, Toporan D, Sima A, Simionescu M. The serum total peroxyl radical trapping potential – an assay to define the stage of atherosclerosis. *J Cell Mol Med*, 5: 285–294, 2001.

35. Naito C, Nakamura M, Yamamoto Y. Lipid peroxides as the initiating factor of atherosclerosis. *Ann NY Acad Sci*, **676:** 27–45, 1993.

36. Skrha J, Prazny M, Haas TV, *et al*. Comparison of laser-Doppler flowmetry with biochemical indicators of endothelial dysfunction related to early microangiopathy in Type I diabetic patients. *J Diabetes Complications,* **15:** 234–240, 2001.

37. Costache G, Popov D, Georgescu A, Simionescu M. Functional-structural alterations of the resistance arteries in experimental hyperlipemia or hyperglycemia. *Proc Rom Acad*, **1:** 31–37, 2000.

38. Costache G, Popov D, Georgescu A, Cenuse M, Jinga VV, Simionescu M. The effects of simultaneous hyperlipemia-hyperglycemia on the mesenteric resistance arteries, myocardium and kidney glomeruli. *J Submicrosc Cytol Pathol*, **32:** 47–58, 2000.

39. Mulvany MJ, Halpern W. Contractile properties of small arterial resistance vessels in spontaneously hypertensive and normotensive rats. *Circ Res*, **41:** 19–26, 1977.

40. Popov D, Costache G, Georgescu A, Enache M. Beneficial effects of L-arginine supplementation in experimental hyperlipemia – hyperglycemia in the hamster. *Cell and Tissue Research*, **308:** 109–120, 2002.

41. Georgescu A, Popov D. The contractile response of the mesenteric resistance arteries to prostaglandin $F_{2\alpha}$; effects of simultaneous hyperlipemia-diabetes. *Fundam Clinical Pharmacology,* **17:** 1–7, 2003.

42. Johnstone MT, Creager SJ, Scales KM, Cusco JA, Lee BK, Creager MA. Impaired endothelium-dependent vasodilatation in patients with insulin-dependent diabetes mellitus. *Circulation*, **88:** 2510–2516, 1993.

43. Panza JA, Quyyumi AA, Brush Jr JE, Epstein SE. Abnormal endothelium-dependent vascular relaxation in patients with essential hypertension. *N Engl J Med*, **323:** 22–27, 1990.

44. Creager MA, Cooke JP, Mendelsohn ME, Gallagher SJ, Coleman SM, Loscalzo J, Dzau V. Impaired vasodilatation of forearm resistance vessels in hypercholesterolemic humans. *J Clin Invest*, **86:** 228–234, 1990.

45. Chauhan A, Mullins PA, Taylor G, Petch MC, Schofield PM. Both endothelium-dependent and endothelium-independent function is impaired in patients with angina pectoralis and normal coronary angiograms. *Eur Heart J*, **18:** 60–68, 1997.

46. Tilton RG, Baier LD, Harlow JE, Smith SR, Ostrow E, Williamson JR. Diabetes-induced glomerular dysfunction: links to a more reduced cytosolic ratio of NADH/NAD+. *Kidney Int*, **41:** 778–788, 1992.

47. Chappey O, Dosquet C, Wautier PM, Wautier JL. AGE products, oxidant stress and vascular lesions. *Eur J Clin Invest*, **27:** 97–108, 1997.

48. Sun M, Yokoyama M, Ishiwata T, Asano G. Deposition of advanced glycation end-products (AGE) and expression of the receptor for AGE in cardiovascular tissue of the diabetic rat. *Int J Exp Path*, **79:** 207–222, 1998.

49. Simionescu M, Sima A, Popov D. The vascular endothelium in diabetes-induced accelerated atherosclerosis. In: Born GVR, Schwarz CJ (eds). *Vascular Endothelium. Physiology, Pathology and Therapeutic Opportunities*, vol. **3**, New Horizon Series, Schattauer, Stuttgart, 1997. 329–344.

50. Sima A, Stancu C. Modified lipoproteins accumulate in human coronary atheroma. *J Cell Mol Med*, **6:** 110–111, 2002.

51. Schmidt AM, Yan SD, Wautier JL, Stern D. Activation of receptor for advanced glycation end-products: a mechanism for chronic vascular dysfunction in diabetic vasculopathy and atherosclerosis. *Circ Res*, **84:** 489–497, 1999.

52. Schmidt AM, Yan SD, Yan SF, Stern D. The multiligand receptor RAGE as a progression factor amplifying immune and inflammatory responses. *J Clin Invest*, **108:** 949–955, 2001.

53. Koya D, King GL. Protein kinase C activation and the development of diabetic complications. *Diabetes*, **47:** 859–866, 1998.

54. King GL. The role of hyperglycaemia and hyperinsulinemia in causing vascular dysfunction in diabetes. *Ann Med*, **28:** 427–432, 1996.

55. Tilton RG. Diabetic vascular dysfunction: links to glucose-induced reductive stress and VEGF. *Microscopy Res Tech*, **57:** 390–407, 2002.

56. Schmidt AM, Vianna M, Gerlach M, Brett J, Ryan J, Kao J, Esposito C, Hegarty H, Hurley W, Clauss M. *et al*. Isolation and characterization of binding proteins for advanced glycation end-products from lung tissue which are present on the endothelial cell surface. *J Biol Chem*, **267:** 14987–14997, 1992.

57. Neeper M, Schmidt AM, Brett J, Yan SD, Wang F, Pan YCE, Ellison K, Stern D, Shaw A. Cloning and expression of a cell surface receptor for advanced glycation end-products of protein. *J Biol Chem*, **267:** 14998–15004, 1992.

58. Stitt AW, He C, Vlassara H. Characterization of the advanced glycation end-product receptor complex in human vascular cells. *Biochem Biophys Res Commun*, **256:** 549–556, 1999.

59. Popov D, Hasu M, Costache G, Stern D, Simionescu M. Capillary and aortic endothelia interact in situ with nonenzymatically glycated albumin and develop specific alterations in experimental diabetes. *Acta Diabetol*, **34:** 285–293, 1997.

60. Popov D, Simionescu M. Structural and transport property alterations of the lung capillary endothelium in diabetes. In: Motta PM, Macchiarelli G and Nottola SA (eds). *Advances in*

Microanatomy of Cells and Tissues, Biophysical and Biochemical Correlates, Marcello Malpighi Symposia Series Vol. 7, Editrice "Il Sedicesimo", Firenze, 2001, 405–412.

61. Dobrian A, Simionescu M. Irreversibly glycated albumin alters the physico-chemical characteristics of low density lipoproteins of normal and diabetic subjects. *Biochim Biophys Acta*, **1270**: 26–35, 1995.

62. Peterson TE, Poppa V, Ueba H, Wu A, Yan C, Berck CB. Opposing effects of oxygen reactive species and cholesterol on endothelial nitric oxide synthase and endothelial cell caveolae. *Circ Res*, **85**: 29–37, 1999.

63. Ceriello A, Quataro A, Caretta F, Varano R, Giugliano D. Evidence for a possible role of oxygen free redicals in the abnormal functional arterial vasomotion in insulin dependent diabetes. *Diab Metab*, **16**: 318–322, 1990.

64. Henning B, Chow CK. Lipid peroxidation and endothelial cell injury: Implications in atherosclerosis. *Free Radic Biol Med*, **4**: 9–106, 1988.

65. Rubanyi GM, Vanhoutte PM. Oxygen-derived free radicals, endothelium, and responsiveness of vascular smooth muscle cells. *Am J Physiol*, **250**: H815–H821, 1986.

66. Pieper GM. Review of alterations in endothelial nitric oxide production in diabetes. Protective role of arginine on endothelial dysfunction. *Hypertension*, **31**: 1047–1060, 1998.

67. Rosen P, Du X, Tschope D. Role of oxygen derived radicals for vascular dysfunction in the diabetic heart: prevention by alpha-tocopherol? *Mol Cell Biochem*, **188**: 103–111, 1998.

68. Annuk M, Zilmer M, Lind L, Linde T, Fellstrom B. Oxidative stress and endothelial function in chronic renal failure. *J Am Soc Nephrol* **12**: 2747–2752, 2001.

69. Garcia Soriano F, Virag L, Jagtap P, Jagtap P, Szabo E, Mabley JG, Liaudet L, Marton A, Hoyt DG, Murty KGK, Salzman AL, Southan GJ, Szabo C. Diabetic endothelial dysfunction: the role of poly (ADP-ribose) polymerase activation. *Nature Medicine*, **7**: 108–113, 2001.

70. Garcia Soriano F, Pacher P, Malbey J, Liaudet L, Szabo C. Rapid reversal of the diabetic endothelial dysfunction by pharmacological inhibition of Poly(ADP-ribose) polymerase. *Circ Res*, **89**: 684–691, 2001.

71. Xia Y, Dawson VL, Snyder SH, Zweiler JL. Nitric oxide synthase generates superoxide and nitric oxide in arginine-depleted cells leading to peroxinitrite-mediated cell injury. *Proc Natl Acad Sci USA*, **93**: 6770–6774, 1996.

72. Warnholtz A, Nickening G, Schultz E, Marcharzina R, Brasen JH, Skatchkov M. Increased NADH-oxidase-mediated superoxide production in the early stages of atherosclerosis: evidence for the involvement of the renin-angiotensin system. *Circulation*, **99**: 2027–2033, 1999.

73. Stralin P, Karlsson K, Johansson BO, Marklund SL. The interstitium of the human arterial wall contains very large amounts of extracellular superoxide dismutase. *Arterioscler Thromb Vasc Biol*, **15**: 2032–2036, 1995.

74. Arnal JF, Dinh-Xuan AT, Pueyo M, Darblade B, Rami J. Endothelium-derived nitric oxide and vascular physiology and pathology. *Cell Mol Life Sci*, **55**: 1078–1087, 1999.

75. Gonzalez-Fernandez F, Jimenez A, Lopez-Blaya A, Velasco S, Arrlero MM, Celdran A, Rico L, Farre J, Casado S, Lopez-Farre A. Cerivastatin prevents tumor necrosis factor-alpha-induced downregulation of endothelial nitric oxide synthase: role of endothelial cytosolic proteins. *Atherosclerosis*, **155**: 61–70, 2001.

76. Pieper GM, Jordan M, Adams MB, *et al*. Syngeneic pancreatic islet transplantation reverses endothelial dysfuncton in experimental diabetes. *Diabetes*, **44**: 1106–1113, 1995.

77. Pieper GM, Dondlinger LA. Plasma and vascular tissue arginine are decreased by diabetes: acute arginine supplementation restores endothelium-dependent relaxation by augmenting cGMP production. *J Pharmacol Exp Ther*, **283**: 684–691, 1997.

78. Georgescu A, Popov D, Simionescu M. Mechanisms of decreased bradykinin-induced vasodilation in experimental hyperlipemia-hyperglycemia: contribution of nitric oxide and Ca^{2+} activated K^+ channels. *Fundam Clinical Pharmacology*, **15**: 1–8, 2001.

79. Böger RH, Bode-Böger SM, Szuba A, Tsao PS, Chan JR, Tangphao O, *et al*. Asymmetric dimethyl arginine (ADMA): a novel risk factor for endothelial dysfunction. *Circulation*, **98**: 1842–1847, 1998.

80. Matsuura A, Yamochi W, Hirata K, Kawashima S, Yokoyama M. Stimulatory interaction between vascular endothelial growth factor and endothelin-1 on each gene expression. *Hypertension*, **32**: 89–95, 1998.

81. Wang W, Dentler WL, Borchardt RT. VEGF increases BMEC monolayer permeability by affecting occludin expression and tight junction assembly. *Am J Physiol Heart Circ Physiol*, **280**: H434–H440, 2001.

82. Dobrian A, Lazar V, Tirziu D, Simionescu M. Increased macrophage uptake of irreversibly glycated albumin modified low density lipoproteins of normal and diabetic subjects is mediated by non-saturable mechanisms. *Biochim Biophys Acta*, **1317**: 5–14, 1996.

83. Simionescu M, Simionescu N. Pro-atherosclerotic events: Pathobiochemical changes occurring in the arterial wall before monocyte migration. *FASEB J,* 7: 1359–1366, 1993.

84. Simon BC, Noll B, Maisch B. Endothelial dysfunction. Update and clinical implications. *Herz,* 24(1): 62–71, 1999.

85. Pierce GN, Beamish RE, Dhalla NS. Heart dysfunction in diabetes. CRC Press, Boca Raton, Fla, 1–245, 1988.

86. Stephenson J, Swerdlow AJ, Devis T, Fuller JH. Recent trends in diabetes mortality in England and Wales. *Diabet Med,* 9: 417–421, 1992.

87. Wilkinson IB, Cockcroft JR. Cholesterol, endothelial function and cardiovascular disease. *Current Opin Lipidol,* 9: 237–242, 1998.

88. Lee ET, Keen H, Bennett PH, Fuller JH, Lu M, WHO Multinational Study Group. Follow-up of the WHO Multinational Study of vascular disease in diabetes: general description and morbidity. *Diabetologia,* 44: S3–S13, 2001.

89. Nurminen ML, Korpela R, Vapaatalo H. Dietary factors in the pathogenesis and treatment of hypertension. *Ann Med,* 30: 143–150, 1998.

90. De Caterina R, Spiecker M, Solaini G, *et al.* The inhibition of endothelial activation by unsaturated fatty acids. *Lipids,* 34: S191–S194, 1999.

91. Popov D, Simionescu M, Shepherd PR. Saturated-fat diet induces moderate diabetes and severe glomerulosclerosis in hamsters. *Diabetologia,* 46: 1408–18, 2003.

92. Brownlee M, Vlassara H, Kooney A, Ulrich P, Cerami A. Aminoguanidine prevents diabetes-induced arterial wall protein crosslinking. *Science,* 232: 1629–1632, 1986.

93. Cooper ME, Thallas V, Forbes J, Scalbert E, Sastra S, Darby I, Soulis T. The cross-link breaker, N-phenacylthiazolium bromide prevents vascular AGE-product accumulation. *Diabetologia,* 43: 660–664, 2000.

94. Wolfenbuttel BH, Boulanger CM, Crijns FR, Huijberts MS, Pottervin P, Swennen GN, Vasan S, Egan JJ, Ulrich P, Cerami A, Levy BI. Breakers of advanced glycation end-products restore large artery properties in experimental diabetes. *Proc Natl Acad Sci USA,* 95: 4630–4634, 1998.

95. Pieper GM, Siebeneich W. Oral administration of the antioxidant, N-acetylcysteine, abrogates diabetes-induced endothelial dysfunction. *J Cardiovasc Pharmacol,* 32: 101–105, 1998.

96. Rajeswari P, Natarajan R, Nadler JC. Glucose induces lipid peroxidation and inactivation of membrane-associated ion-transport enzymes in human erythrocytes *in vivo* and *in vitro.* *J Cell Physiol,* 149: 100–109, 1991.

97. Tesfamarian B, Cohen RA. Free radicals mediate endothelial cell dysfunction caused by elevated glucose. *Am Physiol Soc,* 262: H321–H326, 1992.

98. Jain SK, Palmer M. The effect of oxygen radicals metabolites and vitamin E on glycosylation of proteins. *Free Radic Biol Med,* 22: 593–596, 1997.

99. Ceriello A, Giugliano D, Quatraro A, Donzella C, Dipalo G, Lefebvre PJ. Vitamin E reduction of protein glycosylation in diabetes. *Diabetes Care,* 14: 68–72, 1991.

100. Jain SK, McVie R, Jaramillo JJ, Palmer M, Smith T, Meachum ZD, Little RL. The effect of modest vitamin E supplementation on lipid peroxidation products and other cardiovascular risk factors in diabetic patients. *Lipids,* 31: S87–S90, 1996.

101. Heller FR, Descamps O, Hondekijn JC. LDL oxidation: therapeutic perspectives. *Atherosclerosis,* 137: S25–S31, 1998.

102. Schwenke DC. Antioxidants and atherogenesis. *J Nutr Biochem,* 9: 424–445, 1998.

103. Wascher TC, Posch K, Wallner S, Hermetter A, Kostner GM, Graier WF. Vascular effects of L-arginine: anything beyond a substrate for the NO-synthase? *Biochem Biophys Res Commun,* 234: 35–38, 1997.

104. Servetnick DA, Bryant D, Wells-Knecht KJ, Wiesenfeld PL. L-arginine inhibits *in vitro* nonenzymatic glycation and advanced glycosylated end-product formation of human serum albumin. *Amino Acids,* 11: 69–81, 1996.

105. Hambrecht R, Hilbrich L, Erbs S, *et al.* Correction of endothelial dysfunction in chronic heart failure: Additional effects of exercise training and oral L-arginine supplementation. *J Am Coll Cardiol,* 35: 706–713, 2000.

106. Hornig B, Drexler H. Reversal of endothelial dysfunction in humans. *Coronary Artery Disease,* 12: 463–473, 2001.

107. Chinetti G, Fruchart JC, Staels B. Peroxisomes proliferator-activated receptors (PPARs): nuclear receptors at the crossroads between lipid metabolism and inflammation. *Inflamm Res,* 49: 497–505, 2000.

108. Barbier O, Pineda Torra I, Duguay Y, Blanquart C, Fruchart JC, Glineur C, Staels B. Pleiotropic actions of peroxisome proliferator-activated receptors in lipid metabolism and atherosclerosis. *Arterioscler Thromb Vasc Biol,* 22: 717–726, 2002.

3

PEROXISOME PROLIFERATOR-ACTIVATED RECEPTORS (PPARs) – POTENTIAL TARGETS FOR DIABETIC ATHEROSCLEROSIS

Gabriela ORĂŞANU, Ouliana ZIOUZENKOVA, Jorge PLUTZKY

To an increasing degree, the interface between cardiology and diabetology is broadening. Extensive evidence has established that diabetes mellitus and atherosclerosis are chronic conditions, very often tightly intertwined in patients. Recent data not only from vascular biology, but also from clinical trials show that inflammation significantly contributes to the pathogenesis, progression, and complications in both disorders.

The compelling nature of this evolving story has also promoted considerable interest in biologic mechanisms that may be involved in diabetic atherosclerosis and serve as therapeutic targets. Since their identification, the peroxisome proliferator-activated receptors (PPARs) have been implicated as a molecular pathway involved in diabetes mellitus and atherosclerosis. PPARs, as ligand activated transcription factors, play a central role in many metabolic processes involving glucose control, lipid homeostasis, and adipogenesis. Moreover, PPARs are critical regulators of inflammatory responses, not just through metabolic effects but also through their direct action in vascular and inflammatory cells. These observations have important clinical implications given that the thiazolidinedione class (TZDs) is widely used in diabetic patients at high risk for developing atherosclerotic complications.

The intense basic research on these receptors tries to clarify the molecular mechanism of their complex action through the identification of their key target genes. New PPAR modulators will be specifically useful in the growing prediabetic population that exhibits multiple risk factors for cardiovascular disease.

INTRODUCTION

To an increasing degree, cardiology and diabetology are finding a broadening interface. There is little doubt that atherosclerosis is in many ways a metabolic disorder, just as it is becoming increasingly clear that diabetes mellitus is in many ways a vascular disease. Extensive evidence has established that diabetes mellitus and atherosclerosis are tightly intertwined chronic conditions. Indeed, the prevalence of cardiovascular disease was as high, or even higher, in patients with newly discovered type 2 diabetes than in those whose diabetes mellitus had been present for many years [1].

Stern and colleagues [1] proposed that both diabetes mellitus and cardiovascular disease shared common antecedents, rather than one being a complication of the other. This "common soil" hypothesis is supported by several recent studies that suggest the existence of an atherogenic pre-diabetic state. One unifying component underlying pre-diabetic conditions may be insulin resistance and its associated abnormalities that include central obesity, hypertension, elevated triglyceride and small dense low-density lipoprotein (LDL) cholesterol levels, and decreased high-density lipoprotein (HDL)-cholesterol levels. Insulin resistance may also be characterized by a number of nontraditional risk factors, with increased plasminogen activator inhibitor-1, decreased tissue plasminogen activator, and increased fibrinogen, all of which may promote hypercoagulability. Insulin resistance, diabetes mellitus, and atherosclerosis have also been suggested to be chronic inflammatory conditions, with increased levels of markers of subclinical inflammation such as C-reactive protein (CRP) further supporting cardiovascular disease and diabetes as sharing common genetic, environmental antecedents.

There is a considerable interest in understanding the biologic mechanisms that may be involved in accelerated diabetic atherosclerosis and serve as therapeutic targets. Since their identification, the peroxisome proliferator-activated receptors (PPARs) have been implicated as a molecular pathway involved in diabetes mellitus and atherosclerosis. PPARs, as ligand activated transcription factors, play a central role in many metabolic processes involving glucose control, lipid homeostasis, and adipogenesis.

Recent studies implicate PPARs in inflammation and atherosclerosis. The basic science behind PPAR action has immediate clinical relevance given the ongoing use of PPAR agonists in patients. Interestingly, these synthetic PPAR agonists appear to reduce many of the traditional and nontraditional risk factors that contribute to the pathogenesis, progression, and complications of diabetes mellitus [2].

PPARs

PPARs – BIOLOGY

In 1990 Issemann and Green [3] reported the isolation of a cDNA clone for a ligand-activated transcription factor that interacted with various drugs that induced hepatic peroxisomal proliferation. Of note, this peroxisomal proliferation is only found in rodents and occurs predominantly with PPARα, making it an archaic term in many ways. Since then all three PPAR isoforms – PPAR alpha (PPARα), PPAR beta or delta as it is also called (PPAR β/δ), and PPAR gamma (PPARγ), each of which is encoded by different genes, have been established as playing a critical role in the transcriptional regulation of many aspects of lipid metabolism and implicated as a therapeutic target in diseases such as obesity, diabetes mellitus, and atherosclerosis.

PPARs are members of the nuclear hormone receptor superfamily of ligand-activated transcription factors that are related to retinoid, steroid, and thyroid hormone receptors [4]. In response to specific ligands, PPARs form a heterodimeric complex with another nuclear receptor RXR – activated by its own ligand, 9-cis retinoic acid. This complex then binds to specific DNA sequences known as peroxisome proliferator response elements (PPREs) located in the promoter regions of specific target genes (Plate 3.1). Binding of ligand induces a conformational change in the PPAR protein, resulting in the binding of co-activator molecules, such as PPAR-binding protein, p300, or PPARγ co-activator-1, and/or the release of co-repressors [5]. In this way PPAR ligands can regulate gene expression, either positively or negatively [5]. Interestingly, the mechanisms through which PPAR mediate inhibition of gene expressions, known as trans-repression, remain incompletely understood.

PPARs are characterized by distinct tissue distribution patterns and metabolic functions. PPARα is mostly expressed in brown adipose tissue, liver, kidney, duodenum, heart, and skeletal muscle; PPARγ is mainly found in brown and white adipose tissue and less in the large intestine, retina, and some parts of the immune system, adrenal gland and spleen; PPARβ/δ is the most ubiquitously expressed isotype, it is found in almost all tissues including heart, adipose tissue, brain, intestine, muscle, spleen, lung, and adrenal glands [6].

As will be discussed below, more recent evidence suggests an important role for PPARs in the vasculature and in inflammatory cells.

ROLE IN LIPID AND LIPOPROTEIN METABOLISM

A host of factors combine to determine the unique role each PPAR plays in cellular responses, including the identity of their target genes. Despite these isoform-specific roles, common themes do exist as to PPAR function, including their involvement in energy balance and lipid metabolism. A brief overview of each PPAR will be provided.

PPARγ: key regulator of adipogenesis and insulin sensitivity

PPARγ was first identified as a part of a transcriptional complex integral to adipocyte differentiation. Indeed, transient overexpression of PPARγ in fibroblasts directs those cells toward an adipocyte-like phenotype [7] consistent with high adipose expression of PPARγ [8, 9]. PPARγ also influences lipid metabolism, with target genes such as HMG CoA synthetase, apolipoprotein A-I, and lipoprotein lipase [10, 11].

Through its role in adipocyte differentiation, PPARγ has been considered the "ultimate thrifty gene" [12]. This notion refers to the concept that PPARγ may take part in conserving energy resources during times of starvation, mainly by helping store fatty acids in triglycerides contained in fat. This possibility is supported by reports of several human PPAR mutations and their associated phenotypes. For example, Pro115Gln is thought to lead to a gain of PPAR function, with more active PPARγ, increasing adipocyte differentiation and obesity [13]. The Pro12Ala mutation is thought to render PPARγ less active and is reportedly associated with a lower body mass index (BMI), a decreased risk of diabetes mellitus, and perhaps even a decreased risk of MI [14].

Data from animal studies have shown that PPARγ homozygous deficient mice die as embryos, whereas heterozygous PPARγ-deficient mice appear more, not less, insulin sensitive [15]. The explanation for this increase in insulin sensitivity in these mice is unclear but may reflect greater insulin responsiveness among less differentiated pre-adipocytes.

PPARγ has also been shown to upregulate the expression of the fatty acid transporters FAPT-1 and CD36 in adipocytes [16, 17]. PPARγ modulates a number of many other genes involved in energy storage and utilization. Activation of PPARγ represses the expression of the ob gene, which encodes for leptin [18, 19] and up-regulates expression of the mitochondrial uncoupling proteins UCP1, UCP2, and UCP3 [20, 21].

The increasing list of genes modulated by PPARγ establishes this transcriptional factor as a key regulator of adipocyte function and systemic lipid homeostasis.

PPARα: transcriptional sensor for fatty acid metabolism

PPARα, which is more widely expressed (heart, liver, kidney) than PPARγ, is a key regulator of fatty acid β-oxidation. This is apparent from PPARα control of a host of proteins involved in fatty acid metabolism including acyl-CoA-oxidase (ACO), enoyl-CoA hydratase/3-hydroxyacyl-CoA-dehydrogenase (HD), microsomal fatty acid ω-hydroxylase CYP4A6, mitochondrial HMG-CoA synthase and medium-chain acyl-coA dehydrogenase (MCAD), cytosolic malic enzyme, liver fatty acid binding protein, lipoprotein lipase (LPL), hepatic lipase (HL), lecithin cholesterol acyltransferase (LCAT) [22], and apolipoprotein expression (apolipoprotein A-I, apolipoprotein A-II, and apolipoprotein C-III) [23, 24, 25]. Recent work has established lipoprotein lipase as a pathway for generating endogenous PPAR ligands [26, 27]. Interestingly, several lines of evidence suggest PPARα is a key mediator of energy balance, induced by starvation and activated by LPL action.

The specific nature of PPARα ligands and their pathways suggest PPARα involvement with nutrient-induced gene expression [28]. PPARα agonists may affect body weight through regulation of fatty acid catabolism or energy expenditure [28]. PPARα-/- mice show increased accumulation of body fat as they are ageing [29, 30].

Uncoupling proteins (UCP) 1, 2, 3 are mitochondrial membrane transporters that uncouple substrate oxidation from ATP synthesis, allowing conversion of fuel into heat. Some data indicate that skeletal muscle respiratory uncoupling reverses insulin resistance and lowers blood pressure in genetic mouse models of obesity without affecting thermoregulation [31]. This may decrease the risk of atherosclerosis in type 2 diabetes [31]. Consistent with this, treating rodents with the PPARα agonist bezafibrate increased levels of UCP1 in white adipose tissue (WAT) and increased levels of UCP3 in WAT and skeletal muscle [32]. Expression of UCP3 has been found to be reduced in skeletal muscle from NIDDM subjects compared with healthy control subjects. Furthermore, in NIDDM subjects, UCP3 expression is positively correlated with a whole-body insulin-mediated glucose utilization. These results suggest that UCP3 regulation may be altered in states of insulin resistance [33]. Furthermore, WY14643, a potent PPARα agonist, induces the expression of UCP3 [34]. Rosiglitazone, a PPARγ agonist, activates the UCP1 promoter and increases UCP1 mRNA levels, but a combination of the PPARα and PPARγ agonists does not lead to increased UCP1 expression [33].

PPARβ/δ: key regulator of fat burning in peripheral tissues

Less is known about PPARβ/δ than the other PPARs, perhaps because there is no PPARβ/δ agonist in clinical use. The widespread expression of PPARβ/δ suggests its fundamental role in cellular biology. Recent data suggest that PPARβ/δ is an important regulator of cholesterol metabolism with unique pharmacology that distinguishes it from the other PPAR subtypes. A variety of studies have shown that PPARβ/δ is involved in lipid metabolism and affects more specifically high-density lipoprotein (HDL) levels. Activation of PPARβ/δ *in vivo* led to systematic

metabolic changes including lower levels of triglycerides and free fatty acids, by upregulating fatty acid oxidation and energy expenditure [35]. PPARβ/δ null mutant mice typically die in utero due to placenta defects, but the small number of mice that have survived show decreased adiposity [35].

Interestingly, PPARβ/δ promotes cholesterol accumulation in human macrophages [36] whereas PPARγ increases cholesterol efflux to protect against atherosclerosis [37]. In contrast, in adipose tissue PPARβ/δ stimulates combustion of fatty acids and PPARγ induces free fatty acids influx into adipose tissue [38].

ROLE IN CARBOHYDRATE METABOLISM

Glucose transport across plasma membrane, as the rate-limiting step in glucose metabolism, is a highly regulated process. Facilitated diffusion of glucose into cells is carried out by a family of stereospecific transport proteins known as the glucose transporters GLUT1 through GLUT5 and GLUT7. The insulin-dependent glucose transporter GLUT4 is expressed exclusively in adipose tissue, cardiac muscle, and skeletal muscle, where it regulates glucose uptake into these tissues in response to elevated levels of insulin in the circulation. PPARγ induces GLUT4 suggesting that the thiazolidinedione induction of GLUT4 may be a major mechanism underlying the insulin-sensitizing effects of those agents [39].

PPARγ also regulates the phosphoenolpyruvate carboxykinase, an enzyme of the glyceroneogenesis pathway [40]. The recent finding that the c-Cbl-associated protein, a signaling protein interacting with insulin receptor, is encoded by a PPARγ target gene proves once again the link between this receptor and insulin signaling pathway [41].

ROLE IN THE INFLAMMATION UNDERLYING ATHEROSCLEROSIS

PPARs regulate the expression of key proteins involved in all stages of atherogenesis and atherosclerosis, including targets involved in lipid metabolism and thrombosis as well as the inflammation that is now known to underlie vascular disease. Evidence from a broad range of studies demonstrates that atherosclerosis is a chronic disease that, from its origins to its ultimate complications, involves inflammatory cells including T lymphocytes, monocytes, macrophages, inflammatory proteins like cytokines and chemokines, and inflammatory responses from vascular cells, for example endothelial cell expression of adhesion molecules [42]. Increasing evidence suggests inflammation may also contribute to the development of insulin resistance and diabetes mellitus. Moreover, PPARs modulate the onset and evolution of metabolic disorders like dyslipidemia and diabetes mellitus that predispose to atherosclerosis. Although far from proven, synthetic PPAR agonists are under intense study for their possible vascular effects; responses that could occur indirectly from improved metabolism or directly through changes in gene expression exert at the level of the vascular wall. Thus, PPARs are involved not only in the maintenance of glucose and lipid homeostasis but they are also present in immunological and vascular cells that are implicated in atherosclerotic lesion formation.

Studies have documented that PPARs are present in all critical vascular cells: endothelial cells, vascular smooth muscle cells, and monocyte-macrophages as well as in human atherosclerotic lesions [43, 44]. By modulating transcription of proinflammatory genes such as cytokines, chemokines, endothelial cell adhesion molecules and metalloproteinases, PPAR agonists have emerged as a potential tool to modulate the inception and progression of atherosclerosis. We will consider the evidence of each PPAR isoform in its various vascular settings.

PPARγ in vascular and immune cells

Several laboratories established PPARγ expression in monocytes/macrophages and human atherosclerotic lesions [43, 46]. Jiang *et al.* [45] found that PPARγ agonists decreased production of tumor necrosis factor-α, interleukin-1β, and interleukin-6 by phorbol 13-myristate 12-acetate, but not lipopolysaccharide-stimulated monocyte-like cell lines. Ricote *et al.* [44] reported that PPARγ activators decreased the promoter activity in genes such as inducible nitric oxide synthetase and matrix metalloproteinase-9 (gelatinase B). These studies placed PPARγ action upstream key

macrophage-inflammatory cytokine responses. In concurrent work, direct evidence was reported for PPARγ inhibition of matrix metalloproteinase-9 expression and gelatinolytic activity: effects relevant to arterial remodeling and plaque rupture, as discussed further below [43]. PPARγ activators also may induce apoptosis in monocytes/macrophages, another potential mechanism for limiting inflammation [46].

In contrast to these antiatherosclerotic / antiinflammatory effects, possible proatherosclerotic PPARγ responses were raised, with reports that oxidized LDL; specifically oxidized linoleic acid (9 or 13 monohydroxyoctadecadienoic acid [HODES]) could act as a PPARγ ligand [47, 48] (Plate 3.2). These results suggested that 9 or 13 HODES activated PPARγ in monocytes / macrophages, increasing macrophage scavenger receptor CD36 expression and promoting foam cell differentiation, while inducing PPARγ expression in a proposed metacrine "PPARγ loop." Despite this potential pro-atherosclerotic effect, a possibility exists that these monocytes were taking up triglycerides, and not the cholesterol esters seen in native foam cells, perhaps offsetting some of the implications of these findings. It also possible that CD36 may be induced in other cells and tissues, creating a sink into which oxLDL may be moved. Alternatively, any potential pro-atherosclerotic effect may be offset by the induction of other offsetting responses. Indeed, more recent work from several groups suggests that PPARγ and PPARα ligands also induce cholesterol efflux through adenosine triphosphate-binding cassette protein A1 (ABCA1), offering possible counterbalancing responses that may dominate any CD36 effects [49–51]. Consistent with this, multiple recent studies have found that PPARγ agonists decreased atherosclerosis in either LDL receptor or apolipoprotein E receptor-deficient mice [52–54].

In addition to macrophages, Northern, Western, and immunohistochemical data reveal PPARγ expression in human endothelial cells [55–58]. Examples of identified endothelial cell targets include plasminogen activator inhibitor-1 [55–57], endothelin [58, 59], and vascular endothelial growth factor [60]. PPARγ activators may induce endothelial cell apoptosis, but such effects may be most potent with 15d-PGJ2, a molecule with PPARγ independent effects and questionable *in vivo* relevance [56]. Apoptosis could contribute to the *in vitro* inhibitory effects described above, and it must be considered when evaluating PPARγ responses. Marx *et al.* [61] identified PPARγ-mediated inhibition of certain interferonγ–induced chemokines from the cysteine X-amino acid-cysteine subset of chemokines. These included the interferon-inducible protein of 10 kDa, monokine induced by interferon-γ, and interferon induced T-cell-α chemoattractant [61]. These cysteine X-amino acid-cysteine chemokines, produced by endothelial cells and T cells, are major chemoattractants for T lymphocytes. Of note, PPARγ regulation of monocyte chemoattractant protein-1 was not found, despite its interferon-γ inducibility, consistent with subsequent *in vivo* mouse data. Nevertheless, PPARγ may still regulate monocyte chemoattractant protein-1 responses through downstream regulation of its receptor, cysteine-cysteine chemokine receptor 2 [62, 63]. Indeed, in vitro reports find PPARγ inhibition of monocyte chemoattractant protein-1-directed chemotaxis. PPARγ agonists also inhibit chemokines (interleukin-8) in epithelial cells, suggesting a possible PPARγ agonist use in inflammatory bowel disease [64]. Interestingly, similar PPAR-mediated regulation of chemokine expression in epithelial cells has given rise to a possible role for PPAR agonists in inflammatory bowel disease.

Although Staels *et al.* [65] found limited PPARγ expression in VSMC, numerous other studies report PPARγ expression in VSMC as well as PPARγ ligand effects on established PPARγ target genes and functional VSMC responses [66, 67]. For example, PPARγ regulates matrix metalloproteinase-9 expression in VSMC, inhibiting platelet-derived growth factor-induced VSMC migration and proliferation [67, 69]. Wakino *et al.* [70] subsequently described PPARγ-mediated inhibition of cell cycle G1 to S phase transition. These PPARγ inhibitory effects in VSMC may contribute to decreases seen with troglitazone in carotid intima, including medial thickness [71] and in-stent coronary restenosis [72].

Recent reports have found PPARγ expression in lymphocytes, including B cells [73] and in murine lymphocytes and splenocytes [74–76]. Clark *et al.* [74] found PPARγ agonists 15d-PGJ2 and ciglitazone (40 molμ/L)-mediated inhibition

of murine T-cell and splenocyte proliferation inhibiting interleukin-2 production but not interleukin-2 proliferation of T-cell clones. Yang *et al.* [75] found inhibition of phytohemaglutinin-induced interleukin-2 in response to troglitazone (10 to 25 μmol/L) and 15d-PGJ2 (5 to 10 μmol/L), possibly through the lymphocyte transcription factor, nuclear factor of activated T cells. No effects were seen with PPARα agonist WY14643 [75]. Harris and Phipps [76] studied T cells from a transgenic T-cell receptor mouse (DO11.10), reporting inhibition of proliferation with 15d-PGJ2, but at higher concentrations of ciglitazone (~75 μmol/L). In contrast to Clark *et al.*'s data [74], no proliferation change was evident with ciglitazone at μ40 mol/L. In our own work with T lymphocytes [77] using generally lower concentrations of PPAR agonists, significant inhibition of cytokine induction, including tumor necrosis factor-α, interleukin-1, and interferon-γ, was seen without evidence of apoptosis. These findings further the prospect of PPAR agonists as anti-inflammatory mediators, while also raising the intriguing possibility that they might be of value in the unique atherosclerosis seen among cardiac transplantation patients, a diffuse immune-driven disease that accounts for most transplantation failures.

PPARα in vascular and immune cells

Monocyte/macrophage experiments highlight potential differences between the biologic effects of PPAR isoforms. Whereas PPARγ ligands can induce apoptosis in resting macrophages, PPARα agonists do so only after monocyte/macrophage stimulation with tumor necrosis factor–α or interferon-γ. Tissue factor expression in monocytes/macrophages, a major contributor to plaque thrombogenicity, has also been found to be PPARα regulated [78, 79].

Delerive *et al.* [80] reported PPARα expression in human VSMC, finding that PPARα activators inhibited interleukin-1-induced interleukin-6, as well as expression of cyclooxygenase-2. These investigators went on to demonstrate that interleukin-6 production is increased in aortic explants of PPARα-deficient mice [80]. PPARα activation also inhibits endothelin-1, a potent inducer of smooth muscle cell proliferation [58].

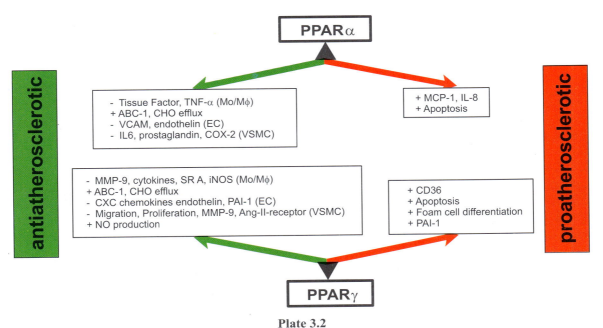

Plate 3.1

The peroxisome proliferator-activated receptors (PPAR) as transcription factor.

As members of the steroid hormone nuclear receptor family, PPARs are thought to control gene expression through a heterodimeric complex with the retinoid X nuclear receptor(RXR). Both PPAR and RXR activation are controlled by binding to specific ligands. The ultimate transcriptional response is determined by the association or release of specific coactivators and corepressors. This complex binds to certain PPAR responseelements (PPRE) in the promoter regions of target genes controlling their expression, either inducing or repressing the transcriptional response. L – ligand; RA – 9-*cis*-retinoic acid.

PPARα

antiatherosclerotic

- Tissue Factor, TNF-α (Mo/Mφ)
+ ABC-1, CHO efflux
- VCAM, endothelin (EC)
- IL6, prostaglandin, COX-2 (VSMC)

+ MCP-1, IL-8
+ Apoptosis

- MMP-9, cytokines, SR A, iNOS (Mo/Mφ)
+ ABC-1, CHO efflux
- CXC chemokines endothelin, PAI-1 (EC)
- Migration, Proliferation, MMP-9, Ang-II-receptor (VSMC)
+ NO production

+ CD36
+ Apoptosis
+ Foam cell differentiation
+ PAI-1

proatherosclerotic

PPARγ

Plate 3.2

PPARs agonists can limit the inflammatory responses and may have proatherosclerotic effects in the vasculature.

A major anti-inflammatory effect of PPARα may occur through its inhibition of cytokine 1-induced endothelial vascular cell adhesion molecule-1 expression, an important early step in atherogenesis. These responses appear to be mediated by decreased nuclear factor-κB assembly, a common theme in PPAR-mediated repression of target gene expression [81]. Although we found this response restricted to PPARα agonists and vascular cell adhesion molecule-1 [81], other researchers have reported PPARγ effects on other adhesion molecules under different conditions [82, 83]. PPARα inhibition of vascular cell adhesion molecule-1 has been seen consistently. Differences may be methodological, even though multiple levels of regulation exist for PPAR pathways. Of note, PPARγ agonists did not alter vascular cell adhesion molecule-1 expression in LDL receptor-deficient mice [52].

PPARα involvement in inflammation is also supported by evidence that lipopolysaccharide-induced inflammatory responses were prolonged in PPARα-deficient mice [65]. Such *in vitro* work would suggest antiatherosclerotic/anti-inflammatory effects through PPARα (see Plate 3.2). Indeed, more recently we have found evidence for such effects *in vivo* with omega-3 fatty acids in the form of oxidized eicosapentaenoic acid, a fatty acid in fish oil. Oxidized eicosapentaenoic acid limited neutrophil adhesion in wildtype but not PPARα–deficient mice [84]. These data suggest that PPARα may be involved in the cardiovascular benefits seen with diets enriched in fish.

In contrast to these anti-inflammatory effects, other reports found evidence for PPARα promoting inflammatory responses in endothelial cells. Lee *et al.* [85] found that certain specific oxidized phospholipids induced inflammation in a PPARα dependent manner. The *in vivo* relevance of these compounds and results is unclear but these observations warrant further study. Studies crossing PPARα-deficient mice with apolipoprotein E atherosclerosis-prone mice and placing them on high-fat diets found less atherosclerosis, despite the PPARα null mice having higher atherogenic lipids [86]. The overall effects at 10 weeks were modest in the arch (25% difference) and greater in the abdomen (65%). Surprisingly, the PPARα null/apolipoprotein E null mice had lower blood pressure and less insulin resistance, a phenotype seen by others as well.

More recently, PPARα agonists were found to decrease atherosclerosis as might have been predicted, especially if these mice carried a human transgene for apolipoprotein AI [87]. This raises a possibility that some species-specific differences may contribute to the results.

PPARs – KEY ROLES IN THE ACCELERATED DIABETIC ATHEROSCLEROSIS

The mechanisms underlying the accelerated atherosclerosis seen in type 2 diabetes mellitus remain unclear. Diabetes is a major risk factor for atherosclerosis, but glucose concentrations in type 2 diabetes are only modestly related to CAD [2]. A possible explanation for the relatively weak effect of glycemia for CAD in diabetes is the existence of broader atherogenic stimuli that exist both in diabetes and over the course of many years before the onset of frank diabetes during the so-called but imprecisely defined prediabetic state. Increased levels of inflammatory markers (*e.g.*, CRP levels and impaired fibrinolysis) and PAI-1 have been shown to be present among patients before the onset of diabetes [2]. Insulin resistance is also related to increased inflammation and PAI-1 concentrations. Emerging evidence suggests that PPARγ agonists may reduce atherosclerosis, which may not be dependent on their effect on glucose concentrations but on decreasing the levels of these markers. Rosiglitazone has, in fact, reduced levels of CRP and PAI-1 in small clinical trials. It remains to be seen if these effects will be borne out in larger studies, many of which are already underway.

But other clinical studies have demonstrated that hyperglycemia is still an independent risk factor for diabetic macrovascular disease [88–91]. Advanced glycation end-products (AGEs) are postulated as possible accelerators of atherosclerosis in patients with diabetes mellitus [92]. AGEs, long-term products of the Maillard reaction, play a causative role in diabetic vasculopathy including atherosclerosis as well as microangiopathy [92]. Interesting findings indicate that AGEs induce enhancement of transcriptional activities of AP-1, NF-kB and PPARγ, being also involved in increased levels of mRNA for some of OxLDL receptors in THP-1-cells treated with PMA. The upregulated surface expression of these receptors on macrophage membranes was closely associated with increased uptake of modified LDL, and culminated in an enhanced foam cell transformation. Thus, AGEs may be involved in the different stages of foam cell formation *via* the increased numbers of OxLDL receptors in accelerated atherosclerotic lesions of individuals with diabetes [92].

Regarding the inflammatory process there is no evidence to suggest that in diabetic patients this is different in non-diabetic individuals. The main difference may be the factors that trigger the inflammation [93]. Sartippour *et al.* [94] identified that the macrophage PPAR genes are response genes for glucose action. They found that macrophage PPAR gene expression is altered in human type 2 diabetes and these changes occur in the vascular wall in the hyperglycemic state that may influence atherogenesis by altering arterial lipid metabolism and inflammatory response. Thus, the high glucose levels regulate PPAR expression in human macrophages in the following manner: PPARα and PPARβ/δ are increased whereas PPARγ is decreased [94].

Atherosclerosis in diabetes can be accelerated due to dysregulation of macrophage PPARs expression in the arterial wall by increasing in vivo the macrophage releasing of LPL and proinflammatory cytokines [94].

PPAR LIGANDS

At the time PPARs were emerging from basic science studies as important transcriptional mediators of metabolism, separate evidence arose that identified specific synthetic agonists as PPAR ligands with potential therapeutic benefit (Table 3.1). These various ligands will be reviewed, with an emphasis on those in clinical use.

Table 3.1

PPARs and their ligands

PPARα	PPARβ/δ	PPARγ
Fibrates: Fenofibrate Gemfibrozil	Carbaprostacyclin GW501516 L165041	Thiazolidinedio-nes: – Pioglitazone – Rosiglitazone – Troglitazone

PPARα LIGANDS – FIBRATES

Specific synthetic PPARα ligands include research agonists such as WY14643 as well as various fibric acids (*e.g.*, bezafibrate, clofibrate, fenofibrate, gemfibrozil) [95,96] in clinical use as lipid-lowering drugs. Although natural PPARα agonists have been suggested to include eicosanoids, certain long-chain fatty acids like docosahexenoic (DHA) and eicosapentenoic acid (EPA), and HODEs, the exact nature and identity of endogenous PPAR ligands remain incompletely defined. Recent work has established lipoprotein lipase as a pathway for generating endogenous PPAR ligands [97, 98].

Fibrates lower triglyceride levels as a result of enhanced lipolysis (by increasing lipoprotein lipase and reducing apolipoprotein CIII gene expression), induction of FA uptake and catabolism, and reduced FA synthesis and VLDL production by the liver [99]. Moreover, fibrates increase the removal of LDL particles by modifying LDL composition with more affinity for LDL receptor [99]. They can reduce the level of fibrinogen, lipoprotein a, PAI-1, uric acid, and the concentration of highly atherogenic small dense LDL3. The prospect that the decrease in cardiovascular events seen with fibrates in clinical trials like VA-HIT may have stemmed from their PPARα activation remains an intriguing possibility.

PPARγ LIGANDS – THIAZOLIDINEDIONES

The thiazolidinedione class of insulin sensitizers are PPARγ ligands. These agents were discovered by empirical screening in rodent models of insulin resistance without prior knowledge of their mechanism of action. Two thiazolidinediones (TZD) are currently available for clinical use in the US: pioglitazone and rosiglitazone. They improve insulin sensitivity and reduce glycemia, lipidemia and insulinemia in patients with type 2 diabetes. The TZDs activate the nuclear receptor PPARγ and improve insulin sensitivity *via* several mechanisms: 1) induce the expression of GLUT4 glucose transporter; 2) regulate release of adipocyte-derived signaling factors that affect insulin sensitivity in muscle, and 3) contribute to a turn-over in adipose tissue inducing production of smaller, more insulin sensitive adipocytes [100]. TZDs affect free fatty acids (FFA) lipotoxicity on islets, improving pancreatic B-cell function. They also lower TNFα and leptin secretion from adipocytes [101, 102]. Early surrogate endpoint data suggest these agonists can decrease the levels of inflammatory markers like C-reactive protein and CD40 ligand.

In clinical trials, thiazolidinediones also modestly but consistently lower blood pressure. Some other studies showed that PPARγ agonists lower blood pressure in diabetic patients and in hypertensive animals [103]. The findings that glitazones also reduce blood pressure in nondiabetic individuals suggest that the antihypertensive effects may be independent of their insulin-sensitizing actions [103]. Given that they are highly expressed in vascular endothelial cells, they may influence blood pressure by regulating the expression of vascular factors that are involved in maintenance of vascular tone such as type C natriuretic peptide, endothelin, and plasminogen activator inhibitor-1 [103, 104].

LOX-1, a novel lectin-like receptor for oxidized LDL (ox-LDL) is expressed in response to ox-LDL, angiotensin II (Ang II), tumor necrosis factor (TNF)-alpha, and other stress stimuli. It is highly expressed in atherosclerotic tissues. A PPARγ ligand, pioglitazone reduced intracellular superoxide radical generation, expression of the LOX-1 gene, and monocyte adhesion to activated endothelium [105]. This effect of PPARγ ligands in atherogenesis may involve the inhibition of LOX-1 and the adhesion of monocytes to endothelium [105].

Rosiglitazone reduces sCD40L serum levels in patients with type 2 diabetes and CAD. It is known that the interaction of CD40L with its receptor CD40 is critically involved in inflammatory cell activation in atherogenesis [106]. Moreover, using a model of accelerated atherosclerosis (male apolipoprotein E (apoE)-deficient mice rendered diabetic by low-dose streptozotocin), rosiglitazone reduced significantly the atherosclerotic aortic plaque area in both diabetic and non-diabetic apoE-deficient mice. Also, rosiglitazone reduced the correlation coefficient between plasma glucose and the degree of atherosclerosis without affecting plasma glucose levels. So, despite higher lipid levels and similar glucose levels rosiglitazone-treated animals showed less atherosclerosis [107].

Also, these compounds lower circulating levels of triglycerides and free fatty acids (FFAs) by increasing lipolysis and clearance of triglyceride-rich lipoproteins in adipose tissue [108].

Together, these findings have important clinical implication given that TZDs are widely used in diabetic patients at high risk for developing atherosclerotic complications. It seems likely that the broad effects of PPARγ agonists result from coordinated indirect and direct actions in multiple tissues. New PPARγ modulators with specific pharmacological profiles may be useful in the treatment of type 2 diabetes associated with atherosclerosis and hypertension without side effects such as weight gain and edema.

PPARα and PPARγ remain attractive therapeutic targets with high potential for the development of new drugs with co-agonistic activity as well as tissue and target gene-selective for the treatment of chronic inflammatory diseases such as diabetes and atherosclerosis.

PPARβ/δ LIGANDS – NOVEL TARGETS IN ATHEROSCLEROSIS

The synthetic PPARβ/δ agonists have revealed an important role for this receptor in lipid metabolism [109, 110]. It is known that PPARβ/δ is a receptor for unsaturated FAs. Recently, it was shown that native VLDL lipoprotein particles might be involved in PPARβ/δ activation pathway [111]. This activation was specific to VLDL and it was produced at a physiologic concentration of VLDL and closely approximated the maximal efficacy of synthetic PPARβ/δ ligands such as carboprostacyclin and GW 501516 [112]. The findings that both PPARβ/δ and PPARα are activated by the triglycerides present in the VLDL suggest that their coupled activation would allow for a coordinated cellular response to incoming fatty acids and triglycerides: the activation of PPARβ/δ might facilitate the "short-term" storage of triglycerides whereas stimulation of PPARα would result in the gene induction, important in fatty acid oxidation [113, 114].

PPARβ/δ is expressed in many tissues that contribute to cholesterol flux [115]. A selective PPARβ/δ agonist, GW501516, that increases cholesterol efflux from cells, in part, through an increase in the expression of the ABCA1 reverse cholesterol transporter. All three PPAR subtypes have the ability to induce ABCA1 expression in the following manner: PPARβ/δ >PPARγ > PPARα.

Hyperinsulinemia and the lipid triad of low HDLc, small LDL particles, and elevated serum triglycerides are characteristics of dyslipidemia associated with the metabolic syndrome X [116, 117]. Individuals with this profile have a higher incidence of premature coronary artery disease [116]. Oliver WR *et al.* [118] demonstrated that PPARβ/δ agonists are likely to have beneficial effects on this lipid triad through a mechanism that increases cholesterol flux from peripheral tissues. These activities, combined with the benefit of lowering serum insulin levels, suggest that PPARβ/δ agonists may be powerful drugs for decreasing the incidence of cardiovascular disease associated with the metabolic syndrome X.

CONCLUSION

Atherosclerosis and diabetes are complex multifactorial diseases that are often intertwined in patients. Inflammation may represent an important contributor to the various processes involved in both atherosclerosis and diabetes, either in response to other known risk factors, or perhaps as its own pathway. It is a story that continues to unfold, and while so doing, holds out the prospect that there may be additional ways to limit atherosclerosis.

Perhaps PPARs will be found to be critical regulators of inflammatory responses, not just through metabolic effects but also through their direct action in vascular and inflammatory cells. If so, PPAR agonists may someday be used as a way of limiting atherosclerosis or its complications. Such future possibilities will be dependent on additional insight into these intriguing receptors, their agonists, and the effects of their activation. Large-scale clinical trials are required to assess their safety and efficacy before they can be added to the clinicians' arsenal of antiatherosclerotic agents.

REFERENCES

1. Stern MP. Diabetes and Cardiovascular Disease: The "Common Soil" Hypothesis. *Diabetes,* **44(4):** 369–74. Review, 1995.

2. Haffner SM. Insulin Resistance, Inflammation, and the Prediabetic State. *Am J Cardiol,* **92(suppl):** 18J–26J, 2003.

3. Issemann I, Green S. Activation of a member of the steroid hormone receptor superfamily by peroxisome proliferators. *Nature,* **347:** 645–650, 1990.

4. Glass CK, Rosenfeld MG. The coregulator exchange in transcriptional functions of nuclear receptors. *Genes Dev,* **14:** 121–141, 2000.

5. Vosper H, Khoudoli GA, Graham TL, Palmer CN. Peroxisome proliferator-activated receptor agonist, hyperlipidaemia, and atherosclerosis. *Pharmacol Ther,* **95(1):** 47–62, 2002.

6. Michalik L, Wahli W. Peroxisome proliferator-activated receptors: three isotypes for a multitude of functios. *Current Opinion in Biotechnology,* **10:** 564–570, 1999.

7. Hu E, Tontonoz P, Spiegelman BM. Transdifferentiation of myoblasts by the adipogenic transcription factors PPAR gamma and C/EBP alpha. *Proc Natl Acad Sci U S A,* **92:** 9856–9860, 1995.

8. Kliewer SA, Forman BM, Blumberg B, Ong ES, Borgmeyer U, Mangelsdorf DJ, Umesono K, Evans RM. Differential expression and activation of a family of murine peroxisome proliferator-activated receptors. *Proc Natl Acad Sci U S A,* **91:** 7355–7359, 1994.

9. Lemberger T, Braissant O, Juge-Aubry C, Keller H, Saladin R, Staels B, Auwerx J, Burger AG, Meier CA, Wahli W. PPAR tissue distribution and interactions with other hormone-signaling pathways. *Ann N Y Acad Sci,* **804:** 231–251, 1996.

10. Auwerx J, Schoonjans K, Fruchart JC, Staels B. Regulation of triglyceride metabolism by PPARs: fibrates and thiazolidinediones have distinct effects. *J Atheroscler Thromb,* **3:** 81–89, 1996.

11. Latruffe N, Vamecq J. Peroxisome proliferators and peroxisome proliferator activated receptors (PPARs) as regulators of lipid metabolism. *Biochimie,* **79:** 81–94, 1997.

12. Auwerx J. PPARgamma, the ultimate thrifty gene. *Diabetologia,* **42:** 1033–1049, 1999.

13. Ristow M, Muller Wieland D, Pffeiffer A, Krone W, Kahn CR. Obesity associated with a mutation in a genetic regulator of adipocyte differentiation. *N Engl Med,* **339:** 953–959, 1998.

14. Deeb SS, Fajas L, Nemoto M, Pihlamaki J, Mykknen L, Kuusisto J, *et al.* A Pro12Ala substitution in PPARgamma2 associated with decreased receptor activity, lower body mass index and improved insulin sensitivity. *Nat Genet,* **20:** 284–287, 1998.

15. Kubota N, Terauchi Y, Miki H, Tamemoto H, Yamauchi T, Komeda K, *et al.* PPARgamma mediates high-fat diet-induced adipocyte hypertrophy and insulin resistance. *Moll Cell,* **4:** 597–609, 1999.

16. Martin G, Schoonjans K, Lefebvre A-M, Staels B, Auwerx J. Coordinate regulation of the expression of the fatty acid transport protein and acyl-CoA synthetase genes by PPARα and PPARγ activators. *J Biol Chem*, **272**: 28210–28217,1997.

17. Sfeir Z, Ibrahimi A, Amri, E, Grimaldi P, Abumrad N. Regulation of FAT/CD36 gene expression: further evidence in support of a role of the protein in fatty acid binding/transport. *Prostaglandins Leukotrienes Essent. Fatty Acids*, **57**: 17–21, 1997.

18. Kallen CB, Lazar MA. Antidiabetic thiazolidinediones inhibit leptin (*ob*) gene expression in 3T3-L1 adipocytes. *Proc Natl Acad Sci USA*, **93**: 5793–5796, 1996.

19. De Vos P, Lefebvre A-M, Miller SG, Guerre-Millo M, Wong K, Saladin R, Hamann LG, Staels B, Briggs MR, Auwerx J. Thiazolidinediones repress *ob* gene expression in rodents *via* activation of peroxisome proliferator-activated receptorγ. *J Clin Invest*, **98**: 1004–1009,1996.

20. Aubert J, Champigny O, Saint-Marc P, Negrel R, Collins S, Ricquier D, Ailhaud G. Up-regulation of UCP-2 gene expression by PPAR agonists in preadipose and adipose cells. *Biochem Biophys Res Commun*, **238**: 606–611, 1997.

21. Cambon B, Reyne Y, Nougues J. *In vitro* induction of UCP1 mRNA in preadipocytes from rabbit considered as a model of large mammals brown adipose tissue development: importance of PPARγ agonists for cells isolated in the postnatal period. *Mol Cell Endocrinol*, **146**: 49–58, 1998.

22. Winegar DA, Su J-L, Kliewer SA. Role of peroxisome proliferator-activated receptors in atherosclerosis. *Current Opinion in Cardiovascular, Pulmonary & Renal Investigational Drugs*, **2(3)**: 233–243, 2000.

23. Auwerx J, Schoonjans K, Fruchart JC, Staels B. Regulation of triglyceride metabolism by PPARs: fibrates and thiazolidinediones have distinct effects. *J Atheroscler Thromb*, **3**: 81–89, 1996.

24. Forman BM, Chen J, Evans RM. Hypolipidemic drugs, polyunsaturated fatty acids, and eicosanoids are ligands for peroxisome proliferator-activated receptors α and γ. *Proc Natl Acad Sci U S A*, **94**: 4312–4317, 1997.

25. Pineda Torra I, Gervois P, Staels B. Peroxisome proliferator-activated receptor in metabolic disease, inflammation, atherosclerosis and aging. *Curr Opin Lipidol*, **10**: 151–159, 1999.

26. Ziouzenkova O, Perrey S, Asatryan L, Hwang J, MacNaul KL, Moller DE, Rader DJ, Sevanian A, Zechner R, Hoefler G, Plutzky J. Lipolysis of triglyceride rich lipoproteins generates PPAR ligands: evidence for an antiinflammatory role for lipoprotein lipase. *Proc Natl Acad Sci USA*, **100**: 2730–2735, 2003.

27. Chawla A, Lee CH, Barak Y, He W, Rosenfeld J, Liao D, Han J, Kang H, Evans RM. PPAR is a very low-density lipoprotein sensor in macrophages. *Proc Natl Acad Sci USA*, **100**: 1268–1273, 2003.

28. Pasceri V, Wu HD, Willerson JT, Yeh ET. Modulation of vascular inflammation in vitro and in vivo by peroxisome proliferator-activated receptor gamma activators. *Circulation*, **101**: 235–238, 2000.

29. Gonzalez FJ. Recent update on the PPARα-null mouse. *Biochimie*, **79**: 139–144, 1997.

30. Costet P, Legendre C, More J, Edgar A, Galtier P, Pineau T. PPARα-isoform deficiency leads to progressive dyslipidemia with sexually dimorphic, obesity and steatosis. J Biol Chem, **273**: 29577–29585, 1998.

31. Bernal-Mizrachi C, Weng S, Li B, Nolte LA, Feng C, Coleman T, Holloszy JO, Semenkovich CF. Respiratory Uncoupling Lowers Blood Pressure Through a Leptin-Dependent Mechanism in Genetically Obese Mice. *Arterioscler Thromb Vasc Biol*, **22**: 961–968, 2002.

32. Timothy MW, Brown PJ, Sternbach DD, Henke BR. The PPARs: From Orphan Receptors to Drug Discovery. Volume 43, Number 4, February 24, 2000.

33. Krook A, Digby J, O'Rahilly S, Zierath JR, Wallberg-Henriksson H. Uncoupling Protein 3 Is Reduced in Skeletal Muscle of NIDDM Patients. *Diabetes*, **47(9)**: 1528–1531, 1998.

34. Brun S, Carmona MC, Mampel T, Vinas O, Giralt M, Iglesias R, Villarroya F. Activators of peroxisome proliferators-activated receptor-R induce the expression of the uncoupling protein-3 gene in skeletal muscle: a potential mechanism for the lipid intake-dependent activation of uncoupling protein-3 gene expression at birth. *Diabetes*, **48**: 1217–1222, 1999.

35. Wang YX, Lee CH, Tiep S, Yu RT, Ham JY, Kang H, Evans RM. PPARβ/δ activates fat metabolism to prevent obesity. *Cell*, **113**: 159–170, 2003.

36. Vosper H, Palel L, Graham TL, Khondoli GA, Hill A, Macphee CH, Pinto I, Smith SA, Suckling KE, Wolf CR, Palmer CN. The PPARβ/δ promotes lipid accumulation in human macrophages. *J Biol Chem*, **276**: 44258–44265, 2001.

37. Lee GH, Provenca R, Montez JM, Carrol KM, Darvishzodeh JG, LeeJI, Friedman JM. Abnormal splicing of the leptin receptor in diabetic mice. *Nature*, **379**: 632–635,1996.

38. Yamanchi T, Kamon J, Waki H, Murakami K, Motojima K, Komed K, Ide T, Kubota N, Terauchi Y, *et al*. The mechanisms by which both heterozygous PPARγ deficiency and PPARγ agonist improve insulin resistance. *J Biol Chem*, **276**: 41245–41254, 2001.

39. Wu Z, Xie Y, Morrison RF, Bucher NLR, Farmer SR. PPARγ Induces the Insulin-dependent Glucose Transporter GLUT4 in the Absence of C/EBPα During the Conversion of 3T3 Fibroblasts Into Adipocytes. *J Clin Invest,* **101(1):** 22–32, 1998.

40. Tononoz P, Hu E, Devine J, Beale EG, Spiegelman BM. PPARγ2 regulates adipose expression of the phosphenolpyruvate carboxykinase gene. *Moll Cell Biol,* **15:** 351–357, 1995.

41. Ribon V, Johnson JH, Camp HS, Saltiel AR. Thiazolidinediones and insulin resistance: PPARγ activation stimulates expression of the CAP gene. *Proc Natl Acad Sci U S A,* **95(25):** 14751–6, 1998.

42. Plutzky J. Inflammatory pathways in atherosclerosis and acute coronary syndromes. *Am J Cardiol,* **88(8A):** 10K–15K, 2001.

43. Marx N, Sukhova G, Murphy C, Libby P, Plutzky J. Macrophages in human atheroma contain PPAR: differentiation-dependent peroxisomal proliferators activate receptor gamma (PPARγ) expression and reduction of MMP-9 activity through PPAR activation in mononuclear phagocytes in vitro. *Am J Pathol,* **153:** 17–23, 1998.

44. Ricote M, Huang J, Fajas L, Li A, Welch J, Najib J, Witztum JL, Auwerx J, Palinski W, Glass CK. Expression of the peroxisome proliferator-activated receptor gamma (PPARγ) in human atherosclerosis and regulation in macrophages by colony stimulating factors and oxidized low density lipoprotein. *Proc Natl Acad Sci USA,* **95:** 7614–7619, 1998.

45. Jiang C, Ting AT, Seed B. PPARγ agonists inhibit production of monocyte inflammatory cytokines. *Nature,* **391:** 82–86, 1998.

46. Chinetti G, Griglio S, Antonucci M, Torra IP, Delerive P, Majd Z, Fruchart JC, Chapman J, Najib J, Staels B. Activation of proliferator-activated receptors and induces apoptosis of human monocyte-derived macrophages. *J Biol Chem,* **273:** 25573–25580, 1998.

47. Nagy L, Tontonoz P, Alvarez JG, Chen H, Evans RM. Oxidized LDL regulates macrophage gene expression through ligand activation of PPAR gamma. *Cell,* **93:** 229–240, 1998.

48. Tontonoz P, Nagy L, Alvarez JG, Thomazy VA, Evans RM. PPARgamma promotes monocyte / macrophage differentiation and uptake of oxidized LDL. *Cell,* **93:** 241–252, 1998.

49. Chawla A, Barak Y, Nagy L, Liao D, Tontonoz P, Evans RM. PPARgamma dependent and independent effects on macrophage-gene expression in lipid metabolism and inflammation. *Nat Med,* **7:** 48–52, 2001.

50. Chinetti G, Lestavel S, Bocher V, Remaley AT, Neve B, Torra IP, Teissier E, Minnich A, Jaye M, Duverger N, *et al.* PPARalpha and PPARgamma-activators induce cholesterol removal from human macrophage foam cells through stimulation of the ABCA1 pathway. *Nat Med,* **7:** 53–58, 2001.

51. Moore KJ, Rosen ED, Fitzgerald ML, Randow F, Andersson LP, Altshuler D, Milstone DS, Mortensen RM, Spiegelman BM, Freeman MW. The role of PPARgamma in macrophage differentiation and cholesterol uptake. *Nat Med,* **7:** 41–47, 2001.

52. Li AC, Brown KK, Silvestre MJ, Willson TM, Palinski W, Glass CK. Peroxisome proliferator-activated receptor ligands inhibit development of atherosclerosis in LDL receptor-deficient mice. *J Clin Invest,* **106:** 523–531, 2000.

53. Chen Z, Ishibashi S, Perrey S, Osuga J, Gotoda T, Kitamine T, Tamura Y, Okazaki H, Yahagi N, Iizuka Y, *et al.* Troglitazone inhibits atherosclerosis in apolipoprotein E-knockout mice: pleiotropic effects on CD36 expression and HDL. *Arterioscler Thromb Vasc Biol,* **21:** 372–377, 2001.

54. Collins AR, Meehan WP, Kintscher U, Jackson S, Wakino S, Noh G, Palinski W, Hsueh WA, Law RE. Troglitazone inhibits formation of early atherosclerotic lesions in diabetic and nondiabetic low-density lipoprotein receptor-deficient mice. *Arterioscler Thromb Vasc Biol,* **21:** 365–371, 2001.

55. Marx N, Bourcier T, Sukhova GK, Libby P, Plutzky J. PPARgamma activation in human endothelial cells increases plasminogen activator inhibitor type-1 expression: PPARgamma as a potential mediator in vascular disease. *Arterioscler Thromb Vasc Biol,* **19:** 546–551, 1999.

56. Bishop-Bailey D, Hla T. Endothelial cell apoptosis induced by the peroxisome proliferator-activated receptor gamma (PPAR gamma) ligand 15-deoxy-12, 14-prostaglandin J2. *J Biol Chem,* **274:** 17042–17048, 1999.

57. Xin X, Yang S, Kowalski J, Gerritsen ME. Peroxisome proliferator-activated receptor ligands are potent inhibitors of angiogenesis in vitro and in vivo. *J Biol Chem,* **274:** 9116–9121, 1999.

58. Delerive P, Martin-Nizard F, Chinetti G, Trottein F, Fruchart JC, Najib J, Duriez P, Staels B. Peroxisome proliferator-activated receptor activators inhibit thrombin-induced endothelin-1 production in human vascular endothelial cells by inhibiting the activator protein-1 signaling pathway. *Circ Res,* **85:** 394–402, 1999.

59. Satoh H, Tsukamoto K, Hashimoto Y, Hashimoto N, Togo M, Hara M, Maekawa H, Isoo N, Kimura S, Watanabe T. Thiazolidinediones suppress endothelin-1 secretion from bovine vascular endothelial cells: a new possible role of PPARgamma on vascular endothelial function. *Biochem Biophys Res Commun,* **254:** 757–763, 1999.

60. Murata T, He S, Hangai M, Ishibashi T, Xi XP, Kim S, Hsueh WA, Ryan SJ, Law RE, Hinton DR. Peroxisome proliferator-activated receptor-gamma ligands inhibit choroidal neovascularization. *Invest Ophthalmol Vis Sci*, **41**: 2309–2317, 2000.

61. Marx N, Mach F, Sauty A, Leung JH, Sarafi MN, Ransohoff RM, Libby P, Plutzky J, Luster AD. Peroxisome proliferator-activated receptor-gamma activators inhibit IFN-gamma- induced expression of the T cell-active CXC chemokines IP-10, Mig, and I-TAC in human endothelial cells. *J Immunol*, **164**: 6503–6508, 2000.

62. Han KH, Chang MK, Boullier A, Green SR, Li A, Glass CK, Quehenberger O. Oxidized LDL reduces monocyte CCR2 expression through pathways involving peroxisome proliferator-activated receptor. *J Clin Invest*, **106**: 793–802, 2000.

63. Kintscher U, Goetze S, Wakino S, Kim S, Nagpal S, Chandraratna RA, Graf K, Fleck E, Hsueh WA, Law RE. Peroxisome proliferator-activated receptor and retinoid X receptor ligands inhibit monocyte chemotactic protein-1-directed migration of monocytes. *Eur J Pharmacol*, **401**: 259–270, 2000.

64. Su CG, Wen X, Bailey ST, Jiang W, Rangwala SM, Keilbaugh SA, Flanigan A, Murthy S, Lazar MA, Wu GD. A novel therapy for colitis utilizing PPAR-gamma ligands to inhibit the epithelial inflammatory response. *J Clin Invest*, **104**: 383–389, 1999.

65. Staels B, Koenig W, Habib A, Merval R, Lebret M, Torra IP, Delerive P, Fadel A, Chinetti G, Fruchart JC, *et al*. Activation of human aortic smooth muscle cells is inhibited by PPARα but not by PPARγ activators. *Nature*, **393**: 790–793, 1998.

66. Benson S, Wu J, Padmanabhan S, Kurtz TW, Pershadsingh HA. Peroxisome proliferator-activated receptor (PPAR)-gamma expression in human vascular smooth muscle cells: inhibition of growth, migration, and c-fos expression by the peroxisome proliferator-activated receptor (PPAR)-activator troglitazone. *Am J Hypertens*, **13**: 74–82, 2000.

67. Law RE, Goetze S, Xi XP, Jackson S, Kawano Y, Demer L, Fishbein MC, Meehan WP, Hsueh WA. Expression and function of PPAR in rat and human vascular smooth muscle cells. *Circulation*, **101**: 1311–1318, 2000.

68. Marx N, Schonbeck U, Lazar MA, Libby P, Plutzky J. Peroxisome proliferator-activated receptor activators inhibit gene expression and migration in human vascular smooth muscle cells. *Circ Res*, **83**: 1097–1103, 1998.

69. Law R, Meehan WP, Xi XP, Graf K, Wuthrich DA, Coats W, Faxon D, Hsueh WA. Troglitazone inhibits vascular smooth muscle cell growth and intimal hyperplasia. *J Clin Invest*, **98**: 1897–1905, 1996.

70. Wakino S, Kintscher U, Kim S, Yin F, Hsueh WA, Law RE. Peroxisome proliferator-activated receptor ligands inhibit retinoblastoma phosphorylation and G13 S transition in vascular smooth muscle cells. *J Biol Chem*, **275**: 22435–22441, 2000.

71. Minamikawa J, Tanaka S, Yamauchi M, Inoue D, Koshiyama H. Potent inhibitory effect of troglitazone on carotid arterial wall thickness in type 2 diabetes. *J Clin Endocrinol Metab*, **83**: 1818–1820, 1998.

72. Takagi T, Akasaka T, Yamamuro A, Honda Y, Hozumi T, Morioka S, Yoshida K. Troglitazone reduces neointimal tissue proliferation after coronary stent implantation in patients with non-insulin dependent diabetes mellitus: a serial intravascular ultrasound study. *J Am Coll Cardiol*, **36**: 1529–1535, 2000.

73. Padilla J, Kaur K, Harris SG, Phipps RP. PPARgamma-mediated regulation of normal and malignant B lineage cells. *Ann N Y Acad Sci*, **905**: 97–109, 2000.

74. Clark RB, Bishop-Bailey D, Estrada-Hernandez T, Hla T, Puddington L, Padula SJ. The nuclear receptor PPARgamma and immunoregulation: PPAR gamma mediates inhibition of helper T cell responses. *J Immunol*, **164**: 1364–1371, 2000.

75. Yang XY, Wang LH, Chen T, Hodge DR, Resau JH, DaSilva L, Farrar WL. Activation of human T lymphocytes is inhibited by peroxisome proliferators-activated receptor gamma (PPARγ) agonists: PPAR co-association with transcription factor NFAT. *J Biol Chem*, **275**: 4541–4544, 2000.

76. Harris SG, Phipps RP. Peroxisome proliferator-activated receptor (PPAR-γ) activation in naive mouse T cells induces cell death. *Ann N Y Acad Sci*, **905**: 297–300, 2000.

77. Marx N, Kehrle B, Kohlhammer K, Grub M, Koenig W, Hombach V, Libby P, Plutzky J. PPAR activators as antiinflammatory mediators in human T lymphocytes: implications for atherosclerosis and transplantation-associated arteriosclerosis. *Circ Res*, **90**: 703–710, 2002.

78. Marx N, Mackman N, Schonbeck U, Yilmaz N, Hombach VV, Libby P, Plutzky J. PPARα activators inhibit tissue factor expression and activity in human monocytes. *Circulation*, **103**: 213–219, 2001.

79. Neve BP, Corseaux D, Chinetti G, Zawadzki C, Fruchart JC, Duriez P, Staels B, Jude B. PPAR agonists inhibit tissue factor expression in human monocytes and macrophages. *Circulation*, **103**: 207–212, 2001.

80. Delerive P, De Bosscher K, Besnard S, Vanden Berghe W, Peters JM, Gonzalez FJ, Fruchart JC, Tedgui A, Haegeman G, Staels B. Peroxisome proliferator-activated receptor α negatively regulates

the vascular inflammatory gene response by negative cross-talk with transcription factors NF-B and AP-1. *J Biol Chem*, **274**: 32048–32054, 1999.

81. Marx N, Sukhova GK, Collins T, Libby P, Plutzky J. PPARα activators inhibit cytokine-induced vascular cell adhesion molecule-1 expression in human endothelial cells. *Circulation*, **99**: 3125–3131, 1999.

82. Jackson SM, Parhami F, Xi XP, Berliner JA, Hsueh WA, Law RE, Demer LL. Peroxisome proliferator-activated receptor activators target human endothelial cells to inhibit leukocyte-endothelial cell interaction. *Arterioscler Thromb Vasc Biol*, **19**: 2094–2104, 1999.

83. Pasceri V, Wu HD, Willerson JT, Yeh ET. Modulation of vascular inflammation in vitro and in vivo by peroxisome proliferator-activated receptor γ activators. *Circulation*, **101**: 235–238, 2000.

84. Sethi S, Ziouzenkova O, Ni H, Wagner DD, Plutzky J, Mayadas TN. Oxidized omega-3 fatty acids in fish oil inhibit leukocyte-endothelial interactions through activation of PPARα. *Blood*, **100**: 1340–1346, 2002.

85. Lee H, Shi W, Tontonoz P, Wang S, Subbanagounder G, Hedrick CC, Hama S, Borromeo C, Evans RM, Berliner JA, Nagy L. Role for peroxisome proliferator-activated receptor α in oxidized phospholipid-induced synthesis of monocyte chemotactic protein-1 and interleukin-8 by endothelial cells. *Circ Res*, **87**: 516–521, 2000.

86. Tordjman K, Bernal-Mizrachi C, Zemany L, Weng S, Feng C, Zhang F, Leone TC, Coleman T, Kelly DP, Semenkovich CF. PPAR-α deficiency reduces insulin resistance and atherosclerosis in apoE-null mice. *J Clin Invest*, **107**: 1025–1034, 2001.

87. Duez H, Chao Y-S, Hernandez M, Torpier G, Poulain P, Mundt S, Mallat Z, Teissier E, Burton CA, Tedgui A, *et al.* Reduction of atherosclerosis by the peroxisome proliferator-activated receptor α agonist fenofibrate in mice. *J Biol Chem*, **277**: 48051–48057, 2002.

88. Singer DE, Nathan DM, Anderson KM, Wilson PW, Evans JC. Association of HbA1c with prevalence of cardiovascular disease in the original cohort of the Framingham Study. *Diabetes,* **41**: 202–208, 1992.

89. Laakso M. Hyperglycemia and cardiovascular disease in type 2 diabetes. *Diabetes*, **48**: 937–942, 1999.

90. Jensen-Urstad KJ, Reichard PG, Rosfors JS, Lindblad LE, Jensen-Urstad MT. Early atherosclerosis is retarded by improved long-term blood glucose control in patients with IDDM. *Diabetes,* **45**: 1253–1258, 1996.

91. Turner RC, *et al.* Risk factors for coronary artery disease in noninsulin dependent diabetes mellitus: United Kingdom Prospective Diabetes Study (UKPDS:23). *BMJ,* **316**: 823–828, 1998.

92. Vlassara H, Bucala R, Striker L. Pathogenic effects of advanced glycosylation: biochemical, biologic, and clinical implications for diabetes and aging. *Lab. Invest,* **70(2)**: 138–151, 1994.

93. Lopes-Virella MF, Virella G. The role of immune and inflammatory processes in the development of macrovascular disease in diabetes. *Front Biosci,* **8**: S750–68, 2003.

94. Sartippour MR, Renier G. Differential Regulation of Macrophage Peroxisome Proliferator–Activated Receptor Expression by Glucose: Role of Peroxisome Proliferator–Activated Receptors in Lipoprotein Lipase Gene Expression. *Arterioscler Thromb Vasc Biol,* **20(1)**: 104–109, 2000.

95. Berthou L, Duverger N, Emmanuel F, Langouet S, Auwerx J, Guillouzo A, Fruchart JC, Rubin E, Denefle P, Staels B, Branellec D. Opposite regulation of human *versus* mouse apolipoprotein A-I by fibrates in human apolipoprotein A-I transgenic mice. *J Clin Invest*, **97**: 2408–2416, 1996.

96. Forman BM, Chen J, Evans RM. Hypolipidemic drugs, polyunsaturated fatty acids, and eicosanoids are ligands for peroxisome proliferator-activated receptors α and γ. *Proc Natl Acad Sci U S A*, **94**: 4312–4317, 1997.

97. Ziouzenkova O, Perrey S, Asatryan L, Hwang J, MacNaul KL, Moller DE, Rader DJ, Sevanian A, Zechner R, Hoefler G, Plutzky J. Lipolysis of triglyceride-rich lipoproteins generates PPAR ligands: evidence for an antiinflammatory role for lipoprotein lipase. *Proc Natl Acad Sci USA*, **100**: 2730–2735, 2003.

98. Chawla A, Lee CH, Barak Y, He W, Rosenfeld J, Liao D, Han J, Kang H, Evans RM. PPARβ/δ is a very low-density lipoprotein sensor in macrophages. *Proc Natl Acad Sci USA*, **100**: 1268–1273, 2003.

99. Wan YJ, Cai Y, Lungo W, *et al.* Peroxisome proliferator-activated receptor α-mediated pathways are altered in hepatocyte-specific retinoid X receptor alpha deficient mice. *J Biol Chem,* **275**: 28285–28290, 2000.

100. Dubois M, Vantyghem MC, Schoonjans K, Pattou F. Thiazolidinediones in type 2 diabetes. Role of peroxisome proliferator-activated receptor gamma (PPARgamma). *Ann Endocrinol (Paris),* **63(6)**: 511–23, 2002.

101. Hallakous S, Foufelle F, Doare L, Kergoat M, Ferre P. Pioglitazone-induced increase of insulin sensitivity in the muscle of the obese Zucker fa/fa rat cannot be explained by local adipocyte differentiation. *Diabetologia,* **41**: 963–968, 1998.

102. Okuno A, Tamemoto H, Tobe K, *et al.* Troglitazone increases the number of small adipocytes without the change of white adipose

tissue mass in obese Zucker rats. *J Clin Invest,* **101:** 1354–1361, 1998.

103. Wilson TM, Brown PJ, Sternbach DD, Henke BR, The PPARs: From Orphan Receptors to Drug Discovery. *J Med Chem,* **43:** 527–50, 2000.

104. Itoh H, Doi K, Tanaka T, Funaka Y, Hosoda K, *et al.* Hypertension and insulin resistance: role of peroxisome proliferator-activated receptor gamma. *Clin. Exp Pharmacol Physiol,* **26:** 558–60, 1999.

105. Mehta JL, Hu B, Chen J, Li D. Pioglitazone Inhibits LOX-1 Expression in Human Coronary Artery Endothelial Cells by Reducing Intracellular Superoxide Radical Generation. *Arterioscler Thromb Vasc Biol,* **23(12):** 2203–8, 2003.

106. Marx N, Imhof A, Froehlich J, Siam L, Ittner J, Wierse G, Schmidt A, Maerz W, Hombach V, Koenig W. Effect of rosiglitazone treatment on soluble CD40L in patients with type 2 diabetes and coronary artery disease. *Circulation,* **107(15):** 1954–7, 2003.

107. Levi Z, Shaish A, Yacov N, Levkovitz H, Trestman S, Gerber Y, Cohen H, Dvir A, Rhachmani R, Ravid M, Harats D. Rosiglitazone (PPARgamma-agonist) attenuates atherogenesis with no effect on hyperglycaemia in a combined diabetes-atherosclerosis mouse model. *Diabetes Obes Metab,* **5(1):** 45–50, 2003.

108. Desverge B, Wahli W. Peroxisome proliferator-activated receptors: nuclear control of metabolism. *Endocr Rev,* **20:** 649–688, 1999.

109. Leibowitz MD, Fievet C, Hennuyer N, Peinado-Onsurbe J, Duez H, Bergera J, Cullinan CA, Sparrow CP, Baffic J, Berger GD, *et al.* Activation of PPARdelta alters lipid metabolism in db/db mice. *FEBS Lett,* **473:** 333–336, 2000.

110. Oliver WR Jr, Shenk JL, Snaith MR, Russell CS, Plunket KD, Bodkin NL, Lewis MC, Winegar DA, Sznaidman ML, Lambert MH, *et al.* A selective peroxisome proliferator-activated receptor delta agonist promotes reverse cholesterol transport. *Proc Natl Acad Sci USA,* **98:** 5306–5311, 2001.

111. Nagy L, Tontonoz P, Alvarez JG, Chen H, Evans RM. Oxidized LDL regulates macrophage gene expression through ligand activation of PPARgamma. *Cell,* **93:** 229–240, 1998.

112. Chawla A, Lee CH, Barak Y, He W, Rosenfeld J, Liao D, Han J, Kang H, Evans RM. PPARβ/δ is a very low-density lipoprotein sensor in macrophages. *Proc Natl Acad Sci U S A,* **100(3):** 1268–73, 2003.

113. Djouadi F, Weinheimer CJ, Kelly DP. The role of PPAR alpha as a "lipostat" transcription factor. *Adv Exp Med Biol,* **466:** 211–220, 1999.

114. Gonzalez FJ. Recent update on the PPAR alpha-null mouse. *Biochimie,* **79:** 139–144, 1997.

115. Braissant O, Foufelle F, Scotto C, Dauca M, Wahli W. Differential expression of peroxisome proliferator-activated receptors (PPARs): tissue distribution of PPAR -alpha, -beta, and -gamma in the adult rat. *Endocrinology,* **137(1):** 354–366, 1996.

116. Grundy SM. Hypertriglyceridemia, atherogenic dyslipidemia, and the metabolic syndrome. *Am J Cardiol,* **81:** 18B–25B, 1998.

117. Ginsberg HN. Insulin resistance and cardiovascular disease. *J Clin Invest,* **106:** 453–458, 2000.

118. Oliver WR Jr, Shenk JL, Snaith MR, Russell CS, Plunket KD, Bodkin NL, Lewis MC, Winegar DA, Sznaidman ML, Lambert MH, Xu HE, Sternbach DD, Kliewer SA, Hansen BC, Willson TM. A selective peroxisome proliferator-activated receptor β/δ agonist promotes reverse cholesterol transport. *Proc Natl Acad Sci U S A,* **98(9):** 5306–11, 2001.

LIPOPROTEINS AND PPAR SIGNALING
IN DIABETES

Ouliana ZIOUZENKOVA, Gabriela ORĂȘANU

Triglyceride-rich lipoproteins (TRL) induce and promote type 2 diabetes. Molecular mechanisms for TRL action include activation of transcription factors that activate or suppress inflammation. This review focuses on the pathways leading to activation of anti-inflammatory transcription factor PPARα that counters pro-inflammatory transcription responses of NFκB and AP-1. The diversity of TRL effects arises from its complex composition as well as the pathway for its uptake. The understanding of TRL transcription function opens new perspectives in the therapeutic and preventive management of lipid levels in patients with type 2 diabetes.

INTRODUCTION

Current care for diabetes includes continuous monitoring of lipid profile in patients with type 2 diabetes [1]. This requirement serves diagnostic and therapeutic purposes and is based on numerous clinical data that show a strict association of lipid abnormalities and cardiovascular complications in patients with type 2 diabetes [1]. Diabetes mellitus progression results in increased triglycerides levels, elevated proportion of atherogenic LDL fractions, and decreased HDL concentrations in plasma [2, 3]. These abnormalities could be improved by diet and exercise at the early stage of the disease and pharmacological treatment later [4]. Effectiveness of each recommendation is largely dependent on understanding of molecular mechanisms leading to pathogenesis.

Findings in the last decade fundamentally changed the view on lipoproteins (LP) as simple lipid carriers and revealed them as powerful regulators of metabolic or pathogenic responses [5–8]. Following LP treatment, cells change activation pattern of transcription factors [8–10], the large group of protein regulating expression of a gene cassette. Transcription factors regulate endothelial inflammatory response [9], vasoconstriction [11], and apoptosis [9] in the vasculature, a primary site for diabetes-related complications. Cytosolic transcription factors like NFκB and AP-1 form nuclear complex upon stimulation with inflammatory cytokines [12]. NFκB and AP-1 are central transcriptional regulators of a variety of inflammatory responses including expression of adhesion molecules (VCAM-1, ICAM-1, E-selectin) [7, 13, 14], cytokines [15], chemokines, and eicosanoid-generating enzymes (cyclooxygenase 2, 15-lipoxygenase) [16, 17]. Interestingly, several lipid mediators in LP augment this action [9, 15, 18]. Nevertheless, in a healthy intact endothelium these transcription factors are repressed. A potent mechanism counteracting NFκB activation has been recently described [7, 19]. NFκB interacts with peroxisome proliferation activating receptor (PPAR) family of nuclear receptors that function as transcription factors upon activation by specific ligand. PPAR was identified in three isoforms – PPARα, PPARβ/δ, and PPARγ – expressed in different tissues [20]. Inflammatory cells as well as vascular cells, endothelium, and SMC express all

PPAR isoforms [21]. Although PPAR were initially characterized as the key regulators of lipid and glucose metabolism [20], their profound anti-inflammatory effect was soon demonstrated in a number of tissues including vasculature [19, 21]. However, the anti-inflammatory action of PPAR is dependent on activation of these nuclear receptors by specific ligands [19, 21]. A major class of synthetic PPARα ligands are fibrates [20]. Large clinical trials revealed their therapeutic action that includes lowering triglycerides and increasing HDL levels [22, 23]. Their major anti-inflammatory effects include inhibition of adhesion molecules [13], C-reactive protein [24], acute phase proteins [25], and IL-6 expression [26, 27]. PPARγ synthetic ligands, thiazolidinediones, improve insulin sensitivity in type 2 diabetes [28]. In vivo thiazolidinediones also exhibit anti-inflammatory effects and inhibit adhesion molecules [29] and chemokines as well as decrease levels of TNFα [30] and CD40 ligand [31] levels in plasma. Notably, novel PPARδ synthetic agonists oppose pro-inflammatory and pro-atherogenic action of unligated PPARδ [32]. The broad beneficial effects of PPAR synthetic activators, discussed in detail in this book by Orăşanu et al., highlight the importance of endogenous PPAR activation. Here we review the role of triglyceride rich lipoproteins (TRL) in transcriptional regulation of vascular inflammation with a major focus on endogenous PPAR activation by TRL that limit inflammation.

TRL ABNORMALITIES IN DIABETES

Lipoprotein profile in diabetes has many specific characteristics [2]. VLDL and chylomicrons levels are often increased in diabetes and considered cardiovascular risk factors, while LDL is recognized as a major pathogenic lipoprotein in atherogenesis [3]. Although, quantitatively, LDL levels in diabetic patients and healthy individuals are similar, the proportion of atherogenic subfractions is markedly elevated in diabetes [2]. These subfractions are represented by dense and electronegative LDL(LDL(-)) [33, Sanchez-Quesada, 1996 #110, 34]. Dense LDL contain a substantial amount of LDL(-) [35]. Chemical and physical composition of these LDL subfractions reveals modification in both protein and lipid part as compared to the native fraction [36, 37]. These changes account for high susceptibility of dense LDL and LDL(-) subfractions to oxidation initializing oxidation of native LDL [35]. Nonetheless, the pathway for dense LDL and LDL(-) uptake and hydrolysis overlaps with that of native LDL [38, 39]. The uptake of modified LDL subfractions through the abundant pathways appears to cause pathologic metabolic changes in cells, *i.e.* LDL(-) plays a role of molecular "Trojan horse" (reviewed in [37]). Such changes in lipid profile can contribute to the different manifestation in vascular pathology in diabetes affecting not only large vessels but also peripheral microvasculature.

TRL MEDIATE PATHOGENESIS OF ARTERIAL WALL

TRL are a primary source for lipid accumulation in the vasculature. All TRL (LDL, VLDL, chylomicrons) have been found in atherosclerotic lesions [40]. However, proatherogenic TRL effects reach beyond lipid accumulation (Plate 4.1) [41]. High TRL levels in diabetes also provoke insulin resistance, which is reversed after lipid lowering approaches [42]. In animal models, as early as one week on a high fat diet, vascular endothelium begins to express vascular adhesion molecule-1 (VCAM-1), a classic marker of early inflammation [43]. Fundamental studies in cultured vascular endothelium show that chylomicrons and VLDL can augment the cytokine-induced expression of VCAM-1 as well as several other adhesion molecules [9]. Moreover, TRL increases expression of cytokines [9] and chemokines like MCP-1 [44] thereby accelerating recruitment of macrophages into the vessel wall. Plate 4.1 shows major aspects of endothelial response to TRL. These processes are interrelated. Inflammation promotes oxidative modification of TRL, while oxidized lipids further accelerate inflammation [41]. In early 80s, the seminal review by D. Steinberg summarized compelling data on oxidation as a major mechanism recruiting LDL into arterial walls due to its potent inflammatory responses and modified uptake by scavenger receptors [6]. In circulation, heavily oxidized LDL may be rapidly scavenged by inflammatory cells. In contrast, pro-inflammatory mildly modified LDL(-) is present in

the circulation of patients with type 2 diabetes [33, 45]. High concentration of TRL and LDL(-) correlated with the number of inflammation markers in diabetic patients in both basic and clinical studies (reviewed in [37]). Interestingly, such a broad pattern of inflammatory TRL responses appears to be activated by a limited number of transcription factors.

TRL-ACTIVATED TRANSCRIPTION FACTORS: CROSSTALK IN THE REGULATION OF INFLAMMATION

Promoter regions of many inflammatory mediators share response elements for cytosolic transcription factor NFκB and AP-1 [12]. In cytosol, NFκB is bound to inhibitory proteins like IκBα that repress its function. Inflammatory signals like lipopolysaccharides (LPS) or cytokines (TNFα) activate a cascade of phosphorylation reactions leading to the degradation of inhibitory proteins and translocation of NFκB to the nucleus [12]. Activated NFκB binds to the cognate response elements in the promoter region of multiple inflammatory genes. NFκB dependent response includes expression of adhesion molecules and chemokines in endothelial cells, integrins in macrophages, and cytokines in vascular cells [12]. These multiple processes in different cell types are sufficient to recruit macrophages to the site of inflammation [41]. The other NFκB and AP-1 regulated proteins affect vasocontractility and coagulation [46]. Beneficial for wound healing, these transcription events are deleterious in atherosclerosis.

Suppression of NFκB pathway is markedly inhibited by an interaction with nuclear receptor PPARα [7, 19]. There are two PPARα–dependent phases of NFκB inhibition. Ligand-activated PPARα directly up-regulates expression of inhibitory IκBα, thereby preventing its translocation to the nucleus [47]. Activated NFκB could also be repressed in the nucleus through physical interaction with activated PPARα [48]. Mechanism for the AP-1 repression by PPARα is less studied but it also involves direct binding between AP-1 and activated PPARα [48]. In support of this observation, synthetic PPARα ligands inhibit activation of various NFκB and AP-1 target genes like VCAM-1 only in the genetic presence of PPARα [7].

Combination of inflammatory cytokines or LPS with TRL markedly augments inflammatory response [49, 50]. Increase in TRL levels leads to concentration-dependent activation of AP-1 and NFκB [51]. This response was stronger in lipoproteins (LP) containing more triglycerides (TG) [9]. TRL oxidation is another process that can augment NFκB/AP-1 activation [8]. For example, native LDL does not induce NFκB activation even in the presence of cytokine, while LDL(-) and oxidized LDL does [10, 50]. The evidence for the pro-inflammatory role of TRL was obtained in cultured endothelial cells [9] and in animals on a high fat diet [43]. However, the feature of endothelium changed during the physiologic postprandial phase, when the concentration of TRL is the highest.

Postprandial phase is characterized by extensive TRL lipolysis and is mediated mainly by lipoprotein lipase (LPL) [52, Goldberg, 1996 #7]. LPL is not expressed by endothelium but it is relocated from peripheral tissue to the endothelial surface during this period [53]. LPL acts on TRL to release (hydrolyse) free fatty acids (FA), which are delivered to the endothelium and peripheral tissue [53]. Interestingly, TRL lipolysis counters also inflammatory response induced by non-hydrolyzed TRL in NFκB- and AP-1-dependent fashion [7, 10]. The inhibition mechanism depends in part on an increased IκBα expression [10]. Of note, TRL treated with LPL resembles anti-inflammatory potential of synthetic PPARα ligands suggesting that this is an endogenous pathway for PPARα generation in healthy endothelium [7, 10]. Anti-inflammatory function of hydrolyzed TRL is evident in response of NFκB and AP-1 target genes [10]. For example, endothelial cells stimulated with TRL and LPL are much less sensitive to inflammation mediated by LPS or TNFα and express less VCAM-1 [7]. Similarly, LPL lipolysis also counters the VCAM-1 expression mediated by atherogenic LDL(-) subfractions. VCAM-1 up-regulated in the presence of LDL(-) and TNFα is decreased below the levels that are seen with TNFα alone [10]. The suppression of VCAM-1 by hydrolyzed TRL and LDL(-) is dependent on genetic presence of PPARα, which underlines the importance of this transcriptional regulator [7]. Taken together, TRL could initiate a crosstalk between transcription factors NFκB, AP-1, or PPARα generating pro- vs.

anti-inflammatory responses. From the clinical standpoint, it is important to define conditions favoring pro- or anti-inflammatory TRL effects. Last decade documented a hypothesis that translation of TRL responses depends on their composition and could be effectively modulated by diet [9, 15, 18]. Next, we will review TRL composition and discuss a novel concept that besides the TRL composition, a mechanism for TRL uptake can discriminate between transcriptional responses in inflammation.

TRL COMPOSITION MODULATES INFLAMMATORY RESPONSE

TRL are a large complex ($> 2.5*10^6$ kD) of several apolipoproteins and lipids (reviewed in [54]). Fatty acids (FA) are predominantly esterified and less than 5% of them are non-esterified (free). FA esters include triglycerides, phospholipids, and cholesterol esters (Plate 4.2). Both saturated and polyunsaturated FA (PUFA) are abundant. Saturated FA are associated mostly with TG while PUFA are essential components of phospholipids [55]. Linoleic acid is the major FA that is easily oxidized to linoleic acid hydroperoxide (HPODE) or linoleic acid hydroxide (HODE). Very long FA such as eicosapentaenoic acid (EPA) and docosahexaenoic acid (DHA) are minor components of TRL. In this large complex of molecules, however, only few compounds can resemble pro-inflammatory effects of native and modified TRL and their transcriptional responses.

Saturated FA are considered major inflammatory mediators in native TRL [56]. Treatment with saturated FA and TNFα increases VCAM-1 expression in endothelium through NFκB and AP-1 dependent mechanisms [56]. Diet containing large amounts of saturated FA is associated with pro-inflammatory and pro-atherogenic changes [57]. Several oxidized lipids, like HPODE [18], lysophosphatidylcholine [50], or some oxidized phospholipids [15] are possible mediators of pro-inflammatory response in modified TRL. In vivo, these compounds have been found in LDL(-) [37]. Moreover, they could be generated enzymatically from native FA [54]. The mechanism for NFκb activation through these TRL lipids is insufficiently studied, but may include induction of specific phosphorylation pathways [18].

A number of TRL compounds have been characterized as anti-inflammatory mediators. In vitro, PUFA suppresses the pro-inflammatory effects of LPS and cytokines [14, 56]. Nonetheless, PUFA, like linoleic and arachidonic acid, could undergo enzymatic conversion to a number of pro-inflammatory mediators – leukotrienes, prostaglandins, and HETE – accounting for the variability of cellular responses to PUFA [58]. Among PUFA, only DHA and EPA could significantly suppress inflammation in vivo and in vitro [58]. Dietary supplementation with EPA and DHA (major components of fish oil) decreases expression of NFκB target genes [57]. Moreover, this supplementation leads to beneficial changes in the lipid profile [59]. Decrease in TRL concentration and increase in HDL concentrations achieved by EPA and DHA was observed in genetic absence of PPARα [59], arguing that the PPARα regulates these responses. In contrast, the genetic presence of PPARα is essential for the anti-inflammatory action of EPA, particularly in its oxidized form [14]. In fact, oxidized EPA is characterized by a higher affinity for binding to PPARα ligand-binding domain [14]. A variety of non-esterified FA has been identified as natural PPARα ligands [60–62]. It is important to mention that all saturated, mono- and poly-unsaturated long-chain FA (more than 12 carbons) can effectively bind to PPARα-LBD in cell free and cell-based assay. The binding of various ligands is due to the unusually large ligand-binding domain of PPARα [20]. Oxidative modifications on FA even increase their affinity for PPARα binding. For example, oxidized EPA has higher affinity for PPARα-LBD than native EPA [14]. The same is true for native and oxidized linoleic acid (HODE) or arachidonic acid and its derivatives HETE and LTB4 [62].

The binding of FA PPARα-LBD in vitro, however, validates them neither as potent PPARα activators in vivo nor as inflammatory suppressors [56, 63]. FA impact on PPARα activation is not evident and lacks clinical benefits seen with synthetic PPARα ligands. The diet rich in saturated fatty acids leads to the increase in triglycerides levels in the blood known for their pro-inflammatory responses [64, 65]. This is unlike the triglyceride-lowering effects of synthetic fibrates, which have an anti-inflammatory effect [27, 66]. The complexity of

FA responses may arise from the different metabolic pathways responsible for the liberation of FA from intracellular sources of esterified FA.

PATHWAY FOR TG-LP UPTAKE INDUCES SPECIFIC TRANSCRIPTION FACTORS

Recently we suggested that the pathway for TRL uptake could be involved in the activation of specific transcription responses [7, 10]. TRL represent a major reservoir for FA, stored in esterified form [54]. The liberation of FA from TRL occurs through two principal pathways (Plate 4.3) [52]. A receptor mediates the uptake of the whole TRL particle, which undergoes hydrolysis in lysosomes. Lipolysis, in contrast, utilizes specific esterified FA in TRL without consumption of the whole particle. This process may deliver selective FA to the specific cell compartment. FA liberated in the lysosomal or lipolytic reactions could be metabolized in various pathways, oxidized to secondary mediators or re-esterified.

TRL are readily taken up by most cells including endothelium, through diverse cellular receptors [7]. In the presence of cytokines, TRL uptake results in an activation of pro-inflammatory transcription factors (NFκB, AP-1) and target molecules (VCAM-1 expression) [49, 50]. Although TRL contains at least 150 molecules of free FA per particle [54], they do not activate PPARα in endothelial cells in vitro [7].

Marked pro-inflammatory responses also cause an uptake of oxidized TRL, which occurs through scavenger receptor [6]. Besides receptor-mediated uptake, phospholipase A2 (PLA2) treatment of TRL also has a marked proinflammatory effect [67]. The PLA2 action of oxidized LDL also leads to PPARα activation [68]. Nevertheless, in the interaction between NFκB and PPARα initiated by oxidized TRL, NFκB cystained activation and pro-inflammatory response prevail [67]. PLA2 lipolysis of oxidized TRL does not match criteria of endogenous pathway for PPARα activation.

In the lipase family, LPL has unique characteristics [53]. LPL selectively utilizes TG in TRL, and markedly activates PPARα. In the endothelium containing LPL, the experimental model of postprandial endothelium, enzymatic

TRL hydrolysis of TRL through LPL can activate PPARα to an extent seen with synthetic PPARα agonists [7]. PPARα activation in the presence of LPL was completely dependent on intact hydrolysis. The mutant LPL was not capable of PPARα activation [7]. Similarly, the uptake of VLDL *via* LDL-receptor pathway does not activate PPARα despite excessive intracellular accumulation of FA. Intact VLDL hydrolysis also reproduces effects of synthetic PPARα ligands on target genes; anti-inflammatory PPARα effects only in the genetic presence of PPARα [7]. LPL hydrolyze also modified LDL subfraction [10]. LDL(-) hydrolysis leads to a marked release of HODE and is associated with both potent PPARα activation and a suppression of inflammatory markers in the presence of cytokines. Thus, lipolysis appears to be a natural anti-inflammatory pathway acting through PPARα activation.

The molecular mechanism of PPARα activation through physiologic lipolysis opens for interpretation and further examination a large number of clinical data on impaired lipolysis in diabetics. In human population, LPL mutations affecting its hydrolytic activity are very common [2, 69]. The mutation lowering hydrolytic LPL activity is associated with high triglycerides and low HDL [69, 70], a phenotype found in PPARα deficient animals [22]. These mutations have been found in patients with hypertriglyceridemia in type 2 diabetes [2] while no association with LPL function was found in type 1 diabetes. Even a stronger relation to hypertriglyceridemia in diabetes was demonstrated for Apo CIII, a natural inhibitor of hydrolytic function of LPL [53]. An increased concentration of Apo CIII or its polymorphisms is associated with dyslipidemia in type 2 diabetes and high risk for coronary disease [71]. Moreover, high levels of TRL represent a cardiovascular risk factor only in combination with plasma Apo CIII levels [72, 73]. Whether impaired LPL function leads to life-long impaired PPARα-mediated transcriptional responses has to be examined to provide a rationale for a preventive or therapeutic treatment of high-risk patients with synthetic PPARα agonists.

Increased LPL activity is associated with atherosclerosis reduction. Mutations increasing hydrolytic LPL activity are potentially athero-protective [74]. A novel pharmacologic lipase activator NO-1886 decreases triglycerides and increases plasma HDL levels leading to the atherosclerotic lesion reduction in rabbit model for atherosclerosis [75]. LPL levels could be effectively increased without pharmacologic treatment. Numerous data show that physical exercise increases LPL levels in muscle four-fold, compared to the basal levels [76]. Of note this LPL expression was experimentally obtained in transgenic mice models [77]. High expression of LPL in the animal model of atherosclerosis was sufficient to abolish development of atherosclerosis even in mice on high fat diet [78]. The regulation of LPL levels through exercise opens a unique opportunity to control the metabolic conditions.

PPARα activation may have hidden dis-advantages in patients with type 2 diabetes with severe complications. Some genetic studies proved that the presence of PPARα increases insulin resistance in animals on a high fat diet [79]. This effect is particularly deleterious and accompanied by hypertension during the administration of dexamethasone in mice genetic studies [80]. This shift in energy metabolism could be of considerable risk in advanced diabetes or combined with dexamethasone. Caloric restriction, particularly decreased carbohydrate proportion in diet may substantially limit the negative consequences of PPARα activation in this pathology.

In specific cell types like macrophages, LPL can also support the action of LDL receptor pathway and promote lesion development in atherosclerosis animal models. In human, whole body LPL dysfunction is strictly associated with pro-atherogenic conditions [81] arguing about the pro-atherogenic role of LPL.

A recent report also shows the principal PPARα role in progression of cardiac hypertrophy in mice model of diabetes [82]. These authors suggest that the PPARα activating drugs may augment hypertrophy in human diabetes. Although the set of PPARα target genes in rodents is substantially different compared to human [83], the careful monitoring of possible hypertrophy in human receiving PPARα agonists should be performed.

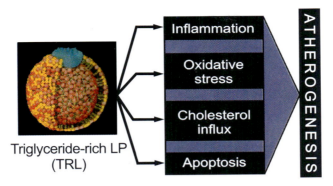

Plate 4.1

Multiple responses mediated through triglyceride-rich lipoproteins (TRL) can induce and accelerate atherosclerosis.

TRL increase oxidative stress leading to TRL oxidation and macrophages recruitment. These are two central events for lipid accumulation in atherosclerotic lesions.

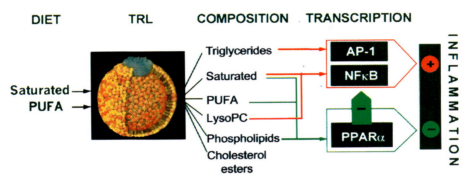

Plate 4.2

Composition of TRL affects inflammation *via* activation of different transcription factors. Diet modulates proportion of different components in TRL. Triglycerides, saturated fatty acids and lysophosphatide choline are potent inducers of proinflammatory transcription factors NFκB and AP-1. On the other hand, polyunsaturated fatty acids (PUFA), certain phospholipids, or even saturated fatty acids delivered through LPL activate PPAR and its proximal antiinflammatory responses.

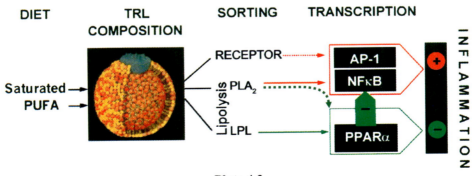

Plate 4.3

The pathway for the TRL delivery to the cell regulates transcription factors affecting inflammation. Besides TRL composition, the pathway for TRL uptake can change transcription responses. Lipoprotein lipase (LPL)-mediated lipolysis of VLDL or electronegative LDL activates PPAR. The uptake of the same VLDL or electronegative LDL through a receptor pathway activates proinflammatory transcription factors NFκB and AP-1. Other lipases, like PLA2, can activate pro-as well as anti-inflammatory transcription factors *in vitro*. The significance of such transcriptional activation on the inflammation *in vivo* remains to be elucidated.

TRL AS PPARγ AND PPARδ ACTIVATORS

TRL also represent a potential source of PPARγ and PPARδ ligands. Synthetic PPARγ ligands are established clinical sensitizers of insulin (reviewed in [20]). Other major physiologic roles include regulation of adipogenesis and cholesterol influx and efflux. PPARγ also supports anti-inflammatory function and decreases expression of adhesion molecules in the presence of TNFα [29]. Moreover, PPARγ also decreases expression of TNFα [84] and cyclooxygenase-2 [16]. Native TRL are weak PPARγ activators *in vitro* without or in the presence of LPL [7, 10]. TRL oxidation increases their affinity to PPARγ [10]. High TRL levels in plasma also increase insulin resistance, arguing against their importance as *in vivo* PPARγ activators [42]. Nonetheless, several potential PPARγ agonists are present in native and oxidized TRL and could be potentially released through an unknown pathway of PPARγ activation. Among FA, the very long chain PUFA are PPARγ activators [20]. PPARγ activators could be formed during inflammation [85]. Identified ligands are HODE [10, 86] and specific oxidized phospholipids [10]. These compounds as well as oxidized LDL induce PPARγ target genes CD36 and ABC transporters participating in both cholesterol influx (CD36) and efflux (ABC) [86, 87]. However, the net effect of oxidized LDL is cholesterol accumulation and inflammation amplification [6]. These responses are not replicating anti-atherogenic and modestly anti-inflammatory effect of PPARγ synthetic agonists [30], suggesting that other pathways mask, prevent, or counter PPARγ activation.

The TRL relevance in PPARδ activation is unclear. TRL are weak PPARδ agonists [7]. Similarly to PPARα, PPARδ-LBD activation *in vitro* increases in the presence of oxidatively modified TRL [7, 10]. The LPL-mediated lipolysis markedly increases PPARδ activation by TRL [7, 88]. This pathway suggests to be a principal pathway for PPARδ activation in macrophages [88]. In animal model of atherosclerosis the genetic presence of PPARδ in macrophages in the presence of TRL promotes lipid accumulation and accelerates atherogenesis [88]. In contrast, a novel synthetic PPARδ agonist decreases atherogenesis and inflammation [32]. The molecular basis for these divergent responses of TRL to natural and synthetic agonists are not clear and may include insufficient generation and delivery of ligands and interference with other pathways.

CONCLUSION

The appreciation of TRL as potent transcription regulators opens new perspectives in the management of dislipidemia. Further studies will need to unite the pathway for TRL uptake with the identification of the specific transcription responses. Given the importance of lipolysis mediated by LPL for PPARα activation, diagnostic screening may include characteristics of metabolic pathway for TRL catabolism along with TRL concentrations. For example, early identification of LPL catalytic activity deficiency (high Apo CIII concentration, mutations in LPL catalytic domain) could be compensated by pharmacologic substitution with synthetic PPARα ligands, physical exercise, or the dietary supplementation with very long chain FA.

REFERENCES

1. Pratley RE, Weyer C, Bogardus C. Metabolic abnormalities in the development of type 2 diabetes mellitus. In: *Diabetes Mellitus: a fundamental and clinical text*. LeRoith D, Taylor SI, Olefsky JM (eds). 2nd ed, Lippincott Williams & Wilkins, Philadelphia, PA, 548–558, 2000.
2. McKenney JM. Understanding and treating dyslipidemia associated with noninsulin-dependent diabetes mellitus and hypertension. *Pharmacotherapy*, 13: 340–352, 1993.
3. Howard BV. Lipoproteins: structure and function. In: *Diabetes and Atherosclerosis: molecular basis and clinical aspects*. Draznin B, Eckel, RH (eds). Elsevier, New York, 3–17, 1993.
4. Gotto AM, Jr. Triglyceride as a risk factor for coronary artery disease. *Am J Cardiol*, 82: 22Q-25Q, 1998.
5. Stemerman MB. Lipoprotein effects on the vessel wall. *Circ Res*, 86: 715–716 , 2000.
6. Steinberg D, Lewis A, Conner Memorial Lecture. Oxidative modification of LDL and atherogenesis. *Circulation*, 95: 1062–1071, 1997.

7. Ziouzenkova O, Perrey S, Asatryan L, Hwang J, MacNaul KL, Moller DE, Rader DJ, Sevanian A, Zechner R, Hoefler G, Plutzky J. Lipolysis of triglyceride-rich lipoproteins generates PPAR ligands: evidence for an antiinflammatory role for lipoprotein lipase. *Proc Natl Acad Sci USA*, **100:** 2730–2735, 2003.

8. Norata GD, Pirillo A, Callegari E, Hamsten A, Catapano AL, Eriksson P. Gene expression and intracellular pathways involved in endothelial dysfunction induced by VLDL and oxidised VLDL. *Cardiovasc Res*, **59:** 169–180, 2003.

9. Dichtl W, Nilsson L, Goncalves I, Ares MP, Banfi C, Calara F, Hamsten A, Eriksson P, Nilsson J. Very low-density lipoprotein activates nuclear factor-kappaB in endothelial cells. *Circ Res*, **84:** 1085–1094, 1999.

10. Ziouzenkova O, Asatryan L, Sahady D, Orasanu G, Perrey S, Cutak B, Hassell T, Akiyama TE, Berger JP, Sevanian A, Plutzky J. Dual roles for lipolysis and oxidation in peroxisome proliferation-activator receptor responses to electronegative low density lipoprotein. *J Biol Chem*, **278:** 39874–39881, 2003.

11. Mallat Z, Gojova A, Sauzeau V, Brun V, Silvestre JS, Esposito B, Merval R, Groux H, Loirand G, Tedgui A. Rho-associated protein kinase contributes to early atherosclerotic lesion formation in mice. *Circ Res*, **93:** 884–888, 2003.

12. Adcock IM. Transcription factors as activators of gene transcription: AP-1 and NF-kappa B. *Monaldi Arch Chest Dis*, **52:** 178–186, 1997.

13. Marx N, Sukhova G, Collins T, Libby P, Plutzky J. PPARalpha activators inhibit cytokine-induced vascular cell adhesion molecule-1 expression in human endothelial cells. *Circulation*, **99:** 3125–3131, 1999.

14. Sethi S, Ziouzenkova O, Ni H, Wagner DD, Plutzky J, Mayadas TN. Oxidized omega-3 fatty acids in fish oil inhibit leukocyte-endothelial interactions through activation of PPARalpha. *Blood*, **100:** 1340–1346, 2002.

15. Yeh M, Leitinger N, de Martin R, Onai N, Matsushima K, Vora DK, Berliner JA, Reddy ST. Increased transcription of IL-8 in endothelial cells is differentially regulated by TNF-alpha and oxidized phospholipids. *Arterioscler Thromb Vasc Biol*, **21:** 1585–1591, 2001.

16. Subbaramaiah K, Lin DT, Hart JC, Dannenberg AJ. Peroxisome proliferator-activated receptor gamma ligands suppress the transcriptional activation of cyclooxygenase-2. Evidence for involvement of activator protein-1 and CREB-binding protein/p300. *J Biol Chem*, **276:** 12440–12448, 2001.

17. Chang WC. Cell signaling and gene regulation of human 12(S)-lipoxygenase expression. *Prostaglandins Other Lipid Mediat*, **71:** 277–285, 2003.

18. Natarajan R, Reddy MA, Malik KU, Fatima S, Khan BV. Signaling mechanisms of nuclear factor-kappab-mediated activation of inflammatory genes by 13-hydroperoxyoctadecadienoic acid in cultured vascular smooth muscle cells. *Arterioscler Thromb Vasc Biol*, **21:** 1408–1413, 2001.

19. Blanquart C, Barbier O, Fruchart JC, Staels B, Glineur C. Peroxisome proliferator-activated receptors: regulation of transcriptional activities and roles in inflammation. *J Steroid Biochem Mol Biol*, **85:** 267–273, 2003.

20. Willson TM, Brown PJ, Sternbach DD, Henke BR. The PPARs: from orphan receptors to drug discovery. *J Med Chem*, **43:** 527–550, 2000.

21. Plutzky J. Peroxisome proliferator-activated receptors in vascular biology and atherosclerosis: emerging insights for evolving paradigms. *Curr Atheroscler Rep*, **2:** 327–335, 2000.

22. Djouadi F, Weinheimer C, Saffitz J, Pitchford C, Bastin J, Gonzalez F, DP.1083-91 K. A gender-related defect in lipid metabolism and glucose homeostasis in peroxisome proliferator-activated receptor alpha- deficient mice. *J Clin Invest*, **102:** 1083–1091, 1998.

23. Montori VM, Farmer A, Wollan PC, Dinneen SF. Fish oil supplementation in type 2 diabetes: a quantitative systematic review. *Diabetes Care*, **23:** 1407–1415, 2000.

24. Kleemann R, Gervois PP, Verschuren L, Staels B, Princen HM, Kooistra T. Fibrates down-regulate IL-1-stimulated C-reactive protein gene expression in hepatocytes by reducing nuclear p50-NFkappa B-C/EBP-beta complex formation. *Blood*, **101:** 545–551, 2003.

25. Anderson SP, Cattley RC, Corton JC. Hepatic expression of acute-phase protein genes during carcinogenesis induced by peroxisome proliferators. *Mol Carcinog*, **26:** 226–238, 1999.

26. Staels B, Koenig W, Habib A, Merval R, Lebret M, Torra I, Delerive P, Fadel A, Chinetti G, Fruchart J, Najib J, Maclouf J, Tedgui A. Activation of human aortic smooth-muscle cells is inhibited by PPARalpha but not by PPARgamma activators. *Nature*, **393:** 790–793, 1998.

27. Cunard R, DiCampli D, Archer DC, Stevenson JL, Ricote M, Glass CK, Kelly CJ. WY14, 643, a PPAR alpha ligand, has profound effects on immune responses *in vivo*. *J Immunol*, **169:** 6806–6812, 2002.

28. Schwartz S, Raskin P, Fonseca V, Graveline JF. Effect of troglitazone in insulin-treated patients with type 2 diabetes mellitus. Troglitazone and Exogenous Insulin Study Group. *N Engl J Med*, **338:** 861–866, 1998.

29. Jackson SM, Parhami F, Xi XP, Berliner JA, Hsueh WA, Law RE, Demer LL. Peroxisome

proliferator-activated receptor activators target human endothelial cells to inhibit leukocyte-endothelial cell interaction. *Arterioscler Thromb Vasc Biol*, 19: 2094–2104, 1999.

30. Li AC, Brown KK, Silvestre MJ, Willson TM, Palinski W, Glass CK. Peroxisome proliferator-activated receptor gamma ligands inhibit development of atherosclerosis in LDL receptor-deficient mice. *J Clin Invest*, 106: 523–531, 2000.

31. Varo N, Vicent D, Libby P, Nuzzo R, Calle-Pascual AL, Bernal MR, Fernandez-Cruz A, Veves A, Jarolim P, Varo JJ, Goldfine A, Horton E, Schonbeck U. Elevated plasma levels of the atherogenic mediator soluble CD40 ligand in diabetic patients: a novel target of thiazolidinediones. *Circulation*, 107: 2664–2669, 2003.

32. Lee CH, Chawla A, Urbiztondo N, Liao D, Boisvert WA, Evans RM, Curtiss LK. Transcriptional repression of atherogenic inflammation: modulation by PPARdelta. *Science*, 302: 453–457, 2003.

33. Sobenin IA, Tertov VV, Orekhov AN. Atherogenic modified LDL in diabetes. *Diabetes*, 45 Suppl 3: S35–39, 1996.

34. Haffner SM. Lipoprotein disorders associated with type 2 diabetes mellitus and insulin resistance. *Am J Cardiol*, 90: 55i–61i, 2002.

35. Sevanian A, Hwang J, Hodis H, Cazzolato G, Avogaro P, Bittolo-Bon G. Contribution of an in vivo oxidized LDL to LDL oxidation and its association with dense LDL subpopulations. *Arterioscler Thromb Vasc Biol*, 16: 784–793, 1996.

36. Sobenin IA, Tertov VV, Orekhov AN. Characterization of chemical composition of native and modified low density lipoprotein occurring in the blood of diabetic patients. *Int Angiol*, 13: 78–83, 1994.

37. Sevanian A, Asatryan L, Ziouzenkova O. Low density lipoprotein (LDL) modification: basic concepts and relationship to atherosclerosis. *Blood Purif*, 17: 66–78, 1999.

38. Avogaro P, Cazzolato G, Bittolo-Bon G. Some questions concerning a small, more electronegative LDL circulating in human plasma. *Atherosclerosis*, 91: 163–171, 1991.

39. Wang X, Greilberger J, Levak-Frank S, Zimmermann R, Zechner R, Jurgens G. Endogenously produced lipoprotein lipase enhances the binding and cell association of native, mildly oxidized and moderately oxidized low-density lipoprotein in mouse peritoneal macrophages. *Biochem J*, Pt 2: 347–353, 1999.

40. Hoff HF, Jackson RL, Gotto AM, Jr. Apolipoprotein localization in human atherosclerotic arteries. *Adv Exp Med Biol*, 67: 109–120, 1976.

41. Libby P. Vascular biology of atherosclerosis: overview and state of the art. *Am J Cardiol*, 91: 3A–6A, 2003.

42. Mingrone G, Castagneto M. Role of lipids in insulin resistance and type 2 diabetes mellitus development. *Nutrition*, 15: 64–66, 1999.

43. Li H, Cybulsky MI, Gimbrone MA, Jr., Libby P. An atherogenic diet rapidly induces VCAM-1, a cytokine-regulatable mononuclear leukocyte adhesion molecule, in rabbit aortic endothelium. *Arterioscler Thromb*, 13: 197–204, 1993.

44. Wang GP, Deng ZD, Ni J, Qu ZL. Oxidized low density lipoprotein and very low density lipoprotein enhance expression of monocyte chemoattractant protein-1 in rabbit peritoneal exudate macrophages. *Atherosclerosis*, 133: 31–36, 1997.

45. Sanchez-Quesada J, Perez A, Caixas A, Ordonmez-Llanos J, Carreras G, Payes A, Gonzalez-Sastre F, de Leiva A. Electronegative low density lipoprotein subform is increased in patients with short-duration IDDM and is closely related to glycaemic control. *Diabetologia*, 39: 1469–1476, 1996.

46. Byrne CD. Triglyceride-rich lipoproteins: are links with atherosclerosis mediated by a procoagulant and proinflammatory phenotype? *Atherosclerosis*, 145: 1–15, 1999.

47. Delerive P, Gervois P, Fruchart JC, Staels B. Induction of IkappaBalpha expression as a mechanism contributing to the anti-inflammatory activities of peroxisome proliferator-activated receptor-alpha activators. *J Biol Chem*, 275: 36703–36707, 2000.

48. Delerive P, De Bosscher K, Besnard S, Vanden Berghe W, Peters JM, Gonzalez FJ, Fruchart JC, Tedgui A, Haegeman G, Staels B. Peroxisome proliferator-activated receptor alpha negatively regulates the vascular inflammatory gene response by negative cross-talk with transcription factors NF-kappaB and AP-1. *J Biol Chem*, 274: 32048–32054, 1999.

49. Moers A, Fenselau S, Schrezenmeir J. Chylomicrons induce E-selectin and VCAM-1 expression in endothelial cells. *Exp Clin Endocrinol Diabetes*, 105: 35–37, 1997.

50. Khan B, Parthasarathy S, Alexander R, Medford R. Modified low density lipoprotein and its constituents augment cytokine-activated vascular cell adhesion molecule-1 gene expression in human vascular endothelial cells. *J Clin Invest*, 95: 1262–1270, 1995.

51. Draczynska-Lusiak B, Chen YM, Sun AY. Oxidized lipoproteins activate NF-kappaB binding

activity and apoptosis in PC12 cells. *Neuroreport*, **9**: 527–532, 1998.

52. Havel RJ. Postprandial lipid metabolism: an overview. *Proc Nutr Soc*, **56**: 659–666, 1997.

53. Goldberg I. Lipoprotein lipase and lipolysis: central roles in lipoprotein metabolism and atherogenesis. *J Lipid Res*, **37**: 693–707, 1996.

54. Esterbauer H, Gebicki J, Puhl H, Jurgens G. The role of lipid peroxidation and antioxidants in oxidative modification of LDL. *Free Radic Biol Med*, **13**: 341–390, 1992.

55. Emken EA, Rohwedder WK, Adlof RO, Rakoff H, Gulley RM. Metabolism in humans of cis-12,trans-15-octadecadienoic acid relative to palmitic, stearic, oleic and linoleic acids. *Lipids*, **22**: 495–504, 1987.

56. De Caterina R, Bernini W, Carluccio MA, Liao JK, Libby P. Structural requirements for inhibition of cytokine-induced endothelial activation by unsaturated fatty acids. *J Lipid Res*, **39**: 1062–1070, 1998.

57. Christon RA. Mechanisms of action of dietary fatty acids in regulating the activation of vascular endothelial cells during atherogenesis. *Nutr Rev*, **61**: 272–279, 2003.

58. Calder PC. Polyunsaturated fatty acids, inflammation, and immunity. *Lipids*, **36**: 1007–1024, 2001.

59. Dallongeville J, Bauge E, Tailleux A, Peters JM, Gonzalez FJ, Fruchart JC, Staels B. Peroxisome proliferator-activated receptor alpha is not rate-limiting for the lipoprotein-lowering action of fish oil. *J Biol Chem*, **276**: 4634–4639, 2001.

60. Forman BM, Chen J, Evans RM. Hypolipidemic drugs, polyunsaturated fatty acids, and eicosanoids are ligands for peroxisome proliferator-activated receptors alpha and delta. *Proc Natl Acad Sci U S A*, **94**: 4312–4317, 1997.

61. Kliewer SA, Sundseth SS, Jones SA, Brown PJ, Wisely GB, Koble CS, Devchand P, Wahli W, Willson TM, Lenhard JM, Lehmann JM. Fatty acids and eicosanoids regulate gene expression through direct interactions with peroxisome proliferator-activated receptors alpha and gamma. *Proc Natl Acad Sci U S A*, **94**: 4318–4323, 1997.

62. Krey G, Braissant O, L'Horset F, Kalkhoven E, Perroud M, Parker M, Wahli W. Fatty acids, eicosanoids, and hypolipidemic agents identified as ligands of peroxisome proliferator-activated receptors by coactivator-dependent receptor ligand assay. *Mol Endocrinol*, **11**: 779–791, 1997.

63. Devchand P, Keller H, Peters J, Vazquez M, Gonzalez F, Wahli W. The PPARalpha-leukotriene B4 pathway to inflammation control. *Nature*, **384**: 39–43, 1996.

64. Bergeron N, Havel RJ. Influence of diets rich in saturated and omega-6 polyunsaturated fatty acids on the postprandial responses of apolipoproteins B-48, B-100, E, and lipids in triglyceride-rich lipoproteins. *Arterioscler Thromb Vasc Biol*, **15**: 2111–2121, 1995.

65. Khosla P, Hayes KC. Comparison between the effects of dietary saturated (16:0), monounsaturated (18:1), and polyunsaturated (18:2) fatty acids on plasma lipoprotein metabolism in cebus and rhesus monkeys fed cholesterol-free diets. *Am J Clin Nutr*, **55**: 51–62, 1992.

66. Havel RJ. Benefits of fibrate drugs in coronary heart disease patients with normal cholesterol levels. *Circulation*, **96**: 2113–2114, 1997.

67. Sonoki K, Iwase M, Iino K, Ichikawa K, Ohdo S, Higuchi S, Yoshinari M, Iida M. Atherogenic role of lysophosphatidylcholine in low-density lipoprotein modified by phospholipase A2 and in diabetic patients: protection by nitric oxide donor. *Metabolism*, **52**: 308–314, 2003.

68. Delerive P, Furman C, Teissier E, Fruchart J, Duriez P, Staels B. Oxidized phospholipids activate PPARalpha in a phospholipase A2-dependent manner. *FEBS Lett*, **471**: 34–38, 2000.

69. Nordestgaard B, Abildgaard S, Wittrup H, Steffensen R, Jensen G, Tybjaerg-Hansen A. Heterozygous lipoprotein lipase deficiency: frequency in the general population, effect on plasma lipid levels, and risk of ischemic heart disease. *Circulation*, **96**: 1737–1744, 1997.

70. Reynisdottir S, Angelin B, Langin D, Lithell H, Eriksson M, Holm C, Arner P. Adipose tissue lipoprotein lipase and hormone-sensitive lipase. Contrasting findings in familial combined hyperlipidemia and insulin resistance syndrome. *Arterioscler Thromb Vasc Biol*, **17**: 2287–2292, 1997.

71. Rigoli L, Raimondo G, Di Benedetto A, Romano G, Porcellini A, Campo S, Corica F, Riccardi G, Squadrito G, Cucinotta D. Apolipoprotein AI-CIII-AIV genetic polymorphisms and coronary heart disease in type 2 diabetes mellitus. *Acta Diabetol*, **32**: 251–256, 1995.

72. Sacks F, Alaupovic P, Moye L, Cole T, Sussex B, Stampfer M, Pfeffer M, Braunwald E. VLDL, apolipoproteins B, CIII, and E, and risk of recurrent coronary events in the Cholesterol and Recurrent Events (CARE) trial. *Circulation*, **102**: 1886–1892, 2000.

73. Lee SJ, Campos H, Moye LA, Sacks FM. LDL Containing Apolipoprotein CIII Is an Independent Risk Factor for Coronary Events in Diabetic Patients. *Arterioscler Thromb Vasc Biol*, **23**: 853–858, 2003.

74. Sawano M, Watanabe Y, Ohmura H, Shimada K, Daida H, Mokuno H, Yamaguchi H. Potentially

protective effects of the Ser447-Ter mutation of the lipoprotein lipase gene against the development of coronary artery disease in Japanese subjects *via* a beneficial lipid profile. *Jpn Circ J*, **65**: 310–314, 2001.

75. Yin W, Tsutsumi K. Lipoprotein lipase activator NO-1886. *Cardiovasc Drug Rev*, **21**: 133–142, 2003.

76. Seip RL, Semenkovich CF. Skeletal muscle lipoprotein lipase: molecular regulation and physiological effects in relation to exercise. *Exerc Sport Sci Rev*, **26**: 191–218, 1998.

77. Levak-Frank S, Radner H, Walsh A, Stollberger R, Knipping G, Hoefler G, Sattler W, Weinstock P, Breslow J, Zechner R. Muscle-specific overexpression of lipoprotein lipase causes a severe myopathy characterized by proliferation of mitochondria and peroxisomes in transgenic mice. *J Clin Invest*, **96**: 976–986, 1995.

78. Shimada M, Ishibashi S, Inaba T, Yagyu H, Harada K, Osuga J, Ohashi K, Yazaki Y, Yamada N. Suppression of diet-induced atherosclerosis in low density lipoprotein receptor knockout mice overexpressing lipoprotein lipase. *Proc Natl Acad Sci USA*, **93**: 7242–7246, 1996.

79. Guerre-Millo M, Rouault C, Poulain P, Andre J, Poitout V, Peters JM, Gonzalez FJ, Fruchart JC, Reach G, Staels B. PPAR-alpha-null mice are protected from high-fat diet-induced insulin resistance. *Diabetes*, **50**: 2809–2814, 2001.

80. Bernal-Mizrachi C, Weng S, Feng C, Finck BN, Knutsen RH, Leone TC, Coleman T, Mecham RP, Kelly DP, Semenkovich CF. Dexamethasone induction of hypertension and diabetes is PPAR-alpha dependent in LDL receptor-null mice. *Nat Med*, **9**: 1069–1075, 2003.

81. Benlian P, De Gennes JL, Foubert L, Zhang H, Gagne SE, Hayden M. Premature atherosclerosis in patients with familial chylomicronemia caused by mutations in the lipoprotein lipase gene. *N Engl J Med*, **335**: 848–854, 1996.

82. Finck BN, Han X, Courtois M, Aimond F, Nerbonne JM, Kovacs A, Gross RW, Kelly·DP. A critical role for PPARalpha-mediated lipotoxicity in the pathogenesis of diabetic cardiomyopathy: modulation by dietary fat content. *Proc Natl Acad Sci U S A*, **100**: 1226–1231, 2003.

83. Staels B, Auwerx J. Regulation of apo A-I gene expression by fibrates. *Atherosclerosis*, **137** **Suppl**:S19-23, 1998.

84. Marx N, Kehrle B, Kohlhammer K, Grub M, Koenig W, Hombach V, Libby P, Plutzky J. PPAR activators as antiinflammatory mediators in human T lymphocytes: implications for atherosclerosis and transplantation-associated arteriosclerosis. *Circ Res*, **90**: 703–710, 2002.

85. Huang JT, Welch JS, Ricote M, Binder CJ, Willson TM, Kelly C, Witztum JL, Funk CD, Conrad D, Glass CK. Interleukin-4-dependent production of PPAR-gamma ligands in macrophages by 12/15-lipooxygenase. *Nature*, **400**: 378–382, 1999.

86. Nagy L, Tontonoz P, Alvarez JG, Chen H, Evans RM. Oxidized LDL regulates macrophage gene expression through ligand activation of PPARgamma. *Cell*, **93**: 229–240, 1998.

87. Chawla A, Boisvert WA, Lee CH, Laffitte BA, Barak Y, Joseph SB, Liao D, Nagy L, Edwards PA, Curtiss LK, Evans RM, Tontonoz P. A PPAR gamma-LXR-ABCA1 pathway in macrophages is involved in cholesterol efflux and atherogenesis. *Mol Cell*, **7**: 161–171, 2001.

88. Chawla A, Lee CH, Barak Y, He W, Rosenfeld J, Liao D, Han J, Kang H, Evans RM. PPARdelta is a very low-density lipoprotein sensor in macrophages. *Proc Natl Acad Sci USA*, **100**: 1268–1273, 2003.

5

INVOLVEMENT OF EICOSANOID METABOLISM IN VASCULAR COMPLICATIONS OF DIABETES MELLITUS

Mihai NECHIFOR

Eicosanoids (prostaglandins, thromboxanes, prostacyclins, lipoxins, hepoxilins, isoprostanes, intermediate hydroperoxides, etc.) and fatty acids precursors (arachidonic, linoleic, eicosapentaenoic and docosahexaenoic acids) are synthesized at the level of blood vessels and blood cells. They have important actions for the normal function of the circulatory system.

Changes in the synthesis of eicosanoid compounds are involved in many pathologic processes with major impact on the human body, *e.g.*, diabetic angiopathy.

PGI_2 (prostacyclin) is one of the main protective factors of vascular endothelium *vs.* hyperglycemia-induced atherogenic action and peroxidic radicals-induced cytotoxic effect. Other eicosanoids, like TxA_2, isoprostanes and leukotrienes, have a proatherogenic effect.

In conditions of hyperglycemia and dyslipidemia, proatherogen eicosanoids (like TxA_2 – with proaggregant action too) are over-synthesized.

We tested, during hyperglycemia in Wistar rats with alloxan-induced diabetes (175 mg/kg alloxan subcutaneously) and during D_2 hypervitaminosis (30 000 UI/kg/day, 42 days), a synthetic prostaglandinic analogue of $PGF_{2\alpha}$ – produced at ICCF Bucharest – optically active cloprostenol (ClPGOA, 50 µg/kg/day). Macroscopic and microscopic examinations of vascular lesions after 6 weeks in Wistar rats with glycemia greater than double *vs.* initial values (before inducing diabetes mellitus) have shown that this $PGF_{2\alpha}$ analogue, without vasoconstrictive action, but with luteolytic action, decreases significantly lesional arterial surface, planimetrically determined.

We consider that some prostaglandin analogues (others than of PGI_2) may have a partially protective vascular action in diabetic angiopathy.

Abbreviations List

AA – arachidonic acid
ClPG – cloprostenol
COX – cyclooxygenase
DHA – docosahexaenoic acid
EPA – eicosapentaenoic acid
ET1 – endothelin 1
HETE – hydroxyeicosatetraenoic acid

HPETE – hydroxyperoxyeicosatetraenoic acid
LO – lipooxygenase
LXA_4 – lipoxin A_4
LXB_4 – lipoxin B_4
NA – noradrenaline
PG – prostaglandin
PGI_2 – prostacyclin
TxA_2 – thromboxane A_2

Eicosanoids represent a huge system of lipid autacoids, largely spread in all living world. All eicosanoids derived from multiple pathways from monocarboxylic polyunsaturated fatty acids: arachidonic acid (AA), linoleic and eicosapentaenoic (EPA) acid. There are recent data that also docosahexaenoic acid (DHA) may be transformed, in specific conditions, in eicosanoids. A general scheme of eicosanoids synthesis is shown in Figure 5.1.

In the normal function of blood vessels and in some pathologic products that appear at this level are involved 4 great eicosanoid groups:

a) Eicosanoids synthesized on cyclooxygenase pathway (COX_1 and COX_2): PGs, PGI_2, TxA_2;

b) Eicosanoids synthesized on lipooxygenase pathway (5-LO, 11-LO, 12-LO, 15-LO): leukotrienes, lipoxins, hepoxilins, trioxilins, 5-HPETE, 12-HPETE, 15-HPETE, etc.;

c) Eicosanoids synthesized on monooxygenase cytochrome P450- dependent pathway;

d) Isoprostanes – synthesized by action of free radicals on some fatty acids, precursors from phospholipids.

All these eicosanoid groups act on receptors at vascular level.

Sources of the above groups of eicosanoids are:
– vascular endothelium,
– vascular smooth muscle,
– blood cells,
– some eicosanoids (e.g., PGI_2) and their metabolites from different tissues and transported by blood plasma.

Endothelial cells produce many eicosanoids. The most known and researched are PGI_2, PGE_2, $PGF_{2\alpha}$, TxB_2 and a multitude of eicosanoids synthesized on the lipooxygenase pathway. Receptors for eicosanoids synthesized on cyclooxygenases pathways are TP receptors (for TxA_2, but also for agonists like intermediate endoperoxides PGG_2 and PGH_2), EP receptors with EP_1, EP_2, EP_3, EP_4 subtypes (for PGE), DP receptors (for PGD_2), FP receptors (for PGF2α) and IP receptors (for PGI_2) [1]. All these receptors are found, in different ratios, at the level of vascular system, but also in blood cells. Genes for these receptors were identified [2]. Receptors for eicosanoids synthesized on COX_1 and COX_2 pathways and transduction mechanisms of biological signals are shown in Table 5.1 (from [3]).

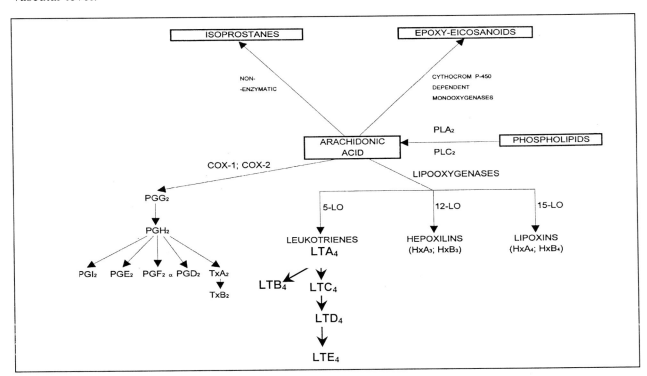

Figure 5.1

Major pathways of synthesis of eicosanoids from arachidonic acid.

Table 5.1

Receptors for eicosanoids synthesized on COX_1 and COX_2 and transduction mechanism of biological signal
(after Robertson, 1998)

Receptor subtype	Mechanism of action
DP	Stimulation of adenylyl cyclase and increased cAMP levels *via* Gs
EP1	Stimulation of phosphatidylinositol turnover and elevation of intracellular free Ca^{2+} *via* Gq
EP2	Stimulation of adenylyl cyclase and increased cAMP levels *via* Gs
EP3	Inhibition of adenylyl cyclase and decreased cAMP levels *via* Gs
EP4	Stimulation of adenylyl cyclase and increased cAMP levels *via* Gs
FP	Stimulation of phosphatidylinositol turnover and elevation of intracellular free Ca^{2+} *via* Gq
IP	Stimulation of adenylyl cyclase and increased cAMP levels *via* Gs
TP	Stimulation of phosphatidylinositol turnover and elevation of intracellular free Ca^{2+} *via* Gq

At the vascular level (in the endothelium and smooth muscle) PGE_2 and $PGF_{2\alpha}$ synthesis takes place and EP and FP receptors for these prostaglandins exist [4]. At vascular endothelium and platelet level receptors were identified for PGD_2 (DP receptors), but the quantity of PGD_2 synthesized in normal conditions, in the vascular wall, is small [5]. Stimulation of FP receptors determines vasoconstriction. It was proved that density of these vascular receptors varies at arterial level with age. It is much lower in new born *vs.* adult, explaining more potent vasoconstrictive action of $PGF_{2\alpha}$ on adult arteries *vs.* newborn arteries [4]. The fact might be involved in developing arterial hypertension associated with diabetic angiopathy in adult. It was observed an age dependent variation of ratio between different types of EP receptors. The ratio between EP1 and EP3 vascular receptors density is 4/1 in adult and is substantially modified in newborn [4]. Consequences of this change in developing of some angiopathic processes are not known yet.

An analysis of the quantitative ratio between different eicosanoids synthesized in the vascular wall, in normal and pathologic conditions, shows that these ratios differ in normal state, in different areas of the vascular bed, and are substantially modified in pathologic conditions. All 4 great eicosanoids groups were identified in the arterial wall. In diabetes mellitus associated or not with dyslipidemic changes appear substantial changes in normal quantitative ratios between different eicosanoids. This fact is considered to be involved in the pathogeny of diabetic arteriopathy.

PGI_2 is considered one of the main antiatheromatose factors produced by vascular endothelium. PGI_2 is, quantitatively, the main eicosanoid synthesized by endothelial cells from arachidonic acid. In the first administration phase of hypercholesterolemic diet (2-4 weeks), PGI_2 synthesis increases moderately (interpreted as an adaptive reaction and as an antiatheromatose defense mechanism) [6, 7]. Endothelial synthesis of PGI_2 is significantly decreased if atherogenic diet is administered a longer period of time. The atherogenic process develops in normal persons with overt atherogenesis in diabetic patients too [8].

Human atherosclerotic arteries generate less PGI_2 than normal ones [6]. An argument for the major role of PGI_2 in the prevention of atherosclerosis emergence and diabetic arteriopathy is the antiatherosclerotic effect of some PGI_2 analogues, like cicaprost, in case of animals that get for a long time atherogenic diets [9, 10]. PGI_2 not only inhibits platelet aggregation, but decreases neutrophils adhesion to endothelial cells [11, 12].

PGI_2 and also some synthetic analogues of prostacycline (*e.g.*, carbacycline) decrease smooth arterial muscle level of cholesteryl ester.

PGI_2 activates cholesteryl ester hydrolysis both in the smooth vascular muscle and in macrophages [13]. The endothelial cell derived eicosanoids have significant paracrine activity, regulating the cholesterol content in smooth muscle cells [14].

At the macrophage level (and possibly of other cells), 5-HETE and leukotrienes stimulate cholesterol deposit (5-LO inhibit this effect) [15].

PGI$_2$ produced especially in the endothelium increases cAMP synthesis, and, cAMP inhibits proliferation of arterial smooth muscle. PGE$_1$ has a similar effect [16]. On this mechanism, PGI$_2$ and PGE$_1$ have a certain antiatherosclerotic effect and a protective role vs. diabetic angiopathy. PGI$_2$ decreases the number of LDL receptors at macrophage level [17].

HDL stimulates PGI$_2$ synthesis at the level of smooth muscle and this is one of the most important antiatherosclerotic mechanisms of HDL [18]. On this way HDL decreases proliferation of smooth muscle cells.

Prostacyclins decrease capillary permeability and decreases capillary filtration coefficient. It is involved in regulation of basal microvascular hydraulic-permeability. Inhibition of prostacyclin synthetase with tranilcipromine increases capillary filtration coefficient [19]. Decreasing PGI$_2$ synthesis in patients with diabetes mellitus has the same effect.

It has been shown that the decreasing activity of prostacyclin synthase is involved in developing atherosclerosis lesions [20]. Also, decreasing PGI$_2$ synthesis leads to a vasorelaxation deficit of these arteries.

It was proved a definite role for arachidonic, linoleic and eicosapentaenoic acids (EPA) and for the quantitative ratio between them, in the normal function of the circulatory system and in developing of different diseases, such as atherosclerosis, diabetic angiopathy, blood hypertension, etc.

Decreasing PGI$_2$, PGE$_1$ and PGE$_2$ synthesis during hyperglycemia increases arterial vaso-constrictive activity of sympathetic nervous system, because PGI$_2$ and especially PGE$_1$ and PGE$_2$ inhibit presynaptic release of NA [21]. PGE$_1$, in i.v. administration in diabetic patients with retinopathy and peripheral vascular disease, manifested by intermittent claudication, leads to an increase of the systolic flow velocity with about 40% and of the diastolic flow velocity with 80%, both in central retinal artery and in at the periphery. PGE$_1$ analogues could be therapeutically used in these situations [22]. PGE$_1$ inhibits endothelial adhesion of neutrophils and decreases the effect of free superoxide radicals generated at the neutrophil level on endothelial cells [23]. In diabetes mellitus, genesis of free peroxides radicals is increased. By this mechanism, PGE$_1$ decreases free radical aggression on vascular endothelium.

An extra argument for the protective role of PGI$_2$ at endothelial level is the experiment of prostacyclin synthase gene transfer, which prevents neointimal formation after experimentally carotid injury in rats. Todaka et al. observed that in this way the proliferative process is decreased and the neointimal formation on rat carotid arteries after experimental balloon injuries is inhibited [24]. PGI$_2$ accelerates re-endothelization at the level of injured vessel [25]. Administration of medium doses of C vitamin (150–600 mg/day) in rabbits bred with atherogenic diet, rich in cholesterol, produced (in the first 4 weeks of diet) increases of PGI$_2$ synthesis. After progression of endothelial lesions, administration of ascorbic acid cannot re-normalize PGI$_2$ synthesis [26]. This fact pleads for a role of peroxide radicals in decreasing endothelial synthesis of PGI$_2$.

PGI$_2$ has numerous actions on all the elements of a blood vessel. Some of the major implications of PGI$_2$ at the endothelial level are: antiatheromatosis effect, increasing lysosomal membrane stability and decreasing platelet aggregation and their adhesion to the endothelium.

The thromboxane A$_2$ (TxA$_2$), that has a short life of 30–40" and is transformed in TxB$_2$ - much more stable, but much less active, is synthesized at the level of vascular endothelium, platelet and circulatory leukocytes [27]. TxA$_2$ has important actions that make the excess synthesis of this eicosanoid to be involved in the pathogeny of atherosclerosis and diabetic vasculopathy i.e.:

– strongly stimulates platelet aggregation,

– has an arterial and venous vasoconstrictive action,

– stimulates proliferation of vascular smooth muscle,

– increases Ca^{2+} in the endothelial cell.

Some eicosanoids and other factors increase TxA$_2$ synthesis. In patients with diabetes mellitus, synthesis and plasmatic level of TxA$_2$ are increased vs. normal subjects. At the same time, endothelial synthesis of PGI$_2$ is decreased [28, 29]. Increasing TxA$_2$ synthesis is an important factor in the pathogeny of diabetic angiopathy. TxA$_2$ excess in diabetic animals or patients at the level of the vascular system leads to:

– platelet hyperaggregation,

– increases sensitivity of small vessels (especially renal vessels) to some vaso-constrictive factors [30],

– stimulates proliferation of smooth vascular muscle,

– increases vascular permeability [31].

Increasing TxA_2 synthesis was observed in rats with alloxan-induced diabetes. Activation of TP receptors at these animals increased the vasoconstrictive effect of serotonin on renal vessels *vs.* normal rats [32].

It was observed that TxA_2 is involved in the pathogeny of many severe diseases like acute myocardial infarct, angina pectoris, bronchial asthma, thrombosis, etc. [33]. Excess of TxA_2 is an important factor in the pathogeny of diabetic angiopathy. TP receptors have been identified in vascular endothelial cells and in vascular smooth muscles, in mammalians [34–36]. It was proved that daltroban (competitive antagonist of TxA_2) decreased experimental-induced atheromatose progression [37].

Basal release of TxB_2 from cells of bovine aorta endothelium is 59 ± 24 pg/10^5 cells at 30 min. If LTB_4 (10^{-8} M) is added, TxB_2 release increases at 571 ± 195 pg/ 10^5 cells at 30 min. If LTD_4 (10^{-8} M) is added, TxB_2 release increases at 355 ± 140 pg/ 10^5 cells at 30 min [38].

Preincubation with dimethylsulfoxide (DMSO) (10^{-5} M), a hydroxyl radical scavenger, decreases LTB_4 induced release of TxA_2. In rats with alloxan-induced diabetes mellitus, sensitivity of the perfused hindquarters vasculature is changing. Perfusion with arachidonic acid determines a strong vasoconstriction by transforming the raised percentage of AA in TxA_2.

Administration of a thromboxane-A_2 mimetic substance (U 46619) determines a raised vasoconstriction in diabetic animals [30]. Stimulation of arterial muscles proliferation produced by platelets in contact with muscular fibers is produced mainly by increased TxA_2 synthesis in diabetic patients. TxA_2 strongly stimulates proliferation of smooth muscular fibers.

The platelets of the patient with hypercholesterolemia incubated with arachidonic acid produce a greater quantity of TxA_2 than the platelets of normal patients [39, 40]. This increase of TxA_2 synthesis is one of the causes of the platelets hyperaggregation met in type 2 diabetic patients with dyslipidemia. Davi *et al.* [40] found a level of TxB_2 in platelet rich plasma (PRP) incubated with AA of 56.7 ± 12.8 ng/10^8 platelets in dyslipidemic patients *vs.* 21.4 ± 5.6 ng/10^8 platelets

in normal subjects ($p < 0.01$). At the same dyslipidemic patients, platelets synthesis of 12 HETE from AA is increased *vs.* normal subjects. Because both synthesis of TxA_2 and 12-HETE are increased in these subjects, the ratio 12-HETE/ TxA_2 remained unchanged *vs.* persons without dyslipidemia. 12-HETE is also an eicosanoid that stimulates platelets aggregation [41].

Stimulation of TxA_2 receptors at the level of vascular smooth muscle potentates pressor response at different other active endogen substances like 5-HT (5 hydroxytryptamine) [42]. Administration in intravenous infusion of U-46619 (an agonist of TP receptors) potentiates significantly a vasoconstrictor response at 5-HT both in non-diabetic and diabetic animals. Calcium channels blockers (*e.g.* nifedipine and verapamil) do not block this effect, suggesting that this effect is not due to Ca^{2+} entrance into the cell. We consider this fact with implications in developing arterial hypertension in diabetic patients with a chronically raised level of TxA_2 in plasma and platelets. De La Cruz *et al.* [43] show that moderate doses of aspirin (2 mg/kg/day *per os*) in persons with diabetes mellitus strongly decrease (almost until suppression) platelet synthesis of TxA_2, but only with 8–10% PGI_2 synthesis and decrease retinal vascular permeability in diabetic patients. It also has a partial protective effect *vs.* emergence of diabetic retinopathy and this fact shows that an excess of TxA_2 is a compound greatly involved in these diabetic complications. Permeability areas on retinal surface decreased in animals with streptozotocin induced diabetes with about 87% after a treatment with aspirin *per os*, 2 mg/kg/day. In diabetic nephropathy, TxA_2 synthesis and endothelin 1 (ET1) play a main pathogenic role. These substances produce vasoconstriction and spasm on afferent glomerular vessels, increase thrombogenesis and decrease glomerular filtration. They are involved in emergence and progression of diabetic nephroangiopathy [44].

Many data show an altered endothelial function in patients with diabetes mellitus. This is a major motif of developing atheromatosis [45]. There are correlations between insulin resistance and subclinical atheromatosis [46].

Increasing insulin resistance is frequently associated with increasing of triglyceride level and with appearance of dyslipidemia, which are atherogenic factors, involved in the emergence of diabetic arteriopathy [47]. In type 2 diabetes, the TxA_2/PGI_2 ratio is increased both by increasing TxA_2 endothelial and platelet synthesis and by decreasing endothelial synthesis of PGI_2 [48, 49]. It is considered that monitorization of TxA_2/PGI_2 plasmatic ratio is necessary for preventing, by therapy, vascular complications of diabetes mellitus [48]. Not only endothelial metabolism of eicosanoids is modified in diabetes mellitus, but also their synthesis in platelets and in other blood cells [50].

During physical exercise, plasmatic concentration of prostacyclin increases both in diabetic patients and in non-diabetic patients [51]. This might be an indication for physical exercise (between some limits) in diabetic patients. Plasmatic concentrations of TxB_2 (the main TxA_2 metabolite) and PGE_2 did not change significantly during physical exercise in diabetes. Analyzing the ratio PGI_2/TxA_2 in the aorta of diabetic animals, Yang *et al.*, 1999 found this ratio decreased with 55% in rat with streptozotocin-induced diabetes [52].

Some eicosanoids (like LTB_4) produced in leukocytes stimulate TxA_2 synthesis in endothelial cells [38].

Leukotrienes. The role of leukotrienes in developing diabetic vasculopathy is complex. In conditions of increased LDL concentrations, synthesis and release of LTB_4 from monocytes increases. LTB_4 is one of the most potent chemotactic agents and attracts a great number of monocytes and other white cells in areas where LDL is greater [53, 54]. On the contrary, LTB_5 synthesized from eicosapentaenoic acid acts on the same LTB receptor and decreases the chemotactic effect of LTB_4. Adhesion of white cells and platelets on vascular endothelium is favored by LTB_4 [41]. This fact is considered by many authors as having a role in developing the atherogenesis process.

Peptidoleukotrienes (LTC_4, LTD_4, LTE_4) from polymorphonuclear cells and from other leukocytes produce plasma leakage and vasoconstriction on terminal arteries.

All these processes are involved in developing diabetic angiopathy.

It was proved that cysteinyl leukotrienes (CysLTS) are involved in AngII-induced vasoconstriction in rats with streptozotocin-induced diabetes. A selective inhibitor of 5-LO (AA861, 10 μM) decreases by 37.6 ± 8.2 % Ang II-induced vasoconstriction in these animals [55].

There is a strong current for an inflammatory component in the genesis of the atheromatosis process [56].

The cells of vascular endothelium do not synthesize leukotrienes, but have receptors for them. Leukotrienes act at the endothelial level and are considered proatherogenic factors.

It is very important that, at the level of the vascular endothelium a transcellular synthesis of some eicosanoids exists. Thus, endothelium converts LTA_4 (synthesized in neutrophils) into LTC_4. LTB_4 and peptidoleukotrienes actions at the level of vascular endothelium are shown in Table 5.2.

Table 5.2

LTB$_4$ and peptidoleukotrienes actions
at the level of vascular endothelium

LTB_4	Peptidoleukotrienes (LTC_4, LTD_4, LTE_4)
– Increases neutrophiles adhesion to vascular endothelium – Increases neutrophiles migration (Lewis *et al.*, 1989) – Increases mastocyte degranulation – Increases free oxygen radicals formation – Increases protein extravasation and transendothelial transport of proteins and lipoproteins – TxA_2 synthesis – Modifies vascular endothelial permeability at macromolecules (Du *et al.*, 1994)	– Are considered pro-atherogenic factors – Increases thrombocyte adhesion to vascular endothelium – Increases Ca^{2+} entrance in the endothelial cell – Increases leukocyte adhesion to endothelium – Increases permeability to vascular endothelium (Lonigro AJ *et al.*, 1988) – Proinflammatory action

Lipoxins (LXA_4 and LXB_4) represent another group of eicosanoids synthesized on the lipooxygenase pathway, namely those synthesized on 15-LO actions. They are synthesized in small quantities at the level of blood vessels.

Through the main implications of lipoxins at the endothelial level we mention:

– LXA_4, LXB_4 are very important for the connection between blood cells and vascular endothelium;

– LXA_4 synthesized by polymorphonuclear leukocytes increases endothelial prostacyclin (PGI_2) synthesis [57].

15-lipooxygenase was identified in the endothelium and in vascular muscular fibers

[58, 59]. This enzyme, involved in lipoxines synthesis, is found in some white cells [60]. The excess synthesis of 15-HETE and 15-HPETE might be involved in developing of diabetic arteriopathy and atheromatosis by at least 4 ways:

a) inhibition of cyclooxygenases and decreasing endothelial synthesis of PGE_2 and PGE_1 [61–63],

b) proinflammatory action,

c) chemoattractant effect,

d) mitogen effect for endothelial cells [63].

An interesting fact, which confirms the idea that eicosanoids form a system and there are numerous interactions between them, which give the possibility of a complex modulation of cell functions, is that 15-HPETE (a lipoxin forerunner) decreases endothelial synthesis of PGI_2. Increasing of endothelial synthesis of 15- HPETE, given by atherogenic factors, contributes to the decreasing endothelial synthesis of PGI_2 and to the development of artheriosclerosis.

There is a very active factor stimulating PGI_2 synthesis: 7-*cis*,1 1-*trans*-lipoxine A_4. We agree with the idea of Brezinski *et al.,* who consider that lipooxygenase-derived eicosanoids, synthesized at the endothelial level, can modulate vascular reactivity [64].

LXA_4 and LXB_4 may determine cerebral arterial dilatation whose meaning is unknown yet.

We consider that the increasing eicosanoids synthesis (including those at the endothelial level) is given by hypoxia [64]. In our opinion, this is a way to maintain a relative normal body function even if over-amounts of some eicosanoids may produce subsequent disorders of endothelial cells functions.

Increasing plasmatic concentrations of LDL is frequent in diabetic patients. Oxidized LDL is involved in the pathogeny of atheromatous vascular lesions [65, 66]. 15-LO, besides its role in 15-HPETE and lipoxins, is also involved in LDL oxidation. This enzyme is presented at the level of atherosclerotic lesions and in macrophages too. Selective inhibition of 15-LO with PD146176 (350 mg/kg/day) has a partial protective effect *vs.* atherosclerotic lesions experimentally-induced, in New Zealand white rabbits, with a diet enriched with cholesterol [67].

LDL oxidation from atherosclerotic lesions by 15-LO is decreased by α-tocopherol and other antioxidant agents [68]. Leukocytes are rich in enzymatic equipment including lipooxygenases involved in eicosanoid synthesis (inclusive 15-LO). Both the increasing of leukocytes adhesion (leukotrienes-induced) at vascular endothelium in diabetic patients and the raise of the 15-LO (from leukocytes) oxidizing activity of LDL (at arterial endothelium level) may facilitate the development of diabetic angiopathy.

Hepoxilins are: A_3 hepoxilin (HxA_3–11, 12, epoxy eicosa 5Z,10E, 14 Z trienoic acid) and B_3 hepoxilin (HxB_3–10, hydroxyl, 11, 12-epoxy-eicosa 5Z, 8Z, 14 Z trienoic acid) synthesized from arachidonic acid on 12-LO pathway [69]. HxA_3, HxB_4 and 12-HPETE are synthesized at arterial level and have a modulator role on vascular tonus and increase permeability of vascular endothelium [70]. They are also involved in the inflammatory process [70]. Endothelial cell may incorporate 12-HETE (synthesized in leukocytes). There are complex relations between eicosanoids.

If LDL concentrations raised, the macrophage synthesis of 12-HETE is 250% higher than in normal conditions [71]. PGE_2, 5-HETE and LTB_4 synthesis in macrophages is not significantly changed by increasing LDL concentrations.

Larger doses (600–1500 mg/d) of C vitamin decrease cholesterol level but also 12-HETE synthesis, *via* 12-LO inhibition [72]. 12-HETE is an important chemotactic agent [73]. 12-HETE, released from aggregated platelets in contact with vascular endothelium, increases white cells infiltration into the vascular smooth muscle.

It was noticed that hydroperoxides produced from arachidonic acid on lipooxygenase pathways (*e.g.*, 12-HPETE, 15-HPETE) inhibit endothelial synthesis of PGI_2 [74].

Eicosanoids synthesized on P450-dependent monooxygenase pathway are produced and act at the level of vascular endothelium.

The metabolism of AA cytochrome P450-monooxygenase dependent results in three types of metabolites:

– epoxyeicosatrienoic acids (EETS) 8, 9–11, 12–14, 15 EETS

– hydroxyacids – 19 hydroxyarachidonic acid
　　　　　　　– 20 hydroxyarachidonic acid

– *cis-trans* hydroxyeicosatetraenoic acids [75].

Epoxyeicosatrienoic acids are converted to dihydroxy-eicosatetraenoic acids in variable percentage and partially released in the blood.

Plasmatic concentration of unesterified EETS, in healthy persons, is about 1nM. EETS are not synthesized only by vascular endothelial cells, but also in platelets. A part of EETS is incorporated in phospholipids from endothelial cells and another part is released in the blood plasma, after transformation in DHETS. At the level of endothelial cells there was identified an epoxydehydrolase that converts EETS into DHETS.

Both plasmatic concentrations of EETS and DHETS and urinary release of DHETS increase in some pathologic conditions, like blood hypertension, hypercholesterolemia, damage of the vascular endothelium by trauma, etc. Atherogen concentrations of LDL stimulate endothelial synthesis of EETS and DHETS.

DHETS are incorporated in membrane phospholipids where there were identified 8,9-DHET and 11,12-DHET. It is considered that the presence in excess of these diols in membrane phospholipids disturbs endothelial cell function.

Other eicosanoids synthesized on cytochrome P450- monooxygenase dependent pathway have actions at vascular level. Thus, 20-HETE, produced on ω-hydroxylase pathway, has a vasodilator action and is involved in hypoxic vasodilatation of arteries from skeletal muscles [76].

Pretreatment with MS-PPOH (N-methylsulfonyl-6-12-propanglyoxy phenyl hexaenoic acid), an inhibitor of EETS synthesis, did not alter hypoxic dilation, but DDMS (dodecenyl-methylsulfimide), a selective inhibitor of 20-hydroeicosatetraenoic acid synthesis (20-HETE), decreases this dilatation. 17-ODYA that inhibits CYP_{450} 4A enzymes decreases hypoxic vasodilatation too.

Metabolites produced by ω/ω-1 oxygenase action (19-OH-AA, 20-OH-AA) modulate ionic flows at the level of vascular endothelium and have prohypertensive effect. At hypertensive rats (SHR) 6 weeks old, inhibition of synthesis of these eicosanoids normalizes blood pressure [77].

Sodium nitroprusiate 10–100 μM inhibits renal microsomal conversion of arachidonic acid in 20-HETE and EETS. NOS inhibition with L-NAME decreases the production of nitric oxide, but increases about 4 times the renal efflux of 20-HETE and other monooxygenase derivatives; sodium chloride 2% increased epoxygenase activity [78].

Miconazole and ketoconazole (relatively largely used drugs) decreased epoxygenase synthesis of eicosanoids from AA. Thus, at a concentration of 1 μM, miconazole decreases epoxygenase activity with about 60% [79].

We consider that decreasing vascular synthesis of EETS (with vasodilatatory actions and the decrease of cytokine-induced endothelial cell adhesion) may be involved in developing diabetic angiopathy [80].

Synthesis of isoprostanes is made by a mechanism involving free radical catalyzed lipid peroxidation. Isoprostanes are synthesized at the vascular level and are present in the blood plasma and in urine. The most studied isoprostane is 8-epi-$PGF_{2\alpha}$ or F-isoprostane. This eicosanoid is very active at vascular level and produces a relative vasoconstriction. Isoprostanes are synthesized both in the endothelium and the smooth vascular muscle. Their formation is preceded by bicyclic endoperoxide (PGH_2-like) intermediates. There were identified isoprostanes E_2 and D_2. Isoprostanes formation is taking place "in situ", at the level of esterified arachidonic acid in phospholipids, independent of cyclooxygenase action. From docosahexaenoic acid it was proved that there are synthesized isoprostane-like substances, named neuroprostanes [81]. Neuroprostanes (F4-NPs) are eicosanoids with a structure related to $PGF_{4\alpha}$ (prostaglandin synthesized from docosahexaenoic acid – DHA). Some quantity of isoprostanes (8-epi-$PGF_{2\alpha}$) was proved to be synthesized in platelets. In situations where oxidative stress is higher or increases the intake of substances that raise lipid oxidation, isoprostane synthesis increases. In heavy smokers, human excretion of 8-epi-$PGF_{2\alpha}$ is 176.5 ± 30.6 pmol/mmol creatinine, in moderate smokers is 112.6 ± 24.9 pmol/mmol creatinine and in non-smokers only 54.1 ± 2.7 pmol/mmol creatinine [82].

Administration of antioxidant substances (e.g., ascorbic acid and vitamin E) decreases synthesis and elimination of isoprostanes. Vascular actions of isoprostanes are important. 8-epi-$PGF_{2\alpha}$ is vasoconstrictor and mutagenic [83]. Besides completely cyclooxygenase independent synthesis of 8-epi-$PGF_{2\alpha}$, there was observed isoprostane COX- dependent formation [84]. From this point of view, isoprostanes synthesis is partially non-enzymatic and in part enzyme-dependent.

8-epi-$PGF_{2\alpha}$ is definitely an agonist on TxA_2 receptors (TP receptors) because vascular effects of 8-epi-$PGF_{2\alpha}$ are blocked by competitive agonists of TxA_2 at receptor level [85].

It is known that $F_{2\alpha}$ isoprostanes (8-iso-PGF2α) produce vasoconstriction by stimulation of TxA_2 receptors (TP receptors). Competitive antagonists on these receptors decrease to a great extent vasoconstriction given by 8-iso-$PGF_{2\alpha}$. On the contrary, E-isoprostanes (8-iso PGE_1 and 8-iso-PGE_2) relax smooth arterial muscles, acting probably on its own receptor.

These isoprostanes are considered important hyperpolarizing and relaxant factors of smooth vascular muscles. The equilibrium between lipidic vasoconstrictive factors (TxA_2, 8-iso-$PGF_{2\alpha}$) and vasorelaxant factors (PGI_2, PGE_1, 8-iso PGE_1, and 8-iso- PGE_2) is very important in modulation of arterial tonus. Prostacyclin and nitric oxide are endothelial factors that inhibit vasoconstriction.

It was identified a membrane hyperpolarization factor present at the vascular endothelial level – endothelium-derived hyperpolarizing factor (EDHF).

This hyperpolarization is obtained by activating K^+ channels. There are many data that EDHFs are metabolites of arachidonic acid [86, 87]. There are data that plead for an isoprostan structure of EDHFs [88]. Blood hypertension, atherosclerosis and hypercholesterolemia (frequently met in diabetes mellitus) were associated with endothelial dysfunction and changes in isoprostanes synthesis. Jansen [88], Momboulli and Vanhoutte [89] consider that a next therapeutic target in all these vascular dysfunctions would be increasing EDHFs synthesis (8-iso-PGE_1 and 8-iso-PGE_2) and decreasing vascular synthesis of vasoconstrictive lipidic factors.

Isoprostane synthesis (by oxidizing phospholipids from vascular endothelium) is considered as an important process that favors development of atherosclerosis. The plasmatic concentration of F_2 isoprostane is a marker for the level of lipidic peroxidation [90].

Analyzing isoprostane synthesis and the ratio between 8-epi-$PGF_{2\alpha}$ (the main isoprostane) and 6-oxo-$PGF_{1\alpha}$ (the main metabolite of PGI_2), Guogho et al. 1999 [91] have shown that this ratio increases in smokers (where it raises the level of isoprostane synthesis and decreases PGI_2 synthesis). Decreasing PGI_2 synthesis and increasing lipidic peroxidation at the level of vascular endothelium with increasing isoprostanes synthesis is considered to be a promoting atherogenic mechanism. Voutilainen et al., 1999

[92] sustain that in the mechanism of hyperhomocysteinemia-induced atherogenesis, stimulation of peroxidation and increasing synthesis of F2 isoprostane are important mechanisms (plasmatic level is about 47% higher than control).

Initially, it was thought that fatty acids, precursors of eicosanoids, are only compounds without biological importance. Nowadays there are data stressing their important role at vascular level.

Peroxidation of eicosapentaenoic acid produces F3-isoprostanes [93]. From DHA are synthesized 8 subfamilies of F4-isoprostanes owing to free radical attack at C6, C9, C12, C15, C18 [94]. Diabetes mellitus is a disease where formation of peroxidic radicals is enhanced. We consider (though data are insufficient) that there is an excess synthesis of F2, and F3-isoprostanes, which are involved in the pathogeny of diabetic angiopathy.

There are some effects of eicosapentaenoic acid (EPA) that prove a vasoprotective, antiatherosclerotic action on the vessel wall. These actions of EPA are:

– decreasing triglyceride levels and plasmatic cholesterol,

– TxA_3 synthesis from EPA under thromboxane-synthase action, that acts also on TP receptors, but is almost lack of proaggregant action (250–400 weaker than TxA_2). TxA_3 prevents TxA_2 binding on its receptors and thus decreases platelet aggregation,

– decreasing stimulation effects of TxA_2 on mitosis and proliferation of vascular smooth muscle.

A repeated administration of eicosapentaenoic acid decreased significantly the level of triglycerides, cholesterol, LDL and plasmatic phospholipids [95]. EPA administration has the advantage of leading to PGI_3 synthesis, with anti-aggregation activity (as PGI_2) and does not decrease PGI_2 action (generated from arachidonic acid) [96]. TxA_3 does neither produce platelet aggregation nor vasoconstriction and occupies TxA_2 receptors, decreasing the action of the last compound. In part, vascular complications of diabetes mellitus may be prevented or diminished by EPA administration. EPA potentates the anti-aggregation platelet effect of PGI_2 and PGE_1 [97].

Administration of EPA for 7 weeks decreased the turnover of phosphoinositides at the level of vascular smooth muscle. Though, this turnover stimulated by LDL decreased with about 10-40% synthesis of IP_3 stimulated by angiotensinogen II (and consequent vasoconstriction) and decreased angiotensinogen II effect on stimulation of TxA_2-synthesis [98]. Stimulation of IP_3 synthesis is involved in increasing Ca^{2+} concentrations, in the vascular muscle and vasoconstriction produced by angiotensin II and, to a lower degree, the excess of LDL.

It is considered that AA/EPA ratio, in serum, is a marker for atherosclerosis risk [99]. In diabetic patients the serum arachidonic acid AA/EPA ratio is increased, fact involved in pathogeny of diabetic arteriopathy.

Percentage of AA transformed in TxA_2 is increased in diabetics *vs.* normal persons and PGI_2 synthesis is decreased.

Hammes *et al.*, [100] show that 750 mg/day of oil fish administered 6 months in rats with experimental diabetes prevent in 75% the appearance of diabetic retinopathy. EPA effect is correlated with a decrease of synthesis and plasmatic concentrations of TxA_2.

Administration of γ-linoleic and /or EPA in patients that already have atherosclerosis in the lower limbs cannot modify significantly the emergence of intermittent claudication but, after 6 months of administration, decreased systolic arterial pressure [101]. This fact pleads for the idea that the protective role of some eicosanoids, mostly prostancyclins, at the endothelial level emerge before and at the start of atheromatosis process. Administration of fatty acids, precursors of eicosanoids, cannot anymore influence significantly vessels state after installation of this pathologic process (even eicosapentoic acid leads to TxA_3 that act on the same receptors as TxA_2 but does not produce platelet aggregation, behaving like an antiaggregant and antithrombotic factor).

There are more data that docosahexaenoic acid (22: 6 ω3, DHA), the most unsaturated biological fatty acid, found usually in the mammalian cell [102], is also involved in the pathogeny of some vascular dysfunction. Permeability of cell membrane and function of mitochondrial membrane is influenced by ω3 fatty acids and especially by DHA [103].

We tested the influence of a prostaglandin analogue on vascular lesions experimentally-induced, in rats with alloxan-induced diabetes.

MATERIAL AND METHOD

It was tested optic active cloprostenol (ClPGOA -Flavoliz[R]) action on arterial lesions induced by hypervitaminosis D_2, in rats with alloxan-induced diabetes. ClPGOA is a synthetic analogue of $PGF_{2\alpha}$, without vasoconstrictive action but with lutheolitic action. The chemical structures are presented in Figure 5.2.

We worked on 5 groups formed by 15 white adult, male, Wistar rats each weighing between 170–200 g, bred in normal laboratory conditions and fed identically.

Group I was control and did not receive any substance.

Group II received ClPGOA 50 µg/kg/d i.p. for 6 weeks.

Groups III, IV and V were with alloxan-induced diabetes (175 mg alloxan (Fluka) s.c., in unique dose).

Group III received D_2 vitamin, 30 000 UI/kg, daily, starting at 72 h after alloxan administration, for 6 weeks.

Group IV received D_2 vitamin, 30 000 UI/kg, as group III but together with ClPGOA 50µg/kg/day i.p.

Group V – rats with alloxan-induced diabetes.

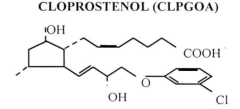

Figure 5.2
Chemical structure of $PGF_{2\alpha}$ and ClPGOA (Flavoliz [R]).

In all groups glycemia was initially determined. There were took into consideration to be included into alloxan-induced groups only animals that, after 7 days of alloxan administration, had *à jeun* glycemia at least double than before alloxan administration. After 6 weeks, rats were anesthetized and sacrificed by cutting carotids.

Aorta and renal arteries were picked up and we followed vascular lesions at these levels. Arterial lesions were macroscopically identified after longitudinal opening of vessels. Aorta was fixed in 10% formalin, stained with Sudan IV. The surface of lesions was quantitatively evaluated by planimetry of sudanophil areas [104]. Lesions at the level of aorta and renal arteries in group with D_2 vitamin and alloxan-induced diabetes (examined in light microscopy according to [26]), were considered for reference (the number of lesions was noted 100%). Data obtained were statistically interpreted with ANOVA test.

RESULTS

The main lesions observed in arterial wall were lipid deposits, ruptures of elastic lamellae and proliferation of smooth muscle cell. Our results show that in alloxan-induced diabetes associated with D_2 hypervitaminosis, prostaglandin analogue tested decreased the incidence of lesions both at

renal arteries level and at the aortic level. The incidence of arterial lesions is significantly raised in the group that received D_2 vitamin *vs.* the group with diabetes only.

The experimental model used for inducing diabetes produced significantly an increase of glycemia *vs.* initial levels (before alloxan administration) and also *vs.* control group (Table 5.3).

Table 5.3

Glycemia levels initially and after 7 days in all groups of rats included into experiment

Group	Glycemia g/l Initial	7 days after alloxan administration	p
I	0.87 ± 0.11	–	
II	0.83 ± 0.09	–	
III	0.84 ± 0.14	1.88 ± 0.15	< 0.01
IV	0.88 ± 0.07	1.99 ± 0.19	< 0.01
V	0.84 ± 0.10	2.02 ± 0.14	< 0.01

Lesions produced both in the aorta and renal arteries were decreased significantly by ClPGOA in animals with alloxan-induced diabetes and D_2 hypervitaminosis. In normal rats (that did not have alloxan-induced diabetes associated with D_2 hypervitaminosis), ClPGOA did not influence significantly vascular endothelium in animals (Figures 5.3 and 5.4).

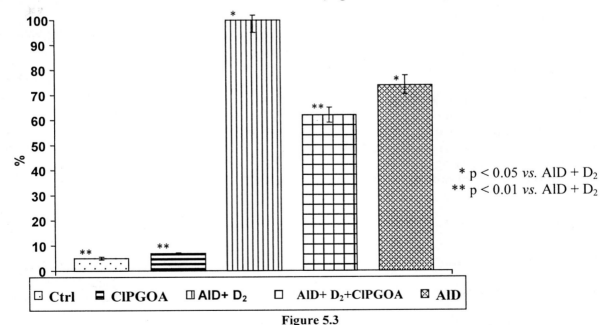

Figure 5.3

ClPGOA influence on aortic lesions in rats with alloxan-induced diabetes.

(Ctrl – control, AlD – alloxan-induced diabetes, D_2 – hypervitaminosis D_2, Lesional area was expressed as percent *vs.* area in group with alloxan-induced diabetes and hypervitaminosis D_2).

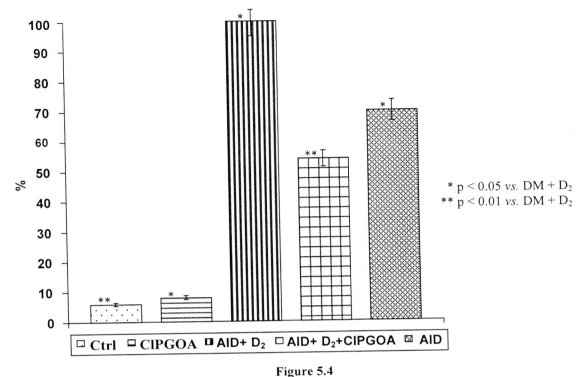

Figure 5.4

ClPGOA influence on renal arteries lesions in rats with alloxan-induced diabetes.
(Ctrl – control, AlD – alloxan-induced diabetes, D_2 – hypervitaminosis D_2, Lesional area was expressed as percent *vs* area in group with alloxan-induced diabetes and hypervitaminosis D_2).

DISCUSSIONS

Prostaglandin analogue tested decreased significantly the vascular lesions in rats with alloxan-induced diabetes associated with D_2 hypervitaminosis. This association increases the incidence of vascular endothelium lesions. Arteriotoxic effect of vitamin D_2 enhances the vascular action of hyperglycemia [105]. A dose of D_2 vitamin administered is sufficient to enhance vascular lesions. In case of association between hypercholesterolemic diet with D_2 vitamin, a dose of 2 000 UI/rat (around 15 000 UI/kg) [106] was sufficient for inducing atheromatosis lesions. In our experiment we administered a normal diet (not hypercholesterolemic).

Diabetes mellitus is usually associated with dyslipidemia even without hypecholesterolemic diet. Our data show that ClPGOA, in daily administration during all 6 weeks of experiment in rats with alloxan-induced diabetes associated with D_2 hypervitaminosis, decreases significantly the incidence of vascular lesions both in the aorta and renal arteries.

The results are in agreement with our previous data that ClPGOA decreases incidence of lesions in D_2 hypervitaminosis-induced in rat and indomethacin (COX-1 inhibitor) enhances these lesions [107, 108]. Our results plead for a partially protective role for other eicosanoids, (PGI_2, PGE_1 and PGE_2) at vascular endothelium, in animals with alloxan-induced diabetes and D_2 hypervitaminosis.

Regarding the mechanism how cloprostenol may decrease the incidence of vascular lesions in alloxan-induced diabetes associated with D_2 hypervitaminosis we consider that, at least in part, this effect can be produced by decreasing formation of free peroxidic radicals [109]. This fact is important in case of increased free radicals formation, as in diabetes mellitus and alloxan treatment.

Therapeutic use of a larger number of synthetic analogues of PGI_2 and other prostaglandins opens the perspective for preventing vascular lesions in diabetic patients.

REFERENCES

1. Negishi M, Sugimoto Y, Ighikawa A. Prostanoid receptors and their biological actions. *Progr Lipid Res,* **32:** 417–434, 1993.
2. Beitz J, Beitz A, Giessler Ch, Mentz P, Orekhov AN, Andreeva ER, Mest HJ. Influence of a cholesterol rich diet in rabbits on the formation of PGI_2 and TXA_2. In: Sinzinger HF, Schror K (Eds). *Prostaglandins in cardiovascular system,* Birkhauser Verlag, Basel, 1992, 235–241.
3. Robertson PR. Dominance of Cyclooxygenase-2 in the Regulation of Pancreatic Islet Prostaglandin Synthesis. *Diabetes,* **47:** 1379–1383, 1998.
4. Li DY, Varna DR, Chemtob S. Ontogenic increase in PGE_2 and $PGF_2\alpha$ receptor density in brain microvessels of pigs. *Br J Pharmacol,* **112:** 59–64, 1994.
5. Left P, Giles H. Classification of platelet and vascular prostaglandin D_2 (DP) receptors: estimation of affinities and relative efficacies for a series of novel bicyclic ligands. *Br J Pharmacol,* **106:** 996–1003, 1992.
6. Sinzinger H, Feigl W, Silberbauer K. Prostacyclin generation in atherosclerotic arteries. *Lancet,* **11:** 469–471, 1979.
7. Martinez-Sales V, Fornas E, Camanas A. Prostacyclin production and lipid peroxidation in the aorta of rats fed with cholesterol antioxidation products. *Artery,* **12:** 213–219, 1983.
8. Betz R, Lagercrantz J, Kedra D, Dumanschi J Nordenskjoed A. Genomic structure 5' flanking sequences and precise localization in 1 p31.1 of the human prostaglandin F receptor gene. *Biochim Biophys Res Commun,* **254:** 413–416, 1999.
9. Braun M, Sarbia M, Kienbaum P, Huhfield Th, Weber A, Schror K. Antiatherosclerotic properties of oral cicaprost in hypercholesterolemic rabbits. In: Sinzinger HF, Schror K. *Prostaglandins in cardiovascular system,* Birkhauser Verlag, Basel, 1992, 282–288.
10. Woditsch I, Hohlfed TH, Strobach H, Schror K. Oral cicaprost protects from hypercholesterolemia impairment of coronary vasodilatation. *Eicosanoids,* **4**(Suppl): pS52, 1991.
11. Boogaerts MA, Vermylen S, Deckmyn H, Roelant C, Vermilghen RL, Jacob HS. Enkephalins modify granulocyte-endothelial interactions by stimulating prostacyclin production. *Thromb Haemost,* **50:** 572–575, 1983.
12. Hennig B, Chow CK. Lipid peroxidation and endothelial cell injury: Implications in atherogenesis. *Free Rad Biol Med,* **4:** 99–106, 1988.
13. Morishita H, Yui Y, Hattori R, Aoyama T, Kawai C. Increased hydrolysis of cholesteryl ester with prostacyclin is potentiated by HDL through prostacyclin stabilization. *J Clin Invest,* **86:** 1885–1891, 1990.
14. Hajjar DP, Pomerantz KB. Spinal transduction in atherosclerosis: integration of cytokines and the eicosanoid network. *FASEB J,* **6:** 2933–2941, 1992.
15. Schroeff J, Havekes L, Weerheim A, Emeis J, Vermeer B. Suppression of cholesteryl ester accumulation in cultured human monocyte-derived macrophages by lipooxygenase inhibitors. *Biochem Biophys Res Commun,* **127:** 366–372, 1985.
16. Southgate K, Newby A. Serum induced proliferation of rabbit aortic smooth muscle cells from the contractile slate is inhibited by γ-Br-cAMP but not by γ-Br-cGMP. *Atherosclerosis,* **82:** 113–123, 1990.
17. Krone W, Klass D, Magele H, Greten H. Effect of prostaglandins on LDL receptor activity and cholesterol synthesis in freshly isolated human mononuclear leukocytes. *J Lipid Res,* **29:** 1663–1669, 1988.
18. Pomerantz K, Tall A, Feinmark S, Cannon P. Stimulation of vascular smooth muscle cell prostacyclin and prostaglandin E_2 synthesis by plasma high and low density lipoproteins. *CircRes,* **54:** 554–565, 1984.
19. Zou MH, Leist M, Uurich V. Selective nitration of prostacyclin synthase and defective vasorelaxation in atherosclerotic bovine coronary arteries. *Am J Pathol,* **154:** 1359–1365, 1999.
20. Chanh PH, Junstad M, Wennmalm A. Augmented Noradrenaline Release Following Nerve Stimulation after Inhibition at Prostaglandin Synthesis with indomethacin. *Acta Physiol Scand,* **86:** 563–567, 1972.
21. Steigerwalt RDJr, Belcaro GV, Christopoulos V, Incandela L, Cesarone MR, De Sanctos MT. Ocular and orbital blood flow velocity in patients with peripheral vascular disease and diabetes treated with intravenous prostaglandin E_1. *J Ocul Pharmacol Ther,* **17:** 529–535, 2001.
22. Jacob HS, Craddock PR, Hammerschmidt DE, Moldow CF. Complement-induced granulocyte aggregation. An unsuspected mechanism of disease. *N Engl JMed,* **302:** 789–794, 1980.
23. Todaka T, Yokoyama C, Yamamoto H, Hashimoto N, Nagata I, Tsukahara T, Hara S, Hatae T, Morishita R, Aoki M, Ogihara T, Kaneda Y, Tanabe T. Gene transfer of human prostacyclin function after carotid balloon injury in rats. *Stroke,* **30:** 419–426, 1999.
24. Numaguchi Y, Naruse K, Harada M, Osanai H, Mokuno S, Murisf K, Matsui H, Toki Y, Ito T, Okumura K., Hayakawa T. Prostacyclin synthase gene transfer accelerates reendothelization and inhibits neointimal formation in rat carotid arteries after balloon injury. *Arteriosclerosis Thrombosis Biol Vasc,* **19:** 727–733, 1999.

25. Beetens JR, Herman AG. Vitamin C increases the formation of prostacyclin by aortic rings from various species and neutralizes the inhibitory effect of 15-hydroperoxy-arachidonic acid. *Br J Pharmacol*, **80**: 249–254, 1983.

26. Goldstein I, Malmsten CL, Kindahl H, Kaplan HB, Radmark O, Samuelsson B, Weissmann G. Thromboxane generation by human peripheral blood polymorphonuclear leukocytes. *J Exp Med*, **148**: 787–792, 1978.

27. Rosen P, Hohl C. Prostaglandins and diabetes. *Ann Clin Res*, **16**: 300–313, 1984.

28. Subbiah MTR, Deitemeyer D. Altered synthesis of prostaglandins on platelet and aorta from spontaneously diabetic Wistar rats. *Biochem Med*, **23**: 231–235, 1980.

29. Boura ALA, Hodgson WC, King RG. Sensitivity changes of the perfused hindquarters vasculature in rats with alloxan-induced diabetes mellitus. *Clin Ex Pharmacol Physiol*, **14**: 481–487, 1987.

30. Colwell JA, Halushka PV, Sarji KE, Lopes-Virella MF, Sagel J. Vascular disease in diabetic pathophysiological mechanisms and therapy. *Arch Intern Med*, **139**: 225–230, 1979.

31. Hodgson WC, King RG, Boura ALA. Augmented Potentiation of Renal Vasoconstrictor Responses by Thromboxane A_2 Receptor Stimulation in the Alloxan-diabetic Rat. *J Pharm Pharmacol*, **42**: 423–427, 1990.

32. Lefer AM. Eicosanoids as mediators of ischemia and shock. *Fed Proc*, **44**: 275–287, 1985.

33. Hanasaki K, Nakano K, Kasai H, Arita H, Ohtami K, Doteuchi K, -Specific receptors for thromboxane A_2 receptor in cultured vascular endothelial cells in rat aorta. *Biochem Biophys Res Commun*, **151**: 1352–1357, 1988.

34. Hunt JA, Merritt JE, Mc Dermot J, Keen M. Characterization of the thromboxane receptor mediatory prostaglandin release from cultured endothelial cells. *Biochem Pharmacol*, **43**: 1747–1752, 1992.

35. Shin Y, Romstedt KJ, Miller DD, Feller DR. Interactions of nonprostanoid trimetoquinol analogs with thromboxane A_2/Prostaglandin H_2 receptors in human platelets, at vascular endothelial cells and rat vascular smooth muscle cells. *J Pharmacol Expt Therap*, **267**: 1017–1023, 1993.

36. Pill J, Metz J, Stegmeier K, Hartig F. Effects of daltroban, a thromboxane (TxA_2) receptor antagonist, on lipid metabolism and atherosclerosis. *Agents Actions Suppl*, **37**: 107–113. 1992.

37. Dunham B, Shepro D, Hechtman HB. Leukotriene induction of TxB_2 in cultured bovine aortic endothelial cells. *Inflammation*, **8**: 313–321, 1984.

38. Tremoli E, Folco G, Agradi E, Gali C. Platelet thromboxane and serum cholesterol. *Lancet*, **1**: 107–109, 1979.

39. Davi G, Averna M, Novo S, Barbagallo CM, Mogavero A, Notarbartolo A, Strano A. Effects of synvinolin on platelet aggregation and thromboxane B_2 synthesis in type 2 hypercholesterolemic patients. *Atherosclerosis*, **79**: 79–83, 1989.

40. Dahlen SE, Bjork J, Hedqvist P, Arfors KE, Hammarstrom S, Lindgren JA, Samuelsson B. Leukotrienes promote plasma leakage and leukocyte adhesion in postcapillary venules: In vivo effects with relevance to the acute inflammatory response. *Proc Natl Acad Sci USA*, **78**: 3887–3891, 1981.

41. Sikorski BW, Hodgson WC, King RC. Thromboxane A_2 receptor stimulation similarly potentates pressor responses to 5-hydroxytryptamine in perfused hindquarters of non-diabetic and alloxan diabetic rats. *Clin Exp Pharmacol Physiol*, **18**: 237–244, 1991.

42. DelaCruz P, Guerrero A, Paniego J, Ananz I, Moreno A, Sanchez-Delacuesta F. Effect of aspirin on prostanoids and nitric oxide production in streptozotocin-diabetic rats with ischemic retinopathy. *Naunyn Schiedebergs Arch Pharmacol*, **365**: 96–101, 2002.

43. Shakhmalova MS, Shestakova MV, Chugunova LA, Dedov II. Vasoactive factors of the vascular endothelium in patients with non-insulin-dependent diabetes mellitus and kidney involvement. *Ter Arkh*, **68**: 43–46, 1996.

44. Biegelsen S, Losalza J. Endothelial function and atherosclerosis. *Coronary Artery Dis*, **10**: 241–256, 1999.

45. Hak AE, Stehouwer CD, Bots ML, Polderman KH, Schalkwijk CG, Westemdorp IC, Hofman A, Witteman JC. Associations of C-reactive protein with measures of obesity insulin resistance, and subclinical atherosclerosis in healthy, middle-age women. *Atherosclerosis Thromb Vasc Biol*, **19**: 1986–1991, 1999.

46. Howard BV. Insulin resistance and lipid metabolism. *Am J Cardiol*, **84**: 28 j-32 j, 1994.

47. Hishinuna T, Tsukamoto H, Suzuki K, Mizugaki M. Relationship between thromboxane prostacyclin ratio and diabetic vascular complications. *Prostaglandins Leuk Essent Fatty Acids*, **65**: 191–196, 2001.

48. Kalogeropoulou K, Mortzos G, Migdalis G, Velentzas C, Mikhailidis DP, Georgiadis E, Cordopatos P. Carotid atherosclerosis in type 2 diabetes mellitus: potential role of endothelin-1, lipoperoxides and prostacyclin. *Angiology*, **53**: 279–285, 2002.

49. Halushka PV, Roger RC, Loadholt CB, Colwell JA. Increased platelet thromboxane synthesis in diabetes mellitus. *J Lab Clin Med*, **97**: 87–96, 1981.

50. Mourits-Andelsen T, Jensen IW, Nohr-Jensen P, Ditzel J, Dyerberg J. Plasma 6-keto-$PGF_{1\alpha}$, thromboxane B_2 and PGE_2 in type 1 (insulinodependent) diabetic

patients during exercise. *Diabetologia,* **30**: 460–463, 1987.

51. Yang JA, Choi JH, Rhee SJ. Effects of green tea catechin on phospholipase A$_2$ activity and antithrombus in streptozotocin diabetic rats. *J Nutr Sci Vitaminol,* **45**: 337–346, 1999.

52. Ford-Hutchinson AW. Leukotrienes: their formation and role as inflammatory mediators. *Fed Proc,* **44**: 25–45, 1985.

53. Sirois P. Pharmacology of the leukotrienes. *Adv Lipid Res,* **21**: 79–95, 1985.

54. Hardy G, Stanke-Labesque F, Peoch M, Hakim A, Devillier P, Caron F, Morel S, Faure P, Halimi S, Bessird G. Cysteinyl leukotrienes modulates angiotensine II constrictor effects on aortas from streptozotocin-induced diabetic rats. *Arterioscler Thromb Vasc Biol,* **21**: 1751–1758, 2001.

55. Whicher J, Biasucci L, Rifai N. Inflammation the acute phase response and atherosclerosis. *Clin Chem Lab Med,* **37**: 495–583, 1999.

56. Uski TK, Hegestatt ED. Effects of various cyclooxygenase and lipoxygenase metabolites on guinea pig cerebral arteries. *General Pharmacology,* **23**: 109–113, 1992.

57. Hopkins NK, Oglesby TD, Bundy GL, Gorman RR. Biosynthesis and metabolism of 15-hydroperoxy-5,8,11,13-eicosatetraenoic acid by human umbilical vein endothelial cells. *J Biol Chem,* **259**: 14048–14053, 1984.

58. Nakao J, Koshihara Y, Ito H, Murota S, Chang W. Enhancement of endogenous production of 12-L hydroxy-5,8,11,13 eicosatetraenoic acid in aortic smooth muscle cells by platelet derived growth factor. *Life Sci,* **37**: 1435–1440, 1985.

59. Turk J, Maas RL, Brash AR, Roberts LJ, Oates JA. Arachidonic acid 15-lipooxygenase products from human eosinophils. *J Biol Chem,* **257**: 7068–7073, 1982.

60. Moncada S, Gryglewski RJ, Bunting S, Vane J. A lipid peroxide inhibits the enzyme in blood vessel microsomes that generates from prostaglandin endoperoxides the substance (prostaglandin X) which prevents platelet aggregation. *Prostaglandins,* **12**: 715–721, 1976.

61. Simon TC, Niakheja AN, Bailey JM. Formation of 15-hydroxyeicosatetraenoic acid (15-HETE) as the predominant eicosanoid in aortas from Watanabe Heritable hyperlipidemic and cholesterol fed rabbits. *Atherosclerosis,* **75**: 31–38, 1989.

62. Setty BNy, Stuart MJ. 15-Hydroxy-5,8,11,13-eicosatetraenoic acid inhibits human vascular cyclooxygenase. Potential role in human diabetic vascular disease. *J Clin Invest,* **77**: 202–207, 1986.

63. Brezinski ME, Gimbrone MA, Nicolaou KC. Lipoxins stimulate prostacyclin generation by human endothelial cells. *FEBS Lett,* **245**: 167–172, 1989.

64. Daugherty A, Zweifel BS, Sobel BE, Schonfeld G. Isolation of low density lipoprotein from atherosclerotic vascular tissue of watanate heritable hyperlipidemic rabbits. *Atherosclerosis,* **8**: 768–777, 1988.

65. Sparrow CP, Doebber TW, Olszewski J, Wu MS, Ventre J, Stevens KA, Chao YS. Low density lipoprotein is protected from oxidation and the progression of atherosclerosis is slowed in cholesterol-fed rabbits by the antioxidant NW-diphenyl-phenylenediamine. *J Clin Invest,* **89**: 1885–1891, 1992.

66. Sendobry MS, Conicelli AJ, Welch K, Bocan T, Tait B, Trivedi B, Colbry N, Dyer RD, Feinmark JS, Daugherty A. Attenuation of diet induced atherosclerosis in rabbits with a highly selective 15-lipooxygenase inhibitor lacking significant antioxidant properties, *Br J Pharmacol,* **120**: 1190–1206, 1997.

67. Upston JM, Neuzil J, Stocker R. Oxidation of LDL by recombinant human 15-lipooxygenase evidence for α-tocopherol-dependent oxidation of esterifield core and surface lipids. *J Lipid Res,* **37**: 2650–2661, 1996.

68. Pace-Asciak CR, Granstrom E, Samuelsson B. Arachidonic acid epoxides isolation and structure of two hydroxy epoxide intermediates in the formation of 8,11,12 -and 10, 11, 12 trihydroxy eicosatrienoic acids. *J Biol Chem,* **258**: 6835–6840, 1983.

69. Laneuville O, Corey EJ, Couture R, Pace-Asciak CR. Hepoxilin A$_3$ (HxA$_3$) is formed by the aorta and is metabolized into HxA$_3$-C a glutathione conjugate. *Biochem Biophys Acta,* **1084**: 60–68,1991.

70. Mathur SN, Field FJ, Spector AA, Armstrong ML. Increased production of lipooxygenase products by cholesterol-rich mouse macrophages. *Biochem Biophys Acta,* 83 A: 13–18, 1985.

71. Ginter E, Bobek P. The influence of vitamin C on lipid metabolism. In : Coursell JN and Hornig DH (eds). *Vitamin C, ascorbic acid.* Applied Science Publishers, London, 1981, 299–347.

72. Nakao J, Oyama T, Ito H, Chang WC, Murota S. Comparative effect of lipooxygenase products of arachidonic acid on rat aortic smooth muscle cell migration. *Atherosclerosis,* **44**: 339–342, 1982.

73. Beetens JR, Coene MC, Verheyen A, Zonnekeyn L, Herman AG. Vitamin C increases the prostacyclin production and decreases the vascular lesions in Experimental Atherosclerosis in rabbits. *Prostaglandins,* **32**: 335–352, 1986.

74. Van Rollins M, Kaduce LT, Fang X, Knapp HR. Arachidonic Acid Diols Produced by Cytochrome P450 Monooxygenases Are Incorporated into Phospholipids of Vascular Endothelial Cells. *J Biol Chem,* **271**: 14001–14009, 1996.

75. Frisbee JC, Roman JR, Krishna UM, Falck RJ, Lomard HJ. Relative contribution of cyclooxygenase and cytochrome P450 ω-hydroxylase dependent pathways to hypoxic dilatation of skeletal muscle resistance arteries. *J Vascular Res,* **38**: 305–314, 2001.

76. Schwartzman ML, McGiff JC. Renal cytochrome P450. *J Lipid Mediat Cell Signal,* **12**(2-3): 229–242, 1995.

77. Oyekan AO, You Seff T, Fulton D, Quilley J, Mc Giff JC. Renal cytochrome P450 omega-hydroxylase and epoxygenase activity are differentially modified by nitric oxide inhibitors and by sodium chloride. *J Clin Invest,* **104**: 1131–1137, 1999.

78. Messer-Letienne I, Bernard N, Roman RJ, Sassard J, Benzoni D. Cytochrome P-450 arachidonate metabolite inhibition improves renal function in Lyon hypertensive rats. *Am J Hypertension,* **12**: 398–404, 1999.

79. Node K, Huo Y, Ruan X, Yang B, Spiecker M, Ley K, Zeldin DC, Liao JK. Antiinflammatory properties of cytochrome P450 epoxygenase-derived eicosanoids. *Science,* **285**: 1276–1279, 1999.

80. Roberts JL, Montine TJ, Markesbeayr WH, Tapaert AR, Hardy P, Chemtodi S, Dettbarn WD, Morrow JD. Formation of Isoprostane-like Compounds (Neoprostanes) *in vivo* from Docosahexaenoic Acid. *Biol Chem,* **278**: 13605–13612, 1998.

81. Reilly M, Delamty N, Lawson JA, Fitzgerald GA. Modulation of Oxidant Stress in Vivo in Chronic Cigarette Smokers. *Circulation,* **94**: 19–25, 1996.

82. Morrow JD, Hill KE, Burk RF, Nammour TM, Badr KF, Roberts LJ 2nd. A series of prostaglandin F2-like compounds are produced *in vivo* in humans by a non-cyclooxygenase, free radical-catalyzed mechanism. *Proc Natl Acad Sci USA,* **87**(23): 9383–9387, 1990.

83. Pratico D, Lawson JA, Fitzgerald GA. Cyclooxygenase dependent formation of 8-iso-prostaglandin F2 alpha by human platelets. *Adv Prostaglandin Thromboxane Leukot Res,* **23**: 229–31, 1995.

84. Banerjee M, Kang KH, Morrow JD, Roberts LJ, Newman JH. Effects of a novel prostaglandin, 8-epi-PGF2 alpha, in rabbit lung *in situ. Am J Physiol,* **263**(3 Pt 2): H660-663, 1992.

85. Mombouli JV, Vanhoutte PM. Endothelium derived hypolarizing factors: updating the unknown. *Trends Pharmacol Sci,* **18**: 252–256, 1997.

86. Campbell WB, Harder DR. Endothelium derived hypolarizing factors and vascular cytochrome P 450 metabolites of arachidonic acid in the regulation of tone. *Circ Res,* **84**: 484–488, 1999.

87. Janssen LJ. Are endothelium-derived hyperpolarizing and contracting factors isoprostanes? *TIPS,* **23**: 59–62, 2002.

88. Mombouli JV, Vanhoutte PM. Endothelial dysfunction from physiology to therapy. *J Mol Cell Cardiol,* **31**: 61–74, 1999.

89. Liu T, Stern A, Roberts LJ, Morrow JD. Isoprostanes: novel prostaglandin-like products of the tree radical-catalysed peroxidation of arachidonic acid. *J Biomed Sci,* **6**(4): 226–235, 1999.

90. Guogho A, Karanikas G, Kritz H, Riehs G, Wagner O, Sinzinger H. 6-oxo-PGF₁ alpha and 8-epi-RGF₂ alpha in human atherosclerotic vascular tissue. *Prostaglandins Leuk Essent Fatty Acids,* **60**: 129–134, 1999.

91. Voutilainen S, Morrow JD, Roberts LJ, Alfthan G, Alho H, Nyssonen K, Salonen JT. Enhanced in vivo lipid peroxidation at elevated plasma total homocysteine levels. *Atherosclerosis Thromb Vasc Biol,* **19**: 1263–1266,1999.

92. Nourooz-Zadeh J, Halliwell B, Anggard EE. Evidence for the formation of F3-isoprostanes during peroxidation of eicosapentaenoic acid. *Biochem Biophys Res Commun,* **236**(2): 467–472, 1997.

93. Nourooz-Zadeh J, Liu EH, Yhlen B, Anggard EE, Halliwell B. F4-isoprostanes as specific marker of docosahexaenoic acid peroxidation in Alzheimer's disease. *J Neurochem,* **72**(2): 734–740, 1999.

94. Willumsen N, Skorve J, Hexeberg S, Rustan AC, Berge RK. The hypotriglyceridemic effect of Eicosapentalinoic Acid in Rats is reflected in Increased Mitochondrial Fatty Acid Oxidation Followed by Diminished Lipogenesis. *Lipids,* **28**: 683–690, 1993.

95. Fischer S, Webe R PC. Prostaglandin I₃ is formed in vivo in man after dietary eicosapentaenoic acid. *Nature,* **307**: 165–168, 1984.

96. Velardo B, Lagarde M, Guichardant M. Decrease of platelet activity after intake of small amounts of eicosapentaenoic acid in diabetics. *Thrombosis Haem,* **48**: 344–351, 1982.

97. Locher R, Sachinidis A, Steiner A, Vogt E, Vetter W. Fish oil affects phosphoinositide turnover and thromboxane A metabolism in cultured vascular muscle cells. *Biochem Biophys Acta,* **1012**: 279–283, 1989.

98. Holler C, Auinger M, Ulberth F, Irsigler K. Eicosanoid precursors potential factors for atherogenesis in diabetic CAPD patient. *Perit Dial Int,* **16**(suppl 1): S250-S253, 1996.

99. Hammes HP, Weiss A, Fuhrel D, Kramer HJ, Papayassillis C, Grimminger F. Acceleration of experimental diabetic retinopathy in the rat by omega-3 fatty acids. *Diabetologia,* **39**: 251–255, 1996.

100. Leng GC, Lee AJ, Fowkes FG, Jepson RG, Lowe GD, Skinner ER, Mowat BE. Randomized controlled trial of gamma-linolenic acid and eicosapentaenoic acid in peripheral arterial disease. *Clin Nutr,* **17**: 265–271, 1998.

101. Stillwell W, Jemski LJ, Crump FT, Ehringer W. Effect of Docosahexaenoic Acid on Mouse Mitochondrial Membrane Properties. *Lipids,* **32**: 497–506, 1997.

102. Stillwell W, Jemski LJ. Membrane Alteration by omega-3 Fatty Acids: Effect of Aging. In: Watson RR. *Handbook of Nutrition in the Aged.* 2nd edition, CRC Press Boca Raton, 1993, 37–55.

103. Zhu BQ, Sievers RE, Isenberg WM, Smith DL, Parmley WW. Regression of Atherosclerosis in Cholesterol-Fed Rabbits Effects of Fish oil and verapamil. *J Am Coll Cardiol,* **15**: 231–237, 1990.

104. Yamanouchi J, Sugawara Y, Itagaki S, Doi K. Ultrastructure of atheromatous lesions experimentally induced in Syrian hamsters of the APA strain. *Histol Histopathol,* **12**: 433–438, 1997.

105. Bennani-Kabchi N, Kehel L, El Bouyadi F, Fdhil H, Amarti A, Saidi A, Marquie G. New model of atherosclerosis in sand rats subjected to a high cholesterol diet and vitamin D_2. *Therapie,* **54**: 559–565, 1999.

106. Nechifor M, Dobrescu G, Adomnicăi M, Teslariu E, Chera G. The influence of Cloprostenol and indomethacin influence on vitamin D_2 vascular lesions. *Proceedings of Third European Congress on Cell Biology,* Firenze, Italy, 675, 1990.

107. Nechifor M, Dobrescu G, Adomnicăi M, Teslariu E, Negru A, Cocu F. The effects of cloprostenol (ClPG) and eicosapentaenoic acid (EPA) on vitamin D_2-induced vascular lesions in rats with alloxanic diabetes, *Proceedings of 66th Congress of the European Atherosclerosis Society, Florence,* 216, 1996.

108. Nechifor M, Păduraru I, Filip C, Teslariu E, Popovici I, Cocu F. Influence of some prostaglandin analogues in free radicals generation in experimental ethanol induced acute intoxication in rats. *ISSX Proceedings,* **11**: 75, 1997.

109. Lewis RE, Miller RA, Granger HJ. Acute microvascular effects of the chemotactic peptide N-formyl-methionyl-leucyl-phenylalanine: comparisons with leukotriene B4. *Microvasc Res,* **37**: 53–69, 1989.

110. Du JB, Zhao B, Zeng HP, Huang LY, Li SZ. Some humoral factors and their interaction on acute hypoxic pulmonary pressor response. *Chin Med J,* **107**: 142–145, 1994.

111. Lonigro AJ, Sprague RS, Stephenson AH, Dahms TE. Relationship of leukotriene C4 and D4 to hypoxic pulmonary vasoconstriction in dogs. *J Appl Physiol,* **64**: 2538–2543, 1988.

GENETIC BASES OF VASCULAR COMPLICATIONS IN DIABETES MELLITUS

Dănuț CIMPONERIU, Pompilia APOSTOL, Irina RADU
Dan CHEȚA, Cristian PANAITE, Bogdan BALAȘ

Diabetes mellitus and its complications have been associated with reducing life quality and expectancy. Micro- (nephropathy, retinopathy and diabetic neuropathy) and macrovascular complications represent important disabilities of those patients.

Diabetic nephropathy is a disease in which haemodynamic and metabolic factors, cytokines, growth factors and antropometric parameters are involved. In addition a genetic component with a particular contribution to disease has been observed, which is independent of the glycaemic control. The investigation of the candidate genes, and the *in vivo, in vitro* and *in silico* studies have provided additional information concerning the genetic component of the diabetic nephropathy. The results of many studies continue to remain contradictory. Therefore, we can say that diabetic nephropathy is a multifactorial and polygenic disease, which appears as a result of the action of environmental factors, on a genetic susceptible background. This background is the result of the balance between the risk and the protective alleles. At present, no polymorphism or genetic test with a predictible value for the appearance or the evolution of diabetic nephropathy is known.

Diabetic retinopathy is the major cause of blindness among diabetic adults. Several factors have been associated to diabetic retinopathy, including: vascular endothelial growth factor, aldose reductase, paraoxonase, α2β1 integrin, IGF-1, angiotensin-converting enzyme, the receptor for advanced glycation end-products, the renin-angiotensin system, TNF genes, the family of NOS enzymes, LDL, endothelin, poly (ADP-ribose) polymerase-1 and GLP-1. The effects of all those factors in diabetic retinopathy (DR) are presented. The role of genetic influences in diabetic retinopathy has been difficult to define due to differences in patient recruitment methods, patient selection criteria, risk factors, variation in ethnicity, and clinical differences in evaluating retinopathy status.

Diabetic neuropathy, with its two major forms, autonomic and peripheral, represents one of the main complications of the nervous system to the patients with diabetus mellitus. Neuropathy is a multifactorial disease, a consequence of the action of the risk factors to the persons with genetic susceptibility. The chain of events is initiated by the chronic perturbance of the glycaemia, which determine preponderantly the formation of the advanced glycosylated products, the activation of the polyol pathway and the increase of the oxidative stress, having as a result the alteration of the structural and functional properties of neurons. The genes which code for proteins involved in these processes, especially those for aldoso-reductase and SOD, have been considered risk genes for neuropathy. Until now, the research studies could not identify markers with true predictible value.

Macrovascular complications. The most common macrovascular complications in diabetic patients are coronary artery disease (CAD), peripheral artery disease (PAD) and cerebrovascular disease. In diabetic patients, the endothelial dysfunction, caused by the general metabolism impairment, represents the major pathway of macrovascular disease (MVD) development. Many studies have demonstrated the involvement of genetic basis in the genesis of these complications. It was established that there is a polygenic predisposition to these complications and the mean candidate genes are those involved in lipidic metabolism.

Abbreviations List

ACE – Angiotensin-Converting Enzyme
AGT – Angiotensinogen
AGEs – Advanced Glycation End-Products
Ang1 – Angiotensin 1
Ang2 – Angiotensin 2
AngR1 – Angiotensin Receptor type I
AngR2 – Angiotensin Receptor type II
ANP – Atrial Natriuretic Peptide
ApoC – Apolipoprotein C
ApoE – Apolipoprotein E
AR – Aldose Reductase
BK – Bradikinin
BKR – Bradikinin Receptor
BMI – Body Mass Index
CAD – Coronary Artery Disease
CCR – Chemokine Receptor
CETP – Cholesteryl Ester Transfer Protein
DM – Diabetes Mellitus
DN – Diabetic Nephropathy
DR – Diabetic Retinopathy
ECM – Extracellular Matrix
ENPP1 – Ecto NucleotidePyrophosphatase / Phosphodiesterase 1
ESRD – End-Stage Renal Disease
ET – Endothelin
GLP-1 – Glucagon-Like Peptide-1
GLP-1R – Glucagon-Like Peptide-1 Receptor
GLUT – Glucose Transporter
HDL – High Density Lipoproteins
HIF – Hypoxia Inducible Factor
HL – Hepatic Lipase
ICAM-1 – Intercellular Adhesion Molecule - 1

IDL – Intermediary Density Lipoproteins
IGF-1 – Insulin-like Growth Factor 1
IGF-1R – Insulin-like Growth Factor 1 Receptor
LDL – Low Density Lipoproteins
LPL – Lipoprotein Lipase
MCP – Monocyte Chemoattractant Protein
MVD – Macrovascular Disease
NO – Nitric Oxide
NOS – Nitric Oxide Synthase
NOS-1 – neural NOS (nNOS)
NOS-2A – inducible NOS (iNOS),
NOS-3 – endothelial NOS (eNOS)
PAI-1 – Plasminogen Activator Inhibitor-1
PARP – Poly(ADP-ribose) polymerase-1
PEDF – Pigment Epithelium-Derived Factor
PON – Paraoxonase
PPAR – Peroxisome Proliferator-Activated Receptor
RAGE – Receptor for Advanced Glycation End-Products
RAS – Renin-Angiotensin System
ROS – Reactive Oxygen Species
SNP – Single Nucleotide Polymorphism
T1DM – DM type 1
T2DM – DM type 2
TG – Triglycerides
TGF β – Transforming Growth Factor β
TNF – Tumor Necrosis Factor
TRL – Triglycerides-Rich Lipoproteins
VEGF – Vascular Endothelial Growth Factor
VLDL – Very Low Density Lipoproteins

Diabetes mellitus (DM) and its complications are associated with reduced life expectancy and quality of life. The permanent increase in number of DM and its complications worldwide, as well as the huge health care costs are well known [1]. The link between diabetes and its vascular alterations is not fully understood, but it was observed that, despite of poor glycaemic control, long term diabetic complications, especially micro- and macrovascular diseases appear only in a part of patients.

DIABETIC MICROVASCULAR COMPLICATIONS

Diabetic microvascular complications are referring to diabetic nephropathy and diabetic retinopathy, and partially to diabetic neuropathy.

DIABETIC NEPHROPATHY

Diabetic nephropathy (DN) is referring to several structural and functional abnormalities of glomeruli with variable rate of decline of glomerular activity [2]. This complication is the most frequent cause of end-stage renal disease (ESRD) and represents almost 40% of starting dialysis patients in the USA [3].

DN has a multifactorial origin [4–7]. The haemodynamic factors (*e.g.*, systemic and glomerular hypertension), metabolic factors (*e.g.*, duration of diabetes, poor glycaemic control, hypercholesterolaemia, oxidative stress), cytokine

and growth factors and anthropometrical parameters (*e.g.*, short stature of men [8]) seem to contribute to DN development (Figure 6.1). The importance of the first two items is supported by the observation that treatment with angiotensin-converting enzyme (ACE) inhibitors and long term normoglycaemia can slow DN evolution. A literature review on DN produced contradictory results on the genetic and environmental factors and the interaction between them, in disease economy. At genetic level, the DN segregation model, the risk and protective alleles, the variable penetrance of some alleles and the quantitative or epistatic effects of some genes were attempted to be identified.

Studies *in vivo* (*e.g.*, animal models), *in vitro* (*e.g.*, cells cultures) and *in silico* (using bioinformatics tools) provided additional information about the involvement of genetic factors in the disease. New techniques used in molecular biology, like microarray (DNA chip), may provide a faster and more accurate image about the pattern of genes expression and allow a systematic analysis of nucleic acids variations, in specific conditions [9].

Many data were gathered regarding diabetes complications. We tried to briefly review only genetic studies done on human population. The contribution of genetic factors to DN was tested especially by candidate gene approach and by positional cloning based on linkage analysis. These studies use the differences in DNA sequences (polymorphisms) – like single nucleotide polymorphism (SNP), micro- and minisatellites – which are tested for associations with the disease. These polymorphisms may be

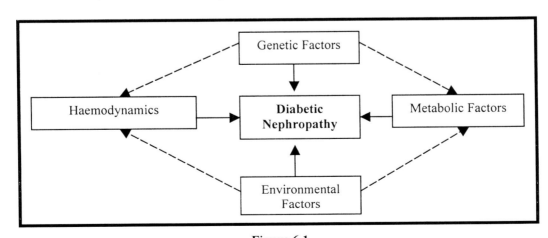

Figure 6.1
The main factors involved in DN.

in linkage with the "real" marker or they may be the "true causes" of disease, if they have a functional effect. In the first case, the real marker is unknown. Until now, no known polymorphism is a certain marker for DN development or evolution.

Evidence for genetic susceptibility in DN. Familial clustering, epidemiological studies, ethnic variation of prevalence and the concordance of glomerular lesions patterns in DM type 1 (T1DM) sibling pairs suggest a genetic component for DN [10–12]. The segregation analysis studies cannot establish a unique model for disease transmission [13]. Although diabetic status, *per se*, favours the development of DN, the genetic bases for both, DM and DN, are not identical. The existence of common elements was suggested after observations that at least in T1DM patients, a familial history of type 2 DM (T2DM) increases susceptibility to DN [14–16].

In the following pages, we will present some of the results obtained by candidate gene approach for DN. The most frequent genes investigated in DN are listed in Table 6.1.

Haemodynamic factors

Renin-angiotensin system. The contribution of haemodynamic factors to DN is well documented, although some results remain contradictory. In mammals, there are two renin-angiotensin systems (RAS), systemic and local. The last one has been found in myocardium, adipose tissue, kidney and skeletal muscle. Primarily, RAS is a blood pressure regulator (modifies vascular tone, salt and water homeostasis) and constitutes an attractive candidate for hypertension. It was observed an association between predisposition to essential hypertension and DN [17]. Increasing of intraglomerular capillary pressure may predispose to diabetic glomerulosclerosis and antihypertensive

Table 6.1
The most frequently investigated genes in diabetic nephropathy

	Gene	Localization	OMIM* ID	DN** Risk	and Protective
1	ACE	17q23	106180	DD	II
2	Aldose reductase	7q35	103880	Z-2	
3	Angiotensin receptor type 1	3q21-q25	106165	1166C	
4	Angiotensinogen	1q42-q43	106150	235T	
5	Atrial natriuretic peptide	1p36.2	108780		
6	Apolipoprotein E	19q13.2	107741	ε2, ε3	ε4
7	Bradykinin receptors type 1	14q32.1-q32.2	600337		-699C
8	Chemokine receptor 5	3p21	601373		
9	ENPP1/PC-1	6q22-q23	173335	121Q	
10	GLUT 1	1p35-p31.3	138140		
11	IGF1	12q22-q24.1	147440		
12	KLKB1	4q35	229000		
13	MTHFR	1p36.3	607093	677TT	
14	NOS-1	12q24	163731		
15	NOS-2A	17cen-q11.2	163730	$(AAAT)_+$	$(CCTTT)_{14}$
16	NOS-3	7q36	163729	4a	
17	Paraoxonase gene 1	7q21.3	168820		
18	Plasminogen activator inhibitor-1	7q21.3-q22	173360	4G/4G	
19	PPARγ 2	3p25	601487		Ala12
20	RAGE	6p21.3	600214		
21	TGF β	19q13.1	190180		
22	VEGF	6p12	192240		

* additional information about the genes can be found, using the ID number, at the following internet address: http://www.ncbi.nlm.nih.gov/Omim/searchomim.html,
** this selection is based on the information known by now.

therapy (*e.g.*, with ACE inhibitors) improves renal activity, especially in the early stage of DN. Therefore, the RAS is a reasonable candidate for DN.

At genetic level, ACE, angiotensinogen (AGT), angiotensin receptor type 1 (AngR1) and renin polymorphisms were more investigated. The contribution of each gene to DN is weak (*e.g.* the renin gene polymorphisms – in T1DM patients [18]), but the cumulative effect of different RAS alleles has been postulated. An interaction between AGT and ACE has been documented in healthy men, regarding blood pressure response to physical exercise, but not in some pathological situations, like early atherosclerosis [19,20]. For a better understanding of RAS implication in DN, complex studies which involve more than two loci have been initiated [21].

Angiotensin-converting enzyme. ACE is a component of both RAS and kallikrein-kinin system. It is involved in hydrolysis of angiotensin 1 (Ang1) to angiotensin 2 (Ang2) and in bradykinin degradation. The most studied ACE polymorphism is located in intron 16 and is represented by the presence (insertion-I) or absence (deletion-D) of a 287 bp of Alu1 repeat sequence. This polymorphism was associated with plasmatic activity of ACE, the II genotype representing a marker for low tissue enzyme activity [22].

The ACE I/D polymorphism was correlated with some diabetes phenotypes [23]. The DD genotype was associated with susceptibility to T2DM [24] and the D allele with more frequent and severe episode of hypoglycaemia, in T1DM [25].

Previous studies suggest that ACE inhibitors treatment may improve insulin sensitivity by decreasing Ang2 and by increasing bradikinin (BK) level. Other beneficial effects may be caused by the reduction of transforming growth factor β (TGFβ) serum level [2,26]. The difference in response of T1DM patients to ACE inhibitors seems to be correlated with ACE I/D polymorphism [27].

In Japanese nondiabetic hypertensive patients, the DD genotype is a risk factor for hypertensive renal disease [28]. In the last decade, the ACE I/D polymorphism has been investigated in patients with DN. The presence of ACE D allele is associated with DN in T2DM patients from South India [29]. T2DM patients presenting microalbuminuria or proteinuria with D allele or DD genotype have a higher risk for an early development of DN and for accelerated decline of renal function [30–32]. The ACE I/D polymorphism may represent an independent determinant of glomerular basement membrane thickening, although duration of diabetes and HbA1c were stronger factors [32].

In T1DM patients with proliferative retinopathy, the ACE I/D polymorphism is correlated with susceptibility to nephropathy and with progression towards renal failure [33]. The correlation between DN and DD genotype is much stronger in patients with duration of DM more than 20 years [34]. Patients with a shorter period of DM, with susceptibility to but without DN, may be missincluded in the control group. In addition, patients with DN have an increased cardiovascular morbidity and mortality, although microalbuminuria itself has a small contribution to mortality [35]. In T2DM with DN, the DD genotype represents a risk factor for premature mortality [31]. All of these may cause some biases in studies which have investigated patients with too short or too long term DN.

In a recent meta-analysis, an association between ACE I/D polymorphism and DN in Japanese T2DM patients was founded. In the same study, the association with DN in Caucasian diabetic patients was weaker, although a trend to protection of II genotype was seen in T1DM patients [36].

In conclusion, the correlation between DN and ACE I/D polymorphism is not very clear, but this is the most constant polymorphism associated with DN. It is unlikely that this intronic polymorphism may be itself the real marker for DN susceptibility. Probably, it is a neutral marker linkated to a functional marker in ACE gene region.

Angiotensinogen. Angiotensinogen (AGT), also called renin substrate, is the first component of RAS. It has an organization characteristic for serpin superfamily (serin protease inhibitor). The last ten aminoacid residues from the amino terminus tail represent Ang1 and the remaining part of protein has an unknown function. Sites for AGT production have been identified in the kidney, adipose tissues and vascular walls.

The human AGT gene has two potential initiation sites and two polyadenylation sites. Two missense mutations, in exon 2, which change codons for threonine and methionine at positions 174 (T174M) and 235 (M235T), in the unknown function region of protein, have been identified.

These alleles have a weak correlation with small changes in AGT plasma levels.

The AGT locus is linked to essential hypertension [37]. In TIDM patients with retinopathy, the cumulative effect of AGT and ACE polymorphisms increases the risk for renal involvement. In some studies, this risk increases progressively, from AGT 235 MM to TT genotype, at the ACE D carriers. These interactions may depend on the genetic background and may differ between populations [33, 38]. In addition, a gender specific effect of the T235 allele in T2DM men, regarding DN, has been postulated [39].

The lack of association between M235T and DN, found in most studies, suggests a small contribution of AGT to disease [40,41]. Because the main point of AGT control is, probably, at transcriptional level, it would be interesting to investigate additional functional polymorphisms.

Angiotensin receptor type 1. Ang2 is a potent regulator of blood pressure, water and electrolytes. Its vascular effects are mediated especially by angiotensin receptor type 1 (AngR1). The function of the second receptor for Ang, angiotensin receptor type II (AngR2), is not fully understood.

The AngR2 A1675 allele, but not AngR1 A1166C SNP, is correlated with reduced receptor expression and with the occurrence of severe hypoglycaemia episodes [42].

AngR1 gene has multiple initiation transcription sites and distinct alternatively spliced sites. The relative abundance of these transcripts in different tissues and the heterodimerisation with bradikinin receptors type II may have functional significance. Therefore, it is difficult to estimate the real contribution of AngR1 to DN susceptibility. In T1DM siblings, a linkage study between RAS regions and DN found a major susceptibility region of 20 cM around AngR1 [43]. The glomerular AngR1 expression is reduced in inflammatory or noninflammatory (*e.g.* DN) glomerular diseases. This may be an adaptative response to high Ang2 intrarenal levels (AngR1 down regulation) [44]. One study has shown that, in T1DM patients with poor glycaemic control, the presence of the AngR1 1166C allele represents a risk factor for DN development [45]. The same polymorphism is associated with changed renal haemodynamics and with increased pressure response to hyperglycaemia, in T1DM patients [46].

Bradykinin receptors. Bradykinin is a functional antagonist of Ang2 and it is considered a protective renal factor. The bradikinin receptors, type I (BKR1) and type II (BKR2), are members of the G-protein coupled receptor superfamily. BKR2 is the principal receptor for kinins, while BKR1 is expressed after tissue injury. BKRs polymorphisms may determine differences in response to kinin peptides, thus influencing disease evolution.

In Caucasian T2DM, the BKR1 promoter polymorphism G-699C and BKR2 C181T, in exon 2, are not associated with DN [47]. Other studies suggest that the less common alleles, BKR1 C and BKR2 T, prevent the progression of DN to ESRD [48,49].

Plasma prekallikrein genes. Kallikreins are a family of serine proteases, which release kinins from kininogens. Kinins are peptides which regulate blood pressure and contribute to the inflammatory process. In human, the kallikrein genes are clustered on 19q13.3–13.4 [50]. KLKB1 (plasma prekallikrein gene, previously known as KLK3) is located 4q34–35 and participates to the vascular bradikinin-dependent response and to the inflammatory processes.

In African American families with DM, the KLKB1 gene may have only a minimal contribution to ESRD susceptibility [51, 52].

Atrial natriuretic peptide. Atrial natriuretic peptide (ANP) is a regulator of systemic and renal circulation and of renal excretory function. Two linked SNPs have been identified in ANP by PCR RFLP, with Bstx1 (C708T) and ScaI (A1/A2 variants). The T708 and A1 alleles seem to be associated with reduced levels of ANP and with the presence of albuminuria, independent of other factors, like diabetes and hypertension [53]. A polymorphism in intron 2 has not been associated with DN, in T1DM and T2DM [54]. The contribution of additional polymorphisms, like T2238C and T2332C, to DN is not clear. However, in T1DM patients, they do not considerably increase the risk for DN [55].

Nitric oxide synthase. Nitric oxide (NO), produced by nitric oxide synthase (NOS) from L-arginine, is an important signalling molecule with many physiological functions, including the modulation of endothelium-derived relaxing factor, renal circulation and renin secretion. The oxidative stress involved in vascular dysfunction may be the result of NO or ACE inappropriate production.

The NOS family has three genes, neuronal NOS (NOS-1), inducible NOS (NOS-2A) and endothelial NOS (NOS-3), with partial homology and distinct functions. These genes have a tissues specific expression, although each of them can be expressed in multiple tissues, including the kidney.

Some polymorphisms of NOS-3 may affect NO production. The most studied polymorphism is a VNTR with 4 (a allele) or 5 (b allele) repeats, located in intron 4. In Japanese T2DM patients, the NOS 4a allele seems to be a risk factor for DN [56]. Recent studies cannot confirm this observation, but suggest that it is a risk factor for progression to ESRD, in nondiabetic patients [57, 58].

The NOS-2A expression is controlled, mainly at transcriptional level. The NOS2 has been less investigated because of the reduced number of known polymorphisms. A promoter polymorphism, represented by insertion (+) or deletion (-) of an AAAT sequence, has been correlated with transcriptional activity. In Caucasian T2DM, the "+" allele contributes to DN, independent of the diabetes duration [59]. Another investigated polymorphism is a (CCTTT)n repeat, located at 2,6 Kb upstream of the gene. In T1DM patients, the variant with 14 repeats seems to be protective for DN development [60]. A recent study cannot confirm the association of the NOS2A +/- and NOS-3 a/b polymorphisms with DN, in Caucasian T1DM patients [61].

Methylenetetrahydrofolate reductase. Methylene-tetrahydrofolate reductase (MTHFR) is involved in the transmethylation pathway, where homocysteine is converted into methionine.

A C677T transition, in exon 4 of MTHFR, which changes a conserved aminoacid (Ala226Val) in the folate binding site, has been associated with disease [62]. The T677 allele has been associated with impaired enzyme activity and middle hyperhomocysteinaemia.

MTHFR polymorphisms may contribute to nephropathy progression, by aggravating renal vascular injury, but results are contradictory [63]. The studies of T1DM and T2DM patients from Germany and Poland, and T1DM from Northern Ireland, did not find any association between C677T polymorphism and DN [64, 65]. In another study, the TT genotype has been strongly associated with DN, in T1DM [66].

Contradictory results have been found in Japanese T2DM patients, regarding the association between MTHFR and DN [63, 67, 68]. In a heterogeneous Israeli population, a relation between MTHFR polymorphism and DN was observed, after stratification for low serum folate levels [69].

β subunit of G proteins. Heterotrimeric GTP-binding proteins (G proteins) are involved in signal transduction from cellular receptors to intracellular components. These G proteins consist of three different subunits: α, β and γ.

In exon 10 of the gene for β3 subunit of G proteins, a C825T substitution has been identified. This polymorphism is associated with an alternative splicing variant and an in-frame deletion of 41 aminoacids, equivalent to 1 WD domain, which is encoded by exon 9 (GNB3s) [70]. The mechanism by which this SNP affects the splicing process is partially understood. The frequencies of 825 C and T alleles have a great variation in different populations [71].

The T825 allele and the GNB3s protein are associated with enhanced signal transduction and with hypertension, left ventricular hypertrophy, obesity, increased aldosterone to renin ratio and decreased kidney allograft survival [72–74]. A study has shown that the T825 allele can contribute to DN susceptibility, in T2DM patients [75]. Recent studies have shown that this allele does not confer an increased risk for DN, in T1DM or T2DM patients [75,76].

Plasminogen activator inhibitor-1. Plasminogen activator inhibitor-1 (PAI-1) is a member of the serpin family. It is a fibrinolysis inhibitor after vascular injury and its level is increased in endothelial dysfunction and in metabolic syndrome. PAI-1 may promote extracellular matrix accumulation, through reducing the activity of matrix degradative enzyme.

A promoter polymorphism, represented by deletion or insertion of one G (4G and 5G variants), affects the local binding of nuclear transcription factors. The G4 homozygous tend to have an increased PAI-1 plasma level. In T1DM Caucasian patients, the 4G/5G polymorphism does not confer a risk for DN [78].

Metabolic factors

Glucose transporter. The members of GLUT family are expressed in a tissue specific manner. In the glomerular and mesangial cells, the major type is glucose transporter 1 (GLUT1). It has been associated with extracellular matrix formation and with renal hypertrophy. The results of some studies suggest a possible link between GLUT1, hyperglycaemia and DN [21]. Nevertheless, the real marker of GLUT1 remains unknown.

In GLUT1 gene some SNPs have been identified: Xba1 (G/T, in intron 2), Hae III (T/C, in exon 2) and another, located in putative enhancer region: enhancer 1 SNP (C/T, located upstream of exon 1); enhancer 3 (C/T, upstream of enhancer 1 SNP); enhancer-2 SNP1 (A/G) and enhancer 2 SNP2 (C/T). A strong linkage disequilibrium between SNPs enhancer 2 SNP1 and Xba1 has been observed.

In Caucasian Mediterranean T2DM population, the XbaI polymorphism has not been correlated with microangiopathic complications, including DN [79].

In T1DM, an association between GLUT1 polymorphism (*e.g.*, Xba1-/-, enhancer 2 SNP1AA) and DN could not be confirmed by several studies [80-82]. The A-2718T substitution, located in the flanking region of GLUT1, has been associated with DN, in Caucasian T1DM [83].

Apolipoprotein E (ApoE) is involved in lipoprotein metabolism. The ApoE gene has three codominant alleles: ε2, ε3 (wild type) and ε4, which encode for proteins with different binding affinity to low density lipoproteins (LDL)-receptor. The ε4 allele has been associated with dyslipidaemia and coronary artery disease.

In T1DM patients, different studies have shown that ApoE alleles are not associated with DN or that they confer only a weak risk for this complication [78, 84, 85].

In Caucasian T2DM patients, the ε2 allele and a lower level of ApoE2 seem to be protective for DN [86]. In contrast, in Chinese T2DM patients, the ε2 allele confers a higher risk for DN; this effect is synergistic with that of the allele T of heparan sulfate proteoglycan [87].

Peroxisome proliferator-activated receptor γ2 (PPAR-γ2) is a ligand activated transcription factor, which controls expressions of genes involved in glucose and lipid metabolisms and in cell differentiation. It reduces the differentiation of preadipocytes into adipocytes and, as a consequence, the levels of several factors implicated in DN, like PAI-1, RAS components and collagen type IV, are diminished [88].

In Caucasian T2DM patients, the Pro12Ala polymorphism has been associated with DN, while the Ala12 allele seems to be the protective one [88].

Ecto-nucleotide pyrophosphatese / phosphodiesterase 1. Insulin resistance has been observed in diabetic patients with microvascular complications. Ecto-nucleotide pyrophosphatase / phosphodiesterase 1 (ENPP1) contributes to insulin resistance, through inhibition of insulin receptor autophosphorylation [89, 90]. ENPP1 is a membrane glycoprotein, expressed in various tissues, like muscle, fat, liver, kidney, mesangial and endothelial cells. Its function is partially understood. The A to C transition, in the first position of codon 121 (or 173, in respect with Bollen M.), changes lysine to glutamine (K121Q). It has been suggested that the Q allele is more potent for binding and inhibiting insulin receptor and it has been correlated with reduced insulin sensitivity, compared to K variant [81, 91]. Additional SNPs, in the 3'UTR, may modify mRNA stability and may predispose to insulin resistance [92].

The contribution of K121Q polymorphism to the development of DN seems to have a minor importance [81,93], but T1DM patients presenting albuminuria with Q allele have a faster rate of DN progression [94] and an increased risk to develop ESRD, early in the course of diabetes [93]. Some discordant reports found in European Caucasian population, referring to an association between ENPP1 and DN, may be the result of a difference in the genetic background and/or environmental conditions or survival bias [95].

Advanced glycosylation end-product-specific receptor. Hyperglycaemia or high levels of other reducing sugars lead to advanced glycation end-products (AGEs) formation. This multisteps process impairs metabolism of proteins and lipids, damages nucleic acids and changes extracellular matrix (ECM) composition and architecture. The specific receptor for AGEs, advanced glycosylation end-product receptor (RAGE), is a member of the immunoglobulin superfamily of the cell surface molecules.

RAGE is involved in the pathogenesis of diabetic vascular complications, *via* activation of NF-kB (an oxidative stress marker) and then, *via* VCAM-1 (an early marker of atherosclerosis). In the vascular system, RAGE is expressed at low level in normal conditions, and at high level in vascular diseases or after increasing AGEs level.

The RAGE T-429C and T-374A polymorphisms, in the promoter region, affect gene transcription and Gly82Ser polymorphism, located in AGEs binding domain, may affect interactions between receptor and ligands [96].

In T1DM patients with poor glycaemic control, there is a link between genetic and environmental factors in the genesis of renal and cardiovascular complications [97]. In another study, this finding has not been confirmed [64].

The RAGE Gly82Ser polymorphism seems not to be associated with susceptibility to T2DM, with or without macrovascular complications [98].

Aldose reductase gene. Aldose reductase (AR) is the first rate limiting enzyme of the polyol pathway, which is involved in diabetic microvascular complications. Its level is moderately increased in white cells from T1DM and T2DM patients and is much higher in erythrocytes from T2DM with nephropathy [99–101]. It was suggested that the AR polymorphisms may influence this level, but only in the presence of diabetes or hyperglycaemic state [102].

The AR gene has a (AC)n microsatellite located at 2,1 kb upstream from the transcription start site. The most common variant of this polymorphism has 24 repeats and is called the Z allele.

In British Caucasian T1DM and in Pima Indians T2DM patients, a linkage between DN and 7q region has been found [103]. This region contains a few presumed risk genes: AR, muscarinic acetylcholine receptor and eNOS.

Some studies on T2DM patients from Poland, Japan and Korea could not show a correlation between (AC)n and susceptibility to DN, but it has been suggested that this polymorphism could contribute to disease progression [101, 104, 105]. In Chinese T2DM patients, the Z-2 allele and the T variant of C/T SNP, located in the promoter region, are associated with severe diabetic microvascular complications [106].

Although a connection between Z-2 allele and the risk for DN has been presumed, in T1DM patients, recent studies from Australia, UK, Germany and a multicenter cross sectional study have not confirmed this association [102, 107–110].

Paraoxonase gene. In diabetic patients, chronic hyperglycaemia and oxidative stress contribute to tissue injury. Paraoxonase (PON) is a high-density lipoproteins (HDL)-associated enzyme, which protects tissue from oxidative damage and has the ability to hydrolyze organophosphorous compounds.

Paraoxonase family has three genes: PON1, PON2 and PON3, located on chromosomes 7 [111].

The PON1 polymorphisms C-107T, in the regulatory region, and Leu55Met, Gln192Arg in the coding region, affect transcription, serum concentration and activity of paraoxonase [112–114].

A case control study of Caucasian T1DM patients has shown that T-107C, Leu54Met, Gln192Arg polymorphisms are not associated with DN [115].

In Caucasian T2DM patients, PON2, but not PON1 polymorphism increases the risk for DN development, and obesity enhances this risk [116]. In turn, the PON1 C-107T polymorphism may influence insulin sensitivity of Japanese T2DM patients [117].

Cytokines and Growth Factors

The transforming growth factor β system has some key components: TGFβ1, latent TGFβ binding protein (LTBP-1), thrombospondin-1 and TGFβ receptors. TGFβ is a member of a dimeric polypeptide growth factors family.

TGFβ1 is widely expressed in endothelial, haematopoetic and connective-tissue cells, and it is secreted as an inactive form. After secretion, the main quantities are stored in ECM, from where they are released especially by trombospondin-1 [118]. TGFβ is involved in tissue repair: it is a chemotactic agent, which controls cellular growth and differentiation, angiogenesis and ECM production (TGFβ up-regulates the genes for ECM proteins and down-regulates the genes for ECM-degrading enzymes). Hyperglycaemia, AGEs and Ang2 change the TGFβ levels. An increase in TGFβ level leads to sclerotic diseases and has an important role in the pathogenesis of DN [26, 119, 120].

The evaluation of TGFβ system in skin fibroblasts from T1DM patients with DN revealed that, in patients who had a slow evolution of the disease, only the LTBP-1 mRNA was reduced [121].

A T29C polymorphism in the signal sequence region, which changes Leu10Pro, can be associated with TGFβ overexpression. In Chinese T2DM patients, the association of this polymorphism with obesity increases the risk of proteinuria [122].

IGF1 has a striking structural homology to proinsulin. It is involved in cell differentiation, glucose homeostasis, intrauterine and postnatal growth controls. A (CA)n polymorphism, located in the promoter region, has a common variant called the Z allele (192 bp). The correlation between this polymorphism and serum IGF1 levels, body height and susceptibility to DM is still contradictory [123–125]. In T1DM patients, plasmatic and urinary IGF1 levels have been associated with DN markers, like kidney volume, microalbuminuria or glomerular filtration rate [125, 126].

Chemokines and chemokine receptors. The inflammatory process is involved in renal diseases [127]. Some chemokines (*e.g.*, RANTES, monocyte chemoattractant protein, ILs) and chemokine receptors (*e.g.*, CCR2, CCR5) have been investigated in DN. Monocyte chemoattractant protein (MCP-1) is a proinflammatory chemokine, which contributes to ECM accumulation and mesangial proliferation. On the monocytes surface, the CCR2 and CCR5 are the main receptors for MCP-1 and RANTES, respectively.

The polymorphisms G59029A, in the promoter region of CCR5 and V64I of CCR2, have been investigated in T2DM patients from Japan. Only the 59029A variant may be an independent risk factor for progression to ESRD [128].

In addition, the adhesion molecules, which mediate leukocyte binding to endothelium, like LECAM-1, can contribute to the renal inflammatory process. The SNP C/T, in exon 6 of LECAM-1, represents an independent risk factor for DN, in Japanese T2DM patients [129].

Vascular endothelial growth factor (VEGF). is a cytokine which induces endothelial cells proliferation and increases the vascular permeability. In human mesangial cells, its levels can be increased by AngR1 stimulation. A polymorphism located in position –2549 of the vascular endothelial growth factor (VEGF) promoter region, represented by an insertion (I) or deletion (D) of 18 bp, has been identified. *In vitro*, the D allele has been associated with enhanced gene expression. This allele contributes to DN susceptibility, and a cumulative effect between VEGF and AR is also possible [130].

Other putative genes involved in DN

Other genes involved in different metabolic or regulatory pathways can contribute to genetic susceptibility for DN.

The β3-adrenergic receptor is predominantly expressed in adipose tissue and is involved in lipid metabolism and regulation of microvascular circulation. The Trp64Arg polymorphism has been correlated with some components of the X metabolic syndrome, like T2DM, insulin resistance, fat accumulation and high BMI. In Japanese T2DM patients, the association of β3-adrenergic receptor with DN is contradictory [131–133]. In Caucasians T1DM and T2DM, a contribution of β3-adrenergic receptor to DN has not been found [134, 135].

The polymorphisms of lipoprotein lipase (Asn291Ser) and cholesteryl ester transfer protein (presence or absence of a restriction site for Taq1B, in intron 1) have been investigated in T1DM, but an association with susceptibility for DN has not been found [85].

The mutations in the haemochromatosis gene have been associated, in some studies, with insulin resistance and T2DM. In T2DM Polish population, the C282Y and H63D mutations in haemochromatosis gene increase the risk for DN [136].

Other genes may have a role in: glomerular or mesangial proliferation (*e.g.*, suppressor of cytokine signalling 2, *via* IGF1 signalling [137]), extracellular matrix accumulation or degradation (*e.g.* ADAMTS 3, 6, 9, matrix metalloproteinases, decorin), fibrosis (*e.g.*, connective tissue growth factor) and glucose toxicity (*e.g.*, GFPT2).

The mitochondrial mutations are associated with complex phenotypes with variable expression. In some cases, these phenotypes include DM and renal diseases. The heteroplasmy makes difficult to estimate the real contributions of these mutations in the disease.

The substitution (*e.g.*, A3243G) or large mitochondrial deletion (*e.g.*, between positions 8214-13991) can contribute to DN development [138, 139]. Initially, the A3243G substitution in the tRNA^{Leu} gene has been associated with MELAS (mitochondrial myopathy, encephalopathy, lactacidosis, stroke) syndrome. This mutation has a frequency of about 1% in diabetic ESRD patients from Japan [140]. Oxidative stress induced by hyperglycaemia increases the conversion of deoxyguanosine to 8-hydroxydeoxyguanosine in DNA, which favours mitochondrial DNA deletions. In the muscle of T2DM patients, the mtDNA deletions of 4977 bp (delta mtDNA 4977) and 8-hydroxydeoxyguanosine levels increase with severity of DN and diabetic retinopathy [141].

In addition, nuclear genes, like poly (ADP-ribose) polymerase-1 (PARP), which encoded for proteins with mitochondrial function, can be involved in DN. Additional putative genes with an uncertain role in DN are presented in Table 6.2.

Table 6.2

Putative genes which may have a role in genetic susceptibility to DN or in disease progression

	GENE	**Localisation**	**OMIM ID**
1	ADAMTS3	4q21	605011
2	ADAMTS6	Chr 5	605008
3	ADAMTS9	3p14.3-p14.2	605421
4	Alkylglycerone phosphate synthase	2q31	603051
5	alpha-4 actinin	19q13	604638
6	Angiotensin receptor type 2	Xq22-q23	300034
7	Cathepsin E	1q31	116890
8	CD2 Associated Protein	6	604241
9	CD37 antigen	19p13-q13.4	151523
10	Chemokine receptor 2	3p21.3	601267
11	COX-2	1q25.2-q25.3	600262
12	Decorin	12q13.2	125255
13	Endothelin 1	6p24-p23	131240
14	Fibronectin 1	2q34	135600
15	Galectin-3	14q21-q22	153619
16	GFPT2	5q34-q35	603865
17	Glycerol-3-phosphate dehydrogenase 1	12q12-q13	138420
18	Growt arrest specific gene 6 (Gas6)	13q34	600441
19	Heparan sulfate proteoglycan/ Syndecan 2	8q22-q24	142460
20	Heparanase-1	4q21.3	604724
21	Hepatic leukemia factor	17q22	142385
22	Hepatocyte growth factor	7q21.1	142409
23	HNF	20q12-q13.1	600281
24	HSD11B2	16q22	218030
25	hSGK	6q23	602958
26	IGF1R	15q25-q26	147370
27	IL6	7p21	147620
28	Interferon regulatory factor 3	19q13.3-q13.4	603734
29	Lactate dehydrogenase C	11p15.5-p15.3	150150
30	Matrix metalloproteinases 9	20q11.2-q13.1	120361
31	MCP-1	17q11.2-q12	158105
32	MnSOD	6q25.3	147460
33	Nephrin (NPHS1)	19q13.1	602716
34	Podocin (NPHS2)	1q25-q31	604766
35	Poly(ADP-Ribose) Polymerase	1q42	173870
36	Protein Kinase Cβ isoform	16p11.2	176970
37	RANTES	17q11.2-q12	187011
38	Renin	1q32	179820
39	SA	16p1311	145505
40	SLC12A3	16q13	600968
41	Spectrin, alpha, erythrocytic 1	1q21	182860
42	SOCS2		605117
43	Uncoupling protein 2	11q13	601693
44	ZNF236	18q22.3-q23	604760

*additional information about the genes can be found, using the ID number, at the following internet address: http://www.ncbi.nlm.nih.gov/Omim/searchomim.html

Conclusions

Epidemiological data show that only a part of DM patients develop DN and these patients have a variable rate of progression to ESRD. The diabetic milieu, genetic susceptibility and environmental factors lead to DN. The genetic base for diabetic vascular complication is polygenic. Every candidate gene may has a small effect and the genetic susceptibility is the result of the balance between the risk ("bad") and the protective ("good") alleles. Until now, there is no known allele or haplotype with major effects on DN susceptibility. This suggests that a large number of genes must be investigated by further studies, for the identification of useful genetic markers.

At the moment, it is impossible to predict, only through genetic means of investigation, which patients will develop DN or how this will progress. Numerous studies have tried to elucidate different pathophysiological components for DN, necessary for the identification of novel possible targets for drugs design and for the development of screening strategies. In most cases, the calculated risk for DN, conferred by genetic polymorphism, is weak and it does not prove a certain pathogenetic relationship. In addition, for the vast majority of investigated polymorphisms, we do not know if these are functional or if they are just in linkage to a true causative marker.

The contradictory results of genetic analysis in diabetic vascular complications are intriguing and provocative. These discordant results, frequently observed in different studies, may reflect:

1) difference in genetic backgrounds and environmental conditions;

2) heterogeneity of DN, at the genetic and phenotypic levels, especially in T2DM;

3) variable contribution of the same allele to DN, in different populations;

4) the strength of linkage between the investigated polymorphisms and the true markers of the disease;

5) some bias caused by study design (*e.g.* inclusion or exclusion criteria, survival bias, selection of control group) or by publication.

For a better understanding of DN susceptibility, more studies are necessary, which will have to extend the investigation to additional genes, which can affect the intraglomerular pressure, glomerular permeability, basement membrane thickening, matrix expansion.

DIABETIC RETINOPATHY

Diabetic retinopathy (DR) is the most common complication of type 1 diabetes and the major cause of new-onset blindness among diabetic adults. The incidence of retinopathy in type 1 diabetes is high, affecting 70–100% of all patients [142].

The main effects of DR are: floaters, blurred and hazy vision, reduced visual acuity, visual field defects, spots and abnormalities in colour vision. DR can be a highly symptomatic disease even before significant visual acuity loss occurs, and these symptoms may not be detected by standard clinical assessments. The visual effects can be categorized, but there is great inter-patient variability in their manifestation. Therefore, qualitative research provides a valuable contribution to the evidence base.

The diagnostic criteria and classification of retinopathy were defined as follows:

1. Non-proliferative retinopathy – microaneurisms, hard exudates, haemorrhages, mild venous dilatation, few "cotton wool" spots;

2. Pre-proliferative retinopathy – same as grade 1 plus venous dilatation;

3. Proliferative retinopathy – retinal proliferation with none of the following: fibrovascular bands, retinal detachment, vitreous haemorrhage;

4. Advanced proliferative retinopathy – retinal proliferation with any of the following: fibrovascular bands, retinal detachment, vitreous haemorrhage.

Two of the complications of DR involve proliferation of endothelial cells and increased retinal vascular permeability. Alterations of the glucose transport system in retinal endothelial cells are involved in the pathogenesis of DR. Retinal hypoxia is responsible for the development of intraocular neovascularization and increased retinal vascular permeability. Although cellular hypoxia correlates with an increased glucose uptake due to elevated glucose transporter mRNA and posttranslational alterations [143], the mechanisms responsible for the hypoxia-induced regulation of the glucose transport system in retinal vascular cells is not completely understood.

According to the DCCT Research Group's (1995) [144], the mean glycosylated haemoglobin (HbAlc) value should be kept below 7% in order to prevent retinopathy. Hyperglycaemia-induced generation of reactive oxygen species (ROS) is linked by three pathological pathways to diabetic complications: the activation of protein kinase C, the formation of advanced glycation end-products, and the sorbitol accumulation. Normalizing mitochondrial ROS production blocks these hyperglycaemia-mediated signalling pathways [145].

Hyperreactive platelets in diabetic patients interact with an exposed subendothelium of damaged vessels and enhance microthrombus formation or small vessel occlusion *in vivo*. This, in turn, might alter retinal blood flow. Moreover, evidence indicating the beneficial effect of antiplatelet therapy [146] on retinopathy suggests the involvement of platelets in the pathogenesis of microangiopathy. The platelet adhesion is a first critical step for primary thrombus formation and leads to intracellular activation processes. There is increased secretion of β-thromboglobulin and platelet factor 4, which are markers of platelet activation *in vivo* [147]. The values of platelet activation markers in diabetic patients without microangiopathy are higher than those in patients without microangiopathy [148].

In proliferative diabetic retinopathy (PDR), initially extensive active proliferation of new vessels occurs [149], followed by visual loss due to vitreous haemorrhage or fluid exudation from fragile new vessels. With time, or after laser photocoagulation, the proliferating vessels become fibrotic and involute, causing traction on the retina that may lead to complications such as retinal detachment [150]. Eventually the disease becomes inactive and further visual loss ceases [151]. The timely inhibition of factors that cause active vascular proliferation may prevent visual loss.

Pericytes isolated from the retina of diabetic eye donors show overexpression of CPP32, a member of the family of interleukin-1β–converting enzymes with caspase activity [152]. Pericytes studied *in situ* in human diabetic retinas show increased levels of Bax – a death-inducing member of the Bcl-2 family – often in association with fragmented chromatin [153]. Bax is also expressed by retinal ganglion cells and cells of the inner nuclear layer, and its levels are increased in preparations of the whole human diabetic retina [153]. Neural cells of the inner retina manifest signs of apoptosis in human and experimental diabetes, even in the absence of retinal microangiopathy [154].

Several genes have been associated to DR, including VEGF, aldose reductase (AR2), PON, α2β1 integrin, IGF-1, ACE, RAGE, RAS, tumor necrosis factor (TNF) genes, the family of NOS enzymes, LDL, ET, PARP and glucagon-like peptide-1 (GLP-1).

Vascular endothelial growth factor

Retinal angiogenesis is a key process for the progression of DR that leads to blindness. Two factors, VEGF, an endothelial cell-specific angiogenic and growth factor, and pigment epithelium-derived factor (PEDF), a potent antiangiogenic factor, play a crucial role in the initiation of retinal angiogenesis. Whereas the increased VEGF level is a major cause responsible for retinal neovascularization, PEDF has a role in maintaining function and structure in retinal capillaries.

Retinal ischaemia induces intraocular neovascularization, which often leads to glaucoma, vitreous haemorrhage, and retinal detachment by stimulating the release of angiogenic molecules. VEGF, a 45-kDa homodimeric glycoprotein [155], is a major mediator of vascular permeability and angiogenesis, and also an important mediator of retinal ischaemia-associated intraocular neovascularization [156]. VEGF's production is increased by hypoxia. VEGF levels are markedly elevated in vitreous and aqueous fluids in the eyes of individuals with PDR [157]. In addition, VEGF induction of vascular permeability may contribute to the development of non-PDR [156].

Seven polymorphisms in the promoter region, 5' untranslated region (UTR) and 3'UTR of the VEGF gene, are associated with DR in type 2 diabetes Caucasian patients [158]. VEGF has at least five isoforms generated through the alternative splicing of mRNA arising from a single gene. The two major prevalent isoforms in the retina are VEGF121 (120) and VEGF165 (164). RNase protection assays have identified VEGF164 as the predominant VEGF isoform expressed in the diabetic retina [159].

Hypoxia regulates VEGF gene transcription by activating the transcription factor, hypoxia inducible factor-1 (HIF-1). HIF-1 is a basic-helix-loop-helix transcription factor, which is composed of two subunits, HIF-1α and HIF-1β. HIF-1β, also known as the arylhydrocarbon nuclear translocator, is constitutively expressed, whereas HIF-1α expression is increased upon hypoxia. In the absence of adequate signals (hypoxia or growth factor stimulation), HIF-1α is rapidly ubiquitinated by the von Hippel-Lindau tumor suppressor E3 ligase complex, and subjected to proteasomal degradation [160]. Under hypoxic conditions or after stimulation with growth factors, HIF-1α is not degraded and accumulates to form an active complex with HIF-1β.

DR is frequently complicated by macular oedema, a pathologic condition that is a direct consequence of blood-retinal barrier breakdown. Macular oedema can appear at any time during the course of DR and is one of the greatest sources of vision loss in diabetes [161]. An effective pharmacological treatment for this complication of diabetes does not currently exist. In the human retinal vasculature, leukocyte counts and intercellular adhesion molecule (ICAM-1) immunoreactivity are both increased in eyes with DR [162]. In experimental diabetes, the inhibition of VEGF suppresses retinal ICAM-1 expression, leukostasis [163] and blood-retinal barrier breakdown [159].

In physiological conditions, pericytes produce high levels of PEDF and prevent abnormal endothelial cell proliferation. Simultaneously, PEDF acts as an autocrine survival factor for pericytes. In hypoxia, PEDF expression by pericytes decreases and contributes to hypoxia-induced angiogenesis in DR.

Aldose reductase

AR2 is the first and rate-limiting enzyme of the polyol pathway and converts glucose to sorbitol in a reduced nicotinamide adenine dinucleotide phosphate (NADPH)–dependent reaction. Sorbitol is subsequently converted to fructose by the sorbitol dehydrogenase enzyme with nicotinamide adenine dinucleotide $(NAD)^+$ as cofactor [164]. Under hyperglycaemic conditions there is increased flux through the polyol pathway, and this in turn leads to a number of metabolic and vascular abnormalities that may ultimately cause tissue ischaemia. *In vivo*, both increased enzyme activity and expression of the AR gene have been reported in patients with diabetic microvascular complications [165].

A (CA)n dinucleotide repeat sequence 2.1 kb upstream of the transcription start site of the AR gene, is strongly associated with human DR [166] and linked to increased expression of the AR gene [167].

A novel polymorphism in the AR gene promoter region located at C-106T is strongly associated with DR in adolescents with type 1 diabetes. Ko *et al.* (1995) [166] studied one of VNTR's, an (AC)n polymorphic marker, located 2.1 kb upstream of the AR gene in the chromosome 7 and found that one of the alleles, the (AC)23 (also called 'Z-2'), was associated to early appearance of retinopathy in type 2 diabetic patients from Hong Kong. The (AC)n polymorphic marker associated to the 5' end of AR gene is also related to an enhanced rate of progression of retinopathy in type 2 diabetic patients [166, 168, 169].

The (AC)23 allele, either by direct binding of transcription factor(s) [170], or by modulating the activation of the promoter [171], could rise the upper limit of the expression of the AR gene. Under that condition, and in the presence of hyperglycaemia, such (AC)23 person would have higher intracellular AR activity than in another diabetic who lacks the allele, then more Diacylglycerol would be formed, and more activation of β2 protein kinase C and faster progression of retinopathy would ensue [172].

The 'Z-2' allelic frequency among 44 type 2 diabetics of Hong Kong was eight times higher than in diabetics without retinopathy, both groups being similar with respect to mean HbA1, duration of the disease, treatment, renal function and prevalence of hypertension [168].

The patients with retinopathy had an increased frequency of the Z-2 allele compared to patients with uncomplicated diabetes (33.6% and 14.3%, respectively). Conversely, the Z+2 allele was decreased in the patients with retinopathy compared to patients with uncomplicated diabetes (13.2% and 33.6%, respectively). The normal control subjects had intermediate Z-2 and Z+2 allelic frequencies compared to those for the uncomplicated diabetes and retinopathy groups.

Chinese and Japanese patients with type 2 diabetes and retinopathy have an increased frequency of the Z-2 5'AR2 allele [173]. Similar findings have been reported for young white adolescents from Australia with T1DM and an early onset of retinopathy [174].

The C/Z-2 haplotype may identify individuals who have enhanced levels of AR mRNA, and the presence of this haplotype may lead to an increased flux through the polyol pathway. In contrast, the C/Z+2 haplotype may be associated with reduced gene expression. Increased gene expression would result in excessive production of sorbitol and fructose, metabolic and vascular abnormalities, and oxidative stress in the cell.

These polymorphisms will provide useful markers for genetic studies of the role of AR and for searching for potential candidate genes in diabetes complications [174].

Paraoxonase

Oxidized low-density lipoprotein (LDL) cholesterol is toxic to the endothelial cells and pericytes in retinal capillaries. An important mechanism contributing to DR may be the oxidation of LDL with consequent injury to retinal endothelia and pericytes. Oxidation of LDL plays an important role in the development and progression of cardiovascular disease, with high-density lipoprotein (HDL) cholesterol potentially protecting LDL from oxidation. The protective effect of HDL is due to serum paraoxonase (PON) [175] – a glycoprotein, which binds HDL and prevents oxidation of LDL by hydrolyzing lipid peroxides. PON is a multigene family. Three of its members, namely PON1, 2 and 3 are all located on chromosome 7.

α2β1 Integrin

The platelet membrane glycoprotein Ia/IIa, α2β1 integrin, a platelet receptor for collagen, mediates platelet primary adhesion to subendothelial tissues, which is an essential first step in thrombus formation. The gene encoding α2 integrin has at least eight polymorphisms, including two silent polymorphisms located within the I domain [149] 224Phe (TTT/TTC) due to a T/C transition at nucleotide 807 (T807C) and 246Thr (ACA/ACG) due to an A/G transition at nucleotide 873 (A873G) [176], and a Bgl II restriction fragment length polymorphism (Bgl II) within intron 7. These three polymorphisms are in linkage disequilibrium, the Bgl II (+) allele being linked to the 807T allele and 873A allele and the Bgl II (-) allele being linked to the 807C allele and 873G allele [177].

The Bgl II polymorphism has been reportedly associated not only with platelet α2β1 density, but also with the extent of platelet adhesion to collagen, and the prevalence of myocardial infarction or stroke [177, 178]. Bgl II (+) containing platelets interacts more easily with nonenzymatically glycosylated collagen and accelerates the occurrence of retinopathy. Patients with the Bgl II (+/-,+/+) genotype might benefit more from antiplatelet therapies.

Insulin-like growth factor 1

Increased growth hormone and insulin-like growth factor 1 (IGF-1) levels accelerate the progress of severe retinopathy. IGF-1 promotes the survival of multiple cell types by activating the IGF-1 receptor (IGF-1R), which signals down-stream to a serine/threonine kinase termed Akt. In the retina of diabetic human donors, IGF-1 mRNA levels are threefold lower than in age-matched nondiabetic controls, whereas IGF-1R activation and signalling are not affected [179].

Both IGF-1 and IGF-1R are expressed in the inner retina [180], and retinal microvascular cells produce [181] and respond to IGF-1 *in vitro* [182]. Activation of the IGF-1R exerts powerful antiapoptotic effects, protecting multiple cell types against a variety of death signals [183]. The phosphorylation of Akt/protein kinase B occurs through the sequential steps of IGF-1R-mediated activation of insulin receptor substrate-1, in turn activating phosphatidylinositol 3-kinase, which activates Akt [183, 184]. Akt promotes cell survival through phosphorylation of several substrates: Bad – a member of the Bcl-2 family – which becomes unable to heterodimerize with, and thus inactivate, prosurvival Bcl-XL [183]; caspase 9, which loses protease activity [185], and members of the Forkhead family of the transcription factors, which are prevented from translocating to the nucleus and activating proapoptotic genes [184].

The efficacy of somatostatin analogues in the treatment of advanced DR has been largely attributed to its effectiveness in lowering serum IGF-1. However, somatostatin may also have a direct antiproliferative effect on human retinal endothelial cells. The inbalance between angiogenic and antiangiogenic factors is crucial for the development of PDR. There is a deficit of somatostatin in the vitreous fluid of diabetic patients with PDR [186].

Haurigot *et al.* (2003) [187] have used transgenic mice as an experimental model in order to study the influence of IGF-1 in DR. Over-expression of IGF-1 in the photoreceptors of the transgenic retina led to protein accumulation in the aqueous humor. Thickening of the basal membrane and loss of pericytes are the first hallmarks of non-PDR. Vascular occlusion, venous dilatation and bleeding, widespread capillary non-perfusion areas and intraretinal microvascular abnormalities were also observed. Neovascularization, the main feature of the proliferative stage, was also detected within the retina. Vascular alterations correlated with VEGF increase. Moreover, IGF-1/VEGF molecular signalling pathways were activated in these eyes, as shown by increased phosphorylation of PKB/Akt. Over-expression of GFAP in Müller cells was also observed. Transgenic mice also developed cataracts and rubeosis iridis, which may be the cause of secondary glaucoma.

The renin-angiotensin system

RAS components such as ACE, prorenin, angiotensinogen, angiotensin I and angiotensin II, renin and specific binding sites for angiotensin II have been identified in human eyes. Because angiotensin II is a potent vasoconstrictor and angiogenic factor, local RAS is also involved in the pathogenesis of proliferative retinopathy found in some diabetic patients. This is evidenced by the fact that prorenin increases in the ocular vitreous fluid [188] and plasma of patients with PDR. Angiotensin II production in the diabetic eye is a causative factor in neovascularization [189]. Therefore, an ocular RAS may be implicated in the proliferation of retinal blood vessels and blindness in diabetic patients.

Angiotensin-converting enzyme

ACE, a key enzyme in the renin-angiotensin system, catalyzes the conversion of angiotensin I to angiotensin II in the liver and inactivates bradykinin in many tissues. ACE insertion / deletion (I/D) polymorphism, characterized by the presence (insertion) or absence (deletion) of a 287-bp AluI-repeat sequence inside intron 16, is associated with coronary artery disease in type 2 diabetic patients [185].

Attenuated fibrinolysis is one of the factors that accelerates the formation of microthrombi in the microcirculation which characterizes PrePDR. Thus, if angiotensin II-induced microvascular occlusion and neovascularization participate in the pathogenic mechanism of ADR (advanced diabetic retinopathy), high ACE content in the retina due to a high frequency of D allele may provide a rationale to explain why ACE inhibitors prevent local conversion of angiotensin I to angiotensin II. Matsumoto *et al.* (2000) [190] detected a significant relationship between the presence of the D allele in the ACE gene polymorphism and ADR in Japanese subjects with type 2 diabetes and normoalbuminuria or early-stage microalbuminuria.

The receptor for advanced glycation end-products

Among several etiopathological mechanisms proposed in DR, AGEs, formed due to nonenzymatic glycation of proteins, is one of the key components causing microvascular complications. Interactions between AGEs and RAGE are implicated in the vascular complications of diabetes. AGEs result from the nonenzymatic glycation of proteins and lipids [191], which form during aging and at an accelerated rate in diabetes as a result of hyperglycaemia.

AGEs produce a plethora of effects through a number of mechanisms. Firstly, AGEs alter vascular structure and trap circulatory proteins, leading to a narrowing of the lumen [191]. Secondly, AGEs modify intracellular proteins and DNA, resulting in cellular changes. Thirdly, the principle means of derangement of AGEs is by specific AGEs-binding receptors, which include the AGEs-receptor complex [192], the macrophage scavenger receptors [193], and RAGE [194], a member of the immunoglobulin superfamily.

During diabetes, the increased concentration of AGEs results in their binding to AGEs-binding proteins. Several AGEs-binding proteins have been identified, including p60 homologous to OST-48, p90 homologous to 80K-H (a PKC substrate), galectin-3, and RAGE [170]. Cell treatment with glycated proteins leads to generation of reactive oxygen species, activation of ERK1/2, and activation of the transcription factor NF-kB [195]. AGEs stimulate VEGF mRNA expression through an increase in HIF-1α accumulation and activation of HIF-1. Moreover, AGEs-induced VEGF expression and HIF-1α accumulation are dependent on ERK. Therefore, blockage of HIF-1 activity by ERK inhibitors could be used as a therapeutic approach to inhibit AGEs-induced neovascularization during diabetes.

The significant suppression of angiogenesis by retinal microvascular endothelial cells during diabetes may be mediated, at least in part, by serum-derived AGEs, with a modulatory role for galectin-3. This may have implications for microvascular repair during the vaso-degenerative stages of DR.

Both excessive formation and accumulation of AGEs and increased interleukin-6 have been implicated in the pathogenesis of diabetic vascular complications. The increased formation of AGEs in the vitreous could promote hyperpermeability of retinal vessels in diabetes through the production of IL-6 from retinal Müller cells.

Glyceraldehyde- and glycolaldehyde-derived advanced glycation end-products (glycer-AGEs and glycol-AGEs), senescent macroproteins formed at an accelerated rate in diabetes, are mainly involved in loss of pericytes, the earliest histopathological hallmark of DR. When human microvascular cultured endothelial cells (EC) were cultured with glycer-AGEs or glycol-AGEs, growth and tube formation of EC, the key steps of angiogenesis, were significantly stimulated. These AGEs increased DNA synthesis and tube formation to about 25% and 50%, respectively. The AGEs-induced growth stimulation was significantly enhanced in RAGE – overexpressed EC, while it was completely blocked by treatments with antisense DNA against RAGE mRNA. Furthermore, AGEs increased transcriptional activity of nuclear factor-kB (NF-kB) and activator protein-1 (AP-1) to about 2-fold, and then up-regulated mRNA levels of VEGF and angiopoietin-2 in EC. Cerivastatin, a hydroxymethylglutaryl CoA reductase inhibitor, significantly inhibited AGEs-induced VEGF mRNA up-regulation, NF-kB and AP-1 transcriptional activation, DNA synthesis and tube formation in microvascular EC. AGEs induced VEGF overproduction through transcriptional activation of NF-kB and AP-1, eliciting angiogenesis. By blocking AGEs-RAGE signalling pathways, Cerivastatin might be a promising remedy for treating patients with PDR, at least in theory [196].

The gene for RAGE is localised on chromosome 6p21.3 in the MHC locus and is composed of a 1.7-kb 59 flanking region and 11 exons [197]. RAGE is normally expressed at low levels by the endothelium, smooth muscle, mesangial, and monocytes [198]. In both animal models and human diabetic subjects, high levels of RAGE expression have been identified in the retina, mesangial and aortic vessels, concomitantly with AGEs accumulation [199].

In normal homeostasis, RAGE binds and internalizes low levels of AGEs for degradation; however, in diabetes, because of the sustained interaction of higher levels of AGEs, this appears to lead to receptor mediated activation and secretion of various cytokines [200]. These induce a cascade of protein expression, among which increased tissue factor [201] and fibrinolytic inhibitor plasminogen-activator inhibitor-1 [202] expression promote a procoagulant state. Further endothelial dysfunction is brought about by the recruitment of monocytes *via* a RAGE-dependent mechanism to these sites of AGEs accumulation [203]. *In vitro* studies have demonstrated that a feedback loop of increasing expression of RAGE, *via* nuclear factor–kβ, results from AGEs-RAGE binding to enhance these effects [200]. Inherited differences in key transcription binding sites involved in RAGE gene regulation could alter this pathway of events by either increasing or decreasing RAGE expression.

Because of the dense nature of genes within the MHC locus, part of the 59 flanking region of RAGE overlaps with the 39 untranslated region (UTR) of the PBX2 gene [197], further complicating the correct identification of the polymorphisms due to the presence of a pseudogene copy of PBX2 on chromosome 3.

Hudson *et al.* [204] have found in the RAGE gene seven polymorphisms in exons and two in introns. Due to this, four functional amino acid changes were detected: Gly82Ser (exon 3), Thr187Pro (exon 6), Gly329Arg (exon 8), and Arg389Gln (exon 10). Gly82Ser polymorphism is particularly interesting because of relatively high prevalence and the polymorphism results in the creation of an Alu1 restriction site (AG↑CT). The nucleotide changes can be rapidly screened by PCR-RFLP method. Ser82 allele in the RAGE gene is a low-risk allele for developing DR in Asian-Indian patients who have type II diabetes [205]. Single nucleotide polymorphisms T-374A, T-429C and a 63 bp deletion in the RAGE promoter region affect the transcriptional repression of RAGE gene.

TNF genes

The TNFα and TNFβ genes on chromosome 6 are 1–2 kilobases apart. TNFβ gene, otherwise known as lymphotoxin α (LTα), is one of the candidate genes involved in the predisposition to DR [206]. TNFβ or LTα is a member of a large family of cytokines with diverse functions, like induction of inflammation, apoptosis, and regulation of lymphocyte proliferation. It binds and signals through members of TNF-Receptor family of cell surface receptors. Monos *et al.* (1995) [207] confirmed the genetic polymorphism of human TNF region in the IDDM. It was also reported that HLA-DR phenotype is a risk factor for the development of PDR independent of glycaemic exposure [208]. From two sets of studies performed in type 2 diabetic patients of South Indian origin, it was inferred that there was an association between human TNF polymorphism and DR. The TNFβ microsatellite marker had 18 alleles and was identified with sizes ranging from 97 to 131 base pairs. Kumaramanickavel *et al.* (2002) [209] found four alleles of size 111, 127, 129 and 131 bp and identified allele 4 (103 bp) with (GT)9 repeat as a low risk allele for developing DR in the Indian population. After separation of the data for North and South Indian patients, the research group found that allele 4 was still significant as a low risk allele. Allele 8 (bp 111) had more risk for developing PDR.

Because low concentrations of TNF increase angiogenesis and high concentrations inhibit angiogenesis, these mechanisms could be playing some role in the presence of allelic polymorphism in making diabetic patients susceptible or protected from developing retinopathy.

The family of NOS enzymes

Most neoangiogenic effects of VEGF in severe forms of DR are mediated by nitric oxide (NO). NO, resulting from NO synthetases (NOS), stimulates vasodilation and modulates endothelial cell proliferation, migration and blood vessel formation. NO has antithrombogenic and antiplatelet regulatory activities, can act both as a free radical scavenger and as a free-radical itself, and has growth regulatory effects on the vascular smooth muscle. Modulation of the NO/NOS pathway alters the phenotype of blood vessels resulting from hemangioblast activity in the retina [210].

Three members of the nitric oxide synthase gene family, namely: NOS1, NOS2A and NOS3 play a role in the diabetic retina. Under normal conditions, NOS2A is not expressed in the retinal vasculature. Exposure to high ambient glucose influences NO release *via* increased NOS2A expression and reduced constitutive endothelial NOS gene (NOS3) expression in cultured retinal vascular endothelial cells [211].

LDL

Capillary leakage is an early feature of DR, and resulting exposure of pericytes to modified LDL, including glycated (G-LDL) and heavily-oxidized-glycated LDL (100 mg protein/l, 24 hr) (HOG-LDL), contribute to pericyte loss. Modified LDL is implicated in apoptotic loss of capillary pericytes in early DR. Exposure to glycated / oxidized LDL increases pericyte diacylglycerol (DAG). DAG activates classical and novel PKCs, regulating a variety of important cellular functions, including apoptosis. In particular, activation of PKC-β has been implicated in processes leading to DR. The activation of PKC is intimately related to translocation and binding to cell membranes. Stimulation of increased DAG levels by modified LDLs induces activation of PKC and contributes to pericyte loss. PKC inhibitors may mitigate DR in part by inhibiting of retinal pericyte death mediated by modified LDL [212].

Endothelin

Changes in retinal blood flow are an early manifestation of DR. Elevation of endothelin-1 (ET-1) is an important mediator of the reduced retinal blood flow. ET-1 was increased in diabetic retina within one week after onset of hyperglycaemia, and remained persistently elevated up to 12 weeks. There was a comparatively delayed and modest increase in ET-3 expression and an increased expression of ET receptor- A, but this was normalized with increasing duration of diabetes. Retinal blood flow was significantly reduced after 2 weeks of diabetes, though this reduction became diminished with increasing duration of diabetes. Using adenoviral transfection studies *in vivo*, Ma *et al.* (2003) [213] showed also that PKC β1, but not PKC δ, mediated the effect of hyperglycaemia on retinal blood flow.

Poly(ADP-ribose) polymerase-1

PARP is a nuclear DNA nick-sensor enzyme involved in the poly(ADP-ribosyl)ation. Potential adverse effects of PARP overactivation include damaging cells *via* energy depletion. Zheng *et al.* (2003) [214] have assessed the effect of a potent PARP inhibitor (PJ34) on diabetes-induced abnormalities of retinal function (ERG), ICAM expression and leukostasis within retinal vessels, and on hyperglycaemia induced death of retinal endothelial cells and pericytes *in vitro*. Elevated glucose caused a significant increase in death of both capillary cell types *in vitro*, and this was inhibited in a dose-dependent manner by PJ34. *In vivo*, diabetes increased activity of PARP in retina and retinal capillary endothelial cells and pericytes. Diabetes also resulted in increased expression of retinal ICAM, abnormal ERG, and leukostasis within retinal vessels. PJ34 significantly inhibited all of these defects. Inhibition of PARP corrects several metabolic and physiologic defects associated with the development of DR.

Glucagon-like peptide-1

GLP-1, an incretin hormone, is released from the intestinal L-cells. GLP-1 binds to the specific receptor (GLP-1R), a member of G-protein-coupled receptor, on the pancreatic β-cell and stimulates glucose-dependent insulin secretion and also growth and proliferation of β-cells. To address the possibility that the partial disruption of GLP-1 signalling could cause diabetes, Tokuyama *et al.* (2003) [180] detect the mutation in GLP-1R gene in the population with type 2 diabetes, and found a rare case with mutated GLP-1R. Five missense mutations were detected: Pro7Leu (CCG > CTG), Arg44His (CGC > CAC), Arg131Gln (CGA > CAA), Thr149Met (ACG > ATG), Lue260Phe (TTA > TTC). Only the proband had Thr149Met mutation in GLP-1R gene. No mitochondrial DNA mutation at positions 3243, 1555, 11778, 3460, 14484, 9101, 9804 and 14498 was detected in peripheral white blood cells. Ophthalmological study showed PDR. Thr149 is located in the first transmembrane domain of GLP-1R and thus this mutation could impair its function, though function analysis remains to be examined. The proband exhibited the severe impairment of both insulin secretion and glucose effectiveness. This diabetic phenotype, in this case, could be partially explained by Thr149Met mutation in GLP-1R.

Conclusion

The role of genetic influences in DR has been difficult to define due to differences in patient recruitment methods, patient selection criteria, risk factors, variation in ethnicity, and clinical differences in evaluating retinopathy status. The coming years promise to be exciting ones in the field of genetics of diabetic complications. Many laboratories throughout the world are taking part in the search for susceptibility genes, and several large initiatives are currently under way to establish large data resources for genetic studies. These activities will provide a tremendous opportunity to improve our understanding of the genetic basis of eye disease among those with diabetes.

DIABETIC NEUROPATHY

Diabetic neuropathy is an extremely common complication in patients with DM, especially in T1DM. The prevalence of diabetic neuropathy, in T1DM patient, was estimated to about 25% in Europe. However, in Romanian patients, the estimated prevalence is much higher than in the rest of Europe, and namely about 70% (Bucharest center) [215]. There are two types of neuropathy: peripheral and autonomic.

Diabetic autonomic neuropathy (AN) affects both T1DM and T2DM patients. Its prevalence is about 20–40% in the patients with long-term diabetes, but those with systemic hypertension, renal complication or peripheral neuropathy, are more probably to have this failure. It was proposed that AN is a consequence of a long-term hyperglycaemia, but it was observed that subclinical AN can appear, also, in the family members of T2DM subjects, in the absence of hyperglycaemia [216, 217]. This can be explained by the inheritance of the susceptibility alleles which, in association with metabolical or environmental factors, leads to neuropathy [218].

Diabetic peripheral neuropathy, the most common form of diabetic neuropathy, is a multifactorial disease which can affect about 30% of diabetic patients [219, 220].

The cause of diabetic peripheral neuropathy is still unknown, but several mechanism believed to be implicated in the pathogenesis of this complication are described. The first event of neuropathy development is represented by metabolical factor alteration, such as hyper-glycaemia, which is considered the major risk factor for this complication [220]. Starting from this, there is a variable number of pathological mechanisms controlled by several genes, which are maybe involved in diabetic neuropathy development. The most studied genes are those involved in polyol pathway and oxidative stress, mechanisms closely related to pathogenesis of diabetic neuropathy. Many factors have implications in DN. Among these, the polymorphism of AR gene, the AR protein level, accumulation of sorbitol and fructose, along with a depletion in the level of myoinositol, responsible for decreased nerve conduction velocity, were shown to be correlated with diabetic neuropathy. A functional osmoregulatory element (AR-ORE) at the 5' end of AR was identified. In over-efficient condition, it leads to accumulation of sorbitol in the nerve [221]. Other two genes, which encode for two antioxidant enzymes, mitochondrial and extracellular superoxide dismutase (Mn-SOD and Ec-SOD), were investigated in a Russian T1DM group. This study has shown that a polymorphism (Ala-9Val) in exon 2 of Mn-SOD is associated with diabetic neuropathy [222]. The Ala-9Val variant affects the processing efficiency of the enzyme, so that the homozygous Val/Val have lower resistance to oxidative stress, which can lead to protein oxidation and damage of mitochondrial DNA, common failures in the pathogenesis of diabetic neuropathy [223, 224].

DIABETIC MACROVASCULAR COMPLICATIONS

Diabetic patients are exposed to a number of cardiovascular risk factors (*e.g.*, abnormal glycaemia, lipidaemia, hypertension, oxidative stress and visceral obesity) which impair endothelial function and predispose to macrovascular disease (MVD). The MVD, represented especially by coronary artery disease (CAD), peripheral artery disease (PAD) and cerebrovascular disease, is the major cause of morbidity and mortality in diabetic patients. All these clinical manifestations increase the mortality rate about three times compared to nondiabetic population [225]. Both environmental and genetic factors are involved in pathogenesis of MVD, but the diabetic status, *per se*, is one of the major risk factors. We will present briefly some of the genes related to endothelial dysfunction.

Lipoprotein metabolism impairments

Lipoprotein lipase (LPL) is a heparin-releasable enzyme, bound to glycosaminoglycan components of the capillary endothelium, and is particularly abundant in the muscle, adipose tissue and macrophages.

LPL plays an important role in lipoprotein metabolism by hydrolyzing triglycerides (TG) in very low-density lipoproteins (VLDL) and chylomicrons -apolipoprotein (Apo) CII as an essential co-factor [226, 227]. A reduction of LPL activity leads to increased levels of TG [226]. In consequence, LPL is regarded as a risk factor for cardiovascular complications, both in diabetic and in non-diabetic populations [227].

The gene for LPL is an obvious candidate for contributing to inherited predisposition for dyslipidaemia and risk of CAD. The human LPL gene has been assigned to chromosome 8p22. The gene spans about 30 kb and contains 10 exons coding for a 475 amino acid protein including a 27 amino acid signal peptide [226].

Three polymorphisms, Asp9Asn (in exon 2), Asn291Ser (in exon 6) and the S447X (in exon 9), in the LPL gene, were identified. The frequencies of Asn9 and Ser291 alleles varied from 1.5 to 5%, in different populations. The X447 allele is found in approximately 20% of healthy European populations [228].

The S447X polymorphism seems to be correlated with changes in TG level and blood pressure, and with vascular disease [229]. In nondiabetic population, this polymorphism has a minor contribution to CAD [230]. The nondiabetic patients, heterozygous for T-93G, Asp9Asn, Gly188Glu or Asn291Ser, have dyslipidaemia and an increased susceptibility to CAD [231, 232]

Additional polymorphisms in LPL, like PvuII (in intron 6), and Hind III (in intron 8), are associated with high TG levels. In diabetic patients, Hind III polymorphism is associated with changes in triglyceride and HDL cholesterol levels and premature CAD. In T2DM, the rare allele of PvuII polymorphism is also associated with elevated triglyceride levels and severity of CAD and it seems to be protective against atherosclerosis [226].

The Ser447Stop mutation localised 635 bp downstream from the HindIII polymorphism is a consequence of a C to G transversion at nucleotide 1595 in exon 9, which converts the serine 447 codon (TCA) to a premature termination codon (TGA). The risk of CAD is decreased by Ser447Stop polymorphism, which underlies increased HDL cholesterol levels and decreased triglyceride levels. Thus, Ser447Stop polymorphism should have a protective effect against the development of atherosclerosis and subsequent CAD, because it seems to be associated with a reduced risk of atherothrombotic cerebral infarction. Asn291Ser polymorphism of the LPL gene is associated with reduced HDL cholesterol levels and premature atherosclerosis [229, 230].

The significant linkage disequilibrium between LPL polymorphisms (*i.e.*, the Ser447Stop mutation is in significant linkage disequilibrium with HindIII and PvuII) make difficult the identification of the real marker for the association with lipid metabolism.

In human LPL promoter has been identified a peroxisome proliferator-activated receptor (PPAR) response element [233]. PPAR-γ is a transcriptional factor that belongs to the nuclear receptor family, and has three isoforms: PPAR-γ1, PPAR-γ2, and PPAR-γ3 [233]. The Pro115Glu substitution in the PPAR-γ2 isoform has been associated with some features of the X metabolic syndrome, such as dyslipidaemia, obesity and insulin resistance. In a Finnish nondiabetic population, the Pro12Ala substitution was correlated with lower BMI, improved insulin sensitivity and increasing HDL cholesterol [234]. The 12Ala allele is very rare in T2DM patients, therefore it is considered a protective factor for diabetes [230, 233].

Hepatic lipase. Human hepatic lipase (HL) is a lipolytic enzyme synthesized primarily in the liver. After secretion from hepatocytes, the enzyme binds to the hepatic sinusoidal endothelial surface, where it hydrolyzes triglycerides and phospholipids contained in plasma lipoproteins. Hepatic lipase is another regulatory factor for plasma lipids level and it is an important enzyme in lipoprotein metabolism, with a role in mediating remnant lipoprotein uptake [235–238].

The human HL gene (LIPC), located on chromosome 15q21, comprises 9 exons and 8 introns, spans about 35 kb of DNA, and encodes for a peptide of 449 amino acids [235].

The HL and LPL have a considerable homology, and they have probably a common ancestral gene. Plasma HDL cholesterol (HDL-C)

levels are inversely correlated with HL activity; specifically, HL promotes the conversion of large, buoyant HDL to small, dense HDL by modulating the phospholipids content of these particles. Epidemiological studies in humans have indicated that a low level of plasma HDL-C is one of the major risk factors for CAD. The plasma HDL concentration is modulated by environmental factors such as obesity, cigarette smoking and a sedentary life-style. Between 40% and 60% of the interindividual variation in HDL-C levels is accounted for by genetic variability. In normolipidaemic subjects, allelic variation at the LIPC locus accounted for 25% of the interindividual variation in plasma HDL-C levels [235].

The genetic polymorphisms affect HL activity, and have been associated with changes in HDL-cholesterol levels [238]. The prevalence of small, dense LDL is associated with an increased risk of premature CAD and is a common trait in the general population. The polymorphism located in the 5' flanking region, like G-250A, C-514T, T-710C and A-763G, are in strong linkage disequilibrium [235, 237]. The alleles: -250A, -514 T, -710C and -763G are associated with decreased HL activity and increased HDL cholesterol levels [237].

The G-250A, C-514T and S267F (splice site mutation in intron 1) polymorphisms were associated with CAD in Korean patients without DM [238].

The C-480T polymorphism is associated with higher HDL (HDL2) and less small, dense LDL levels, which, in turn, increases the risk for CAD in T2DM patients [239, 240].

The -514T HL allele, which is associated with low HL activity and increased plasma HDL-C concentrations is more common among African-Americans than among white Americans [236].

Men have twice the HL levels of women and have smaller, more dense LDL particles. A polymorphism in the promoter region of the HL gene accounts for 20% of the variation in HL activity among normal subjects and for 32% among coronary disease patients and contributes to the modulation of the LDL buoyancy in these two groups [235].

HL activity represents a potential therapeutic target by which LDL density and coronary disease risk may be favourably affected. HL activity may be inhibited directly at its site of action or indirectly by modulation of the gene promoter region. HL is a potential key mediator of beneficial therapeutic effects on lipoprotein composition and coronary risk. These insights may help to improve substantially on the 20% to 35% cardiovascular risk reduction seen with treatment strategies focused on LDL-C lowering [235].

Apolipoprotein C. Apolipoprotein CIII (ApoCIII) participates in the regulation of the metabolism of triglyceride-rich lipoproteins (TRL) and it is a constituent of VLDL, which binds to syalic acid and glucidic residues. ApoCIII inhibits the activity of HL, affecting TRL metabolism [241, 242]. Diabetic patients have a higher plasma ApoCIII and TG levels than nondiabetic subjects, and a higher risk for CAD [242].

The APOC3 gene is located in the highly polymorphic APOA1-C3-A4 gene cluster on chromosome 1 [240]. APOC3 gene has an insulin response element (IRE), a proximal promoter and a distal regulatory region, that acts as a common enhancer for the three genes of the cluster [243].

The -455 and -482 polymorphisms, located in the putative IRE of APOC3 gene, are responsible for the loss of insulin regulation of APOC3 and for overexpression of the APOC3 gene, which contributes to the development of hypertriglycerides (HTG) and CAD [244].

The C3238G polymorphism, in the 3'UTR, also known as SstI polymorphism, is a CAD risk factor in T2DM and in nondiabetic populations. The SstI polymorphism accounts for approximatively 5% of LDL-C variability in response to changes in dietary fat in men. The least common allele of this polymorphism, named S2, has a variable frequency in different ethnic groups: 0.08% in Caucasian and 0.25% in Japanese populations [245, 246]. In nondiabetic populations, S2 allele has been associated with higher TG levels, lower concentration of HDL-C and increased apoCIII non HDL in men, and with increased ApoB levels and LDL cholesterol in women. Despite these observations, in a Framingham study it was observed that the S2 allele is a weak risk factor for CAD [241]. The men carriers of the S2 allele showed increased fasting insulin plasma levels, compared to non-carriers [241].

The mild association of the S2 allele with decreased HDL-C levels could be attributed to linkage disequilibrium of the S2 allele with other polymorphisms at the APOA1 locus, which may affect the expression of the APOA1 gene. Moreover, the APOA1 and APOC3 genes share common regulatory elements and mutations at these regions could also affect the expression of APOA1 [241].

Apolipoprotein E. Apolipoprotein E (ApoE) – a glycoprotein composed of 299 amino acids, is a constituent of VLDL, intermediary density lipoproteins (IDL) and HDL. It binds with high affinity to the LDL receptor-related protein, starting intracellular lipid metabolism [230, 247, 248].

Three isoforms for ApoE have been identified. They are encoded by three alleles: ε2, ε3 and ε4, differentiated by substitutions in codons 112 and 158 [247, 249, 250]. The ε3 isoform has cysteine and arginine at position 112 and 158, respectively. The ε4 has arginine and the ε2 has cysteine at both sites. The presence of the ε4 allele tends to associate with higher serum total cholesterol level, and in contrast the ε2 allele seems to be related to the lower serum total cholesterol values in normolipidaemic subjects. The cholesterol modulating effect of ApoE has been attributed to regulation of the LDL-receptor.

In T2DM, the ε2 allele can provide protection to, while the ε4 allele tends to increase the risk against macrovascular complications [247].

Carriers of Apoε4 have higher plasma levels of total and LDL cholesterol than Apoε2 or Apoε3 homozygotes. Apoε4 is a significant risk factor for different diseases (*i.e.* Alzheimer) but confers only a moderate risk for CAD.

The binding of ApoE2 to lipoprotein receptors is defective in comparison with that of ApoE3 or ApoE4 and results in delayed clearance of triglyceride lipoproteins. ApoE2 has been strongly associated with the development of type III hyperlipoproteinaemia and subsequent CAD as well as with rare forms of lipoprotein glomerulopathy [250].

The mechanisms by which ApoE isoforms may influence the development of diabetic microvascular complications are unclear. ApoE isoforms are associated with lipid abnormalities. Compared with ApoE3, individuals with ApoE2 have lower cholesterol and higher triglyceride levels. Dyslipidaemia caused by the ApoE2 isoform may promote the development of vascular complications. A high level of ApoE localizes to the extracellular matrix after nerve injury, suggesting that ApoE has some role on the tissue repair system. ApoE2 accumulates in the mesangial area under diabetic conditions and changes the properties of mesangial matrix or cell functions [250].

Dysfunction of ApoE leads to HTG, supporting the idea that ApoE is involved in the development of atherosclerosis in diabetic patients [251, 252]. The ε2 allele and the lower seric LDL cholesterol levels seem to confer protection, and the ε4 allele tends to be a risk factor for macrovascular complications in diabetic subjects [230, 247].

Cholesteryl ester transfer protein. The cholesteryl ester transfer protein (CETP), a hydrophobic glycoprotein composed of 476 aminoacids, mediates the transfer of cholesteryl ester from HDL-LDL and VLDL in exchange for triglycerides and plays an important role in the reverse cholesterol transport system. High plasma levels of CETP are associated with reduced HDL cholesterol levels and increased LDL cholesterol levels. The increase in cholesteryl ester transfer rate in plasma of patients with T2DM is due to alterations in the composition and concentration of endogenous lipoproteins [253–255]. The CETP is another factor thought to contribute to the development of macrovascular complications, including atherosclerosis. HDL cholesterol concentration is inversely related to the risk of CAD [256].

Several mutations in the gene for CETP have been reported, and most of them affect plasma HDL cholesterol levels, resulting in an increased risk for atherosclerosis. The substitution of the 227 nucleotide in the first intron of CETP gene was identified by RFLP with TaqI. This polymorphism seems to affects lipid-transfer activity and HDL cholesterol concentrations [257, 258]. The two alleles of TaqI (B1 and B2) have a different effect in T2DM patients. B1 allele seems to be associated with progression of CAD, while men with B2B2 genotype have a lower incidence of ischaemic disease [230].

In Japanese T2DM patients, TaqIB polymorphism was found to be an important risk factor for macroangiopathy [253]. The association of CETP gene polymorphism with increased risk for atherosclerosis, in T1DM patients, is not sufficiently studied [259].

Paraoxonase (PON) is a serum enzyme, HDL-associated, with a molecular mass of 43 kDa and 354 amino acids, which protects LDL against oxidation, through the hydrolysis of lipid peroxides. This antioxidant effect is one of the natural antiatherogenic mechanisms. It represents the basis for assessment of PON in CAD. [230, 260–262].

Serum PON activity, based on the capacity of the enzyme to hydrolyze paraoxon, varies among individuals and populations. The PON gene family has three known members, PON1, PON2 and PON3, located on the long arm of chromosome 7 between q21.3 and q22.1. In humans, all PON are capable of impeding lipid peroxidation and could therefore act in an antiatherosclerotic manner. Within a given mammalian species, PON1, PON2 and PON3 share approximately 60% identity at the amino acid level and about 70% identity at the nucleotide level. Between mammalian species, each of the three genes shares 79–90% identity at the aminoacid level and 81–91% identity at the nucleotide levels. Codon 106 (lysine) present in PON1 is missing in all PON2 and PON3 cDNA's sequenced to date [230, 261, 263].

The M55L substitution is correlated with PON1 serum levels and the Q192R substitution affects enzyme activity [230, 261, 263–265]. The carrier for Q192 allele exhibits lower concentrations of total TGs and ApoB, and higher concentrations of Apo AII than those with R allele [261]. RR genotype, compared with RQ and QQ genotype, manifests the lowest capacity for protecting LDL against oxidative modification and is correlated with an increased risk of CAD [263, 266]. This effect was observed in a nondiabetic population. The involvement of PON1 activity in diabetic patients with macrovascular disease is still contradictory. In T1DM patients from Japan a significant association of R allele with CAD was detected [267]. Also, diabetic patients with R allele had about a three time higher risk for myocardial infarction than QQ genotype [268]. In T1DM populations, the R192Q polymorphism can be an independent risk factor for CAD [267].

The contradictory results of association of PON1 55L allele with atherosclerosis could be explained by a greater interindividual variation in the enzymatic activity of PON1 [261]. This polymorphism, located in the NH2- terminal region of the peptide, affects the binding ability of paraoxonase to HDL [269]. *In vivo*, the PON1 55L allele is more effective for protecting LDL against oxidation than M allele [261].

In the 5' upstream region of the PON1 gene, five polymorphisms (-107/-108, -126, -160/-162, -824/-832 and -907/-909) which affect the transcription of the gene were detected. The allele frequencies for PON1 polymorphisms differ among ethnic groups. Only the allele frequency of -108 polymorphism does not differ between white and Japanese populations. This may be a coincidence, or selection pressures may have acted on this polymorphism to maintain specific allele frequencies across different ethnic groups [261].

The C-108T polymorphism is located in a putative site for transcriptional binding factor Sp1 [263, 270]. The -108T, -824G and -907C alleles are associated with lower expression, serum concentration and activity of PON1, therefore, are regarded as risk factors for CAD in T2DM [264].

The effect of G-909C, C-108T and A-162G polymorphisms on PON1 activity is caused by linkage disequilibrium with the functional polymorphisms, like L55M and Q192R [270]. Linkage disequilibrium between -108C and 192R PON1 alleles can also explain the lower capacity of protection against atherosclerosis. -107T, -824G and -907C were associated with lower serum PON levels, whereas -107C, -824A and -907G were correlated with the highest concentrations and activities [270].

The correlation of PON1 allele with myocardial infarction is still unclear. There is a possiblity that a particular allele, in particular conditions, may confer a risk for CAD [268]. The diabetes status increases the risk of association between an individual gene and macrovascular complications [230].

Endothelial vascular impairment

Smoking, hypertension, dyslipidaemia and T2DM are associated with endothelial dysfunction. Through impaired NO and free radicals production, hyperglycaemia mediates endothelial dysfunction, which is regarded as an initial event in the development of diabetic macrovascular complications [271].

Nitric oxide synthase. There are three distinct isoforms of NOS: neural NOS-1 (nNOS), inducible NOS-2 (iNOS) and endothelial NOS-3 (eNOS), transcribed from a separate gene. Each NOS enzyme has its own unique aminoacid structure sharing some 50 percent homology. NO is an extremely important signalling molecule in the cardiovascular system. Atheroscleropathy is related to the underproduction and/or the excessive consumption of eNO by redox stress [271].

The eNOS is a 1203 aminoacid protein enzyme and it is constitutively expressed in vascular endothelium and is responsible for arterial vasodilatation. In the vascular complications of diabetes, NO has an opposing impact. This paradoxal effect is the result of a different biological context and involvement of various NOS isoforms.

The gene encoding eNOS is located on chromosome 7q35-36 and comprises 26 exons spanning 21 kb. Several polymorphisms in the NOS3 have been associated with susceptibility to CAD in T2DM patients.

Two alleles in intron 4 of the eNOS gene have been identified. The larger 4b allele consists of five tandem 27-bp repeats. In the 4b allele, the first three repeats have A and the last two G at the 19th base of the 27-bp repeat, and in the 4a allele the first two repeats have A and the last two G at the 19th base of the repeat. The 4a/b polymorphism located in intron 4 of the eNOS has been associated with CAD. The 4a allele has been associated with elevated blood pressure, and it may contribute to hypertension in T2DM. The 4a/a genotype increases the risk for smoking-dependent CAD and endothelial dysfunction in T2DM patients [272, 273]. In T2DM patients, the 4a/b heterozygous could influence the endothelium-dependent vasodilatation, but not endothelium independent vasodilatation, through NO production or release [274].

The polymorphism identified at position 1917 (Glu298Asp), in exon 7 of the eNOS gene seems to play a major role in the development of T2DM and in accelerating atherosclerosis, but the association with CAD is still contradictory [271, 272–276].

Tumor necrosis factor. Tumor necrosis factor (TNF)-α is a proinflammatory cytokine produced by macrophages associated with the atheroma plaque, with effects on endothelial function, coagulation, lipid metabolism and insulin resistance. TNFα affects lipid metabolism by decreasing LPL activity and, therefore, it is considered an important risk factor for CAD [277, 278]. Its action is characterized by the stimulation of adhesion molecule production, thrombogenesis, smooth muscle proliferation, platelet activation and release of vasoactive agents.

Variable expression of TNFα in humans, as a consequence of the variability of the TNFα gene, has been demonstrated by *in vitro* studies, showing a different transcription rate in lymphocytes according to a polymorphism located in the promoter of the gene at position -308. Because the presence of an A allele (related to a greater -308 TNFα mRNA transcription rate) is associated with a greater insulin resistance, the carriage of an A allele could represent a link between T2DM and increased CAD risk [277].

TNFα gene is in linkage disequilibrium with lymphotoxin α (TNFβ or LTα) gene, another proinflammatory cytokine which plays a key role in the initiating of local vascular inflammatory response [279]. The genes for these cytokines are located in tandem within the MHCIII region on the short arm of chromosome 6 [278].

The contribution of two polymorphisms, the G-308A (with A1 and A2 allele) in the TNFα promoter region and the G252A (with B1 and B2 allele) in the first intron of TNFβ gene, in the progression of atherosclerosis is still unclear [278].

The TNFA2 allele is associated with increased gene transcription rate and higher TNFα levels, which predispose to inflammatory diseases, such as atherosclerosis [279].

Similarly to TNFA2 allele, TNFB1 is associated with an increased level of LTα, related to increased gene transcription [279].

Vendrell *et al.* (2003) have studied the G-308A and found that the -308A variant could increase CAD risk especially in T2DM women, whereas Keso *et al.* (2001) showed that TNFA and B polymorphism have a minimal effect on CAD in non diabetic middle-aged men [277, 278].

Since atherosclerosis is an inflammatory process and TNFα is a mediator of inflammatory response, it could be speculated that in diabetic patients with CAD, TNFα has a high level.

Advanced glycation end-products. Advanced glycation end-products (AGEs) play a major role in diabetic complications by inducing oxidative stress, inflammation and vascular dysfunction. These accelerated effects in DM patients may represent the main cause of endothelial dysfunction in DM [280].

RAGE has been studied in diabetic vascular complications. The Gly82Ser polymorphism, in the AGEs-binding domain, was not found to be related to macrovascular complications in diabetic populations [281, 282]. The common promoter polymorphisms, T-429C and T-374A, were thought to be associated with macrovascular complications. Additional studies did not show any correlations between these polymorphisms and macrovascular complications in nondiabetic population [282].

Other putative genes

Plasminogen activator inhibitor-1. PAI-1 produced by the liver, adipose tissue, and vascular cells, is the main fibrinolytic system inhibitor. Elevated circulating levels of PAI-1 represent an increased risk factor for CAD in patients with insulin resistance [283]. A deletion-insertion polymorphism (4G/5G) in the promoter region was shown to be associated with myocardial infarction and, also, with an increased level of PAI-1 in T2DM. In diabetic patients with CAD, the 4G/4G genotype was encountered more frequently than 5G/5G [230, 283].

MTHFR. A C677T transition in MTHFR, in TT form is associated with enzyme thermolability and decreased activity, higher levels of total homocysteine and increased risk of CAD in Japanese population [284, 249]. The frequency of the thermolabile MTHFR phenotype in the nondiabetic population is about 5% [284].

Apolipoprotein AI (ApoAI) is the major protein constituent of HDL cholesterol [230]. In the presence of normal HDL-cholesterol level, low serum ApoAI concentrations could represent an important factor for CAD development [285]. The polymorphisms in the apo(a1) gene can affect apo(a) and HDL levels [286, 287]. Therefore, the T83C polymorphism is associated with increased HDL cholesterol in nondiabetic subjects, but not in T2DM patients [288].

Elevated levels of HDL cholesterol and apo(a1) are associated with a reduced risk of developing CAD, probably because of the ability of HDL particles to promote cholesterol efflux from the cells [288].

Lipoprotein a [Lp(a)] differs from LDL by the presence of apo(a), which confers the unique structural and functional properties to Lp(a) [289]. High Lp(a) concentrations and the apo(a) isoforms are the risk factor for MVD. The apo(a) isoforms present differences in Kringle-IV (K-IV) numbers repeats [290]. The apo(a) gene is located in a region which contains IDDM8 locus [291]. The number of K-IV repeats is inversely correlated with Lp(a) plasma concentrations and is associated with T1DM and with T1DM life expectancy [292].

Variants in the apo(a1) gene have been recently reported that potentially could modify HDL cholesterol and apo(a1) levels. A G-to-A transition in the promoter region of the apo(a1) gene (-75 bp) is relatively common, occurring in approximately 20% of normal Caucasians. Hypomethylation which occurs in the T and/or A substitution at the 5' region of the apo(a1) gene increases apo(a1) gene expression. The T and/or A substitutions which are located in the 5'-end leader region of the apo(a1) mRNA could be important for the initiation of mRNA translation. The apo(a1) gene (+83 bp) is less common than the G-for-A substitution in the promoter region (-75 bp), but it could be an important marker for the risk of CAD if it significantly affects HDL cholesterol levels [288].

Renin-Angiotensin System. In addition to poor glycaemic control, additional factors controlling blood pressure could increase the risk for development of MVD in DM patients [293]. From this point of view, genetic RAS polymorphisms are an intensely studied marker linked to susceptibility to macrovascular complications in diabetes.

The 1166C allele of angiotensin-II type 1 receptor was associated with hypertension, severity of coronary artery stenosis in a population with artery disease, and in another study, with lower office blood pressures, compared to AC or AA genotype [294, 295].

Several studies show that ACE DD-genotype is associated with an increased risk for CAD in T1DM, myocardial infarction in T2DM, and hypertensive cardiovascular disease with endothelial cell damage [296–299]. The presence of the I allele of the ACE-ID polymorphism was associated with protection against CAD in T1DM patients with nephropathy [300]. In addition, it has been shown that in patients with atherosclerosis and D allele, acute administration of ACE inhibitor improves coronary epicardial and microvascular endothelium-dependent vasomotility [301]. In patients with CAD, the ACE DD genotype increased the risk for myocardial infarction [302].

Conclusions

The genetic polymorphisms in the genes which encode for enzymes and proteins which are involved in lipid metabolism, such as LPL, HL, apolipoproteins, CETP, etc., have been shown to affect plasma lipid concentrations and to be correlated with susceptibility to macrovascular complications.

REFERENCES

1. Cheţa DM. *Preventing diabetes: theory, practice, and new approaches*, John Wiley&Sons, Chichester, pp 1–4, 1999.
2. Remuzzi G, Betani T. Pathophysiology of progressive nephropathies. *N Engl J Med*, **12:** 1448–1456, 1998.
3. Nelson RG, Knowler WC, Pettitt DJ, Bennett PH. Kidney Diseases in Diabetes. Chapter 16. http://diabetes.niddk.nih.gov/dm/pubs/america/pdf/chapter16.pdf.
4. Trevisan R, Viberti G. Pathophysiology of diabetic nephropathy. In: LeRoit D, Taylor SI, Olefsky JM (eds). *Diabetes Mellitus: a fundamental and clinical text,* 2nd edition, Lippincott, Williams & Wilkins, Philadelphia, 2000, 898–910.
5. Chowdhury TA, Dyer PH, Kumar S, Barnett AH, Bain SC. Genetic determinant of diabetic nephropathy. *Clinical Science*, **96:** 221–230, 1996.
6. Rippin JD, Patel A, Bain SC. Genetics of diabetic nephropathy. *Best Pract Res Clin Endocrinol Metab*, **15:** 345–358, 2001.
7. Ibrahim HA, Vora JP. Diabetic nephropathy. *Best Pract Res Clin Endocrinol Metab*, **3:** 345–358, 2001.
8. Rossing P, Tarnow L, Nielsen FS, Boelskifte S, Brenner BM, Levine SA, Parving HH. Short stature and diabetic nephropathy. *BMJ*, **310:** 296–297, 1995.
9. Rao PV, *et al.* Genetic basis for nephropathy phenotype in Asian Indians with type 2 diabetes mellitus. *Diabetologia*, **46**(S2): A337, 2003.
10. Canani LH, Gerchman F, Gross JL. Familial clustering of diabetic nephropathy in Brazilian type II diabetic patients, *Diabetes*, **48:** 909–913, 1999.
11. Fava S, Hattersley AT. The role of genetic susceptibility in diabetic nephropathy: evidence from family studies. *Nephrol Dial Transplant*, **17:** 1543–1546, 2002.
12. Fioretto P, Steffes MW, Barbarosa J, Rich SS, Miller ME, Mauer M. Is Diabetic nephropathy inherited? Studies of glomerular structure in type 1 diabetic sibling pairs. *Diabetes*, **48:** 865–869, 1999.

13. Imperatore G, Knowler WC, Pettitt DJ, Kobes S, Bennett PH, Hanson RL. Segregation analysis of diabetic nephropathy in Pima Indians. *Diabetologia*, **49**: 1049–1056, 2000.

14. Chowdhury TA, Dyer PH, Mijovic CH, Dunger DB, Barnett AH, Bain SC. Human leukocyte antigen and insulin gene regions and nephropathy in type 1 diabetes. *Diabetologia*, **42**: 1017–1020, 1999.

15. Perez-Luque E, Malacara JM, Olivo-Diaz A, Alaez C, Debaz H, Vazquez-Garcia M, Garay ME, Nava LE, Burguete A, Gorodezky C. Contribution of HLA class II gene to end stage renal disease in Mexican patients with type 2 diabetes mellitus. *Hum Immunol*, **61**: 1031–1038, 2000.

16. Fagerudd JA, Pettersson-Fernholm KJ, Grönhagen-Riska C, Groop PH. The impact of a family history of type II diabetes mellitus and the risk of diabetic nephropathy in patients with type I diabetes mellitus. *Diabetologia*, **42**: 519–526, 1999.

17. Fagerudd JA, Tarnow L, Jacobsen P, Stenman S, Nielsen FS, Pettersson-Fernholm KJ, Gronhagen-Riska C, Parving HH, Groop PH. Predisposition to essential hypertension and development of diabetic nephropathy in IDDM patients. *Diabetes*, **47**: 439–444, 1998.

18. Deinum J, Tarnow L, Gool JM, Bruin RA, Derkx FH, Schalekamp MA, Parving HH. Plasma renin and prorenin and renin gene variation in patient with insulin dependent diabetes mellitus and nephropathy. *Nephrol Dial Transplant*, **14**: 1904–1911, 1999.

19. Rankinen T, *et al*. AGT M235 and ACE ID polymorphism and exercise blood pressure in the Heritage family study. *Am J Physiol Heart Circ Physiol*, **279**: H368–H374, 2000.

20. Arnett DK, Borecki IB, Ludwig EH, Panakow JS, Myers R, Evans G, Folsom AR, Heiss G, Higgins M. Angiotensinogen and angiotensin converting enzyme genotypes and carotid atherosclerosis: the atherosclerosis in communities and the NHLBI family heart studies. *Atherosclerosis*, **138**: 111–116, 1998.

21. Pettersson K, *et al*. Analyses of genotype combinations in genes of the Renin-Angiotensin-Aldosterone system and diabetic nephropathy in type 1 diabetic patients. *Diabetes*, **52**(S1): A49, 2003.

22. Montgomery H, Clarkson P, Barnard M, Bell J, Brynes A, Dollery C, Hajnal J, Hemingway H, Mercer D, Jarman P, Marshall R, Prasad K, Rayson M, Saeed N, Talmud P, Thomas L, Jubb M, World M, Humphries S. ACE gene I/D polymorphism and response to physical training. *Lancet*, **353**: 541–545, 1999.

23. Crisan D, Carr J. Angiotensin I-converting enzyme. Genotype and disease association. *J Mol Diagnostic*, **3**: 105–115, 2000.

24. Feng Y, Niu T, Xu X, Chen C, Li Q, Qian R, Wang G, Xu X. Insertion/Deletion polymorphism of the ACE gene is associated with type 2 diabetes. *Diabetes*, **51**: 1986–1988, 2002.

25. Pedersen-Bjergaard U, Agerholm-Larsen B, Pramming S, Hougaard P, Thorsteinsson B. Prediction of severe hypoglycaemia by ACE activity and genotype in type I diabetes. *Diabetologia*, **46**: 89–96, 2003.

26. Blobe GC, Schiemann WP, Lodish HF. Role of Transforming Growth Factors β in human disease. *N Engl J Med*, **342**: 1350–8, 2000.

27. Penno G, Chaturvedi N, Talmud PJ, Cotroneo P, Manto A, Nannipieri M, Luong L, Fuller JH, EUCLID study group. Effect of angiotensin-converting enzyme gene polymorphism on progression of renal disease and the influence of ACE inhibition in IDDM patients. *Diabetes*, **47**: 1507–1511, 1998.

28. Kario K, Kanai N, Nishiuma S, Fujii T, Saito K, Matsuo T, Matsuo M, Shimada K. Hypertensive Nephropathy and the gene for ACE. *Arterioscler Thromb Vasc Biol*, **17**: 252–256, 1997.

29. Viswanathan V, Zhu Y, Bala K, Dunn S, Snehalatha C, Ramachandran A, Jayaraman M, Sharma K. Association between ACE gene polymorphism and diabetic nephropathy in South Indian patients. *JOP*, **2**: 83–87, 2001.

30. Canani L *et al*. The Association of Angiotensin Converting Enzyme (ACE) Insertion/Deletion (I/D) polymorphism and the presence of diabetic nephropathy in patients with type 2 diabetes mellitus according to the duration of diabetes. *Diabetes*, **52**(S1): A479, 2003.

31. Fava S, Azzopardi J, Ellard S, Hattersley TA. ACE gene polymorphism as a prognostic indicator in patients with type 2 diabetes and established renal disease. *Diabetes Care*, **24**: 2115–2120, 2001.

32. Solini A, Dalla Vestra M, Saller A, Nosadini R, Crepaldi G, Fioretto P. The Angiotensin – converting enzyme DD genotype is associated with glomerulopathy lesions in type 2 diabetes. *Diabetes*, **51**: 251–255, 2002.

33. Marre M, Jeunemaitre X, Gallois Y, Rodier M, Chatellier G, Sert C, Dusselier L, Kahal Z, Chaillous L, Halimi S, Muller A, Sackmann H, Bauduceau B, Bled F, Passa P, Alhenc-Gelas F. Contribution of genetic polymorphism in the renin angiotensin system to the development of renal complications in insulin dependent diabetes. *J Clin Invest*, **99**: 1585–1595, 1997.

34. Barnas U, Schmidt A, Illievich A, Kiener HP, Rabensteiner D, Kaider A, Prager R, Abrahamian H, Irsigler K, Mayer G. Evaluation of risk factors for the development of nephropathy in patient with IDDM: insertion/deletion angiotensin converting enzyme gene polymorphism, hypertension and metabolic control. *Diabetologia*, **40**: 327–331, 1997.

35. Rossing P, Hougaard P, Borch-Johnsen K, Parving HH. Predictors of mortality in insulin dependent diabetes: 10 year observational follow up study. *BMJ,* **313**: 779–84, 1996.

36. Tarnow L, Gluud C, Parving HH. Diabetic nephropathy and the insertion/deletion polymorphism of the angiotensin-converting enzyme gene. *Nephrol Dial Transplant*, **13**: 1125–1130, 1998.

37. Caulfield M, Lavender P, Farrall M, Munroe P, Lawson M, Turner P, Clark AJ. Linkage of the angiotensinogen gene to essential hypertension. *N Engl J Med,* **330**: 1629–1633, 1994.

38. Ittersum FJ, Man AM, Thijssen S, Knijff P, Slagboom E, Smulders Y, Tarnow L, Donker AbJM, Bilo HJG, Stehouwer CDA. Genetic polymorphisms of the renin-angiotensin system and complication of insulin-dependent diabetes mellitus. *Nephrol Dial Transplant*, **15**: 1000–1007, 2000.

39. Freire MB, Ji L, Onuma T, Orban T, Warram JH, Krolewski AS. Gender-specific association of M235T polymorphism in angiotensinogen gene and diabetic nephropathy in NIDDM. *Hypertension*, **31**: 896–899, 1998.

40. Doria A, Onuma T, Gearin G, Freire MB, Warram JH, Krolewski AS. Angiotensinogen polymorphism M235T, hypertension, and nephropathy in insulin dependent diabetes. *Hypertension*, **27**: 1134–1139, 1996.

41. Corvol P, Jeunemaitre X. Molecular genetics of human hypertension: role of angiotensinogen. *Endocr Rev,* **18**: 662–677, 1997.

42. Pedersen-Bjergaard U *et al.* Angiotensin II receptor gene polymorphisms and occurrence of severe hypoglycemia in type 1 diabetes. *Diabetes*, **52**(S1): A29, 2003.

43. Moczulski DK, Rogus JJ, Antonellis A, Warram JH, Krolewski AS. Major susceptibility locus for nephropathy in type 1 diabetes on chromosome 3q: results of novel discordant sib-pair analysis. *Diabetes*, **47**: 1164–1169, 1998.

44. Wagner J, Gehlen F, Ciechanowicz A, Ritz E. Angiotensin II receptor type I gene expression in human glomerulonephritis and diabetes mellitus. *J Am Soc Nephrol*, **10**: 545–551, 1999.

45. Doria A, Onuma T, Warram JH, Krolewski AS. Synergistic effect of angiotensin II type I receptor genotype and poor glycaemic control on risk of nephropathy in IDDM. *Diabetologia*, **40**: 1293–1299, 1997.

46. Miller JA, Thai K, Scholey JW. Angiotensin II type 1 receptor gene polymorphism and the response to hyperglycemia in early type 1 diabetes. *Diabetes*, **49**: 1585–1589, 2000.

47. Zychma MJ, Gumprecht J, Trautsolt W, Szydlowska I, Grzeszczak W. Polymorphic genes for kinin receptors, nephropathy and blood pressure in type 2 diabetic patients. *Am J Nephrol*, **23**: 112–116, 2003.

48. Zychma MJ, *et al.* Polymorphisms in the gene encoding for human kinin receptors and the risk of end stage renal failure: results of transmission/disequilibrium test. *J Am Soc Nephrol*, **10**: 2120–2124, 1999.

49. Knigge H, Bluthner M, Bruntgens A, Sator H, Ritz E. G-699/C polymorphism in the bradykinin-1 receptor gene in patients with renal failure. *Nephrol Dial Transplant*, **15**: 586–588, 2000.

50. Diamandis EP, Yousef GM, Luo LY, Magklara A, Obiezu CV. The new human Kallikrein gene family: implication in carcinogenesis. *Trends Endocrinol Metab*, **11**: 54–60, 2000.

51. Yu H, Bowden DW, Spray BJ, Rich SS, Freedman BI. Identification of human plasma kallikrein gene polymorphism and evaluation of their role in end-stage renal disease. *Hypertension*, **31**: 906–911, 1998.

52. Yu H, Anderson PJ, Freedman BI, Rich SS, Bowden DW. Genomic structure of the human plasma prekallikrein gene, identification of allelic variants, and analysis in end stage renal disease. *Genomics*, **69**: 225–234, 2000.

53. Nannipieri M, Posadas R, Williams K, Politi E, Gonzales-Villalpando C, Stern MP, Ferrannini E. Association between polymorphism of the Atrial Natriuretic Peptide gene and proteinuria: a population-base study. *Diabetologia*, **46**: 429–432, 2003.

54. Schmidt S, Bluthner M, Giessel R, Strojek K, Bergis KH, Grzeszczak W, Ritz E and the Diabetic Nephropathy Study Group. A polymorphism in the gene for the atrial natriuretic peptide and diabetic nephropathy. *Nephrol Dial Transplant,* **13**: 1807–1810, 1998.

55. Roussel R *et al.* Atrial natriuretic peptide gene and nephropathy in type 1 diabetes. *Diabetologia*, **46**(S2): A335, 2003.

56. Neugebauer S, Baba T, Watanabe T. Association of nitric oxide synthase gene polymorphism with an increased risk for diabetic nephropathy in type 2 diabetes. *Diabetes,* **49**: 500–503, 2000.

57. Shimizu T, Onuma T, Kawamori R, Makita Y, Tomino Y. Endothelial nitric oxide synthase gene and the development of diabetic nephropathy. *Diabetes Res Clin Pract*, **58**: 179–185, 2002.

58. Wang Y, Kikuchi S, Suzuki H, Nagase S, Koyama A. Endothelial nitric oxide synthase gene polymorphism in intron 4 affects the progression of renal failure in non-diabetic renal disease. *Nephrol Dial Transplant*, 14: 2898–2902, 1999.

59. Morris BJ, Markus A, Glenn CL, Adams DJ, Colagiuri S, Wang L. Association of a functional inducible nitric oxide synthase promoter variant with complications in type 2 diabetes. *J Mol Med*, 80: 96–104, 2002.

60. Johannesen J, Tarnow L, Parving HH, Nerup J, Pociot F. CCTTT-repeat polymorphism in the human NOS2 promoter confers low risk of diabetic nephropathy in type 1 diabetic patients. *Diabetes Care*, 23: 560–562, 2000.

61. Rippin JD, Patel A, Belyaev ND, Gill GV, Barnett AH, Bain SC. Nitric oxide synthase gene polymorphisms and diabetic nephropathy. *Diabetologia*, 46: 426–428, 2003.

62. Födinger M, Hörl WH, Sunder-Plassmann G. Molecular biology of 5,10-methylenetetrahydrofolate reductase. *J Nephrol*, 13: 20–33, 2000.

63. Neugebauer S, Baba T, Watanabe T. Methylenetetrahydrofolate reductase gene polymorphism as a risk factor for diabetic nephropathy in NIDDM patients. *Lancet*, 352: 454, 1998.

64. Blüthner M, Brüntgens A, Schmidt S, Strojek K, Grzeszczak W, Ritz E. Association of methylenetetrahydrofolate reductase gene polymorphism and diabetic nephropathy in type 2 diabetes? *Nephrol Dial Transplant*, 14: 56–57, 1999.

65. Smyth JS, Savage DA, Maxwell AP. MTHFR gene polymorphism and diabetic nephropathy in type 1 diabetes. *Lancet*, 353: 1156–1157, 1999.

66. Shcherbak NS, Shutskaya ZV, Sheidina AM, Larionova VI, Schwartz EI. Methylenetetrahydrofolate reductase gene polymorphism as a risk factor for diabetic nephropathy in IDDM patients. *Mol Genet Metab*, 68: 375–378, 1999.

67. Fujita H, Narita T, Meguro H, Ishii T, Hanyu O, Sozuki K, Kamoi K, Ito S. No association between MTHFR gene polymorphism and diabetic patients with proliferative diabetic retinopathy. *J Diabet Complications*, 13: 284–287, 1999.

68. Odawara M, Yamashita K. A common mutation of the methylenetetrahydrofolate reductase gene as a risk factor for diabetic nephropathy. *Diabetologia*, 42: 631–632, 1999.

69. Shpichinetsky V, Raz I, Friedlander Y, Goldschmidt, Wexler DI, Yehuda AB, Friedman G. The association between two common mutations C677T and A1298C in human methylentetrahydrofolate reductase gene and the risk for diabetic nephropathy in type II diabetic patient. *J Nutr*, 130: 2493–2497, 2000.

70. Rosskopf D, Busch S, Manthey I, Siffert W. G protein β3 gene. Structure, promoter, and additional polymorphisms. *Hypertension*, 36: 33–41, 2000.

71. Siffert W *et al.* Worldwide ethnic distribution of the G Protein β3 subunit 825T allele and its association with obesity in Caucasian, Chinese, and Black African individuals. *J Am Soc Nephrol*, 10: 1921–1930, 1999.

72. Schunkert H, Hense HW, Döring A, Riegger GAJ, Siffert W. Association between a polymorphism in the G protein β3 subunit gene and lover renin and elevated diastolic blood pressure levels. *Hyperthension*, 32: 510–513, 1998.

73. Dzida G, Siekierska-Golon P, Puźniak A, Sobstyl J, Bilan A, Mosiewicz J, Hanzlik J. G-protein β3 subunit gene C825T polymorphism is associated with type 2 diabetes mellitus. *Med Sci Monit*, 8: 597–602, 2002.

74. Beige J, Engeli S, Ringel J, Offermann G, Distler A, Sharma AM. Donor G-protein β3 subunit 825TT genotypes associated with reduced kidney allograft survival. *J AM Soc Nephrol*, 10: 1717–21, 1999.

75. Bluthner M, Schmidt S, Siffert W, Knigge H, Nawroth P, Ritz E. Increased frequency of G-protein beta 3-subunit 825 T allele in dialyzed patients with type 2 diabetes. *Kidney Int.* 55: 1247–1250, 1999.

76. Beige J, Ringel J, Distler A, Sharma AM. G-protein beta3 subunit C825T genotype and nephropathy in diabetes mellitus. *Nephrol Dial Transplant*, 15: 1384–1387, 2000.

77. Shcherbak NS, Schwartz EI. The C825T polymorphism in the G-protein beta3 subunit gene and diabetic complications in IDDM patients. *J Hum Genet*, 46: 188–191, 2001.

78. Tarnow L, Stehouwer CD, Emeis JJ, Poirier O, Cambien F, Hansen BV, Parving HH. Plasminogen activator inhibitor-1 and apolipoprotein E gene polymorphism and diabetic angiopathy. *Nephrol Dial Transplant*, 15: 625–630, 2000.

79. Gutierrez C, Vendrell J, Pastor R, Broch M, Aguilar C, Llor C, Simon I, Richart C. GLUT1 gene polymorphism in non insulin dependent diabetes mellitus: genetic susceptibility relationship with cardiovascular risk factors and microangiopathic complication in a Mediterranean population. *Diabetes Res Clin Pract*, 41: 113–120, 1998.

80. Daniel PK, *et al.* Polymorphisms in GLUT1 are associated with the development of diabetic nephropathy in diabetes mellitus. *Diabetes*, 51(S2): A36, 2002.

81. Tarnow L, Grarup N, Hansen T, Parving HH, Pedersen O. Diabetic microvascular complications are not associated with two polymorphisms in the

GLUT-1 and PC-1 genes regulating glucose metabolism in Caucasian type 1 diabetic patients. *Nephrol Dial Transplant*, **16**: 1653–1656, 2001.

82. Ng PKD, Canani L, Araki S, Smiles A, Moczulski D, Warram JH, Krolewski AS. Minor effect of GLUT 1 polymorphism on susceptibility to diabetic nephropathy in type 1 diabetes. *Diabetes*, **51**: 2264–2269, 2002.

83. Hodgkinson A, Page T, Millward BA, Demaine AG. Polymorphism in the flanking region of the Glucose Transporter Gene-1 is associated with nephropathy in patients with type 1 diabetes mellitus. *Diabetes*, **52**(S1): A186, 2003.

84. Shcherbak NS. Apolipoprotein E gene polymorphism is not a strong risk factor for diabetic nephropathy and retinopathy in type I diabetes: case-control study. *BMC Med Genet*, **2**: 8, 2001.

85. Hadjadj S *et al*. Lack of relationship in long-term type 1 diabetic patients between diabetic nephropathy and polymorphisms in apolipoprotein ε, lipoprotein lipase and cholesteryl ester transfer protein. *Nephrol Dial Transplant*, **15**: 1971–1976, 2000.

86. Boize R, Benhamou PY, Corticelli P, Valenti K, Bosson JL, Halim S. ApoE polymorphism and albuminuria in diabetes mellitus: a role for LDL in the development of nephroapthy in NIDDM?. *Nephrol Dial Transplant*, **13**: 72–75, 1998.

87. Liu L *et al*. Synergistic effect between HSPG and ApoE gene polymorphism in type 2 diabetic nephropathy. *Diabetes*, **52**(S1): A188, 2003.

88. Herrmann SM, Ringel J, Wang JG, Staessen JA, Brand E. Peroxisome Proliferator – Activated Receptor γ2 polymorphism pro12Ala is associated with nephropathy in type 2 diabetes. The Berlin Diabetes Mellitus Study. *Diabetes*, **51**: 2653–2657, 2002.

89. Rasmussen SK, Urhammer SA, Pizzuti A, Echwald SM, Ekstrøm CT, Hansen L, Hansen T, Johnsen Borch K, Frittitta L, Trischitta V, Pedersen O. The K121Q variant of the human PC-1 gene is not associated with insulin resistance or type 2 diabetes among Danish Caucasians. *Diabetes*, **49**: 1608–1611, 2000.

90. Gu HF, Almgren P, Lindholm E, Frittitta L, Pizzuti A, Trischitta V, Groop LC. Association between the human glycoprotein PC-1 gene and elevated glucose and insulin levels in a paired-sibling analysis. *Diabetes*, **49**: 1601–1603, 2000.

91. Costanzo BV, Trischitta V, Di Paola R, Spampinato D, Pizzuti A, Vigneri R, Frittitta L. The Q allele variant (GLN121) of membrane glycoprotein PC-1 interacts with the insulin receptor and inhibits insulin signaling more effectively than the common K allele variant (LYS121). *Diabetes,* **50**: 831–836, 2001.

92. Frittitta L, *et al*. A cluster of three single nucleotide polymorphisms in the 3'-untanslated region of human glycoprotein PC-1 gene stabilizes PC-1 mRNA and is associated with increased PC-1 protein content and insulin resistance-related abnormalities. *Diabetes*, **50**: 1952–1955, 2001.

93. Canani LH, Ng Daniel PK, Smiles A, Rogus JJ, Warram JH, Krolewski AS. Polymorphism in Ecto-Nucleotide Pyrophosphatase / Phosphodiesterase 1 gene (ENPPP1/PC-1) and early development of advanced diabetic nephropathy in type 1diabetes. *Diabetes*, **51**: 1188–1193, 2002.

94. DeCosmo S *et al*. A PC-1 amino acid variant (K120Q) is associated with faster progression of renal disease in patients with type 1 diabetes and albuminuria. *Diabetes*, **49**: 521–524, 2000.

95. Michel Marre. A KQ121 variant in the PC-1 gene and diabetic nephropathy: discrepant results between North and South Europe. *Nephrol Dial Transplant*, **17**: 1546–1547, 2002.

96. Hudson BI, Stickland MH, Futers TS, Grant PJ. Effect of novel polymorphism in the RAGE gene on transcriptional regulation and their association with diabetic retinopathy. *Diabetes*, **50**: 1505–1511, 2001.

97. Petterson-Fernholm K, Forsblom C, Hudson BI, Perola M, Grant PJ, Groop PH. The functional -374 T/A RAGE gene polymorphism is associated with proteinuria and cardiovascular disease in type I diabetic patients. *Diabetes*, **52**: 891–894, 2003.

98. Hudson BI, Stickland MH, Grant PJ. Identification of polymorphisms in the receptor for advanced glycation end-products (RAGE) gene. Prevalence in type 2 diabetes and ethnic groups. *Diabetes*, **47**: 1155–1157, 1998.

99. Kicic E, Palmer TN. Increased white cell aldose reductase mRNA levels in diabetic patients. *Diabetes Res Clin Prac*, **33**: 31–36, 1996.

100. Hasegawa G, Obayashi H, Kitamura A, Hashimoto M, Shigeta H, Nakamura N, Kondo M, Nishimura CY. Increased levels of aldose reductase in peripheral mononuclear cells from type 2 diabetic patients with microangiopathy. *Diabetes Res Clin Prac*, **45**: 9–14, 1999.

101. Maeda S, Haneda M, Yasuda H, Tachikawa T, Isshiki K, Koya D, Terada M, Hidaka H, Kashiwagi A, Kikkawa R. Diabetic nephropathy is not associated with the dinucleotide repeat polymorphism upstream of the aldose reductase (ALR2) gene but with erythrocyte aldose reductase content in Japanese subjects with type 2 diabetes. *Diabetes*, **48**: 420–422, 1999.

102. Shah VO, *et al*. Z-2 microsatellite allele is linked to increased expression of aldose reductase gene in diabetic nephropathy. *J Clin Endocrinol Metab*, **83**: 2886–2891, 1998.

103. Patel A, Hibberd ML, Millward BA, Demaine AG. Chromosome 7q35 and susceptibility to diabetic microvascular complications. *J Diabetes Complications*, **10**: 62–67, 1996.

104. Mockzulski DK, Burak W, Doria A, Zychma M, Szczechowaska- Zukowska E, Warram JH, Grzeszczak W. The role of aldose reductase gene in the susceptibility to diabetic nephropathy in type II diabetes mellitus. *Diabetologia*, **42**: 94–97, 1999.

105. Park HK, Ahn CW, Lee GT, Kim SJ, Song YD, Lim SK, Kim KR, Huh KB, Lee HC. (AC)n polymorphism of aldose reductase gene and diabetic microvascular complication in type 2 diabetes mellitus. *Diabetes Res Clin Prac*, **55**: 151–157, 2002.

106. Wang Y, *et al.* The association between a CA repeat and a promoter polymorphism of aldose reductase gene and diabetic complications. *Diabetes*, **51**(S2): A184, 2002.

107. Ng DP, Conn J, Chung SS, Larkins RG. Aldose reductase (AC)(n) microsatellite polymorphism and diabetic microvascular complications in Caucasian type 1 diabetes mellitus. *Diabetes Res Clin Pract*, **52**: 21–27, 2001.

108. Dyer PH, Chowdhury TA, Dronsfield MJ, Dunger D, Barnett AH, Bain SC. The 5'-end polymorphism of aldose reductase gene is not associated with diabetic nephropathy in Caucasian type I diabetic patients. *Diabetologia*, **42**: 1030–1031, 1999.

109. Isermann B *et al.* (CA)n dinucleotide repeat polymorphism at the 5'-end of the aldose reductase gene is not associated with microangiopathy in Caucasians with long-term diabetes mellitus 1. *Nephrol Dial Transplant*, **15**: 919, 2000.

110. Fanelli A *et al.* The aldose reductase promoter gene –106C/T mutations is not associated with nephropathy but is a determinant of retinopathy in type 1 diabetic patients. *Diabetes*, **51**(S2): A512, 2002.

111. Primo-Parmo SL, Sorenson RC, Teiber J, Du La BN. The human serum paraoxonase/ arylesterase gene (PON1) is one member of a multigene family. *Genomics*, **33**: 498–507, 1996.

112. Suehiro T, Nakamura T, Inoue M, Shiinoki T, Ikeda Y, Kumon Y, Shindo M, Tanaka H, Hashimoto. A polymorphism upstream from the human paraoxonase (PON1) gene and its association with PON1 expression. *Atheroscleorsis*, **150**: 295–298, 2000.

113. Mackness B, Mackness MI, Arrol S, Turkie W, Julier K, Abuasha B, Miller J, Boulton AJ, Durrington PN. Serum paraoxonase (PON1) 55 and 192 polymorphism and paraoxonase activity and concentration in non-insulinodependent diabetes mellitus. *Atherosclerosis*, **139**: 341–349, 1998.

114. Brophy VH, Jampsa RL, Clendenning JB, McKinstry LA, Jarvik GP, Furlong CE. Effects of 5' regulatory region polymorphisms on paraoxonase gene (PON1) expression. *Am J Hum Genet*, **68**: 1428–1436, 2001.

115. Araki S, Makita Y, Canani L, Ng D, Warram JH, Krolewski AS. Polymorphism of human paraoxonase 1 gene (PON1) and susceptibility to diabetic nephropathy in type 1 diabetes mellitus. *Diabetologia*, **43**: 1540–1543, 2000.

116. Pinizzotto M, Castillo E, Fiaux M, Temler E, Gaillard RC, Ruiz J. Paraoxonase 2 polymorphisms are associated with nephropathy in type II diabetes. *Diabetologia*, **44**: 104–107, 2001.

117. Ikeda Y, Suehiro T, Ohsaki F, Arii K, Kumon Y, Hashimoto K. Relationships between polymorphisms of the human serum paraoxonase gene and insulin sensitivity in Japanese patients with type 2 diabetes. *Diabetes Res Clin Prac*, **60**: 79–85, 2003.

118. Hugo C. The thrombospondin 1-TGF-β axis in fibrotic renal disease. *Nephrol Dial Transplant*, **18**: 1241–1245, 2003.

119. Border WA, Noble NA. Transforming growth factor β in tissue fibrosis. *N Engl J Med*, **331**: 1286–1292, 1994.

120. Reeves WB, Andreoli TE. Transforming growth factor β contributes to progressive diabetic nephropathy. *Proc Natl Acad Sci* USA, **97**: 14, 2000.

121. Huang C, Kim Y, Caramori MLA, Fish AJ, Rich SS, Miller ME, Russell GB, Mauer M. Cellular basis of diabetic nephropathy. The transforming growth factors-β system and diabetic nephropathy lesions in type I diabetes. *Diabetes*, **51**: 3577–3581, 2002.

122. Ronald C, *et al.* Obesity, T29→C Polymorphism of the Transforming Growth Factor- β 1 gene and susceptibility to diabetic nephropathy in subject with type 2 diabetes. *Diabetes*, **51**(S2): A188, 2002.

123. Vaessen N, *et al.* A polymorpism in the gene for IGF-1. Functional properties and risk for type 2 diabetes and myocardial infarction. *Diabetes*, **50**: 637–642, 2001.

124. Frayling TM, Hattersley AT, McCarthy A, Holly J, Mitchell SMS, Gloyn AL, Owen K, Davies D, Smith GD, Shlomo YB. A putative functional polymorphism in the IGF-1 gene: association studies with type 2 diabetes, adult height, glucose tolerance, and fetal growth in UK population. *Diabetes* **51**: 2313–2316, 2002.

125. Janssen JA, Jacobs ML, Derkx FH, Weber RF, Lely AJ, Lamberts SW. Free and total insulin like growth factors1 and IGFBP-1, and IGFBP-3 and their relationship to the presence of diabetic retinopathy and glomerular hyperfiltration in

insulin dependent diabetes mellitus. *JCEM*, **82**: 2809–2815, 1997.

126. Cummings EA, Sochett EB, Dekker MG, Lawson ML, Danemin D. Contribution of growth hormone and IGF-1 to early diabetic nephropathy in type 1 diabetes. *Diabetes*, **47**: 1341–1346, 1998.

127. Segerer S, Nelson PJ, Schlöndorff D. Chemokines, chemokine receptors, and renal disease: from basic science to pathophysiologic and therapeutic studies. *J Am Soc Nephrol*, **11**: 152–176, 2000.

128. Nakajima K, Tanaka Y, Nomiyama T, Ogihara T, Piao L, Sakai K, Onuma T, Kawamori R. Chemokine receptor genotype is associated with diabetic nephropathy in Japanase with type 2 diabetes. *Diabetes*, **51**: 238–242, 2002.

129. Kamiuchi K, Hasegawa G, Obayashi H, Kitamura A, Ishii M, Yano M, Kanatsuna T, Yoshikawa T, Nakamura N. Leucocyte-endothelial cell adesion molecule 1 (LECAM-1) polymorphism is associated with diabetic nephropathy in type 2 diabetes mellitus. *J Diabet Complications*, **16**: 333–337, 2002.

130. Yang B, Cross DF, Ollerenshaw M, Millward BA, Demaine AG. Polymophisms of the vascular endothelial growth factor and susceptibility to diabetic microvascular complications in patients with type 1 diabetes mellitus. *J Diabet Complications*, **17**: 1–6, 2003.

131. Nakajima S, Baba T. Trp64Arg polymorphism of the β3-adrenergic receptor is not associated with diabetic nephropathy in Japanese patients with type 2 diabetes. *Diabetes Care*, **23**: 862–863, 2000.

132. Sakane N, Yoshida T, Yoshioka K, Nakamura Y, Umekawa T, Kogure A, Takakura Y, Kondo M. Trp64Arg mutation of beta3-adrenoceptor gene is associated with diabetic nephropathy in type II diabetes mellitus. *Diabetologia*, **41**: 1533–1534, 1998.

133. Yamauchi T, Kuno T, Takada H, Mishima K, Nagura Y, Takahashi S, Kanmatsuse K. The impact of Trp64Arg mutation in the β3-adrenegic receptor gene on haemodialysis patients. *Nephrol Dial Transplant*, **16**: 641, 2001.

134. Tarnow L, Urhammer SA, Mottlau B, Hansen BV, Pedersen O, Parving HH. The Trp64Arg amino acid polymorphism of the β3-adrenergic receptor gene does not contribute to the genetic susceptibility of diabetic microvascular complications in Caucasian type 1 diabetic patients. *Nephrol Dial Transplant*, **14**: 895–897, 1999.

135. Grzeszczak W, Saucha W, Zychma MJ, Zukowska-Szczechowska E, Labuz B, Lacka B, Szydlowska I. Is Trp64Arg polymorphism of beta3-adrenergic receptor a clinically useful marker for the predisposition to diabetic

nephropathy in type II diabetic patients? *Diabetologia*, **42**: 632–633, 1999.

136. Moczulski DK, Grzeszczak W, Gawlik B. Role of hemochromatosis C282Y and H63D mutation in HFE gene in development of type 2 diabetes and diabetic nephropathy. *Diabetes Care*, **24**: 1187–1191, 2001.

137. Isshiki K, *et al.* Identification of SOCS2's potential roles in the development of diabetic nephropathy by DNA Microarray and its regulation by insulin and islet cell transplantation. *Diabetes*, **52**(S1): A49, 2003.

138. Nakamura S, Yoshinari M, Doi Y, Yoshizumi H, Katafuchi R, Yokomizo Y, Nishiyama K, Wakisaka M, Fujishima M. Renal complications in patients with diabetes mellitus associated with an A to G mutation of mitochondrial DNA at the 3243 position of leucine tRNA. *Diabetes Res Clin Prac*, **44**: 183–189, 1999.

139. Liu CS, Ko LY, Lim PS, Kao SH, Wei YH. Biomarker of DNA damage in patients with end stage renal disease: mitochondrial DNA mutations in hair follicles. *Nephrol Dial Transplant*, **16**: 561–565, 2001.

140. Yamagata K, Tomida C, Umeyama K, Urakami K, Ishizu T, Hirayama K, Gotoh M, Iitsuka T, Takemura K, Kikuchi H, Nakamura H, Kobayashi M, Koyama A. Prevalence of Japanese dialysis patients with an A-to-G mutation at nucleotide 3243 of the mitochondrial tRNA $^{Leu(UUR)}$ gene. *Nephrol Dial Transplant*, **15**: 385–388, 2000.

141. Suzuki S, Hinokio Y, Komatu K, Ohtomo M, Onoda M, Hirai S, Hirai M, Hirai A, Chiba, M, Kasuga S, Akai H, Toyota T. Oxidative damage to mitochondrial DNA and its relationship to diabetic complications. *Diabetes Res Clin Prac*, **45**: 161–168, 1999.

142. Levy AP, Levy NS, Goldberg MA. Hypoxia-inducible protein binding to vascular endothelial growth factor mRNA and its modulation by the von Hippel-Lindau protein. *J Biol Chem*, **271**: 25492–25497, 1996.

143. Sjolie AK, Stephenson J, Aldington S, Kohner E, Janka H, Stevens L, Fuller JH. Retinopathy and vision loss in insulin-dependent diabetes in Europe. The EURODIAB IDDM. Complications Study Group. *Ophthalmology*, **104**: 252–260, 1997.

144. The DCCT Research Group. Effect of intensive diabetes management on macrovascular events and risk factors in the diabetes control and complication trial. *Am J Cardiol*, **75**: 894–903, 1995.

145. Hinokio Y, *et al.* Oxidative DNA damages and the development of diabetic retinopathy: 6 years prospective study. *Diabetes*, **51**(S2): A209, 2002.

146. Giustina A, *et al.* Long-term treatment with the dual antithromboxane agent Picotamide decreases microalbuminuria in normotensive type II diabetic patients. *Diabetes*, **47**: 423, 1998.

147. Mustard JF, Packham MA. Platelets and diabetes mellitus. *N Engl J Med*, **311**: 665, 1987.

148. Dallinger KJC, Jennings PE, Toop MJ, Clyde OHB, Barnet AH. Platelet aggregation and coagulation factors in insulin dependent diabetes with and without microangiopathy. *Diabet Med*, **4**: 44, 1987.

149. Rand LI. Recent advances in diabetic retinopathy. *Am J Med*, **70**: 595–602, 1982.

150. Early Treatment Diabetic Retinopathy Study Research Group Results from the Early Treatment Diabetic Retinopathy Study. *Ophthalmology*, **98**: 741–840, 1991.

151. Blankenship GW. Fifteen-year argon laser and xenon photocoagulation results of Bascom Palmer Eye. Institute's patients participating in the diabetic retinopathy study. *Ophthalmology*, **98**: 125–128, 1991.

152. Li W, Yanoff M, Jian B, He Z. Altered mRNA levels of antioxidant enzymes in preapoptotic pericytes from human diabetic retinas. *Cell Mol Biol*, **45**: 59–66, 1999.

153. Podestà F, Romeo G, Liu WH, Krajewski S, Reed JC, Gerhardinger C, Lorenzi M. Bax is increased in the retina of diabetic subjects and is associated with pericyte apoptosis *in vivo* and *in vitro*. *Am J Pathol*, **156**: 1025–1032, 2000.

154. Barber AJ, Lieth E, Khin SA, Antonetti DA, Buchanan AG, Gardner TW. Neural apoptosis in the retina during experimental and human diabetes: early onset and effect of insulin. *J Clin Invest*, **102**: 783–791, 1998.

155. Ferrara N, Davis-Smyth T. The biology of vascular endothelial growth factor. *Endocr Rev*, **18**: 4-25, 1997.

156. Duh E, Aiello LP. Vascular endothelial growth factor and diabetes: the agonist *versus* antagonist paradox. *Diabetes*, **48**: 1899–1906, 1999.

157. Aiello LP, Avery RL, Arrigg PG, Keyt BA, Jampel HD, Shah ST, Pasquale LR, Thieme H, Iwamoto MA, Park JE, Nguyen HV, Aiello LM, Ferrara N, and King GL. Vascular endothelial growth factor in ocular fluid of patients with diabetic retinopathy and other retinal disorders. *N Engl J Med*, **22**: 1480–1487, 1994.

158. Awata T, Inoue K, Kurihara S, Ohkubo T, Watanabe M, Inukai K, Inoue I, Katayama S. A common polymorphism in the 5'-untranslated region of the VEGF gene is associated with diabetic retinopathy in type 2 diabetes. *Diabetes*, **51**: 1635–1639, 2002.

159. Qaum T *et al.* VEGF-initiated blood-retinal barrier breakdown in early diabetes. *Invest Ophthalmol Vis Sci*, **42**: 2408–2413, 2001.

160. Jaakkola P, Mole DR, Tian YM, Wilson MI, Gielbert J, Gaskell SJ, Kriegsheim A, Hebestreit HF, Mukherji M, Schofield CJ, Maxwell PH, Pugh CW, Ratcliffe PJ. Targeting of *HIF*-alpha to the von Hippel-Lindau ubiquitylation complex by O_2 -regulated prolyl hydroxylation. *Science*, **292**: 468–472, 2001.

161. Moss SE, Klein R, Klein BE. The 14-year incidence of visual loss in a diabetic population. *Ophthalmology*, **105**: 998–1003, 1998.

162. McLeod DS, Lefer DJ, Merges C, Lutty GA. Enhanced expression of intracellular adhesion molecule-1 and P-selectin in the diabetic human retina and choroid. *Am J Pathol*, **147**: 642–653, 1995.

163. Joussen AM *et al.* Retinal vascular endothelial growth factor induces intercellular adhesion molecule-1 and endothelial nitric oxide synthase expression and initiates early diabetic retinal leukocyte adhesion *in vivo*. *Am J Pathol*, **160**: 501–509, 2002.

164. Williamson JR *et al.* Hyperglycaemic pseudo-hypoxia and diabetic complications. *Diabetes*, **42**: 801–813, 1993.

165. Shah VO, Dorin RI, Sun Y, Braun M, Zager PG. Aldose reductase gene expression is increased in diabetic nephropathy. *J Clin Endocrinol Metab*, **82**: 2294–2298, 1997.

166. Ko BC-B, Lam KS-L, Wat NM-S, Chung SS-M. An (A-C)n dinucleotide repeat polymorphic marker at the 5' end of the aldose reductase gene is associated with early-onset diabetic retinopathy in NIDDM patients. *Diabetes*, **44**: 727–732, 1995.

167. Shah VO, Scavini M, Nikolic J, Sun Y, Vai S, Griffith JK, Dorin RI, Stidley C, Yacoub M, Vander Jagt DL, Eaton RP, Zager PG. Z-2 microsatellite allele is linked to increased expression of the aldose reductase gene in diabetic nephropathy. *J Clin Endocrinol Metab*, **83**: 2886–2891, 1998.

168. Olmos P, Futers S, Acosta AM, Siegel S, Maiz A, Schiaffino R, Morales P, Diaz R, Arriagada P, Claro JC, Vega R, Vollrath V, Velasco S, Emmerich M. (AC)23 [Z-2] polymorphism of the aldose reductase gene and fast progression of retinopathy in Chilean type 2 diabetics. *Diabetes Res Clin Pract*, **47**: 169–176, 2000.

169. Heesom AK, Hibberd ML, Millward A, Demaine AG. Polymorphism in the 5' end of the aldose reductase gene is strongly associated with the development of diabetic nephropathy in type 1 diabetes. *Diabetes*, **46**: 287–291, 1997.

170. Li YM, Mitsuhashi T, Wojciechowicz D, Shimizu N, Li J, Stitt A, He C, Banerjee D, Vlassara H.

Molecular identity and cellular distribution of advanced glycation endproduct receptors: relationship of p60 to OST-48 and p90 to 80K-H membrane proteins. *Proc Natl Acad Sci* USA, **93:** 11047–11052, 1996.

171. Krontiris TG. Minisatellites and human disease. *Science,* **269:** 1682–1683, 1995.

172. Larkins RG, Dunlop ME. The link between hyperglycemia and diabetic nephropathy. *Diabetologia,* **35:** 499–504, 1992.

173. Ichikawa F, Yamada K, Ishiyama-Shigemoto S, Yuan X, Nonaka K. Association of an (A-C)n dinucleotide repeat polymorphic marker at the 59-region of the aldose reductase gene with retinopathy but not with nephropathy or neuropathy in Japanese patients with type 2 diabetes mellitus. *Diabet Med,* **16:** 744–748, 1999.

174. Kao YL, Donaghue K, Chan A, Knight J, Silink M. A novel polymorphism in the aldose reductase gene promoter region is strongly associated with diabetic retinopathy in adolescents with type 1 diabetes. *Diabetes,* **48:** 1338–1340, 1999.

175. Watson AD, Berliner JA, Hama SY, La Du BN, Faull KF, Fogelman AM, Navab M. Protective effect of high density lipoprotein associated paraoxonase. Inhibition of the biological activity of minimally oxidized low density lipoprotein. *J Clin Invest,* **96:** 2882–2891, 1995.

176. Takada Y, Hemler ME. The primary structure of the VLA-2/collagen receptor α2 subunit (platelet GPIα): homology to other integrins and the presence of a possible collagen-binding domain. *J Cell Biol,* **109:** 397, 1989.

177. Kritzik M, Savage B, Nugent DJ, Santoso S, Ruggeri ZM, Kunicki TJ. Nucleotide polymorphism in the *a2* genes define multiple alleles that are associated with differences in platelet α2β1 density. *Blood,* **92:** 2382, 1998.

178. Moshfegh K *et al.* Association of two silent polymorphisms of platelet glycoprotein Iα/IIα receptor with risk of myocardial infarction: a case-control study. *Lancet,* **353:** 351, 1999.

179. Burren CP, Berka JL, Edmondson SR, Werther GA, Batch JA. Localization of mRNAs for insulin-like growth factor-I (IGF-I), IGF-I receptor, and IGF binding proteins in rat eye. *Invest Ophthalmol Vis Sci,* **37:** 1459–1468, 1996.

180. Tokuyama Y *et al.* A case of type 2 diabetes with Thr149Met mutation in glucagon-like peptide-1 receptor gene. *Diabetologia,* **46**(S2): A130, 2003.

181. Moriarty P, Boulton M, Dickson A, McLeod D. Production of IGF-I and IGF binding proteins by retinal cells *in vitro. Br J Ophthalmol,* **78:** 638–642, 1994.

182. King GL, Goodman AD, Buzney S, Moses A, Kahn CR. Receptors and growth promoting effects of insulin and insulin-like growth factors on cells from bovine retinal capillaries and aorta. *J Clin Invest,* **75:** 1028–1036, 1985.

183. Peruzzi F, Prisco M, Dews M, Salomoni P, Grassilli E, Romano G, Calabretta B, Baserga R. Multiple signaling pathways of the insulin-like growth factor 1 receptor in protection from apoptosis. *Mol Cell Biol,* **19:** 7203–7215, 1999.

184. Brunet A, Bonni A, Zigmond MJ, Lin MZ, Juo P, Hu LS, Anderson MJ, Arden KC, Blenis J, Greenberg ME. Akt promotes cell survival by phosphorylating and inhibiting a forkhead transcription factor. *Cell,* **96:** 857–868, 1999.

185. Huang XH, Rantalaiho V, Wirta O, Pasternack A, Koivula T, Hiltunen TP, Nikkari T, Lehtimaki T. Angiotensin-converting enzyme gene polymorphism is associated with coronary heart disease in non-insulin-dependent diabetic patients evaluated for 9 years. *Metabolism,* **47:** 1258–1262, 1998.

186. Simo R, *et al.* CD4/CD8 and CD28 expression in T cells infiltrating the vitreous fluid in diabetic patients with proliferative diabetic retinopathy: a flow cytometric analysis. *Diabetes,* **52**(S1): A203, 2003.

187. Haurigot VA, *et al.* Transgenic mice overexpressing IGF-I in the retina develop diabetic eye disease. *Diabetologia,* **46**(S2): A11, 2003.

188. Danser AH, van den Dorpel MA, Deinum J, Derkx FH, Franken AA, Peperkamp E, de Jong PT, Schalekamp MA. Renin, prorenin, and immunoreactive renin in vitreous fluid from eyes with and without diabetic retinopathy. *J Clin Endocrinol Metab,* **68:** 160–167, 1989.

189. Schalekamp M. Renin-angiotensin system components and endothelial proteins as markers of diabetic microvascular disease. *Clin Invest,* **71:** S3–6, 1993.

190. Matsumoto A, Iwashima Y, Abiko A, Morikawa A, Sekiguchi M, Eto M, Makino I. Detection of the association between a deletion polymorphism in the gene encoding angiotensin I-converting enzyme and advanced diabetic retinopathy. *Diabetes Res Clin Pract,* **50:** 195–202, 2000.

191. Brownlee M. Advanced protein glycosylation in diabetes and aging. *Annu Rev Med,* **46:** 223–234, 1995.

192. Stitt AW, He C, Vlassara H. Characterisation of the advanced glycation end-product receptor complex in human vascular endothelial cells. *Biochem Biophys Res Commun,* **256:** 549–556, 1999.

193. Horiuchi S, Higashi T, Ikeda K, Saishoji T, Jinnouchi Y, Sano H, Shibayama R, Sakamoto T, Araki N. Advanced glycation end-products and their recognition by macrophage and macrophage-derived cells. *Diabetes,* **45:** S73–S76, 1996.

194. Schmidt AM, Hori O, Brett J, Yan SD, Wautier JL, Stern D. Cellular receptors for advanced glycation end-products: implications for induction of oxidant stress and cellular dysfunction in the pathogenesis of vascular lesions. *Arterioscler Thromb,* **14**: 1521–1528, 1994.

195. Lander HM, Tauras J M, Ogiste JS, Hori O, Moss RA, Schmidt. Activation of the receptor for advanced glycation end-products triggers a p21(ras) -dependent mitogen-activated protein kinase pathway regulated by oxidant stress. *J Biol Chem,* **272**: 17810–17814, 1997.

196. Yamagishi SI *et al.* Cerivastatin blocks the AGE-RAGE signaling pathways in microvascular endothelial cells. *Diabetologia,* **46**(S2): A13, 2003.

197. Sugaya K, Fukagawa T, Matsumoto K, Mita K, Takahashi E, Ando A, Inoko H, Ikemura T. Three genes in the human MHC class III region near the junction with the class II: gene for receptor of advanced glycosylation end-products, PBX2 homeobox gene and a notch homolog, human counterpart of mouse mammary tumor gene int-3. *Genomics,* **23**: 408–419, 1994.

198. Brett J, Schmidt AM, Yan SD, Zou YS, Weidman E, Pinsky D, Nowygrod R, Neeper M, Przysiecki C, Shaw A, Migheli A, Stern D. Survey of the distribution of a newly characterized receptor for advanced glycation end-products in tissues. *Am J Pathol,* **143**: 1699–1712, 1993.

199. Soulis T, Thallas V, Youssef S, Gilbert RE, McWilliam BG, Murray-McIntosh RP, Cooper ME. Advanced glycation end-products and their receptors co-localise in rat organs susceptible to diabetic microvascular injury. *Diabetologia,* **40**: 619–628, 1997.

200. Schmidt AM, Yan SD, Wautier JL, Stern D. Activation of receptor for advanced glycation end-products: a mechanism for chronic vascular dysfunction in diabetic vasculopathy and atherosclerosis. *Circ Res,* **84**: 489–497, 1999.

201. Bierhaus A, Illmer T, Kasper M, Luther T, Quehenberger P, Tritschler H, Wahl P, Ziegler R, Muller M, Nawroth PP. Advanced glycation end-product (AGE)-mediated induction of tissue factor in cultured endothelial cells is dependent on RAGE. *Circulation,* **96**: 2262–2271, 1997.

202. Yamagishi S, Fujimori H, Yonekura H, Yamamoto Y, Yamamoto H. Advanced glycation end-products inhibit prostacyclin production and induce plasminogen activator inhibitor-1 in human microvascular endothelial cells. *Diabetologia,* **41**: 1453–1441, 1998.

203. Schmidt AM, Yan SD, Brett J, Mora R, Nowygrod R, Stern D. Regulation of human mononuclear phagocyte migration by cell surface-binding proteins for advanced glycation end-products. *J Clin Invest,* **91**: 2155–2168, 1993.

204. Hudson BI, Stickland MH, Grant BJ. Identification of polymorphisms in the receptor for advanced glycation end-products (RAGE) gene. *Diabetes,* **47**: 1155–1157, 1998.

205. Kumaramanickavela G, Ramprasada VL, Sripriyaa S, Upadyayb NK, Paulc PG, Sharmab T. Association of *Gly82Ser* polymorphism in the RAGE gene with diabetic retinopathy in type II diabetic Asian Indian patients. *J Diabetes Complicat,* **16**: 391-394, 2002.

206. Hawrami K, *et al.* An association in non-insulin-dependent diabetes mellitus subjects between susceptibility to retinopathy and tumour necrosis factor polymorphism. *Hum Immunol,* **46**: 49–54, 1996.

207. Monos DS, *et al.* Genetic polymorphism of the human tumor necrosis factor region in insulin-dependent diabetes mellitus. Linkage disequilibrium of TNFab microsatellite alleles with HLA haplotypes. *Hum Immunol,* **44**: 70–79, 1995.

208. Hitman GA, Niven MJ. Genes and diabetes mellitus. *Brit Med Bull,* **45**: 191–205, 1989.

209. Kumaramanickavel G, Sripriya S, Vellanki RN, Upadyay NK, Badrinath SS, Arokiasamy T, Sukumar B, Vidhya A, Joseph B, Sharma T, Gopal L. Tumor necrosis factor allelic polymorphism with diabetic retinopathy in India. *Diabetes Res Clin Pract,* **2**: 89–94, 2001.

210. Grant Maria B, *et al.* Hemangioblast activity of stem cells as promoted by injury and modulated by nitric oxide in a model of retinal neovascularization. *Diabetes,* **52**(S1): A20, 2003

211. Chakravarthy U, Hayes RG, Stitt AW, McAuley E, and Archer DB. Constitutive nitric oxide synthase expression in retinal vascular endothelial cells is suppressed by high glucose and advanced glycation end-products. *Diabetes,* **47**: 945–952, 1998.

212. Song W, *et al.* Modified LDL stimulation of PKC translocation in human retinal pericytes. *Diabetes,* **52**(S1): A203, 2003.

213. Ronald CMa *et al.* Overexpression of endothelin-1 and protein kinase c β1 isoform *in vivo* mimic abnormal retinal hemodynamics of diabetes. *Diabetes,* **52**(S1): A20, 2003.

214. Zheng L, *et al.* PARP inhibitor corrects diabetes-induced alterations in retinal function and leukostasis. *Diabetes,* **52**(S1): A205, 2003.

215. Tesfaye S, *et al.* Prevalence of diabetic peripheral neuropathy and its relation to glycaemic control and potential risk factors: the EURODIAB IDDM complications study. *Diabetologia,* **39**: 1377–1384, 1996.

216. .*. Understanding diabetic neuropathy (Editorial). *Lancet,* **338**: 1496–1497, 1991.

217. Greene DA, Sima AA, Stevens MJ, Feldman EL, Lattimer SA. Complications: neuropathy, pathogenetic considerations. *Diabetes Care*, **15**: 1902–1925, 1992.

218. Hauerslev Foss C, Vestbo E, Frøland A, Gjessing HJ, Mogensen CE, Damsgaard EM. Autonomic neuropathy in nondiabetic offspring of type 2 diabetic subjects is associated with urinary albumin excretion rate and 24-h ambulatory blood pressure. *Diabetes,* **50**: 630–636, 2001.

219. Veves A, King GL. Can VEGF reverse diabetic neuropathy in human subjects? *J Clin Invest,* **10**: 1215–1218, 2001.

220. Greene DA, Stevens MJ, Obrosova I, Feldman EL. Glucose-induced oxidative stress and programmed cell death in diabetic neuropathy. *Eur J Pharmacol*, **375**: 217–223, 1999.

221. Heesom AE, Millward A, Demaine AG. Susceptibility to diabetic neuropathy in patients with insulin diabetes mellitus is associated with a polymorphism at the 5' end of the aldose reductase gene. *J Neurol Neurosurg Psychiatry*, **64**: 213–216, 1998.

222. Chistyakov DA, Savost'anov KV, Zotova EV, Nosikov VV. Polymorphisms in the Mn-SOD and EC-SOD genes and their relationship to diabetic neuropathy in type 1 diabetes mellitus. *BMC Med Gene*, **1: 4**, 2001.

223. Low PA, Nickander KK, Tritschler HJ. The roles of oxidative stress and antioxidant treatment in experimental diabetic neuropathy. *Diabetes*, **46**: S38–S42, 1997.

224. Zhu M, Spink DC, Yan B, Bank S, DeCaprio AP. Formation and structure of cross-linking and monomeric pyrrole autooxidation products in 2,5-hexanedione-treated amino acids, peptides, and protein. *Chem Res Toxicol*, **7**: 551–558,1994.

225. Hassanin MM, Azeez M. Macrovascular disease in people with type 2 diabetes in Conwy and Denbighshire: are we achieving the treatment targets? *Diabetes Metab*, **29**: 4S39, 2003.

226. Ukkola O, Savolainen MJ, P I Salmela, von Dickhoff K, Kesäniemi YA. DNA polymorphism at the lipoprotein lipase gene is associated with macroangiopathy in type 2 (non-insulin-dependent) diabetes mellitus. *Atherosclerosis*, **115**: 99–105, 1995.

227. Shimo-Nakanishi Y, Urabe T, Hattori N, Watanabe Y, Nagao T, Yokochi M, Hamamoto M, Mizuno Yoshikuni. Polymorphism of the lipoprotein lipase gene and risk of atherothrombotic cerebral infarction in the Japanese. *Stroke,* **32**: 1481–1486, 2001.

228. Fisher RM, Humphries SE, Talmud PJ. Common variation in the lipoprotein lipase gene: effects on plamsa lipids and risk of atherosclerosis. *Atherosclerosis*, **135**: 145–159, 1997.

229. Clee SM, Loubser O, Collins J, Kastelein JJ, Hayden MR. The LPL S447X cSNP is associated with decreased blood pressure and plasma triglycerides, and reduced risk of coronary artery disease. *Clin Genet*, **4**: 293–300, 2001.

230. Barakat K, Hitman GA. Genetic susceptibility to macrovascular complications of type 2 diabetes mellitus. *Best Pract Res Clin Endocrinol Metab*, **3**: 3259–370, 2001.

231. Wittrup HH, Tybjaerg-Hansen A, Steffensen R, Deeb SS, Brunzell JD, Jensen G, Nordestgaard BG. Mutations in the lipoprotein lipase gene associated with ischemic heart disease in men. *Arterioscler Thromb Vasc Biol,* **19**: 1535–1540, 1999.

232. Gilbert B, Rouis M, Griglio S, de Lumley L, Laplaud P. Lipoprotein lipase (LPL) deficiency: a new patient homozygote for the preponderant mutation Gly188Glu in the human LPL gene and review of reported mutations: 75% are clustered in exons 5 and 6. *Ann Genet*, **1**: 25–32, 2001.

233. Schneider J, Kreuzer J, Hamann A, Nawroth PP, Dugi KA. The proline 12 alanine substitution in the peroxisome proliferator-activated receptor-γ2 gene is associated with lower lipoprotein lipase activity *in vivo*. *Diabetes,* **51**: 867–870, 2002.

234. Deeb SS, Fajas L, Nemoto M, Pihlajamaki J, Mykkanen L, Kuusisto J, Laakso M, Fujimoto W, Auwerx J. A Pro12Ala substitution in PPAR-gamma2 associated with decreased receptor activity, lower body mass index and improved insulin sensitivity. *Nat Genet*, **20**: 284–287, 1998.

235. Zambon A, Hokanson JE, Brown GB, Brunzell JD. Evidence for a new pathophysiological mechanism for coronary artery disease regression. Hepatic lipase – mediated changes in LDL density. *Circulation,* **99**: 1959–1964, 1999.

236. Vega GL, Clark LT, Tang A, Marcovina S, Grundy SM, Cohen JC. Hepatic lipase activity is lower in African American men than in white American men: effects of 5' flanking polymorphism in the hepatic lipase gene (LIPC). *J Lipid Res*, **39**: 228–32, 1998.

237. van't Hooft FM, Lundahl B, Ragogna F, Karpe F, Olivecrona G, Hamsten A. Functional characterization of 4 polymorphisms in promoter region of hepatic lipase gene. *Arterioscler Thromb Vasc Biol*, **20**: 1335–1339, 2000.

238. Hong SH, Song J, Kim JQ. Genetic variations of the hepatic lipase gene in Korean patients with coronary artery disease. *Clinical Biochem*, **33** (4): 291–296, 2000.

239. Tan KCB, Shiu SWM, Chu BYM. Roles of hepatic lipase and cholesteryl ester transfer protein in determining low density lipoprotein subfraction distribution in Chinese patients with non-insulin-dependent diabetes mellitus. *Atherosclerosis,* **145**: 273–278, 1999.

240. Hokanson JE, Cheng S, Snell-Bergeon JK, Fijal BA, Grow MA, Hung C, Erlich HA, Ehrlich J, eckel RH, Rewers M. A common promoter polymorphism in the hepatic lipase gene (*LIPC-480C>T*) is associated with an increase in coronary calcification in type 1 diabetes. *Diabetes*, **51**: 1208–1213, 2002.

241. Russo GT, *et al.* Association of the Sst-I polymorphism at the APOC3 gene locus with variations in lipid levels, lipoprotein subclass profiles and coronary heart disease risk: the Framingham offspring study. *Atherosclerosis*, **158**: 173–181, 2001.

242. Lee SJ, Moye LA, Campos H, Williams GH, Sacks FM. Hypertriglyceridemia but not diabetes status is associated with coronary heart disease. *Atherosclerosis*, **167**: 293–302, 2003.

243. Zannis VI, Kan HY, Kritis A, Zanni EE, Kardassis D. Transcriptional regulatory mechanisms of the human apolipoprotein genes *in vitro* and *in vivo*. *Curr Opin Lipid*, **12**: 181–207, 2001.

244. Li WW, Dammerman MM, Smith JD, Metzger S, Breslow JL, Left T. Common genetic variation in the promoter of the human apoCIII gene abolishes regulation by insulin and may contribute to hypertriglyceridemia. *J Clin Invest*, **96**: 2601–2605, 1995.

245. Dammerman M, Sandkujil LA, Hlaas JL, Chung W, Breslow JL. An apolipoprotein CIII haplotype protective against hypertriglyceridemia is specified by promoter and 3'untranslated region polymorphisms. *Proc Natl Acad Sci*, **90**: 4562–4566, 1993.

246. Zeng Q, Dammerman M, Takada Y, Matsunaga A, Breslow JL, Sasaki J. An apolipoprotein CIII marker associated with hypertriglyceridemia in Caucasians also confers increased risk in a west Japanese population. *Hum Genet*, **95**: 371–375, 1995.

247. Kalina A, Szalai C, Prohászka Z, Reiber I, Császár A. Association of plasma lipid levels with apolipoprotein E polymorphism in type 2 diabetes. *Diabetes Res Clin Pract*, **56**: 63–68, 2000.

248. Powell DS, Maksoud H, Chargé SBP, Moffitt JH, Desai M, Da Silva Fihlo RL, Hattersley AT, Stratton IM, Matthews DR, Levy JC, Clark A. Apolipoprotein E genotype, islet amyloid deposition and severity of type 2 diabetes. *Diabetes Res Clinical Pract*, **60**: 105–110, 2003.

249. Ou T, Yamakawa-Kobayashi, Arinami T, Amemiya A, Fujiwara H, Kawata K, Saito M, Kikuchi S, Noguchi Y, Sugishita, Hamaguchi H. Methylenetetrahydrofolate reductase and apolipoprotein E polymorphisms are independent risk factors for coronary heart disease in Japanese: a case-control study. *Atherosclerosis*, **137**: 23–28, 1998.

250. Araki S, Moczulski DK, Scott LJ, Warram JH, Krolewski AS. APOE polymorphisms and the development of diabetic nephropathy in type 1 diabetes. *Diabetes*, **49**: 2190–2195, 2000.

251. Shcherbak NS. Apolipoprotein E gene polymorphism is not a strong risk factor for diabetic nephropathy and retinopathy in type 1 diabetes: case-control study. *BMC Medical Genetics*, **2**: 8, 2001.

252. Chen G, Paka L, Kako Y, Singhal P, Duan W, Pillarisetti S. A protective role for kidney apolipoprotein E. *J Biol Chem*, **52**: 49142–49147, 2001.

253. Meguro S, Takei I, Murata M, Hirose H, Takei N, Mitsuyoshi Y, Ishii K, Oguchi S, Shinohara J, Takeshita E, Watanabe K, Saruta T. Cholesteryl ester transfer protein polymorphism associated with macroangiopathy in Japanese patients with type 2 diabetes. *Atherosclerosis*, **156**: 151–156, 2001.

254. Kawasaki I, Tahara H, Shoji T, Nishizawa Y. Relationship between *Taq*IB cholesteryl ester transfer protein gene polymorphism and macrovascular complications in Japanese patients with type 2 diabetes. *Diabetes*, **51**: 871–874, 2002.

255. Ordovas JM, Cupples LA, Corella D, Otvos JD, Osgood D, Martinez A, Lahoz C, Coltell O, Wilson PWF, Schaefer EJ. Association of cholesteryl ester transfer protein – *Taq*IB polymorphism with variations in lipoprotein subclasses and coronary heart disease risk. *Arterioscler Thromb Vasc Biol*, **20**: 1323–1329, 2000.

256. Kuivenhoven JA, Jukema JW, Zwinderman AH, de Knijff P, McPherson R, Bruschke AVG, Lie KI, Kastelein JJP. The role of a common variant of the cholesteryl ester transfer protein gene in the progression of coronary atherosclerosis. *New Eng J Med*, **338**: 86–93, 1998.

257. Hannuksela ML, Liinamaa MJ, Kesaniemi YA, Savolainen MJ. Relation of polymorphisms in the cholesteryl ester transfer protein gene to transfer protein activity and plasma lipoprotein levels in alcohol drinkers. *Atherosclerosis*, **1**: 35–44, 1994.

258. Freeman DJ, Griffin BA, Holmes AP, Lindsay GM, Gaffney D, Packard CJ, Shepherd J. Regulation of plasma HDL cholesterol and subfraction distribution by genetic and environmental factors: associations between the TaqI B RFLP in the CETP gene and smoking and obesity. *Arterioscler Thromb*, **14**: 336–344, 1994.

259. Colhoun HM, Scheek LM, Rubens MB, Gent TV, Underwood RS, Fuller JH, van Tol A. Lipid transfer protein activities in type 1 diabetic patients without renal failure and nondiabetic control subjects and their association with coronary artery calcification. *Diabetes*, **50**: 652–659, 2001.

260. Leviev I, James RW. Promoter polymorphisms of human paraoxonase PON1 gene and serum activities and concentrations. *Arterioscler Thromb Vasc Biol,* **20**: 516–521, 2000.

261. Mackness MI, Mackness B, Durrington P. Paraoxonase and coronary heart disease. *Atheroscler Suppl,* **3**: 49–55, 2002.

262. Osei-Hyiaman D, Hou L, Mengbai F, Zhiyin R, Zhiming Z, Kano K. Coronary artery disease risk in Chinese type 2 diabetics: is there a role for paraoxonase 1 gene (Q192R) polymorphism? *Eur J Endocrinol,* **144**: 639–644, 2001.

263. Suehiro T, Nakamura T, Inoue M, Shiinoki T, Ikeda Y, Kumon Y, Shindo M, Tanaka H, Hashimoto K. A polymorphism upstream from the human paraoxonase (PON1) gene and its association with PON1 expression. *Atherosclerosis,* **150**: 295–298, 2000.

264. James RW, Leviev I, Ruiz J, Passa P, Froguel P, and Garin MC. Promoter polymorphism T(-107)C of the paraoxonase PON1 gene is a risk factor for coronary heart disease in type 2 diabetic patients. *Diabetes,* **49**: 1390–1393, 2000.

265. Durrington PN, Mackness B, Mackness M. Paraoxonase and Atherosclerosis. *Arterioscler Thromb Vasc Biol,* **21**: 473–480, 2001.

266. Mackness B, Mackness MI, Arrol S, *et al.* Effect of the human serum paraoxonase 55 and 192 genetic polymorphisms on the protection by high density lipoprotein against low density lipoprotein oxidative modification. *FEBS* (Letters) **423**: 57, 1998.

267. Odawara M, Tachi Y, Yamashita K. Paraoxonase polymorphism (Gln^{192}-Arg) is associated with coronary heart disease in Japanese noninsulin-dependent diabetes mellitus. *J Clin Endocrinol Metab,* **7**: 2257–2260, 1997.

268. Aubo C, Senti M, Marrugat J, Tomas M, Vila J, Sala J, Masia R. Risk of myocardial infarction associated with Gln/Arg 192 polymorphism in the human paraoxonase gene and diabetes mellitus. The REGICOR Investigators. *Eur Heart J,* **21**: 33–38, 2000.

269. Garin MC, James RW, Dussoix P, Blanché H, Passa P, Froguel P, Ruiz J. Paraoxonase polymorphisms. Met-Leu54 is associated with modified serum concentrations of the enzyme. A possible link between the paraoxonase gene and increased risk of cardiovascular disease in diabetes. *J Clin Invest,* **1**: 62–66, 1997.

270. Brophy VH, Jampsa RL, Clendenning JB, McKinstry LA, Jarvik GP, Furlong CE. Effects of 5' regulatory-region polymorphisms on paraoxonase gene (PON1) expression. *Am J Hum Genet,* **68**: 1428–1436, 2001.

271. Komatsu M, Kawagishi T, Emoto M, Shoji T, Yamada A, Sato K, Hosoi M, Nishizawa Y. ecNOS gene polymorphism is associated with endothelium-dependent vasodilatation in type 2 diabetes. *Am J Physiol Heart Circ Physiol,* **283**: H557–H561, 2002.

272. Odawara M, Sasaki K, Tachi Y, Yamashita K. Endothelial nitric oxide synthase gene polymorphism and coronary heart disease in Japanese NIDDM. *Diabetologia* (Letters), **41**: 365–367, 1998.

273. Pulkkinen A, Viitanen L, Kareinen A, Lehto S, Vauhkonen I, Laakso M. Intron 4 polymorphism of the endothelial nitric oxide synthase gene is associated with elevated blood pressure in type 2 diabetic patients with coronary heart disease. *J Mol Med,* **78**: 372–379, 2000.

274. Hayden MR, Tyagi SC. Is type 2 diabetes mellitus a vascular disease (atheroscleropathy with hyperglycemia a late manifestation? The role of NOS, NO and redox stress. *Cardiovasc Diabetol,* **2**: 2, 2003.

275. Nassar BA, Bevin LD, Johnstone DE, O'neill BJ, Bata IR, Kirkland SA, Title LM. Relationship of the Glu298Asp polymorphism of the endothelial nitric oxide synthase gene and early-onset coronary artery disease. *Am Heart J,* **145**: 586–589, 2001.

276. Cai H, Wang X, Colagiuri S, Wilcken DEL. A common Glu^{298}→Asp (894G→T) mutation at exon 7 of the endothelial nitrc oxide synthase gene and vascular complications in type 2 diabetes. *Diabetes Care* (Letters), **12**: 2195, 1998.

277. Vendrell J, Fernandez-Real JM, Gutierrez C, Zamora A, Simon I, Bardaji A, Ricart W, Richart C. A polymorphism in the promoter of tumor necrosis factor-α gene (-308) is associated with coronary heart disease in type 2 diabetic patients. *Atherosclerosis,* **167**: 257–264, 2003.

278. Keso T, Perola M, Laippala P, Ilveskoski E Kunnas, TA, Mikkelsson J, Pentillä A, Hurme M, Karhunen PJ. Polymorphisms within the tumor necrosis factor locus and prevalence of coronary artery disease in middle-aged men. *Atherosclerosis,* **154**: 691–697, 2001.

279. Padovani JC, Pazin-Filho A, Simões MV, Marin-Neto JA, Zago MA, Franco RF. Gene polymorphisms in the TNF locus and the risk of myocardial infarction. *Thromb Res,* **100**: 263–269, 2000.

280. Tan KCB, Chow WS, Ai VHG, Metz C, Bucala R, Lam KSL. Advanced glycation end-products and endothelial dysfunction in type 2 Diabetes. *Diabetes Care,* **25**: 1055–1059, 2002.

281. Hudson BI, Stickland MH, Grant PJ. Identification of polymorphisms in the receptor for advanced glycation end-products (RAGE) gene: prevalence in type II diabetes and ethnic groups. *Diabetes,* **47**: 1155–1157, 1998.

282. Hudson BI, Stickland MH, Futers TS, Grant PJ. Study of the −429T/C and −374T/A receptor for advanced glycation end-products promoter polymorphisms in diabetic and nondiabetic subjects with macrovascular disease. *Diabetes Care*, **11**: 2004, 2001.

283. Tarnow L, Stehouwer CDA, Emeis JJ, Poirier O, Cambien F, Hansen BV, Parving HH. Plasminogen activator inhibitor-1 and apolipoprotein E gene polymorphism and diabetic angiopathy. *Nephrol Dial Transplant*, **15**: 625–630, 2000.

284. Kang SS, wong PWK, Susmano A, Sora J, Norusis M, Ruggie N. Thermolabile methylene-tetrahydrofolate reductase: an inherited risk factor for coronary artery disease. *Am J Hum Genet*, **48**: 536–45, 1991.

285. Francis CM, Frohlich JJ. Coronary artery disease in patients at low risk − apolipoprotein AI as an independent risk factor. *Atherosclerosis*, **155**: 165–170, 2001.

286. Wang XL, Badenhop R, Humphrey KE, Wilcken DE. C to T and/or G to A transitions are responsible for loss of a *MspI* restriction site at the 5'-end of the human apolipoprotein AI gene. *Human Genet*, **95**: 473–474, 1995.

287. Wang XL, Badenhop R, Humphrey KE, Wilcken DE. New *MspI* polymorphism at +83 pb of the human apolipoprotein AI gene: association with increased circulating high density lipoprotein cholesterol levels. *Genet Epidemiol*, **13**: 1–10, 1996.

288. Pulkkinen A, Viitanen L, Kareinen A, Lehto S, Laakso M. *MspI* polymorphism at +83 pb in intron 1 of the human apolipoprotein A1 gene is associated with elevated levels of HDL cholesterol and apolipoprotein A1 in nondiabetic subjects but not in type 2 diabetic patients with coronary heart disease. *Diabetes Care*, **23**: 791–796, 2000.

289. Gabel BR, May LF, Marcovina SM, Koschinsky ML. Lipoprotein(a) assembly. Quantitative assessment of the role of Apo(a) Kringle IV types 2–10 in particle formation. *Arterioscler Thromb Vasc Biol*, **12**: 1559–1567, 1996.

290. van der Hoek YY, Wittekoek, Beisiegel U, Kastelein JJ, Koschinsky ML. The apolipoprotein(a) kringle IV repeats which differ from the major repeat kringle are present in variably-sized isoforms. *Hum Mol Genet*, **4**:361–366, 1993.

291. Kronenberg F, Auinger M, Trenkwalder E, Irsigler K, Utermann G, Dieplinger H. Is apolipoprotein(a) a susceptibility gene for type I diabetes mellitus and related to long-term survival? *Diabetologia*, **42**: 1021–1027, 1999.

292. Gazzaruso C, Garzaniti A, Buscaglia P, *et al.* Association between apolipoprotein(a) phenotypes and coronary heart disease at a young age. *J Am Coll Cardiol*, **33**: 157–163, 1999.

293. van Ittersum FJ, de Man AME, Thijssen S, de Knijff P, Slagboom E, Smulders Y, Tarnow L, Donker AJM, Bilo HJG, Stehouwer CDA. Genetic polymorphisms of the renin-angiotensin system and complications of insulin-dependent diabetes mellitus. *Nephrol Dial Transplant*, **15**: 1000–1007, 2000.

294. Keavney BD, Dudley CR, Stratton IM, *et al.* UK prospective diabetes study (UKPDS) 14: association of angiotensin-converting enzyme insertion/deletion polymorphism with myocardial infarction in NIDDM. *Diabetologia*, **8**: 948–952, 1995.

295. Nakauchi Y, *et al.* Significance of angiotensin I-converting enzyme and angiotensin II type 1 receptor gene polymorphisms as risk factors for coronary heart disease. *Atherosclerosis*, **125**: 161–169, 1996.

296. Benetos A, *et al.* Influence of the angiotensin II type 1 receptor gene polymorphism on the effects of perindopril and nitrendipine on arterial stiffness in hypertensive individuals. *Hypertension*, **28**: 1081–1084.

297. Lindpaintner K, Pfeffer MA, Kreutz R, Stampfer MJ, Grodstein F, LaMotte F, Buring J, Hennekens CH. A prospective evaluation of an angiotensin-converting-enzyme gene polymorphism and the risk of ischemic heart disease. *N Engl J Med*, **11**: 706–711, 1995.

298. Zak I, Niemiec P, Sarecka B, Balcerzyk A, Ciemniewski Z, Rudowska E, Dylag S. Carrier-state of D allele in ACE gene insertion/deletion polymorphism is associated with coronary artery disease, in contrast to the C677T transition in the MTHFR gene. *Acta Biochim Pol*, **2**: 527–534, 2003.

299. Kario K, Matsuo T, Kobayashi H, Kanai N, Hoshide S, Mitsuhashi T, Ikeda U, Nishiuma S, Matsuo M, Shimada K. Endothelial cell damage and angiotensin-converting enzyme insertion / deletion genotype in elderly hypertensive patients. *J Am Coll Cardiol*, **2**: 444–450, 1998.

300. Parving HH, Andersen AR, Smidt UM, Svendsen PA. Early aggressive antihypertensive treatment reduces rate of decline in kidney function in diabetic nephropathy. *Lancet*, **1**: 1175–1179, 1983.

301. Prasad A, Narayanan S, Husain S, Padder F, Waclawiw M, Epstein N, Quyyumi AA. Insertion-Deletion polymorphism of the ACE gene modulates reversibility of endothelial dysfunction with ACE inhibition. *Circulation*, **1**: 35–41, 2000.

302. Naber CK, Husing J, Wolfhard U, Erbel R, Siffert W. Interaction of the ACE D allele and the GNB3 825T allele in myocardial infarction. *Hypertension*, **6**: 986–989, 2000.

7

THE ROLE OF HYPERGLYCEMIA IN THE DEVELOPMENT OF DIABETIC COMPLICATIONS, INVESTIGATED IN TRANSGENIC MOUSE MODEL

Doina POPOV, Dorel Lucian RADU

Double transgenic mice (dTg) were obtained by crossing insulin-hemagglutinin (Ins-HA) Tg mice, expressing hemagglutinin of PR8 influenza virus in the pancreatic β-cells under the rat insulin promotor, with Tg mice expressing the T-cell receptor-hemagglutinin (TCR-HA), specific for immunodominant epitope HA110-120 of the same virus. These mice were introduced as an experimental model of fulminant type 1 insulin-dependent diabetes mellitus. In this study, we investigated the morphological changes of heart ventricle, kidney glomeruli and aortic wall, in diabetic dTg mice (comparatively with their age-matched non-diabetic mice). The main cardiovascular alterations of diabetic dTg mice are: left ventricular hypertrophy (at circulating glucose concentration 365 to 475 mg/dl) followed by dilatative cardiomyopathy (at glucose concentration over 600 mg/dl), interstitial fibrosis of the heart, narrowing of the coronary capillaries under the pressure exerted by the hyperplasic pericapillary extracellular matrix, lipid loading of the epicardium (as a new attribute of diabetes), renal hypertrophy associated with glomerulopathy and the activation of endothelium and smooth muscle cells within the aortic wall. At present, understanding the molecular mechanisms underlying the morphological changes in diabetic dTg mice is an exciting challenge for the current research.

Abbreviations List

AGEs – advanced glycation end-products
AGE-Rs – AGE-receptors
dTg – Double transgenic
GH – growth hormone
GBM – glomerular basement membrane

IGF-I – insulin growth factor I
MAPK – mitogen-activated protein kinase
NO – nitric oxide
TCR-HA – T-cell receptor-hemagglutinin

Animal models that mimic some aspects of the pathophysiology of diabetes have been developed. These models have increased our understanding of the roles of immunologic, environmental and genetic factors in the generation, activation and expansion of self-reactive cells. In addition, transgenic models of particular genes, with certain genetic backgrounds, have also contributed to the understanding of single gene function and its possible contribution to pathogenesis.

Transgenic (Tg) mice have been used to study human disease, to understand and study physiological as well as physiopathological aspects. The advantages of using genetically engineered mouse models are that fewer mice are needed, the time to develop disease is greatly reduced and may provide useful experimental models for fundamental or pharmacological research. An area of current interest is the use of transgenic mice as experimental models for diabetes.

Patients with diabetes frequently suffer from a complex dyslipidemia which is characterized, in part, by defective lipoprotein uptake and metabolism. Diabetic patients have been found to exhibit high circulating levels of protein-bound advanced glycation end-products (AGEs). Mice transgenic for the human LDL receptor, under control of the mouse metallothionein I promoter have been used to study how AGE-modified LDL forms rapidly by the direct reaction of native LDL with circulating reactive AGE-peptides. LDL modified by AGE-peptides exhibited markedly impaired clearance kinetics when injected into transgenic mice expressing the human LDL receptor [1–3].

Diabetes causes cardiovascular complications, including direct cardiac muscle weakening known as diabetic cardiomyopathy, which occurs in the absence of ischemic heart disease and hypertension. Diabetic cardiomyopathy is characterized by disturbances in both cardiac contraction and relaxation, which are maintained by calcium homeostasis in cardiac cells. To investigate if AGE and AGE-Rs (AGE-receptors) may directly affect the myocardial Ca^{2+} homeostasis, transgenic mice that overexpressed human AGE-Rs in the heart were produced. Using these mice there were analyzed the Ca^{2+} transients in cultivated cardiac myocytes (CM) from the AGE-Rs transgenic and non-transgenic control fetuses. Compared with CM from the control

mice, CM from transgenic mice showed a reduced systolic and diastolic intracellular calcium concentration. Exposure to AGE caused a significant prolongation of the decay time of calcium in CM from control mice, and this response was augmented in CM from the AGE-Rs transgenic mice. These results suggest that the AGE and AGE-Rs could play an active role in the development of diabetes-induced cardiac dysfunction [4].

Clinically, diabetes mellitus is often accompanied by elevated GH (growth hormone), which is followed by reduced IGF-I (insulin growth factor I) levels, possibly due to hepatic resistance to GH, which is followed by reduced IGF-I production that, in turn, lowers feedback inhibition over further GH production. These changes were most evident when glycemia is poorly controlled and diabetogenic effects of excess GH have been also demonstrated in humans with acromegaly, as well as in dogs that were given GH injections [5].

A growing body of evidence for a role of GH in nephropathy has come from studies of transgenic mice expressing GH. In addition to displaying a giant phenotype, transgenic mice expressing either bovine GH or human (h) GH-releasing hormone (GHRH) developed progressive glomerulosclerosis. In contrast, transgenic mice expressing hIGF-I did not develop renal damage, although their glomeruli were enlarged. Also, transgenic mice expressing GH antagonists' transgenes (dwarf animals) did not develop glomerulosclerosis. These results strengthen the hypothesis of a direct role of GH in nephropathy, independent of IGF-I activation [6].

There is a general agreement on the involvement of immune reactions in type 1 diabetes. Performed during insulitis phase, the gene transfer of calcitonin-related peptide was reported to selectively suppress the proinflammatory T lymphocytes (Th 1 subsets) and to promote the anti-inflammatory Th 2 subsets, resulting in amelioration of beta-cell destruction in streptozotocin-injected mice [7].

Recently, the transgenic mice that expressed human semicarbazide-sensitive amine oxidase in smooth muscle cells were used to understand to what extent inhibition of this enzyme can prevent the development of vascular complications in diabetes [8].

The double transgenic mouse (dTg), expressing the hemagglutinin of influenza virus under the insulin promoter and the TCR specific for the immunodominant CD4 T cell epitope of hemagglutinin was introduced as an experimental model of fulminant type 1 insulin-dependent diabetes mellitus [9–11]. In this study, the diabetic dTg mice were examined for the occurrence of microvascular complications (in myocardium and kidney glomeruli) and for the macrovascular changes (in the aorta).

Experiments were performed on dTg mice at 7, 8, 10 and 13 weeks of biological age. At each time point pairs from the same litter were selected: one animal that develop type 1 insulin-dependent diabetes mellitus and an age-matched pair that did not develop the disease. The criteria used for selection of the animals were: the body weight, the blood glucose after fast, and the heart hypertrophy (expressed by the ratio of heart weight to body weight). Throughout the experiment, mice selected as diabetics had a reduced body weight (7.5 to 15 g), significantly lower as compared to that of the age-matched pairs (22 to 25 g), and their blood glucose was higher than 365 mg/dl, while that of mice without diabetes was at the normal levels (92 ± 12 mg/dl).

At 7, 8, 10 and 13 weeks into the experiment, mice were perfused *in situ* until free of blood (*via* abdominal aorta), the tissues fixed by perfusion and processed for standard electron microscopy. The thin sections were reacted with uranyl acetate (7.6 % in distilled water) and lead citrate (0.4% in 0.1N NaOH) and examined with the Philips 201C electron microscope (Eindhoven, The Netherlands).

The main cardiovascular changes observed in the diabetic dTg mice (as compared to the age-matched controls) consisted in: glucose-dependent left ventricular hypertrophy, interstitial fibrosis of the heart, lipid loading of the epicardium, activation of endothelium and smooth muscle cells within the aortic wall, and microangiopathic changes similar to those reported for both human and experimental diabetes.

LEFT VENTRICULAR HYPERTROPHY

Compared to normal mice (non-diabetic, age-matched), there was a glucose-dependent response of the left ventricle of the diabetic dTg mice. Thus,

at circulating glucose levels between 365 and 475 mg/dl, left ventricular hypertrophy was a constant occurrence (Plate 7.1a, b), while at glucose levels over 600 mg/dl, the ventricular wall became thinner and the heart cavity became enlarged (Plate 7.1c).

As in humans [12], the cardiomyocytes of the diabetic dTg mice with circulating glucose concentration 365 to 475 mg/dl respond with hypertrophy to the metabolic insult (since the cardiomyocytes are nondividing cells, unable to generate additional cellular mass to face the increased metabolic demands) (Plate 7.1b). Comparing with the data in age-matched controls, higher values of the heart to body weight ratio were found in diabetic dTg mice, *i.e.* at 7 weeks and plasma glucose 475 mg/dl, the ratio was 0.714×10^{-2} in diabetic dTg mice *vs.* 0.511×10^{-2} in controls. The left ventricular hypertrophy was also reported for hamsters with spontaneous hypertension and is a characteristic pattern of hypertensive heart disease in humans [13, 14]. It is generally agreed that left ventricular hypertrophy involves growth of cardiomyocytes, as well as remodeling of the extracellular matrix proteins [15]. Interestingly, the pressure overload was reported to transiently induce the expression of several genes (including hsp70 and the oncogenes c-myc, c-fos and c-jun) that participate in the cardiac adaptative response [16].

At the extremely high glucose levels (over 600 mg/dl), the left ventricle appeared thinner (Plate 7.1c) and the structure of the cardiomyocytes was severely damaged (see bellow). In addition, at 13 weeks and plasma glucose 760 mg/dl, the heart to body weight ratio was 0.430×10^{-2} in diabetic dTg mice *vs.* 0.549×10^{-2} in the age-matched controls. To the thinner ventricular wall several factors may contribute, such as a very high overload that can not be compensated by hypertrophy and damage /or apoptosis of cardiomyocytes [17]. Although apoptosis is known to characterize the diabetic heart, using a model of transgenic mice Kajstura *et al.* reported that IGF-1 interferes with the development of myopathy by attenuating p53 function, Ang II production and AT(1) activation [18]. The latter event might be responsible for the decrease in oxidative stress and myocytes death induced by IGF-1.

Taken together, the results of our study assess that in diabetic dTg mice, the left ventricular hypertrophy is controlled by the circulating

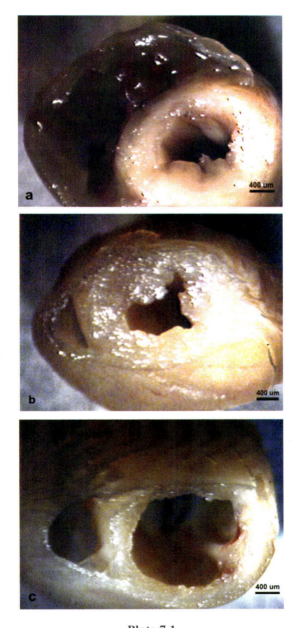

Plate 7.1
A comparative illustration of the thickness of the left ventricle.
a – control group, mice with circulating glucose ~ 133 mg/dl), b – type 1 diabetic
dTg mice with circulating glucose ~ 475 mg/dl and c – ~ 760 mg/dl.

glucose levels, rather than by the biological age of the diabetic animals.

THE STRUCTURE OF THE MYOCARDIUM AND OF THE CORONARY CAPILLARIES

In the group of control mice, the myocardium of the left ventricle showed a normal structure with the usual alignment of the contractile fibrils in cardiomyocytes (Figure 7.1). In contradistinction, in the enlarged left ventricular wall of diabetic dTg mice (blood glucose 475 mg/dl) frequent areas of extracellular matrix containing membranary materials apparently separated the cardiomyocytes (Figure 7.2), supporting for interstitial fibrosis of the heart. Interruption of the Z bands and replacement of the contractile fibers by extracellular matrix containing lipid droplets were also evident (Figure 7.3); all these features may eventually affect the heart contractility. The dTg mice with blood glucose 725 mg/dl showed frequent lysosomes within the cardiomyocytes (data not shown), a structural feature indicative for the degradation processes, associated with a thinner ventricular wall (and in turn, with the enlargement of the heart cavity).

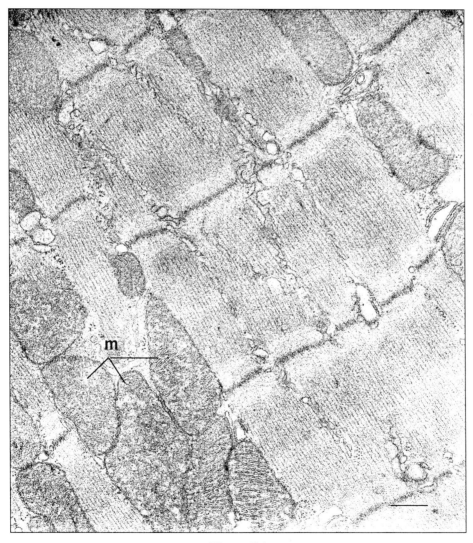

Figure 7.1

The structure of the ventricular myocardium in a non-diabetic mouse at 7 weeks biological age.

m: mitochondria, Bar: 0.38μm.

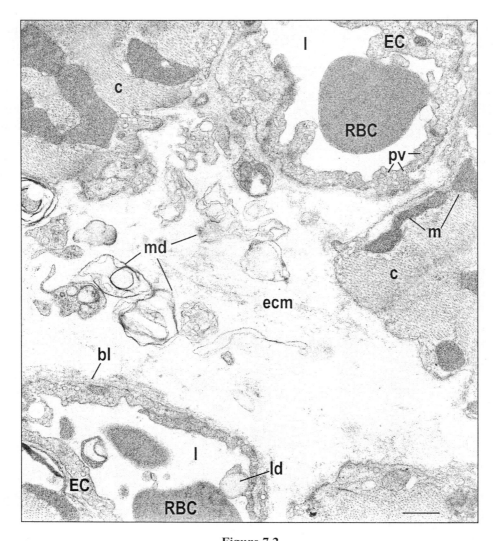

Figure 7.2
Ultrastructure of left ventricle myocardium in a diabetic dTg mouse (7 weeks biological age).

The capillaries are endowed with numerous plasmalemmal vesicles (pv), contained lipid droplets (ld) and produced a multilayered basal lamina (bl) and abundant extracellular matrix (ecm). The latter may be the site of intense degradative processes since it is rich in membranary debris (md). EC: endothelial cell; l: capillary lumen; c: cardiomyocyte; RBC: red blood cell; m: mitochondria. Bar: 0.52μm.

In diabetic dTg mice the endothelial cells of the coronary capillaries showed a secretory phenotype enriched in the rough endoplasmic reticulum with dilated cisternae (Figure 7.3), lipid droplets and a multilayered basal lamina (Figure 7.2). The pericapillary extracellular matrix may impede the oxygen transport to the cardiomyocytes, inducing locally hypoxic phenomena.

Taken together, the structural alterations of the capillary endothelium in diabetic dTg mice were similar to the microangiopathic complications of diabetes reported for humans and for animal models of chemically-induced disease [19, 20]. To this similarity contribute the high level of circulating glucose, hemodynamic factors and mediators that may induce inflammatory mechanisms in endothelial cells [21, 22]. Recently, Romano *et al.* [23] reported a correlation between the inflammatory reactions and the endothelial perturbations.

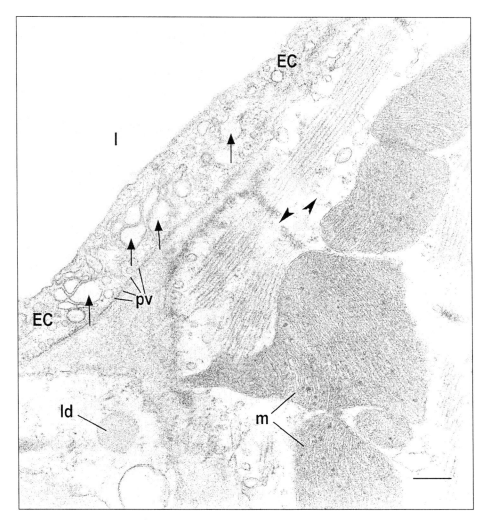

Figure 7.3

A typical electron micrograph showing the disorganization of the contractile fibers (arrow heads)
and occurrence of lipid droplets (ld) within the myocardium
in a diabetic dTg mouse (10 weeks biological age).

Note the secretory phenotype of the capillary endothelium (EC) containing enlarged rER cisternae (arrow).
l: capillary lumen; pv: plasmalemmal vesicles, m: mitochondria. Bar: 0.27 μm.

THE STRUCTURE OF THE EPICARDIUM (LAMINA VISCERALIS PERICARDII)

The heart specimens of diabetic dTg mice showed that the epicardium has a hyperplasic extracellular matrix enriched in collagen fibers and beneath it large lipid deposits that included cholesterol crystals, were evident (Figure 7.4). To our knowledge, this feature was not reported so far in the literature. The endocardium has an important role for the development of coronaries; recently, a hypothesis was advanced, claiming that epicardium – derived cells give instructive signals to the myocardium for the proper differentiation of the compact and the trabeculated compartments [24].

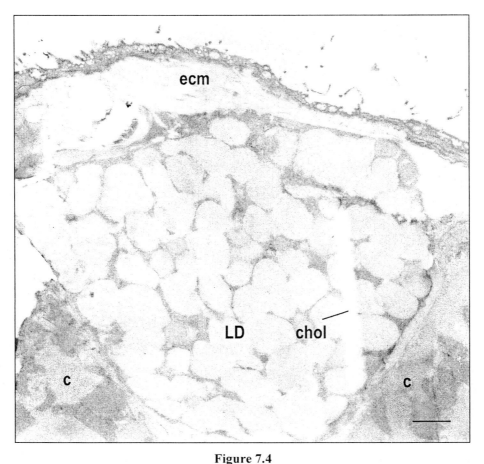

Figure 7.4

A huge lipid deposit (LD) containing a prominent cholesterol crystal (Chol) beneath the epicardium in the heart of a diabetic dTg mouse (7 weeks of biological age).

Note also the large amount of extracellular matrix (ecm) made of collagen fibers. c: cardiomyocyte. Bar: 0.75 μm.

THE STRUCTURE OF THE GLOMERULAR CAPILLARIES

A first observation on the kidneys of diabetic dTg mice was their increased dimensions and weight, compared to the age-matched non-diabetics. Thus, in diabetics at 7 and 10 weeks biological age, the ratio kidney weight/body weight was 0.924×10^{-2} and 1.306×10^{-2}, respectively (*vs.* 0.598×10^{-2} and 0.668×10^{-2} in controls). Renal hypertrophy was also reported for the nonobese diabetic mouse, a model of spontaneous insulin-dependent diabetes mellitus [25].

Examined by electron microscopy, the kidney glomeruli of dTg diabetics showed numerous, partially or totally collapsed capillaries and the thickening of the glomerular basement membrane (GBM) that double the normal value, *i.e.* 190 to 342 nm in diabetics, *versus* 106 to 152 nm in controls. In some locations, GBM became folded (Figure 7.5) and the mesangial area significantly increased (Figure 7.6). Morphometric estimations revealed an increase of the mesangial fractional volume to 37% (compared to ~ 10% in control mice) ($p < 0.002$).

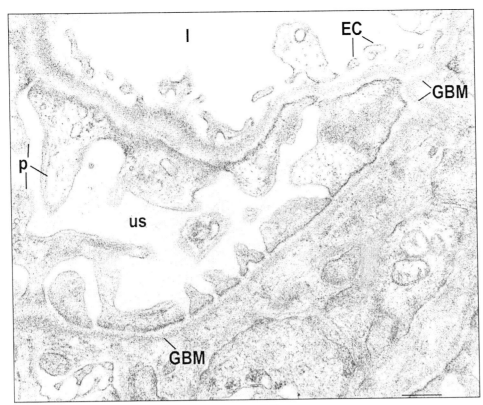

Figure 7.5

Electron micrograph of a segment of a glomerulus from a diabetic dTg mouse at 8 weeks of biological age.

Note the folding of the thickened glomerular basement membrane (GBM) and the narrowing of the urinary space (us). EC: endothelial cell; l: capillary lumen; p: podocyte. Bar: 0.38 μm.

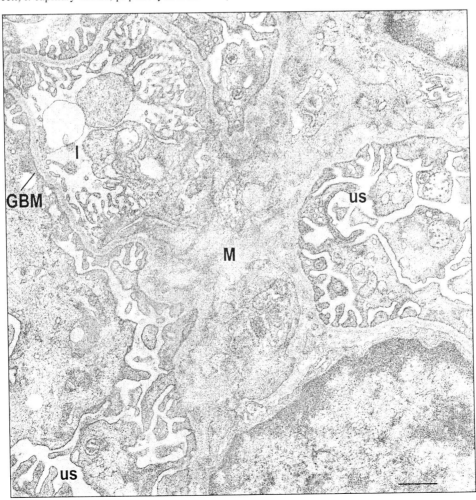

7.6a

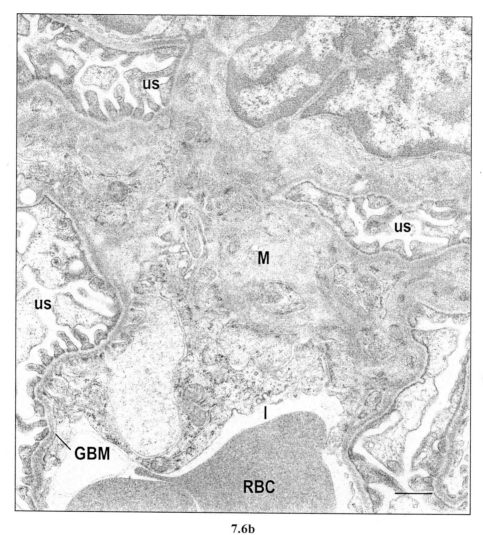

7.6b

Figure 7.6

The mesangial area.

(a) – a non-diabetic mouse at 7 weeks biological age; b – a diabetic dTg mouse, age-matched. Note in (b) the enlargement of the mesangium (M), and the narrowing of the urinary space (us). GBM: glomerular basement membrane, l: capillary lumen; RBC: red blood cell. Bars: (a, b) 0.52 μm.

The results obtained show that diabetic dTg mice developed alterations similar to those described for diabetic glomerulopathy, including the "smooth muscle cell phenotype"-like of mesangial cells [26]. Recent reports advanced the idea that kinin receptors contribute to the development of glomerular injury in diabetes and that amelioration of glomerular lesions occurred after administration of OPB-9195, an inhibitor of advanced glycation end-products formation [27, 28]. In mesangial cells, the high glucose was reported to activate several mitogen-activated protein kinase (MAPK) pathways, which, in turn, regulate transcription factors and control the mesangial cells growth and extracellular matrix gene expression [29]. Recently, Wilmer *et al.* showed that the reactive oxygen species were involved in glucose-activation of p38 MAPK pathway in human mesangial cells [30]. The strong relationship between glomerular structure and renal function was recently reported for patients with long standing type 1 diabetes [31].

THE STRUCTURE OF THE AORTIC ARCH

Since aortic arch is one of the atherosclerotic-prone areas, we considered worth to investigate it in non-diabetic and diabetic mice. In the non-diabetic mice there were no alterations of the normal structure of the endothelium and smooth muscle cells, *i.e.* both cells showed the non-secretory phenotype typical for the quiescent condition. The pathological alterations were obvious in diabetic dTg mice and indicated cellular activation. Thus, endothelial cells were endowed with abundant secretory and degradative compartments and hyperplasia of the basal lamina was often interposed between the endothelium and the subjacent lamina elastica interna (Figure 7.7a).

The smooth muscle cells turned from the contractile to the secretory phenotype and were enriched in rough endoplasmic reticulum (Figure 7.7b). At the time intervals studied, no lipid deposits or foam cells were detected within the wall of the aortic arch of diabetic dTg mice. In further studies, it will be interesting to investigate the vascular reactivity and the associated signal transduction pathways in aorta of diabetic dTg mice. Recent reports showed that in the aorta of diabetic animals the lipid peroxidation was increased, the glutathione levels were decreased, the bioavailability of NO was reduced and that diets enriched in primrose oil prevented the development of deficits in endothelium-dependent relaxation [32–34].

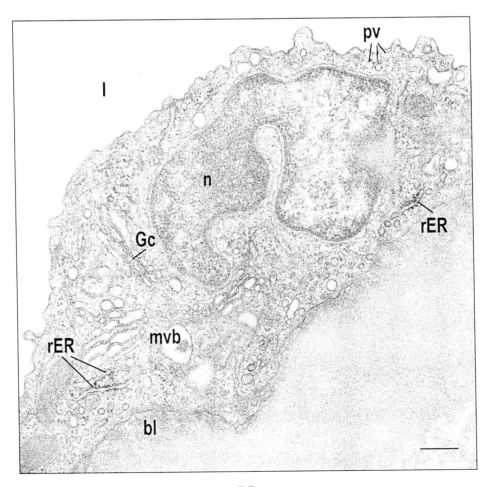

7.7a

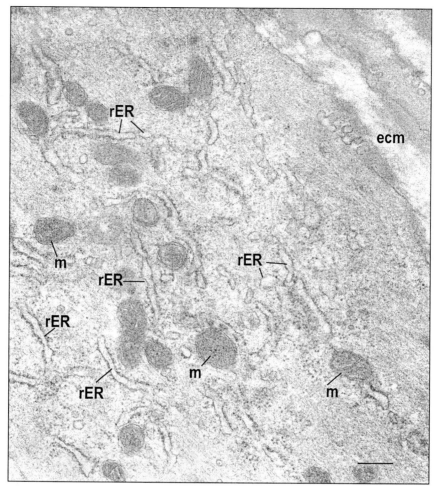

7.7b

Figure 7.7

The structure of the aortic arch in a diabetic dTg mouse at 10 weeks biological age.

a – the secretory phenotype of the endothelium enriched in biosynthetic organelles, such as rough endoplasmic reticulum (rER) and Golgi complex (Gc) and with degradative compartments, such as the multivesicular body (mvb); b – the secretory phenotype of the smooth muscle cells enriched in rER, and apparently with a reduced amount of contractile fibers. n: nucleus; pv: plasmalemmal vesicles; m: mitochondria. Bar: 0.27 μm.

PERSPECTIVES

The study of the morphological changes of heart ventricle, kidney glomeruli and aortic wall of diabetic dTg mice indicates features in common with human disease, such as the left ventricular hypertrophy (a potentially useful bioassay of strategies of global cardiovascular prevention [35, 36]), the glomerulopathy, the activated phenotype of the cells within the aortic vascular wall and the lipid loading of epicardium, as a new attribute of diabetes. At present, understanding the molecular mechanisms underlying the morphological changes in diabetic dTg mice represents an exciting challenge for the basic research.

Acknowledgements. The authors acknowledge the expert technical assistance of M. Misici (microtomy) and the valuable help of Dr. E. Constantinescu with the electronic processing of the illustrations in the Institute of Cellular Biology and Pathology "N. Simionescu" of the Romanian Academy. This work is the "Partner" (Dr. D. Popov) section of the project of Dr. DL Radu (Project Director) that was awarded with the "VIASAN" Grant no. 068/2001 of the Ministry of Education and Research, Romania.

REFERENCES

1. Vlassara H. The AGE-receptor in the pathogenesis of diabetic complications. *Diabetes Metab Res Rev,* **17**: 436–443, 2001.

2. Schnider SL, Kohn RR. Effects of age and diabetes mellitus on the solubility and nonenzymatic glucosylation of human skin collagen. *J Clin Invest,* **67**: 1630–1635, 1981.

3. Bucala R, Makita Z, Vega G, Grundy S, Koschinsky T, Cerami A, Vlassara H. Modification of low density lipoprotein by advanced glycation end-products contributes to the dyslipidemia of diabetes and renal insufficiency. *Proc Natl Acad Sci USA,* **91**: 9441–9445, 1994.

4. Petrova R, Yamamoto Y, Muraki K, Yonekura H, Sakurai S, Watanabe T, Hui Li, Takeuchi M, Makita Z, Kato I, Takasawa S, Okamoto H, Imaizumi Y, Yamamoto H. Advanced glycation endproduct-induced calcium handling impairment in mouse cardiac myocytes. *J Mol Cell Cardiol,* **34**: 1425–1431, 2002.

5. Bellush LL, Doublier S, Holland AN, Striker LJ, Striker GE, Kopchick J. Protection against diabetes-induced nephropathy in growth hormone receptor/binding protein gene-disrupted mice. *Endocrinology,* **141**: 163–168, 2000.

6. Esposito C, Liu ZH, Striker GE, Phillips C, Chen NY, Chen WY, Kopchick JJ, Striker LJ. Inhibition of diabetic nephropathy by a GH antagonist: a molecular analysis. *Kidney Int,* **50**: 506–514, 1996.

7. Sun W, Wang L, Zhang Z, Chen M, Wang X. Intramuscular transfer of naked calcitonin gene-related peptide gene prevents autoimmune diabetes induced by multiple low-dose streptozotocin in C57BL mice. *Eur J Immunol,* **33**: 233–242, 2003.

8. Göktürk C, Garpenstrand H, Nilsson J, Nordquist J, Oreland L, Forsberg-Nilsson K. Studies on semicarbazide-sensitive amine oxidase in patients with diabetes mellitus and in transgenic mice. *Biochim Biophys Acta,* **1647**: 88–91, 2003.

9. Radu DL, Brumeanu T-D, McEvoy RC, Bona CA, Casares S. Escape from self-tolerance leads to neonatal insulin-dependent diabetes mellitus. *Autoimmunity,* **30**: 199–207, 1999.

10. Radu DL, Noben-Trauth N, Hu-Li J, Paul WE, Bona CA. A targeted mutation in the IL-4Rα gene protects mice against autoimmune diabetes *Proc Natl Acad Sci USA,* **97**: 12700–12704, 2000.

11. Radu DL, Bona C. Experimental models to study Type I diabetes using transgenic mice. In Cheța D (ed) *New insights into experimental diabetes.* Editura Academiei Romăniei, Bucharest, 2002, 15–34.

12. Cotran RS, Kumar V, Robbins SL. Cellular growth and differentiation: normal regulation and adaptation. In: Cotran RS, Kumar V, Robbins SL (eds). *Pathologic basis of disease,* 5th edition, WB Saunders Comp, Philadelphia, 1994, p 46.

13. Thomas CL, Artwohl JE, Suzuki H, Gao XP, White E, Saroli A, Bunte RM, Rubinstein I. Initial characterization of hamsters with spontaneous hypertension. *Hypertension,* **30**: 301–304, 1997.

14. Leonetti G, Cuspidi C. The heart and vascular changes in hypertension. *J Hypertens,* **13**: S29–S34, 1995.

15. Grimm D, Jabusch HC, Kossmehl P, Huber M, Fredersdorf S, Griese DP, Krämer BK, Kromer EP. Experimental diabetes and left ventricular hypertrophy: effects of beta-receptor blockade. *Cardiovasc Pathol,* **11**: 229–237, 2002.

16. Schneider MD, Roberts R, Parker TG. Modulation of cardiac genes by mechanical stress. The oncogene signalling hypothesis. *Mol Biol Med,* **8**: 167–183, 1991.

17. Teiger E, Dam TV, Richard L, Wisnewsky C, Tea BS, Gaboury L, Tremblay J, Schwarz K, Hamet P. Apoptosis in pressure overload-induced heart hypertrophy in the rat. *J Clin Invest,* **97**: 2891–2897, 1996.

18. Kajstura J, Fiordaliso F, Andreoli AM, Li B, Chimenti S, Medow MS, Limana F, Nadal-Ginard B, Leri A, Anversa P. Igf-1 overexpression inhibits the development of diabetic cardiomyopathy and angiotensin II- mediated oxidative stress. *Diabetes,* **50**: 1414–1424, 2001.

19. Gavin JB, Maxwell L. Pathogenic involvement of the microvasculature in cardiovascular disease. *Eur Heart J,* **1**: L26–L31, 1999.

20. Popov D, Hasu M, Costache G, Stern D, Simionescu M. Capillary and aortic endothelia interact in situ with nonenzymatically glycated albumin and develop specific alterations in experimental diabetes. *Acta Diabetol,* **34**: 285–293, 1997.

21. Fujii S. Advances in the understanding of diabetic vascular disease. *Journal of Cardiovascular Risk,* **4**: 67–69, 1997.

22. Hansen PR.. Inflammatory alterations in the myocardial microcirculation. *J Mol Cell Cardiol,* **12**: 2555–2559, 1998.

23. Romano M, Pomilio M, Vigneri S, Falco A, Chiesa PL, Chiarelli F, Davi G. Endothelial perturbation in children and adolescents with type 1 diabetes: association with markers of the inflammatory reaction. *Diabetes Care,* **24**: 1674–1678, 2001.

24. Poelmann RE, Lie-Venema H, Gittenberger-de Groot AC. The role of the epicardium and neural crest as extracardiac contributors to coronary vascular development. *Tex Heart Inst J,* **29**: 255–261, 2002.

25. Maeda M, Yabuki A, Suzuki S, Matsumoto M, Taniguchi K, Nishinakagawa H. Renal Lesions in Spontaneous Insulin-dependent Diabetes Mellitus in the Nonobese Diabetic Mouse: Acute Phase of Diabetes. *Vet Pathol*, **40**: 187–195, 2003.

26. Schleicher E, Nerlich A. The role of hyperglycaemia in the development of diabetic complications. *Horm Metab Res*, **28**: 367–373, 1996.

27. Christopher J, Jaffa AA. Diabetes modulates the expression of glomerular kinin receptors. *Int Immunopharmacol*, **2**: 1771–1779, 2002.

28. Nakamura S, Tachikawa T, Tobita K, Aoyama I, Takayama F, Enomoto A, Niwa T. An inhibitor of advanced glycation end-product formation reduces N epsilon-(carboxymethyl)lysine accumulation in glomeruli of diabetic rats. *Am J Kidney Dis*, **41**: S68–S71, 2003.

29. Haneda M, Araki S, Togawa M, Sugimoto T, Isono M, Kikkawa. Mitogen-activated protein kinase cascade is activated in glomeruli of diabetic rats and glomerular mesangial cells cultured under high glucose conditions. *Diabetes*, **46**: 847–853, 1997.

30. Wilmer WA, Dixon CL, Herbert C. Chronic exposure of human mesangial cells to high glucose environments activates the p38 MAPK pathway. *Kidney International*, **60**: 858–871, 2001.

31. Caramori ML, Kim Y, Huang C, Fish AJ, Rich SS, Miller ME, Russell G, Maurer M. Cellular basis of diabetic nephropathy: 1. Study design and renal structural-functional relationships in patients with long-standing type 1 diabetes. *Diabetes*, **51**: 506–513, 2002.

32. Sener G, Saçan O, Yanardağ R, Ayanoğlu-Dülger G. Effects of chard (Beta vulgaris L. var. cicla) extract on oxidative injury in the aorta and heart of streptozotocin-diabetic rats. *J Med Food*, **5**: 37–42, 2002.

33. Shukla N, Thompson CS, Angelini GD, Mikhailidis DP, Jeremy JY. Homocysteine enhances impairment of endothelium-dependent relaxation and guanosine cyclic monophosphate formation in aortae from diabetic rabbits. *Diabetologia*, **45**: 1325–1331, 2002.

34. Jack AM, Keegan A, Cotter MA, Cameron NE. Effects of diabetes and evening primrose oil treatment on responses of aorta, corpus cavernosum and mesenteric vasculature in rats. *Life Sci*, **71**: 1863–1877, 2002.

35. de Simone G, Palmieri V, Bella JN, Celentano A, Hong Y, Oberman A, Kitzman DW, Hopkins PN, Arnett DK, Devereux RB. Association of left ventricular hypertrophy with metabolic risk factors: the HyperGEN study. *J Hypertens*, **20**: 323–231, 2002.

36. Radu DL, Georgescu A, Stavam C, Carale A, Popov D. Double transgenic mice with Type 1 diabetes mellitus develop somatic, metabolic and vascular disorders. *J Cell Mol Med*, **8**: 349–358, 2004.

EXCITABILITY OF THE HUMAN NERVE: BASIC MECHANISMS AND EFFECTS OF HYPERGLYCAEMIA, HYPOXIA AND ISCHAEMIA

Gordon REID

The aetiology of diabetic neuropathy is as yet poorly understood, however hypoxia and hyperglycaemia are clearly important contributory factors. The present review will describe some of the direct effects of hypoxia and hyperglycaemia on nerve conduction and excitability. I begin by explaining our present understanding of axonal excitability in terms of "classical" voltage-dependent ion channels as well as more recently discovered channels whose activity depends on the metabolic state of the axon. In the past our understanding of these channels came from studies in other species, but in the lastest decade we have begun to study them directly in human axons. I will then describe an *in vitro* model of diabetes, the application of hypoxic and hyperglycaemic solutions to excised nerve; this work has shown that intracellular acidosis is a major factor in inducing axonal depolarisation under these conditions, which may lead to death of axons. Finally, I will describe attempts to understand ischaemic and post-ischaemic spontaneous activity by recording directly from human subjects; spontaneous impulse generation in axons is likely to underlie neuropathic pain. Although it may be too early to say how far this work clarifies the causes of diabetic neuropathy, a number of candidate mechanisms have been revealed which suggest some sensible directions for further experimental work in this area.

BACKGROUND

Neuropathy is a widespread complication of diabetes, and its commonest form is a symmetrical impairment of both sensory and motor function, mostly affecting distal extremities, and involving axonal loss [1]. A rarer, but very distressing manifestation is severe pain, often with a burning quality [2].

The pathophysiology of diabetic neuropathy is poorly understood. Strict glycaemic control largely prevents the onset of neuropathy, although recent animal studies suggest that the lack of insulin could itself be a causal factor [3]. Biochemical changes following directly from hyperglycaemia have been implicated in animal models, but this is not always supported by studies in patients. In human diabetic neuropathy, nerve hypoxia or ischemia – secondary to microvascular changes – emerges as the most likely underlying mechanism [4]. One major post-mortem study concluded that the patchy, multifocal nature of nerve fibre loss in diabetic neuropathy indicates an ischaemic mechanism [5]. For this reason, the present review will concentrate on the effects of hypoxia or ischaemia, combined with hyperglycaemia, on nerve excitability.

The origin of neuropathic pain, in diabetic or other neuropathies, is also obscure. Although structural and functional alterations are found in the spinal cord, which lead to nociceptive pathways becoming potentiated ("wind-up") and to non-nociceptive peripheral axons becoming connected to nociceptive pathways, these changes are largely secondary to ongoing activity in nociceptive peripheral axons [6, 7]. In neuropathic pain, this ongoing spontaneous activity presumably arises at a site where the primary sensory neurone itself is abnormal, either the soma in the dorsal root ganglion (DRG), or more distally in the axon [8–10]. Spontaneous activity in primary sensory neurones has been recorded in a rat model of diabetic neuropathy [11]. Because abnormal spontaneous activity is likely to be an important causal factor in neuropathic pain, this review will investigate the known mechanisms by which nerve axons can become spontaneously active, especially as a result of ischaemia.

Although we cannot as yet give a clear overall picture of how diabetes leads to nerve fibre loss and to spontaneous activity in nerve fibres, recent neurophysiological research has shed light on some aspects of the process. We now understand how ion channels in normal nerve axons are modulated by ischaemia and hypoxia; how reproducing *in vitro* some of the conditions likely to be found in diabetic nerve can lead to axonal dysfunction; and how ischaemia and the release of ischaemia can lead to spontaneous activity in axons. In this review I will describe the work that has illuminated these three aspects of axonal function. But first, it is necessary to describe the mechanisms that underlie normal excitation and conduction in human nerve.

HUMAN NERVE: EXCITATION AND CONDUCTION

In student physiology textbooks, myelinated axons are generally treated in a very simple way. An action potential is generated at a node of Ranvier, where there are sodium channels of the classic type to create the depolarisation, and potassium channels of the classic type to ensure repolarisation. It then "jumps" to the next node (saltatory conduction), and the length of nerve fibre between the nodes is treated as a simple cable insulated with myelin to ensure efficient conduction. This simple model spawned a fertile research programme on frog axons in the 1960s and 1970s (reviewed in [12]). It can explain, in good quantitative detail, the conduction of an impulse along an axon. So, the reader might wonder, why bother to go into any more depth? If the "job" of an axon is to take an impulse from one end and deliver it to the other without losing it along the way or generating spurious impulses, and we can explain how it does that, is that not enough?

In this section, I will show that the myelinated axon is more intriguing than was previously realised. Its complement of ion channels is larger and more varied than first thought, and its structural complexity endows the channels with functions that are not obvious at first sight. This does not mean that an axon modulates its message. As far as we can tell, the role of an axon is to transport an impulse unchanged from one end to the other, but it is becoming clear that this is not always an easy task. The theme of this section and the next will be that each type of ion channel found in the axon has a role in ensuring that the axon can keep doing that job under sometimes stressful conditions. These ion channels, particularly those found in human myelinated axons, will be described in some detail.

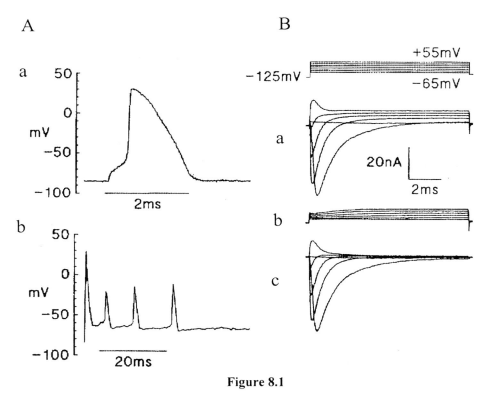

Figure 8.1

Action potentials (A) and membrane currents (B) in isolated human nodes of Ranvier.

A, a – Action potential in a human node at 25 °C, in response to a 0.5 ms stimulus; A, b – repetitive activity in the same node in response to a long-lasting depolarising current. B, a – Membrane currents in a different node at 20 °C; B, b – currents in the same node in 300 nM tetrodotoxin, which blocks the Na$^+$ current; B, c – subtraction of (b) from (a) reveals the Na$^+$ current. From Schwarz, Reid and Bostock (1995), ref. [15].

Na$^+$ channels are the predominant type in mammalian (including human) nodes of Ranvier, and there are very few K$^+$ channels [13–15] (see Figure 8.1). However, in demyelinated nerve, K$^+$ channel blockers prolong the action potential duration [16], indicating that the axonal membrane under the myelin contains K$^+$ channels. This is confirmed by acute demyelination, which exposes K$^+$ currents that are not present in the node [17, 18]. This seems, at first sight, paradoxical – how could these channels have any effect on axonal excitability if they are hidden under the myelin? – but the paradox is resolved by the finding that the myelin is not a perfect insulator. The periaxonal space (under the myelin sheath) is connected to the extracellular space at the node through a high-resistance pathway [19], which is largely contributed by the very complex axoglial junction area [20]. This means that the time constant of the internodal axon is long, of the order of hundreds of milliseconds, which means that the internode plays very little role in excitability on the time scale of the action potential (this is why the "classical" model works

well as an explanation of action potential initiation and conduction). On longer time scales, however, the role of the internode is very important. In particular, the internode and not the node generates the greater part of the axonal resting potential. Blocking nodal K$^+$ channels causes only a very small depolarisation and, indeed, the importance of the internode in generating the resting potential could have been predicted on theoretical grounds even with knowledge gained in the 1950s [21]. In addition, the internode repolarises the node after the action potential. Although the earlier idea that repolarisation depends on nodal K$^+$ channel activation is still met in textbook accounts (and is indeed valid in the preparation where it was first described, the squid axon, and in other unmyelinated axons), this model is not valid for mammalian myelinated axons. In these axons, repolarisation results from current flowing from internode to node, through the axoglial junction resistance. Because the internodal axon is depolarised very little during the action potential, no channel activation is required for the large internodal axon to bring the

137

tiny nodal membrane, less than a thousandth of its area, back to resting potential (see ref. [22] for a more detailed explanation).

The location of axonal ion channels and not only their properties is, thus, an essential determinant of their function. The role of paranodal and internodal K$^+$ channels in generation of the resting potential has already been mentioned. During nerve activity, nodal Na$^+$ channels generate the fast depolarisation during the action potential "upstroke", as in the classical model. The role of internodal K$^+$ channels during nerve activity is primarily to "short-circuit" the action potential and prevent excessive depolarisation of the internode. In normal conditions, the internodal axon depolarises by less than 2 mV during a single action potential; most of the action potential appears as a potential change across the *myelin*, and not the axonal membrane itself. If the internodal axon were allowed to depolarise more than a few millivolts, it would re-excite the node.

This is precisely what happens when paranodal and internodal K$^+$ channels are blocked: after a single action potential, a burst of action potentials follows [23]. Internodal axonal K$^+$ channels, therefore, have two major roles: to generate the resting potential and to prevent repetitive activity that would result from excessive internodal depolarisation.

Until just over a decade ago, the excitability of human axons was understood primarily from recordings that had been made in other species. No recordings at the membrane level had ever been made from human axons. In 1990 we began to apply the techniques that had recently been developed for patch clamping *Xenopus* axons [24] to record ion channels in acutely demyelinated human internodes (Figure 8.2. and ref. [25]). The outcome of this work confirmed that our understanding of human nerve excitability was fairly well-founded, because the ion channels we found were very similar to those already described in *Xenopus* [24] and rat [26].

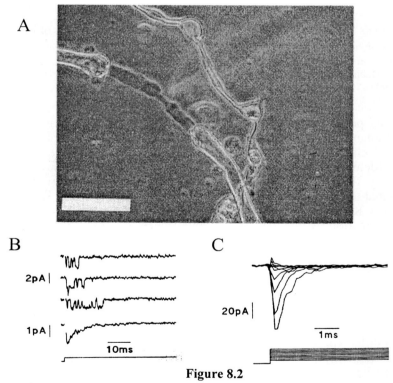

Figure 8.2

A – Human axon prepared for patch clamp recording. The site of the former node of Ranvier is visible as a constriction in the axon, and retracted myelin can be seen at either end of the exposed area of membrane. Phase contrast, scale bar 50 μm. From Scholz, Reid, Vogel and Bostock (1993), ref. [28]. B – Single Na$^+$ channel currents in an excised patch from a human axon, in response to a depolarising pulse to -60 mV. Three individual traces are shown, and the fourth trace is the average of 24 such recordings (compare with the multi-channel current in C). The bottom trace shows the timing of the voltage pulse. C – Multi-channel Na$^+$ current in an excised patch from a different axon in response to pulses to between -80 mV and +100 mV (as shown below the current traces). Compare with macroscopic Na$^+$ currents from the whole node in Figure 8.1. From Reid (1996), ref. [22].

However, quantitative differences between human and rat Na^+ channels do exist and have been shown to be functionally important [27]. Initially, we described one type of voltage-gated Na^+ channel and three major types of voltage-gated K^+ channel with different kinetics (F, I and S for fast, intermediate and slow; see ref. [28]); in addition to these, we also found two other voltage-gated K^+ channels distinct from those already described in other species [29]. In the first voltage-clamp recordings from human nodes of Ranvier, we showed that the macroscopic properties of the currents through these channels and their distribution in the node and paranode are similar to that already described in other mammalian species (Figure 8.1 and ref. [15]).

AXONAL ION CHANNELS MODULATED BY METABOLIC STATE OR INTRACELLULAR LIGANDS

As well as "classical" voltage-gated channels, a number of other channel types exist in myelinated axons, which are likely to be activated during metabolic disturbances. Others are probably active under more normal conditions, but with their activity depending on intracellular modulation rather than membrane potential. Again the roles of these can be understood in terms of ensuring the safety of conduction while preventing a single action potential from becoming a burst of impulses.

THE HYPERPOLARISATION-ACTIVATED CURRENT I_H

On injecting hyperpolarising current into an axon, the membrane potential initially shifts toward a more negative value within less than 1 ms due to nodal hyperpolarisation, then continues to become more negative over a period of some hundreds of milliseconds as the internodal axonal membrane potential also hyperpolarises. However, this hyperpolarisation deviates from its expected exponential timecourse and begins to "sag" towards the resting potential again [23, 30]. This is because hyperpolarisation activates an inward current (carried largely by Na^+ ions), which acts to limit the extent of the hyperpolarisation. This current, termed I_h (for hyperpolarisation-activated current) is carried by channels of the HCN family [31].

The function of this current is primarily to prevent conduction block during strong hyperpolarisation (for instance, that induced by Na^+/K^+ ATPase activation during the post-ischaemic period, as described below). In this situation, the risk would arise that the currents generated by an action potential would not be sufficient to ensure its further conduction along the axon. Normally, an action potential generates 6–10 times as much current as is necessary for propagation [32], but during extreme hyperpolarisation this "safety factor" could drop below 1 and, thus, conduction would be blocked. This happens in some nociceptive C-fibre axons even at low action potential frequencies, around 4 Hz [33]. Activation of I_h prevents hyperpolarisation from becoming so extreme: for instance post-tetanic hyperpolarisation (also due to Na^+/K^+ ATPase activation) is limited by I_h and augmented greatly by caesium, which blocks I_h. In the presence of caesium, post-tetanic hyperpolarisation can become strong enough to block conduction [23].

Ca^{2+}-ACTIVATED K^+ CHANNELS

In inside-out patches from *Xenopus* axons, it was found that application of a raised Ca^{2+} concentration induced activity of a large-conductance K^+ channel [34, 35]. This is termed BK (for big K^+ channel) and is expressed in a wide range of tissues. BK activation appears at intracellular Ca^{2+} concentrations ($[Ca^{2+}]_i$) of around 1 μM, which is well above the normal resting neuronal $[Ca^{2+}]_i$ of below 50 nM. Activation is voltage dependent, being greater at more positive membrane potentials. We have also described this channel in human axons (Figure 8.3.A and ref. [28]). It was suggested that ischaemia would cause BK channels to open, increasing K^+ conductance and stabilising the resting potential [34]. However, the BK channel only has significant open probability near the resting potential when $[Ca^{2+}]_i$ reaches levels above 10 μM, which would only occur globally in a dead axon or one very close to death; it is perhaps more likely that its activation depends on a high *local* $[Ca^{2+}]_i$, such as might be reached during normal tetani [36]. It should also be pointed out that during ischaemia, when BK channels are proposed to be active, the raised extracellular $[K^+]$ would cause them to generate a regenerative *inward* current, probably exacerbating paraesthesiae [37] rather than stabilising the resting potential. The voltage-gated activation of BK channels is fast, so all that can safely be concluded is that BK channels would increase the fast voltage-gated K^+ current (normally contributed by the F channel described above) at times when the $[Ca^{2+}]$ near their inner mouth is raised (as might happen during long periods of persistent activity). Their function might then be similar to that of the F channel, to reduce

the probability of a burst of action potentials being generated by a single impulse.

ATP-SENSITIVE K^+ CHANNELS

An ATP-sensitive K^+ channel (K_{ATP}) is also present in *Xenopus* axons (Figure 8.3.B, C and refs. [34, 35]). This channel, in excised patches, is inhibited by micromolar concentrations of ATP, leading initially to the suggestion that it could never be active except under the most extreme metabolic stress. In recent years, the modulation

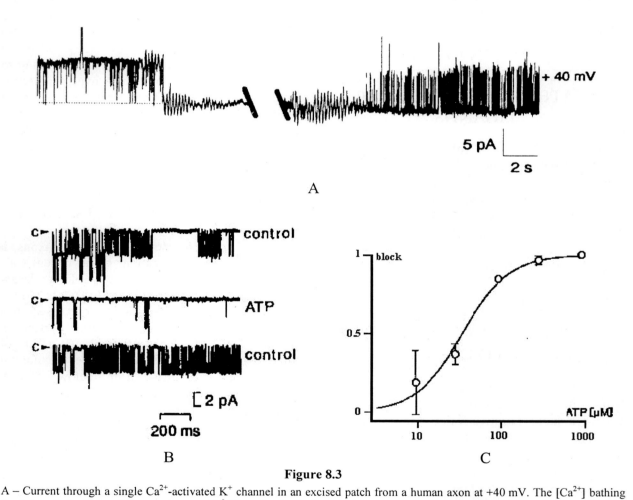

Figure 8.3

A – Current through a single Ca^{2+}-activated K^+ channel in an excised patch from a human axon at +40 mV. The $[Ca^{2+}]$ bathing the intracellular face of the patch was 10^{-5} M at the beginning of the recording; briefly exposing the channel to 10^{-7} M intracellular $[Ca^{2+}]$ caused the channel to close (middle part of recording), and it re-opened on returning to 10^{-5} M intracellular $[Ca^{2+}]$ (end of recording). From Scholz, Reid, Vogel & Bostock (1993), ref. [28]. B – Currents through ATP-sensitive K^+ channels in an excised patch from a *Xenopus* axon. Moving from control solution to an intracellular solution containing 96 μM ATP strongly inhibited channel activity (middle trace). C – Fractional block of ATP-sensitive K^+ channel activity by ATP; the curve is a least-squares fit to the Hill equation $f(c) = \left[1 + \left(IC_{50}/c\right)^a\right]^{-1}$ with half-maximal inhibitory concentration $IC_{50} = 35$ μM and Hill coefficient $a = 1.5$. B and C from Jonas, Koh, Kampe, Hermsteiner and Vogel (1991), ref. [34].

of K_{ATP} channels has attracted intense interest, related to their important role in controlling insulin secretion in the pancreas: for many years it was considered paradoxical that a channel that could only be active at improbably low ATP concentrations was, nevertheless, clearly the main mechanism regulating insulin secretion. The resolution of this paradox was the revelation of the role of PIP_2 (phosphatidylinositol 4,5-bisphosphate) in modulating the K_{ATP} channel. By competing with ATP for its binding site on the channel, PIP_2 effectively makes K_{ATP} channels much less sensitive to ATP *in situ* than they are in excised patches, so that their activity can be regulated by changes in ATP concentration in the normal millimolar range found in healthy cells [38, 39]. It is, therefore, quite probable that mild ischaemia increases the activity of axonal K_{ATP} channels, thus stabilising the resting potential and also (since K_{ATP} channels are voltage-independent) flattening the current-voltage curve and counteracting any tendency to develop a region of negative slope [37], therefore reducing the tendency to generate paraesthesiae during ischaemia. The K_{ATP} channel has not yet been described in mammalian axons, but this is probably because of the small number of studies that have been made; it is unlikely to be absent in mammals.

Na^+-ACTIVATED K^+ CHANNELS

Near the node of Ranvier, a population of K^+ channels has been found in *Xenopus* axons which are activated by relatively high concentrations (EC_{50} = 33 mM) of intracellular Na^+ [40]. Calculations of the likely diffusion of Na^+ ions entering the axon during an action potential suggest that these channels would be activated even by a single action potential, because they are closely co-localised with nodal Na^+ channels. This suggests a likely role in spike-frequency adaptation. Although spike-frequency adaptation can be simulated by adding only a conventional slow K^+ conductance to a nodal model, the limitation on the number of action potentials is always more robust in the real axon than in the model [15], suggesting that an additional mechanism is operating in the real axon. The Na^+-dependent K^+ channel would be a good candidate for this additional mechanism: activation of K^+ channels by Na^+ entry during a spike would

provide a strong negative feedback to limit the number of spikes generated. It may also be involved in setting the resting potential [40].

AN *IN VITRO* MODEL OF DIABETES: EFFECTS ON NERVE FUNCTION

The likelihood that hyperglycaemia is the root cause of diabetic neuropathy and ischaemia is the main mechanism by which it acts, prompted *in vitro* studies on the acute effects of this combination, of treatments on nerve conduction and excitability [41]. This work has led to a clearer understanding of potential mechanisms of ischaemic damage and, in particular, has revealed an unexpected involvement of intracellular acidosis.

Diabetic nerve has the paradoxical property of being resistant to ischaemic conduction block (one of the earliest effects of diabetes on nerve conduction) while being unusually highly sensitive to ischaemic damage. In a normal subject, compression of a limb with a cuff at above arterial pressure (cutting off the blood supply to the nerve) leads to numbness in the affected limb within less than 30 minutes because axonal conduction is blocked. In diabetic subjects, the time until numbness ensues is extended to over an hour [42]. A more rapid test can be made by using the change in threshold during ischaemia. In normal nerve, the application of an ischaemic cuff is followed within less than 10 seconds by a marked depolarisation, which can be detected, *in vivo*, in human subjects, as a reduction in the threshold stimulus required to elicit an action potential [43]; the method and its interpretation are described in ref. [44]. This depolarisation progresses as ischaemia is maintained. In diabetic subjects, the threshold change is virtually abolished, and the post-ischaemic hyperpolarisation normally observed after release of ischaemia (which is due to increased activation of the Na^+/K^+ ATPase) is also greatly attenuated [45].

Remarkably, resistance to ischaemia can be induced, in normal nerve, by only brief exposure to high glucose concentrations. Rat spinal roots incubated in 25 mM D-glucose for 8 hours reduced the depolarisation recorded during a subsequent 30-minute period of hypoxia by 90 %, and had a similar effect on the fall in peak action potential amplitude (Figure 8.4A and ref. [46]); both are clear indications of resistance to ischaemia. This *in vitro* model also reproduces the increased sensitivity to ischaemic damage in diabetic nerve: while dorsal roots incubated in normal glucose concentrations (5 mM) recovered completely from 30 min hypoxia, roots incubated in 25 mM glucose recovered less than 40 % of their pre-hypoxic action potential amplitude [46].

The possible involvement of glycolysis in this phenomenon was tested by blocking glycolysis with iodoacetate (IAA, 10 mM). IAA exacerbated the effects of hypoxia on action potential amplitude and membrane potential (Figure 8.4A), but in spite of this, recovery after 30 minutes of hypoxia was greatly improved by IAA [47]. This observation therefore suggested that increased glycolytic activity could underlie both resistance to ischaemia and sensitivity to ischaemic damage.

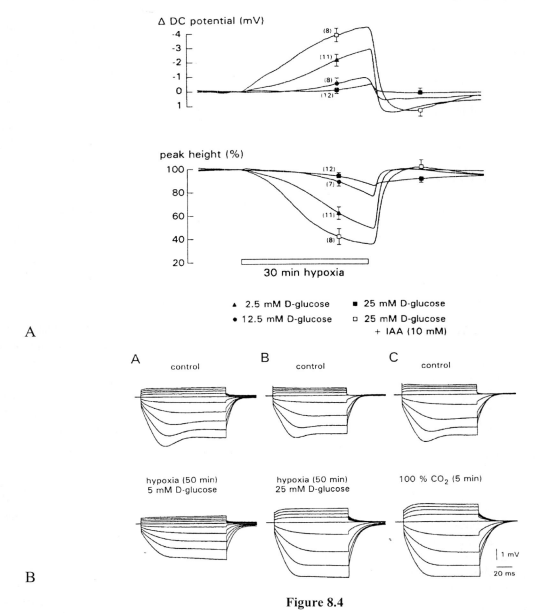

Figure 8.4

A – Effect of hypoxia on resting membrane potential (top) and action potential amplitude (bottom) in ventral spinal root from rat. High glucose concentrations induce resistance to hypoxia, which is abolished by iodoacetate (IAA). B – Changes in electrotonus in rat dorsal spinal roots in tetrodotoxin-containing solutions. Voltage changes induced by currents up to ±10 μA are shown. In normal glucose concentration, hypoxia decreases input resistance (left); in high glucose, hypoxia increases input resistance (centre). The effect of hyperglycaemic hypoxia is imitated by acidosis (right). From Grafe (1996), ref. [41].

The mechanism by which increased glycolytic activity induces nerve damage was investigated by measuring extracellular pH during hypoxia [48]; increased glycolytic activity, by increasing lactate production, would be expected to lower tissue pH. This situation could be exacerbated by the exhaustion of tissue HCO_3^- supplies in ischaemia, so that a depleted buffer system would be put under a greater than normal load [49]; for this reason, the effects of reduced buffering were also investigated.

Recovery in action potential amplitude after 30 minutes of hypoxia following incubation in 25 mM glucose was clearly worsened by reducing buffering capacity, either by reducing bicarbonate concentration or by substituting HEPES for bicarbonate buffering. Hypoxia was accompanied by acidosis and the pH change was prevented by blocking glycolysis with 2-deoxyglucose; like IAA (above), 2-deoxyglucose led to a greater reduction in peak action potential amplitude during ischaemia, but better recovery afterwards [48]. These observations indicate that glycolysis acidifies nerve during hypoxia and that increased levels of glycolytic activity produce greater acidosis; this acidification can be blocked by blocking glycolysis.

How could intracellular acidosis lead to conduction abnormalities and to axonal loss? Here, the first clue came from the depolarising afterpotential (DAP) which is seen after each action potential. The DAP is caused by depolarisation of the axonal membrane in the internode [19] and manoeuvres that reduce internodal K^+ conductance increase the DAP amplitude [50]. During normoglycaemic hypoxia, DAP amplitude remains constant; however, in hyperglycaemic hypoxia (25 mM glucose), the DAP amplitude increases greatly. This suggested that internodal K^+ conductance may be reduced during hyperglycaemic, but not normoglycaemic, hypoxia. The possibility that intracellular acidification may be involved in this was tested by adding sodium propionate to the extracellular solution; intracellular acidification similarly increased DAP amplitude [51]. More direct evidence that hyperglycaemic hypoxia reduces axonal K^+ conductance through intracellular acidification was provided by measurements of electrotonus (membrane potential changes due to current injection): hyperglycaemic hypoxia increased the amplitude of slow electrotonus during depolarising pulses (*i.e.* reduced internodal K^+ conductance) and reducing intracellular pH by increasing CO_2 concentration had the same effect (Figure 8.4B and ref. [52]).

The search for the ion channels involved in this phenomenon was done directly at the level of the internodal axon membrane using the patch-clamp technique. In inside-out membrane patches from rat spinal roots, recordings were chosen in which either the I channel or the F channel component dominated the patch. On reducing pH on the intracellular face of the patch from 7.4 to 6.0, the I channel current was reduced by only 30 %, while the F channel current was reduced by about 80 % (Figure 8.5 and ref. [51]). The conclusion was that hyperglycaemic hypoxia reduces internodal K^+ conductance by a direct inhibition of internodal F channels. As explained in the first section of this chapter, internodal K^+ channels are the main determinant of the resting potential of myelinated axons: if these are blocked, the axon will depolarise, which will directly induce conduction abnormalities, but more importantly in the long term, is likely to lead to axonal death by increasing Ca^{2+} entry into the axon.

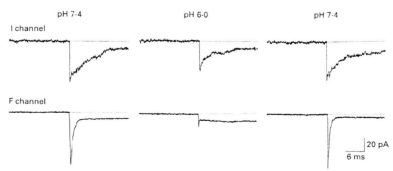

Figure 8.5

Effects of intracellular acidification on multi-channel rat axonal I and F channel currents in excised patches. Patches were depolarised to +50 mV then stepped to −80 mV; raised extracellular $[K^+]$ allowed the inward K^+ current to be recorded. Note the inhibition of F channel currents by low pH, which left I channel currents relatively unaffected. From Schneider, Quasthoff, Mitrovic and Grafe (1993), ref. [51].

Interestingly, a similar mechanism was later shown to be operating in a different neuro-degenerative disease, amyotrophic lateral sclerosis (ALS). Changes in threshold electrotonus (explained in the next section) showed reduced K^+ conductance and, in those patients showing fasciculations (indicative of axonal death), depolarisation rapidly induced conduction block. All these changes, including the conduction block (due to Na^+ channel inactivation secondary to depolarisation), could be reproduced by blocking nodal and internodal K^+ channels [53]. This study thus provides evidence of K^+ channel block associated with ongoing axonal loss, in human patients recorded *in vivo*.

SPONTANEOUS ACTIVITY DURING AND AFTER ISCHAEMIA

Ongoing spontaneous activity in peripheral axons leads to central changes that are associated with persistent pain [6]. If this spontaneous activity is in nociceptive axons, it will directly be perceived as pain. Spontaneous activity in peripheral axons is a feature of experimental diabetic neuropathy [11], as well as other forms of experimental axonal damage [54]. Peripheral axons are not normally spontaneously active – indeed, spontaneous activity would be a very undesirable attribute and evolution has produced a complement of axonal ion channels whose function is largely to inhibit spontaneous activity (see first section of this chapter). The generation of spontaneous activity in axons thus requires some abnormality. The most common situation in everyday life that induced spontaneous activity in axons is ischaemia, induced simply by sitting or lying in a position that presses on a nerve and blocks its blood supply. When the blood supply is restored (by moving, on noticing that an extremity has become numb), "pins and needles" result – bursts of action potentials in several types of axons that induce uncomfortable tingling or sharp prickling sensations. Since ischaemia is also a feature of diabetic nerve, understanding the mechanisms of ischaemia-induced spontaneous activity may be relevant to understanding spontaneous activity in diabetic nerve. The analogy cannot be carried too far, however, because of the resistance to ischaemic conduction block of diabetic nerve. It is nevertheless instructive to look at the basic mechanisms of generation of spontaneous activity in human axons *in vivo*, under one well defined and easily studied set of conditions.

Early attempts to develop an *in vitro* model using rat axons proved unsuccessful, because rats have a different complement of axonal ion channels from humans: their electrotonus differs in ways that suggest a different population of K^+ channels [55], and it is surprisingly difficult to make rat axons spontaneously active. For this reason it was decided to go directly to human subjects. Membrane potential and conductance changes, in human axons, can be indirectly inferred from changes in threshold [44]. Ischaemia, in these experiments, was induced by applying a standard cuff as used for measuring blood pressure and inflating it above arterial pressure (to 200 mmHg). The ulnar nerve was stimulated either directly under the cuff or distal to it, and muscle action potentials recorded from the abductor digiti minimi or first dorsal interosseus muscles. This allows the activity of all motor axons in the nerve to be followed, or of a single motor axon if a selective recording is made from a single muscle fibre [56]; we used motor axons because both single- and multi-unit activity can be measured much more easily in humans *in vivo* in motor than in sensory axons.

Nerve excitability, during ischaemia and after ischaemia, changes in opposite directions depending on how it is measured (Figure 8.6). Using short depolarising pulses – the conventional measure of threshold – axons become more excitable during ischaemia and rapidly much less excitable after ischaemia. However, if ramp stimuli are used, the opposite effect is seen: the axon accommodates strongly during ischaemia (ramp threshold increases) and becomes more excitable after ischaemia (ramp threshold decreases). These effects can be reproduced accurately simply by injecting polarising current: depolarising current reproduces all the changes during ischaemia and hyperpolarising current reproduces the changes seen after ischaemia [43]. From this we concluded that ischaemia depolarises axons, easily explained by the inhibition of the Na^+/K^+ ATPase, while during the post-ischaemic period axons are hyperpolarised, also simply explained by the stimulation of Na^+/K^+ ATPase activity by the sodium load accumulated during ischaemia. This finding was initially rather paradoxical, because it is precisely during the period immediately after ischaemia, when axons were most strongly hyperpolarised and excitability in response to a short pulse was at its lowest, that post-ischaemic paraesthesiae are strongest.

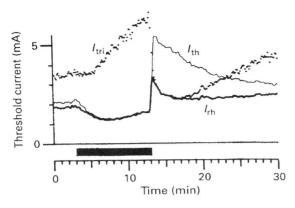

Figure 8.6

Excitability changes during ischaemia in a single motor
axon in the ulnar nerve of the author,
recorded using an intramuscular needle electrode
in first dorsal interosseus muscle.

Three thresholds are shown: rheobase (I_{rh}), threshold to a
brief 2 ms pulse (I_{th}) and threshold to a triangular stimulus
(I_{tri}). From Bostock, Baker, Grafe and Reid (1991), ref. [43].

This paradox was resolved by Hugh Bostock
in a powerful and elegant combination of

experimental work, mostly with himself as the
subject, and simulation studies. Firstly, it was
necessary to use longer periods of ischaemia,
sufficient to induce motor fasciculations and not
only sensory paraesthesiae. In this situation, the
post-ischaemic period was distinguished not by a
uniform hyperpolarisation, as with shorter periods
of ischaemia, but by a bimodal distribution of
thresholds with some axons being hyperpolarised
and others depolarised (Figure 8.7). The period of
actual motor fasciculations, shown by integrated
EMG activity, coincided exactly with this bimodal
distribution of thresholds. The number of axons in
each of the two states changed during this period,
indicating that axons were moving or "flipping"
between the two states [37].

How could axons have two stable threshold
states? Since threshold is primarily determined by
axonal resting potential [44], this indicates that
axons have two possible stable resting potentials.
If we consider the steady-state current-voltage
curve of the axon (see [57]), the resting potential

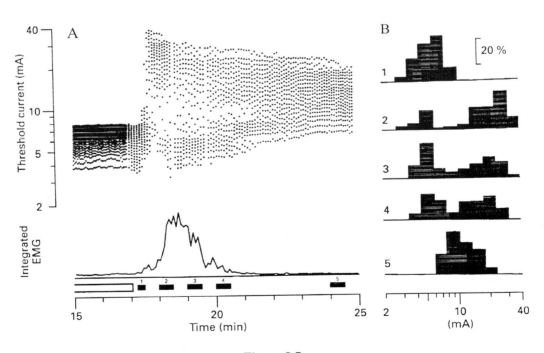

Figure 8.7

A – Bimodal distributions of multi-unit threshold after 15 min ischaemia in human ulnar nerve. Each dot represents fibres
contributing 5 % of the maximal motor action potential. The integrated EMG trace (bottom) shows the period during which
muscle fasciculation (due to spontaneous nerve activity) was taking place. B – Threshold distributions calculated from the
recording in A for five time periods indicated by numbered black bars in A. Note the increase in the number of fibres in the low-
threshold group between 2 and 4 (18 – 20 min), while spontaneous activity was taking place. From Bostock, Baker and Reid
(1991), ref. [37].

is a point where membrane current is zero and the slope of the current-voltage curve is positive (in this case, depolarisation will result in an outward current and hyperpolarisation in an inward current, both of which will tend to return the axon's membrane potential to the point of zero current). This point is therefore stable. If the current-voltage curve has two points of zero current with positive slope, there must be an intervening region of negative slope; regions of negative slope in the current-voltage curve indicate instability [57]. The region of negative slope results from extracellular K^+ accumulation that occurs during ischaemia and is cleared slowly after ischaemia: it is contributed by voltage-gated K^+ channels which are open at potentials that are now negative to the K^+ equilibrium potential. As extracellular $[K^+]$ returns to normal, this negative slope region disappears (Figure 8.8A).

Why should axons "flip" between these two stable states? This can be explained on the basis that Na^+/K^+ ATPase activity is not constant: the Na^+/K^+ ATPase produces an outward current, and when this current changes the membrane potential follows the curve shown in Figure 8.8B. An increase in Na^+/K^+ ATPase activity may reach the point where the more depolarised resting potential is no longer stable, and the axon is forced to shift to the more hyperpolarised one (e in Figure 8.8B); conversely, when Na^+/K^+ ATPase activity falls, the resting potential shifts in the opposite direction until eventually the more hyperpolarised resting potential is no longer stable and the axon "flips" to the more depolarised state (g in Figure 8.8B). This phenomenon is capable of explaining the bimodal distribution of thresholds recorded after ischaemia (Figure 8.7), and the "flip" to a more depolarised state is sufficient to explain a burst of action potentials (Figure 8.9 and ref. [37]).

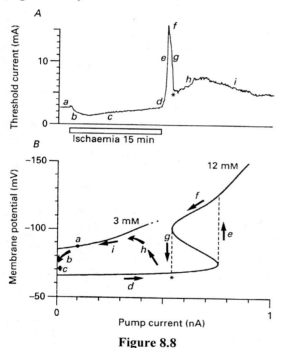

Figure 8.8

Interpretation of ischaemic and post-ischaemic excitability changes in terms of changes in Na^+/K^+ ATPase current and ionic gradients.

A – changes in threshold of human ulnar nerve for 25 % of maximal motor action potential during and after 15 min ischaemia. B – dependence of membrane potential on Na^+/K^+ ATPase current at 12 mM and 3 mM extracellular $[K^+]$, simulated using a Hodgkin-Huxley type model [37]. Lower case letters indicate the suggested correspondence between membrane potential (B) and threshold (A). Note the "flip" from hyperpolarised to depolarised state at g. From Bostock, Baker and Reid (1991), ref. [37].

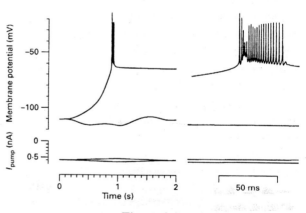

Figure 8.9

Spontaneous burst discharge of the human nerve model [37] in high extracellular $[K^+]$.

A – The simulation starts with the axon in the more hyperpolarised of two stable states (12 mM $[K^+]$, Na^+/K^+ ATPase "pump" current 0.6 nA). Increasing pump current has little effect, but reducing it induces a "flip" to the more depolarised state (corresponding to **g** in Figure 8). This "flip" induces a burst of action potentials. B – Expansion of period from 0.85 to 0.95 s in A. From Bostock, Baker and Reid (1991), ref. [37].

In sensory axons, which are more prone to spontaneous activity than motor axons, all axons appear to follow the more depolarised course shown in Figure 8.7 [58]. Since the most prominent difference between sensory and motor axons is a larger hyperpolarisation-activated current (I_h) in sensory axons, the simplest explanation for the sensory-motor difference would be that a "flip" to the more hyperpolarised state in a sensory axon immediately activates a large I_h, which rapidly causes a "flip" to the more depolarised resting potential, in a time that is too short for axons to be recorded while at the more hyperpolarised resting potential; these "flips" from hyperpolarised to depolarised resting potential, which are capable of explaining the bursts of action potentials that underlie post-ischaemic paraesthesiae and post-ischaemic motor fasciculations, would thus be predicted to be very frequent in sensory axons but much less frequent in motor axons, causing a lower level of spontaneous activity in motor axons, as is indeed the case.

CONCLUSION

Although the pathological mechanisms of diabetic neuropathy are still unclear, it is becoming increasingly evident that hypoxia or ischaemia plays an important role. Understanding the effects of these insults on the function of normal axons can give some clues to areas that could be investigated in an attempt to clarify how diabetes damages axons. The present chapter has reviewed some of the known effects of metabolic disturbance, hypoxia and ischaemia on nerve function, at several levels: single ion channels, whole nerves *in vitro*, and single axons and whole nerves *in vivo* in human volunteers. Some insights have been offered into how simulated diabetes *in vitro* may cause axonal loss, and how ischaemia and recovery from ischaemia can lead to spontaneous firing in axons. Important areas that are just beginning to emerge, for instance the possibility that insulin withdrawal may directly underlie some nerve damage, have not been covered in detail. It is too early to make firm conclusions based on this work that could lead to practical conclusions on treatment and prevention of diabetic neuropathy – as yet we can offer only clues and pointers for future work – but the field of work is developing fast, and I would hope that a similar review written ten years from now would tell a very different story.

Acknowledgements. Work in the author's laboratory is supported by the Volkswagen Foundation, the Physiological Society and the Wellcome Trust.

REFERENCES

1. Perkins BA, Bril V. Diabetic neuropathy: a review emphasizing diagnostic methods. *Clin Neurophysiol*, **114**: 1167–1175, 2003.
2. Archer AG, Watkins PJ, Thomas PK, Sharma AK, Payan J. The natural history of acute painful neuropathy in diabetes mellitus. *J Neurol Neurosurg Psychiatry*, **46**: 491–499, 1983.
3. Huang TJ, Price SA, Chilton L, Calcutt NA, Tomlinson DR, Verkhratsky A, Fernyhough P. Insulin prevents depolarization of the mitochondrial inner membrane in sensory neurons of type 1 diabetic rats in the presence of sustained hyperglycemia. *Diabetes*, **52**: 2129–2136, 2003.
4. Low PA. Recent advances in the pathogenesis of diabetic neuropathy. *Muscle and Nerve*, **10**: 121–128, 1987.
5. Dyck PJ, Karnes JL, O'Brien P, Okazaki H, Lais A, Engelstad J. The spatial distribution of fiber loss in diabetic polyneuropathy suggests ischemia. *Ann Neurol*, **19**: 440–449, 1986.
6. Yaksh TL, Hua XY, Kalcheva I, Nozaki-Taguchi N, Marsala M. The spinal biology in humans and animals of pain states generated by persistent small afferent input. *Proc Natl Acad Sci USA*, **96**: 7680–7686, 1999.
7. Woolf CJ, Mannion RJ. Neuropathic pain: aetiology, symptoms, mechanisms, and management. *Lancet*, **353**: 1959–1964, 1999.
8. Wall PD, Gutnick M. Properties of afferent nerve impulses originating from a neuroma. *Nature*, **248**: 740–743, 1974.
9. Wall PD, Devor M. Sensory afferent impulses originate from dorsal root ganglia as well as from the periphery in normal and nerve injured rats. *Pain*, **17**: 321–339, 1983.
10. Burchiel KJ. Effects of electrical and mechanical stimulation on two foci of spontaneous activity which develop in primary afferent neurons after peripheral axotomy. *Pain*, **18**: 249–265, 1984.
11. Burchiel KJ, Russell LC, Lee RP, Sima AA. Spontaneous activity of primary afferent neurons in diabetic BB/Wistar rats. A possible mechanism of chronic diabetic neuropathic pain. *Diabetes*, **34**: 1210–1213, 1985.
12. Stämpfli R, Hille B. Electrophysiology of the peripheral myelinated nerve. In: R. Llinas and W. Precht (Eds). *Frog Neurobiology*, Springer-Verlag, Berlin, 1976, 3–32.
13. Chiu SY, Ritchie JM, Rogart RB, Stagg D. A quantitative description of membrane currents in rabbit myelinated nerve. *J Physiol*, **292**: 149–166, 1979.

14. Brismar T. Potential clamp analysis of membrane currents in rat myelinated nerve fibres. *J Physiol*, **298**: 171–184, 1980.

15. Schwarz JR, Reid G, Bostock H. Action potentials and membrane currents in the human node of Ranvier. *Pflugers Arch*, **430**: 283–292, 1995.

16. Sherratt RM, Bostock H, Sears TA. Effects of 4-aminopyridine on normal and demyelinated mammalian nerve fibres. *Nature*, **283**: 570–572, 1980.

17. Chiu SY, Ritchie JM. Evidence for the presence of potassium channels in the paranodal region of acutely demyelinated mammalian single nerve fibres. *J Physiol*, **313**: 415–437, 1981.

18. Brismar T. Potential clamp experiments on myelinated nerve fibres from alloxan diabetic rats. *Acta Physiol Scand*, **105**: 384–386, 1979.

19. Barrett EF, Barrett JN. Intracellular recording from vertebrate myelinated axons: mechanism of the depolarizing afterpotential. *J Physiol*, **323**: 117–144, 1982.

20. Berthold CH, Rydmark M. Anatomy of the paranode-node-paranode region in the cat. *Experientia*, **39**: 964–976, 1983.

21. Chiu SY, Ritchie JM. On the physiological role of internodal potassium channels and the security of conduction in myelinated nerve fibres. *Proc R Soc Lond B Biol Sci*, **220**: 415–422, 1984.

22. Reid G. Ion channels in human axons. In: H. Bostock, P. Kirkwood and A.H. Pullen (Eds). *The Neurobiology of Disease – Contributions from Neuroscience to Clinical Neurology*, Cambridge University Press, Cambridge, 1996, 47–60.

23. Baker M, Bostock H, Grafe P, Martius P. Function and distribution of three types of rectifying channel in rat spinal root myelinated axons. *J Physiol*, **383**: 45–67, 1987.

24. Jonas P, Bräu ME, Hermsteiner M, Vogel W. Single-channel recording in myelinated nerve fibers reveals one type of Na channel but different K channels. *Proc Natl Acad Sci USA*, **86**: 7238–7242, 1989.

25. Reid G, Kampe K, Scholz A, Birch R, Bostock H, Vogel W. Single channel currents in internodes of human axons. *Eur J Neurosci*, **Supp. 4**: 254, 1991.

26. Safronov BV, Kampe K, Vogel W. Single voltage-dependent potassium channels in rat peripheral nerve membrane. *J Physiol*, **460**: 675–691, 1993.

27. Bostock H, Rothwell JC. Latent addition in motor and sensory fibres of human peripheral nerve. *J Physiol*, **498**: 277–294, 1997.

28. Scholz A, Reid G, Vogel W, Bostock H. Ion channels in human axons. *J Neurophysiol*, **70**: 1274–1279, 1993.

29. Reid G, Scholz A, Bostock H, Vogel W. Human axons contain at least five types of voltage-dependent potassium channel. *J Physiol*, **518**: 681–696, 1999.

30. Eng DL, Gordon TR, Kocsis JD, Waxman SG. Current-clamp analysis of a time-dependent rectification in rat optic nerve. *J Physiol*, **421**: 185–202, 1990.

31. Clapham DE. Not so funny anymore: pacing channels are cloned. *Neuron*, **21**: 5–7, 1998.

32. Hodgkin AL. Evidence for electrical transmission in nerve. Part 2. *J Physiol*, **90**: 211–232, 1937.

33. Serra J, Campero M, Ochoa J, Bostock H. Activity-dependent slowing of conduction differentiates functional subtypes of C fibres innervating human skin. *J Physiol*, **515**: 799–811, 1999.

34. Jonas P, Koh DS, Kampe K, Hermsteiner M, Vogel W. ATP-sensitive and Ca-activated K channels in vertebrate axons: novel links between metabolism and excitability. *Pflugers Arch*, **418**: 68–73, 1991.

35. Wu J, Rubinstein C, Shrager P. Single channel characterization of multiple types of potassium channels in demyelinated Xenopus axons. *J Neurosci*, **13**: 5153–5163, 1993.

36. Lev-Ram V, Grinvald A. Ca^{2+}- and K^+-dependent communication between central nervous system myelinated axons and oligodendrocytes revealed by voltage-sensitive dyes. *Proc Natl Acad Sci U S A*, **83**: 6651–6655, 1986.

37. Bostock H, Baker M, Reid G. Changes in excitability of human motor axons underlying post-ischaemic fasciculations: evidence for two stable states. *J Physiol*, **441**: 537–557, 1991.

38. Shyng SL, Nichols CG. Membrane phospholipid control of nucleotide sensitivity of KATP channels. *Science*, **282**: 1138–1141, 1998.

39. Baukrowitz T, Schulte U, Oliver D, Herlitze S, Krauter T, Tucker SJ, Ruppersberg JP, Fakler B. PIP_2 and PIP as determinants for ATP inhibition of K_{ATP} channels. *Science*, **282**: 1141–1144, 1998.

40. Koh D-S, Jonas P, Vogel W. Na^+-activated K^+ channels localized in the nodal region of myelinated axons of *Xenopus*. *J Physiol*, **479**: 183–197, 1994.

41. Grafe P. An *in vitro* model of diabetic neuropathy: electrophysiological studies. In: H. Bostock, P. Kirkwood and A.H. Pullen (Eds). *The Neurobiology of Disease – Contributions from Neuroscience to Clinical Neurology*, Cambridge University Press, Cambridge, 1996, 61–68.

42. Thomas PK, Tomlinson DR. Diabetic and hypoglycemic neuropathy. In: PJ Dyck, PK Thomas, JW Griffin, PA Low and JF Poduslo (Eds). *Peripheral Neuropathy*, W.B. Saunders, Philadelphia, 1993, 1219–1250.

43. Bostock H, Baker M, Grafe P, Reid G. Changes in excitability and accommodation of human motor axons following brief periods of ischaemia. *J Physiol*, **441**: 513–535, 1991.

44. Bostock H, Cikurel K, Burke D. Threshold tracking techniques in the study of human peripheral nerve. *Muscle Nerve*, **21**: 137–158, 1998.

45. Weigl P, Bostock H, Franz P, Martius P, Muller W, Grafe P. Threshold tracking provides a rapid indication of ischaemic resistance in motor axons of diabetic subjects. *Electroencephalogr Clin Neurophysiol*, **73**: 369–371, 1989.

46. Schneider U, Jund R, Nees S, Grafe P. Differences in sensitivity to hyperglycemic hypoxia of isolated rat sensory and motor nerve fibers. *Ann Neurol*, **31**: 605–610, 1992.

47. Schneider U, Niedermeier W, Grafe P. The paradox between resistance to hypoxia and liability to hypoxic damage in hyperglycemic peripheral nerves: evidence for glycolysis involvement. *Diabetes*, **42**: 981–987, 1993.

48. Strupp M, Jund R, Schneider U, Grafe P. Glucose availability and sensitivity to anoxia of isolated rat peroneal nerve. *Am J Physiol*, **261**: E389–394, 1991.

49. Kraig RP, Pulsinelli WA, Plum F. Carbonic acid buffer changes during complete brain ischemia. *Am J Physiol*, **250**: R348–R357, 1986.

50. David G, Modney B, Scappaticci KA, Barrett JN, Barrett EF. Electrical and morphological factors influencing the depolarizing after-potential in rat and lizard myelinated axons. *J Physiol*, **489**: 141–157, 1995.

51. Schneider U, Quasthoff S, Mitrović N, Grafe P. Hyperglycaemic hypoxia alters after-potential and fast K^+ conductance of rat axons by cytoplasmic acidification. *J Physiol*, **465**: 679–697, 1993.

52. Grafe P, Bostock H, Schneider U. The effects of hyperglycaemic hypoxia on rectification in rat dorsal root axons. *J Physiol*, **480**: 297–307, 1994.

53. Bostock H, Sharief M, Reid G, Murray N. Axonal ion channel dysfunction in amyotrophic lateral sclerosis. *Brain*, **118**: 217–225, 1995.

54. Boucher TJ, Okuse K, Bennett DLH, Munson JB, Wood JN, McMahon SB. Potent analgesic effects of GDNF in neuropathic pain states. *Science*, **290**: 124–127, 2000.

55. Bostock H, Baker M. Evidence for two types of potassium channel in human motor axons *in vivo*. *Brain Research*, **462**: 354–358, 1988.

56. Stålberg E, Trontelj JV. *Single fibre electromyography*, Mirvalle Press Ltd., Old Woking, Surrey, U.K., 1979.

57. Hodgkin AL, Huxley AF, Katz B. Measurement of current-voltage relations in the membrane of the giant axon of *Loligo*. *J Physiol*, **116**: 424–448, 1952.

58. Bostock H, Burke D, Hales JP. Differences in behaviour of sensory and motor axons following release of ischaemia. *Brain*, **117**: 225–234, 1994.

9

INSULIN GLYCATION AND ITS POSSIBLE ROLE IN THE PATHOGENESIS OF DIABETES

Elena GANEA

There is now a consensus that hyperglycemia plays an important role in the development of diabetes complications. Sustained hyperglycemia induces continuous accumulation of glycation products in various tissues of the body, including blood vessels walls, being associated with diabetic micro- and macrovascular complications. The deleterious cumulative effects of AGEs are felt after months or years, whereas insulin plasma half-life under normal conditions is less than 4–5 min, which may explain why insulin glycation has been ignored so long time. Due to the development of the modern techniques, insulin glycation has been demonstrated: a) *in vitro,* under hyperglycemic conditions, b) in pancreatic and islet extracts from various animal models of type 2 diabetes, c) in clonal insulin-secreting cells maintained in culture under hyperglycemic conditions and more recently, d) in diabetic plasma.

Experimental data suggest that both insulin and proinsulin are glycated *in vivo* in diabetic animals, glycation occurring in pancreatic β-cells during synthesis and storage, before the mature granules fuse with the plasma membrane and discharge their content onto the extracellular fluid. The hyperglycemic extracellular environment in diabetes may induce a high intracellular concentration of glucose, which is transported into β-cell by the GLUT2 transporter. The insulin may be glycated in the cell by glucose, but also by its metabolite, glucose 6-phosphate (G6P), which is a much more reactive glycating agent than glucose.

The main glycation site of *in vitro* glycated human insulin was identified as β-chain NH$_2$-terminal Phe[1] residue and the second, minor glycation site has been detected as Gly[1] in the α-chain. The insulin monomer is stabilized by disulfide bridges and by a network of bonds such as van der Waals contacts, hydrogen bonding and salt bridges. Glycation reaction alters the surface charge of the molecules, which affects the protein-protein and protein-water interactions, and could destabilize the native conformation.

The insulin glycation of results in reducing of its biological activities: the ability of the glycated insulin to regulate plasma glucose metabolism, to stimulate glucose uptake by the cell, as well as glucose oxidation and glycogen synthesis are reduced as compared with the native peptide. Although many studies have shown that biological activity of insulin (glucose transport and metabolism, cell growth and mitogenesis) correlates with receptor binding, recent data suggest that post-receptor events might be involved.

In conclusion, glycated insulin has been detected and characterized in human diabetic plasma. Glycation significantly impairs its biological activity, which may contribute to glucose intolerance and insulin resistance in type 2 diabetes.

There is now a consensus that hyperglycemia plays an important role in the development of diabetes complications. Non-enzymatic glycosylation of proteins (glycation) provides an attractive hypothesis to link hyperglycemia with major patho-physiological processes involved in these complications, especially vascular disease, neuropathy and cataract. Sustained hyperglycemia induces continuous accumulation of glycation products in various tissues of the body, included blood vessels walls. The first protein glycation product is a Schiff base, formed over a period of hours in a non-enzymatic condensation of a reducing sugar with protein free amino groups; this is an unstable compound, which may either dissociate or may be converted over several days into a stable Amadori product (AP). The next steps of the glycation process consisting of a series of complex reactions, where the free sugar is no more involved, lead to the advanced glycation end-products (AGEs) formation. The accumulation of AGEs in various tissues is known to progress during normal aging and at an accelerated rate in diabetes mellitus, being associated with diabetic micro- and macro-vascular complications [1–3]. The deleterious cumulative effects of AGEs are felt after months or years, which explains the increased interest in the study of glycated long-lived structural proteins, such as collagen, myelin or crystalline. However, functional changes induced by glycation in proteins with shorter half-life have been reported over the past decade. Studies on serum albumin AP isolated from diabetic patients suggested that tissue changes in diabetic nephropathy may be initiated by AP rather soon after hyperglycemia was installed [4]. Progressive inactivation of several enzymes during *in vitro* glycation for short periods of time (from few hours to few days) support the idea that also the first stages of glycation, not only the advanced one, may induce conformational changes in proteins, compromising their function [5–8].

INSULIN GLYCATION

Insulin has no plasma carrier protein and, as a consequence, its plasma half-life is less than 4–5 min, under normal conditions. This may explain why insulin glycation has been ignored for too long, the process of non-enzymatic glycosylation occurring in stages of hours, days or weeks. However, due to the development of the modern techniques, insulin glycation has been demonstrated: a) *in vitro,* under hyperglycemic conditions or when insulin was incubated with reducing sugars other than glucose [9–11], b) in pancreatic and islet extracts from various animal models of type 2 diabetes [12], c) in clonal insulin-secreting cells maintained under hyperglycemic conditions in culture [13, 14] and more recently, d) in diabetic plasma [15, 16].

a) Covalent incorporation of glucose and mannose into insulin molecule was shown earlier, by incubation of bovine insulin with D-[1-^{14}C]-glucose and D-[1-^{3}H]-mannose, at 37°C (9). The *in vitro* glycation of human insulin was characterized by reversed-phase HPLC, 15 years later. It has been found that the rate and the extent of insulin glycation increase with the ambient glucose concentration over the range from 0 to 220mM and with time over the period from 0 to 24 hours [10]. Glycation occurred even faster when insulin was incubated with phosphorylated reducing sugars, such as glucose-6-phosphate (G6P) or fructose-6-phosphate (F6P). After 2 hours of incubation with 220 mM G6P, 17.1% of insulin has been glycated [11]. It has been found that G6P was more potent in glycating insulin than glucose, fructose and F6P, all of them at high and at low concentrations (6.9 and 13.8 mM), closer to the physiological ones. These data suggest that intracellular glycation of insulin and proinsulin by G6P may occur in the pancreatic β-cells, more efficiently than *in vitro* glycation by glucose.

b) The glycation of immunoreactive insulin (IRI) has been demonstrated in pancreatic extracts from diabetic animals, separating the glycated and non-glycated insulin by affinity chromatography and estimating their amount by radioimmunoassay. A significant increase in glycated pancreatic IRI content was found at different animal models with varying levels of hyperglycemia, such as diabetic obese mouse, displaying many characteristics of NIDDM, streptozotocin (SZT)-induced diabetic mouse, displaying characteristics of IDDM and hydrocortisone-treated rats, showing a severe insulin resistance [12]. Similar results were reported for islets isolated from obese hyperglycemic mice, as well as for islets isolated from normal mice and cultured in a hyperglycemic medium. Separation by RP HPLC of the glycated IRI extracted from pancreatic islets indicated that 28% of the total IRI content corresponded to glycated proinsulin, suggesting that glycation of proinsulin may be associated with a defective cleavage of proinsulin to insulin by the specific endoproteases [12].

c) New pancreatic β-cell lines, created by molecular biology techniques, very similar to normal insulin-secreting cells, help to overcome the limitations of usefulness of many β-cell lines for the study of insulin secretion. Three new clonal glucose-responsive insulin-secreting cells were created by the electrofusion of normal NEDH rat pancreatic β-cells with immortal RINm5F, namely BRIN BG5, BRIN BG7 and BRIN BD11 [13]. BRIN BD11 cells exhibited a superior glucose responsiveness compared to the other two cell lines, which was associated with an increased expression of the glucose transporter GLUT2 and an increased glucokinase activity. Experiments performed on these pancreatic cells cultured under hyperglycemic conditions, some of them present in diabetes, indicate that the cells readily secreted glycated insulin.

The secretion of glycated insulin after culture of BRIN BD11 cells for 72 hours at glucose concentrations between 1.4 and 33.3 mM was almost six fold increased for hyperglycemic concentrations, compared to lower glucose concentrations. Besides, compared with the *in vitro* glycation, the intracellular glycation of insulin in BRIN BD11 cells was higher, for the same glucose concentration and time of exposure, suggesting that glycation of insulin may occur in pancreatic β-cells during synthesis and storage [14].

d) Despite the results indicating the presence of glycated insulin in the pancreatic and islets extract, as well as in clonal insulin-secreting cells cultured in the presence of a high concentration of glucose, the technology for the evaluation of a glycated insulin in plasma has not been sensitive or reliable enough until recently. The successful production of polyclonal antisera with high specificity and affinity for glycated insulin made possible to demonstrate the presence of glycated insulin in the plasma and islets of diabetic animal models. The specific antibodies to glycated insulin were raised in rabbits and guinea pigs, by using two glycated, synthetic sequences from the insulin β-chain [15]. The highest titre antisera were obtained in animals immunized with glycated

insulin β-chain (1-6)Tyr^7 and Lys^8, coupled to ovalbumin, using glutaraldehyde. Glycated insulin in the plasma of hydrocortisone treated diabetic rats, measured by radioimmunoassay, using these immune sera, indicated values corresponding to 16% of total circulating insulin concentration, compared to 4% glycated insulin in the plasma of the control animals [15].

More recently, the glycated insulin was estimated in human plasma by high-pressure liquid chromatography (HPLC), electrospray ionization-mass spectrometry (ESI-MS) and radioimmunoassay (RIA) techniques, showing for type 2 diabetic patients values corresponding to 9% of total circulating insulin [16]. Using a novel, specific radioimmunoassay it has been found that the circulating concentration of glycated insulin in a combined group of type 2 diabetic patients (well, moderately and poorly controlled) was increased about 3-fold compared with control subjects [17].

THE POSSIBLE MECHANISM FOR THE *IN VIVO* GLYCATION OF INSULIN

Although it seems unlikely that plasma circulating insulin is glycated during its 5–10 minutes half-life, the experimental data suggest that insulin glycation occurs in pancreatic β-cells during synthesis and storage, before the mature granules fuse with plasma membrane and discharge their content onto the extracellular fluid (emiocytosis) [12]. The hyperglycemic extracellular environment in diabetes may induce a high intracellular concentration of glucose, transported into β- cell by the GLUT2 transporter. The insulin may be glycated in the cell by glucose, but also by its metabolite glucose-6-phosphate (G6P), which is produced in a reaction catalyzed by glucokinase and it is a much more reactive glycating agent than glucose. Thus, the elevation of glucose in the cytosol of pancreatic β-cell, coupled with specific transport to ER, by glucose-6-phosphatase system transport proteins may facilitate a rapid glycation of proinsulin and insulin where these are most concentrated, and incorporated into vesicles, transported to Golgi and packed into secretory granules. The presence, in diabetic pancreatic tissue, of insulin containing phosphate group remains to be clarified by future characterization of the glycated insulin.

The above-mentioned data also showed that both insulin and proinsulin were glycated *in vivo,* in diabetic animals. The cleavage of proinsulin to insulin by two specific endopeptidases, which recognizes dibasic sequences in the proinsulin molecule, may be impaired by conformational modifications induced by glycation in the neighboring areas. Therefore, the glycation of proinsulin may be associated with impaired processing of the prohormone.

THE SITES OF INSULIN GLYCATION

The identification of the precise site of glycation within such a functionally important protein-like-insulin has a great importance. By a combination of specific enzymatic digestion, followed by RP-HPLC purification and mass spectrometry, the main glycation site of *in vitro* glycated human insulin was identified as β-chain NH_2-terminal Phe[1] residue [18]. A second, minor glycation site has been detected more recently, as Gly[1] in the α-chain of human insulin, glycated insulin, glycaticemic reducing conditions [19].

The diglycated human insulin (Phe[1] β and Gly[1] α) has been purified and characterized by reversed-phase HPLC, digestion by endoproteinase Glu-C, a highly specific serine protease which cleaves peptide bonds at the carboxyl side of glutamic acid and by mass spectrometry and automated Edman degradation.

The nonenzymatic covalent binding of a reducing sugar (*e.g.,* glucose) to the free amino groups of amino terminal residues of both α and β chains may influence insulin stability and its biological activity. It has been shown that the glycation reaction alters the surface charge of the molecules, which affects the protein-protein and protein-water interactions and could destabilize the native conformation [20]. Proteins are mainly glycated at the ε-amino group of lysine and / or α-amino group of the N-terminal amino acid and the glycation at α-amino residue alters the pK of the protein much more than at lysine residues [21]. Insulin contains only one lysyl residue (B29) among the 51 amino acids present in α (21 residues) and β-chains (30 residues). However, insulin glycation occurs at the β-chain

amino terminal phenylalanine (B1) and α-chain amino terminal glycine (A1), as mentioned above, suggesting that disruption of the inter- or intrachain bonding, as a consequence of the surface charge alteration, may induce conformational changes and modified biological activity.

INSULIN STRUCTURE AND REGIONS REQUIRED FOR BIOLOGICAL ACTIVITY

Insulin monomer is stabilized by two interchain disulfide bridges at A7-B7 and A20-B19, which link covalently α- and β chain, and one intrachain disulfide bond at A6-A11. These bridges have an important contribution to the correct folding of insulin into the native, biologically active conformation [22, 23].

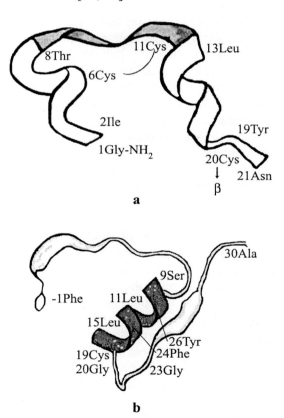

Figure 9.1

Structure of insulin.

a – α-chain, consisting of two alpha helices (A2Ile-A8Thr and A13Leu-A19Tyr), stabilized by the A6-A11 disulfide); b – β-chain, consisting of an α-helix (B9Ser-B19Cys); the folding B20 and B23 allows the contacts between B24Phe with B15Leu and B26Tyr with B11Leu.

The three dimensional structure of insulin, studied by X-ray crystallography and NMR spectroscopy, shows that insulin molecule is a compact globular structure, with a hydrophobic core, containing three α-helical regions, two of the α-chain, at A2 Ile-A8 Thr and A13 Leu-A19Tyr, and a central α-helix in the β chain, at B9 Ser-B19 Cys (Figure 9.1a and b). In the insulin fold, β-chain is wrapped around the compact α chain (Figure 9.2) and a network of bonds stabilize the monomer (Figure 9.3):

– *van der Waals* contacts between A2 Ile-A19 Tyr connect the N and C termini of the α-chain and also connect C terminal residues B24 Phe and B26 Tyr with the α-helix residues B15 Leu and B11 Leu, respectively;

– *hydrogen bonding* at A13 Leu-B4 Gln, A7 Cys-B5 His, A19 Tyr-B25 Phe;

– *salt bridges* at B29 Lys-A4 Glu, B22 Arg-A21 Asn, A11 Cys-B4 Gln.

Some of these links involve amino acids fully conserved during evolution, such as A2 Ile, A3 Val, A19 Tyr, B11 Leu and B24 Phe, suggesting the importance of these interactions for the integrity of insulin molecule.

– *hydrophobic interactions* involving residues B8 Gly, B9 Ser, B12 Val, B13 Glu, B16 Tyr, B24 Phe, B25 Phe, B26 Tyr, B27 Thr and B28 Pro mediate dimer formation.

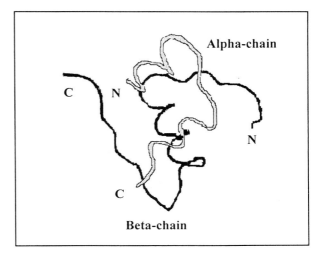

Figure 9.2

Insulin monomer, the active form of the hormone: grey, α-chain; black, β-chain.

Insulin, at physiological concentration (1 ng/ml), in solutions at neutral pH, exists as monomer, which is the active form. At a higher concentration, at acid or neutral pH (in the absence of Zn ions) the hydrophobic surfaces of two monomers come together, forming an antiparallel β-strand between residues B23 Gly and B30 Thr of each monomer.

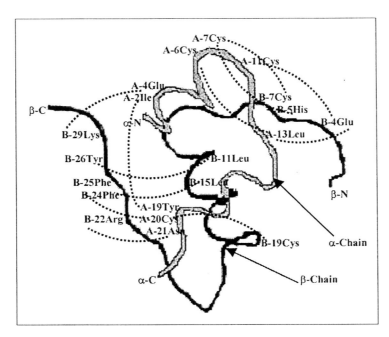

Figure 9.3

Interactions between α-chain (grey) and β-chain (black), stabilizing the insulin monomer molecule.

The dimer obtained is stabilized by intermolecular hydrogen bonds, as well as by van der Waals contacts between B28 Pro and residues B20 Gly-B23 Gly of the adjacent monomer. The residues B26-B30 are essential for dimer formation, but they are not involved in receptor binding. In the presence of zinc ions, insulin has an inherent tendency to form hexamers, soluble globular structures, consisting of three dimers and two zinc atoms coordinated by B10 His from each of the dimers, plus three water molecules. Insulin hexamers, present in the mature secretory granules of pancreatic β-cells, suggest that 2Zn hexamer is the storage form of insulin, which also protects insulin molecule from physical and chemical degradation, as well as from fibril formation [24].

These interactions have important clinical effects. Monomers and dimers readily diffuse into the blood, whereas hexamers diffuse very poorly. Hence, absorption of insulin preparations containing a high proportion of hexamers is delayed and slow. This problem, among others, has stimulated development of a number of recombinant insulin analogs. The first of these molecules to be marketed – called insulin lispro – is engineered such that lysine and proline residues on the C-terminal end of the B chain are reversed; this modification does not alter receptor binding, but minimizes the tendency to form dimers and hexamers.

Our *in vitro* experiments on insulin glycation, in the presence of fructose, ribose and glyceraldehyde, respectively showed an increase in the negative electrical charge of the molecule, as well as formation of high molecular weight aggregates (Plate 9.1), suggesting that such changes may induce disruption of intra- or intermolecular interactions, altering the stability of insulin molecule (Ganea E., unpublished data).

Glycation could also influence the insulin activity by altering the hormone interaction with its receptor. Insulin actions are initiated at the plasma membrane, by the response of insulin receptor binding to the ligands. It has been shown that the N-terminal region of insulin α-chain is important in the receptor interaction, with a special contribution of the amino group of A1 Gly, the peptide bond A1 Gly-A2 Ile and the side chains of both A2 Ile and A3 Val to confer affinity on this interaction [25]. The mechanism suggested involves a partial unfolding of N-terminal α-helix, facilitating the access of the insulin molecule to the receptor binding site and the refolding after binding; before the interaction takes place, a detachment of the C-terminal end of β-chain from the rest of the molecule (Figure 9.4) enhances the accessibility of A3 Val to the receptor, with which it realizes a direct contact [26]. It has been suggested that at physiological insulin concentrations, one molecule of insulin binds to two different binding sites on the two α-subunits of the receptor, with high affinity; at high insulin concentrations, a second molecule will bind to only one receptor site, with low affinity (Plate 9.2). The residue A1 Gly undergoes multiple close contacts, such as hydrogen bonding and salt bridge between its α-amino group and γ-carbonyl group of A4 Glu; as A1 is the second glycation site detected, it seems very likely that the covalent binding of a reducing sugar to its α-amino group could alter the interaction with the receptor.

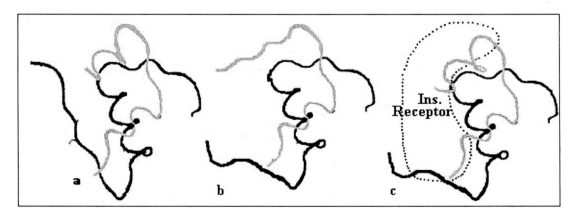

Figure 9.4

Conformational changes in insulin molecule during the receptor binding: a – native insulin monomer, b – unfolding of the α-chain and detachment of β-chain, c – refolding of α-chain and binding to the receptor.

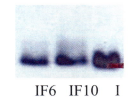

a

IF6 IF10 I

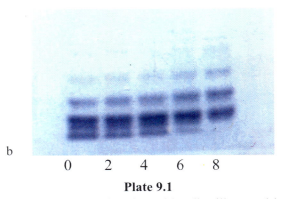

b

0 2 4 6 8

Plate 9.1

Changes induced by *in vitro* glycation of insulin, illustrated by SDS-PAGE.
a – glycation with fructose for 6 (IF6) and 10 (IF10) days; I – native insulin; b – glycation
with glyceraldehyde for 0, 2, 4, 6 and 8 hours.

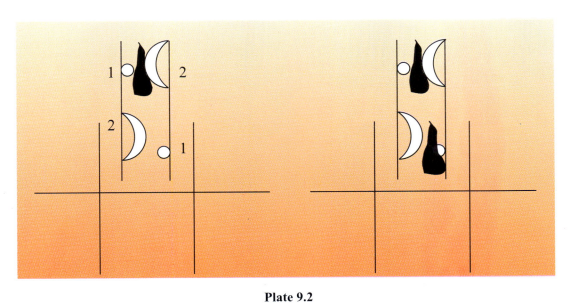

Plate 9.2
Insulin receptor binding sites 1 and 2 (white).
Left, high-affinity binding of the first insulin molecule (black) and right, low-affinity
binding of the second insulin molecule.

A structural model realized in a very recent study on three-dimensional structural interactions between insulin and its receptor, by STEM (scanning transmission electron microscopy), coupled with 3D reconstruction and fitting of atomic subdomains offers an understanding of insulin binding at the atomic level [27]. The model can explain the biological activity of the naturally occurring insulin and insulin analogues, as well as the effect of receptor mutations on insulin binding. The altered activity of several insulins such as that of chicken, guinea pig or hagfish, when assayed using mammalian insulin receptor could be explained by the structural fitting of insulin into the IR binding sites. Sequence changes in hagfish insulin Phe(B1) Arg, Ser(B9)Lys, Thr(A8)His, Ser(A9)Lys, and Ile(A10)Arg reduce its biological activity with more than 95%.

Although the most studies have shown that biological activity of insulin (glucose transport and metabolism, cell growth and mitogenesis) correlates with receptor binding, the lack of such correlation has been demonstrated for insulin effects on protein degradation, suggesting that post-receptor events might be involved [28]. The influence of glycation on insulin activity of protein degradation inhibition has not been studied so far, and the factors beyond receptor binding in the insulin actions deserve evaluation.

GLYCATION OF INSULIN RESULTS IN REDUCED BIOLOGICAL ACTIVITY

In order to understand the glycation of pancreatic insulin in diabetes and its significance to the pathology of the disease, the effects of the glycated insulin on the glucose uptake, transport and metabolism have been studied in animals and man.

Earlier studies reported that *in vitro* glycated insulin has a reduced biological activity when assayed for stimulation of glucose oxidation, lipogenesis and antilipolysis in adipose tissue [9]. Similar conclusions can be found in more recent worws which, unlike previous studies using mixtures of glycated and non glycated insulin,

employed pure, stable glycated insulin for *in vitro* or *in vivo* experiments [16, 19, 29–31].

Effects of insulin glycation on plasma glucose homeostasis.

It has been shown that plasma glucose lowering activity of the glycated insulin administered in 39% (w/v) glucose, by intraperitoneal injections to normal mice, was significantly reduced compared with that of the non-glycated hormone, and the compromised action of insulin was directly related to the degree of glycation [30].

The ability of the glycated insulin to regulate plasma glucose homeostasis, in mice, was also evaluated by the administration of monoglycated and diglycated insulin, respectively. Monoglycated insulin is the major fraction of glycated insulin, containing a single glucitol adduct substituted at the Phe1 of the amino-terminus of the β-chain, while the diglycated fraction contains a glucitol adduct bound at both N-terminal Phe1 of the β-chain and at Gly1 of the insulin α-chain. The results showed that both fractions of glycated insulin are significantly less potent than native insulin in inducing hypoglycemia in mice, 20% and 30% reduction of activity being exhibited by mono- and diglycated insulin, respectively, compared with the control insulin [19, 31].

The possible significance of circulating glycated insulin in type 2 diabetes was evaluated in human healthy volunteers, using a two-steps euglycemic hyperinsulinemic clamp technique, with pure monoglycated insulin. The amount of glucose needed to maintain normoglycemia during the steady state was significantly lower with infusion of glycated insulin than with control insulin, and a 70% greater dose of glycated insulin was required to induce a similar effect to that of the control hormone. These results indicate that the ability of glycated insulin to lower plasma glucose concentration was significantly impaired compared with that of the control peptide [16].

THE ACTIVITY OF THE GLYCATED INSULIN AT THE CELLULAR LEVEL

The effect of glycation on insulin activity, at the cellular level, was evaluated by studies of glucose uptake, transport and insulin-receptor binding.

Insulin stimulates fat and muscle cell to take up glucose. Experiments performed on the isolated mouse abdominal muscle showed that both monoglycated and diglycated insulin also induce an increase of the intracellular glucose uptake, but 19% and respectively 38% less than the native form [19, 31]. The decreased insulin mediated glucose uptake has been suggested to indicate a receptor binding abnormality. However, an early study using human monocytes and a mixture of glycated and nonglycated insulin suggested that insulin glycation compromised the insulin action at a postreceptor level [32]. More recent data demonstrate that the exposure of 3T3-L1 adipocytes to high glucose and glucosamine concentrations, in the presence of low insulin, caused resistance of glucose transport by different mechanisms: glucosamine inhibited GLUT4 translocation, whereas high glucose impaired GLUT4 "intrinsic activity"; interestingly, this occurred without detectable changes in total expression of GLUT4 or GLUT2 [33].

Receptor interaction studies of native and glycated insulin binding to the Chinese hamster ovary (CHO)-T cells, transfected with human insulin receptor, revealed no changes in binding affinity for the glycated hormone [16]. The authors suggest that glycation may modify the charge density or insulin tertiary structure, affecting postreceptor signaling. This explanation is supported by several recent studies, such as those on glucagon-like peptide1, which demonstrate that very simple structural modifications, like glycation, can induce important agonist or antagonist properties, independent of changes in receptor binding [34]. It is also possible that intracellular signaling proteins, known as insulin receptor substrates (IRS-1 and IRS-2), could be involved, but the identification of signaling molecules that mediate many of the insulin specific actions, such as GLUT4 translocation to the cell surface, remain an important challenge [35].

EFFECTS OF GLYCATED INSULIN ON METABOLISM

Biological activity of the modified insulin in the regulation of glucose metabolism was assessed by the evaluation of hormone ability to stimulate glucose oxidation and glycogen synthesis in isolated muscle [19, 29–31]. Glucose oxidation, evaluated by measuring $^{14}CO_2$ production in experiments performed on isolated mouse diaphragm muscle or abdominal muscle have demonstrated that glycation of insulin significantly reduced its ability to promote glucose oxidation, compared with the native peptide. The percent of the activity reduction was related to the extent of glycation, insulin amount and purity of the preparation of glycated insulin (mixture of glycated and native, pure glycated insulin or pure mono- and diglycated fractions). These results are in agreement with earlier observations that insulin glycated for a longer period, in vitro, exhibits a reduced ability to stimulate glucose oxidation and lipogenesis, in isolated rat adipocytes [9].

Studies on the capacity of insulin to stimulate glycogen production in isolated mouse abdominal muscle showed a similar decrease of the ability of glycated insulin compared with the control insulin [19, 31]. Interestingly, the activity of the diglycated insulin decreased more than that of the monoglycated peptide (22–38% and 20% respectively).

Lipogenetic and antilipolytic effects, studied on adipocytes, were also decreased in the presence of glycated insulin compared with the native hormone, although the effect of glycation on antilipolytic activity was relatively small [9]. However, a recent study on biological activity of insulin assessed by euglycemic hyperinsulinemic clamp technique, in humans, found that glycation of insulin did not affect the suppression of lipolysis effect, or the concentrations of plasma nonesterified free fatty acids and glycerol [16]. It has been also suggested that the effect of glycation on biological activity does not extend on the hepatic insulin action, as the suppression of endogenous glucose production (as an index of hepatic insulin action) during the experiment mentioned above was similar for glycated and native insulin.

In conclusion, these data demonstrate that glycation of insulin under hyperglycemic conditions significantly impair its biological activity at the cellular level and this may contribute to glucose intolerance and insulin resistance in type 2 diabetes. The scientists are working to finding and synthesizing compounds to prevent or delay the deleterious effects of insulin glycation.

REFERENCES

1. Kiuchi K, Nejima J, Takano T, Ohta M, Hashimoto H. Increased serum concentrations of advanced glycation end-products: a marker of coronary artery disease activity in type 2 diabetic patients. *Heart*, **85(1)**: 87–91, 2001.
2. Yamagishi S, Inagachi Y, Okamoto T, Amano S, Koga K, Takeuchi M, Makita Z. Advanced glycation end-product-induced apoptosis and overexpression of vascular endothelial growth factor and monocyte chemoattractant protein-1 in human-cultured mesangial cells. *J Biol Chem*, **277(23)**: 20309–20315, 2002.
3. Aso Y, Inukai T, Tayama K, Takemura Y. Serum concentration of advanced glycation end-products is associated with the development of atherosclerosis as well as diabetic microangiopathy in patients with type 2 diabetes. *Acta Diabetol*, **37**: 87–92, 2000.
4. Furth AJ. Glycated proteins in diabetes. *Br J Biomed Sci*, **54**: 192–200, 1997.
5. Ganea E, Harding JJ. Molecular chaperones protect against glycation-induced inactivation of glucose-6-phosphate dehydrogenase. *Eur J Biochem*, **231**: 181–185, 1995.
6. Heath MM, Rixon KC, Harding JJ. Glycation-induced inactivation of malate dehydrogenase protection by aspirin and a lens molecular chaperone, α-crystallin. *Biochim Biophys Acta*, **1315**: 176–184, 1996.
7. Yan H, Harding JJ. Glycation-induced inactivation and loss of antigenicity of catalase and superoxide dismutase. *Biochem J*, **328**: 599–605, 1997.
8. McCarty AD, Cortizo AM, Gimenez Segura G, Bruzzone L, Etcheverry SB. Non-enzymatic glycosylation of alkaline phosphatase alters its biological properties. *Mol Cel Biochem*, **181**: 63–69, 1998.
9. Dolhofer R, Wieland OH. Preparation and biological properties of glycosylated insulin. *FEBS Lett*, **100**: 133–136, 1979.
10. O'Harte FP, Boyd AC, Abdel-Wahab YH, Barnett CR, Flatt PR. Characterization of the glycation of human insulin by reversed-phase HPLC. *Biochem Soc Trans*, **22**: 239S, 1994.
11. O'Harte FP, Penney AC, Flatt PR. Glycation of insulin by phosphorylated and nonphosphorylated reducing sugars. *Biochem Soc Trans*, **25**: 150S, 1997.
12. Abdel-Wahab YH, O'Harte FP, Ratcliff H, McClenaghan NH, Barnett CR, Flatt PR. Glycation of insulin in the Islet of Langerhans of normal and diabetic animals. *Diabetes*, **45**: 1489–1496, 1996.
13. McClenaghan NH, Flatt PR. Engineering cultured insulin-secreting pancreatic B-cell lines. *J Mol Med*, **77**: 235–243, 1999.
14. Abdel-Wahab YH, O'Harte FP, Barnett CR, Flatt PR. Glycation of insulin in a cultured insulin-secreting cell line. *Biochem Soc Trans*, **25**: 128S, 1997.
15. McKillop AM, McCluskey JT, Boyd AC, Mooney MH, Flatt PR, O'Harte FP. Production and characterization of specific antibodies for evaluation of glycated insulin in plasma and biological tissues. *J Endocrinol*, **167**: 153–163, 2000.
16. Hunter SJ, Boyd AC, O'Harte FP, McKillop AM, Wiggam MI, Mooney MH, McCluskey JT, Lindsay JR, Ennis CN, Gamble R, Sheridan B, Barnett CR, McNulty H, Bell PM, Flatt PR. Demonstration of glycated insulin in human diabetic plasma and decreased biological activity assessed by euglycemic- hyperinsulinemic clamp technique in humans. *Diabetes*, **52**: 492–498, 2003.
17. Lindsay JR, McKillop AM, Mooney MH, O' Harte FP, Bell PM, Flatt PR. Demonstration of increased concentrations of circulating glycated insulin in human Type 2 diabetes using novel and specific radioimmunoassay. *Diabetologia*, **46**: 475–478, 2003.
18. O'Harte PM, Hojrup P, Barnett CR, Flatt PR. Identification of the site of glycation of human insulin. *Peptides*, **17**: 1323–1330, 1996.
19. O'Harte PM, Boyd AC, McKillop AM, Abdel-Wahab YH, McNulty H, Barnett CR, Conlon JM, Hojrup P, Flatt PR. Structure, antihyperglycemic activity and cellular actions of a novel diglycated human insulin. *Peptides*, **21**: 1519–1526, 2000.
20. Beswick HT, Harding JJ. Conformational changes induced in lens α- and γ-crystallins by modification with glucose-6-phosphate. Implications for cataract. *Biochem J*, **246**: 761–769, 1987.
21. Schleicher E, Wieland OH. Protein glycation: measurement and clinical relevance. *J Clin Chem Clin Biochem*, **27**: 577–587, 1989.
22. Yan H, Guo ZY, Gong XW, Xi D, Feng YM. A peptide model of insulin folding intermediate with one disulfide. *Protein Sci*, **12**: 768–75, 2003.
23. Hua QX, Chu YC, Jia W, Phillips NF, Wang RY, Katsoyannis PG, Weiss MA. Mechanism of insulin chain combination. Asymmetric roles of A-chain alpha-helices in disulfide pairing. *J Biol Chem*, **277**: 43443–43453, 2002.
24. Whittingham JL, Edwards DJ, Antson AA, Clarkson JM, Dodson GG. Interactions of phenol and m-cresol in the insulin hexamer, and their effect on the association properties of B28 Pro→Asp insulin analogues. *Biochemistry*, **37**: 11516–11523, 1998.

25. Nakagawa SH, Tager HS. Importance of aliphatic side-chain structure at position 2 and 3 of the insulin A chain in insulin-receptor interactions. *Biochemistry*, **31**: 3204–3214, 1992.
26. Keller D, Clausen R, Josefsen K, Led JJ. Flexibility and bioactivity of insulin: an NMR investigation of the solution structure and folding of an unusually flexible human insulin mutant with increased biological activity. *Biochemistry*, **40**: 10732–10740, 2001.
27. Yip CC, Ottensmeyer P. Three dimensional structural interactions of insulin and its receptor. *J Biol Chem*, **278**: 27329–27332, 2003.
28. Fawcett J, Hamel FG, Bennett RG, Vajo Z, Duckworth WC. Insulin and analogue effects on protein degradation in different cell types. Dissociation between binding and activity. *J Biol Chem*, **276**: 11552–11558, 2001.
29. Abdel-Wahab YH, O´Harte FP, Barnett CR, Flatt PR. Studies of the effect of glycation of insulin on glucose metabolism in isolated mouse diaphragm muscle. *Biochem Soc Trans*, **22**: 238S, 1994.
30. Abdel-Wahab YH, O'Harte FP, Boyd AC, Barnett CR, Flatt PR. Glycation of insulin results in reduced biological activity in mice. *Acta Diabetol*, **34**: 265–270, 1997.
31. Boyd AC, Abdel-Wahab YH, McKillop AM, McNulty H, Barnett CR, O'Harte FP, Flatt PR. Impaired ability of glycated insulin to regulate plasma glucose and stimulate glucose transport and metabolism in mouse abdominal muscle. *Biochim Biophys Acta*, **1523**: 128–134, 2000.
32. Lapolla A, Tessari P, Poli T, Valerio A, Duner E, Iori E, Fedele D, Crepaldi G. Reduced *in vivo* biological activity of *in vitro* glycosylated insulin. *Diabetes*, **37**: 787–791, 1988.
33. Nelson BA, Robinson KA, Buse MG. High glucose and glucosamine induce insulin resistance via different mechanisms in 3T3-L1 adipocytes. *Diabetes*, **49**: 981–991, 2000.
34. O'Harte FP, Abdel-Wahab YH, Conlon JM, Flatt PR. Glycation of glucagon-like peptide-1(7–36) amide: characterization and impaired action on rat insulin secreting cells. *Diabetologia*, **41**: 1187–1193, 1998.
35. Clarck SF, Molero J-C, James DE. Release of insulin receptor substrate protein from an intracellular complex coincides with the development of insulin resistance. *J Biol Chem*, **275**: 3819–3826, 2000.

10

MOLECULAR MECHANISMS OF INSULIN TRANSDUCTION AND ROLE OF METFORMIN IN INSULIN RESISTANCE

Florin GRIGORESCU

Insulin action at the cellular level is initiated by binding to a specific plasma membrane insulin receptor (IR), followed by activation of the IR tyrosine kinase, and phosphorylation of insulin receptor substrates (IRSs). Association of intracellular signaling proteins leads ultimately to the stimulation of mitogenic and metabolic functions of insulin. Alterations at every steps in this cascade of events may produce insulin resistance (recognized as primary mechanism), although insulin resistance in various clinical conditions (*e.g.*, obesity, type 2 diabetes or polycystic ovary syndrome) may involve other regulatory (secondary) tissue specific mechanisms. This distinction is important in targeting insulin resistance by pharmacological agents. Metformin (N_1N_1-dimethylbiguanide), a drug currently used in the treatment of diabetes, has beneficial effects by lowering blood glucose, improving lipid metabolism and providing cardioprotective actions, although molecular mechanisms remain unknown. To understand molecular mechanism of metformin, we set up an experimental rat model able to study transduction events in the liver after bolus injection of insulin in the portal vein, under acutely or chronically *per os* administration of metformin. Results from various experimental protocols, including the study of phosphorylation events and activation of PtdIns 3' kinase, suggested that metformin acts at transductional level by changing kinetics of IR/IRS association and using IRS-2 as a preferential substrate in the liver. These data reinforce our current knowledge on the particular role of IRS-2 in hepatic glucose homeostasis and give a new insight into understanding mechanisms involving IRS-2 in other tissues, including effects of leptin in the hypothalamus or vascular effects of insulin.

Abbreviations List

HGP – Hepatic glucose production
IR – Insulin Receptor
IRS– Insulin Receptor Substrate
PtdIns 3'-kinase – Phosphatidylinositol 3'-kinase

PCOS – Polycystic Ovary Syndrome
T2DM – Type 2 Diabetes Mellitus
TNF – Tumor Necrosis Factor

INTRODUCTION

Insulin resistance characterizes several genetic syndromes in humans and, albeit in a moderate form, in current diseases such as type 2 diabetes mellitus (T2DM), syndrome X, obesity or, in women, the polycystic ovary syndrome (PCOS). It is generally accepted that insulin resistance plays a major role in the pathogenesis of diabetes as indicated by the fact that insulin resistance precedes the occurrence of hyperglycemia in predisposed individuals [1, 2]. Moreover, insulin resistance appears to be the best predictor for subjects who will develop diabetes later in their life [3]. These features explain our major interest in deciphering molecular mechanisms of insulin resistance and new targets for anti-diabetic drugs.

The concept of insulin resistance dramatically changed during years. Initially, the term was designated for resistance to the injected insulin. The discovery of genetic syndromes of severe insulin resistance with *Acanthosis nigricans* rapidly pointed out towards a more pathophysiological definition, similar to that of other hormone-resistant states [4, 5]. The recognition of the pivotal role of defects in the insulin receptor (IR) in genetic syndromes, permitted to conceptualize a so-called primary mechanism of insulin resistance, in opposition to secondary mechanism, which involves downstream insulin metabolic effects in various tissues [6–9]. This distinction was important, particularly in considering genetic aspects (*e.g.* searching for genetic markers or candidate genes) as well as in understanding less classical actions of insulin, such as vascular effects. To date, two major scientific discoveries contributed to the understanding of molecular mechanisms of insulin resistance. One major contribution was the discovery of insulin receptor substrate (IRS), which provided the link between IR tyrosine-kinase activation and intracellular signaling events, such as the stimulation of phosphatidylinositol 3'-kinase (PtdIns 3'-kinase) and glucose transport [10, 11]. In contrast to the well-recognized role of IR in insulin resistance, the contribution of IRS to insulin inaction has remained elusive for many years. Although transgenic animals offered new experimental models for the study of IRS, the knockout mouse model of IRS-1 (the principal substrate of IR) was unable to demonstrate dramatic changes in glucose homeostasis, since disruption of this gene did not induce diabetes [12]. One possible explanation for this behavior of IRS-1 was its redundant role at the cellular level in face of other IRS genes. From then, transgenic mice with tissue specific disruption of IR or IRS provided a second major progress [13, 14]. Thus, many aspects of the role of these two genes were reconsidered after these animal models. The most striking observation was that IR knockout in the muscle (MIRKO), formally considered as a major site of insulin resistance, was not associated with alterations in glucose transport and diabetes, but rather with alterations in the lipid metabolism [15]. These animal models as well as cells from various tissues of transgenic mice are now currently used for both genetic and pharmacological studies.

In this chapter we will review some aspects in the molecular mechanism of insulin transduction as a basis for understanding insulin resistance. In the first part, we will focus particularly on very early events in insulin action occurring in the first minute after insulin stimulation. In a second part, we will present how our laboratory approached pharmacological aspects of insulin resistance, with particular emphasis on the mechanism of action of metformin in the rat liver. Metformin (N_1N_1-dimethylbiguanide) is a drug currently used in the treatment of T2DM, acting as a potent insulin-sensitizing agent. Beneficial effects are recognized particularly in T2DM obese individuals by lowering blood glucose, but also as a cardiovascular protective drug by improving lipid metabolism, clotting factors and platelet function [16–18]. Despite these multiple beneficial effects, recognized from more than 50 years in the clinical practice, the molecular mechanism of action of metformin remains unknown.

MOLECULAR MECHANISMS OF INSULIN ACTION

The insulin action at the cellular level is initiated by binding of the hormone to a specific plasma membrane receptor. The IR was firstly identified by specific binding of labeled ^{125}I – insulin to the plasma membrane [19]. The receptor is a hetero-tetrameric protein ($\alpha_2\beta_2$) composed of two α and two β subunits [5]. The α-subunit of 135 kDa contains the specific binding site for insulin. The β-subunit is a *trans*-membrane protein of 95 kDa, containing a tyrosine-specific protein kinase [20]. The tyrosine kinase is similar to other proto-oncogenes or receptors for growth factors, such as EGF (epidermal growth factor), PDGF (platelet-derived growth factor) or CSF-1 (colony stimulating growth-factor-1) [21, reviewed in Ref. 22]. In humans, the IR is encoded by a gene located on chromosome 19p13.2 [23, 24]. Major progress in understanding transduction mechanism was provided by deciphering the three dimensional (3D) structure of the receptor. The α-subunit was constructed by homology modeling from the crystal structure of the IGF-1 receptor, while the β-subunit was resolved by crystallography with 2.1 Å resolution [25, 26].

The activation of the IR kinase is a complex involving several molecular steps. The specific binding of insulin represents the first step [5]. One molecule of insulin binds asymmetrically to two α- subunits, followed immediately by a conformational change. This, in turn, induces the activation of the kinase. In fact, the tyrosine kinase of β subunit is constitutive, that is, it is permanently activated. The association with α-subunit in the absence of the ligand exerts an inhibitory effect. Binding of insulin induces conformational changes which unmask this inhibition, thus dictating the full kinase activation

through phosphorylation. IR activation involves the autophosphorylation on several specific endogenous sites: Y^{1158}, Y^{1162} and Y^{1163}, all contained in the particular hydrophilic domain of the β-subunit (T loop).

The phosphorylation of three tyrosine residues is progressive and ordered, starting with residue 1162, continuing with 1158 and then 1163 [25, 27]. Using synthetic peptides corresponding to the sequence of the T-loop, our laboratory has shown that phosphorylation of tyrosine induces conformational changes, which may explain the further activation of the receptor [28]. The effect of autophosphorylation is the 100-fold increase in the exogenous activity towards specific substrates. The mechanism is not known, but it likely involves a better positioning of the substrate. Thus, the transfer of the γ-phosphate from the ATP is possible when the tyrosine from the substrate is sufficiently close (2.8 Å) for esterification. The overall activity of the IR is regulated by dephosphorylation by tyrosine specific phosphatases (such as LAR), but also by transmodulation [29]. The best-known mechanism of transmodulation involves the serine kinase PKC, which is able to phosphorylate residues S^{967} and S^{968} in the juxta-membrane region, and S^{1327} and S^{1348} at the C-terminal domain (Figure 10.1).

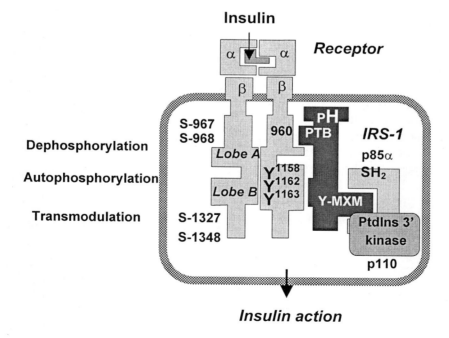

Figure 10.1

Major functional domains involved in insulin receptor activation and association to intracellular substrates.

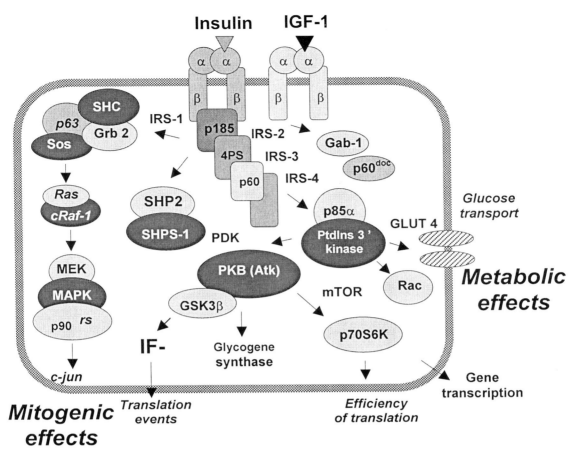

Figure 10.2

Insulin and IGF-1 signaling at intracellular level.

A major progress in understanding the molecular mechanism of insulin action was provided by the discovery of IRS protein [10, 11]. The first protein described was IRS-1, of 135 kDa, but with an apparent molecular weight of 185 kDa during migration in SDS-PAGE [11, 30]. (Figure 10.2) IRS-1 gene is located on human chromosome 2q36 (mouse chromosome 1). A second member of this family was described in ^{32}D cells, the protein 4PS or IRS-2 of 145 kDa, which is slightly longer than IRS-1 [31]. IRS-2 gene is located on chromosome 13q34 (mouse chromosome 8) [31]. Alignment of these proteins revealed several homologous domains. At N-terminal, a domain of 100 residues is homologous to pleckstrine (PH domain or IH-1) while downstream, another domain is found in interaction with the IR and designated PTB (phospho-tyrosine-binding) domain [11]. The C-terminal is less conserved (35% homology) among IRSs, but contains multiple tyrosine phosphorylation sites with crucial role in binding to SH_2 (src homology) domains of signaling proteins. Tyrosine acceptor sites of IRS are located within particular structural motifs Y-M-X-M or Y-X-X-M with a high affinity for SH_2 domains [11].

The IRS family of proteins contains other members such as IRS-3, IRS-4 or several smaller proteins, Gab-1 and p62^{doc} or APS [32, 33]. Human gene of IRS-4 is located on chromosome Xq22.3 and encodes for a 160-kDa protein. IRS-3 was cloned from rat adipocytes and corresponds to the previously described protein-substrate pp60 in these cells. In the human genome this gene is deleted and thus remains unexpressed [34]. IRS-3 contains both PH and PTB domains, but the C-terminal portion is shorter, containing however all potential sites for binding to PtdIns 3' kinase, SHP_2 and Grb$_2$ [35]. In adipocyte, IRS-3 binds better than IRS-1 the p85α subunit of PtdIns 3' kinase and in cells with IRS$^{(-/-)}$ disruption, IRS-3 is the predominant substrate of the IR. The Gab-1 is a protein that possesses a PH domain, but does not contain PTB domain [11]. Gab-1 is apparently a good substrate of the IR only at supra-physiological concentrations of insulin. The p62^{doc} seems to be identical to p62^{rasGAP} previously described as substrate of *v-Abl* and *v-src* kinases. p62^{doc} contains both PH and PTB domains, although the PTB domain is different from that of IRS-1. This protein does not contain at C-terminal the binding sites for PtdIns 3' kinase. All IRSs possess a highly homologous structure and have a redundant role at the cellular level. The association with the IR through the PTB domain is very specific since constructions of IRS-1 with heterologous PTB domain do not translate the insulin signal. The PTB domain in substrate binds to NPEY motif of the juxta-membrane domain of the IR. To date, in IRS-2, another motif KRLB domain binds to the T-loop of the receptor kinase [36].

These structural considerations helped the understanding of the mechanism of signal transduction upon insulin stimulation of a cell. The fundamental mechanism requires the association with several intracellular signaling proteins. The formation of these macromolecular complexes involves proteins such as PtdIns 3' kinase, SHP2, Fyn, Grb-2, nck and Crk, which allow transmission of the signal towards two major pathways: (a) the PtdIns 3' kinase pathway, implicated in glucose transport and (b) the Raf1/MAP kinase pathway, involved in cell proliferation and mitogenesis. Among signaling proteins, the SHPTP$_2$ acts as a protein phosphatase while GRB$_2$, protein homologous of Sem5 in *C. elegans*, acts as an adaptor in the association with mSos in the ras pathway [37–39]. In the same ras pathway of activation, SHC protein (Src and Human Collagen homology) represents an alternative way of insulin stimulation, which is different from IRS [37–41].

Progressive identification of multiple intracellular proteins in insulin action gives a new insight into understanding insulin resistance. It was hypothesized that defects at various levels of insulin transduction may determine the insulin resistant state. Thus, at transductional level, insulin action and inaction are thought as a balance between positive and negative regulators.

Obviously, positive regulators involve insulin itself and the amplification of the signal through IRSs leading ultimately to the stimulation of the glucose transport. Among negative regulators, the best known are: a) the down-regulation of IR in the presence of insulin, b) the dephosphorylation of the IR as turnoff mechanism, c) the phosphorylation on serine residues, mainly by the PKC [41]. Other inhibitory mechanisms invoked molecules such as glycoprotein PC-1, the pp63 and the tumor necrosis factor (TNF)-α [42–45]. This last cytokine, secreted by adipocytes, favors the serine phosphorylation of the IR in balance with that of another adipocyte hormone, the leptin. The relative importance of these regulators in the pathogenesis of diabetes is not known. One major mechanism thought to operate in T2DM is the activation of PKC at high glucose concentrations, through the serine phosphorylation of IR. However, many aspects of pathogenesis of insulin resistance are not limited to the regulation of signal transduction (see below). More recent genetic studies lay emphasis on regulation of gene expression, which may alter the level of intracellular proteins. There are many deleterious mutations or polymorphisms located in regulatory regions (*e.g.*, promoters) which may induce alterations in the gene expression in insulin resistance.

IN VIVO MECHANISMS OF INSULIN RESISTANCE AND HUMAN PATHOLOGY

Insulin resistance is defined as impaired metabolic response to either endogenous or exogenous insulin and involves all cellular actions of insulin, although the hallmark is the chronic hypeinsulinemia. WHO consensus defines insulin resistance as the lowest quartile of insulin sensitivity during the euglycemic clamp [46, 47]. Beside this "gold standard" technique, the insulin resistance can be assessed *in vivo* by other methods such as ITT (insulin tolerance test), Minimal model calculations from IVGTT, or, simply by the HOMA$_{IR}$ index (homeostasis model assessment) [48, 49]. The HOMA$_{IR}$ index is a robust parameter in epidemiological studies, but useless in T2DM with fasting hyperglycemia [49].

It is now recognized that insulin resistance characterizes the normal population. Thus, the WHO consensus estimated a prevalence rate of 25% in the general population, data confirmed by a recent survey of a large population [47]. The phenotype associated with insulin resistance is variable and includes features such as low birth weight, short stature, increased upper to lower body ratio, *Acanthosis Nigricans*, hyper-androgenemia, hirsutism (or PCOS), dyslipidemia and hypertension. All these manifestations characterize complex diseases, such as obesity, PCOS and T2DM [50]. Studies of these diseases at cellular level revealed various additional mechanisms that may explain insulin resistance [51].

In obesity, insulin resistance is pending on the proportion of visceral (central) adiposity. The mechanisms involved are: a) increase of triglyceride (TG) content in insulin target organs, including deleterious effects on β-cell function (lipotoxicity); b) release of free fatty acids (FFA) with the stimulation of protein kinase C-isoforms; c) down regulation of IR in peripheral tissues. There are several other potential mediators of insulin action (*e.g.*, TNF-α, adiponectin, resistin or leptin). Recently, the leptin, which is produced by adipocyte cells, received particular attention in relation with IRS function. Thus, IRS-2 gene appears to interact with leptin action in the hypothalamus at the level of STAT-3 [51–53].

PCOS is another complex condition associated with insulin resistance together with chronic anovulation and hyperandrogenism [54]. There is a compelling evidence for considering insulin resistance in PCOS as a primary defect, which induces hyperandrogenism since, in castrated women (chemically or surgically), high androgen levels are still persistent [55, 56]. Although almost 60% of PCOS patients are obese, the insulin resistance in this syndrome is independent from obesity. Studies in twins also indicated that despite the discordance in appearance of PCO at ultrasonography, twin adolescent females present concordant levels of fasting insulin, indicating again a primary defect in insulin action [57]. The treatment of insulin resistance with troglitazones or metformin ameliorates insulin resistance as well as hyperandrogenemia and ovarian function

in PCOS, consistent with the effects of these drugs on insulin resistance [58].

T2DM is a complex disease associated with profound insulin resistance. Beside insulin resistance, this disorder recognizes in its pathogenesis additional factors, such as increased hepatic glucose production (HGP) and pancreatic β-cell dysfunction [59]. This form of diabetes is also characterized by strong gene-gene and gene-environment interactions [59]. Insulin resistance is closely tied with epidemic of T2DM, again suggesting a primary defect before installation of altered insulin secretion [3]. Cross-sectional studies in early stage of diabetes, first-degree relatives of diabetic patients or offspring of diabetic parents have suggested that the insulin resistance might represent a valuable predictive abnormality in the later development of T2DM [2, 3]. All these suggest that the research on the genetic background of T2DM may conceivably begin with insulin resistance and that the pharmacological agents should primarily focus the insulin resistance. The expert committee of ADA (American Diabetes Association) proposed to introduce insulin resistance in the definition of T2DM, hence the prevalence should be considered at 100%. The survey of 479 diabetics in Bruneck Study estimated the prevalence of insulin resistance at 84% in T2DM [46].

TARGETING INSULIN ACTION WITH ANTI-DIABETIC DRUGS

Metformin (N_1N_1-dimethylbiguanide) is an oral anti-hyperglycemic drug currently used in the T2DM treatment [16–18]. It was used in Europe from 1957 and introduced in the US in 1995. In contrast to a high number of pharmacodynamic and clinical studies, the molecular mechanism of metformin action remains poorly understood. From the clinical point of view, metformin appears effective either as monotherapy or in combination with sulfonylureas or thiazolidindiones (TZD). The major effect is to decrease the blood glucose, thus reducing fasting glucose as well as chronic levels of HbA1c in diabetics. Metformin appears particularly beneficial in obese individuals with T2DM [16, 60]. The weight loss is attributed to reduced appetite and subsequent reduction in caloric intake, but other mechanisms may be involved [61]. This feature enormously complicates *in vivo* experiments since reduced insulin levels and upregulation of the IR in various tissues follow the weight loss. More recently, metformin showed additional cardioprotective actions. Thus, in the UKPDS study, patients treated with metformin had an almost 40% reduced risk of myocardial infarction and, to the same extent, of diabetes-related mortality compared to conventional therapy [62].

Many studies were devoted to the understanding of *in vivo* mechanisms of metformin action. It was recognized that metformin acts at both hepatic and peripheral levels [63–65]. The major effect appears to be the reduction in the HGP through the inhibition of neoglucogenesis (90%) and, to a lesser extent, of glycogenolysis (10%) as elegantly demonstrated by *in vivo* nuclear magnetic resonance spectroscopy [64]. In *in vitro* experiments, the decrease in neoglucogenesis was attributed to the increase in pyruvate influx, inhibition of PEPCK and hepatic lactate uptake as well as to decreased concentrations of adenosine triphosphate [66–68]. No clear molecular mechanisms were provided for these actions, but compelling evidence suggests that mitochondria may be a privileged site of action through the disruption of respiratory chain oxidation of glutamate [69].

More directly related to the insulin-sensitizing action of metformin, many studies suggested the involvement of increased translocation of glucose transporters at the cellular level [70–73]. Our laboratory showed for the first time that metformin in *Xenopus laevis* oocyte has a role in maturation, either in the presence of insulin alone or after microinjection of the pp60[src] kinase [74, 75]. The overall role of metformin in insulin transduction remains however elusive. Many *in vitro* or humans studies indicated an increase in insulin binding, although these data were not confirmed. Contradictory results concerning the effect on the IR tyrosine kinase were also provided. Using adipocytes, HepG2 cells or vascular smooth muscle cells (VSMC) several studies reported minor effects, including increase in the basal activity of the receptor. More consistent results were obtained in adipocytes, hepatocytes and muscle cells from *in vivo* treatment of animals or humans [76–81]. One explanation for these contradictory results is that the insulin transduction events may be studied with difficulty because of the rapid interactions among signaling proteins upon insulin stimulation. As indicated above, in mechanistic terms, insulin transduction involves: a) activation of the IR kinase through phosphorylation; b) subsequent association with substrates (such as IRS-1 and IRS-2); c) phosphorylation of tyrosine residues in these substrates and d) association with signaling proteins as multimolecular complexes; e) activation of PtdIns 3' kinase and f) redistribution of signaling proteins in various sub-cellular compartments. No ideal model to study all these molecular events was described.

SETTING UP
THE RAT EXPERIMENTAL MODEL

Our laboratory has been for a long time involved in the study of cellular mechanisms of metformin action, since this drug specifically treats insulin resistance. We have used progressively several cellular *in vitro* models, such as human erythrocytes, rat adipocytes and *Xenopus laevis* oocytes. The erythrocyte model was used because of the accuracy of insulin binding measurements. In these cells we have shown no modification in insulin binding under the effect of metformin (data not shown). The *X. laevis* oocytes were useful since these cells allow the microinjection of active molecules, although they contain a very few number of insulin receptors. More recently, interesting results regarding the tyrosine phosphorylation of the IR were obtained in the rat model, particularly in solubilized receptors from the liver. The major advantage of the rat model was that metformin can be administered *per os*, in either acute (bolus) or chronic treatment, situation which is similar to therapeutics in humans. The disadvantage was that insulin transduction events might be assessed with difficulty. Thus, the preparation of rat tissues requires a long time for extraction, homogenization and solubilization, rendering experiments unable to detect very early events in insulin action. In collaboration with Lipha-Merck Laboratories (Lyon, France) we ended up with an experimental model using anesthetized rats, *per os* administration of metformin, injection of insulin in the portal vein and rapid extraction of liver tissue for examination of IR cascade of events (Figure 10.3).

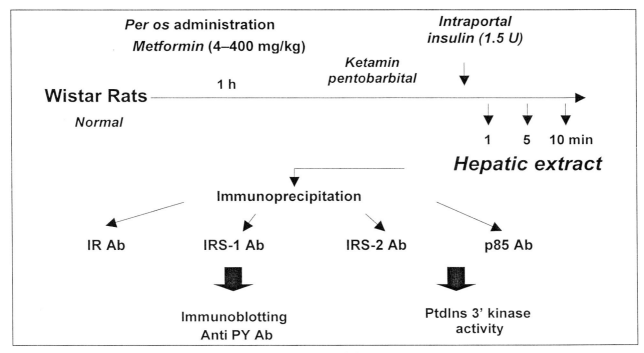

Figure 10.3
Experimental rat model for the study of metformin.

In these experiments, we have used Wistar rats (150–200 g) at *fast* or at *post absorptive* state, treated with metformin 1-h before the experiment at doses of 4, 40 and 400 mg/kg. The rats were anesthetized with ketamin/pentobarbital mixture and the abdomen was open to obtain access to the portal vein. The stimulation with insulin was performed by a bolus injection (1.5 U) of insulin and then pieces of liver were excised at 1, 5 and 10 min and rapidly frozen in liquid nitrogen. The tissue was firstly homogenized in the presence of anti-proteases at 4°C and then solubilized in the extraction buffer containing either 1% Triton or NP-40 as detergent, a phosphotyrosine "stopp solution" and anti-proteases. The extract was usually cleared by centrifugation at 16 000 x g and the supernatant was used for various analyses.

This experimental model allowed the study of various events in insulin transduction. In one set of experiments, the IR was immunoprecipitated with anti-IR antibodies (AB-3 Ab) and protein G (fast flow) by incubation 3 h at 4°C, followed by mild wash.

The proteins were resolved by SDS-PAGE and transferred on nitrocellulose paper for immunoblotting. By this procedure, we were able to measure the degree of phosphorylation and to identify proteins the associated to the IR. The

same IR-immunoprecipitates may be used for the measurement of kinase activity on exogenous substrate, Raytide (experiments not shown). The Western blotting was performed with anti phospho-tyrosine Ab (RC-20) for detection of phosphorylation (membranes were blocked with 3% PVP or 3% BSA). Immunoblotting was also used for identification of PtdIns 3'-kinase with anti-PtdIns 3'-kinase (p85α) (membranes were blocked with 5% milk) while detection of IRS-1 and IRS-2 proteins was performed with specific antibodies. In another set of experiments, the PtdIns 3'-kinase activity was measured after immunoprecipitation of IRS-1 (with C-terminal Ab) or IRS-2, chromatography of phospholipids on thin layer plates (TLC) and autoradiography.

The first interesting observation was that the hepatic IR, solubilized and partially purified by wheat germ agglutinin (WGA), displayed an increase in both autophosphorylation and kinase activity after chronic administration (3 weeks) of metformin. The effect was dose dependent, although, at a low statistical significance. This was explained by the high variability between individual animals during extraction procedure (Figure 10.4). The ED_{50} of the dose-response curve was not changed between groups and the effect was observed mainly at high insulin concentrations, suggesting a modification in the V_{max} rather than K_m. These preliminary experiments in animals treated *in vivo* with metformin prompted us to further investigate the acute effect of this drug in the liver IR, particularly in association of signaling proteins with IR-IRS complexes.

As is shown in Figure 10.5, liver IR was rapidly autophosphorylated after insulin stimulation and then, progressively decreased up to 10 min. A series of experiments have indicated that metformin, at high doses (400 mg/kg), slightly increases the phosphorylation of the IR, but the results remained quite variable.

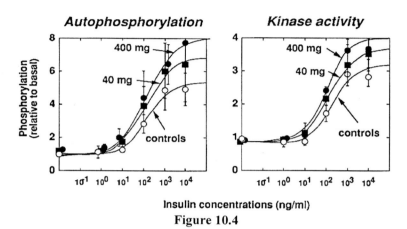

Figure 10.4

Effect of metformin on "*ex in vivo*" enzymatic activity of the liver insulin receptors.

Wistar rats were chronically treated with metformin (*in vivo*), sacrified and then IR were extracted from the liver tissue, solubilized with Triton X-100 and partially purified on Wheat germ agglutinin (WGA) coupled on agarose. IR (about 5 μg protein) was stimulated with insulin and the phosphorylation was determined after incubation with ^{32}P-ATP (50 μM, 0.2 μCi/ml). Proteins were submitted to SDS-PAGE and autoradiography at −80°C on X-O-MAT AR films. Autoradiograms were scanned on, with a Dual-Wavelength scanner. The kinase activity was measured on random peptide poly (Glu,Tyr) (4:1) at 2 mg/ml final concentration.

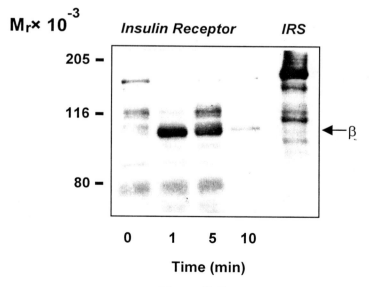

Figure 10.5

Kinetics of the rat liver insulin receptor phosphorylation.

IR was extracted from the liver of Wistar rats, solubilized in the presence of Triton X-100 and "stopp solution" and proteins were resolved on SDS-PAGE, transferred on nitrocellulose and immunoblotted with anti-phosphotyrosine antibodies. Lanes 1–4 indicate the IR kinetics and lane 5 contain purified IRS-1 protein which was phosphorylated *in vitro* in the presence of IR and used as positive control for phosphorylation.

We concluded that metformin has only moderate effect on IR phosphorylation at 1 min, but the drug rather maintained the tyrosine phosphorylation at a higher degree of phosphorylation by 5 and 10 min (data not shown). Thus, the variable effects of metformin as function of rapid kinetics of IR phosphorylation perhaps explain our difficulties in establishing the dose-response curve in this model. During similar experiments, we have also demonstrated that a 10-times more potent analogue of metformin (phenformin) dramatically increased the IR activation. However, this drug is not used in clinical practice any more and, thus, remains of poor interest in understanding the anti-diabetic effect in humans.

The most interesting observation was the effect of metformin on the association of signaling proteins, upon insulin stimulation. A typical experiment is shown in Figure 10.6. After insulin stimulation by injection in the portal vein, both IRS-1 and IRS-2 are associated with immunoprecipitated IR. This association was possible, because the antibodies used did not interfere with the substrate association. Interestingly, metformin was able to potentiate this IR-IRS association. The effect was more pronounced for IRS-2 than IRS-1, strongly suggesting that IRS-2 protein represents a more specific target for metformin than IRS-1.

These data are concordant with similar experiments performed by Gunton *et al.* [80]. In another series of experiments, the immuno-precipitations were performed with Ab against IRS-1, IRS-2 and p85α subunit of the PtdIns 3'- kinase and similar results were obtained (data not shown). Precipitation with anti-IRS-1, -IRS-2 and -PtdIns 3'-kinase antibodies seems to indicate more association and phosphorylation of IRS-1 and IRS-2 after metformin treatment. This was confirmed by the activity of PtdIns 3'-kinase in various immunoprecipitates. Thus, precipitation of PtdIns 3'-kinase indicated a potentialisation by metformin of the enzymatic activity by almost 10-fold (data not shown). Moreover, the activity of PtdIns 3'-kinase was higher under metformin treatment when precipitation was performed with IRS-2 compared to IRS-1 antibodies (Figure 10.7).

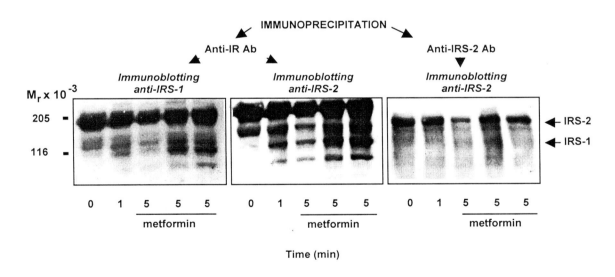

Figure 10.6

Effect of metformin on insulin receptor association with IRS proteins in the rat liver.

Extracts of liver tissue were obtained as indicated in legends of Figures 3 and 5. Immunoprecipitation of IR was performed with anti-IR antibodies and immunoblotting was performed with antibodies against IRS-1 (left panel) or IRS-2 (middle panel). As a control experiment (right panel) in the same extract, IRS-2 was firstly immunoprecipitated with specific antibodies, proteins resolved on SDS-PAGE and transferred on nitrocellulose paper and IRS-2 was revealed with anti-IRS-2 antibodies. In all experiments metformin (40 mg/kg) was studied in the absence of insulin and within 5 min (at 40 and 400 mg/kg) after insulin stimulation. Note that association of IRS in the presence of metformin after 5 min of insulin stimulation was similar to the association at 1 min after insulin stimulation in the absence of the drug.

IMMUNOPRECIPITATION

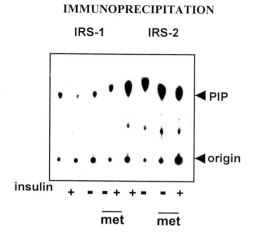

Figure 10.7

Effect of metformin on the activity of PtdIns 3'-kinase
in the rat liver.

Liver extracts obtained after insulin stimulation were immunoprecipitated with antibodies against IRS-1 or IRS-2 and the lipid kinase activity was measured after this layer plates chromatography and autoradiography. Note the higher level of phospholipids obtained by IRS-2 precipitation compared to IRS-1.

The major question was whether these data are explained by the intrinsic quality of antibodies (IRS-1 *versus* IRS-2) or signify indeed that IRS-2 was more operative and sensitive to metformin than IRS-1.

We concluded from these data that metformin may acts at transductional level of insulin by changing kinetics of IR/IRS association. IRS-2 appears as a preferential substrate in the liver, although further experiments are necessary to confirm these initial observations and to explain, in mechanistic terms, the overall anti-diabetic effect of metformin. Obviously, the most interesting aspect revealed in our model was the particular role of IRS-2 in the liver tissue. Indeed, it was recently shown that IRS-2 plays a central role in insulin regulation of hepatic glucose production, since mice with IRS-2 gene disruption present an increased gluconeogenesis with a consequent resistance to insulin in mediating suppression of HGP [82–84]. Similarly, in insulin resistance states which characterize *ob/ob* and lipodystrophic mice, the level of IRS-2 (mRNA) is downregulated in face of the chronic hyper-insulinemia [85]. This downregulation appears not to be limited to the liver tissue. In PCOS, for instance, another disease characterized by insulin resistance, recent studies in the granulosa cells suggested a down regulation of IRS-2 gene expression concomitantly with increased IRS-1 [86]. In these cells, thiazolidindiones as anti-diabetic drugs reverse the IRS-2 down regulation and this was considered as a sign of reversing insulin resistance at the ovarian level in PCOS.

Although all these data suggest in a concordant manner the major role of IRS-2 in insulin resistance and the regulation by insulin of HGP, the mechanisms involved at molecular level and the potential role of metformin remain poorly understood. Insulin acts at the hepatic level by stimulation of the IR kinase, increasing phosphorylation of IRS substrates association with signaling proteins including PtdIns 3' kinase. Through Akt stimulation, insulin is able to inhibit the transcription of several genes involved in neoglucogenesis, such as PEPCK [85].

To date, positive regulators (*e.g.*, glucocorticoids) appear to operate through the SREBP-1c (sterol regulatory element-binding protein 1c). It is expected that an anti-diabetic drug such as metformin, would potentate insulin action in the liver (increased level of mRNA of IRS-2) and thus reduce the HGP and blood glucose. However, an intriguing effect of insulin in the liver is the inhibition of IRS-2 expression itself. This mechanism involves a transcriptional regulation in a similar way as for PEPCK, the presence of an IRE (insulin responsive element) in the promoter. Indeed, it was recently shown that FKHR and FKHRL1 (members of forkhead/wingled-helix family) might interact with expression of IRS-2 through the binding to a hepta-nucleotide in IRS-2 promoter [87–89]. By this mechanism, insulin would down regulate the expression of IRS-2 and this may explain, eventually, the long effect of chronic hyperinsulinemia. Thus, it remains unclear at what level metformin would potentate the action of insulin in the liver. Our data suggest that metformin potentates insulin at the level of insulin signal transduction, but this effect should be produced in such a manner that do not down regulate IRS-2 expression (which would be similar to an insulin resistant state). This complex regulation of transduction (involving first minute of insulin stimulation) concomitantly with transcriptional events (in hours) may explain some contradictory results on metformin action. Establishing *in vivo* models that allow, at the same time, to explore rapid transductional events may be of high value in understanding molecular mechanisms of metformin action.

Specific actions of insulin are now recognized at the arterial wall, where insulin has in general a protective effect. The relationship between insulin resistance and endothelial dysfunction (*e.g.*, vascular tone, platelet aggregation, coagulation process) is complex. Interestingly, metformin was recently recognized as a potential cardioprotective agent in diabetics, although, it remains unclear whether the beneficial effect is explained by improving insulin resistance or by specific action at vascular level [16–18, 90–95]. Development of *in vitro* models to study vascular smooth muscle (VSMC) or endothelial cells represents a good opportunity to investigate the specific role of metformin at the vascular level, which may give a new insight into understanding the complex role of IRS proteins in insulin action and insulin resistance.

REFERENCES

1. DeFronzo RA, Bonadonna RC, Ferrannini E. Pathogenesis of NIDDM. A balanced overview. *Diabetes Care,* **15:** 318–368, 1992.
2. Warram JH, Martin BC, Krolewski AS, Soldner JS, Kahn CR. Slow glucose removal rate and hyperinsulinemia precede the development of type II diabetes in offspring of diabetic parents. *Ann Intern Med,* **113:** 909–915, 1990.
3. Martin BC, Warram JH, Krolewski AS *et al.* Role of glucose and insulin resistance in development of type 2 diabetes mellitus: results of a 25-year follow-up study. *Lancet,* **340:** 925–929, 1992.
4. Kahn CR, Flier JS, Bar RS, Archer JA, Gorden P, Martin NM, Roth J. The syndromes of insulin resistance and *Acanthosis nigricans*: insulin receptor disorders in man. *N Engl J Med,* **294:** 739–745, 1976.
5. Kahn CR, White MF. The insulin receptor and the molecular mechanism of insulin action. *J Clin Invest,* **82:** 1151–1156, 1988.
6. Taylor SI, Kadowaki T, Kadowaki H, Accili D, Cama A, McKeon C. Mutations in insulin receptor gene in insulin-resistant patients. *Diabetes Care,* **13:** 257–279, 1990.
7. Accili D, Cama A, Barbetti F, Kadowaki H, Kadowaki T, Taylor SI. Insulin resistance due to mutations of the insulin receptor gene: an overview. *J Endocrinol Invest,* **15:** 857–864, 1992.

8. Grigorescu F, Flier JS, Kahn CR. Defect in insulin receptor phosphorylation in erythrocytes and fibroblasts associated with severe insulin resistance. *J Biol Chem,* **259:** 15003–15006, 1984.
9. Grigorescu F, White MF, Kahn CR. Insulin binding and insulin-dependent phosphorylation of the insulin receptor solubilized from human erythrocytes. *J Biol Chem,* **258:** 13708–13716, 1983.
10. White MF, Maron R, Kahn CR. Insulin rapidly stimulates tyrosine phosphorylation of a Mr-185,000 protein in intact cells. *Nature* (Lond), **318:** 183–186, 1985.
11. White MF. The IRS-signaling system: a network of docking proteins that mediate insulin action. *Mol Cell Biochem,* **182:** 3–11, 1998.
12. Araki E, Lipes MA, Patti ME, Bruning JC, Haag B 3rd, Johnson RS, Kahn CR. Alternative pathway of insulin signaling in mice with targeted disruption of the IRS-1 gene. *Nature,* **372:** 186–190, 1994.
13. Brüning JC, Winnay J, Bonner-Weir S, Taylor SI, Accili D, Kahn CR. Development of a novel polygenic model of NIDDM in mice heterozygous for IR and IRS-1 null alleles. *Cell,* **88:** 561–572, 1997.
14. Baudler S, Krone W, Bruning JC. Genetic manipulation of the insulin signalling cascade in mice - potential insight into the pathomechanism of type 2 diabetes. *Best Pract Res Clin Endocrinol Metab,* **17:** 431–443, 2003.
15. Brüning JC, Michael MD, Winnay JN, Hayashi T, Horsch D, Accili D, Goodyear LJ, Kahn CR. A muscle-specific insulin receptor, knockout exhibits features of the metabolic syndrome of NIDDM without altering glucose tolerance. *Molecular Cell,* **2:** 559–569, 1998.
16. Kirpichnikov D, McFarlane SI, Sowers JR. Metformin: An update. *Ann Intern Med,* **137:** 25–33, 2002.
17. Wiernsperger NF, Bailey CJ. The antihyperglycaemic effect of metformin: therapeutic and cellular mechanisms. *Drugs,* **58** (*Suppl* 1) : 31–39, 1999.
18. Bailey CJ. Biguanides and NIDDM. *Diabetes Care,* **15:** 755–772, 1992.
19. Freychet P, Roth J, Neville DM. Insulin receptors in the liver: specific binding of (125I) insulin to the plasma membrane and its relation to insulin bioactivity. *Proc Natl Acad Sci* USA, **68:** 1833–1837, 1971.
20. Kasuga M, Zick Y, Blithe DL, Crettaz M, Kahn CR. Insulin stimulates tyrosine phosphorylation of the insulin receptor in cell-free system. *Nature,* **298:** 667–669, 1982.
21. Hanks SK, Quinn AM, Hunter T. The protein kinase family: conserved features and deduced

phylogeny of the catalytic domains. *Science* **241:** 42–52, 1988.

22. Wei L, Hubbard SR, Smith RF, Ellis L. Protein kinase superfamily – comparison of sequence data with three-dimensional structure. *Curr Opin Struct Biol,* **4:** 450–455, 1994.

23. Ullrich A, Bell JR, Chen EY, Herrera R, Petruzzelli LM, Dull TJ, Gray A, Coussens L, Liao YC, Tsubokawa M, Mason A, Seeburg PH, Grunfeld C, Rosen OM, Ramachandran J. Human insulin receptor and its relationship to the tyrosine kinase family of oncogene. *Nature,* **313:** 756–761, 1985.

24. Ebina Y, Ellis L, Jarnagin K, Edery M, Graff L, Clauser E, Ou J, Masiarz F, Kan YW, Goldfine ID, Roth R, Rutter W. Human insulin receptor cDNA: the structural basis for hormone activated transmembrane signalling. *Cell,* **40:** 747–758, 1985.

25. Garrett TP, McKern NM, Lou M, Frenkel MJ, Bentley JD, Lovrecz GO, Elleman TC, Cosgrove LJ, Ward CW. Crystal structure of the first three domains of the type-1 insulin-like growth factor receptor. *Nature,* **394:** 395–399, 1998.

26. Hubbard SR, Wei L, Ellis L, Hendrickson WA. Crystal structure of the tyrosine domain of the human insulin receptor. *Nature,* **372:** 746–754, 1994.

27. Levine BA, Clack B, Ellis L. A soluble insulin receptor kinase catalyzes ordered phosphorylation at multiple tyrosines of dodecapeptide substrates. *J Biol Chem,* **266:** 3565–3570, 1991.

28. Keane NE, Levine BA, Quirk P, Calas B, Chavanieu A, Grigorescu F, Ellis L. Substrate specificity of the insulin receptor tyrosine kinase domain. *Biochem Soc Trans,* **21** (Pt3) : 266S, 1993.

29. Zabolotny JM, Kim YB, Peroni OD, Kim JK, Pani MA, Boss O, Klaman LD, Kamatkar S, Shulman GI, Kahn BB, Neel BG. Overexpression of the LAR (*leukocyte antigen-related*) protein-tyrosine phosphatase in muscle causes insulin resistance. *Proc Natl Acad Sci* USA, **98:** 5187–92, 2001.

30. Sun XJ, Rothenberg P, Kahn CR, Backer JM, Araki E, Wilden PA, Cahill DA, Goldstein BJ, White MF. Structure of the insulin receptor substrate IRS-1 defines a unique signal transduction protein. *Nature,* **352:** 73–77, 1991.

31. Sun XJ, Wang LM, Zhang Y, Yenush L, Myers MG, Glasheen E, Lane WS, Pierce JH, White MF. Role of IRS-2 in insulin and cytokine signalling. *Nature,* **377:** 173–177, 1995.

32. Lavan B, Lane WS, Leinhard G. The 60-kDa phosphotyrosine protein in insulin treated adipocytes is a new member of the insulin receptor substrate family. *J Biol Chem,* **272:** 11439–11443, 1997.

33. Lavan BE, Fantin VR, Chang ET, Lane WS, Keller SR, Leinhard GE. A novel 160-kDa phosphotyrosine protein in insulin-treated embryonic kidney cells is a new member of the insulin receptor substrate family. *J Biol Chem,* **272:** 21403–21407, 1997.

34. Bjornholm M, He AR, Attersand A, Lake S, Liu SC, Lienhard GE, Taylor S, Arner P, Zierath JR. Absence of functional insulin receptor substrate-3 (IRS-3) gene in humans. *Diabetologia,* **45:** 1697–702, 2002.

35. Smith Hall J, Pons S, Patti ME, Burks DJ, Yenush L, Sun XJ, Kahn CR. White MF. The 60 kDa insulin receptor substrate functions like an IRS protein (pp60^{IRS3}) in adipose cells. *Biochemistry,* **36:** 8304–10, 1997.

36. Sawka-Verhelle D, Tartare-Deckert S, White MF, Van Obberghen E. Insulin receptor substrate-2 binds to the insulin receptor through its phosphotyrosine-binding domain and through a newly identified domain comprising amino acids 591–786. *J Biol Chem,* **271:** 5980–5983, 1996.

37. Hall A. Ras and GAP – who's controlling whom? *Cell,* **61:** 921–923, 1990.

38. Nishida E, Gotoh Y. The map kinase cascade is essential for diverse signal transduction pathways. *TIBS,* **18:** 128–131, 1993.

39. Bokoch GM, Der CJ. Emerging concepts in Ras superfamily of GTP-binding proteins. *FASEB,* **7:** 750–759, 1993.

40. Skolnik EY, Lee CH, Batzer A, Vicentini LM, Zhou M, Daly R, Myers MJ Jr, Backer JM, Ullrich A, White MF, Schlessinger J. The SH2/SH3 domain-containing protein GRB2 interacts with tyrosine-phosphorylated IRS1 and Shc: implications for insulin control of ras signalling. *EMBO J,* **12:** 1929–1936, 1993.

41. Virkamaki A, Ueki K, Kahn CR. Protein-protein interaction in insulin signaling and molecular mechanism of insulin resistance. *J Clin Invest,* **103:** 931–943, 1999.

42. Maddux BA, Sbraccia P, Kumakura S, Sasson S, Youngren J, Fisher A, Spencer S, Grupe A, Henzel W, Stewart TA, Reaven GM, Goldfine ID. Membrane glycoprotein PC-1 and insulin resistance in non-insulin- dependent diabetes mellitus. *Nature,* **373:** 448–451, 1995.

43. Auberger P, Falquefho L, Contreres JO, Pages G, Le Cam G, Rossi B, Le Cam A. Characterization of a natural inhibitor of the insulin receptor tyrosine kinase: cDNA cloning purification, and anti-mitogenic activity. *Cell,* **58:** 631–640, 1989.

44. Hotamisligil GS, Budavari A, Murray D, Spiegelman BM. Reduced tyrosine kinase activity of the insulin receptor in obesity-diabetes: central role of tumor necrosis factor-alpha. *J Clin Invest,* **94:** 1543–1549, 1994.

45. Barzilai N, Wang J, Massilon D, Vuguin P, Hawkins M, Rossetti L. Leptin selectively decreases visceral adiposity and enhances insulin action. *J Clin Invest,* 12: 3105–3110, 1997.

46. ⁎⁎ World Health Organisation (WHO). Definition, diagnosis and classification of diabetes mellitus and its complications. Report of a WHO Consultation, Part 1: diagnosis and classification of diabetes mellitus. Geneva, Switzerland: WHO, 1999.

47. Akinmokun A, Selby PL, Ramaiya K, Alberti KG. The short insulin tolerance test for determination of insulin sensitivity: a comparison with the euglycemic clamp. *Diabet Med,* 9: 432–437, 1992.

48. Bergman RN, Finegood DT, Ader M. Assessment of insulin sensitivity in vivo. *Endocrine Rev,* 6: 45–86, 1985.

49. Matthews DR, Hosker JP, Rudenski AS, Naylor BA, Treacher DF, Turner RC. Homeostasis model assessment: insulin resistance and b-cell function from fasting plasma glucose and insulin concentration in man. *Diabetologia,* 28: 412–419, 1985.

50. Ovalle F, Azziz R. Insulin resistance, polycystic ovary syndrome, and type 2 diabetes mellitus. *Fertil Steril,* 77: 1095–1105, 2002.

51. Goldstein BJ. Insulin resistance as the core defect in type 2 diabetes mellitus. *Am J Cardiol,* 90 (5A): 3G-10G, 2002.

52. Ferrannini E, Natali A, Bell P, Cavallo-Perin P, Lalic N, Mingrone G. Insulin resistance and hypersecretion in obesity. European Group for the Study of Insulin Resistance (EGIR). *J Clin Invest,* 100: 1166–1173, 1997.

53. Withers DJ. Insulin receptor substrate proteins and neuroendocrine function. *Biochem Soc Trans,* 29 (Pt 4): 525–529, 2001.

54. Azziz R, Ehrmann D, Legro RS, Whitcomb RW, Hanley R, Fereshetian AG, O'Keefe M, Ghazzi MN. Troglitazone improves ovulation and hirsutism in the polycystic ovary syndrome: a multicenter, double blind, placebo-controlled trial. *J Clin Endocrinol Metab,* 86: 1626–1632, 2001.

55. Dunaif A, Segal KR, Futterweit W, Dobrjansky A. Profound peripheral insulin resistance, independent of obesity, in polycystic ovary syndrome. *Diabetes,* 38: 1165–1174, 1989.

56. Geffner ME, Kaplan SA, Bersch N, Golde DW, Landaw EM, Chang RJ. Persistence of insulin resistance in polycystic ovarian disease after inhibition of ovarian steroid secretion. *Fertil Steril,* 45: 327–33, 1986.

57. Jahanfar S, Eden JA, Warren P, Seppala M, Nguyen TV. A twin study of polycystic ovary syndrome. *Fertil Steril,* 63: 478–86, 1995.

58. Giannarelli R, Aragona M, Coppelli A, Del Prato S. Reducing insulin resistance with metformin: the

evidence today. *Diabetes Metab,* 29 (4 Pt 2): 6S28–6S35, 2003.

59. DeFronzo RA. Pathogenesis of type 2 diabetes: metabolic and molecular implications for identifying diabetes genes. *Diabetes Reviews,* 5: 177–269, 1997.

60. Bailey CJ. Insulin resistance and antidiabetic drugs. *Biochem Pharmacol,* 58: 1511–1520, 1999.

61. Yki-Jrvinen H, Nikkila K, Sowers JR. Metformin prevents weight gain by reducing dietary intake during insulin therapy in patients with type 2 diabetes mellitus. *Drugs* 58 (Suppl 1): 53–54, 1999.

62. ⁎⁎ Effect of intensive blood-glucose control with metformin on complications in overweight patients with type 2 diabetes (UKPDS 34). UK Prospective Diabetes Study (UKPDS) Group. *Lancet,* 352: 854–865, 1998.

63. Hundal RS, Krssak M, Dufour S, Laurent D, Lebon V, Chandramouli V, Inzucchi SE, Schumann WC, Petersen KF, Landau BR, Shulman GI. Mechanism by which metformin reduces glucose production in type 2 diabetes. *Diabetes,* 49: 2063–2069, 2000.

64. Inzucchi SE, Maggs DG, Spollett GR, Page SL, Rife FS, Walton V, Shulman GI. Efficacy and metabolic effects of metformin and troglitazone in type II diabetes mellitus. *N Engl J Med,* 338: 867–872, 1998.

65. Hundal RS, Inzucchi SE. Metformin: new understandings, new uses. *Drugs,* 63: 1879–1894, 2003.

66. Radziuk J, Bailey CJ, Wiernsperger NF, Yudkin JS. Metformin and its liver targets in the treatment of type 2 diabetes. *Curr Drug Targets Immune Endocr Metabol Disord,* 2: 151–169, 2003.

67. Radziuk J, Zhang Z, Wiernsperger N, Pye S. Effects of metformin on lactate uptake and gluconeogenesis in the perfused rat liver. *Diabetes,* 46: 1406–1413, 1997.

68. Argaud D, Roth H, Wiernsperger N, Leverve XM. Metformin decreases gluconeogenesis by enhancing the pyruvate kinase flux in isolated rat hepatocytes. *Eur J Biochem,* 213: 1341–1348, 1993.

69. El-Mir MY, Nogueira V, Fontaine E, Averet N, Rigoulet M, Leverve X. Dimethylbiguanide inhibits cell respiration *via* an indirect effect targeted on the respiratory chain complex I. *J Biol Chem,* 275: 223–228, 2000.

70. Hundal HS, Ramlal T, Reyes R, Leiter LA, Klip A. Cellular mechanism of metformin action involves glucose transporter translocation from an intracellular pool to the plasma membrane in L6 muscle cells. *Endocrinology,* 131: 1165–1173, 1992.

71. Kozka IJ, Holman GD. Metformin blocks downregulation of cell surface GLUT4 caused by chronic insulin treatment of rat adipocytes. *Diabetes,* 42: 1159–1165, 1993.

72. Matthaei S, Reibold JP, Hamann A, Benecke H, Haring HU, Greten H, Klein HH. *In vivo* metformin treatment ameliorates insulin resistance: evidence for potentiation of insulin-induced translocation and increased functional activity of glucose transporters in obese (fa/fa) Zucker rat adipocytes. *Endocrinology,* **133**: 304–311, 1993.

73. Matthaei S, Hamann A, Klein HH, Benecke H, Kreymann G, Flier JS, Greten H. Association of Metformin's effect to increase insulin-stimulated glucose transport with potentiation of insulin-induced translocation of glucose transporters from intracellular pool to plasma membrane in rat adipocytes. *Diabetes,* **40**: 850–857, 1991.

74. Grigorescu F, Laurent A, Chavanieu A, Capony JP. Cellular mechanism of metformin action. *Diabete Metab,* **17**: 146–149, 1991.

75. Stith BJ, Goalstone ML, Espinoza R, Mossel C, Roberts D, Wiernsperger N. The antidiabetic drug metformin elevates receptor tyrosine kinase activity and inositol 1,4,5-trisphosphate mass in *Xenopus* oocytes. *Endocrinology,* **137**: 2990–2999, 1996.

76. Klip A, Leiter LA. Cellular mechanism of action of metformin. *Diabetes Care,* **13**: 696–704, 1990.

77. Dominguez LJ, Davidoff AJ, Srinivas PR, Standley PR, Walsh MF, Sowers JR. Effects of metformin on tyrosine kinase activity, glucose transport, and intracellular calcium in rat vascular smooth muscle. *Endocrinology,* **137**: 113–121, 1996.

78. Fulgencio JP, Kohl C, Girard J, Pegorier JP. Effect of metformin on fatty acid and glucose metabolism in freshly isolated hepatocytes and on specific gene expression in cultured hepatocytes. *Biochem Pharmacol,* **62**: 439–46, 2001.

79. Sarabia V, Lam L, Burdett E, Leiter LA, Klip A. Glucose transport in human skeletal muscle cells in culture. Stimulation by insulin and metformin. *J Clin Invest,* **90**: 1386–95, 1992.

80. Gunton JE, Delhanty PJ, Takahashi S, Baxter RC. Metformin rapidly increases insulin receptor activation in human liver and signals preferentially through insulin-receptor substrate-2. *J Clin Endocr Metab,* **88**: 1323–32, 2003.

81. Michael MD, Kulkarni RN, Postic C, Previs SF, Shulman GI, Magnuson MA, Kahn CR. Loss of insulin signaling in hepatocytes leads to severe insulin resistance and progressive hepatic dysfunction. *Mol Cell,* **6**: 87–97, 2000.

82. Withers DJ, Burks DJ, Towery HH, Altamuro SL, Flint CL. White MF. Irs-2 coordinates Igf-1 receptor-mediated beta-cell development and peripheral insulin signalling. *Nature Genet,* **23**: 32–40, 1999.

83. Kido Y, Burks DJ, Withers D, Bruning JC, Kahn CR, White MF, Accili D. Tissue-specific insulin resistance in mice with mutations in the insulin receptor, IRS-1, and IRS-2. *J Clin Invest,* **105**: 199–205, 2000.

84. Withers DJ. Insulin receptor substrate proteins and neuroendocrine function. *Biochem Soc Trans,* **29** (Pt 4): 525–529, 2001.

85. Shimomura I, Matsuda M, Hammer RE, Bashmakov Y, Brown MS, Goldstein JL. Decreased IRS-2 and increased SREBP-1c lead to mixed insulin resistance and sensitivity in livers of lipodystrophic and ob/ob mice. *Mol Cell,* **6**: 77–86, 2000.

86. Wu XK, Zhou SY, Liu JX, Pölanën P, Sallinen K, Mäkinen M, Erkkola R. Selective ovary resistance to insulin signaling in women with polycystic ovary syndrome. *Fertil Steril,* **80**: 954–965, 2003.

87. Zhang J, Ou J, Bashmakov Y, Horton JD, Brown MS, Goldstein JL. Insulin inhibits transcription of IRS-2 gene in rat liver through an insulin response element (IRE) that resembles IREs of other insulin-repressed genes. *Proc Natl Acad Sci* USA, **98**: 3756–3761, 2001.

88. Anai M, Funaki M, Ogihara T, Kanda A, Onishi Y, Sakoda H, Inukai K, Nawano M, Fukushima Y, Yazaki Y, Kikuchi M, Oka Y, Asano T. Enhanced insulin-stimulated activation of phosphatidylinositol 3-kinase in the liver of high-fat-fed rats. *Diabetes,* **48**: 158–69, 1999.

89. Anai M, Ono H, Funaki M, Fukushima Y, Inukai K, Ogihara T, Sakoda H, Onishi Y, Yazaki Y, Kikuchi M, Oka Y, Asano T. Different subcellular distribution and regulation of expression of insulin receptor substrate (IRS)-3 from those of IRS-1 and IRS-2. *J Biol Chem,* **273**: 29686–29692, 1998.

90. Hsueh WA, Law RE. Insulin signaling in the arterial wall. *Am J Cardiol,* **84** (1A): 21J–24J, 1999.

91. Hsueh WA, Quinones MJ. Role of endothelial dysfunction in insulin resistance. *Am J Cardiol,* **92** (4A): 10J–17J, 2003.

92. Yki-Jarvinen H. Insulin resistance and endothelial dysfunction. *Best Pract Res Clin Endocrinol Metab,* **17**: 411–430, 2003.

93. Nolan BP, Senechal P, Waqar S, Myers J, Standley CA, Standley PR. Altered insulin-like growth factor-1 and nitric oxide sensitivities in hypertension contribute to vascular hyperplasia. *Am J Hypertens,* **16** (5 Pt 1): 393–400, 2003.

94. Velloso LA, Folli F, Sun XJ, White MF, Saad MJ, Kahn CR. Cross-talk between the insulin and angiotensin signaling systems. *Proc Natl Acad Sci* USA, **93**: 12490–12595, 1996.

95. Carvalheira JB, Ribeiro EB, Folli F, Velloso LA, Saad MJ. Interaction between leptin and insulin signaling pathways differentially affects JAK-STAT and PI 3-kinase-mediated signaling in rat liver. *Biol Chem,* **384**: 151–159, 2003.

CLINICAL ASPECTS
AND
THERAPEUTICAL APPROACHES

11

RELATIONSHIP BETWEEN DIABETES AND ATHEROSCLEROSIS – THE ROLE OF INFLAMMATION

Eduard APETREI, Ruxandra CIOBANU-JURCUȚ

Cardiovascular disease is the major cause of death in the patients with diabetes mellitus. Atherosclerosis accounts for approximately 80% of all mortality in patients with diabetes, and more than 75% of hospitalizations for complications of diabetes are attributable to cardiovascular disease.

In recent years, it has been firmly established that inflammation not only plays a role in the development of acute coronary syndromes, but also it is a key factor in the initiation, progression and the final pathophysiological steps of atherosclerosis, plaque erosion or fissure, and eventually plaque rupture. Important evidence comes from prospective studies, which have identified several markers of systemic inflammation that are predictors of the clinical outcome of future cardiovascular events, not only in healthy subjects, but mainly in patients with stable and unstable coronary disease (acute coronary syndromes with or without ST elevation).

While impressive evidence has already been accumulated regarding the pivotal pathogenic role of inflammation in atherosclerosis, insulin resistance has also been increasingly recognized as having an important correlation with inflammatory pathways. Defects in insulin action on the main insulin-sensitive tissues (adipose tissue, muscle, and liver) are proposed to lead to a worsening of the chronic, low-grade inflammatory state. Independent of the triggering agent and of the initial events, the relationship is bidirectional; any process linked to chronic inflammation will decrease insulin action, and insulin resistance will lead to worsening of inflammation in a vicious cycle.

Thus, reducing inflammation may have beneficial effects on the development of diabetes and prevention of the accelerated atherogenesis present in diabetic patients. Future investigations are clearly needed to further examine this possibility.

BACKGROUND

Cardiovascular disease is the major cause of death in patients with diabetes mellitus. Atherosclerosis accounts for approximately 80% of all mortality in patients with diabetes, and more than 75% of hospitalizations for complications of diabetes are attributable to cardiovascular disease [1]. Mortality from coronary artery disease is approximately 3 to 10 fold higher in patients with type 1 diabetes mellitus and about 2-fold higher in men and 4-fold higher in women with type 2 diabetes mellitus.

Morbidity from atherosclerosis in patients with diabetes is increased even more than mortality is. Several observations showed that the carotid intima – media thickening is significantly increased in patients with newly diagnosed type 2 diabetes [2]. Coronary artery disease, stroke, and peripheral vascular disease are approximately 2.5 times more prevalent in white and Hispanic men with diabetes than in nondiabetic men [3]. In women, there is a 3.5 to 4.5 fold greater risk for these complications associated with diabetes. Diabetes is also the most common cause of heart disease in young people. At the time of first diagnosis of type 2 diabetes, more than 50% of patients are found to have preexisting coronary heart disease (CHD).

Explained in part by these observations on close associations between type 2 diabetes and CHD, recent efforts focused on the elucidation of shared etiological mechanisms. One of the human clinical models that permitted studies of these hypotheses is the metabolic syndrome (alternatively called the insulin resistance syndrome), which is characterized by the simultaneous occurrence of several cardiovascular risk factors: abdominal obesity, dyslipidemia (elevated triglycerides, small dense LDL particles, low HDL cholesterol), hypertension and insulin resistance, with or without overt hyperglycemia. Although the mechanisms that underlie this clustering are complex and not fully understood, their statistical association is remarkably consistent. Furthermore, the strong correlation between glucose metabolic disorders and the incidence of coronary artery disease has raised the question of the existence of common antecedents for atherosclerosis and type 2 diabetes [4, 5].

INFLAMMATION AND ATHEROSCLEROSIS

PATHOPHYSIOLOGICAL CONSIDERATIONS

In recent years, it has been firmly established that inflammation not only plays a role in the development of acute coronary syndromes, but also it is a key factor in the initiation, progression and the final pathophysiological steps of atherosclerosis, plaque erosion or fissure, and eventually plaque rupture [6]. The observation that atherosclerosis has an important histological inflammatory component first came from animal models. Thus, the administration of an atherogenic diet to animals leads to increased monocyte adhesion to the endothelial cells, especially at the level of vessel regions predisposed to atheroma development (arterial branches and curves) [7]. Also, histological analysis of atherosclerotic coronary arteries taken from patients who died of acute coronary syndromes has shown that unstable or ruptured atherosclerotic plaques are characterized by the presence of foam cells, macrophages, lymphocytes and mast cells. Macrophages and to a lesser extent T lymphocytes were the dominant cell types at the site of plaque rupture or erosion [4]. Specific arterial sites, such as branches, bifurcations and curvatures, cause characteristic alterations in the blood flow, including decreased shear stress and increased turbulence. At these sites, specific molecules formed on the endothelium are responsible for the adherence, migration and accumulation of monocytes and T cells. Hence, one of the first steps in atherogenesis is the adhesion of circulating leukocytes to the endothelium. Normally, leukocytes do not adhere to the intact endothelium, but there is increased adherence associated with endothelial dysfunction. That is why adhesion molecules play a central role in this setting [9]. Many observations showed that, while vascular cell adhesion molecule-1 (VCAM-1) is not a constitutive molecule of the endothelial cell, it can be induced by proatherogenic and proinflammatory stimuli (ex. shear stress forces, oxidized LDL, several cytokines, *e.g.*, tumor necrosis factor-α or interleukin 1). During the atherogenesis and plaque activation processes, several other adhesion molecules play a central role – for example intercellular adhesion molecules (ICAM-1), E- and P-selectins [10, 11]. Whereas endothelial adhesion molecules are probably released into the blood stream, recent clinical studies suggest that circulating levels of these molecules can be used as disease activity markers and, hence, could have a predictive value [12, 13].

The antigens that promote the inflammatory response are incompletely elucidated. Several have been discussed in the literature: oxidized LDL, infections (*e.g.*, *Cytomegalovirus*, *C. pneumoniae*, *H. Pylori*) [14].

The differentiation of macrophages from monocytes takes place under the influence of the monocytes colony stimulation factor (MCSF-1). Several recent studies showed that macrophages, and to a lesser extent vascular smooth muscle derived foam cells, synthesize a variety of enzymes called metalloproteinases which degrade the extracellular matrix (matrix metalloproteinases – MMP). These enzymes degrade the matrix component of the fibrous cap in the atheroma, hence leading to its thinning and increased predisposition to rupture.

Monocytes and macrophages also synthesize tissue factors, which induce a hypercoagulable state when the lipid core of the vulnerable plaque comes in direct contact with the blood flow, leading to thrombus formation [15].

In plaque disruption, the fibrous cap of a plaque tears, is exposing the highly thrombogenic lipid-rich core to blood in the lumen of artery. The mechanical strength of the plaque cap is therefore a vital component of plaque stability, and depends on the thickness, collagen content and the amount of other tissue proteins. A decline in smooth muscle cells density inevitably leads to a decline in collagen synthesis and thinning of the cap,

making it more susceptible to rupture [16]. The exact mechanism that contributes to the loss of smooth muscle cells from the fibrous cap is not entirely understood. It could include an inhibition of their replication or an increase of cell death, *i.e.* apoptosis or necrosis. It was shown that interferon-γ, a cytokine derived from activated T lymphocytes, inhibits the expression of collagen synthesizing genes in the smooth muscle cells, as well as their growth and proliferation [17].

Several pivot genes involved in the inflammatory pathway of the atherogenic process are activated by the nuclear transcription factor κB (NF-κB). NF-κB is necessary in activating the transcription process of proinflammatory cytokines, adhesion molecules, growth factors and metalloproteinases [18]. Multiple observations showed that NF-κB is selectively and intensely activated in leucocytes from patients with unstable angina. Its presence was proven in human vessels intima and media, and its concentration was correlated with the extension of the atherosclerosis process, with low levels in normal arteries wall.

All these facts represent only a part of the histopathological and biochemical evidence that inflammation is a critical pathogenic component of the atherosclerotic process.

INFLAMMATORY MARKERS AND ATHEROSCLEROSIS

Prospective studies have identified several markers of systemic inflammation that are predictors of the clinical outcome of future cardiovascular events, not only in healthy subjects, but mainly in patients with stable and unstable coronary disease (acute coronary syndromes with or without ST elevation) [19]. This represents indirect evidence to the role of the inflammatory pathways in atherosclerosis (Table 11.1).

Beginning with the classical inflammation markers, the number of leukocytes has been known to be associated with coronary heart disease, the first studies being published as early as 1974 [20]. More specifically, in one study, monocyte count was an independent predictor of

Table 11.1

Acute phase reactants with prospective studies in coronary disease (adapted from [19])

Non-protein markers	Protein markers – frequently studied	Protein markers – unfrequently studied
WBC ESR Plasma viscosity	Fibrinogen C-reactive protein Serum amyloid A Albumin Plasminogen PAI-1 von Willebrand factor Cytokines (interleukins, TNF-α) Cellular adhesion molecules (VCAM, ICAM, P and E selectins)	Orosomucoid α1 – antitrypsine Haptoglobin Ceruloplasmin C3, C4 Ig A, G, M, and E Sialic acid CIC Lipoprotein (a) Lp-assoc phospholipase A2
WBC, white blood count; ESR, erythrocyte sedimentation rate; PAI-1, plasminogen activator inhibitor; TNF-α, tumour necrosis factor-α; VCAM, vascular cell adhesion molecule; ICAM, intercellular adhesion molecule; CIC, circulating immune complexes; Lp-assoc, lipoprotein associated		

premature myocardial infarction in middle-aged men [21]. Further investigations into the role of leukocytes in acute coronary syndromes have shown that circulating neutrophils in patients with unstable angina and acute myocardial infarction have a low myeloperoxidase content (enzyme which is promptly released after activation by various agonists). Moreover, the resolution of unstable angina is associated with return to normal of neutrophils myeloperoxidase content to concentrations similar to those of patients with stable angina and controls [22].

Erythrocyte sedimentation rate (ESR) is influenced by the size and number of erythrocytes, but also by the presence of large asymmetrical plasma proteins like fibrinogen, immunoglobulins, lipoproteins and α2-macroglobulin. A recent analysis of 2014 apparently healthy men aged 40 to 60 years and followed for 23 years reported a strong association between ESR and cardiovascular mortality (in particular through coronary heart disease) [23].

In an attempt to improve global cardiovascular risk prediction, considerable interest has been focused on C-reactive protein (CRP), a marker of inflammation that has been shown in multiple prospective epidemiological studies to predict incident myocardial infarction, stroke, peripheral arterial disease and sudden cardiac death (Figure 11.1 from [24]). CRP levels have also been

shown to predict risk of both recurrent ischemia and death among those with stable and unstable angina, those undergoing percutaneous angioplasty and those presenting to emergency rooms with acute coronary syndromes [25].

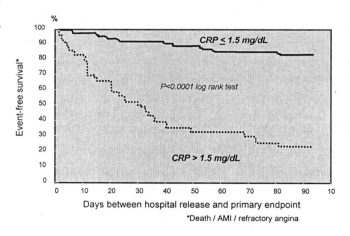

Figure 11.1

Prognostic value of CRP in patients with acute coronary syndromes (adapted from [24]).

During the last decade, CRP was studied as a marker of subtle and persistent systemic alterations, generally known under the name of "low-level inflammation" [26]. Indeed, high sensitive (hs)-CRP assays have recently been used in several prospective studies in initially clinically healthy studies, but also patients with stable and unstable coronary heart disease. For example, an analysis of data from the Physicians' Health Study showed that those in the highest quartile of CRP had a twofold higher risk of future stroke, a threefold risk of future myocardial infarction and a fourfold higher risk of peripheral vascular disease [27]. In most cases, this association has proved independent of age, smoking, cholesterol levels, blood pressure and diabetes, the major "traditional" risk factors evaluated in daily practice. In our experience, plasma levels of CRP in patients with acute coronary syndromes, at the first coronary episode, predict an unfavorable mid-term prognosis, independent of the association with classic cardiovascular risk factors [28]. Despite its lack of specificity, CRP has now emerged as one of the most powerful predictors of cardiovascular risk. Even more remarkable, the predictive power of CRP when measured with a high-sensitivity test (hs-CRP) resides in the range between 1 to 5 μg/mL, which was previously regarded to be normal in the era preceding the hs-CRP test (Figure 11.2). In fact, tests showing serum CRP levels greater than 10 μg/mL, in apparently healthy men or women, should be repeated to exclude occult infection or other systemic inflammatory process [29].

In our studies, both the inflammatory status (quantified by the CRP plasma levels) and the endothelial toxicity (induced by homocystein) are correlated significantly with the cardiovascular risk, as evaluated by the TIMI risk score in patients with unstable angina.

The statistical significance was more important for CRP that is for the implication of inflammation in the pathogeny of the vulnerable "guilty" plaque (Figure 11.3). As demonstrated in our study, plasma levels of CRP above the superior reference limit predict with high accuracy a cardiovascular TIMI risk score above 3, hence a worse prognosis for patients with unstable angina [30].

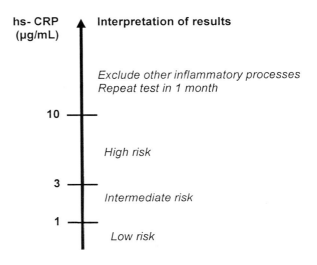

Figure 11.2

Interpretation of the high-sensitivity C-reactive protein test values. Links with the cardiovascular risk (from [29]).

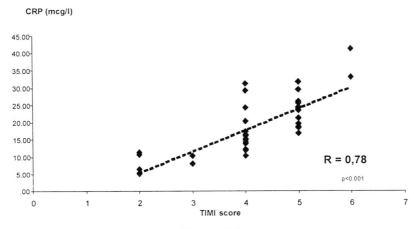

Figure 11.3

Correlation between the CRP plasma levels and the TIMI risk score in patients with unstable angina (adapted from [54]).

Quantitative measurements of a large array of inflammatory and immune markers (orosomucoid, α1-antitrypsin, haptoglobin, fibrinogen, ceruloplasmin, complement factors C3 and C4, and immunoglobulins G, A, M) were carried out and related to cardiac events both in several small separate studies, and in a large prospective study, in which 6384 initially healthy men, mean age 46.8 years at entry, were followed for 16 years [31]. For all these proteins (except C3), from the lowest to the highest quartile, a stepwise increase in cardiac events was observed.

Moreover, serum concentrations of interleukin (IL)-6 proved a useful local and circulating marker of atherosclerotic plaque inflammation. Ubiquitously produced by human cells, including lymphocytes, monocytes, fibroblasts, smooth muscle cells and endothelial cells, IL-6 stimulates the expression of tissue factor, monocyte chemotactic protein-1 (MCP-1), matrix metalloproteinases and LDL receptors on macrophages. It also stimulates platelet aggregation, hepatic CRP and fibrinogen synthesis. The actions of IL-6 are synthesized in Figure 11.4. Several studies showed that circulating IL-6 levels are increased in unstable coronary syndromes, bringing a negative prognostic value both in apparently healthy individuals and in patients with unstable angina [32, 33].

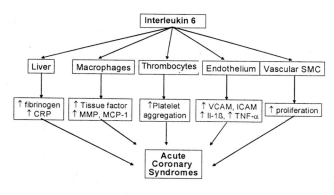

Figure 11.4

Mechanisms of action of interleukin-6.

Tumor necrosis factor-α (TNF-α) is a pleiotropic cytokine produced by several of the cells involved in the atherogenic process, including macrophages, endothelial cells and smooth muscle cells [34]. TNF-α stimulates the endothelial synthesis of E-selectin and also ICAM-1 expression in macrophages and endothelial cells, while it increases the synthesis of IL-6 by fibroblasts. A recent analysis of a cohort of men in the stable phase of myocardial infarction demonstrated that elevated levels of TNF-α are associated with an increased risk of coronary events recurrence [35].

Finally, attention was drawn to the fact that in response to injury the endothelium promotes coagulation and mediates the binding and transendothelial migration of activated leukocytes. These processes are mediated by cell adhesion molecules (ICAM-1, VCAM-1, P-selectin, E-selectin, integrins and cadherins) [36]. Although increased cell surface expression of these molecules is difficult to quantify in vivo, soluble forms have been identified and can be measured in the serum. Hence, increased levels of soluble ICAM-1, VCAM-1, P-selectin were shown in several studies to have a predictive role for future cardiovascular events in both apparently healthy individuals and patients with established coronary heart disease [37, 38, 39].

A special mention should also be made to the results of the recently published PREDICT study, which showed that, in patients with acute coronary syndromes and normal cardiac Troponin I levels, the concurrent determination of D-dimers and several inflammatory markers (CRP, P- and E-selectins, VCAM and ICAM) provide further insight into the risk stratification of these patients [40].

Although a direct, causal relationship between markers of inflammation and subsequent cardiovascular events remains to be proved, various plausible mechanisms do exist for a number of these markers suggesting their involvement in atherogenesis and its complications (for a complete review see Koenig and Rosenson, 2002). However, future studies are required to address these associations, in order to completely explain the mechanisms of the inflammatory response in atherogenesis.

INFLAMMATION, INSULIN RESISTANCE AND DIABETES

Insulin resistance and progressive pancreatic beta cell failure are key factors in the development of type 2 diabetes. Insulin resistance precedes the onset of overt hyperglycemia in approximately

80% of patients. The recently updated NCEP guidelines recognize insulin resistance as an important and modifiable cardiovascular risk factor, and define the clinical components of the syndrome (Table 11.2 from [41]).

Table 11.2

Clinical definition of Insulin Resistance
(adapted from [41])

At least any Three of the Following	
Fasting glucose	> 110 mg/dl
Triglycerides	> 150 mg/dl
HDL Male Female	< 40 mg/dl < 50 mg/dl
Waist circumference Male Female	> 102 cm > 99 cm
Hypertension	> 130/> 85 mm Hg
HDL, high density lipoprotein	

While impressive evidence has already been accumulated regarding the pivotal pathogenic role of inflammation in atherosclerosis (see above), insulin resistance has also been increasingly recognized as having an important correlation with inflammatory pathways [42, 43, 44, 45]. Initially, in the late '80s, active chronic inflammatory disease was found to lead to peripheral insulin resistance [46]. After achieving remission of the inflammatory process, normalization of the glucose handling and insulin sensitivity was observed. The data were interpreted as follows: "The linkage between inflammatory indices and glucose metabolism might reflect a special consequence of inflammation" [47].

Defects in insulin action on the main insulin-sensitive tissues (adipose tissue, muscle and liver) are proposed to lead to a worsening of the chronic, low-grade inflammatory state. Independent of the triggering agent and of the initial events, the relationship is bidirectional; any process linked to chronic inflammation will decrease insulin action, and insulin resistance will lead to worsening of inflammation in a vicious cycle [48].

Several studies also suggested a positive association between components of the insulin resistance syndrome and acute – phase reactants, including CRP and fibrinogen [43, 49].

Thus, inflammatory markers appear to predict the development of type 2 diabetes, as shown in the Atherosclerosis Risk in Communities (ARIC) study [50]. These data showed that higher levels of fibrinogen, white cells count and lower serum albumin predicted later development of type 2 diabetes. A high leukocyte index also predicted evolution to NIDDM in Pima Indians [51].

Moreover, CRP levels appeared to be associated with body mass index and obesity, serum lipids and fasting glucose. Elevated levels of inflammatory markers (including CRP) were also found in type 2 diabetic patients with features of the insulin resistance syndrome, as well as associated with the risk of type 2 diabetes in otherwise healthy middle-aged women [52]. In the study of Festa et al., CRP was independently related to insulin sensitivity, hence proving a place for chronic subclinical inflammation as part of the insulin resistance syndrome. In the Insulin Resistance Atherosclerosis Study (IRAS), among 1008 non-diabetic subjects with no prior history of coronary disease, CRP levels were independently associated with insulin sensitivity as measured by a frequently sampled glucose tolerance test. More recently, several large studies confirmed that CRP and other inflammatory markers predict the development of type 2 diabetes mellitus, metabolic syndrome, and, at the same time, cardiovascular events [53]. Han et al. even suggested that measurement of CRP alone or combined with BMI or waist circumference could be used instead of complicated measures (e.g., fasting insulin, which requires a fasting state) as a risk factor for developing diabetes and the metabolic syndrome.

A study conducted by our group also showed a strong association between CRP levels and the number of components of the metabolic syndrome (Figures 11.5, 11.6) [54]. At the same time, high CRP levels appeared to be linked with a worse prognosis in patients with metabolic syndrome and acute coronary syndromes (unstable angina or acute myocardial infarction). These results suggested not only that CRP reveals the inflammatory pathogenic component in the development of the metabolic syndrome, but it also plays an important role in the development of acute coronary syndromes in patients with metabolic syndrome and coronary

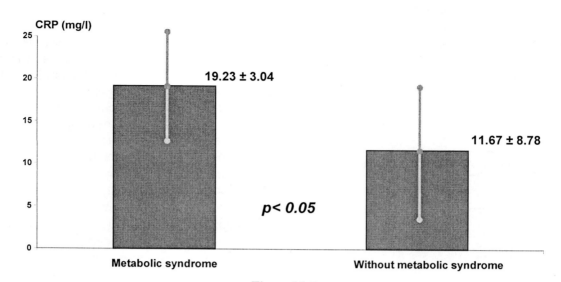

Figure 11.5

Correlations between level of low grade subclinical inflammation (CRP) and the presence of the metabolic syndrome (adapted from [30]).

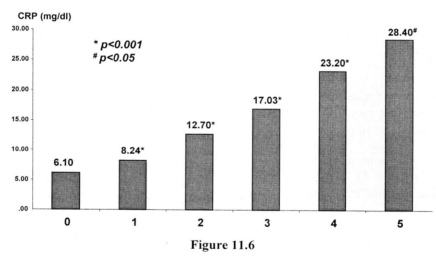

Figure 11.6

Correlations between CRP level and the number of components of the metabolic syndrome (adapted from [30]).

heart disease. This goes along with the histological observations that coronary tissue from diabetic patients has larger areas of lipid-rich plaques and a higher degree of macrophage infiltration (more prone to rupture – "vulnerable" plaques) than non-diabetic coronary tissue [55].

All these data bring the hypothesis that an enhanced acute phase response is associated with insulin resistance and may presage the development of type 2 diabetes.

These rich epidemiological findings are strengthened by experimental studies, which demonstrate the hyperglycemic effects of several proinflammatory cytokines, including IL-6 and TNF-α, both of which derive mainly from the liver and the adipose tissue. Mohamed-Ali *et al.* have estimated that approximately one third of the total circulating IL-6 originates from the subcutaneous adipose tissue in healthy adults [56]. It is not yet well delineated if this reflects the fact that IL-6 is an adipocyte-signaling molecule, which acts in the complex process of diabetogenesis, or if the inflammatory markers are simply co-released in parallel with other truly pathogenic substances.

In rodent models of glucose homeostasis, IL-6 modifies glucose stimulated insulin release from isolated pancreatic beta-cells and diminishes insulin stimulated glycogen synthesis by hepatocytes in culture [57]. In humans, the exogenous administration of IL-6 induces dose-dependent hyperglycemia and concordant elevations in circulating levels of glucagon.

TNF-α may promote insulin resistance by several complex mechanisms, including direct inhibitory effects on glucose transporter GLUT4, on the insulin receptor and its substrates (*e.g.*, serine phosphorylation of the insulin receptor substrate, decreasing the tyrosine kinase activity of the receptor) [58]. Numerous studies addressed the importance of TNF-α receptors polymorphism in the development of diabetes mellitus – increased sTNFR2 levels circulate in association with insulin resistance in healthy volunteers and in nondiabetic offsprings of type 2 diabetic subjects.

Nuclear factor kappa-beta, the key transcription factor responsible for the expression of numerous proinflammatory cytokines, as mentioned above, was shown to be chronically activated in the peripheral monocytes of patients with type 2 DM, which is known to be different from circulating monocytes among nondiabetic patients [59].

Moreover, Simionescu *et al.* published very interesting experimental data showing that high glucose promotes adhesion of monocytes to endothelial cells, which expressed in this setting significantly more ICAM-1 and E/P–selectins [60]; these adhesion molecules thus preparing the endothelial cells for increased monocytes adhesion as a known step in the development of atherosclerosis. A study conducted by Schmidt *et al.* also found that the interaction between advanced glycation end-products (the modified proteins occurring in diabetes) and their endothelial receptors induces the expression of VCAM-1 on cultured endothelial cells of human and mice [61].

Dyslipidemia is an important component of both the insulin resistance syndrome and the biological profile of diabetic patients. Patients with type 2 DM have a characteristic lipoprotein profile. These patients have a tendency for hypertriglyceridemia, low levels of HDL cholesterol and modestly elevated LDL cholesterol, with a disproportionate elevated level of small-oxidized LDL particles. As mentioned above, oxidized LDL functions as a chemotactic factor for leukocytes at the level of the atherosclerotic plaque, as well as a stimulator for the proliferation of macrophages. Hence, high level of circulating LDL (especially the small dense fraction, which is the most prone to oxidation) appears to be associated to an increased inflammatory response by recruiting leukocytes to atherosclerotic lesions and inducing the proliferation of macrophages at the site of the plaque, thus starting the inflammatory response cascade, responsible not only for its development, but also for plaque fissuring and rupture.

More recent study results also suggest that inflammatory markers might predict not only the development of diabetes mellitus or metabolic syndrome, but also diabetic-associated complications. The time-related development of microalbuminuria was significantly and independently determined by increased baseline CRP and fibrinogen in type 2 diabetics and nondiabetic individuals (for example in the IRAS study population). Also, in earlier studies conducted by McMillan, elevated plasma levels of CRP, α-1 glycoprotein, haptoglobin, and plasma viscosity significantly correlated with development of microangiopathy in type 2 diabetic subjects [62]. Interestingly, TNFα polymorphisms also seem to modulate the risk of diabetic retinopathy [63].

DIABETES AND ATHEROSCLEROSIS – IS INFLAMMATION THE STRONGEST LINK?

Risk factors for atherosclerosis, insulin resistance and the development of type 2 diabetes closely overlap, and the three disorders may share a mutual inflammatory and genetic basis. Given that abnormalities in the immune system function and inflammatory pathways have been demonstrated to influence several of the classical cardiovascular risk factors (such as hypertension, dyslipidemia, obesity, insulin resistance, endothelial dysfunction and prothrombotic activation – for a thorough review also see Fernandez-Real and Ricart, 2003), it could be that cardiovascular disease, and mainly atherosclerosis, is the common endpoint of both metabolic and inflammatory pathways.

From a pragmatic point of view, this pathogenic theory would serve to find new therapeutic targets in the prevention and treatment of type 2 diabetes mellitus. It is already known that both statins and ACE inhibitors have anti-inflammatory properties, and preliminary findings have suggested that they may lower the risk of diabetes [64, 65]. In addition, insulin-sensitizing agents, such as thiazolidinediones and physical exercise also appear to have anti-inflammatory properties [66, 67]. More recent animal data suggest that salicylates prevent obesity and diet-induced insulin resistance [68].

A discussion on inflammation, diabetes and atherosclerosis would not be complete without shortly discussing the very interesting issue of the nuclear receptors named "peroxisome proliferator-activated receptors" (PPARs) and of their modern developed ligands – the thiazolidinediones (TZD) (also known as glitazones). There are currently two available agents: rosiglitazone and pioglitazone. The use of these pharmacological agents brought deeper insight in the mechanisms of endothelial dysfunction and inflammation in diabetic patients. Thus, the PPAR family consists of three distinct receptors: PPAR-α, PPAR-β and PPAR-γ. The TZDs' binding affinity for PPAR-γ appears to correlate with their glucose-lowering ability. At the same time, the expression of PPAR-γ is well established in human endothelial cells, vascular smooth muscle cells, monocytes, macrophages and macrophage-derived foam cells in the atherosclerotic plaque [69]. PPAR-γ modifies transcriptional factors such as NF-κB, and inhibits the activation of several cytokines (IL-6, TNFα), which, as shown above, are responsible for the plaque progression and rupture [65]. In addition, PPAR-γ inhibits the expression of MCP-1 and reduces the expression of matrix metalloproteinases by activated plaque macrophages [70, 71]. These findings suggest that TZD could inhibit the inflammatory component of atherosclerosis, thus contributing to plaque stability.

Thus, reducing inflammation may have beneficial effects on the development of diabetes and other metabolic disorders, as well as on the prevention of the accelerated atherogenesis present in diabetic patients. Future investigations are clearly needed to further examine this possibility and, maybe, to bring spectacular advances in the therapeutic field of diabetes prevention and treatment.

REFERENCES

1. Garber AJ. Vascular disease and lipids in diabetes. *Med Clin North Am*, **82(4)**: 931–948, 1998.

2. Temelkova-Kurktschiev TS, Koehler C, Leonhardt W, *et al*. Increased intimal-media thickness in newly detected type 2 diabetes: risk factors. *Diabetes Care*, **22**: 333–338, 1999.

3. Kannel WB. Lipids, diabetes, and coronary heart disease: insights from the Framingham Study. *Am Heart J*, **110**: 1100–1107, 1985.

4. Stern MP. Diabetes and cardiovascular disease. The "common soil" hypothesis. *Diabetes*, **44**: 369–374, 1995.

5. Pradhan AD, Ridker PM. Do atherosclerosis and type 2 diabetes share a common inflammatory basis?. *Eur Heart J*, **23**: 831–834, 2002.

6. Ross R. Atherosclerosis – an inflammatory disease. *N Engl J Med*, **340**: 115–126, 1999.

7. Keaney JF, Vita JA. The value of inflammation for predicting unstable angina. *N Engl J Med*, **347**: 55–57, 2002.

8. Kohchi K, Takebayashi S, Hiroki T, *et al*. Significance of adventitial inflammation of the coronary artery in patients with unstable angina: results at autopsy. *Circulation*, **71**: 709–716, 1985.

9. Poston RN, Johnson-Tidey RR. Localized adhesion of monocytes to human atherosclerotic plaques demonstrated *in vitro*: implications for atherogenesis. *Am J Pathol*, **149**: 73–80, 1996.

10. Johnson-Tidey RR, McGregor JL, Taylor PR, *et al*. Increase in the adhesion molecule P-selectin in the endothelium overlying atherosclerotic plaques. Coexpression with intracellular adhesion molecule-1. *Am J Pathol*, **144**: 952–961, 1994.

11. Poston RN, Haskard DO, Coucher JR, *et al*. Expression of intercellular adhesion molecule-1 in atherosclerotic plaques. *Am J Pathol*, **140**: 665–673, 1992.

12. Ridker PM. Inflammation, infection and cardiovascular risk management : how good is the clinical evidence? *Circulation*, **97**: 1671–1674, 1998.

13. Mulvihill NT, Foley JB, Crean P, Walsh M. Prediction of cardiovascular risk using soluble cell adhesion molecules. *Eur Heart J*, **23(20)**: 1569–1574, 2002.

14. Hansson GK. Immune responses in atherosclerosis. In: Hanssen GK, Libby P (eds): *Immune functions of the vessel wall*, Harwood Academic, Amsterdam, 1996.

15. Libby P. Changing concepts of atherogenesis. *J Intern Med*, **247**: 349–358, 2000.

16. Ravn HB, Falk E. Histopathology of plaque rupture. *Cardiol Clin*, **17(2)**: 263–270, 1999.

17. Libby P. Molecular bases of the acute coronary syndromes. *Circulation*, **91**: 2844–2850, 1995.

18. Barnes PJ, Karin M. Nuclear factor- κB: a pivotal transcription factor in chronic inflammatory disease. *N Engl J Med*, **336**: 1066–1071, 1997.

19. Koenig W, Rosenson RS. Acute phase reactants and coronary heart disease. *Sem Vasc Med*, **2(4)**: 417–428, 2002.

20. Friedman GD, Klatsky AL, Siegelaub AB. The leukocyte count as a predictor of myocardial infarction. *N Engl J Med*, **290**: 1275–1278, 1974.

21. Olivares R, Ducimetiere P, Claude JR. Monocyte count: a risk factor for coronary heart disease? *Am J Epidemiol*, **137**: 49–53, 1993.

22. Biasucci LM, D'Onofrio G, Liuzzo G, *et al*. Intercellular neutrophil myeloperoxidase is reduced in unstable angina and acute myocardial infarction, but its reduction is not related to ischemia. *J Am Coll Cardiol*, **27**: 611–616, 1996.

23. Erikssen G, Liestol K, Bjornholt JV, *et al*. Erythrocyte sedimentation rate: a possible marker of atherosclerosis and a strong predictor of coronary heart disease mortality. *Eur Heart J*, **21**: 1614–1620, 2000.

24. Ferreirós ER, Boissonnet CP, Pizarro R, *et al*. Independent prognostic value of elevated C-Reactive Protein in unstable angina. *Circulation*, **100**: 1958–1963, 1999.

25. Ridker PM. Clinical application of C-reactive protein for cardiovascular disease detection and prevention. *Circulation*, **107**: 363–369, 2003.

26. Danesh J, Collins R, Appleby P, Peto R. Association of fibrinogen, C-reactive protein, albumin, or leukocyte count with coronary heart disease: meta-analysis of prospective studies. *JAMA*, **279**: 1477–1482, 1998.

27. Ridker PM, Cushman M, Stampfer M, Tracy RP, Hennekens C. Inflammation, aspirin, and the risk of cardiovascular disease in apparently healthy men. *N Engl J Med*, **336**: 973–979, 1997.

28. Gavrila A, Ciobanu-Jurcut RO, Rugina M, *et al*. Plasmatic levels of homocysteine and C-reactive protein: which one correlates better with TIMI score in unstable angina patients? *Arch Mal Coeur Vaiss*, **96** (suppl.II): 62, 2003.

29. Yeh ETH, Willerson JT. Coming of age of C-reactive protein. Using inflammation markers in cardiology. *Circulation*, **107**: 370–371, 2003.

30. Apetrei E, Ciobanu-Jurcut RO, Gavrila A, *et al*. Linking the proinflammatory status to the dysmetabolic syndrome in patients with acute coronary syndromes. *Arch Mal Coeur Vaiss*, **96** (suppl II): 111, 2003.

31. Lindgarde F, Lind P, Heldblad B, *et al*. Incidence of myocardial infarction and death in relation to plasma levels of inflammatory sensitive proteins. A long term cohorte study. *Circulation*, **98**: 357–364, 1998.

32. Ridker PM, Rifai N, Stampfer MJ, Hennekens CH. Plasma concentration of interleukin-6 and the risk of future myocardial infarction among apparently healthy men. *Circulation*, **101**: 1767–1772, 2000.

33. Biasucci LM, Vitelli A, Liuzzo G, *et al*. Elevated levels of interleukin-6 in unstable angina. *Circulation*, **94**: 874–877, 1996.

34. Blake GJ, Ridker PM. Tumour necrosis factor - α, inflammatory biomarkers and atherogenesis. *Eur Heart J*, **23**: 345–347, 2002.

35. Ridker PM, Rifai N, Pfeffer M, *et al*. Elevation of TNF-α and increased risk of recurrent coronary events after myocardial infarction. *Circulation*, **101**: 2149–2153, 2000.

36. Mulvihill NT, Foley JB, Crean P, Walsh M. Prediction of cardiovascular risk using soluble cell adhesion molecules. *Eur Heart J*, **23**: 1569–1574, 2002.

37. Ridker PM, Hennekens CH, Roitman-Johnson B, Stampfer MJ, Allen J. Plasma concentration of soluble intercellular adhesion molecule-1 and risk of future myocardial infarction in apparently healthy men. *Lancet*, **351**: 88–92, 1998.

38. Ridker PM, Buring JE, Rifai N. Soluble P-selectin and the risk of future cardiovascular events. *Circulation*, **103**: 491–495, 2001.

39. Malik I, Danesh J, Whincup P, *et al*. Soluble adhesion molecules and prediction of coronary heart disease: a prospective study and meta-analysis. *Lancet*, **358**: 971–975, 2001.

40. Menown IBA, Mathew TP, Gracey HM, *et al*. Prediction of Recurrent Events by D-dimer and Inflammatory Markers in Patients with Normal Cardiac Troponin I (PREDICT) study. *Am Heart J*, **145**(6): 986–992, 2003.

41. Executive Summary of the Third Report of the National Cholesterol Education Program (NCEP) Expert Panel on Detection, Evaluation, and Treatment of High Blood Cholesterol in Adults (Adult Treatment Panel **III**). *JAMA*, **285**: 2486–2497, 2001.

42. Pickup JC, Mattock MB, Chusney GD, Burt D. NIDDM as a disease of the innate immune system: association of the acute-phase reactants and interleukin 6 with metabolic syndrome X. *Diabetologia*, **40**: 1286–1292, 1997.

43. Pickup JC, Crook MA. Is type II diabetes a disease of the innate immune system? *Diabetologia*, **41**: 1241–1248, 1998.

44. Fernandez-Real JM, Ricart W. Insulin resistance and inflammation in an evolutionary perspective: the contribution of cytokine genotype/phenotype to thriftiness. *Diabetologia*, **42**: 1367–1374, 1999.

45. Festa A, D'Agostino RJr, Howard G, Mykkanen L, Tracy RP, Haffner SM. Chronic subclinical inflammation as part of the insulin resistance syndrome: the Insulin Resistance Atherosclerosis Study (IRAS). *Circulation*, **102**: 42–47, 2000.

46. Svenson KL, Pollare T, Lithell H, Hallgren R. Impaired glucose handling in active rheumatoid arthritis: relationship to peripheral insulin resistance. *Metabolism*, **37**: 125–130, 1988.

47. Svenson KL, Lundqvist G, Wide L, Hallgren R. Impaired glucose handling in active rheumatoid arthritis: relationship to the secretion of insulin and counter-regulatory hormones. *Metabolism,* **36:** 940–943, 1987.

48. Fernandez-Real JM, Ricart W. Insulin resistance and chronic Cardiovascular Inflammatory Syndrome. *Endocrine Reviews* **24**(3): 278–301, 2003.

49. Yudkin JS, Stehouwer CDA, Emeis JJ, Coppack SW. C-reactive protein in healthy subjects: associations with obesity, insulin resistance, and endothelial dysfunction. A potential role for cytokines originating from adipose tissue? *Arterioscler Thromb Vasc Biol*, **19:** 972–978, 1999.

50. Schmidt MI, Duncan BB, Sharrett AR *et al.* Markers of inflammation and prediction of diabetes mellitus in adults (Atherosclerosis Risk in Community Stuy): a cohort study. *Lancet,* **353:** 1649–1652, 1999.

51. Vozarova B, Weyer C, Lindsay RS, Pratley RE, Bogardus C, Tataranni PA. High white blood cell count is associated with worsening of insulin sensitivity and predicts the development of type 2 diabetes. *Diabetes,* **51:** 455–461, 2002.

52. Pradhan AD, Manson JE, Rifai N, Buring JE, Ridker PM. C-reactive protein, interleukin 6, and risk of developing type 2 diabetes mellitus. *JAMA,* **286:** 327–334, 2001.

53. Han TS, Sattar N, Williams K, Gonzalez-Villapando C, Lean ME, Haffner SM. Prospective study of C-reactive protein in relation to the development of diabetes and metabolic syndrome in the Mexico City Diabetes Study. *Diabetes Care,* **25:** 2016–2021, 2002 .

54. Jurcut RO, Gavrila A, Rugina M, *et al.* Inflammation and endothelial dysfunction – correlations with TIMI risk score in unstable angina patients. *Eur Heart J,* **24**(20) : 160, 2003.

55. Moreno PR, Murcia AM, Palacios IF, *et al.* Coronary composition and macropahge infiltration in atherectomy specimens from patients with diabetes mellitus. *Circulation,* **102:** 2180–2184, 2000.

56. Mohamed-Ali V, Goodrick S, Rawesh A, *et al.* Subcutaneous adipose tissue releases interleukin – 6, but not tumor necrosis factor-alpha, *in vivo. J Clin Endocrinol Metab,* **82:** 4196–4200, 1997.

57. Sandler S, Bendtzen K, Euzirik DL, Welsh M. Interleukin-6 affects insulin secretion and glucose metabolism of rat pancreatic islets *in vivo. Endocrinology,* **126:** 1288–1294, 1990.

58. Hotamisligil GS, Spiegelman BM. Tumor necrosis factor-alpha: a key component of the obesity-diabetes link. *Diabetes,* **43:** 1271–1278, 1994.

59. Bierhaus A, Schiekofer S, Schwaninger M *et al.* Diabetes-associated sustained activation of the transcription factor nuclear factor-kappa β. *Diabetes,* **50:** 2792–2808, 2001.

60. Simionescu M, Sima A, Popov D. The vascular endothelium in diabetes-induced accelerated atherosclerosis, In: Born GVR, Schwartz CJ (eds.). *Vascular Endothelium. Physiology, Pathology and Therapeutic Opportunities,* Schattauer, Stuttgart,1997, 329–344.

61. Schmidt AM, Hasu M, Popov D, *et al.* Receptor for advanced glycation end-products (AGEs) has a central role in vessel wall interactions and gene activation in response to circulating AGE proteins. *Proc Natl Acad Sci USA,* **91:** 8807–8812, 1994.

62. McMillan DE. Increased levels of acute-phase proteins in diabetes. *Metabolism,* **38:** 1042–1046, 1989.

63. Hawrami K, Hitman GA, Rema M, *et al.* An association in non-insulin-dependent diabetes mellitus subjects between susceptibility to retinopathy and tumor necrosis factor polymorphism. *Hum Immunol,* **46:** 49 –54, 1996.

64. Palinski W. New evidence for beneficial effects of statins unrelated to lipid lowering. *Arterioscler Thromb Vasc Biol,* **21:** 3–5, 2001.

65. Gullestad L, Aukrust P, Ueland T, *et al.* Effect of high- versus low-dose angiotensin converting enzyme inhibition on cytokine levels in chronic heart failure. *J Am Coll Cardiol,* **34:** 2061–2067, 1999.

66. Jiang C, Ting AT, Seed B. PPAR-gamma agonists inhibit production of monocyte inflammatory cytokines. *Nature,* **391:** 82–86, 1998.

67. Smith JK, Dykes R, Douglas JE, Krishnaswamy G, Berk S. Long-term exercise and atherogenic activity of blood mononuclear cells in persons at risk of developing ischemic heart disease. *JAMA,* **281:** 1722–1727, 1999.

68. Yuan M, Konstantopoulos N, Lee J, *et al.* Reversal of obesity- and diet-induced insulin resistance with salicylates or targeted disruption of Ikkbeta. *Science,* **293:** 1673–1677, 2001.

69. Khamaisi M, Symmer L, Raz I. Thiazolidinediones in cardiovascular risk in type 2 diabetes mellitus. In: Hancu N. (ed). *Cardiovascular risk in type 2 diabetes mellitus,* Springer-Verlag, Berlin, 2003, 193–203.

70. Ricote M, Li AC, Willson TM, Kelly CJ, Glass CK. The PPAR-γ is a negative regulator of macrophage activation. *Nature,* **391:** 79–82, 1998.

71. Marx N, Sukhova G, Murphy C, Libby P, Plutzky J. Macrophages in human atheroma contain differentiation dependent peroxisomal proliferator-activated receptor gamma expression and reduction of MMP-9 activity through PPAR-γ activation in mononuclear phagocytes *in vitro. Am J Pathol,* **153:** 17–23, 1998.

12

INSULIN RESISTANCE
AND ENDOTHELIAL DYSFUNCTION

Amorin-Remus POPA, Katalin BABEŞ, Petru Aurel BABEŞ

Relevant to the syndrome of insulin resistance, this chapter will discuss the evidence and functional implications of the endothelium as a target tissue for insulin action. The vascular endothelium responds to insulin by increasing the release of nitric oxide and this action is impaired when insulin resistance develops.

Insulin has a dose-dependent effect of dilating the skeletal muscle vasculature. Resistance to insulin's action to stimulate glucose metabolism, which characterizes clinical states of obesity, type 2 diabetes, and hypertension is associated with impaired insulin-mediated vasodilation. The data suggest that insulin vasodilates skeletal muscle vasculature *via* the net release of endothelium-derived NO. Insulin-mediated vasodilation appears to augment insulin's action to stimulate skeletal muscle glucose uptake. Insulin-mediated vasodilation is NO dependent and insulin-mediated vasodilation is impaired in states of insulin resistance. Insulin resistance is associated with day-long elevations in FFA and these chronic elevations can be the cause of endothelial dysfunction in states of insulin resistance. These are evidences of a mechanism linking insulin resistance disease such as diabetes and obesity, with defects in vasodilator actions of insulin and endothelial dysfunction that may predispose to macrovascular disease and hypertension. The importance of eNOS to the regulation of vascular tone and hemodynamics has been unequivocally demonstrated. Endothelial dysfunction may represent an early and central pathogenic event leading to macrovascular disease in patients with insulin resistance.

INTRODUCTION

The endothelium is a diaphanous cellular monolayer lining the lumen of the vasculature throughout the body and weighing approximately 1.8 kg in a 70 kg man. This large organ has long been recognized for its barrier and transport functions and is thought to be in most of the cases passive for these values. In the past decade, the endothelium has been shown to have many other diverse biological functions. These include the active control of the vascular tone [1–3], regulation of blood fluidity [4], modulation of monocyte adhesion [5, 6], and lipid peroxidation [7–10], to name but a few. More recently, the endothelium is also being recognized as an endocrine and humoral-responsive organ. The endothelium produces a variety of hormones acting in a paracrine fashion to regulate vascular tone as

well as growth and remodeling of the vascular wall [11–14]. In addition, the endothelium possesses receptors for humoral ligands. These receptors, whose predominant role was thought to be transendothelial transfer of hormones, are now known to have downstream signal transduction mechanisms resident in the endothelium.

Relevant to the syndrome of insulin resistance, this chapter will discuss the evidence and functional implications of the endothelium as a target tissue for insulin action. The vascular endothelium responds to insulin by increasing the release of nitric oxide and this action is impaired when insulin resistance develops. The pathophysiological implications of these observations to the increased risk of macrovascular disease associated with insulin resistance will be discussed (Figure 12.1).

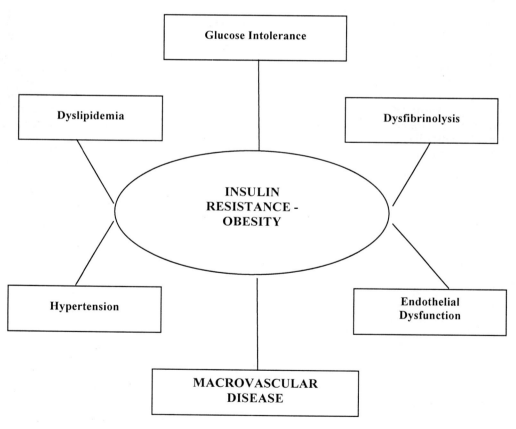

Figure 12.1

Conceptual representation of the syndrome of insulin resistance.

Insulin resistance is associated with a clustering of cardiovascular risk factors. These risk factors are: increased blood pressure, dyslipidemia, glucose intolerance, dysfibrinolysis, and endothelial dysfunction.

IN VIVO PERSPECTIVE

DOSE-DEPENDENT EFFECTS OF INSULIN ON VASODILATATION IN SKELETAL MUSCLE VASCULATURE

Insulin has a dose-dependent effect of enlarging the skeletal muscle vasculature [15]. This vasodilation occurs at physiological insulin concentrations with an EC50 (concentration to reach half-maximal effect) of 44 µU/ml and with a t1/2 (time to reach half-maximal vasodilation) of approximately 35 min [16]. A physiologic concentration of insulin causes an approximately twofold increase in leg blood flow above baseline in lean insulin-sensitive individuals (measured by thermodilution). Because these studies were performed during euglycemic clamp conditions, it follows that this insulin effect is independent of changes in glycemia. The magnitude of the vasodilation appears to be related not only to the insulin concentration but also to the rate of insulin-stimulated glucose metabolism.

Resistance to insulin's action to stimulate glucose metabolism, which characterizes clinical states of obesity, type 2 diabetes, and hypertension is associated with impaired insulin-mediated vasodilation [1, 16]. The dose-response curves for insulin-mediated glucose uptake in subjects of varying degrees of insulin resistance are largely parallelled by the dose response curves for insulin's action to vasodilate. The most insulin-resistant subjects display the greatest impairment in insulin-mediated vasodilation. Insulin administration is also accompanied by important increase in cardiac output and a modest fall in mean arterial blood pressure, consistent with the effect of insulin to reduce systemic vascular resistance. The fall in systemic vascular resistance (~40%) suggests a differential and specific effect of insulin to vasodilate skeletal muscle vasculature [17].

In summary, insulin action, to vasodilate skeletal muscle vasculature, differs in its function of stimulating glucose metabolism and occurs predominantly at the level of resistance vessels. It appears that insulin-mediated vasodilation and the insulin-sensitivity towards its action to stimulate glucose metabolism are tightly coupled in some yet to be determined fashion.

NITRIC OXIDE AND INSULIN-MEDIATED VASODILATION

Nitric oxide (NO) is a gas that is continuously released from the endothelium where it is synthesized from its precursor, L-arginine, in a reaction catalyzed by nitric oxide synthase (eNOS isoform in endothelium). NO released from the endothelium diffuses via the subendothelial space to the smooth muscle where it binds to the heme group of guanylate cyclase and stimulates the generation of cyclic GMP which then transduces its effects to cause smooth muscle relaxation resulting in vasodilation. In vivo, one can probe: 1) endothelium-dependent vasodilation by the use of agents which cause the release of NO from the endothelium such as the muscarinic agonist methacholine chloride; 2) endothelium-independent vasodilation by the use of NO donor compounds such as sodium nitroprusside and, 3) NO-dependent vascular tone with the use of an inhibitor of NO synthase such as the arginine analog N G-monomethyl-L-arginine (L-NMMA). Vascular responses at infusing these agents directly into femoral artery can be assessed by measuring changes in limb blood flow. These methods allow one to assess endothelial-dependent and -independent vasodilation as well as NO-dependent vascular tone in humans.

To determine whether insulin-mediated vasodilation is dependent on the release of endothelium-derived NO, intrafemoral artery infusions of the NO synthase inhibitor L-NMMA were performed after a period of euglycemic hyperinsulinemia designed to cause maximal vasodilation. Infusion of L-NMMA completely abrogated the insulin induced vasodilation, suggesting that insulin-mediated vasodilation is entirely NO-dependent. Other studies have confirmed the NO reliance on insulin-mediated vasodilation in the forearm [18]. To further test whether insulin-mediated vasodilation occurs *via* a direct effect of insulin to enhance the release of NO from vascular endothelium rather than merely enhance the action of NO on the vascular smooth muscle cell, other experimental approaches have been taken. One approach is to examine the effects of subvasodilatory insulin doses (~ 25µU/mL) to enhance the vasodilatory response to an endothelium-dependent vasodilator such as methacholine chloride [19]. Studies performed in the leg and forearms have shown that endothelium-dependent vasodilation is enhanced in the presence of insulin. [19, 20]. In contrast, the response to the NO donor sodium nitroprusside was unaltered by co-infusion of insulin, suggesting that insulin is sensitizing the endothelial response to the endothelium-dependent vasodilator methacholine chloride [19, 21]. To establish if insulin increases NO release from the endothelium, studies were recently undertaken to measure femoral venous efflux of the stable oxidative end-products of nitric oxide, nitrate (NO_3) and nitrite (NO_2) together (commonly referred to as NO_x). NO_x concentrations were measured by a chemoluminescence technique and NO_x flux was calculated as the product of the NO_x concentration × the rate of the leg blood flow. Femoral venous NO_x fluxes were measured under basal conditions and after a period of euglycemic hyperinsulinemia designed to stimulate NO production. Insulin was found to cause a net increase in NO_x release from the leg [22]. Moreover, when L-NMMA was infused concomitantly with insulin, venous NO_x flux fell rapidly and could not be overcome by continued hyperinsulinemia [22].

Together, these data suggest that insulin vasodilates skeletal muscle vasculature *via* the net release of endothelium-derived NO. While it is possible for insulin to cause the production of NO *via* the stimulation of NOS isoforms residing in cells other than the endothelium [22, 23], it is unlikely that vasodilation in response to intraarterial methacholine chloride (an endothelium-dependent vasodilator) was enhanced by insulin [24] but had no effect on the response to sodium nitroprusside. Together these data are consistent with a direct *in vivo* effect of insulin to stimulate NO release from the endothelium.

SKELETAL MUSCLE VASODILATION, TISSUE PERFUSION, AND INSULIN SENSITIVITY

Given the importance of tissue perfusion for substrate and hormone delivery, it is reasonable to examine the contribution of insulin-mediated vasodilation to insulin overall effect to stimulate glucose uptake into skeletal muscle. To this end, euglycemic hyperinsulinemic clamp studies achieving high, but physiologic, prevailing insulin

levels (~75 µU/mL) were performed in lean healthy subjects. Leg glucose uptake (LGU) was measured 1) under near steady-state conditions after 4 h of hyperinsulinemia during which rates of insulin stimulated glucose uptake and vasodilation were fully expressed and 2) during a subsequent 30 min intrafemoral artery infusion of L-NMMA designed to inhibit NO production and reduce leg blood flow rates to basal rates. LGU was calculated by the balance technique, LGU= Femoral arteriovenous glucose difference × Flow or LGU = AVGΔ×F.L-NMMA infusion caused a complete abrogation of the insulin-mediated vasodilation, thus returning rates of leg blood flow back to baseline values. With the reduction in limb blood flow (LBF), glucose extraction (AVGΔ) rose approximately 50% from ~30 mg/dL to 44 mg/gL. However, this rise in extraction was not sufficient to overcome the fall in perfusion rate and LGU decreased by ~ 25%, $p < 0.0001$ [25]. Thus, insulin-mediated vasodilation appears to augment insulin's action to stimulate skeletal muscle glucose uptake and may account for approximately one-fourth of insulin's overall stimulating effect on glucose uptake. The corollary of this finding is that impairment of insulin's normal ability to vasodilate could in turn contribute to insulin resistance. A mechanism has been proposed to account for the insulin resistance associated with essential hypertension that occurs independently of other factors like obesity [1].

INSULIN SENSITIVITY AND NITRIC OXIDE PRODUCTION

Insulin-mediated vasodilation is NO dependent and insulin-mediated vasodilation is impaired in states of insulin resistance. Thus, it follows logically that insulin-mediated NO release may be impaired in states of insulin resistance. Recent studies have examined the effects of maximally effective doses of insulin to stimulate femoral venous NO_x flux in subjects exhibiting a wide range of insulin sensitivity [22]. Basal NO_x flux rates were not different between subject groups exhibiting insulin-stimulated rates of whole-body glucose uptake ranging from 4 mg/kg/min in obese type 2 diabetic subjects to 15 mg/kg/min in endurance-trained athletes. In contrast, during insulin stimulation, athletes exhibited a significant

130% increase in NO_x production above baseline while diabetic subjects exhibited no change in NO_x production above basal level. Thus, the data are consistent with the notion that insulin-mediated NO production appears as a function of insulin sensitivity, with insulin resistant subjects exhibiting reduced NO production. In sum, insulin resistance is associated with impairment of the endothelial NO system as reflected by reduced stimulated NO_x production and, thus, may be associated with more generalized endothelial dysfunction.

INSULIN SENSITIVITY AND ENDOTHELIAL FUNCTION

To test whether insulin resistance is associated with more generalized endothelial dysfunction, studies have examined endothelial-dependent vasodilation to various endothelial-dependent vasodilators [19] and flow mediated vasodilation [26] in insulin resistant states. Endothelium-dependent vasodilation to the agent metacholine chloride is markedly impaired in obese insulin resistant subjects ($\geq 28\%$ body fat) compared to lean insulin sensitive subjects ($< 28\%$ body fat). This endothelial dysfunction was independent of factors known to be associated with endothelial impairment such as high blood pressure, elevation in low-density lipoprotein (LDL) or total cholesterol, and smoking, suggesting that the simple state of obesity/insulin resistance is associated with endothelial dysfunction. It is important to point out that more recent data suggest that the relationship between obesity and endothelial dysfunction is stronger in men than in premenopausal women [27]. Interestingly, obese subjects of either gender, with type 2 diabetes, exhibit endothelial dysfunction that is similar to obese male non-diabetic counterparts. Vasodilatory responses to the administration of intra-arterial sodium nitroprusside were identical in lean, obese, and type 2 diabetic subjects indicating normal endothelium-independent vasodilation [19]. Thus, simple obesity/insulin resistance is associated with marked endothelial dysfunction, independent of hyperglycemia. In summary, obesity / insulin resistance is associated with endothelial dysfunction independent of other known clinical factors that modulate endothelial function.

Importantly, hyperglycemia does not appear to further impair endothelial function over that observed with simple obesity/insulin resistance alone. Hyperglycemia *per se* has been shown to impair endothelium-dependent vasodilation in animal models [28, 29] and humans [30]. Therefore, the mechanism(s) for insulin resistance and hyperglycemia-induced endothelium dysfunction do not appear additive and may be quite different.

POTENTIAL MECHANISMS FOR ENDOTHELIAL CELL DYSFUNCTION ASSOCIATED WITH INSULIN RESISTANCE

Role of fatty acids

Recent studies have explored potential mechanisms linking insulin resistance (independent of hyperglycemia, hypertension, and hyper-cholesterolemia) with endothelial dysfunction. Subjects with insulin resistance exhibit impaired antipolytic actions of insulin and, thus, exhibit daylong elevation of circulating concentrations of free fatty acids (FFA) [31]. Based on *in vitro* data suggesting that FFA impair NO synthase activity in cultured endothelial cells [32], we tested the hypothesis that elevated circulating FFA levels can impair endothelial cell function *in vivo*. To this end, graded intrafemoral artery infusions of methacholine chloride were performed to establish the full dose-response curve for endothelium-dependent vasodilation during an infusion of saline or an infusion of two hours of a lipid emulsion in conjunction with heparin to enhance hydrolysis of the triglyceride particle and elevate circulating FFA concentrations to approximately $1\,200\ \mu M$. Raising FFA concentrations caused a marked impairment of endothelium-dependent vasodilation. Similar endothelial dysfunction was also induced by inhibition of endogenous insulin secretion with somatostatin, thereby enhancing the release of endogenous FFA to achieve circulating levels approximating those achieved with exogenous infusions. Thus, elevating circulating FFA concentrations from both endogenous and exogenous sources causes marked endothelial cell dysfunction. Given that insulin resistance is associated with day-long elevations in FFA, it is logical to suggest that chronic elevations of these substrates may be instrumental in causing endothelial dysfunction in states of insulin resistance.

Role of altered insulin signaling

The precise defects in insulin signal transduction pathways underlying insulin resistance in common diseases such as diabetes, obesity and hypertension have not been elucidated for the majority of patients. However, it is clear that abnormalities in signaling molecules involved in metabolic insulin signaling pathways can cause insulin resistance. For example, many patients with syndromes of extreme insulin resistance have been found to have functionally significant mutations in their insulin receptor gene [33]. Similarly, transgenic mice homozygous for a null allele of the insulin receptor substrate-1 (IRS-1) gene are mildly insulin resistant [34, 35], and transgenic mice heterozygous for null alleles of both the insulin receptor and IRS-1 develop diabetes [36]. Since it was established the insulin sensitivity with respect to glucose metabolism and insulin sensitivity with respect to vasodilation, it is conceivable that metabolic insulin signaling pathways share elements in common with insulin signaling pathways in endothelium involved with vasodilator actions. Thus, signaling defects that contribute to insulin resistance with respect to glucose metabolism may also affect the vasodilator actions of insulin. This would provide a plausible mechanism linking insulin resistant diseases such as diabetes and obesity with defects in the vasodilator actions of insulin and endothelial dysfunction that may predispose to macrovascular disease and hypertension.

IN VITRO PERSPECTIVES

REGULATED PRODUCTION OF NO IN ENDOTHELIUM

The major isoform of NO synthase expressed in the endothelium is endothelial nitric oxide synthase (eNOS). eNOS is a heme-containing enzyme that catalyzes the synthesis of NO by hydroxylation of the substrate L-arginine to NG-hydroxy-L-arginine followed by oxidation of this intermediate to the products NO and L-citrulline.

Cofactors that participate in the transfer of electrons required for the production of NO by eNOS include NADPH, FAD, FMN, tetrahydrobiopterin, and molecular oxygen. The eNOS protein contains a linker region with a calmodulin binding site which links the amino-terminal oxygenase domain (containing heme and binding sites for L-arginine and tetrahydrobiopterin) to the carboxy- terminal reductase domain (containing FAD, FMN, and NADPH binding sites homologous to P450 reductase). Treatment of endothelial cells with classical cholinergic agonists such as acetylcholine causes an influx of calcium mediated by activation of the acetylcholine receptor (a seven transmembrane G protein-coupled receptor) that results in stimulation of eNOS activity via interaction of calcium/calmodulin with the calmodulin binding site on eNOS. Endothelial-derived NO diffuses into vascular smooth muscle cells causing vasorelaxation. The importance of eNOS to the regulation of vascular tone and hemodynamics has been unequivocally demonstrated by the presence of hypertension in transgenic mice that are homozygous for a null allele of the eNOS gene [37].

INSULIN SIGNALING PATHWAYS RELATED TO PRODUCTION OF NO IN ENDOTHELIUM

In vivo studies implicate endothelial-derived NO as a mediator of vasodilator actions of insulin [24]. Most, if not all, of the biological actions of insulin are initiated by the binding of insulin to its cell surface receptor [38]. The insulin receptor belongs to a large family of receptor tyrosine kinases. Cytokines and other growth factors that signal through tyrosine kinase dependent mechanisms are known to greatly induce transcription of the iNOS isozyme found in macrophages (resulting in increased production of NO for cytotoxic functions) [39]. However, a clearly defined mechanism linking signaling by tyrosine kinase receptors such as the insulin receptor with activation of eNOS in endothelial cells has not been well established.

It has been appreciated for some time that insulin receptors are expressed at low levels in endothelial cells (~40,000 receptors/cell) [40, 41]. One function of endothelial insulin receptors is to transport insulin across the endothelium to classical targets such as muscle, adipose tissue, and liver where insulin can exert its metabolic effects [42]. It is also possible that signal transduction by endothelial insulin receptors plays an important physiological role and contributes to metabolic effects of insulin. Endothelial cells themselves are not very responsive to insulin with respect to glucose uptake because they do not express the insulin responsive glucose transporter GLUT4. However, if activation of the insulin receptor mediates production of NO in endothelium, this may contribute to whole body glucose disposal by resulting in increased blood flow to muscle (a major determinant of glucose uptake). Furthermore, this would imply that defects in insulin-stimulated production of NO are capable of contributing to insulin resistance with respect to glucose metabolism.

In order to elucidate specific insulin signal transduction pathways responsible for the production of NO in endothelial cells, it is necessary to investigate this novel action of insulin at the cellular and molecular level. Because NO has a short half-life (~5s) and is present at nanomolar concentrations *in vivo*, it has been difficult to establish methods for directly measuring NO in cell culture models that are amenable to cellular and molecular manipulations. Recently, a commercially available NO-selective amperometric electrode has been used to directly measure NO production in response to insulin in primary cultures of human umbilical vein endothelial cells (HUVEC) [41]. This has made it possible to begin the characterization of insulin signal transduction pathways related to production of NO in a physiologically relevant cell type.

Insulin causes a dose-dependent, saturable increase in the production of NO in HUVEC [41]. Of note, the production of NO in response to insulin is an acute effect that occurs within a few minutes. This is in contrast to the vasodilator effects of insulin *in vivo* which occur on a time scale of 15–20 min to hours [15, 43]. This discrepancy between the time-scale for in vitro endothelial NO production and *in vivo* vasodilator response suggests that other effects of insulin may also be contributing to the hemodynamic actions of insulin. For example, insulin may stimulate the release of compounds such as endothelin that may oppose effects of NO [44]. In addition, activation of sympathetic activity by insulin may also modulate vasodilator responses [45]. Finally, because vasodilation appears to be coupled to the

rate of insulin-stimulated glucose uptake (which during insulin infusions appears within hours), it follows that insulin's *in vivo* vasodilatory effects parallel the time course of insulin's action on glucose metabolism.

The concentrations of insulin required to stimulate the production of NO *in vitro* are significantly higher than those required for vasodilator effects of insulin *in vivo*. This is likely due to technical limitations of the direct measurement method. For example, the *in vitro* experiments are carried out at room temperature because the NO electrode is extremely sensitive to temperature variations and it is difficult to carry out experiments at physiological temperature (37°C). Furthermore, HUVEC may not be as sensitive to insulin with respect to production of NO as endothelial cells from small vessels perfusing the muscle beds. Finally, it is possible that the NO electrode is simply not sensitive enough to detect significant production of NO in response to insulin concentrations in the low physiological range. Nevertheless, this model system has proven useful for understanding insulin signal transduction pathways related to production of NO.

Similar to the vasodilator response *in vivo*, insulin-stimulated production of NO in HUVEC can be completely blocked by preincubation of cells with L-NAME (a competitive inhibitor of eNOS). Furthermore, preincubation of the cells with genestein (a tyrosine kinase inhibitor) also completely blocks the production of NO in response to insulin. Taken together, these data suggest a necessary role for the receptor tyrosine kinase in activation of eNOS by insulin. More direct evidence that the insulin receptor tyrosine kinase is necessary to mediate the effect of insulin on production of NO has been obtained using HUVEC that were transfected with either wild-type insulin receptors or kinase-deficient mutant insulin receptors [46]. Overexpression of wild-type insulin receptors leads to a threefold increase in the level of NO produced in response to maximal insulin stimulation while cells overexpressing kinase-deficient insulin receptors respond like the untransfected control cells.

Interestingly, the number of insulin receptors present in HUVEC is ~ 10 times less than the number of related insulin growth factors (IGF-1) receptors [41]. The binding affinity of insulin for the IGF-1 receptor is ~100 times less than for the insulin receptor. Therefore, high concentrations of insulin may signal, in part, through the more abundant IGF-1 receptor. However, the level of NO produced in response to a maximally stimulating concentration of insulin is approximately twice than that seen with maximal IGF-1 stimulation. In addition, incubating HUVEC with a blocking antibody against the IGF-1 receptor only partially inhibits the production of NO in response to insulin while completely blocking the response to IGF-1. Therefore, while some of insulin's effects on production of NO may be mediated through the IGF-1 receptor, there is a significant effect mediated specifically by the insulin receptor.

PARALLELS BETWEEN METABOLIC INSULIN SIGNALING PATHWAYS AND INSULIN SIGNALING PATH- WAYS RELATED TO PRODUCTION OF NO IN ENDOTHELIUM

After the binding of insulin to its receptor and activation of the receptor tyrosine kinase, cellular substrates such as IRS-1, -2, -3, -4, and Shc are phosphorylated [47–53]. Phosphotyrosine impulses on these substrates then engage and activate multiple downstream signaling molecules [38]. In some cases, specific downstream signaling molecules have been associated with particular biological actions of insulin. For example, phosphatidylinositol 3-kinase (PI-3K) has been shown to be a necessary mediator of metabolic actions of insulin such as the translocation of the insulin responsive glucose transporter GLUT4 to the cell surface in adipose cells [54]. Interestingly, wortmannin (an inhibitor of PI-3K) is able to partially block the production of NO in response to insulin in HUVEC [41]. Therefore, insulin signaling pathways involved with production of NO in the endothelium may share elements in common with insulin signaling pathways related to glucose transport in classical insulin target cells. These data also imply that defects in signaling resulting in insulin resistance with respect to glucose metabolism have the potential to cause insulin resistance with respect to vasodilator actions of insulin. Thus, insulin resistance may contribute to a relative increase in

peripheral vascular tone. This is an attractive hypothesis that provides a mechanism by which one can relate insulin resistance and diabetes with commonly associated diseases such as hypertension and abnormalities associated with endothelial dysfunction. Indeed, consistent with this hypothesis is the *in vivo* observation that insulin sensitivity with respect to glucose metabolism is positively correlated with insulin sensitivity with respect to vasodilatory actions of insulin [1, 15, 16, 17].

Another parallel between metabolic insulin signaling pathways in classical insulin targets such as adipose cells and insulin signaling pathways related to production of NO in endothelium is the fact that activation of PI-3K *per se* is not sufficient to elicit an insulin-like response. For example, stimulation of adipose cells with platelet-derived growth factor (PDGF) results in activation of PI3K at a level comparable to that seen with insulin stimulation but does not result in the translocation of GLUT4 [55, 56]. Similarly, PDGF stimulation of endothelial cells results in activation of PI-3K [57] but does not result in measurable production of NO [41]. These results suggest that the biological specificity of insulin action is dependent on more than simply activating a particular signaling molecule. Perhaps subcellular localization of signaling molecules or the formation of specific signaling complexes are both providing data for specificity.

As progress is made in the elucidation of insulin signaling pathways related to production of NO in the endothelium, it will be interesting to determine the extent of overlap between metabolic signaling pathways in classical insulin targets such as muscle and adipose tissue and signaling pathways related to production of NO in the endothelium. For example, a physiological role for Akt (a serine-threonine kinase downstream of PI-3K) in insulin-stimulated translocation of GLUT4 was recently identified in rat adipose cells [58]. Does Akt also play a role in insulin-stimulated production of NO in endothelium or will this represent a point of divergence in the insulin signaling pathway? Another important avenue of investigation that remains is to determine mechanisms linking insulin signaling pathways with the activation of eNOS. Recently, tyrosine phosphorylation of eNOS was reported in endothelial cells treated with phosphatase inhibitors [59]. However, the physiological significance of this phenomenon and its relationship to insulin signaling are unclear. Other recent studies demonstrating interactions of calmodulin with IRS-1 and PI-3K are also intriguing since calmodulin is a major regulator of eNOS activity [60, 61]. Although there is still a great deal to be learned, it is clear that insulin signal transduction pathways in endothelium are mediating important and novel physiological actions related to the regulation of hemodynamics and metabolism.

CLINICAL IMPLICATIONS OF ENDOTHELIAL DYSFUNCTION IN STATES OF INSULIN RESISTANCE

Over a decade ago, Gerald Reaven coined Syndrome X or Insulin Resistance Syndrome (IRS) [62]. While the definition of this syndrome is one of debate and in constant evolution, there is much consensus about its existence and its core features. The greater than chance clustering of insulin resistance (particularly in the context of central obesity) with elevated FFA, elevated triglycerides and reduced high-density lipoprotein (HDL), elevated fasting glucose (also known as impaired fasting glucose or dysglycemia), impaired glucose tolerance, abnormalities in blood fluidity, and elevations of blood pressure are common clinical findings [63]. The syndrome's clinical importance stems from the consistent observation that IRS is associated with a 2–3 fold increased risk of coronary heart disease mortality [62, 64]. That insulin resistance is the central factor accounting for the clustering of cardiovascular risk factors is suggested by numerous studies demonstrating amelioration of these risk factors with therapeutic maneuvers directed at improving insulin sensitivity such as weight reduction [65, 66] and exercise [67, 68]. Perhaps some of the most compelling evidence that insulin resistance is central to the syndrome comes from studies utilizing the insulin action enhancing family-drug thiazolidindiones in obese patients with impaired glucose tolerance that exhibit many features of the syndrome [69]. Thiazolidindiones therapy was shown to enhance (but not normalize) insulin sensitivity in these patients and this effect was accompanied by moderate but significant reductions in circulating triglycerides, increases in

HDL and lowering of blood pressure independent of changes in weight or adiposity. Thus, while a number of issues remain to be resolved about the genetics, molecular, biochemical and metabolic basis of IRS, features of the syndrome appear to be at least partially reversible with therapeutic strategies that are directed towards reversing the abnormality in the action of insulin.

It is important to underline that the cardiovascular risk factors (abnormal lipoproteins, blood pressure, dysglycemia) associated with insulin resistance do not fully account for the increase in the cardiovascular risk. Therefore, other factors associated with insulin resistance are likely to be involved. The endothelium plays a critical role in maintaining the health of the vascular wall, blood pressure, blood fluidity, and redox state [70]. In turn, endothelial dysfunction is suspected to play a critical and initiating role in the pathogenesis of the atherosclerotic plaque [71–74]. Through the coordinate production of vasodilating and growth inhibiting factors and counterbalancing vaso-constricting growth promoting factors, the endothelium plays a key role in maintaining the health of the vascular wall [11, 12]. For example, NO decreases vascular smooth muscle cell proliferation and lowers vascular resistance [75] while endothelin I promotes smooth muscle cell growth and increases vascular tone [75]. In addition, NO inhibits monocyte adhesion to endothelial cells, enhances fibrinolysis, reduces platelet adhesiveness and lipid peroxidation thus protecting the vascular wall from plaque formation [11]. Given that insulin resistance is associated with dysfunction of the endothelium derived NO system, it follows logically that endothelial dysfunction likely contributes significantly to the increased risk of macrovascular disease in insulin resistant states. Dysfunction of the endothelium derived NO system has been shown to be associated with accelerated atherosclerosis in a variety of animal models [76, 77]. Conversely, maneuvers directed at elevating endothelium derived NO production appear to protect against atherosclerotic plaque formation [78–80]. Thus, it follows logically from these lines of evidence that endothelial dysfunction may represent an early and central pathogenic event leading to macrovascular disease in patients with insulin resistance. This hypothetical construct will undoubtedly be the focus of future research.

REFERENCES

1. Baron AD, Brechtel-Hook G, Johnson A, Harding D. Skeletal muscle blood flow. A possible link between insulin resistance and blood pressure. *Hypertension,* **21:** 129–135, 1993.
2. Vallance P, Collier J, Moncada S. Effects of endothelium-derived nitric oxide on peripheral arteriolar tone in man. *Lancet,* **2:** 997–1000, 1989.
3. Stammler JS, Loh E, Roddy M-A, Currie KE, Creager MA. Nitric oxide regulates basal systemic and pulmonary vascular resistance in healthy humans. *Circulation,* **89:** 2035–2040, 1994.
4. Wu KK, Thiagarajan P. Role of endothelium in thrombosis and hemostasis. *Ann Rev Med,* **47:** 315–331, 1996.
5. Adams MR, McCredie R, Jessup W, Robinson J, Sullivan D, Celermaje DS. Oral L-arginine improves endothelium-dependent dilatation and reduces monocyte adhesion to endothelial cells in youngs with coronary artery disease. *Atherosclerosis,* **129:** 261–269, 1997.
6. Lefer AM. Nitric Oxide: nature's naturally occurring leucocyte inhibitor. *Circulation,* **95:** 553–554, 1997.
7. Bruckdorfer KR, Jakobs JM, Rice-Evans C. Endothelium-derived relaxing factor (nitric oxide), lipoprotein oxidation and atherosclerosis. *Biochem. Soc. Trans.,* **18:** 1061–1063, 1990.
8. Hoog N, Kalyanaraman B, Joseph J, Struck A, Parthasarathy S. Inhibition of low-lipoprotein oxidation by nitric oxide. *FEBS Lett.,* **334:** 170–174, 1993.
9. Jessup W, Dean RT. Autoinhibition of murine macrophage mediated oxidation of low density lipoprotein by nitric oxide synthesis. *Atherosclerosis,* **101:** 145–155, 1997.
10. Jessup W. Cellular modification of low-density lipoproteins. *Biochem. Soc. Trans.,* **21:** 321–325, 1993.
11. Moncada S, Higgs A. The L-arginine - nitric oxide pathway. *N Engl J Med,* **1329:** 2002–2012, 1993.
12. Cooke JP, Tsao PS. Endothelium-derived relaxing factor. In: Sowers JR, (ed). *Endocrinology of the Vasculature.* Humana, Totowa, NJ, 1996, 3–20.
13. Cohen RA. The role of nitric oxide and other endothelium-derived vasoactive substances in vascular disease. *Prog Cardiovasc Dis,* **38:** 105–128, 1995.
14. Lloyd-Jones DM, Bloch KD. The cardiovascular biology of nitric oxide and its role in atherogenesis. *Annu Rev Med,* **47:** 365–375, 1996.
15. Laakso M, Edelman SV, Brechtel G, Baron AD. Decreased effect of insulin to stimulate skeletal muscle blood flow in obese men: A novel mechanism for insulin resistance. *J Clin Invest,* **85:** 1844–1852, 1990.
16. Laakso M, Edelman SV, Brechtel G, Baron AD. Impaired insulin mediated skeletal muscle blood flow in patients with NIDDM. *Diabetes,* **41:** 1076–1083, 1992.
17. Baron AD, Brechtel G. Insulin differentially regulates systemic and skeletal muscle vascular resistance. *Am J Physiol,* **265:** E61–E67, 1993.
18. Scherrer U, Randin D, Vollenweinder L, Nicod P. Nitric oxide release accounts for insulin's vascular effects in humans. *J Clin Invest,* **94:** 2511–2515, 1994.
19. Steinberg H, Chaker H, Leaming R, Johnson A, Brechtel G, Baron AD. Obesity/insulin resistance is associated with endothelial dysfunction. Implications for the syndrome of insulin resistance. *J Clin Invest,* **97:** 2601–2610, 1996.
20. Taddei S, Virdis A, Mattei P, Natali A, Ferrannini E, Salvetti A. Effects of insulin on acetylcholine-induced vasodilation in the forearm of normotensive subjects. *Hypertension,* **25:** 552, 1995.
21. Nagao T, Illiano S, Vanhoutte PM. Heterogeneous distribution of endothelium-dependent relaxations resistant to Ng-nitro-L-arginine in rats. *Am J Physiol,* **263:** H1090–H1094, 1992.
22. Steiberg HO, Cresssman Y, Wu G, Hook J, Cronin A, Johnson A, Baron AD. Insulin mediated nitric oxide production is impaired in insulin resistance. *Diabetes,* **46 (Suppl 1):** 24A, 1997.
23. Madar Z, Zierrath J, Nollte L, Thorne A, Voet H, Walberg-Henriksson H. Human skeletal muscle nitric oxide synthase-characterization and its activity in obese subjects. *Diabetes,* **46 (Suppl 1):** 24A, 1997.
24. Steiberg HO, Brechtel G, Johnson A, Fineberg N, Baron AD. Insulin mediated skeletal muscle vasodilation is nitric oxide dependent. A novel action of insulin to increase nitric oxide release. *J Clin Invest,* **94:** 1172–1179, 1994.
25. Baron AD, Steinberg HO, Chaker H, Leaming R, Johnson A, Brechtel G. Insulin-mediated skeletal muscle vasodilation contributes to both insulin sensitivity and responsiveness in lean humans. *J Clin Invest* **96:** 786–792, 1995.
26. Natali A, Taddei S, Galvan AQ, Camastra S, Baldi S, Frascerra S, Virdis A, Sudano I, Salvetti A, Ferrannini E. Insulin sensitivity, vascular reactivity, clamp-induced vasodilatation in essential hypertension. *Circulation,* **96:** 8498–855, 1997.
27. Steiberg HO, Hook G, Cronin J, Johnson A, Baron AD. Endothelial function is preserved in obese premenopausal women but not in obese men. *Hypertension,* **30(3):** 503, 1997.
28. Bohlen HG, Last JM. Topical hyperglycemia rapidly suppresses EDRF-mediated vasodilation of normal rat arterioles. *AM J Physiol,* **265:** H219–H225, 1993.

29. Jin JS, Bohlen HG. Non-insulin-dependent diabetes and hyperglycemia impair rat intestinal flow-mediated regulation. *Am J Physiol*, **272**: H728–H734, 1997.

30. Williams SB, Cusco JA, Roddy M-A, Johnstone MA, Creager MT. Impaired nitric oxide-mediated vasodilation in non-insulin-dependent diabetes. *Circulation*, **90**: 1–513, 1994.

31. Jeng C-Y, Fuh MM-T, Sheu WH-H, Chen Y-DI, Reaven GM. Hormone and substrate modulation of plasma triglyceride concentration in primary hypertriglyceridaemia. *Endocrinol Metab*, **1**: 15–21, 1994.

32. Davda RK, Stepniakowski KT, Lu G, Ullian E, Goodfriend TL, Egan BM. Oleic acid inhibits endothelial nitric oxide synthase by a protein kinase C-independent mechanism. *Hypertension*, **26**: 764–770, 1995.

33. Taylor SI. Lilly Lecture: Molecular mechanisms of insulin resistance. Lessons from patients with mutations in the insulin-receptor gene. *Diabetes*, **41**: 1473–1490, 1992.

34. Araki E, Lipes MA, Patti M-E, Bruning JC, Haag BIII, Johnson RS, Kahn CR. Alternative pathway of insulin signaling in mice with targeted disruption of the IRS-1 gene. *Nature*, **372**: 186–190, 1994.

35. Tamemoto H, Kadowaki T, Tobe K, Yagi T, Sakura H, Hayakawa T, Terauchi Y, Kaburagi Y, Satoh S, Sekihara H, Yoshika S, Horikoshi H, Furuta Y, Kasuga M, Aizawa S. Insulin resistance and growth retardation in mice lacking insulin receptor substrate-1. *Nature*, **372**: 182–186, 1994

36. Bruning JC, Winnay J, Bonner-Weir S, Taylor SI, Accili D, Kahn CR. Development of a novel polygenic model of NIDDM in mice heterozygous for IR and IRS-1 null alleles. *Cell*, **88**: 561–572, 1997.

37. Huang PL, Huang Z, Mashimo H, Bloch KD, Moskwitz MA, Bevan JA Fishman MC. Hypertension in mice lacking the gene for endothelial nitric oxide synthase. *Nature*, **377**: 239–242, 1995.

38. Quon MJ, Butte AJ, Taylor SI. Insulin signal transduction pathways. *Trends Endocrin Metab*, **5**: 369–376, 1994.

39. Nathan C, Xie QW. Nitric oxide synthase: roles, tolls, controls. (Review) (30refs). *Cell*, **78**: 915–918, 1994.

40. Bar RS, Hoak JC, Peacock ML. Insulin receptors in human endothelial cells: identification and characterization, *J Clin Endicrinol Metab*, **47**: 699–702, 1978.

41. Zeng G, Quon MJ. Insulin-stimulated production of nitric oxide is inhibited by wortmannin. Direct measurement in vascular endothelial cells. *J Clin Invest*, **98 (4)**: 894–898, 1996.

42. King GL, Johnson SM. Receptors-mediated transport of insulin across endothelial cells. *Science*, **227**: 1583–1586, 1985.

43. Baron AD. Hemodynamic actions of insulin. *Am J Physiol*, **267**: E187–E202, 1994.

44. Ferri C, Pittoni V, Piccoli A, Laurenti O, Cassone MR, Bellini C, Properzi G, Valesini G, De Mattia G, Santucci A. Insulin stimulates endothelin-1 secretion from human endothelial cells and modulates its circulating levels *in vivo*. *JH Clin Endocrinol Metab*, **80**: 829–835, 1995.

45. Saruta T, Kumagai H. The sympathetic nervous system in hypertension and renal disease. *Curr Opin Neph Hypert*, **5**: 72–79, 1996.

46. Zeng GB, Clinton K, Kirby M, Mostowski H, Quon MJ. Tyrosine kinase-deficient mutant insulin receptors overexpressed in vascular endothelial cells fail to mediate production of nitric oxide. *Hypertension*, **30**: 504, 1997.

47. Myers MG Jr, White MF. Insulin signal transduction and the IRS proteins. *Annu Rev Pharmacol Toxicol*, **36**: 615–618, 1996.

48. Sun XJ, Wang LM, Zhang Y, Yenush L, Myers MG Jr, Lane WS, Pierce JH, White Mf. Role of IRS-2 in insulin and cytokine signaling. *Nature*, **377**: 173–177, 1995.

49. Lavan BR, Lane WS, Lienhard Ge. The 60-kDa phosphotyrosine protein in insulin-treated adipocyte is a new member of the insulin receptor substrate family. *J Biol Chem*, **272**: 11439–11443, 1997.

50. Holgado-Madruga M, Emlet DR, Moscatello DK, Godwin AK, Wong AJ. A-Grb2-associated docking protein in EGF-and insulin-receptor signaling. *Nature*, **379**: 560–564, 1996.

51. Ricketts WA, Rose DW, Shoelson S, Olefsky JM. Functional roles of the Shc phosphotyrosine binding and Src homology 2 domains and epidermal growth factor signaling. *J Biol Chem*, **271**: 26165–26169, 1996.

52. Sasaoka T, Draznin B, Leitner JW, Olefsky JM. Shc is the predominant signaling molecule coupling insulin receptors to activation of guanine nucleotide releasing factor and p21ras-GTP formation. *J Biol Chem*, **269**: 10734–10738, 1994.

53. Lavan BE, Fantin VR, Chang ET, Lane WS, Keller SR, Lienhard GE. A novel 160-kDa phosphotyrosine protein in insulin treated embryonic kidney cells is a new member receptor substrate family. *J Biol Chem*, **272**: 21403–21407, 1997.

54. Quon MJ, Chen H, Ing BL, Zarnowski MJ, Yonezawa K, Kasuga M, Cushman SW, Taylor SI. Roles of 1-phosphatidylinositol 3-kinase and ras in regulating of GLUT4 in transfected rat adipose cells. *Mol Cell Biol*, **15**: 5403–5411, 1995.

55. Quon Mj, Chen H, Lin CH, Zhou L, Zarnowski MJ, Kazlauskas A, Cushman SW, Taylor SI.

Effects of overexpressing wild-type and mutant PDGF receptors on translocation of GLUT4 in transferred rat adipose cells. *Biochem Biophys Res Commun*, **226**: 587–594, 1996.

56. Isakoff SJ, Taha C, Rose E, Marcusohn J, Klip A, Skolnik EY. The inability of phosphatidylinositol 3-kinase activation to stimulate GLUT4 translocation indicates additional signaling pathways are required for insulin-stimulated glucose uptake. *Proc Natl Acad Sci USA*, **92**: 10247–10251, 1995.

57. Wennstrom S, Hawkins P, Cooke F, Yonezawa K, Jackson T, Claeson-Welsh L, Stephens L. Activation of phosphoinositide 3-kinase for PDGF-stimulated membrane ruffling. *Curr Biol*, **4**: 385–393, 1994.

58. Cong L, Chen H, Li Y, Zhou L, McGibbon MA, Taylor SI, Quon MJ. Physiologic role of Akt in insulin-stimulated translocation of GLUT 4 in transfected rat adipose cells. *Mol Endocrinol*, **11**: 1881–1890, 1997.

59. Garcia-Cardena G, Fan R, Stern DF, Liu J, Sessa WC. Endothelial nitric oxide synthase is regulated by tyrosine phosphorylation and interacts with caveolin-1. *J Biol Chem*, **271**: 27237–27240, 1996.

60. Munshi HG, Burks DJ, Joyal JL, White MF, Sacks DB. Ca^{2+} regulates calmodulin binding to IQ motifs in IRS-1. *Biochemistry*, **35**: 15883–15889, 1996.

61. Joyal JL, Burks DL, Pons S, Matter WF, Vlahos CJ, White MF, Sacks DB. Calmodulin activates phosphatidylinositol 3 kinase. *J Biol Chem*, **272**: 28183–28186, 1997.

62. Reaven GM. Role of insulin resistance in human disease. *Diabetes*, **37**: 1595–1607, 1988.

63. Laakso M, Lehto S. Epidemiology of macrovascular disease in diabetes. *Diabetes Rev*, **5(4)**: 294–315, 1997.

64. Chen Y-DI, Reaven GM. Insulin resistance and atherosclerosis. *Diabetes Rev*, **5(4)**: 331–342, 1997.

65. Henry RR, Wallace P, Olefsky JM. Effects of weight loss on mechanisms of hyperglycemia in obese non-insulin dependent diabetes mellitus. *Diabetes*, **35**: 990–998, 1986.

66. Henry RR, Gumbiner B. Benefits and limitations of very-low-calorie diet therapy in obese NIDDM. [Review] [151 refs]. *Diabetes Care*, **14**: 802–823, 1991.

67. Devlin JT. Effects of exercise on insulin sensitivity in humans. [Review] [25 refs]. *Diabetes Care*, **15**: 1690–1693, 1992.

68. Holloszy JO, Schultz J, Kusnierkiewicz J, Hagberg JM, Ehsani AA. Effects of exercise on glucose tolerance and insulin resistance. Brief review and some preliminary results. [Review] [25 refs] *Acta Medica Scand-Supplementum*, **711**: 55–65, 1986.

69. Nolan J, Ludvik B, Beerdsen P, Joyce M, Olefsky J. Improvement in glucose tolerance and insulin resistance in obese subjects treated with troglitazone. *N Engl J Med*, **331**: 1188–1193, 1994.

70. Hsueh WA, Quinones MJ, Creager MA. Endothelium in insulin resistance and diabetes. *Diabetes Rev*, **5(4)**: 343–352, 1997.

71. Von der Leyen HE, Gibbons GH, Morishita R, Lewis NP, Zhang L, Nakajima M, Kaneda Y, Cooke JP, Dzau VJ. Gene therapy inhibiting neointimal vascular lesion: In vivo transfer of endothelial cell nitric oxide synthase gene. *Proc Natl Acad Sci USA*, **92**: 1137–1141, 1995.

72. Marks DS, Vita JA, Fots JD, Keaney JF Jr, Welch GN. Inhibition of neointimal proliferation in rabbits after vascular injury by a single treatment with a protein adduct of nitric oxide. *J Clin Invest*, **96**: 2630–2638, 1995.

73. De Caterina R, Libby P, Peng HB, Thannickal VJ, Gimbrone MA, Shin WS, Liao JK. Nitric oxide decreases cytokine-induced endothelial activation. Nitric oxide selectively reduces endothelial expression of adhesion molecules and proinflammatory cytokines. *J Clin Invest*, **96**: 60–681995.

74. Zeiher AM, Fisslthaler B, Schray-Utz B, Buse R. Nitric oxide modulates the expression of monocyte chemoattractant protein 1 in cultured human endothelial cells. *Circ Res*, **76**: 980–986, 1995.

75. Vanhoutte PM, Rubanyi GM, Miller VM, Houston DS. Modulation of vascular smooth muscle contraction by the endothelium. [Review] [97 refs] *Ann Rev Physiol*, **48**: 307–320, 1986.

76. Cayatte AJ, Palacino JJ, Horten K, Cohen RA. Chronic inhibition of nitric oxide production accelerates neointima formation and impairs endothelial function in hypercholesterolemic rabbits. *Arterioscl Thromb*, **14**: 753–759, 1994.

77. Naruse K, Shimizu K, Muramatsu M, Toki Y, Miyazaki Y, Hashimoto H, Ito T. Long-term inhibition of NO synthesis promotes atherosclerosis in the hypercholesterolemic rabbit thoracic aorta. PGH2 does not contribute to impaired endothelium-dependent relaxation [see comments]. *Arterioscl Thromb*, **14**: 746–752, 1994.

78. Girerd XJ, Hirsch AT, Cooke JP, Dzau VJC. L-arginine augments endothelium-dependent vasodilation in cholesterol-fed rabbits. *Circ Res*, **67**: 1301–1308, 1990.

79. Cooke JP, Singer AH, Tsao P, Zera P, Rowan RA. Antiatherogenic effects of L-arginine in the hypercholesterolemic rabbit. *J Clin Invest*, **90**: 1168–1172, 1992.

80. Tsao PS, McEvoy LM, Drexler H, Butcher EC, Cooke JP. Enhanced endothelial adhesiveness in hypercholesterolemia is attenuated by L-arginine. *Circulation*, **89**: 2176–2182, 1994.

13

ENDOTHELIAL DYSFUNCTION AND TYPE 2 DIABETES MELLITUS

Cristian GUJA, Constantin IONESCU-TÎRGOVIŞTE

Considerable amount of data accumulated during the latest years sustains the central role played by endothelial dysfunction in the pathogenesis of micro and macrovascular complications of diabetes mellitus. Endothelium is metabolically a very active tissue, secreting a great number of active molecules with the aim of maintaining a balance between opposing forces, such as vasodilatation and vasoconstriction; thrombosis and fibrinolysis; cell growth and its inhibition, etc.

Endothelial dysfunction consists in the decrease or loss of normal endothelial activity and represents an early functional marker of increased cardiovascular risk. Since the regulation of vascular tone is the most widely studied aspect of endothelial function, Endothelial Dysfunction is frequently defined as the loss of the endothelium-dependent (NO mediated) vasodilatory response. A lot of factors contribute to the genesis of endothelial dysfunction, more studied being the decrease of NO bio-availability (reduction of NO synthesis due to decreased expression of endothelial Nitric Oxide Synthase and increased NO destruction, mainly superoxide anion mediated), increased endothelin-1 and angiotensin II production, etc.

Multiple mechanisms contribute to the genesis of endothelial dysfunction in type 2 diabetes, the main being chronic hyperglycaemia. This acts by increased synthesis of diacylglycerol, which activates protein kinase C signaling, increased aldose reductase activity with accumulation of polyol pathway products, and formation of advanced glycation end-products. All these mechanisms may have a common precursor: increased oxidative stress, characteristic of the "diabetic internal milieu". Other mechanisms are represented by insulin resistance *per se*, oxidative stress, dyslipidemia, prothrombotic status, over expression of growth factors, etc.

Due to the major role of endothelial dysfunction in the genesis of diabetic vascular complications, therapeutic intervention with the aim of improving endothelial function is essential. It is obvious the importance of obtaining a good metabolic control, of treating diabetic dyslipidemia and hypertension. In addition, taking into account the link between endothelial dysfunction and insulin resistance, improving insulin sensitivity (lifestyle changes, Metformin, Thiazolidindiones, etc.) seems to be equally important. Finally, there is strong evidence regarding the direct beneficial effects on endothelial function of treatment with gliclazide, statins, fibrates, ACE inhibitors and antioxidants.

Abbreviations List

ACE – Angiotensin Converting Enzyme
ACEI – ACE Inhibitors
AGE – Advanced Glycation End-Products
ARB – Angiotensin Receptor Blockers
DAG – Diacylglycerol
EDRF – Endothelial Derived Relaxing Factor
FFA – Free Fatty Acid
GSH – Glutathione
ICAM-1 – Intercellular Adhesion Molecule 1
IGF – Insulin-like Growth Factor
IRS – Insulin Receptor Substrate
MAPK – Mitogen Activated Protein Kinase
MCP-1 – Monocyte Chemo-Attractant Protein 1
NF-κB – Nuclear Factor κB
NO – Nitric Oxide
NOS – Nitric Oxide Synthase

PAI-1 – Plasminogen Activator Inhibitor 1
PDGF – Platelet Derived Growth Factor
PI-3K – Phosphatidyl Inositol 3 Kinase
PKC – Protein Kinase C
PPAR α(γ) – Peroxisome Proliferator Activated Receptor α(γ)
RAGE – Receptors for Advanced Glycation End-Products
RAS – Renin Angiotensin System
ROS – Reactive Oxygen Species
T2DM – Type 2 Diabetes Mellitus
TNFα – Tumor Necrosis Factor α
t-PA – tissue Plasminogen Activator
VCAM-1 – Vascular Cell Adhesion Molecule 1
VEGF – Vascular Endothelial Growth Factor
VSMC – Vascular Smooth Muscle Cells

INTRODUCTION

Diabetes (and especially Type 2 Diabetes – T2DM) represents one of the main health care problems that modern society confronts with. It is predicted that T2DM will reach epidemic proportions in this century, with an estimated number of diabetic patients of 240 million by the year 2010, the worst hit being the developing countries. [1] Much of the health burden related to T2DM is due to the complications of the disease, both macro-vascular and micro-vascular. These complications lead to an increased mortality and a decrease of the life expectancy, which, in T2DM patients, can be of at least 10 years. It is of interest to note that pathogenic processes that lead to these complications begin early in the evolution of the disease, quite often before the actual diagnosis of T2DM is made. This is why, in newly diagnosed T2DM patients, the prevalence of diabetic neuropathy or retinopathy reached up to 20–30% in some datasets.

The prevalence of diabetic chronic complications is quite high and increasing with disease duration. For information, we are presenting in Table 13.1 data regarding the prevalence of the main diabetic complications in T2DM patients according with the duration of the disease. The data are based on the analysis of around 12 000 cases registered at the "Ion Pavel" Bucharest Diabetes Center between 1992 and 2001 [C. Ionescu-Tîrgovişte unpublished data]. Interestingly, analyzing 16 000 newly diagnosed T2DM patients registered at the same Diabetes Center, we found a prevalence of diabetic retinopathy of 23% (proliferative retinopathy 2%) and 24% for diabetic neuropathy [C. Ionescu-Tîrgovişte unpublished data].

Table 13. 1

Prevalence of Chronic Diabetic Complications (according with disease duration) in T2DM patients from "I. Pavel" Diabetic Center, Bucharest

	< 5 yrs	5–9 yrs	10–19 yrs	> 20 yrs
Neuropathy	15%	25%	48%	65%
Retinopathy				
– Background	18%	35%	49%	52%
– Proliferative	4%	6%	8%	10%
– Blindness	1.5%	2.5%	5.5%	8.5%
Renal Disease	7%	14%	22%	25%
Cardiovascular Disease	26%	41%	56%	71%

The costs associated with treatments for the vascular complications of diabetes are huge. It is sufficient to remind that in the USA and Western Europe, end stage renal disease diabetic patients represent more than 50% of those currently receiving renal substitution therapy, approximate half being T2DM patients. For example, from the 932 patients currently on dialysis at the Renal Disease and Dialysis Unit of "N. Paulescu" Institute Bucharest, 456 (48.92%) are T2DM patients.

All these data highlight the importance of the primary prevention of these complications, one essential step in this regard being the complete elucidation of their pathogenic mechanisms.

Many genetic, metabolic and hemodynamic factors are involved in the genesis of diabetic "angiopathy". Considerable biochemical and clinical evidence indicates that the endothelium is the "target" tissue and that endothelial dysfunction is a critical part of the pathogenesis of micro and macrovascular complications both in T1DM and T2DM [2]. This is not at all surprising since the endothelium has both the anatomical and physiological characteristics for this. First of all, the endothelium lines all the blood vessels, thus it is the "first line of contact" with the noxious "diabetic milieu". Second, endothelium is also the front-line tissue in the response to hemodynamic changes – flow, shear rate and pressure. Thirdly, it should be noticed that the endothelium is not just an "inert barrier" isolating the vessel wall matrix from the plasma compartment. In fact it is a very active metabolic tissue. Thus, in the latest years, as detailed in Table 13.2, it has been shown that endothelial cells produce a great number of active molecules [3, 4].

Through these molecules, endothelium is involved in the regulation of the vascular tone and the permeability of the vascular wall, in the production of the extra-cellular matrix proteins (that are increased in diabetes and lead to capillary membrane thickening), in the tuning of the balance between pro-thrombotic and fibrinolytic mechanisms. It also plays a key role in tissue repair and defense, in the maintenance of tissue fluid economy and it is the tissue from which new blood vessels arise.

Thus, as summarized in Table 13.2, the endothelium maintains a balance of opposing physiological and molecular effects, *i.e.* a balance of opposing forces with the end result of maintaining a proper blood supply to tissues and regulating inflammation and coagulation.

Table 13.2

Physiological Active Molecules Produced by Endothelial Cells
(Adapted after Calles-Escandon *et al.* 2001 [3] and James RW 2002 [4])

Function	Molecule
Vasodilatation	Nitric Oxide (NO), Prostacyclin (PGI2), Bradykinin, Endothelium-Derived Hyperpolarizing Factor (EDHF)
Vasoconstriction	Endothelin-1, Angiotensin-II, Thromboxane A2, Reactive Oxygen Species (ROS)
Anti-Proliferating	NO, PGI2
Pro-Proliferating	Endothelin-1, Angiotensin-II, TGFβ, ROS, Platelet Derived Growth Factor (PDGF), Basic Fibroblast Growth Factor (FGF), Insulin-like Growth Factor (IGF)
Anti-thrombotic	NO, PGI2, Tissue Plasminogen Activator (t-PA), Protein C, Thrombomodulin
Pro-thrombotic	Plasminogen Activator Inhibitor 1 (PAI-1), Endothelin-1, ROS, von Willebrand's Factor, Fibrinogen, Thromboxane A2
Adhesion Molecules	Vascular Cell Adhesion Molecule (VCAM), Intercellular Adhesion Molecule 1 (ICAM1), L Selectin, P Selectin, Platelet Endothelial Cell Adhesion Molecule 1 (PECAM1)
Permeability	Receptors for Advanced Glycation End-Products (RAGE)
Angiogenesis	Endothelial Derived Growth Factor

ENDOTHELIAL DYSFUNCTION

No single definition of endothelial dysfunction covers the whole array of possible disruption in normal function. Since the regulation of vascular tone is the most widely studied aspect of endothelial function, a restrictive definition (but widely accepted) is that endothelial dysfunction is the loss of the endothelium-dependent vasodilatory response to acetylcholine or hyperemia (both of which are known to produce NO-dependent vasodilation) [3]. However, as we have shown above, endothelium has much more physiological functions than the regulation of vasomotricity alone. This is why a more correct definition is that endothelial dysfunction consists in the decrease or loss of normal endothelial activity, decrease that represents an early functional marker of increased risk for cardiovascular events [4].

Endothelial dysfunction is manifested by a variety of abnormalities, including:
– Impaired endothelium-dependent vasodilation [5, 6, 7];
– Reduced synthesis and release of nitric oxide [6, 8], which is associated with less inhibition of platelet aggregation [9];
– Elevated levels of endothelin, which cause abnormal vasoconstriction [10];
– Elevated levels of asymmetric dimethylarginine (an endogenous competitive inhibitor of nitric oxide synthase) in hypercholesterolemic young adults [11];
– Increased endothelial production of oxygen free radicals, which may bind to and inactivate nitric oxide [12];
– Increased endothelial permeability for various macromolecules [13];
– Increased prothrombotic and/or procoagulant activity [14];
– Increased endothelial production of adhesion molecules, PAI-1 and von Willebrand's factor [15].

Endothelial dysfunction is present in a variety of pathological conditions, including diabetes and the insulin resistance syndrome, but also atherosclerosis, hypercholesterolemia, hypertension, cigarette smoking and aging.

We shall review first the characteristics of some of the main effectors produced by endothelial cells that are involved in the genesis of endothelial dysfunction and finally we shall present the pathogenic mechanisms of endothelial dysfunction in T2DM.

THE ROLE OF NITRIC OXIDE (NO)

The modern history of "endothelial biology" was revolutionized at the beginning of 1980's by a study of Robert Furchgott and John Zawadski which showed that vasodilatation produced by acetylcholine is dependent on a mediator produced by the endothelial cells – the Endothelial Derived Relaxing Factor (EDRF) [16]. Subsequently, EDRF was proved to be the molecule of Nitric Oxide [17, 18]. Nitric oxide is synthesized from the nitrogen molecule provided by the precursor L-arginine during its conversion to L-citrulline [19]. In the endothelium, the reaction is mediated by the specific (type III – endothelial) isoform of Nitric Oxide Synthase (eNOS). NOS type I (isolated from the brain) and type III (isolated from endothelial cells) are termed "constitutive NOS" and are Ca^{++}-calmodulin dependent. Types II and IV NOS (isolated from macrophages) are Ca^{++}-calmodulin independent and are termed "inducible NOS" since their activation is only promoted under pathophysiological situations in which macrophages exert cytotoxic effects in response to cytokines.

eNOS is a multimeric protein comprising oxygenase and reductase domains and catalyses a reaction in which NO and L-citrulline are produced from L-arginine, molecular oxygen and NADPH [20]. Essential co-factors of eNOS are the vitamin-derived molecules: tetrahydrobiopterin, flavin adenine dinucleotide (FAD) and flavin mononucleotide (FMN). eNOS has a high degree of homology with the amino acid sequence of cytochrome P450 reductase within the C-terminal domain [3]. Interestingly, under circumstances in which the relative abundance of L-arginine and tetrahydrobiopterin are disrupted, eNOS may itself produce superoxide anion [21]. eNOS is regulated by local concentrations of bradykinin which interacts with β2 receptors on the endothelial cell surface membrane, increasing the generation of NO *via* NOS activation [22]. NO has a very short half-life (just a few seconds), being rapidly oxidized to nitrate by oxi-hemoglobin, O_2 and superoxide anion (O_2^-).

Nitric oxide released by the endothelial cells targets many cells, including smooth muscle cells, nerve cells and fibroblasts from the vascular wall, leukocytes and platelets from the blood stream. The main effect of NO is represented by the regulation of vascular tone. In addition, NO released from endothelial cells is a potent inhibitor of platelet aggregation and adhesion to the vascular wall. Endothelial NO also controls the expression of genes involved in atherogenesis. It decreases expression of the chemo-attractant protein MCP-1, and of surface adhesion molecules such as CD11/CD18, P-Selectin, Vascular Cell Adhesion Molecule-1 (VCAM-1), and Intercellular Adhesion Molecule-1 (ICAM-1). Endothelial cell NO also reduces vascular

permeability and decreases the rate of oxidation of low-density lipoprotein (LDL) to its proatherogenic form. Finally, endothelial cell NO inhibits proliferation of vascular smooth muscle cells [23, 24]. NO may therefore be considered to be an antiatherogenic molecule, and the conditions characterized by reduced NO bioavailability represent a hallmark of the proatherogenic state.

Most of the actions of NO have been attributed to the stimulation of the enzyme guanylyl cyclase and, consecutively, the increase of cellular concentrations of cyclic guanosine 3', 5'-monophosphate (cGMP) [25]. In vascular smooth muscle cells cGMP leads to relaxation, the subsequent vasodilation being used as a simple and reproducible marker for endothelial cell function [4].

Because NO accounts for the majority of the vasodilator function of the endothelium, the impaired vasodilator function in diabetes may be viewed as an impairment of NO generation / activity. It is documented now that NO occupies a key position in the genesis of endothelial dysfunction in diabetes [26]. In diabetic patients, the bioavailability of NO is markedly decreased due to: a) insufficient production; b) excessively rapid inactivation/degradation or decreased NO activity in the target cells.

a) *Reduced NO production.* The basis for the theory that NO production is reduced in diabetic states was the experimental observation that there is decreased vasodilation in response to agonists, such as acetylcholine, metacholine or increased blood flow (shear stress) which act endothelium-dependent by NO generation (endogenous NO), but the responses to a NO donor such as sodium nitroprusside or nitroglycerin (exogenous NO) are unchanged [7]. A possible mechanism for reduced NO production in diabetes could be a decreased expression of eNOS gene. This hypothesis is sustained both by animal and human data. Thus, culturing endothelial cells in a highly elevated glucose environment reduce the expression of eNOS, a change that may be related to the formation of AGE (advanced glycation end-products) [27] and reduced endothelium-dependent relaxation of diabetic arteries may be restored when eNOS is over-expressed in the artery *in vitro* with an adenoviral vector [28]. Moreover, diabetic patients with neuropathy and vascular disease have decreased expression of the eNOS in their skin [29].

b) *Increased NO destruction.* As mentioned above, NO has a very short half-life, being very susceptible to oxidation by ROS. The combination of superoxide anion and nitric oxide (reaction that occurs immediately after the contact of NO with O_2^-) leads to the generation of a highly toxic species, the peroxynitrite. Peroxynitrite chemically oxidizes proteins, lipids and DNA and leads to the loss of NO biological activity. Furthermore, peroxynitrite inhibits the biosynthesis of NO by oxidizing tetrahydrobiopterin (and subsequently inactivating the eNOS) [30]. Thus, increased oxidative stress (a *sine qua non* of the diabetic state) leads – by generating peroxynitrite – to a reduced availability of biological active NO via a dual mechanism. *In vivo*, the endothelial dysfunction caused by NO deficiency can be (at least partially) reversed experimentally by antioxidants such as vitamins A, C and E [31]. A family of enzymes termed "superoxide dismutases" (SOD's) has evolved to scavenge most of the superoxide anion produced by enzymatic reactions in cells, the major isoform in blood vessels being Cu^{2+}/Zn^{2+} SOD. There is now considerable evidence that a reduction in SOD activity decreases NO bioavailability in diabetes. The reduction of SOD activity in the diabetic tissues [32] has been attributed to the glycation of the enzyme by chronic exposure to hyperglycemia [33]. Moreover, addition of SOD to isolated arteries ameliorates abnormalities in NO-dependent vasodilatation caused by diabetes [34].

THE ROLE OF ENDOTHELIN-1

Endothelin-1 (ET-1) is the strongest endogenous vasoconstrictor and is secreted by the endothelium in response to insulin and other agonists. Endothelin can bind to two receptors: ET-A which exists in vascular smooth muscle and mediates vasoconstriction; and ET-B which is found predominately in endothelial cells and mediates vasodilatation through the release of NO and prostacyclin [35]. In one study in healthy subjects, for example, selective antagonism of the ET-A receptor caused vasodilatation associated with an increase in nitric oxide generation; this response was attenuated by inhibition of NO synthesis or antagonism of the ET-B receptor [36].

ET-1 blockade improves insulin-mediated vasorelaxation in rats, implying that insulin-mediated vascular responses reflect, in part, a balance between NO and ET-1 production [37]. There is also evidence that ET-1 impairs calcium-dependent endothelial responses. Chronic ET-1 blockade improves acetylcholine-mediated vasodilatation in hyperinsulinemic rats, but has no effect in control animals [38]. In addition, ET-1 may mediate the cardiovascular and renal effects of angiotensin II. A further way in which ET-1 may impair endothelial function is by inducing NADPH oxidase activity in endothelial cells and finally increasing the production of superoxide anion [26]. Interestingly, circulating ET-1 levels are elevated in diabetic and insulin-resistant subjects [39], while ET-1 inhibits glucose uptake and administration of exogenous ET-1 induces insulin resistance in humans [26], suggesting a possible dual pathogenic link.

All these data suggest that hyperinsulinemia enhances ET-1 production by endothelial cells and that this may consequently worsen insulin resistance and promote endothelial dysfunction by decreasing the production of (and competing with) NO.

THE ROLE OF RENIN ANGIOTENSIN SYSTEM

As mentioned above (Table 13.1), the endothelium produces mediators that induce vasoconstriction, including angiotensin II [40] and regulates vascular tone by maintaining a balance between vasodilatation (NO production) and vasoconstriction (Angiotensin-II generation). Angiotensin-II is produced in local tissues by the endothelium, the key enzyme being the angiotensin-converting enzyme (ACE) [3]. Locally, angiotensin-II binds to and regulates the tone of vascular smooth muscle cells (VSMC) via specific angiotensin-II receptors. Depending upon the specific receptor activated, angiotensin-II can exert regulatory effects upon several VSMC functional activities including vasoconstriction, growth, proliferation, and differentiation. Overall, the actions of angiotensin-II oppose those of NO. Interestingly, high local ACE concentrations will antagonize NO activity not only by increasing angiotensin-II generation but also, and possibly most importantly, by decreasing concentrations of bradykinin, a NO-generating vasodilator [41]. In addition to its vasoconstrictor properties, angiotensin-II promotes endothelin production and stimulates superoxide anion production from vascular NADPH oxidase [42].

A model of regulation of vascular tone (and lumen regulation) in which ACE plays a key role has emerged in recent years. This model predicts that high ACE activity will result in vasoconstriction because of a decrease in NO generation and increased generation of angiotensin-II. This results in contraction of VSMC and a decrease in lumen diameter. Moreover, sustained activity of this enzyme will presumably be associated with an increase in the growth, proliferation, and differentiation of the VSMC as well as a decrease in the antiproliferative action of NO coupled with a decrease in local fibrinolysis and an increase in platelet aggregation [3].

T2DM, insulin resistance and atherosclerosis are all associated with activation of the renin-angiotensin system, with high ACE activity and, as shown above, deleterious effects on normal endothelial function. This is why the inhibition of this system would be expected to be beneficial. Indeed, ACE inhibitors and angiotensin-II receptor antagonists have been shown to improve endothelial function in T2DM patients [43, 44].

MECHANISMS OF ENDOTHELIAL DYSFUNCTION IN T2DM AND INSULIN RESISTANCE

The proposed mechanisms by which diabetes causes endothelial dysfunction are diverse, and multiple changes in cellular enzymatic activity, levels of metabolites and changes in ionic and redox homeostasis occur in the vessel walls of the "target tissues".

THE ROLE OF HYPERGLYCEMIA

Hyperglycemia leads to endothelial dysfunction by at least three major mechanisms: a) synthesis of diacylglycerol (DAG) which activates protein kinase C (PKC), b) increased aldose reductase metabolism and c) formation of advanced glycation end-products (AGE).

a) *Increased DAG/PKC Signaling.* Hyperglycemia increases the flux of glucose through the glycolytic pathway, increasing *de novo* synthesis of DAG [45]. Increased DAG has been shown to occur in both endothelial cells and VSMC, leading to increased PKC activity. Both DAG and PKC are important intracellular signaling molecules involved in a wide variety of cellular responses, including promoting the synthesis and/or action of prostanoids, limiting NO production, increasing superoxide anion and endothelin-1 production and modulating the contraction of VSMC, *i.e.* vasoconstriction [46]. Activation of PKC will also contribute to the depletion of the cellular NADPH pool [3].

b) *Increased Aldose Reductase Activity.* Aldose Reductase is a cytosolic, monomeric oxidoreductase that catalyzes the NADPH-dependent reduction of a wide variety of carbonyl compounds including glucose. When cells are exposed to hyperglycemia, metabolism is shifted increasingly through the polyol pathway and this may lead to the increased conversion of reduced NADPH to its oxidized form ($NADP^+$). Depletion of NADPH may limit the conversion of oxidized glutathione (GSSG) to its reduced form (GSH). GSH is a major cellular antioxidant, and its depletion leads to increased oxidative stress, which in turn decreases the bioavailability of NO. Depletion of NADPH may also directly reduce eNOS activity, for which it is also a co-factor [47]. Moreover, increases in NADH (which result from enhanced sorbitol dehydrogenase activity) have been cited as stimulating the activity of NADPH oxidases that produce superoxide anion [48] and also inhibiting activity of the enzyme glyceraldehyde-3-phosphate dehydrogenase and increasing concentrations of triose phosphate [49]. Elevated triose phosphate concentrations in turn, could increase formation of both methylglyoxal, a precursor of AGEs, and DAG, thus activating PKC.

c) *Increased AGE formation.* Chronic hyperglycemia leads to non-enzymatic glycation of proteins and macromolecules finally generating the AGE. Intracellular production of AGE precursors damages target cells by three general mechanisms: 1) Intracellular proteins modified by AGEs have altered function; 2) Extracellular matrix components modified by AGE precursors interact abnormally with other matrix components and with matrix-receptors (integrins) on cells; and 3) Plasma proteins modified by AGE precursors bind to AGE receptors on cells such as macrophages, inducing receptor-mediated ROS production. The interaction AGE with their receptors activates also the pleiotrophic nuclear transcription factor NF-κB, causing pathologic changes in gene expression.

Basic fibroblast growth factor (bFGF) is one of the major AGE-modified proteins in endothelial cells, consequently the endothelial cell mitogenic activity being reduced 70% by AGE formation [50]. For endothelial cells, plasmatic AGE binding to its receptor (RAGE) induces changes in gene expression that include alterations in thrombomodulin, tissue Plasminogen Activator (t-PA), and VCAM-1 [51, 52].

These changes induce procoagulatory changes in the endothelial surface and increase the adhesion of inflammatory cells to the vessel wall. In addition, endothelial RAGE binding mediates, at least in part, the hyper-permeability induced by diabetes, probably through the induction of vascular endothelial growth factor (VEGF) [53]. AGE might also induce endothelial dysfunction by increasing superoxide anion production and scavenging NO [27]. In addition, AGE (and also hyperglycemia-induced activation of PKC) have been shown to mediate the activation of the pleiotrophic nuclear transcription factor NF-κB in endothelial cells and vascular smooth muscle cells [54, 55]. Increasing evidence suggests that NF-κB transcription factor may play important roles in atherosclerosis *via* regulation of genes encoding (between others) TNFα, IL-1, VCAM-1, and ICAM-1 [55].

The seemingly diverse mechanisms listed above may have a common precursor related to a single hyperglycemia induced process: over-production of superoxide anion by the mitochondrial electron transport chain. Preventing this increase on experimental models (bovine aortic endothelial cells) also prevents glycation of intracellular proteins, stimulation of PKC and hyperactivity of polyol pathway with sorbitol accumulation [56]. Thus, the varied mechanisms of diabetic endothelial cell dysfunction may have a common root in the increased production of superoxide anion.

Another issue is the role of acute hyperglycemia (postprandial hyperglycemia) in the pathogenesis of endothelial dysfunction. There is compelling evidence showing that a rapid increase of the blood glucose might alter the physiologic homeostasis of various organs, acting through non-enzymatic labile glycation and production of free radicals [31]. The endothelium is freely permeable to glucose and, as a result, it has almost free glucose supply correlated with its circulating concentration, glucose that will be transformed into energy at the mitochondrial level [56]. This implies that the free glucose influx is transformed not only into energy but also in production of superoxide anion. This led to the hypothesis that an acute increase of glucose serum concentration can equally produce acute oxidative stress and, subsequently, endothelial dysfunction, activation of coagulation and increase of ICAM-1 in the plasma [31].

THE ROLE OF INSULIN RESISTANCE/HYPERINSULINEMIA

There is a growing body of evidence accumulating to demonstrate the coexistence of insulin resistance and endothelial dysfunction. Thus, the vasodilatory responses to acetylcholine (or insulin) were reduced and high levels of plasma endothelin-1 (ET-1), vWF, soluble intercellular adhesion molecule (sICAM), and soluble vascular cell adhesion molecule (sVCAM) were described in non-diabetic but insulin-resistant obese individuals, women with previous gestational diabetes, women with polycystic ovary syndrome, prediabetic, glucose intolerant patients and also in non-diabetic first-degree relatives of patients with diabetes [3, 15, 57, 58].

There is compelling evidence now that insulin itself has important direct effects on the blood vessels. In insulin sensitive individuals and at physiologic concentrations, insulin acts as a vasodilator, an effect that is largely endothelium-dependent through NO production [59]. Insulin promotes NO synthesis and release via a PI-3-kinase dependent signaling pathway [60], and thus has a major anti-atherogenic effect. In contrast, in insulin-resistant individuals, insulin stimulates the release of vasoconstrictor endothelin-1 [26]. Moreover, two other major proatherogenic effects of insulin are the modulation of PDGF-induced VSMC proliferation and the stimulation of VSMC plasminogen activator inhibitor 1 (PAI-1) production [61, 62]. It is worth noticing that the effects of insulin on smooth muscle cells are mediated by the Ras-Raf-MEKK-Mitogen-Activated Protein (MAP) Kinase signal transduction pathway [63, 64].

These observations led to the hypothesis that the disruption of the IRS1/IRS2 – PI3-kinase signaling pathway in the insulin-resistant state leads to endothelial dysfunction. This observation was confirmed by a study in which insulin signaling on the PI3-kinase and MAP-kinase pathways was compared in vascular tissues of lean and obese Zucker rats [65]. Insulin resistant rats showed down-regulation of IRS-1, PI-3K and Akt activity in the vessels. Interestingly, the MAPK pathway, which promotes gene expression and cell growth, remains intact in the insulin resistant animals. These data suggest that in the insulin-resistant state, insulin's vasodilatory and antiatherogenic functions, mediated by PI-3K, may be impaired, whereas proatherogenic actions, mediated through MAPK cascade, may continue and even be enhanced.

Whether this hypothesis is valid in humans and whether hyperinsulinemia per se contributes to endothelial dysfunction in insulin-resistant states, still remains a matter of debate [26].

THE ROLE OF OXIDATIVE STRESS

As discussed above, the endothelium is very susceptible to damage by oxidative stress and the diabetic state is typified by an increased tendency for oxidative stress [66]. The role of oxidant stress in endothelial dysfunction has been the subject of intense debate and research in the recent years. The major sources of ROS in the vessel wall are represented by NADPH oxidase [67] and alterations of eNOS function which, as previously discussed, in the absence of its critical cofactor tetrahydrobiopterin, generates superoxide anion rather than NO [21]. Data supporting the role of oxidant stress in the genesis of endothelial dysfunction in T2DM are offered not only by animal data but also by human studies. For example, in human blood vessels, superoxide anion production by NADPH oxidase is associated with impaired endothelium-dependent vasodilatation and is correlated with the presence of clinical risk factors [68].

THE ROLE OF DYSLIPIDEMIA

Diabetic hyperlipidemia is associated with a characteristic lipoprotein profile that includes a high very-low-density lipoprotein (VLDL) with a correspondent high triglyceride level, a low high-density lipoprotein (HDL), and small, dense LDL. This profile arises (in conditions of insulin resistance and/or hyperglycemia) as a direct result of increased net free fatty acid (FFA) release by insulin resistant adipocytes [24]. Both low HDL and high small, dense LDL (and to some extent high tryglyceride) are each independent risk factors for macrovascular disease.

Small, dense LDL is very prone to oxidation. Oxidized LDL is a major cause of injury to the endothelium and underlying VSMC. In addition to its ability to injure these cells, modified LDL is chemotactic for other monocytes and can up-regulate the expression of genes for macrophage colony stimulating factor (MCSF) and monocyte chemotactic protein (MCP-1) derived from endothelial cells. Thus, it may help expand the inflammatory response by stimulating the replication of monocyte-derived macrophages and the entry of new monocytes into the vascular wall lesions [69].

Regarding the role of FFA, high levels of these molecules have been shown to induce an increased level of oxidation of phospholipids as well as proteins. A proposed hypothesis suggests that this might be one of the etiological factors in inducing endothelial dysfunction in type 2 diabetes [3]. To confirm this hypothesis, a number of studies have assessed the effects of FFA on vascular function. In healthy volunteers, transient increases in circulating FFA led to impairment of endothelium-dependent responses to metacholine [70]. At the cellular level, there is evidence that FFA reduce NO bioavailability by inhibiting eNOS activity and stimulate the production of ROS by NADPH oxidase [71].

OTHER POSSIBLE MECHANISMS

a) *The prothrombotic/antifibrinolytic state.* The diabetic state in humans is associated with a prothrombotic tendency as well as increased platelet aggregation. This may be related to several factors, including diminished NO production [72] and decreased fibrinolytic activity related to high levels of PAI-1 found in the blood of T2DM patients [73]. Remarkably, this defect may be an acquired one. Thus, it has been demonstrated that mimicking the diabetic environment in normal individuals by simultaneous infusion of glucose and intravenous fat emulsion induces an increase in the blood concentrations of PAI-1 [3].

In addition to decreased fibrinolysis, the diabetic state is also associated with an increase in the activation of the coagulation cascade by various mechanisms such as non-enzymatic glycation, formation of advanced glycation end-products (AGE), and decreased heparan sulfate synthesis [24, 63]. Although there is no direct link between activation of the coagulation cascade and endothelial dysfunction in humans, it is possible to speculate that repeated activation of the coagulation cascade may cause over-stimulation of the endothelial cells, and finally induce endothelial dysfunction.

b) *Abnormalities in arachidonic acid metabolism.* This kind of abnormalities have long been recognized in diabetes and are characterized by a reduction in the vasodilator prostaglandin I2 (PGI2 – prostacyclin) and increases in vasoconstrictor eicosanoids including thromboxane A2, prostaglandin endoperoxide, hydroxyeicosotetraenoic acids and F2-isoprostanes [74]. When the levels of these eicosanoids are increased by diabetes, they contribute to reduce NO activity, direct stimulation of vasoconstriction through thromboxane A2 receptors and generation of the oxidative stress [74].

c) *The role of TNFα.* Tumor Necrosis Factor α (TNFα) has been implicated as a link between insulin resistance, diabetes, and endothelial dysfunction [75]. TNFα also can induce the synthesis of other cytokines, which alone or in concert with others, may alter endothelial function. There are several ways in which TNFα might contribute to the genesis of endothelial dysfunction. *In vitro* experiments showed that TNFα impairs insulin signaling by stimulating phosphorylation of IRS proteins, which then inhibit insulin receptor kinase activity, and thus insulin mediated NO genesis [26]. In fact, it was proved that TNFα reduces NO bioavailability in cultured endothelial cells and impairs endothelium dependent dilatation in both animal and human studies [76]. Possible mechanisms include TNFα mediated reduction in eNOS and increased superoxide anion production by vascular NADPH oxidase [77, 78]. TNFα may also promote apoptotic cell death in endothelial cells thereby contributing to endothelial injury, effect that is counteracted by insulin in insulin-sensitive individuals [79].

d) *Overexpression of growth factors and adhesion molecules* has also been implicated as a link between diabetes and proliferation of both endothelial cells and VSMC, possibly promoting neo-vascularization [3].

e) *The role of adiponectin.* Adipocytes are a rich source of biologic active molecules that modulate cardiovascular and metabolic risk, including leptin, resistin and adiponectin [80]. Adiponectin, (also known as AdipQ) has a high homology to complement factor C1q and its plasmatic levels are decreased in obesity, insulin resistance, type 2 diabetes, dyslipidemia and particularly in patients with coronary artery disease [81]. At the same time, weight loss and improved insulin sensitivity are associated with increased adiponectin levels [82, 83]. Thus adiponectin, in contrast to other adipocyte-derived molecules like resistin, seems to have protective metabolic and anti-inflammatory properties. Some experimental and human data sustain this hypothesis.

In vitro, adiponectin suppressed adhesion molecule expression on endothelial cells [84] and reduced vascular inflammatory responses mediated by NF-κB signaling [85]. *In vivo*, adiponectin adhered to endothelial lesions [86] and prevented neointimal formation and atherosclerosis in mice [87]. In addition, administration of adiponectin reversed insulin resistance as a result of obesity [88] and ameliorated hepatic glucose metabolism in mice [89]. In humans, an inverse association between decreased plasma adiponectin levels and increased plasma levels of C reactive Protein (CRP) and IL-6 (both known mediators of vascular wall inflammation) was noted in obese women [81].

All these data suggest a possible protective effect of adiponectin for the endothelium (perhaps mainly mediated by decreased insulin resistance) and a possible link between decreased plasma adiponectin levels and endothelial dysfunction.

THERAPEUTIC PERSPECTIVES

It is obvious that since hyperglycemia is the main cause of endothelial dysfunction in diabetic patients, specific treatment (the aim being near normal blood glucose levels and HbA1c < 7%) with diet/exercise, oral hypoglycemic agents or insulin is a must. However, it should be noted that given the long period of insulin resistance with normal glucose tolerance which precedes the clinical onset of T2DM in most patients, the endothelium may be exposed to a "noxious", pro-atherogenic milieu for many years before the diagnosis of a clinical relevant cardiovascular disease. The close link between insulin resistance and endothelial dysfunction raises the possibility that treatments that primarily target insulin resistance might be equally effective in improving endothelial function. The therapeutic approach could include: life style changing interventions, insulin sensitizers (Metformin and Thiazolidindiones) and maybe ACE inhibitors and Angiotensin Receptor Blockers (ARBs).

On the other hand, there is important evidence regarding a direct beneficial effect of the sulphonylurea drug gliclazide, lipid lowering drugs, antioxidants and ACE inhibitors / ARBs on endothelial function in T2DM patients.

LIFE STYLE CHANGES

There are reports that regular physical exercise and dietary intervention (including reduction in saturated fats and cholesterol and an increase of carbohydrates, especially with a low glycaemic index, and dietary fibres) lead to improvements not only in insulin sensitivity (mainly by inducing weight loss), but also in endothelial function [90].

INSULIN SENSITIZERS

As discussed above, insulin resistance is closely linked with endothelial dysfunction, even before the clinical onset of T2DM. This is why, at least theoretically, improvement of insulin sensitivity will lead to an improvement of endothelial function. The main pharmacological classes are represented by biguanides and thiazolidindiones.

a) *Biguanides*. Metformin is widely used in the treatment of T2DM and, in addition to the glucose lowering action, it has been shown to lower triglyceride and FFA levels reduce insulin resistance and hyperinsulinemia and help with weight reduction [91]. Metformin treatment has been shown to improve endothelial function in T2DM patients by reducing insulin resistance, the correlation between these two parameters being

very strong [92]. In addition, Metformin also reduces PAI-1 levels in obese T2DM patients and may reduce the formation of AGEs by reacting with dicarbonyl compounds such as methylglyoxal and glyoxal [93]. Thus, it is not surprising that Metformin treatment was associated with a more favorable outcome with respect to development of diabetes-related end-points, all-cause mortality and stroke in the UKPDS [94].

b) *Thiazolidindiones*. The thiazolidindiones are a novel class of insulin sensitizing drugs, which act by interacting with the nuclear transcription factor, Peroxisome Proliferator Activated Receptor (PPAR) γ, interaction which leads to increased (or decreased) expression of different "target" genes. Thiazolidindiones improve insulin sensitivity, action explained (among others) by an increased expression of GLUT1, GLUT4, Glucokinase and PI3-K genes and decreased levels of TNFα, FFAs, leptin and resistin [95, 96]. Finally, there are reports of increased plasma adiponectin levels after treatment with PPARγ agonists, associated with improved insulin sensitivity [97].

Thiazolidindiones have some anti-atherogenic effects on the vascular wall, including inhibition of VSMC proliferation and migration [96], reduction of VCAM-1 and ICAM-1 expression on endothelial cells [98], and inhibition of TNFα and MCP1 expression [99]. Regarding the direct effect of PPARγ agonists on endothelial function, there are reports about improvements in endothelial function with these agents both *in vitro* and *in vivo*. These include suppression of endothelin-1 secretion and increased endothelium-derived C-type natriuretic peptide production [100], and improved endothelial-dependent vasodilatation of brachial artery [101]. There are also reports regarding significant decreases of PAI-1 synthesis in the vascular wall in individuals with insulin resistance syndrome [102].

GLICLAZIDE

Gliclazide is an oral hypoglycemic agent from the second-generation sulphonylurea class. In addition to its proved long-term efficacy in maintaining glycemic control, gliclazide has unique properties in improving endothelial function and providing vascular protection in T2DM patients

[103]. All these will be addressed in detail in another chapter of this book.

LIPID LOWERING THERAPY

As previously discussed, hyperlipidemia, in addition to its major pro-atherogenic effect, has an important role in the genesis of endothelial dysfunction in T2DM. Hence, lipid-lowering therapy in T2DM has proven beneficial effects on prevention of cardiovascular disease and, at least theoretically, it might improve endothelial function. The major classes of drugs used today include HMG-CoA reductase inhibitors (statins) and Peroxisome Proliferator Activated Receptor (PPAR) α agonists (fibrates).

This is not the objective of this chapter to discuss either the mechanism of lipid lowering action of these drugs or the algorithm for hyperlipidemia treatment, which is the subject of internationally widely accepted guidelines [104, 105]. We shall focus here only on the direct effect of statins and fibrates on endothelial function, irrespective of their lipid lowering action.

a) *Statins*. It is well established the role of 3-hydroxy-3-methyl-glutaryl-coenzyme A (HMG-CoA) reductase inhibitors (statins) in the primary and secondary prevention of cardiovascular disease due to their cholesterol lowering action. In addition, it is increasingly apparent that statins have some other cardio-protective properties, the so-called "pleiotrophic effects". Recently, this was indirectly proved by the results of the Heart Protection Study [106]. This study showed beyond doubt that statin treatment (simvastatin 40 mg qid) significantly reduces the rates of major cardiovascular events irrespective of the initial lipid profile of the patients.

Statins increase NO bioavailability and improve endothelial function in patients with atherosclerosis [107]. At the cellular level, statins stimulate NO production by up-regulating expression of eNOS mRNA, and increasing protein levels [108]. In addition, statins scavenge superoxide anion in a dose-dependent manner and inhibit superoxide anion production by inhibition of NADPH oxidase, independently of their lipid lowering actions [109].

b) *Fibrates*. This class of drugs exerts its pharmacological actions *via* interaction with the group of nuclear transcription factors represented by PPARα, interaction which leads to increased (or decreased) expression of different genes. A lot of data have accumulated recently regarding the direct role of fibrates in improving endothelial function, mainly by interfering with various pro-inflammatory mechanisms involved in the genesis of atherosclerosis. These include inhibition of NFκB signal pathway and consecutively a reduction in adhesion molecule production (VCAM1, ICAM1); inhibition of IL-1β induced expression of Cyclooxygenase-2 in VSMCs, lowering of plasma IL-6 and C Reactive Protein (CRP) and inhibition of endothelin-1 production by interfering with AP-1 transcription factor [110]. In addition, PPARα activators inhibit thrombin induced ET-1 secretion in human endothelial cells [111] and negatively regulate fibrinogen-β expression [112].

ACE INHIBITORS AND ANGIOTENSIN RECEPTOR BLOCKERS (ARB)

Mediators of the Renin Angiotensin System (RAS) are associated with the insulin resistance syndrome and Angiotensin-II locally produced by endothelial cells is one important mediator of endothelial dysfunction. Thus, it is expected that drugs which block the RAS may be of benefit. An indirect proof was provided by large-scale prevention trials, such as the Heart Outcomes Prevention Evaluation Study (HOPE), which showed that ACE inhibitors significantly reduce cardiovascular mortality and morbidity, particularly in T2DM patients [113]. Interestingly, perhaps as a consequence of improved insulin sensitivity, treatment with Ramipril in the HOPE Study did reduce the incidence of new cases of diabetes [114].

Two effects may be taken into account. First, ACE inhibitors improve insulin sensitivity and, thus, may indirectly ameliorate endothelial function. The effect on insulin sensitivity was shown both in animals [115] and humans [116]. This effect could be explained by increased IRS-1 tyrosine phosphorylation and PI-3K activity and inhibition of bradykinin degradation. Second, ACE inhibitors may directly improve endothelial function, perhaps by blocking local endothelial Angiotensin-II production. This was first shown in non-diabetic, normotensive, coronary disease patients, in which 6 months treatment with quinapril led to a significant net improvement, in the vasodilatory response to acetylcholine – The TREND (Trial on Reversing Endothelial Dysfunction) Study [117]. The hypothesis was also confirmed in T2DM patients, for which treatment with ACE inhibitors improved endothelial function [43].

Quite few data are available regarding the efficacy of Angiotensin-II Receptor Blockers (ARBs) in improving endothelial function. Some human studies showed improvements in endothelial function in patients with T2DM [44].

ANTIOXIDANTS

As previously discussed, there are a lot of data supporting the important role of the ROS in the genesis of endothelial dysfunction in T2DM. Antioxidant therapy has been shown to improve endothelial function in experimental studies [118]. Although epidemiological studies suggest a strong inverse correlation between dietary consumption of antioxidants (mainly different vitamin supplements) and cardiovascular disease [119], randomized trials of antioxidants provided conflicting and disappointing results. Even though early small scale studies showed a reduction in the frequency of cardiovascular events [120], a recent large-scale trial [121] could not find any evidence of a protective effect for vitamins E, C, and A. Another issue is related to the dietary supplements of L-arginine. Given that L-arginine is a substrate for NOS, it was assumed that L-arginine supplementation would activate NOS and produce more NO with greater vasodilatation. This hypothesis has been tested and there is some evidence regarding reversal of endothelial dysfunction associated with diabetes by administration of L-Arginine [122], but these data require reconfirmation.

REFERENCES

1. Amos AF, McCarty DJ, Zimmet P. The rising global burden of diabetes and its complications: estimates and projections to the year 2010. *Diabet Med*, **14**: S1–S85, 1997.

2. Wiltshire EJ, Gent R, Hirte C, Pena A, Thomas DW, Couper JJ. Endothelial dysfunction relates to folate status in children and adolescents with type 1 diabetes. *Diabetes*, **51**: 2282–2286, 2002.

3. Calles-Escandon J, Cipolla M. Diabetes and endothelial dysfunction: a clinical perspective. *Endocr Rev*, **22**: 36–52, 2001.

4. James RW. The pathogenesis of cardiovascular disease in diabetes. In: Mogensen CE (ed) *Hypertension and Diabetes* Vol. 1, Lippincott Williams & Wilkins, London, UK, 2002, pp 43–56.

5. Kuhn FE, Mohler ER, Satler N *et al*. Effects of high density lipoprotein on acetylcholine induced coronary vasoreactivity. *Am J Cardiol*, **68**: 1425–1428, 1991.

6. Quyyumi AA, Dakak N, Andrews NP, Husain S, Arora S, Gilligan DM, *et al*. Nitric oxide activity in the human coronary circulation: Impact of risk factors for coronary atherosclerosis. *J Clin Invest*, **95**: 1747–1755, 1995.

7. Hogikyan RV, Galecki AT, Pitt B, Halter JB, Greene DA, Supiano MA. Specific impairment of endothelium-dependent vasodilation in subjects with type 2 diabetes independent of obesity. *J Clin Endocrinol Metab*, **83**: 1946–1952, 1998.

8. Boger RH, Bode-Broger SM, Thiele W, Junker W, Alexander K, Frolich JC *et al*. Biochemical evidence for impaired nitric oxide synthesis in patients with peripheral arterial occlusive disease. *Circulation*, **95**: 2068–1074, 1997.

9. Diodati JG, Dakak N, Gilligan DM, Quyyumi AA. Effect of atherosclerosis on endothelium-dependent inhibition of platelet activation in humans. *Circulation*, **98**: 17–24, 1998

10. Wenzel RR, Duthiers N, Noll G, Bucher J, Kaufmann U, Luscher TF. Endothelin and calcium antagonists in the skin microcirculation of patients with coronary artery disease. *Circulation*, **94**: 316–322, 1996.

11. Boger RH, Bode-Boger SM, Szuba A, Tsao PS, Chan JR, Tangphao O, *et al*. Asymmetric dimethylarginine (ADMA): A novel risk factor for endothelial dysfunction: Its role in hypercholesterolemia. *Circulation*, **98**: 1842–1847, 1998.

12. Mangin EL Jr, Kugiyama K, Nguy JH, Kerns SA, Henry PD. Effects of lysolipids and oxidatively modified low density lipoproteins on endothelium-dependent relaxation of rabbit aorta. *Circ Res*, **72**: 161–166, 1993.

13. Antonetti DA, Barber AJ, Khin S, Lieth E, Tarbell JM, Gardner TW. Vascular permeability in experimental diabetes is associated with reduced endothelial occludin content: vascular endothelial growth factor decreases occludin in retinal endothelial cells. Penn State Retina Research Group. *Diabetes*, **47**:1953–1959, 1998.

14. Kario K, Matsuo T, Kobayashi H, Matsuo M, Sakata T, Miyata T. Activation of tissue factor-induced coagulation and endothelial cell dysfunction in non-insulin-dependent diabetic patients with microalbuminuria. *Arterioscler Thromb Vasc Biol*, **15**: 1114–1120, 1995.

15. Caballlero AE, Arora S, Saouaf R, Lim SC, Smakowski P, Park JY, *et al*. Microvascular and macrovascular reactivity is reduced in subjects at risk for type 2 diabetes. *Diabetes*, **48**: 1856–1862, 1999.

16. Furchgott RF, Zawadzki JV. The obligatory role of endothelial cells in the relaxation of arterial smooth muscle by acetylcholine. *Nature* **288**: 373–376, 1980.

17. Palmer RMJ, Ferrige AG, Moncada S. Nitric oxide release accounts for the biological activity of endothelium-derived relaxing factor. *Nature*, **327**:524–526, 1987.

18. Ignarro LJ, Buga GM, Wood KS, Byrns RE, Chaudhuri G. Endothelium-derived relaxing factor produced and released from artery and vein is nitric oxide. *Proc Natl Acad Sci USA*, **84**: 9265–9269, 1987.

19. Schmidt HH, Nau H, Wittfoht W *et al*. Arginine is a physiological precursor of endothelium-derived nitric oxide. *Eur J Pharmacol*, **154**: 213–216, 1988.

20. Andrew P, Mayer B. Enzymatic function of nitric oxide synthases. *Cardiovasc Res*, **43**: 521–531, 1999.

21. Xia Y, Dawson VL, Dawson TM, Snyder SH, Zweier JL. Nitric oxide synthase generates superoxide and nitric oxide in arginine depleted cells leading to peroxynitrite-mediated cellular injury. *Proc Nat Acad Sci USA*, **93**: 6770–6774, 1996.

22. Busse R, Fleming I, Hecker M Signal transduction in endothelium-dependent vasodilatation. *Eur Heart J*, **14[Suppl I]**: 2–9, 1993.

23. Harrison DG. Cellular and molecular mechanisms of endothelial cell dysfunction. *J Clin Invest*, **100**: 2153–2157, 1997.

24. Brownlee M, Aiello LP, Friedman E, Vinik AI, Nesto RW, Boulton AJM. Complications of diabetes mellitus. In: Larsen PR, Kronenberg HM, Melmed S and Polonsky KE (ed). *Williams Textbook of Endocrinology*, 10'th ed, Saunders, Philadelphia, Pennsylvania, USA, 2003, pp 1510–1583.

25. Arnold W, Mittal C, Katsuki S, Murad F. Nitric oxide activates guanylate cyclase and increases guanosine 3,5-cyclic monophosphate in various tissue preparations. *Proc Nat Acad Sci USA*, **74**: 3203–3207, 1977.

26. Wheatcroft SB, Williams IL, Shah AM, Kearney MT. Pathophysiological implications of insulin resistance on vascular endothelial function. *Diabetic Med*, **20**: 255–268, 2003.

27. Chakravarthy U, Hayes RG, Stitt AW, McAuley E, Archer DB. Constitutive nitric oxide synthase expression in retinal vascular endothelial cells is suppressed by high glucose and advanced glycation end-products. *Diabetes*, **47**: 945–952, 1998.

28. Lund DD, Faraci FM, Miller FJ Jr, Heistad DD. Gene transfer of endothelial nitric oxide synthase improves relaxation of carotid arteries from diabetic rabbits. *Circulation*, **101**: 1027–1033, 2000.

29. Veves A, Akbari CM, Primavera J *et al*. Endothelial dysfunction and the expression of endothelial nitric oxide synthetase in diabetic neuropathy, vascular disease and foot ulceration. *Diabetes*, **47**: 457–463, 1998.

30. Laursen JB, Somers M, Kurz S, McCann L, Warnholtz A, Freeman BA, *et al*. Endothelial regulation of vasomotion in apoE-deficient mice: implications for interactions between peroxynitrite and tetrahydrobiopterin. *Circulation*, **103**: 1282–1288, 2001.

31. Ceriello A. The possible role of postprandial hyperglycemia in the pathogenesis of diabetic complications. *Diabetologia*, **46[Suppl.1]**: M9–M16, 2003.

32. Loven D, Schedl H, Wilson H, *et al*. Effect of insulin and oral glutathione on gluthatione levels and superoxide dismutase activities in organs of rats with streptozotocin-induced diabetes. *Diabetes*, **35**: 503–507, 1986.

33. Oda A, Bannai C, Yamaoka T, Katori T, Matsushima T, Yamashita K. Inactivation of Cu,Zn-superoxide dismutase by in vitro glycosylation and in erythrocytes of diabetic patients. *Horm Metab Res*, **26**: 1–4, 1994.

34. Vallejo S, Angulo J, Peiro C, *et al*. Highly glycated oxyhemoglobin impairs nitric oxide relaxations in human mesenteric microvessels. *Diabetologia*, **43**: 83–90, 2000.

35. Fujise K, Stacy L, Beck P, Yeh ET, Chuang A, Brock TA, Willerson JT. Differential effects of endothelin receptor activation on cyclic flow variations in rat mesenteric arteries. *Circulation*, **96**: 3641–3646, 1997.

36. Verhaar MC, Strachan FE, Newby DE, Cruden NL, Koomans HA, Rabelink TJ, Webb DJ. Endothelin-A receptor antagonist-mediated vasodilatation is attenuated by inhibition of nitric oxide synthesis and by endothelin-B receptor blockade. *Circulation*, **97**: 752–756, 1998.

37. Verma S, Yao L, Stewart DJ, Dumont AS, Anderson TJ, McNeill JH. Endothelin antagonism uncovers insulin-mediated vasorelaxation in vitro and in vivo. *Hypertension*, 37:328–333, 2001.

38. Verma S, Skarsgaard P, Bhanot S, Yao L, Laher I, McNeill JH. Reactivity of mesenteric arteries from fructose-hypertensive rats to endothelin-1. *Am J Hypertens*, 10: 1010–1019, 1997.

39. Piatti P, Monti LD, Galli L, Fragasso G, Valescchi G, conti M, *et al*. Relationship between endothelin-1 concentration and metabolic alterations typical of the insulin resistance syndrome. *Metabolism*, 49: 748–752, 2000.

40. McFarlane R, McCredie RJ, Bonney MA, Molyneaux L, Zilkens R, Celermajer DS, Yue DK. Angiotensin converting enzyme inhibition and arterial endothelial function in adults with type 1 diabetes mellitus. *Diabetic Med*, 16: 62–66, 1999.

41. Mombouli JV. ACE inhibition, endothelial function and coronary artery lesions. Role of kinins and nitric oxide. *Drugs*, 54 [Suppl 5]: 12–22, 1997.

42. Luscher TF, Barton M. Endothelins and endothelin receptor antagonists: therapeutic considerations for a novel class of cardiovascular drugs. *Circulation*, 102: 2434–2440, 2000.

43. O'Driscoll G, Green D, Maiorana A, Stanton K, Colreavy F, Taylor R. Improvement in endothelial function by angiotensin-converting enzyme inhibition in non-insulin-dependent diabetes. *J Am Coll Cardiol*, 33: 1506–1511, 1999.

44. Cheetham C, Collis J, O'Driscoll G, Stanton K, Taylor R, Green D. Losartan, an angiotensin type 1 receptor antagonist, improves endothelial function in non-insulin-dependent diabetes. *J Am Coll Cardiol*, 36: 1461–1466, 2000.

45. Wolf BA, Williamson JR, Easom RA, Chang K, Sherman WR, Turk J. Diacylglycerol accumulation and microvascular abnormalities induced by elevated glucose levels. *J Clin Invest*, 87:31–38, 1991.

46. Cipolla MJ. Elevated glucose potentiates contraction of isolated rat resistance arteries and augments protein kinase C-induced intracellular calcium release. *Metabolism*, 48:1015–1022, 1999.

47. Okuda Y, Kawashima K, Suzuki S, *et al*. Restoration of nitric oxide production by aldose reductase inhibitor in human endothelial cells cultured in high-glucose medium. *Life Sci*, 60: L53–L56, 1997.

48. Ido Y, Kilo C, Williamson JR. Cytosolic NADH/NAD$^+$, free radicals, and vascular dysfunction in early diabetes mellitus. *Diabetologia*, 40: S115–S117, 1997.

49. Williamson JR, Chang K, Frangos M, *et al*. Hyperglycemic pseudohypoxia and diabetic complications. *Diabetes*, 42: 801–813, 1993.

50. Giardino I, Edelstein D, Brownlee M, Nonenzymatic glycosylation in vitro and in bovine endothelial cells alters basic fibroblast growth factor activity: a model for intracellular glycosylation in diabetes. *J Clin Invest*, 94: 110–114, 1994.

51. Schmidt AM, Hori O, Chen JX, Li JF, Crandall J, Zhang J, *et al*. Advanced glycation end-products interacting with their endothelial receptor induce expression of vascular cell adhesion molecule-1 (VCAM-1) in cultured human endothelial cells and in mice: a potential mechanism of the accelerated vasculopathy of diabetes. *J Clin Invest*, 96: 1395–1403 1995.

52. Sengoelge G, Fodinger M, Skoupy S, Ferrara I, Zangerle C, Rogy M, *et al*. Endothelial cell adhesion molecule and PMNL response to inflammatory stimuli and AGE-modified fibronectin. *Kidney Int*, 54: 1637–1651 1998.

53. Lu M, Kuroki M, Amano S, Tolentino M, Keough K, Kim I, *et al*. Advanced glycation end-products increase retinal vascular endothelial growth factor expression. *J Clin Invest*, 101: 1219–1224, 1998.

54. Lander HM, Tauras JM, Ogiste JS, Hori O, Moss RA, Schmidt AM. Activation of the receptor for advanced glycation end-products triggers a p21(ras)-dependent mitogen-activated protein kinase pathway regulated by oxidative stress. *J Biol Chem*, 272: 17810–17814, 1997.

55. Yerneni KK, Bai W, Khan BV, Medford RM, Natarajan R. Hyperglycemia-induced activation of nuclear transcription factor kappa B in vascular smooth muscle cells. *Diabetes*, 48: 855–864, 1999.

56. Nishikawa T, Edelstein D, Du XL, *et al*. Normalizing mitochondrial superoxide production blocks three pathways of hyperglycaemic damage. *Nature*, 404: 787–790, 2000.

57. Laws A, Stefanick ML, Reaven GM., Insulin resistance and hypertriglyceridemia in nondiabetic relatives of patients with non-insulin-dependent diabetes mellitus. *J Clin Endocrinol Metab*, 69:343-347, 1989.

58. Cleland SJ, Petrie JR, Small M, Elliott HL, Connell JM. Insulin action is associated with endothelial function in hypertension and type 2 diabetes. *Hypertension*, 35: 507–511, 2000.

59. Kearney MT, Cowley AJ, Stubbs TA, Evans A, Macdonald IA. Depressor action of insulin on skeletal muscle vasculature: a novel mechanism for postprandial hypotension in the elderly. *J Am Coll Cardiol*, 31: 209–216, 1998.

60. Kuboki K, Jiang ZY, Takahara N, Ha SW, Igarashi M, Yamauchi T, *et al*. Regulation of endothelial constitutive nitric oxide synthase gene expression in endothelial cells and in vivo: a specific vascular action of insulin. *Circulation*, 101: 676–681, 2000.

61. Stolar MW. Atherosclerosis in diabetes: the role of hyperinsulinemia. *Metabolism*, **7[Suppl 1]**: 1–9, 1988.

62. Banskota NK, Taub R, Zellner K, King GL. Insulin, insulin-like growth factor I, and platelet-derived growth factor interact additively in the induction of the protooncogene *c-myc* and cellular proliferation in cultured bovine aortic smooth muscle cells. *Mol Endocrinol*, **8**: 1183–1190, 1989.

63. King G, Brownlee M. The cellular and molecular mechanisms of diabetic complications. *Endocrinol Metab Clin North Am*, **25**: 255–270, 1996.

64. Hsueh WA, Law RE. Cardiovascular risk continuum: implications of insulin resistance and diabetes. *Am J Med*, **105**: S4-S14, 1998.

65. Jiang ZY, Lin YW, Clemont A, Feener EP, Hein KD, Igarashi M, *et al.* Characterization of selective resistance to insulin signaling in the vasculature of obese Zucker (fa/fa) rats. *J Clin Invest*, **104**: 447–457, 1999.

66. Giugliano D, Ceriello A, Paolisso G. Oxidative stress and diabetic vascular complications. *Diabetes Care*, **19**: 257–267, 1996.

67. Griendling KK, Sorescu D, Ushio-Fukai M. NAD(P)H oxidase. Role in cardiovascular biology and disease. *Circulation Res*, **86**: 494–501, 2000.

68. Guzic TJ, West NEJ, Black E, McDonald D, Ratnatunga C, Pillai R, *et al.* Vascular superoxide production by NAD(P)H oxidase. Association with endothelial dysfunction and clinical risk factors. *Circulation Res*, **86**: E85-E90, 2000.

69. Ross R. Atherosclerosis: an inflammatory disease. *N Engl J Med*, **340**: 115–126, 1999.

70. Steinberg HO, Tarshoby M, Monestel R, Hook G, Cronin J, Johnson A, *et al.* Elevated circulating free fatty acid levels impair endothelium-dependent vasodilation. *J Clin Invest*, **100**: 1230–1239, 1997.

71. Inoguchi T, Li P, Umeda F, Yu HY, Kakimoto M, Imamura M, *et al.* High glucose level and free fatty acid stimulate reactive oxygen species production through protein kinase C-dependent activation of NAD(P)H oxidase in cultured vascular cells. *Diabetes*, **49**: 1939–1945, 2000.

72. Cipolla MJ, Harker CT, Porter JM. Endothelial function and adrenergic reactivity in human type-II diabetic resistance arteries. *J Vasc Surg*, **23**: 940–949, 1996.

73. Schneider DJ, Nordt TK, Sobel BE. Attenuated fibrinolysis and accelerated atherogenesis in type II diabetic patients. *Diabetes*, **42**: 1–7, 1993.

74. Cohen RA. Nitric oxide bioavailability and diabetic endothelial cell dysfunction. In: Tooke J (ed) *Vascular Disease in Diabetes*, Wells Healthcare Communications Ltd, Kent, UK, 2001, pp 87–106.

75. Peraldi P, Spiegelman B. TNFα and insulin resistance: summary and future prospects. *Mol Cell Biochem*, **182**:169–175, 1998.

76. Bhagat K, Vallance P. Inflammatory cytokines impair endothelium-dependent dilatation in human veins *in vivo*. *Circulation*, **96**:3042–3047, 1997.

77. Yoshzumi M, Perella M, Burnett J, Lee M. Tumor necrosis factor downregulates endothelial nitric oxide synthase mRNA by shortening its half-life. *Circulation Res*, **73**: 205–209, 1993.

78. DeKeulenaer GW, Alexander RW, Ushio-Fukai M, Ishizaka N, Griendling KK. Tumor necrosis factor alpha activates a p22 phox-based NADH oxidase in vascular smooth muscle. *Biochem J*, **329**: 653–657, 1998.

79. Hermann C, Assmus B, Urbich C, *et al.* Insulin-mediated stimulation of protein kinase Akt: a potent survival signaling cascade for endothelial cells. *Arterioscler Thromb Vasc Biol*, **20**: 402–409, 2000.

80. Frühbeck G, Gomez-Ambrosi J, Muruzabal FJ, Burrell MA. The adipocyte: a model for integration of endocrine and metabolic signaling in energy metabolism regulation. *Am J Physiol*, **280**: E827–E847, 2001

81. Engeli S, Feldpausch M, Gorzelniak K, Hartwig F, Heintze U, Janke J, *et al.* Association between adiponectin and mediators of inflammation in obese women. *Diabetes*, **52**:942–947, 2003.

82. Maeda N, Takahashi M, Funahashi T, Kihara S, Nishizawa H, Kishida K, *et al.* PPARγ ligands increase expression and plasma concentrations of adiponectin, an adipose-derived protein. *Diabetes*, **50**: 2094–2099, 2001.

83. Tschritter O, Fritsche A, Thamer C, Haap M, Shirkavand F, Rahe S *et al.* Plasma adiponectin concentrations predict insulin sensitivity of both glucose and lipid metabolism. *Diabetes*, **52**:239–243, 2003.

84. Ouchi N, Kihara S, Arita Y, Maeda K, Kuriyama H, Okamoto Y, *et al.* Novel modulator for endothelial adhesion molecules: adipocyte – derived plasma protein adiponectin. *Circulation*, **100**: 2473–2476, 1999.

85. Ouchi N, Kihara S, Arita Y, Okamoto Y, Maeda K, Kuriyama H, *et al.* Adiponectin, an adipocyte-derived plasma protein, inhibits endothelial NF-κB signaling through a cAMP-dependent pathway. *Circulation*, **102**: 1296–1301, 2000.

86. Okamoto Y, Arita Y, Nishida M, Muraguchi M, Ouchi N, Takahashi M, *et al.* An adipocyte-derived plasma protein, adiponectin, adheres to injured vascular walls. *Horm Metab Res*, **32**: 47–50, 2000.

87. Okamoto Y, Kihara S, Ouchi N, Nishida M, Arita Y, Kumada M, *et al.* Adiponectin reduces

atherosclerosis in apolipoprotein E-deficient mice. *Circulation*, **106**: 2767–2770, 2002.

88. Yamauchi T, Kamon J, Waki H, Terauchi Y, Kubota N, Hara K, *et al*. The fat-derived hormone adiponectin reverses insulin resistance associated with lipoatrophy and obesity. *Nat Med*, 7:941–946, 2001.

89. Berg AH, Combs TP, Du X, Brownlee M, Scherer PE. The adipocyte-secreted protein Acrp30 enhances hepatic insulin action. Nat Med, 7: 947–953, 2001.

90. Goodyear LJ, Kahn BB. Exercise, glucose transport, and insulin sensitivity. *Annu Rev Med* 49: 235–261, 1998.

91. DeFronzo RA. Pathogenesis of type 2 diabetes: implications for metformin. *Drugs*, **58[Suppl1]:** 29–30, 1999.

92. Mather KJ, Verma S, Anderson TJ. Improved endothelial function with metformin in type 2 diabetes mellitus. *J Am Coll Cardiol*, **37**:1344–1350, 2001.

93. Beisswenger PJ, Howell SK, Touchette AD, Lal S, Szwergold BS. Metformin reduces systemic methylglyoxal levels in type 2 diabetes. *Diabetes*, **48**: 198–202, 1999.

94. UK Prospective Diabetes Study (UKPDS) Group. Effect of intensive blood-glucose control with metformin on complications in over-weight patients with type 2 diabetes (UKPDS 34). *Lancet*, **352**: 854–865, 1998.

95. Kahn CR, Chen L, Cohen SE. Unraveling the mechanism of action of thiazolidindiones. *J Clin Invest*, **106**: 1305–1307, 2000.

96. Khamaisi M, Symmer L, Raz I. Thiazolidindiones in cardiovascular risk in type 2 diabetes mellitus. In: Hâncu N (ed). *Cardiovascular Risk in Type 2 Diabetes Mellitus. Assessment and Control.* Springer-Verlag, Berlin, Heidelberg, New York, 2003, pp 191–203.

97. Phillips SA, Ciaraldi TP, Kong AP, Bandukwala R, Aroda V, Carter L, *et al*. Modulation of circulating and adipose tissue adiponectin levels by antidiabetic therapy. *Diabetes*, **52**: 667–674, 2003.

98. Pasceri V, Wu H, Willerson JT, Yeh ET. Modulation of vascular inflammation *in vitro* and *in vivo* by peroxisome proliferator-activated receptor-γ activators. *Circulation*, **101**: 235–238, 2000.

99. Murao K, Imachi H, Momoi A, Sayo Y, Hosokawa H, Sato M, *et al*. Thiazolidindione inhibits the production of monocyte chemoattractant protein-1 in cytokine treated human vascular endothelial cells. *FEBS*, **454**: 27–30, (Letter) 1999.

100. Fukunaga Y, Itoh H, Doi K, Tanaka T, Yamashita J, Chun TH, *et al*. Thiazolidinediones, peroxisome proliferator-activated receptor gamma agonists, regulate endothelial cell growth and secretion of vasoactive peptides. *Atherosclerosis*, **158**: 113–119, 2001.

101. Avena R, Mitchell ME, Nylen ES, Curry KM, Sidawy AN. Insulin action enhancement normalizes brachial artery vasoactivity in patients with peripheral vascular disease and occult diabetes. *J Vasc Surg*, **28**: 1024–1031, 1998.

102. Fonseca VA, Reynolds T, Hemphill D, Randolph C, Wall J, Valiquet TR *et al*. Effect of Troglitazone on fibrinolysis and activated coagulation in patients with non-insulin-dependent diabetes mellitus. *J Diabetes Complications*, **12**: 181–186, 1998.

103. Weeks AJ. Gliclazide and diabetic angiopathy. In: Hâncu N (ed). *Cardiovascular Risk in Type 2 Diabetes Mellitus. Assessment and Control.* Springer-Verlag, Berlin Heidelberg New York, 2003, pp 28–36.

104. National Cholesterol Education Program Expert Panel. Executive summary of the third report of the National Cholesterol Education Program (NCEP) Expert Panel on Detection, Evaluation, and Treatment of High Blood Cholesterol in Adults (Adult Treatment Panel III). *JAMA*, **285**: 2486–2497, 2001.

105. American Diabetes Association. Management of dyslipidemia in adults with diabetes. *Diabetes Care*, **26[Suppl.1]**: S83–S86, 2003

106. Heart Protection Study Collaborative Group. MRC/BHF Heart protection study of cholesterol lowering with simvastatin in 20536 high-risk individuals: a randomised placebo-controlled trial. *Lancet*, **360**: 7–22, 2002.

107. Treasure CB, Llein JL, Weintraub WS, Talley JD, Stillabower ME, Kosinski AS *et al*. Beneficial effects of cholesterol-lowering therapy on the coronary endothelium in patients with coronary artery disease. *N Engl J Med*, **332**: 481–487, 1995.

108. Laufs U, LaFata V, Plutzky J, Liao J. Upregulation of endothelial nitric oxide synthase by HMG CoA reductase inhibitors. *Circulation*, **97**: 1129–1135, 1998.

109. Wagner AH, Kohler T, Ruckschloss U, Just I, Hecker M. Improvement of nitric oxide-dependent vasodilatation by HMG-CoA reductase inhibitors through attenuation of endothelial superoxide anion formation. *Arterioscler Thromb Vasc Biol*, **20**: 61–69, 2000.

110. Fruchart JC. Physiology of lipids and lipoproteins. *Prev Cardiol*, **11**: 119–125, 1999.

111. Singaraje RR, Fievet C, Castro G, James ER, Hennuyer N, Clee SM, *et al.* Increased ABCA-1 activity protects against atherosclerosis. *J Clin Invest*, **110**: 35–42, 2001.

112. Raspe E, Duez H, Gervois P, Fievet C, Fruchart JC, Besnard S, *et al.* Transcriptional regulation of apolipoprotein C-111 gene expression by the orphan nuclear receptor RORa. *J Biol Chem*, **276**: 2865–2871, 2001.

113. Heart Outcomes Prevention Evaluation Study Investigators. Effects of ramipril on cardiovascular and microvascular outcomes in people with diabetes mellitus: results of the HOPE study and MICRO-HOPE substudy. *Lancet*, **355**: 253–259, 2000.

114. Yusuf S, Sleight P, Pogue J, Bosch J, Davies R, Dagenais G. Effects of an angiotensin-converting enzyme inhibitor, ramipril, on cardiovascular events in high-risk patients. The Heart Outcomes Prevention Evaluation Study Investigators. *N Engl J Med*, **342**: 145–153, 2000.

115. Nawano M, Anai M, Funaki M, Kobayashi H, Kanda A, Fukushima Y, *et al.* Imidapril, an angiotensin-converting enzyme inhibitor, improves insulin sensitivity by enhancing signal transduction via insulin receptor substrate proteins and improving vascular resistance in the Zucker fatty rat. *Metabolism*, **48**: 1248–1255, 1999.

116. DeMattia G, Ferri C, Laurenti O, Cassone-Faldetta M, Picolli A, Santucci A. Circulating catecholamines and metabolic effects of captopril in NIDDM patients. *Diabetes Care*, **19**: 226–230, 1996.

117. Mancini GB, Henry GC, Macaya C, O'Neill BJ, Pucillo AL, Carere RG *et al.* Angiotensin-converting enzyme inhibition with quinapril improves endothelial vasomotor dysfunction in patients with coronary artery disease. The TREND (Trial on Reversing Endothelial Dysfunction) Study. *Circulation*, **94**: 258–265, 1996.

118. Ting HH, Timimi FK, Boles KS, Creager SJ, Ganz P, Creager MA. Vitamin C improves endothelium-dependent vasodilation in patients with non-insulin-dependent diabetes mellitus. *J Clin Invest*, **97**: 22–28, 1996.

119. Rimm EB, Stampfer MJ, Ascherio A, Givannucci E, Colditz GA, Willett WC. Vitamin E consumption and the risk of coronary heart disease in men. *N Engl J Med*, **328**: 1450–1456, 1993.

120. Stephens NG, Parsons A, Schofield PM, Kelly F, Cheeseman K, Mitchinson MJ. Randomised controlled trial of vitamin E in patients with coronary disease: Cambridge Heart Antioxidant Study (CHAOS). *Lancet*, **347**: 781–786, 1996.

121. Heart Protection Study Collaborative Group. MRC/BHF Heart Protection Study of antioxidant vitamin supplementation in 20536 high-risk individuals: a randomised placebo-controlled trial. *Lancet*, **360**: 23–33, 2002.

122. Pieper GM, Dondlinger L. Plasma and vascular tissue arginine are decreased in diabetes: acute arginine supplementation restores endothelium-dependent relaxation by augmenting cGMP production. *J Pharmacol Exp Ther*, **238**: 684–691, 1997.

14

RENAL HAEMODYNAMICS IN DIABETES

Tudor NICOLAIE, Dana M. NEDELCU

Diabetic nephropathy, the main cause of morbidity and mortality in diabetes mellitus, represents one of the frequent aethiologies of chronic renal failure. In many countries, diabetic nephropathy is the main reason of substitution therapy.

Related to different factors implicated in initiation, maintaining and progression of nephropathy, we analyzed the contribution of renal haemodynamics in diabetes mellitus related kidney injury.

During the evolution of diabetes, no matter what type, even at the beginning of disease, modifications of renal haemodynamics were identified. Using animal models and groups of diabetic patients were proved glomerular hyperperfusion, increased pression at glomerular capillaries level and hyperfiltration. These events stimulate increasing of matrix production at mesangial cells levels, thickening of basement membrane and expression of sclerosis, enhancement production factors as TGF-β and type IV collagen. We analyzed metabolical and hormonal factors, which acting on systemic and local haemodynamics, at kidney level, initiate and maintain diabetic nephropathy.

We presented the influence of hyperglycaemia, ketone bodies, diet type, insulin, glucagon, growth hormone, atrial natriuretic peptide and somatostatin-like hormone-octreotid-acting, directly or through mediators with haemodynamic effects, on glomerular filtration and plasmatic renal flow.

The implication of prostaglandines and pressor hormones, like angiotensin II, is emphasized on losing the harmony of vasodilatator and vasoconstrictor systems that deal with vascular resistance.

The important participation of angiotensin II at initiation and development of diabetic nephropathy is demonstrated using presentation of some studies (UKPDS, MICRO-HOPE, AIPRI, RENAAL), which prove the renoprotective effect of angiotensin converting enzyme inhibitors and angiotensin II type 1 receptor antagonists, delivered altogether or individually.

The endothelial dysfunction and high level of endothelin 1, which were studied intensively related to diabetes mellitus, act also through the haemodynamic chain on the initiation and the development of diabetic nephropathy.

Personal studies on the evaluation of sensitivity and predictability of Doppler ultrasonography, related to the early detection of haemodynamic renal injury, are presented.

All this data sustain the idea that renal haemodynamics represents the key point of pathogenic chains implicated on initiation, maintaining and progression of diabetic nephropathy.

Abbreviations List

ACE – Angiotensin converting enzyme
ACEI – Angiotensin converting enzyme inhibitors
Ang II – Angiotensin II
ARA – Antagonist of receptors 1 of angiotensin II
ANP – Atrial natriuretic peptide
HMG-Co reductase – Hydroxy-3-methyl-glutaryl-
    -coenzyme A reductase

PI – Intrarenal pulsatility index
AT1 – Receptor 1 of angiotensin II
AT2 – Receptor 2 of angiotensin II
RI – Resistive index
TGF-β – Transforming growth factor β
VEGF – Vascular endothelial growth factor

The consequences on the kidney of type 1 and type 2 diabetes mellitus are expressed both in specific glomerular lesions (known under the generic term of diabetic nephropathy – 20–30 % of diabetic individuals) and in non-specific ones, similar to other nephropathies (pielonephritis, intra-renal and peri-renal abscesses, papillary necrosis, nephroangiosclerosis); the latter conditions (together with the atherosclerosis of the renal artery) occur more frequently in diabetes, running a specific course.

Renal involvement in diabetes mellitus was identified in the 18th century by Contunnius (1764) and Rollo (1798) who signaled the presence of proteins in the urine of diabetic patients. In 1936, Kimmelstiel and Wilson described the development of some glomerular intercapillary nodular lesions. Subsequently, due to the special concern towards diabetes and its problems (including costs), mostly in the latest 10 years, an accumulation of data has occurred, the extent and importance of which will be rightly appreciated in the future.

Renal involvement in diabetes mellitus generates at present high costs caused by the necessity to substitute the renal function due to the progress of the disease. Diabetic nephropathy caused by type 2 diabetes mellitus is the most frequent cause of end-stage renal disease in many national registries [1, 2]. Diabetic nephropathy is the major cause of morbidity and mortality in diabetes mellitus.

Clinical diagnosis of diabetic nephropathy can be made in diabetic patients having persistent microalbuminuria (< 300 mg/24 h or > 20 µg/min) – Table 14.1 – associated with diabetic retinopathy, in the absence of any clinical or paraclinical signs suggestive for another kidney or urinary tract disease [3].

Table 14.1

Abnormalities in albumin excretion can be measured using different protocols

Category	24 h collection (mg/24 h)	Timed collection (µg/min)	Spot collection (µg/mg creatinine)
Normal	< 30	< 20	< 30
Microalbumin-uria	30–300	20–200	30–300
Clinical albuminuria	> 300	> 200	> 300

Microalbuminuria represents an important and independent risk factor both in the general population and in the diabetic or hypertensive patients [4]. The natural history of diabetic nephropathy has several stages: normoalbuminuria, microalbuminuria, macroalbuminuria and end-stage renal disease. The strategies for lowering proteinuria and consequently for stabilizing renal failure, can have positive consequences on cardiovascular and general mortality and also on the costs required by diabetic nephropathy.

Glomerular involvement in diabetes mellitus is predominant, but the other structures of the nephrons, as well as the remainder of the renal parenchyma are affected by the aggressive mechanisms specific for diabetes.

Multiple factors were identified to contribute to the initiation and progress of diabetic nephropathy [3]:

– genetic and racial predisposition;
– anomalies in the metabolism of glucides, together with other metabolic anomalies specific to diabetes mellitus;
– alteration of the systemic and renal haemodynamics;
– intervention of numerous cytokines and growth factors.

Arterial hypertension and smoking, with their known aggressivity, are added to these factors.

The following main factors are considered to be the promoters of the diabetic nephropathy evolution:

– the degree of albuminuria;
– arterial hypertension;
– the level of serum lipids.

In animals, diabetes determines glomerular hyperperfusion, a rise in the glomerular capillary pressure and hyperfiltration; in animal diabetes, the rise in the intra-glomerular pressure induces the appearance and evolution of nephropathy. In 1996, Nelson et al. [5] noticed that glomerular hyperfiltration was present and persistent in patients with normoalbuminuria and in those with microalbuminuria, while examining the natural evolution of nephropathy in the history of Pima Indians with altered tolerance to glucose or type 2 diabetes mellitus with variable duration and various degrees of albuminuria. The same study showed the preservation of glomerular filtration in patients with macroalbuminuria. The alteration rhythm of glomerular filtration is dependent upon the level of proteinuria (3–10 ml/min/year) [6] and race (10–4 mL/min/year) [3, 5]. Renal failure is increased by hypertension both in type 1 and type 2 diabetes mellitus [7]. Normalization of arterial blood pressure in diabetic patients usually slows down the progress of nephropathy, suggesting the interference of systemic haemodynamics in the renal haemodynamics and the involvement of both in diabetic nephropathy.

Renal haemodynamic involvement is present in diabetes mellitus, but, until now, it is not very clear whether this problem is a pathogenic component in the development of diabetic nephropathy or its consequence.

Twenty years ago it was found that haemodynamic disturbances at the glomerular level, causing an increase in flux and pressure, appear early in the course of the disease. This suggested the fact that glomerular haemodynamics disturbances might be directly responsible for glomerulosclerosis and accompanying proteinuria [8]. Numerous and consistent observations demonstrate the glomerular lesion in diabetes mellitus as being induced by a rise in the glomerular filtration rate, of the renal plasmatic flux and of the glomerular capillary hydraulic pressure [9–13]. The rise in intraglomerular pressure may lead to an increased matrix production in the mesangial cells and to a thickening of the basal membrane [8, 14]. Physical stress and scissoring forces induce damages to the endothelium and epithelial surface, affecting the glomerular barrier; these elements seem to determine the expression of certain sclerosis contributing factors, such as transforming growth factor β (TGF-β) and type IV collagen [15]. Alterations of local physical forces at the glomerular level determine, in time, the development of sclerotic modifications characteristic of diabetes; the interference of these modifications delays the development of nephropathy [16–19]. Decreased intraglomerular pressure alleviates the glomerular capillary wall stress – a promoter of glomerulosclerosis.

Glomerular involvement determines the initiation and progress of diabetic nephropathy set on by hyperfiltration, in the absence of any changes at the level of the structures that make up the glomerulus; no glomerular lesions have been identified up to now to be concomitant to hyperfiltration. It may be considered that hyperfiltration is the consequence of some events within the pre- and postglomerular territories. These territories become the target of numerous types of aggressions which are characteristic of diabetes mellitus as concerns the vascular system, with specific features for type 1 as compared to type 2, which have initially had functional effects on the tuft of glomerular capillaries. It is hard to believe that only the tuft of glomerular capillaries, the afferent and efferent arterioles are affected by the complex events with vascular targets in diabetes mellitus. In time, modifications of glomerular structures set on, emphasizing the glomerular filtration disjunction and determining the progress of diabetic nephropathy to end-stage renal disease.

Glomerular hyperfiltration is the first dysfunctional element identified in the development of diabetic nephropathy. The filtration fraction accounts for the sum of haemodynamic effects on the tuft of glomerular capillaries and it is not strictly a measure of intraglomerular pressure. Glomerular filtration rate is determined by:
– renal plasmatic flow;
– oncotic systemic pressure;
– the difference in hydraulic pressure of transcapillary glomeruli;
– the coefficient of glomerular ultrafiltration;
– hormonal and metabolic mediators.

The renal plasmatic flow is increased in both types of diabetes mellitus. It has been proved that improvement of glycaemic control in type 2 diabetes mellitus does not influence the renal plasmatic flow and filtration fraction. There is a growth in the renal plasmatic flow in type 1 diabetes mellitus, even under the conditions of an intensification of insulin treatment and of a good metabolic control.

Oncotic systemic pressure was found normal in type 1 and type 2 diabetes both in human subjects and in experimental animals.

The difference in glomerular transcapillary hydraulic pressure influences the glomerular filtration rate. The studies on diabetic rats made by micropunctures identified an increase in the transglomerular pressure gradient [20, 21]. It was found in experimental diabetic animals that the increased glomerular flow and pressure are caused by a decrease in the arteriolar vascular resistance, which is more marked on the afferent than on the efferent arteriole [20].

The glomerular ultrafiltration coefficient is the result of the capillary hydraulic conductivity and of the capillary surface available for filtration.

At present, numerous data are available to account for the appearance of hyperfiltration as an element identified at the beginning of the onset of diabetic nephropathy.

A series of hormonal and metabolic factors intervenes in the glomerular filtration rate which, acting systemically and locally at the level of diabetic kidney, determines glomerular filtration alterations, initiating the renal involvement specific to diabetes.

Glucose can bring about glomerular filtration modifications by changing the glomerular ultrafiltration coefficient under certain circumstances [22, 23]. Hyperfiltration occurs in the conditions of a moderate hyperglycaemia. The elevation of blood glucose may induce vasodilatation at the level of retinal circulation [24]; a similar mechanism is found at the level of the glomerular arterioles. In patients with renal insufficiency, hyperglycaemia may lower the glomerular perfusion rate by 30%, an effect mediated by the change in intrarenal production of prostaglandin (by route of blocking the cyclooxygenase) [23].

Infusion of ketonic bodies in supraphysiological doses in diabetic patients determines an increase by 33% in the glomerular filtration rate [25]; this is accompanied by a 16% increase in the renal plasmatic flow and a 14% increase of the filtration rate. Severe decrease of the serum glucose level through insulin infusion in diabetic patients reduces glomerular filtration rate in 30–60 minutes, but only by 6% [26]. The fall in the serum glucose level in diabetic patients by insulin perfusion lowers the increased glomerular pressure, suggestive for a complex interaction of insulin on the changes in renal haemodynamics, independent of the insulin effects on the blood glucose.

Hyperproteic diet in diabetic individuals may contribute to the glomerular hyperfiltration; the decrease of protein intake normalizes the glomerular filtration irrespective of the variations of glycaemia and arterial pressure [27, 28].

Part of the rise in the glomerular filtration rate in diabetes mellitus is accounted for by the increased renal plasmatic flow.

In early diabetes, there is a lack of balance between the systems of vasodilatation and vasoconstriction, regulating the glomerular vascular resistance in favour of vasodilatation. Prostaglandins, by their preferential vasodilatation effect on the afferent arteriole, increase the renal blood flow, the glomerular ultrafiltration coefficient and the glomerular capillary pressure, determining an increased glomerular filtration rate [29]. Pressor hormones, such as angiotensin II (Ang II), act preferentially on the efferent arteriole, attenuating the vasodilatation effects of prostaglandins which lead to an increase in the glomerular filtration rate.

In diabetic rats, the elevation of atrial natriuretic peptide (ANP) is associated with glomerular hyperfiltration. ANP receptors blockade or administration of ANP antagonists lower the glomerular filtration rate [30–32].

Growth hormone daily administration brings about an increase in the glomerular filtration rate and renal plasmatic inflow, both in healthy and in diabetic individuals, the intensification of response being related to hyperfiltration [33]. Most physiological actions of the growth hormone are mediated by the insulin-like growth factors; this is the reason why the insulin-like growth factor plays a role in the renal haemodynamics [34]. Octreotide – a somatostatin analogue – may reduce the hyperfiltration irrespective of the glycaemic control [35].

Perfused glucagon increases the glomerular filtration rate and the renal plasmatic flow in healthy and diabetic individuals. Glucagon has effects on renal haemodynamics by directly mediating the renal production of prostaglandin [36].

Renal production of prostaglandins is important for the appearance of glomerular hyperfiltration and for the vasodilatation which occurs in response to hyperglycaemia; these effects are blocked by the perfusion of indomethacin. Indomethacin reduces the renal plasmatic flow and significantly lowers the glomerular filtration rate [37]. Administration of aspirin to rats with streptozotocin-induced diabetes prevents the early onset of hyperfiltration [38]. The inhibition of prostaglandins in diabetic subjects reduces the glomerular filtration rate and the urinary excretion of albumin [39].

Renin-angiotensin system is involved in diabetic nephropathy. The most efficient method, demonstrated on experimental animals, to delay the glomerular involvement is represented by antihypertensive therapy combined with hypolipaemiant medication [40, 41]. This finding demonstrates that effects on other cell functions within this territory are obtained by the renal haemodynamic effect of pharmacological intervention. The data supplied by clinical studies on and meta-analyses of the evolution of diabetic nephropathy in human subjects reveal the efficiency of the interference of renin-angiotensin system by means of enzyme conversion inhibitors (ACEI); antagonist of receptors 1 of angiotensin II (ARA) or the association of these categories of therapeutic agents have a salutary influence on the progress of diabetic nephropathy.

Ang II, besides its known haemodynamic effect (vasoconstriction), also demonstrates other important non-haemodynamic effects at the level of the kidneys [42, 43]:
− stimulation of mesangial cells and macrophage infiltration of the mesangium;
− proliferation of sclerogenic cytokine-secretory cells (TGF, PDGF);
− formation and liberation of collagen and of extracellular matrix by mesangial and renal cells;
− stimulation of the hypertrophy of the renal vessels smooth muscles.

The beneficial effect of the renin-angiotensin system blockade in diabetic nephropathy is obvious, being demonstrated by numerous studies which used conversion-enzyme inhibitors or blockers of the receptor 1 of Ang II (AT1). The conversion-enzyme inhibitors proved to be more efficient in the treatment of diabetic nephropathy [44] − MICRO-HOPE study [45], AIPRI study [46] − as compared to beta-blockers − UKPDS study [47].

The physiological functions carried out by the receptor 2 of Ang II (AT2) are now partially known, but this seems to be responsible for counteracting the effects of vasoconstriction and proliferation of the AT1 and induces apoptosis. The use of sartans proved to have similar effects on ACEI as regards renal protection in the course of diabetic nephropathy as shown by several studies with losartan and enalapril, with candesartan and lisinopril [48, 49]. The RENAAL study [50] demonstrated the renoprotective role of losartan. Receptor 1 antagonists of Ang II fight the effects mediated by AT1 receptor which is stimulated by another route than by the activation of the angiotensin-converting enzyme (ACE). The majority of circulating Ang II is derived from the activity of ACE, but the alternative pathways also could play an important role, especially the chimase derived production of Ang II. The ACEI − ARA association would increase the serum levels of angiotensin (1–7), which definitely plays a vasodilatation role. The blockade achieved by using the two classes of drugs proves much more efficiency than by using them separately [43, 49, 51]. ARA administered together with inhibitors of hydroxy-3-methyl-glutaryl-coenzyme A (HMG-CoA) reductase, in experimental diabetes, reduce kidney injury and the renal expression of TGF-β and of vascular endothelial growth factor (VEGF) [52]. TGF-β is involved in the pathogenesis of some kidney diseases characterized by glomerulosclerosis [53]. Diabetic nephropathy is associated with an increase in the production of TGF-$β_1$ [54]. The therapy of the renin–angiotensin system by drugs which have no organ selectivity works efficiently upon diabetic nephropathy (having a salutary influence on the level of proteinuria and on lowering the rhythm at which this develops). This action is certainly not only due to the haemodynamic systemic activity, but also to the effects on the intrarenal vessels flowing into or out of the glomerulus.

In diabetes mellitus, there is an endothelial dysfunction [55] demonstrated both in experimental animals and in diabetic patients; diabetic nephropathy is a specific manifestation of the endothelial dysfunction [56] exacerbated by hypertension [57]. Endothelial function in diabetes is affected by numerous mediators: glucotoxicity, polyol pathway, protein kinase C system, prostaglandins, advanced glycosylation end-products, growth factors. To these is added a risk in nitric oxide production and sensitivity which may be important for the onset of hyperfiltration in the diabetic kidney [58], alongside with a rise in endothelin renal production. Nitric oxide vasodilatation role in glomerular hyperfiltration was first demonstrated in experimental diabetes [59]. Nitric oxide excessive synthesis participates in the glomerular hyperfiltration [60].

The most potent vasoconstrictors known so far, endothelins, are produced by the endothelium. Endothelins show, besides a powerful vaso-constrictive role, a profibrotic effect, especially at the level of the kidneys, by an increase in the production of extracellular matrix brought about by mesangial cells. Diabetic nephropathy is associated with an increased production of endothelin 1. Endothelin 1 may act in a paracrine way at the level of the kidney [61]. Together with lisinopril, nonselective endothelin antagonists alleviate the exaggerated expression of endothelin 1 renal gene in induced animal diabetes [62]. Endothelin receptor antagonists administered in animal models of diabetes mellitus (streptozotocin-diabetic rats) reduce proteinuria and normalize the expression of renal matrix proteins, being demonstrated to have an antifibrotic effect [63]. At the level of the kidney, endothelin causes mesangial cells hypertrophy characteristic for diabetic nephropathy as it influences the kinetics of certain genes involved in the mesangial cells hypertrophy [64].

The importance of the role-played by these hormonal and metabolic mediators and the sequence in which they intervene, as well as the identification of the moment in which they act to generate diabetic nephropathy, are not known yet. The combined action of metabolic and hormonal mediators in diabetes mellitus induces renal haemodynamic modifications, resulting in the initiation and development of diabetic nephropathy.

The blood supply to the kidneys is provided by the renal arteries emerging from the aorta and having a larger diameter, according to the function of filtration. In the renal hilum, the renal artery is divided in arteries for each of the kidney parts: the superior polar arteries, the median arteries for the middle part of the kidney and the inferior polar arteries for the inferior pole. In the renal parenchyma these arteries pass between the pyramids (between the renal lobes) and are termed interlobar arteries. At the basis of the pyramid and at the level of the medullar and cortical junction, the interlobar arteries give off the archiform arteries from which the interlobular arteries arise piercing the cortical. The interlobular artery gives off the afferent vessel which ramifies forming a tuft of capillaries, the glomerulus, which becomes invaginated in the initial portion of the renal tubule, the Bowman capsule. From the glomerulus, the efferent vessel emerges, being distributed into a new capillary network which surrounds the renal tubes and is continued with the veins. The veins accompany the corresponding arteries, leaving the kidney at the level of the hilum where they form a common trunk, called the renal vein emptying into the inferior cava vein. The venous blood from the cortical part is initially collected in the stellate veins, then in the interlobular veins (which accompany the homonymous arteries and subsequently the arcuate veins). The venous blood from the medullar is collected by the right veins. The outflowing veins unite forming the renal vein.

Many data have been gathered concerning the involvement of the glomerular capillaries, the afferent and efferent arteries and of the nonvascular structures neighbouring the glomerulus in diabetes mellitus.

Lesions have been histologically identified at the level of the arcuate and interlobular arteries, being more marked by arteriosclerosis in diabetes mellitus as compared to other conditions in which the internal elastic lamina is duplicated.

Afferent and efferent arterioles are more frequently identified to show arteriosclerotic lesions; subendothelial PAS positive hyaline deposits are identified at this level (Plates 14.1, 14.2).

Within the accelerated atherogeneous process in diabetes mellitus, the renal artery sclerosis is more frequent than in the general population, causing hypertension which may take an accelerated course towards renal insufficiency by the administration of angiotensin enzyme-conversion inhibitors.

Nephroangiosclerosis (renal arteriosclerosis) is characterized by the hyalization of the intima and media of the renal arterioles which occurs much earlier, more frequently and more severely in diabetes as compared to non-diabetic population, and in type 2 diabetes as compared to type 1 diabetes (Plate 14.3). There are no histopathological, clinical or biological particularities in diabetes mellitus (irrespective of its type).

PERSONAL FINDINGS

Starting from the assumption that the numerous vascular disturbances in diabetes mellitus concomitantly affect the vessels transporting blood to and from the glomerulus, we have analyzed the functional parameters during the progress of diabetes mellitus. This assumption is also supported by the beneficial effect of the pharmacological approach with a general vascular and not a strictly glomerular target, which slows down the progress of diabetic nephropathy.

The studies carried on by us aimed at evaluating Doppler sensitivity and degree of predictability in detecting the renal haemodynamics premature involvement in patients with diabetic nephropathy (Plate 14.4).

We have investigated the arterial and venous circulation about: flow, velocity, intrarenal arterial pulsatility index (PI) and resistive index (RI) at the medium and great renal arterial and venous divisions. We have focused on the resistive index, which we consider could estimate the vascular activity better than other haemodynamic parameter. The results were assessed using the statistical analysis of the data from patients and control subjects.

Several clinical and biochemical criteria were monitorized, such as: microalbuminuria, plasmatic insulinaemia, creatinine and creatinine clearance, blood urea nitrogen, arterial blood pressure (those results described several groups). We also take into consideration the gender of patient, age, occupation and various treatments. We analyzed renal haemodynamics parameters on a group of 233 patients, of which 133 with diabetes mellitus and compared the results with those from our own database (normal subjects). Even on the Internet, we were not able to find some recent data concerning normal renal haemodynamic parameters, so we were supposed to build our own database (especially on Resistive Index) (Plates 14.5–14.11).

Our subjects were:
– 100 non-diabetic patients with normal renal function (control group);
– 60 newly discovered diabetic patients;
– 73 diabetic patients with more than five-year evolution of the disease.

According to the level of 24-hour urinary albumin excretion, the diabetic subjects were divided in the following three groups:
– with microalbuminuria under 20 mg/L;
– with microalbuminuria between 21 and 40 mg/L;
– with microalbuminuria over 41 mg/L.

We monitored several biochemical and clinical parameters:
– microalbuminuria;
– plasmatic insulinaemia;
– glycosylated haemoglobin;
– blood urea nitrogen;
– creatinine and creatinine clearance;
– arterial blood pressure (with and without ACEI treatment).

We studied renal haemodynamics using 2D, color duplex Doppler, pulsed Doppler, power Doppler and 3D imaging ultrasonography.

The parameters of interest were:
– parenchyma/sinus index;
– flow;
– velocity;
– Resistive Index (RI) – this was the target parameter;
– intrarenal arterial pulsatility index.

Statistical correlation between ultrasonographical parameters (RI) and biochemical data (microalbuminuria) was done using several mathematical formulae:

Arithmetic mean:

$$\overline{X} = \sum_{i=1}^{n} \frac{X_i}{n}$$

Median standard deviation:

$$\Gamma = \sqrt{\frac{\sum_{i=1}^{n}(X_i - \overline{X})^2}{n}}$$

Correlation coefficient:

$$\Re_{xy} = \frac{\sum(X_i - \overline{X})(Y_i - \overline{Y})}{n\Gamma_x\Gamma_y}$$

The correlation coefficient can have values between −1 and +1. If the coefficient is over 0, the relation between variables is direct (*e.g.*, the increase of one is associated with the increase of the other). When the coefficient is under 0, the relation between variables is inverse (*e.g.*, the increase of one is associated with the decrease of the other). The relationship is very strong with the correlation coefficient closer than ±1.

Because this is an undergoing study, we consider that it is not the right moment to present our detailed data. Instead, we will show only the statistical correlation between microalbuminuria and resistive index (Tables 14.2 and 14.3).

We realized that, according to the correlation coefficient, the resistive index (RI) was inversely correlated with mean microalbuminuria values in the diabetic patients.

However, the statistical interpretation showed that RI directly correlated with urinary albumin excretion in the group of patients with microalbuminuria under 20 mg/L. These values were not statistically significant in the overall view.

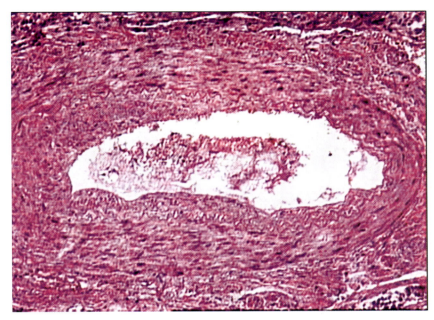

Plate 14.1
Arteriosclerotic lesions – intrarenal arteries – HE ob. ×10.

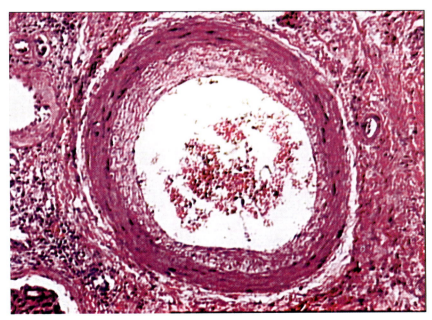

Plate 14.2
Arteriosclerotic lesions – intrarenal arteries – HE ob. ×10.

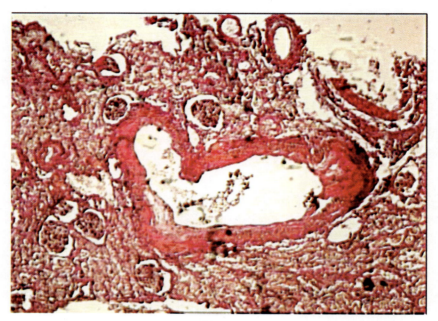

Plate 14.3
Atherosclerotic lesions, atheroma in intrarenal arteries – V.G. ob. ×4.

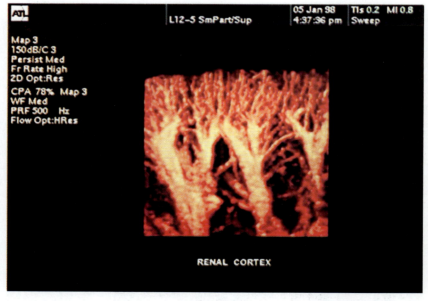

Plate 14.4
Medial third level vascularisation of the left kidney – 3D Power Doppler

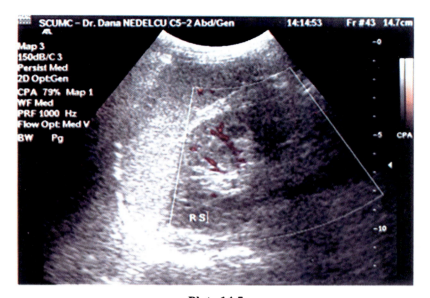

Plate 14.5

Left Kidney – arterial branches II and III degree; 2B and Power Doppler
ultrasonography in sagittal – oblic section.

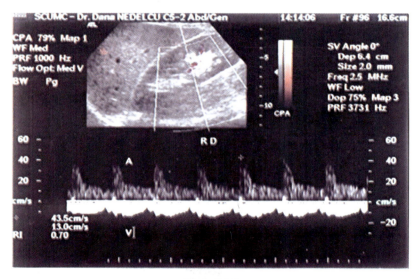

Plate 14.6

Right Kidney – arterial spectrogram of III degree branch suggesting high
velocity (double value in comparison with normal velocity); lower resistivity
index; medium stenosis.

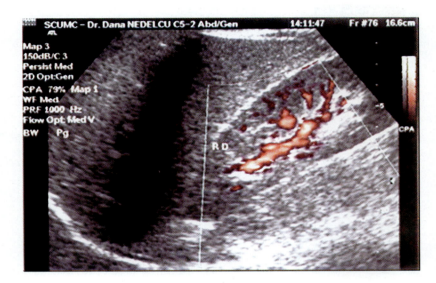

Plate 14.7

2B and Power Doppler ultrasonography.

Right Kidney with II and III degree branches of arterial vessels. Normal echographical aspect.

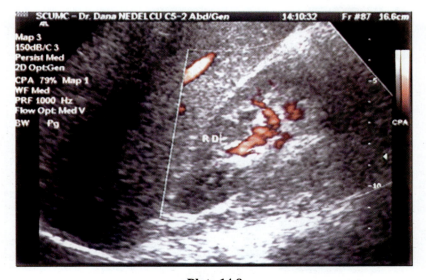

Plate 14.8

2B and Power Doppler ultrasonography.

II degree arterial branches with disappearance of III degree arterial branches.

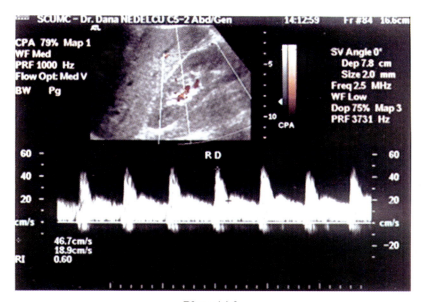

Plate 14.9
Arterial spectrogram of right Kidney (high velocity) suggesting II degree
stenosis (low resistivity index).

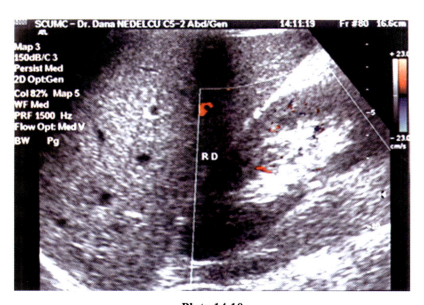

Plate 14.10
Right Kidney – arterial branches of II and III degree, thinner and filiform.

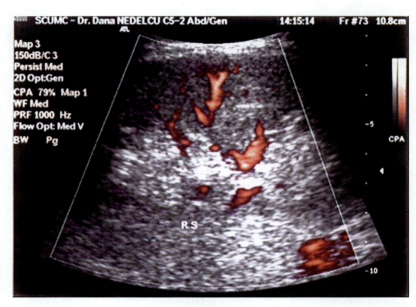

Plate 14.11
Repermeabilisation of II and III degree arterial branches
after diabetes treatment.

Table 14.2

The statistical correlation between microalbuminuria
and resistive index (in the three groups)

Statistical parameter	Micro-albuminuria	Resistive Index
First group (urinary albumin < 20 mg/l)		
Mean	13	0.997
Median standard deviation	4.58	0.006
Correlation coefficient	0.307	–
Second group (urinary albumin 21–40 mg/l)		
Mean	35	0.927
Median standard deviation	5	0.018
Correlation coefficient	– 0.502	–
Third group (urinary albumin > 41 mg/l)		
Mean	73.08	0.880
Median standard deviation	20.53	0.023
Correlation coefficient	0.065	–

Table 14.3

The statistical correlation between microalbuminuria
and resistive index (in all the 133 patients)

Statistical parameter	Micro-albuminuria	Resistive Index
Mean	43.33	0.93
Median standard deviation	28.78	0.05
Correlation coefficient	– 0.802	–

We considered those results only the first step
of a developing study, which will show that
complex Doppler ultrasonography is a really
helpful tool in assessing the renal haemodynamics.
Furthermore, renal haemodynamic alterations are
most valuable in predicting the outcome of
diabetic nephropathy.

Thus, we consider that this is only a
qualitative interpretation of our thought (that
besides microalbuminuria, there is a more precise

and predictive sign in the outcome of diabetic
nephropathy – the altered values of resistive
index). After studying a greater number of cases,
we will be able to offer also a quantitative
interpretation of resistive index values, which will
represent the real proof of this idea. From the view
of our results, we can estimate that the use of the
Doppler ultrasonography is more helpful (*e.g.*,
cheaper, affordable, noninvasive and precise) in
evaluating the diabetic nephropathy, than the
measurement of urinary albumin excretion.

CONCLUSIONS

The clinical diagnosis of diabetic nephropathy
made as early as possible due to the sustained
control of the factors determining the progress of
renal involvement in diabetes can contribute to
lower the costs determined by the progress towards
end-stage renal disease. The modifications
identified at the level of the intra-renal vessels in
the course of diabetes mellitus contribute to a
certain extent – which has to be correctly
evaluated in the future – to the activity of the
glomerulus and to the onset and progress of
diabetic nephropathy. Additional data provided by
our non-invasive and relatively cheap method,
which is sure to be improved in the future, can
contribute to the early identification and
sanctioning of the onset and evolution of diabetic
nephropathy.

The data presented above are in favour of the
hypothesis that renal haemodynamics represents
the turning point in the activity of diabetes
mellitus pathogenic vectors as regards the onset
and progress of diabetic nephropathy.

REFERENCES

1. Van Dijk PC, Jager KJ, de Charro F, *et al*. Renal
   replacement therapy in Europe: the results of a
   collaborative effort by the ERA-EDTA registry and
   six national or regional registries. *Nephrol Dial
   Transplant*, **16**: 1120–1129, 2001.
2. US Renal Data System. *Annual Data Report.
   National Institutes of Health; National Institute of
   Diabetes and Digestive and Kidney Diseases,*
   Bethesda, MD, 2000. http://www.usrds.org/
   2kpdf/01_incid_&_prev.pdf

3. Parving H-H, Østerby R, Anderson PW, Hsueh WA. Diabetic nephropathy. In: Brener BM (ed). *The Kidney,* 5th ed, Vol.2. WB Saunders, Philadelphia, 1996, 1864–1892.

4. Gerstein HC, Mann JFE, Qilong Y, *et al.* Albuminuria and risk of cardiovascular events, death, and heart failure in diabetic and nondiabetic individuals. *JAMA,* **286:** 421–426, 2001.

5. Nelson RG, Bennettt PH, Beck GJ, *et al.* Development and progression of renal disease in Pima Indians with non-insulin-dependent diabetes mellitus. *N Engl J Med,* **335:** 11636–1642, 1996.

6. Hunsicker LG, Adler S, Caggiula A, *et al.* Predictors of the progression of renal disease. Modification of Diet in Renal Disease Study. *Kidney Int,* **51:** 1908–19, 1997.

7. Ritz E, Stefanski A. Diabetic nephropathy in type II diabetes. *Am J Kidney Dis,* **27:** 167–194, 1996.

8. Hostetter TH, Rennke HG, Brenner BM. The case for intrarenal hypertension in the initiation and progression of diabetic and other glomerulopathies. *Am J Med,* **72:** 375–380, 1982.

9. Steffes MW, Brown DM, Mauer SM. Diabetic glomerulopathy following unilateral nephrectomy in the rat. *Diabetes,* **27:** 35–41, 1978.

10. Mauer SM, Steffes MW, Azar S, Sandberg SK, Brown DM. The effects of Goldblatt hypertension on development of the glomerular lesions of diabetes mellitus in the rat. *Diabetes,* **27:** 738–744, 1978.

11. Béroniade VC, Lefèbvre R, Falardeau P. Unilateral nodular diabetic glomerulosclerosis: recurrence of an experiment of nature. *Am J Nephrol,* **7:** 55–9, 1987.

12. Zatz R, Dunn BR, Meyer TW, Anderson S, Rennke HG, Brenner BM. Prevention of diabetic glomerulopathy by pharmacologic amelioration of glomerular capillary hypertension. *J Clin Invest,* **77:** 1925–30, 1986.

13. Anderson S, Rennke HG, Brenner BM. Therapeutic advantages of converting-enzyme inhibitors in arresting progressive renal disease associated with systemic hypertension in the rat. *J Clin Invest,* **77:** 1925–1930, 1986.

14. Webb RC, Bohr DF. Recent advances in the pathogenesis of hypertension: consideration of structural, functional, and metabolic vascular abnormalities resulting in elevated arterial resistance. *Am Heart J,* **102:** 251–264, 1981.

15. Cortes P, Riser BL, Zhao X, Narins RG. Glomerular volume expansion and mesangial cell mechanical strain: mediators of glomerular pressure injury. *Kidney Int Suppl,* **45:** S11–S16, 1994.

16. Orloff MJ, Yamanaka N, Greenleaf GE, Huang YT, Huang DG, Leng XS. Reversal of mesangial enlargement in rats with long-standing diabetes by whole pancreas transplantation. *Diabetes,* **35:** 347–354, 1986.

17. Bank N, Klose R, Aynedjian HS, Nguyen D, Sablay LB. Evidence against increased glomerular pressure initiating diabetic nephropathy. *Kidney Int,* **31:** 898–905, 1987.

18. Kasiske BL, O'Donnell MP, Cleary MP, Keane WF. Treatment of hyperlipidaemia reduces glomerular injury in obese Zucker rats. *Kidney Int,* **33:** 667–72, 1988.

19. O'Donnell MP, Kasiske BL, Katz SA, Schmitz PG, Keane WF. Lovastatin but not enalapril reduces glomerular injury in Dahl salt-sensitive rats. *Hypertension,* **20:** 651–658, 1992.

20. Hostetter TH, Troy JC, Brenner BM. Glomerular haemodynamics in experimental diabetes mellitus. *Kidney Int,* **19:** 410–415, 1981.

21. Jensen PK, Christiansen JS, Steven K, Parving HH. Renal function in streptozotocin-diabetic rats. *Diabetologia,* **21:** 409–414, 1981.

22. Remuzzi A, Viberti GC, Ruggenenti P, Battaglia C, Pagai R, Remuzzi G. Glomerular response to hyperglycaemia in human diabetic nephropathy. *Am J Physiol,* **259:** F545–552, 1990.

23. DeCosmo S *et al.* Glucose-induced changes in renal haemodynamics in proteinuric type 1 (insulin-dependent) diabetic patients: inhibition by acetylsalicylic acid infusion. *Diabetologia,* **36:** 622–627, 1993.

24. Atherton A, Hill DW, Keen H, Young S, Edwards EJ. The effect of acute hyperglycaemia on the retinal circulation of the normal cat. *Diabetologia,* **18:** 233–237, 1980.

25. Trevisan R, *et al.* Ketone bodies increase glomerular filtration rate in normal man and in patients with type 1 (insulin-dependent) diabetes mellitus. *Diabetologia,* **30:** 214–221, 1987.

26. Mogensen CE, Christensen NJ, Gundersen HGJ. The acute effect of insulin on renal haemodynamics and protein excretion in diabetics. *Diabetologia,* **15:** 153–157, 1978.

27. Pedersen MM, Winther E, Mogensen CE. Reducing protein in the diabetic diet. *Diabete Metab,* **16:** 454–459, 1990.

28. Humphreys M, Cronin CC, Barry DG, Ferriss JB. Are the nutritional recommendations for insulin-dependent diabetic patients being achieved? *Diabet Med,* **11:** 79–84, 1994.

29. Noth RH, Krolewski AS, Kaysen GA, Meyer TW, Schambelam M. Diabetic nephropathy: hemodynamic basis and implications for disease management. *Ann Int Med,* **110:** 795–813, 1989.

30. Zhang PL, MacKenzie HS, Troy JL, Brenner BM. Effects of an atrial natriuretic peptide receptor antagonist on glomerular hyperfiltration in diabetic rats. *J Am Soc Nephrol*, 4: 1564–1570, 1994.

31. Sakamoto K, Kikkawa R, Haneda M, Shigeta Y. Prevention of glomerular hyperfiltration in rats with streptozotocin-induced diabetes by an atrial natriuretic peptide receptor antagonist. *Diabetologia*, 38: 536–542, 1995.

32. Ortola FV, Ballermann BJ, Anderson S, Mendez RE, Brenner BM. Elevated plasma atrial natriuretic peptide levels in diabetic rats. Potential mediators of hyperfiltration. *J Clin Invest*, 80: 670–674, 1987.

33. Blankestijn PJ, et al. Glomerular hyperfiltration in insulin-dependent diabetes mellitus is correlated with enhanced growth hormone secretion. *J Clin Endocrinol Metab*, 77: 498–502, 1993.

34. Hirschberg R, Kopple JD. Evidence that IGF-I increases renal plasma flow and glomerular filtration rate in fasted rats. *J Clin Invest*, 83: 326–330, 1991.

35. Serri O, et al. Somatostatin analogue, octreotide, reduces increased glomerular filtration rate and kidney size in insulin-dependent diabetes. *JAMA*, 265: 888–892, 1991.

36. Fioretto P, et al. Impaired renal response to a meat meal in insulin-dependent diabetes: role of glucagon and prostaglandins. *Am J Physiol*, 258: F675–683, 1990.

37. Jensen PK, Steven K, Blæhr H, Christiansen JS, Parving HH. Effects of indomethacin on glomerular haemodynamics in experimental diabetes. *Kidney Int*, 29: 490–495, 1986.

38. Moel DI, Safirstein RL, McEvoy RC, Hsueh W. Effect of aspirin on experimental diabetic nephropathy. *J Lab Clin Med*, 110: 300–307, 1987.

39. van den Berg BW, Kruseman AC, van Geel JL, Cornelissen P, Mulder AW. Effect of short-term inhibition of prostaglandin synthesis on glomerular filtration rate and microalbuminuria in patients with incipient nephropathy. *Neth J Med*, 33: 106–112, 1988.

40. Rubin R, Silbiger S, Sablay L, Neugarten J. Combined antihypertensive and lipid-lowering therapy in experimental glomerulonephritis. *Hypertension*, 23: 92–95, 1994.

41. Lee SK, Jin SY, Han DC, Hwang SD, Lee HB. Effects of delayed treatment with enalapril and/or lovastatin on the progression of glomerulosclerosis in 5/6 nephrectomized rats. *Nephrol Dial Transplant*, 8: 1338–1343, 1993.

42. Ruggenenti P, Aros C, Remuzzi G. Renin-angiotensin system, proteinuria and tubulointerstitial damage. *Contrib Nefrol*, 135: 187–199, 2001.

43. Hilgers KF, Man JFE. ACE inhibitors versus AT1 receptor antagonists in patients with chronic renal disease. *J Am Soc Nephrol*, 13: 1100–1108, 2002.

44. The Microalbuminuria Captopril Study Group. Captopril reduces the risk of nephropathy of patients with microalbuminuria. *Diabetologia*, 39: 587–593, 1996.

45. ⁂ Effects of ramipril on cardiovascular and microvascular outcomes in people with diabetes; the results of the HOPE study and MICRO-HOPE substudy. Heart Outcomes Prevention Evaluation – Report of investigators. *Lancet*, 355: 253–259, 2000.

46. Maschio G, Alberti D, Janin G, et al. Effect of the angiotensin-converting-enzyme on the progression of chronic renal insufficiency. The Angiotensin-Converting-Enzyme Inhibitors in Progressive Renal Insufficiency Study Group. *N Engl J Med*, 334: 939–945, 1996.

47. ⁂ UK Prospective Diabetes Study Group. Efficacy of atenolol and captopril in reducing macrovascular and microvascular complications in type 2 diabetes: UKPDS 39. *BMJ*, 317: 729–738, 1998.

48. Lacourciere Y, Balanger A, Godin C, et al. Long-term comparison of losartan and enalapril on renal function in hypertensive type 2 diabetics with early nephropathy. *Kidney Int*, 58: 762–769, 2000.

49. Mogensen CE, Neldam S, Tikkanen I, et al. Randomised controlled trial of dual blockade of renin angiotensin system in patiens with hypertension, microalbuminuria and non-insulin diabetes: the candesartan and lisinopril microalbuminuria (CALM) study. *BMJ*, 321: 1440–1448, 2000.

50. Brenner BM, Cooper ME, de Zeeuw D, et al. Effects of losartan on renal and cardiovascular complications in patients with type 2 diabetes and nephropathy. *N Engl J Med*, 345: 861–869, 2001.

51. Jacobsen P, Andersen S, Rossing K, Handen BV, Parving HH. Dual blockade of the renin angiotensin system in type 1 patients with diabetic nephropathy. *Nephrol Dial Transplant*, 22: 1017–1024, 2002.

52. Qin J, Zhang Z, Liu J, Sun L, Hu L, Cooper ME, Cao Z. Effects of the combination of an angiotensin II antagonist with an HMG-CoA reductase inhibitor in experimental diabetes. *Kidney International*, 64 (2): 565–571, 2003.

53. Gilbert RE, Wilkinson-Berka J, Johnson DW, Cox A, Soulis T, Wu LL, Kelly DJ, Jerums G, Pollock CA, Cooper ME. Renal expression of transforming

growth factor-β inducible gene h3 (βig-h3) in normal and diabetic rats. *Kidney Int*, **54 (4):** 1052–1062, 1998.

54. Sharma K, Ziyadeh FN, Alzahabi B, McGowan TA, Kapoor S, KurniK BR, Kurnik PB, Weisberg LS. Increased renal production of transforming growth factor-beta1 in patients with type II diabetes. *Diabetes*, **46 (5):** 854–859, 1997.

55. Lorenzi M, Cagliero E. Pathobiology of endothelial and other vascular cells in diabetes mellitus: call for data. *Diabetes,* **40:** 653–659, 1991.

56. Hseuh WA, Anderson PW. Hypertension, the endothelial cell, and the vascular complications of diabetes mellitus. *Hypertension,* **20:** 253–263, 1992.

57. Henrich WL. The endothelium – a key regulator of vascular tone. *Am J Med Sci,* **302:** 319–328, 1991.

58. Komers R, Allen TJ, Cooper ME. Role of endothelium-derived nitric oxide in the pathogenesis of the renal hemodynamic changes of experimental diabetes. *Diabetes,* **43:** 1190–1197, 1994.

59. King AJ, Zayas MA, Troy JL, Downes SJ, Brenner BM. Inhibition of diabetes-induced hyperfiltration and hyperemia by N-monomethyl-l-arginine (l-NMMA). *J Am Soc Nephrol*, **1:** 665A. 1990.

60. Bank N, Aynedjian HS. Role of EDRF (nitric oxide) in diabetic renal hyperfiltration. *Kidney Int,* **43:** 1306–1312, 1993.

61. Masood AKhan, Mick RD, Faiz HM, Cecil ST, Dimitri PM, Robert JM. Upregulation of endothelin A receptor sites in the rabbit diabetic kidney: potential revleance to the early pathogenesis of diabetic nephropathy. *Nephron,* **83 (3):** 261–267, 1999.

62. Benigni A, Colosio V, Brena C, Bruzzi I, Bertani T, Remuzzi G. Unselective inhibition of endothelin receptors reduces renal dysfunction in experimental diabetes. *Diabetes.* **47 (3):** 450–456, 1998.

63. Hocher B, Schwarz A, Reinbacher D, Jacobi, Lun A, Priem F, Bauer C, Neumayer HH, Raschack M. Effects of endothelin receptor antagonist on the progression of diabetic nephropathy. *Nepfron,* **87(2):** 161–169, 2001.

64. Goruppi S, Bonventre J, Kyriakis M. Signaling pathways and late-onset gene induction associated with renal mesangial cell hypertrophy. The *EMBO J*, **21 (20):** 5427–5432, 2002.

15

MICROALBUMINURIA AND CARDIOVASCULAR DISEASE

Cristian SERAFINCEANU

Microalbuminuria, defined as the persistent presence of an amount of 30–300 mg/24h (20–200 µg/min) albumin in the urine of diabetic patients, was initially described as closely linked to the incipient stage of diabetic renal disease. Although this assumption remains almost entirely true for type 1 diabetic patients, further developments emphasized the independent association between MA and hypertension, insulin resistance and cardiovascular morbidity/mortality, mainly in type 2 diabetic patients and in non-diabetic subjects too. In fact, the presence of MA seems to double the cardiovascular risk for these individuals, thus MA must be considered as an early sign (marker) of damage not only of the kidney but also of the cardiovascular system.

The epidemiological studies brought new data about the familial clustering of MA, its association with hypertension and the possible predictive genetic markers. The presence of MA itself showed a good predictive power for future cardiovascular events, in type 2 diabetic, as well as in non-diabetic populations.

The possible mechanisms through which MA can produce the cardiovascular injury are complex and not fully understood yet. MA appears like a marker of a "disadvantageous" alteration in the conventional cardiovascular risk factors individual pattern, with a special type of association between MA and hypertension ("bad companions").

On the other hand, there is a strong intrinsic relationship between MA and the so-called "non-conventional" cardiovascular risk factors, such as markers of endothelial dysfunction, insulin resistance and low-grade inflammation. MA might be considered as a marker of widespread microvascular lesion, or a direct manifestation of endothelial dysfunction. The association of MA with markers of inflammation seems to confer to MA its significance as a cardiovascular risk marker.

In the light of these recent data, it is of great importance to define a correct multifactorial approach for the prevention of cardiovascular disease in microalbuminuric diabetic as well as non-diabetic patients. The new strategies for this intervention necessarily include the insulin-sensitizers (thiazolidinediones), the blockade of renin-angiotensin system and statins as essential components.

INTRODUCTION

The term "microalbuminuria" was first used by Keen and Chlouverakis in "Guy's Hospital Resorts", 1969, when following the determination of subclinical urinary albumin excretion by a radioimmunoassay in a cohort of type 2 diabetic patients.

Microalbuminuria (MA), as subclinical persistent presence of an amount of albumin between 30–300 mg/day (20–200μg/minute) in urine, was initially described as closely linked with diabetic renal disease [1, 2, 3] (defining the incipient stage of renal involvement in diabetic patients); further developments emphasized the association between MA and antecedent hyperfiltration [4], increasing blood pressure [5] and cardiovascular events [6]. MA was also found in non-diabetic patients, usually associated with essential hypertension [7] and dyslipidemia [8].

In practical terms, it has now been proposed to screen for microalbuminuria by using an early morning urine sample or a random urine sample and to measure albumin/ creatinine excretion ratio (ACR) [9]. The normal value is usually indicated as being below 2.5 mg/mmol (30 mg/g), with the MA between 2.5 and 25 mg/mmol (30–300 mg/g) (Table 15.1).

Viberti *et al.* [10] reported in 1982 an association between MA and mortality in patients with T1DM; two years later, Mogensen *et al.* [11] found an increase in cardiovascular and total mortality in T2DM microalbuminuric patients. In a meta-analysis of 11 longitudinal studies that included 2,138 T2DM patients with MA, Dinneen and Gerstein [12] found an odds ratio for cardiovascular mortality and/or morbidity of 2.0 (95% CI = 1.4–2.7) and an odds ratio for global mortality of 2.4 (95% CI = 1.8–3.1). In other words, MA doubled the risk of having a cardiovascular event, even after adjustments for other cardiovascular risk factors.

These data indicate that MA is involved in early renal and vascular disorders that can predict the advancing renal disease as well as progression of cardiovascular disease, with high risk for cardiovascular events [13, 14, 15, 16]. This concept of prediction however is becoming increasingly difficult to pursue because many patients are treated with anti-hypertensive drugs or other types of medical interventions at the moment when MA is diagnosed, since such measures return MA to normal or slow its progression to clinical proteinuria.

It is an actual controversy, which must be separately discussed later in this chapter, if MA should be considered as a part of the metabolic syndrome X, although in population-based studies the presence of MA in non-diabetic subjects, especially in the elderly, showed a strong association with cardiovascular disease and mortality [17, 18]. However, in these studies MA was more specifically related to high blood pressure and dyslipidemia rather than to insulin resistance and obesity [19].

Thus, MA can be considered as an early sign or risk marker of damage not only of the kidney but also of the cardiovascular system (Figure 15.1). It is crucial, for preventive or curative interventional strategies in diabetic patients, to identify and fight against the pathogenetic risk factors and it is

Table 15.1

Diagnostic definitions for normo-, micro- and macroalbuminuria
(Adapted from: Mogensen CE, *Microalbuminuria in perspectives*, 2002 [22])

	24h AER	Overnight AER	A/C ratio
Normoalbuminuria	< 30mg	< 20μg/min	< 2.5mg/mmol (men) < 3.5mg/mmol (women) < 30mg/g
Microalbuminuria	30–300mg	20–200μg/min	2.5 (3.5)–25mg/mmol 30–300mg/g
Macroalbuminuria	> 300mg	> 200μg/min	> 25mg/mmol > 300mg/g

AER: albumin excretion rate.
A/C ratio: urinary albumin/creatinine ratio (random sample).

RISK FACTORS	PRE-CLINICAL DISEASE	CLINICAL DISEASE
High blood pressure	Left ventricular hypertrophy	Coronary heart disease
Diabetes mellitus		
Obesity	**Microalbuminuria**	Overt renal disease
Dyslipidemia		
Non-conventional (insulin resistance)	Retinopathy	Vision loss
SCREENING	**"SURROGATE" ENDPOINTS**	**CLINICAL ENDPOINTS**

Figure 15.1

The progression of cardiovascular, ocular and renal disease.
(Adapted from: Damsgaard ME and Mogensen CE, 1986 [16]).

equally important to diagnose the presence of MA and monitor its evolution. Very early risk factors to be questioned about could be pre-natal, such as genetic markers, birth weight and familial predisposition to renal and vascular disease. After the clinical onset of diabetes mellitus (DM), there are two fundamental risk factors, which must be considered together, namely high blood glucose and high blood pressure ("bad companions"-parving) [20]; associated hyperlipidemia in DM patients (especially type 2 DM) could be also of great importance [21].

THE SCREENING FOR MICROALBUMINURIA

Microalbuminuria has emerged in the latest two decades as a strong and highly significant predictor of renal and cardiovascular disease in the diabetics [22] and also in the general population. It should be stressed that to some extent the definition is arbitrarily defined in the original consensus paper [20]; however, the consensus level of 20–200 µg/min has proved quite relevant and useful over the years and has gained significant general acceptance.

An important study that has recently been published [23], after an 8-year follow-up of a cohort of 599 diabetic normoalbuminuric patients, showed that there is an increasing risk for progression from normo- to microalbuminuria according to the baseline level of albuminuria. The patients with a baseline albumin excretion rate in the upper normal range ("upper normal" albuminuria, 20–30 mg/24 h [24, 25]) have accelerated rates of decline in GFR, elevated relative risk for microalbuminuria and cardiovascular events, compared to those with a baseline albumin excretion rate under 20 mg/24 h. So, the authors conclude that albuminuria is a continuous variable and the definition threshold should be reconsidered for specific categories of subjects, such as high risk individuals for cardiovascular events.

This data points out also for the need of population microalbuminuria screening studies. It is noteworthy that the WHO criteria for screening are completely fulfilled by microalbuminuria (Table 15.2).

Table 15.2

WHO screening criteria for microalbuminuria in diabetic patients and non-diabetic population
(Adapted from: Mogensen CE, 2002, [22])

Generally accepted criteria	Criteria fulfilled by MA (Y/N)	Significance
The condition should be an important public health problem	Y	Predicts cardiovascular and renal morbidity/mortality
There should be a generally accepted specific treatment if the disease is recognized	Y	Blocking the renin-angiotensin system
Diagnosis and treatment facilities should be available for the specified population	Y	Available in most countries
There should be a recognizable latent or early symptomatic stage	Y	Related both to cardiovascular and renal disease
There should be a suitable test or examination, acceptable for the population use	Y	Related to other risk factors; urine samples usually convenient
The natural evolution/ progression of the disease should be adequately understood	Y	Relationship with cardiovascular disease not completely understood
There should be an agreed policy about whom to treat (as patients)	Y	Best medical care should be offered
The cost/case found should be balanced to possible expenditure on medical care as a whole	Y	Difficult to calculate
Case finding should be a continuing process and not a "once-and-for-all" project	Y	Almost generally accepted

FAMILIAL AND GENETIC RISK FACTORS

RACIAL DIFFERENCES

There are many reports showing that familial clustering of renal and cardiovascular disease in diabetic patients may be accounted for by racial background. The prevalence of MA associated with high blood pressure (HBP) and cardiovascular events, as well as diabetic renal disease (DRD) appears to be 5 to 6 times higher among black Americans and Mexican Americans than in white non-Hispanic Americans [26, 27, 28]. The reasons for these differences remain unclear; the argument that cost barriers to medical care for black and Hispanic Americans [29] may impede early detection of MA and further medical intervention is not consistent for other populations with equally higher rates of HBP and DRD, such as Pima Indians.

However, other aspects of access to medical care, such as cultural barriers, should be evaluated for some specific ethnic groups.

SIBLINGS OF AFFECTED INDIVIDUALS

MA was found among 83% of the diabetic siblings of type 1 diabetic probands [30] with DRD, but in only 17% of diabetic siblings of type 1 diabetic probands without DRD (Figure 15.2); these data were confirmed by recent studies for type 2 diabetic patients also (71.5% *vs.* 24.5%) [31, 32].

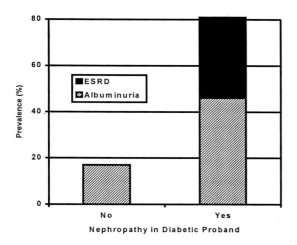

Figure 15.2

Prevalence of microalbuminuria and end stage renal disease in diabetic siblings of diabetic probands with or without diabetic renal disease.

(Adapted from Seaquist, *et al.*, *N Engl J Med,* 1989, [30], modified).

OFFSPRINGS OF AFFECTED INDIVIDUALS

An important study conducted in Pima Indians showed that proteinuria occurred among 14% of the diabetic offsprings of diabetic parents if neither parent had proteinuria, 23% if one parent had proteinuria and 46% if both parents had proteinuria [33] (Figure 15.3).

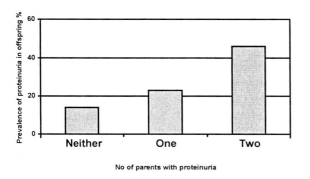

Figure 15.3

Prevalence of proteinuria in diabetic offsprings of diabetic individuals by number of parents with proteinuria in Pima Indians with T2DM.

(Adapted from Pettitt D, *et al.,* Diabetologia, 1990, [33]).

As with the siblings concordance described above, the inheritance could be to a larger extent due to shared environment, but since the environments of parents and of their children is very likely to differ more than those of siblings, a genetic inheritance is a strong possibility. The segregation analysis of the above data supported a major gene effect on the prevalence of DRD when duration of diabetes was accounted for, suggesting that individuals homozygous or heterozygous for the putative high risk allele have a high risk for MA (or proteinuria), particularly after a long diabetes duration, while those heterozygous for low risk allele have a low risk for DRD regardless of diabetes duration.

These conclusions were confirmed afterwards in a segregation analysis of albumin excretion rate conducted in Caucasian type 2 diabetic patients, which was consistent with the deleterious effect of a single gene [34].

FAMILIAL HYPERTENSION AND DRD

The examination of blood pressure in non-diabetic family members of diabetic patients with MA or proteinuria found that both systolic and diastolic blood pressures were significantly higher in the parents of diabetic subjects with proteinuria than in the parents of diabetic subjects without proteinuria [35], the differences in mean blood pressure averaging 15 mmHg [36].

The reported risk for developing MA for type 1 diabetic patients is about three times higher if they have one parent with HBP than in those without such a parental history [37]; approximately same values for the relative risk were found in T2DM patients with paternal history of hypertension [38].

Among type 2 diabetic Pima Indians whose parents did not have proteinuria, those with hypertensive parents had a significantly higher prevalence of proteinuria than those with normotensive parents, irrespective of the presence of parental diabetes [38] (Figure 15.4).

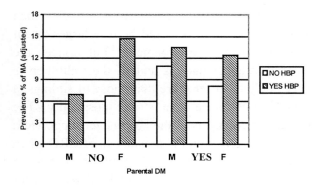

Figure 15.4

Prevalence of proteinuria according to parental hypertension and diabetes, adjusted for sex, DM duration and post load plasma glucose.

(Adapted from Nelson, *et al.*, Diabetologia, 1996 [38]).

GENETIC MARKERS

A biochemical marker with a clear genetically transmitted background, which was related in several studies with higher risk for essential hypertension and DRD, in diabetic patients, is the sodium-lithium countertransport (SLC) activity in red blood cells membrane [39].

A higher SLC activity, consecutive to a congenitally higher "set-up point" of the transporter rate, was detected in proteinuric diabetic patients [40] as well as in parents of type 2 diabetic proteinuric patients, compared with normoalbuminuric patients, respectively with parents of type 1 diabetic normoalbuminuric patients [41].

Familial clustering studies [42] reported a higher prevalence of HBP among siblings of subjects with type 2 diabetes mellitus than in siblings of type 1 diabetes mellitus subjects and the presence of HBP in siblings was not related to the BP of the probands.

Among Pima Indians, the presence of HBP measured one-year prior the onset of type 2 diabetes predicted the MA after the diagnosis of diabetes [43].

A number of studies aimed to detect a significant relationship between MA and the genes of the major histocompatibility system (HLA), but the results are still conflictual. A recent evaluation

of a large cohort of type 1 diabetic patients [44] found no association between HLA loci and DRD; however, in another study [45], authors have detected an association between specific phenotypes of heavy chains of immunoglobulins and the presence of MA, suggesting an immunogenetic predisposition for DRD.

A larger number of association studies for DRD were conducted with candidate genes selected for their possible pathogenetic role, the most prominent in this category being the angiotensin 1-converting enzyme (ACE) gene, on chromosome 17. The ACE gene displayed an insertion/deletion (I/D) type polymorphism, located in the intron 16 of the gene, which is related to the variable expression of the enzyme [46]: the presence of D allele increases the ACE activity with about 50% [47]. In a prospective study conducted in type 1 diabetic patients [48] the prevalence and severity on renal and vascular involvement was found dependent in a dominant manner on the presence of D allele (the relative risk for DRD attributable to D allele is 1.9) [48] Table 15.3.

Table 15.3

Diagram of the renin-angiotensin system, and its components which display genetic polymorphisms with clinical impact

(Adapted from Marre M, *et al.*, *J Clin Invest* 1997, [48])

Protein	Polymorphism	Clinical association
Angiotensinogen ↓← renin Angiotensin I ↓← ACE Angiotensin II ↓ ATR 1	M235T, T174M I/D A1166C	Essential hypertension Myocardial infarction Renal failure Essential hypertension

ACE: angiotensin converting enzyme
ATR 1: angiotensin receptor type 1
I/D : insertion/deletion (polymorphism)

Another genetic polymorphism of renin-angiotensin system (RAS) is caused by a M235T translocation located at the level of angiotensinogen gene (chromosome 3), which is related to an increased amount of substrate for ACE and thus an increased activity of RAS [49]; the angiotensin II receptor type 1 (ATR 1) structure might be also affected by a similar type of polymorphism (A1166C), which was related to the presence of MA and poor glycemic control in type 1 diabetic patients [50].

A recent study conducted in Pima Indians [51] with type 2 diabetes found suggestive linkage for DRD and cardiovascular disease with a region located on chromosome 7, which contains three possible candidate genes: the aldose reductase (ALDR 1), endothelial nitric oxide synthase (NOS 3) and the T-cell receptor b-chain (TCRBC). The results of studies with the polymorphism caused by the dinucleotide-repeat variability of ALDR1 are equivocal [52], but the a-deletion allele of NOS3 gene was strongly associated with an increased risk of rapid deterioration of renal and vascular functions in type 1 diabetic patients [53] and also Caucasian T2DM patients [54].

EPIDEMIOLOGICAL DATA

TYPE 2 DIABETIC PATIENTS

The suspicion that MA is not only a marker of renal involvement, but rather is indicative for a systemic cardiovascular alteration associated with diabetes mellitus, was first raised by studies which found a two to four times higher cardiovascular mortality in type 2 microalbuminuric diabetic patients with the same "classic" risk factors (plasma lipids, blood pressure levels) as normoalbuminuric patients [55].

Several prospective studies have shown microalbuminuria to be an independent predictor of mortality [56, 57, 58] (Table 15.4). In a 8 year follow-up study conducted in a type 2 diabetic patients cohort [56], MA was the best predictor of long-term mortality; the increase in risk was detectable at an albumin excretion rate (AER) of 10.6 µg/min and the relative risk (RR) for cardiovascular death in these patients was 1.7 [57]. The above data led to the suggestion that in T2DM patients MA should be defined as an AER of more than 10µg/min [59].

Table 15.4

Multivariate analysis of risk factors for coronary heart disease mortality in type 2 diabetes
(Adapted from Mattock, *et al.*, *Diabetes*, 1998, discussed in [59])

	CHD mortality (RR)
Age	2.0 (0.94 – 4.3)
Sex	3.8 (1.16 – 12.6)
Pre-existent CHD	2.7 (093 – 7.94)
HbA1$_c$	1.5 (1.01 – 2.32)
Microalbuminuria	**1.8 (0.56 – 6.04)**
Serum cholesterol	2.5 (1.5 – 4.17)

CHD: coronary heart disease.
RR: relative risk (95% confidence level).

In a 9 year follow-up prospective study [60] conducted in type 2 diabetic Caucasian patients, the global mortality was 28.4%, 68% of the deaths were caused by cardiovascular disease (CVD); the baseline predictors of death were higher HbA1c, higher LDL-cholesterol, lower HDL-cholesterol, higher non-esterified fatty acids concentrations and MA. 45% of the patients who died in the follow-up period had MA, as opposed to 6% of the survivors.

In a recent 7-year prospective study of a hospital-based cohort of type 2 diabetic patients [61], coronary heart disease (CHD) was the cause of death in 72% of patients with MA, as compared with 39% of normoalbuminuric patients. In this study, MA was an independent predictor of mortality only if plasma cholesterol and HbA1c levels were entered as categorical variables, suggesting that the cardiovascular risk associated with MA is, at least in part, related to a "disadvantageous" alteration in conventional cardiovascular risk factors. These data confirmed previous results of a 10 year prospective study conducted in a cohort of newly diagnosed type 2 diabetic patients [62]. In this study, the levels of AER after 5 years of follow-up predicted the 10-year CVD mortality independently of plasma lipids levels, but the presence of MA was not an independent predictor when adjusted for blood glucose levels.

TYPE 1 DIABETIC PATIENTS

MA is strongly predictive for the development of proteinuria (overt DRD), chronic renal failure, (Table 15.5) and is also associated with excess of risk for coronary, cerebrovascular and peripheral vascular disease in type 1 diabetic patients [63].

Table 15.5

Risk factors for the development of chronic renal failure in diabetic patients. The WHO-MSVDD Study

(Adapted from Colhoun, *et al.*, *Diabetologia*, 2001, cited by [59])

	Type 1 DM (RR)	Type 2 DM (RR)
TAs (>140 mmHg)	1.5 (1.1–1.9)	0.9 (0.7–1.1)
Microalbuminuria	**2.8 (1.6–5.1)**	**1.9 (1.2–3.1)**
Hypertriglyceridemia	0.9 (0.6–1.4)	1.3 (1.1–1.5)
Hyperglycaemia	1.4 (0.8–2.4)	2 (1.6–2.5)
Diabetic retinopathy	2.3 (1.3–4.4)	4 (2.5–6.4)

RR: relative risk (95% confidence level).

An important prospective study [64] found that after 23 years of follow-up the RR of cardiovascular mortality for insulin-dependent diabetic patients with MA, compared with those without MA at the baseline was 2.94 (95% CI = 1.18–7.34). A recent 10 year observational follow-up study [65], conducted in 939 type 1 diabetic patients, confirmed the above data, MA appearing as an independent risk factor for cardiovascular mortality, as well as age, smoking and overt proteinuria.

There are other two specific risk factors, which are independently associated with MA in increasing the CVD risk in T1DM patients: significant neuropathy [66] and left ventricular hypertrophy [67, 68].

ESSENTIAL HYPERTENSION

There is an intrinsic strong relationship between diabetes mellitus (high blood glucose) and HBP in the determination of high cardiovascular risk associated with DRD ("bad companions"). MA, as a marker of cardiovascular damage, is independently associated with both hyperglycemia and hypertension, and also with lipid abnormalities. MA is now widely considered the link between the metabolic and hemodynamic pathogenic processes that are leading to the CVD in diabetic patients. Recent data are suggesting that the endothelial dysfunction may be the underlying explanation for these defects [69].

The studies conducted in hypertensive non-diabetic subjects have found that the presence of MA (25% in treated and 40% in untreated patients, [70]) is associated with some specific clinical features: an altered blood pressure circadian rhythm, with less nocturnal reduction in arterial pressure [71], phenomenon called "non-dipper"; salt-sensitivity, a condition whereby a salt intake results in raised glomerular pressure [72], which itself is associated with a higher CVD risk. Generally speaking, the microalbuminuric hypertensive patients have a higher mean 24 h BP, lower day/night ratio and greater variability of pressure readings (Table 15.6).

Table 15.6

The relationships between urinary albumin excretion rate and ambulatory blood pressure in young type 1 diabetic patients.
(Adapted from Lafferty, *et al.*, *Diabetes Care*, **23**: 533–538, 2000)

	Non-diabetic	Normoalbuminuria	MA intermittent	MA persistent	P
BPs/24h	119.7±8.3	122.4±5.1	125.3±8.9	**128.1±11.4***	0.009
BPd/24h	68.2±6.5	69.2±3.5	72.7±7.1	**76.5±7.3****	>0.001
BPm/24h	85.5±7.0	87.7±3.4	91,2±6.1	**94.5±7.2****	>0.001
BPs n	109.2±8.2	111.6±10.2	114.9±10.2	**117.7±10.1***	0.008
BPd n	57.8±6.5	59.2±4.1	61.8±7.2	**66.8±8.5****	>0.001
BPm n	76.5±5.9	78.8±7.4	81.3±7.0	**85.3±7.3****	>0.001
BPs d	122.2±8.5	124.8±5.2	127.7±9.4	**130.4±11.8***	0.012

Table 15.6

(continued)

	Non-diabetic	Normoalbuminuria	MA intermittent	MA persistent	P
BPd d	70.7±7.0	71.6±4.3	75.4±7.6	**78.6±7.7****	0.002
BPm d	88.2±6.4	89.6±4.0	93.5±6.6	**96.6±7.9****	>0.001

n – nocturnal.
d – diurnal.
* – statistically significant compared with non-diabetics.
** – statistically significant compared with non-diabetics and normoalbuminuric diabetics.
BPs – systolic blood pressure.
BPd – diastolic blood pressure.
BPm – mean blood pressure.

The microalbuminuric patients showing this particular profile of HBP are more prone to develop increased carotid artery thickness [73], left ventricular hypertrophy [74] and coronary events [75]. Interestingly, in hypertensive non-diabetic patients, the few morphological studies have failed to prove any association between MA and renal structural alterations [76].

THE POSSIBLE MECHANISMS OF CARDIOVASCULAR DAMAGE

The debate on the possible involvement of MA in the pathogenesis of cardiovascular disease is focused on several topics which must be separately discussed: the role of "traditional" cardiovascular risk factors, which are strongly associated with the development of the progressive renal failure; the significance of the association between MA and some specific features in the evolution of systemic hypertension; the intrinsic relationship between MA and glycemic control; the relevance of the "non-conventional" risk factors which are clustering with MA (insulin resistance, endothelial dysfunction, inflammation).

THE RELATIONSHIP BETWEEN MA AND ATHEROSCLEROTIC RISK FACTORS

As we emphasized in the first part of this chapter, MA doubles the risk of major cardiovascular events and this risk level is similar or even higher than that conferred by established atherosclerotic risk factors. These findings held even after adjustments for the factors frequently associated with MA, such as age, current smoking, dyslipidemias, left ventricular hypertrophy and abdominal obesity [11] (Table 15.7).

The relevance of the deterioration of the renal function (predicted by MA) for the cardiovascular risk is quite different in type 1 *vs.* type 2 diabetes mellitus. A substudy of the HOPE (Heart Outcomes Prevention Evaluation) Study [77] found that MA was a strong predictor for cardiovascular disease in type 2 diabetic patients, even after adjustment for renal function. These data are particularly noteworthy, because MA has not been clearly demonstrated to predict overt nephropathy in type 2 diabetes patients; hence, the reason for the high cardiovascular risk in this population is not necessarily related to the later development of renal failure.

On the other hand, in type 1 diabetic patients MA is the best predictor of progressive renal disease [78]; other significant correlations of MA in these patients are with hypertension, long-term diabetes and poor glycemic control. Based on these data, the relation between MA and cardiovascular morbidity and mortality has been mainly attributed to the later development of renal failure, although some studies [79, 80] found that MA alone has been associated with excess cardiovascular mortality in type 1 diabetic adult patients. However, these findings were not confirmed in the DCCT (Diabetes Control and Complications Trial, [81]), where the 40% lower incidence of MA in the intensive treated group was not associated with significant changes in the incidence of cardiovascular morbidity. Nevertheless, nobody expected to have a significant incidence of macrovascular problems in the DCCT patients because their average age was about 27 years and they have had diabetes for only 5.6 years when the study began.

Table 15.7

The relationship between microalbuminuria and atherosclerosis risk factors (meta-analysis, discussed by [20])

	Winocour (1992)	Woo 1992	Metcalf (1992)	Gould (1993)	Dimmitt (1993)	Beatty (1993)	Mykannen (1994)	Jensen (1997)
Sex(M)				↑	↑			↑
Age				↑	↓		↑	
BP	↑	↑	↑	↑			↑	↑
Insulinemia		↑					↑	
Plasma lipids			↑		↑	↑	↑	
Body mass index			↑					↑
Current smoking			↑					↑
Glycemia				↑		↑		

↑ – the association between microalbuminuria and the specified risk factor increased the cardiovascular risk comparing with the presence of the risk factor without microalbuminuria.

The specific pathogenic mechanisms behind the associations between "classic" cardiovascular risk factors and MA are still poorly understood; it was previously shown that healthy individuals with MA, as well as diabetic patients, have a generalized increase in transvascular escape rate of albumin, so MA could be considered as a marker of widespread microvascular damage (the Steno hypothesis). Experimental studies demonstrated that increased transvascular albumin transport is associated with an increased transport of lipoproteins into the vascular wall and therefore was speculated that MA might be a marker of increased susceptibility to the atherogenic effect of the established ("classic") risk factors.

Thus, individuals with other atherosclerotic risk factors such as smoking, dyslipidemia or high blood pressure should have their urinary albumin excretion measured, because this piece of information might contribute to the classification of the subject as a high-risk (or high-susceptibility) individual.

MICROALBUMINURIA AND ARTERIAL BLOOD PRESSURE

MA occurs in about 30% of non-diabetic hypertensive subjects (ranging between 10 to 40%), depending on age and ethnic group [82, 83]; in hypertensive patients MA correlates with conventional and non-conventional markers of cardiovascular disease. After adjustment for these factors, MA has been shown to be an independent risk factor for cardiovascular disease and mortality in hypertensive patients (p = 0.001), [84].

In an analysis [85] performed on the initially untreated hypertensive patients group from a larger population prospective study of more than 2000 non-diabetic patients followed for 10 years (WHO-Monitoring Trends and Determinants of Cardiovascular Disease, MONICA Study), the authors found a relative risk (in the final model, (Table 15.8) for developing ischemic heart disease in microalbuminuric patients of 5.4 (95%

CI = 1.8–15.7, p = 0.002). MA was also, in a 5 year follow-up of the Hoorn Study population [86], a good predictor for cardiovascular mortality, with an overall adjusted relative risk of 2.8 (95% CI= = 1.15–7.16) and even higher for the diabetic population, 5.20 (1.57–12.03), Table 15.9.

In the Copenhagen City Heart Study [87] also, the clinically "healthy" individuals with a urinary albumin excretion level higher than 90th percentile (≥ 7μg/min) were characterized by higher blood pressure, lower plasma HDL-cholesterol,

concentrations but MA was independently related to the incidence of CVD.

In hypertensive population MA seems to result from an increased filtered albumin load, rather from decreased tubular reabsorption [88]. The systemic blood pressure levels have a good correlation with intraglomerular pressure and MA [89]. In hypertensive patients, MA correlates with salt sensitivity, absence of nocturnal dip in blood pressure and higher mean 24h blood pressure measurements [90].

Table 15.8

Final model for prediction of ischemic heart disease in 204 subjects with arterial hypertension

(Adapted from: Jensen JS, *et al.*, *Hypertension*, 2000, [85])

Variables in final model	Relative risk (95% CI)	P
Microalbuminuria	5.4 (1.8–15.7)	**0.002**
Male gender	3.9 (1.2–12.8)	0.005
Plasma total cholesterol	1.6 (1.2–2.3)	0.004

All variables were initially entered in the model and, if insignificant (p ≥ 0.05), they were successively excluded by the conditional backward elimination method.

Table 15.9

Relative risk of 5-year cardiovascular mortality associated with the presence of MA after adjusting for potential confounding risk factors

(Adapted from: Jager A, *et al.*, *Arterioscl Thromb Vasc Biol,* 1999, [86])

Added variables	Non-diabetic subjects (n = 458)*	Diabetic subjects (n = 173)*	All subjects (n = 631)*
Model 1 and MA**	1.84 (0.20–16.5)	5.5 (1.91–15.84)	4.31 (1.79–10.36)
Model 2 and MA***	2.30 (0.15–34.56)	5.23 (1.66–16.48)	**2.87 (1.15–7.16)**
Model 3 and MA****	0.99 (0.04–26.57)	5.20 (1.57–12.03)	**2.86 (1.11–7.34)**

    * – relative risk ratio (95% confidence interval level).

    ** – stratification variables: age, sex, type 2 diabetes (IGT).

   *** – as model 1, plus all risk factors associated with cardiovascular mortality: hypertension, low HDL-cholesterol, triglyceride level and pre-existent ischemic heart disease.

  **** – as model 2 plus risk factors that were non-significant: obesity, current smoking and total cholesterol level.

   MA – Albumin/creatinine ratio ≥ 2mg/mmol.

THE RELATIONSHIP BETWEEN GLYCEMIA AND MICROALBUMINURIA

A recent evaluation of the Framingham Offspring Study population was aimed to assess current and long term associations between glycemia (in non-diabetic subjects) and MA (considered as a marker of generalized endothelial injury) [91]. MA was detected in 9.5% of men and 13.4% of women; the age-adjusted odd ratios for MA associated with each 5mg/dl increase in baseline and time-integrated 24h glucose levels were 1.12 (95% CI = 1.00–1.16), respectively 1.16 (95% CI = 1.11–1.21). These effects persisted after adjustments for systolic blood pressure levels and other possible confounders.

Higher glucose levels (baseline and time-integrated) were also predictive for the development of MA, diabetes mellitus and cardiovascular disease (CVD). The type of association suggests that the risk for MA, like risk for CVD, may increase in a graded fashion across the spectrum of glucose tolerance [92]. Further work is required to determine whether there is any glycemic threshold below, which there is no risk for increased urinary albumin excretion or CVD.

These long-term associations are consistent with the hypothesis that type 2 diabetes mellitus, CVD and MA arose together over the course of decades and they may be caused by a common pathogenetic antecedent (the "common soil"), putatively insulin resistance and the consecutive endothelial dysfunction. Apart of this association, the other specific mechanisms that could produce glycemia-related MA include glycation of basement membrane proteic components, with loss of charge selectivity and the glomerular hyperperfusion/hyperfiltration, with increased intraglomerular pressure.

Chronic hyperglycemia (long-term type 1 diabetic patients) is well established as an important cause of microalbuminuria. Moreover, as results of a recent study [93] have shown, given the long duration of diabetes in these patients, it is therefore

Table 15.10

Molecular mechanisms of insulin resistance and their relationship to insulin-resistant states in humans
(Adapted from: Makimattila, *et al.*, *Circulation*, 1996, [93])

Type	Etiology	Proteins involved	Mechanism	Insulin resistant human state
Sequence alterations	Genetic	Insulin receptor	Over 100 mutations described	Leprechaunism ++
		IRS-1	G972R, S892G, A513P etc	Type 2 diabetes ++
		PI3-kinase	M326I	Type 2 diabetes ++
Level of expression	Genetic	Insulin receptor	Promoter mutations, half-life effects	Leprechaunism ++
Decreased protein level	Acquired	Insulin receptor	Degradation	Obesity ++ Type 2 diabetes ++
		IRS-1, IRS-2	Degradation	Obesity++ Type 2 diabetes ++
Decreased tyrosine phosphorylation	Acquired	Insulin receptor	PTB-1B, PC-1	Obesity++ Type 2 diabetes ++
		IRS-1	unknown	Obesity++ Type 2 diabetes ++
Increased serine phosphorylation	Acquired	Insulin receptor	PKC	Obesity+ Type 2 diabetes + Type 1 diabetes +
		IRS-1	TNFα	Obesity++ Type 2 diabetes ++
O-glycosylation	Acquired	Transcription factors	Hexosamine pathway	Obesity+ Type 2 diabetes + Type 1 diabetes + Hyperlipidemia +

possible that another important mechanism responsible for MA might lead to secondary (acquired) insulin resistance (Table 15.10) due to long term effects of hyperglycemia and caused by a defect in insulin stimulation of glucose extraction and not blood flow dependent (as in endothelial dysfunction).

Together, these data imply that hyperglycemia can determine MA via at least three different mechanisms: lesions of the basement membranes, raised intraglomerular pressure and insulin resistance (primary or secondary); these mechanisms might be of distinct importance in different situations: type 1 vs. type 2 diabetes, or recent vs. long term diabetes.

MICROALBUMINURIA AND THE ENDOTHELIAL DYSFUNCTION

Since the functions of endothelial cells are multiple and involve several systems, (Table 15.11) no single definition of endothelial dysfunction (ED) covers the whole array of possible disruption in normal function [94]. Pragmatically defined, ED includes any modification (increase or decrease out of normal range) of the endothelium-related chemical messengers and/or alteration of any known endothelial function: vascular permeability to macromolecules [95], vascular tonus [96] and coagulant activity of plasma.

Table 15.11

Endothelial cells functions
(Adapted from: Calles-Escandon J, *et al.*,
Endocrine Rev, 2001, [94])

Functional targets	Specific cellular or physiological actions and mediators	
Vascular lumen	*Vasoconstriction* endothelin-1 angiotensin II	*Vasodilatation* NO Bradykinin
Cellular growth and proliferation	*Stimulation* PGDF FGF IGF-1	*Inhibition* NO PGI 2 TGF
Inflammation	*Proinflammatory* VCAM ICAM	*Antiinflammatory?*
Hemostasis	*Prothrombotic* PAI-1	*Antithrombotic* Prostacyclin

According to this view, MA is a direct manifestation of ED (either widespread or at the glomerular level), reflecting increased capillary permeability.

ED in type 1 diabetes mellitus is not a constant finding and is not clear from the literature whether it is a consequence of the diabetic milieu or a marker of CVD that independently associated with diabetes.

In experimental models [97], the most commonly accepted ED manifestation, namely decrease of endothelium-dependent vasodilatation is not significantly impaired by hyperglycemia. A depression of acetylcholine-stimulated vasodilatation was found in human type 1 diabetic patients, relative to healthy control subjects, directly related with the presence of MA and inversely related with diabetic retinopathy [98]. Flow-mediated vasodilatation was significantly impaired in type 1 diabetic patients *vs.* non-diabetic controls [99], the difference being directly related to the diabetes duration and low density lipoprotein (LDL) cholesterol levels and inversely related to insulin concentration [100]. No relationship was found between endothelial function alterations and glycosylated hemoglobin levels.

These data suggest that ED in type 1 diabetic patients is an early marker of CVD and not a direct consequence of the diabetic milieu; although the diabetic state predisposes to ED, it seems to be not sufficient to cause it. MA, if not associated with major ED manifestations in these patients, is more likely a sign of diabetic renal disease than a marker of cardiovascular risk.

ED in type 2 diabetes mellitus plays a more complicated role than that in type 1, because the effect of aging, hypertension, dyslipidemia and other factors add to the complexity of the problem. In fact, markers of ED are often present in type 2 diabetic patients years before any manifestation of microvascular involvement, such as MA, becomes evident [101, 102].

Insulin resistant subjects like type 2 diabetic patients, by definition, are defective in insulin-dependent intracellular glucose transport, which is mediated through the phosphatidylinositol 3-kinase (PI3-K) pathway. This pathway also mediates the vasodilator and NO production stimulator insulin effects. Mounting evidence suggests that insulin resistance is associated with a defect in insulin-stimulated NO production. On the other hand, the MAPK-dependent insulin effects (cell proliferation and migration) seem to be not affected by insulin resistance; moreover, due to hyperinsulinemia, these effects are enhanced, contributing to the proatherogenic action of insulin resistance.

Recent data provide evidence about the strong intrinsic relationship between hyperinsulinemia / insulin resistance (which is the main feature of type 2 diabetes mellitus) and ED, even before the clinical onset of diabetes (persistent hyperglycemia). Thus, the obese state, a model of human insulin resistance, is associated with impaired basic and acetylcholine-stimulated [103] NO-dependent vasodilatation [104] and with significant elevations of endothelin-1 [105] and PAI-1, whose decreasing was particularly noted in response to moderate weight loss [106].

Table 15.12

Cellular and molecular basis for endothelial dysfunction in diabetes
(Adapted from: Calles-Escandon J, *et al.*, *Endocrine Rev*, 2001, [94])

Molecular mechanism	Results
Increased activation of PKC	Vessels proliferation, altered contraction and signal transduction
Over expression of growth factors	Increased growth and phenotypic changes of VSMC
Non-enzymatic glycation of proteins, lipids and other molecules (DNA)	Changes in function and antigenicity (immune mediated damage)
Increased synthesis of DAG (glycemia-induced)	Impaired vasodilatation, enhanced proliferation of VSMC and activation of PKC
Impaired insulin activation of PI3-kinase but normal activation of MAP-kinase	Increased growth of vessels and proliferation of VSMC, in response to hyperinsulinemia
Increased production of PAI-1	Decreased fibrinolysis, pro-coagulant state
Oxidative stress	Decreased synthesis of NO, hyperreactivity of VSMC to vasoconstrictor stimuli, inflammation

The insulin resistance syndrome encompasses more than truncal obesity and a subnormal response to insulin-mediated glucose disposal, but frequently associates high blood pressure, dyslipidemia (higher triglycerides levels and lower HDL-cholesterol levels), dysfibrinolysis and MA. Therefore, it is tempting to speculate that loss of endothelial-dependent vasodilatation and increased vasoconstrictors activity, like endothelin-1, might be etiologic factors of hypertension. Moreover, decreased activity of endothelium-bound protein lipase may contribute to dyslipidemia. Some recent studies [107–109] suggested also that PAI-1 increased activity, which is a marker of ED present in insulin resistance syndrome, plays a major role in the progression of CVD.

Highlights of some cellular molecular mechanisms (Table 15.12) that were involved in ED pathogenesis in type 2 microalbuminuric diabetic patients are:

– increase of intracellular glucose disposal results in abnormal activation of protein kinase C (PKC) pathway through increased *de novo* synthesis of diacylglycerol (DAG); both DAG and PKC are important signaling molecules involved in a wide variety of cellular metabolic processes, including modulation of NO release. Activation of PKC induces a depletion of NADPH pool (hyperglycemic pseudohypoxia, [110]), changing the redox state of the cell with a consecutive decrease in NO production and vasoconstriction [111];

– overexpression of growth factors, including insulin, insulin-like GF (IGF), vascular endothelial GF (VEGF), platelet-derived GF (PDGF), etc., which is characteristic for the diabetic milieu, might be a necessary link between diabetes and the proliferation of endothelial and vascular smooth muscle cells (VSMC) observed in early stages of CVD [112];

– non-enzymatic glycation of proteins and other macromolecules, such as LDL particles or membrane phospholipids, induces changes in the properties of proteins as well as antigenic changes and generates oxidative stress through overproduction of reactive oxygen species (ROS). The endothelial cells are particularly susceptible to damage by oxidative stress [113], the main manifestations being the diminished production of NO [114], a prothrombotic tendency and increased platelet aggregation [115].

MICROALBUMINURIA
AND INFLAMMATION

Phenotypic heterogeneity of MA. The associations between MA and ED may underlie its clustering with hypertension and CVD; nevertheless, there is increasing evidence of heterogeneity among these relationships [116–118].

The EURODIAB IDDM Complications Study [119] detected a significant correlation between urinary albumin excretion rate, hypertension and ED markers (von Willebrand factor), but only in subjects with evidence of diabetic retinopathy (about 50% in the study group). Renal histology in microalbuminuric type 1 diabetic patients with hypertension and retinopathy shows increase in both mesangial volume and basement membrane width [120], but these changes do not usually appear in normotensive patients with MA; this variability is in keeping with the observation that not all type 1 diabetic patients with MA progress to proteinuria [121].

Type 2 diabetic patients show a more significant association between the presence of MA, hypertension and ED markers than in type 1 diabetes; however, there is an important heterogeneity among these associations as well as in the renal morphology [117]. Two recent papers analyzed renal biopsies performed in type 2 diabetic patients with MA; in the first study [122], typical diabetic renal disease lesions were found in 77% of 35 patients, two-thirds of them having diabetic retinopathy *vs.* none in the non-diabetic renal histological abnormalities group. The other study [123] found typical renal disease changes in only 30% of 34 microalbuminuric patients; the remaining 70% of the patients show either near-normal renal structure (30%) or other type of lesions, mainly tubulo-interstitial (40%). The ED markers (von Willebrand factor) were present only in those patients with typical or atypical renal lesions, but not in the patients with near-normal renal structure.

Thus, both in type 1 diabetes and, even more in type 2 diabetes, the relationships of MA with renal and vascular lesions are clearly heterogeneous and such different patterns may imply heterogeneity of etiology and prognosis.

Low-grade inflammation. Based on the above data, it was further speculated [118] that MA in diabetes mellitus may have at least two different etiologies: one etiology that involves a close link with generalized ED and one that does not. Only MA associated with ED ("malignant" MA, [118]) seems to confer an increased risk of CVD and/or chronic renal failure (Table 15.13). Some genetic and environmental factors might predispose to the ED-related MA, such as early growth retardation, abnormalities of cationic membrane transport, polymorphisms of specific enzymes like angiotensin converting enzyme or endothelial nitric oxide synthase, etc.

Table 15.13

Prognostic implications of heterogeneity of microalbuminuria in diabetes mellitus

(Adapted from Stehouwer, *et al.*, *Nephrol Dial Transplant*, 1998 [118])

	Normoalbuminuria	MA without EC dysfunction markers ("benign")	MA with EC dysfunction markers ("malignant")
Severe retinopathy	–	+	+++
Renal failure	–	+/++	+++
Cardiovascular disease	–	+	+++

MA – microalbuminuria.

EC – endothelial cells.

Table 15.14

The cross-sectional associations between elevated levels of sVCAM and cardiovascular risk factors or risk indicators

(Adapted from: Jager A, *et al.*, *Diabetes,* 2000, [126])

Risk factor	Mean (SD) or %	RR (95% CI)* for CV mortality	P**
Fasting insulin (pmol/l)	84 (21)	1.35 (0.73–2.48)[++]	0.009
Type 2 diabetes (Y/N)	27	2.76 (1.35–5.65)	< 0.0005
Total cholesterol (mmol/l)*	6.6 (1.2)	1.23 (0.97–1.56)	< 0.0005
LDL-cholesterol (mmol/l)*	4.5(1.1)	1.27 (0.97–1.65)	< 0.0005
HDL- cholesterol (mmol/l)*	1.3 (0.4)	2.74 (1.31–5.71)[++]	0.03
vWF(IU/ml)[+]	1.37 (0.7)	1.95 (1.04–3.64)	< 0.0005
CRP(mg/l)[+]	1.75	2.02 (1.08–3.80)	0.004
Microalbuminuria (Y/N)[+++]	11	3.38 (1.71–6.68)	0.002

*   – RR (95% CI) was obtained with Cox regression analysis, after adjustment for age, sex and glucose tolerance, for cardiovascular mortality associated with continuous or dichotomous variables.

**   – p values were obtained by linear regression analysis, with sVCAM levels as dependent variable and risk factors as independent variables.

*** – *per* 1 mmol/l increase.

[+]   – upper tertile *vs.* lower tertiles (>1.56 IU/ml for vWF and >2.84 mg/l for C-reactive protein).

[++]   – upper tertile *vs.* lower tertile (log-transformed values); < 0.9 *vs.* ≥ 0.9 mmol/l.

[+++] – albumin-to-creatinine ratio < 2 *vs.* ≥ 2 mg/mmol.

Y/N: yes *vs.* no.

The nature of link between MA and ED in diabetes needs to be clarified; as we mentioned before, ED might directly cause MA through synthesis of a leaky basement membrane, or ED and MA might develop together because of a common underlying pathophysiological process. A support for the later hypothesis is in a recent study [124] that demonstrates that the occurrence of "traditional" risk factors (hypertension, dyslipidemia, and hyper-glycaemia) could not explain the excess of cardiovascular risk due to impairment of endothelial functions in diabetic patients with progressive renal disease.

On the other hand, a large number of recent epidemiological and observational studies have shown an association between low-grade inflammation (subclinical) markers, MA and CVD (risk of cardiovascular events) [125]. It was further demonstrated that exposure of endothelial cells to inflammatory cytokines, which have 8 to 10 times higher plasma levels in microalbuminuric diabetic patients in the presence of ED markers [126], leads to expression of cell-surface adhesion molecules and impairs endothelium-dependent vascular relaxation. The soluble adhesion molecules high plasmatic levels are directly and independently related to cardiovascular mortality (RR = 1.10, 95% CI = 1.05–1.15, for every 100 ng/ml increase in soluble vascular cell adhesion molecule, sVCAM, [126]), to fasting insulinemia [127], von Willebrand factor (vWF) levels and presence of MA too [128]. (Table 15.14) These associations are highly suggestive for a unique etiology of ED and MA, having as common background hyperinsulinemia / insulin resistance and the progressive low-grade vessel wall inflammation.

Noteworthy, the fact that sVCAM (and other adhesion molecules, like sICAM or E-selectin) association with cardiovascular mortality is independent of the levels of ED markers, like vWF, raises the possibility that sVCAM is not a marker of ED, or it might reflect another "facet" of ED, different from that reflected by increased levels of vWF or the presence of microalbuminuria.

A recent study [129] aimed to verify if insulin resistance *per se* is associated with inflammation in non-diabetic subjects with insulin resistance syndrome (IRS). All three studied inflammatory markers (C-reactive protein, fibrinogen and white cell count) were correlated with several components of IRS; strong correlations were found between CRP and body mass index, fasting insulin/proinsulin plasma levels, systolic blood pressure and insulin sensitivity index, in a multivariate linear regression model.

Conclusions. The above data suggest that chronic subclinical (low-grade) inflammation is the fundamental pathophysiological process that underlies the development of insulin resistance and widespread endothelial dysfunction in diabetic patients. The systemic inflammatory response might be triggered by infectious and non-infectious factors; its evolution and intensity is modulated by a multitude of metabolic and hemodynamic factors, hyperglycemia and high systemic blood pressure being the most important. Different biologic markers, such as vWF, soluble adhesion molecules or CRP are useful in monitoring this process, but MA is the best independent predictor of future cardiovascular events and mortality in diabetic as well as in non-diabetic patients, because it reflects a global and generalized microvascular wall lesion. These findings strongly argue in favor of initiating new anti-inflammatory and insulin-sensitizing treatment strategies in IRS patients, even before the clinical onset of diabetes.

NEW STRATEGIES TO REDUCE CARDIOVASCULAR RISK IN MICROALBUMINURIC DIABETIC PATIENTS

Recent epidemiological trials [130] have shown that mortality from cardiovascular disease is increased by a factor of two to three in persons with diabetes mellitus and MA, as compared with the general population. To reduce this increased risk, a multifactorial approach to the management of type 2 diabetes has been advocated, including not only a better glycemic control, but also aggressive treatment of associated "traditional" and non-traditional cardiovascular risk factors with more stringent target levels for lipids and blood pressure than those recommended for the general population.

Such a multifactorial intensive intervention was provided for a cohort of type 2 micro-albuminuric diabetic patients (Table 15.15), followed-up for a period of 7.8 years in a recent study [131], which were compared with a cohort of type 2 diabetic patients "conventionally" treated and followed-up for the same period.

Table 15.15

Treatment goals for the conventional- and intensive-therapy group
(Adapted from: Gaede P, *et al., N Engl J Med,* 2003, [131])

	Conventional therapy group (n = 63)		Intensive therapy group (n = 67)	
	1993–1999	2000–2001	1993–1999	2000–2001
Systolic BP (mmHg)	<160	<135	<140	<130
Diastolic BP (mmHg)	<95	<85	<85	<80
Glycosylated hemoglobin (%)	<7.5	<6.5	<6.5	<6.5
Fasting serum total cholesterol (mg/dl)	<250	<190	<190	<175
Fasting serum triglycerides (mg/dl)	<195	<180	<150	<150
ACE-I treated (irrespective of BP)	No	Yes	Yes	Yes

The intensive treatment consists of lifestyle and dietetic counseling, an intensified metabolic control, aiming for HbA1c levels of less than 7%, a tight blood pressure control (targeting to 130/80 mmHg) and lowering the lipids levels into the recommended range (LDL-cholesterol ≤ 100 mg/dl; triglycerides ≤ 150 mg/dl). The groups differed significantly with respect to HbA1c values, fasting serum lipids concentrations, systolic and diastolic blood pressure and albumin excretion rates; these differences were maintained throughout the follow-up period (Table 15.16). From a total of 118 cardiovascular events occurred during the follow-up period, there were 85 events among the patients in the conventional-therapy group and only 33 events among the patients in the intensive-therapy group, with an adjusted hazard ratio for the intensive-therapy group of 0.47 (95% CI = 0.22–0.74, p = 0.01). The differences were significant for the incidence of diabetic complications (diabetic retinopathy and neuropathy) and for the incidence rate of overt diabetic renal disease.

These results showed that a targeted, long-term and intensive intervention involving multiple risk factors reduction produced an absolute 20% reduction in the risk of cardiovascular events in microalbuminuric type 2 diabetic patients; taken together the risk for macro- and microvascular complication, the overall risk reduction was about 50%. The global risk reduction was significantly higher than those obtained in studies applying a single-factor intervention strategy [132–135] and this finding might have considerable implications for the future management of type 2 diabetes. This type of focused multifactorial intervention, with continuous education/motivation, should be offered to type 2 diabetic patients with MA, who are at increased risk for cardiovascular complications, representing about one third of the population with type 2 diabetes mellitus.

Several specific therapeutic interventions have been tested in clinical trials aimed at improving endothelial function in diabetic patients with MA, such as those testing insulin sensitizers, renin-angiotensin system blockade and antioxidants; other trials have shown that hypolipidemic agents or estrogen replacement therapy improved endothelial functions, but these works were not focused directly on the effects in diabetic patients.

Table 15.16

Significant changes in clinical, behavioral and biochemical variables at the end of the follow-up period

(Adapted from: Gaede P, *et al., N Engl J Med*, 2003, [131])

Variable	Conventional therapy group	Intensive therapy group	P value
Systolic BP (mmHg)	−3±3	−14±2	<0.001
Diastolic BP (mmHg)	−8±2	−12±2	0.006
Carbohydrates (% of energy intake)	4.8±0.9	9.3±0.9	0.002
Fat (% of energy intake)	−6.8±0.9	−10.4±0.9	<0.001
Fasting plasma glucose (mg/dl)	−18±11	−52±8	<0.001
Fasting serum total cholesterol (mg/dl)	−3±7	−50±4	<0.001
Fasting serum LDL cholesterol (mg/dl)	−13±6	−47±5	<0.001
Urinary albumin excretion rate (mg/24h)	30	−20	0.007
Glycosylated hemoglobin (%)	0.2±0.3	−0.5±0.2	<0.001

Values are expressed as mean ± SD.

INSULIN SENSITIZERS

The thiazolidinediones (TZD) are a class of compounds that improve insulin action *in vivo* and have recently been introduced as therapeutic agents for the treatment of type 2 diabetes.

TZD have been administered in animal studies to a variety of insulin-resistant obese and diabetic animal models [136–137], showing significant improvements in insulin-stimulated glucose disposal as well as inhibition of hepatic glucose production. Experimental data [138, 139] also showed that activators of peroxisome proliferator receptors-γ, like troglitazone and other TZD, significantly reduced monocyte/macrophage homing to atherosclerotic plaques and also reduced in a dose-dependent manner the expression of adhesion molecules (VCAM-1, ICAM-1 and E-selectin) induced by different amounts of oxidized LDL and a tumor necrosis factor.

Based on these data, some clinical trials have been conducted to investigate the effects of this new class of antidiabetic drugs on endothelial functions in human diabetic subjects. These studies demonstrated beneficial effects, like amelioration of flow-dependent vasodilatation [140], insulin-induced vasodilatation [141] and whole-body and forearm glucose uptake [141]. This combination of findings is consistent with the presumed action of these compounds as insulin-sensitizing agents, as was therefore directly demonstrated by performing glucose clamps in type 2 diabetic patients before and after a period of TZD treatment.

TZD have also been used in the treatment of non-diabetic human insulin-resistant states, like non-complicated obesity, impaired glucose tolerance and polycystic ovarian syndrome [142, 143]. Since the mechanisms of insulin resistance are almost certainly heterogeneous across all these human conditions, the effectiveness of TZDs provides pharmacologic evidence about their capacity to ameliorate insulin resistance regardless of the diverse underlying genetic and acquired mechanisms. Treatment with TZDs seems to have beneficial effects on most, if not all, of the components of syndrome X [144]: reduction in circulating triglyceride levels, modest increase in HDL levels and reductions in PAI-1 levels [145].

The molecular mechanisms which can explain these pharmacologic actions remained relatively obscure until Ibrahimi *et al.* [146] discovered that these agents behave as agonists for the peroxisome proliferator-activated receptors γ (PPAR γ), which is a member of the PPAR family of nuclear receptors [147], directly involved in the regulation of genes controlling glucose and lipid metabolism.

A recent trial evaluated the efficacy and safety of rosiglitazone (a potent TZD) monotherapy in patients with type 2 diabetes. The results showed a reduction of HbA1c levels by 1.2 to 1.5%, compared to placebo; plasma insulinemia decreased significantly too. Homeostasis model assessment (HOMA) estimates indicate that rosiglitazone treatment reduced insulin resistance by about 25% and improved beta-cell function by 60%. Urinary albumin excretion rate in the microalbuminuric patients was reduced by approximate 21%; this decrease is probably the result of either improved glycemic control or a different effect of TZD on mesangial cell function.

CARDIOVASCULAR PROTECTION BY RENIN-ANGIOTENSIN SYSTEM BLOCKADE

A large number of recent trials [148] demonstrated the superiority of therapy with inhibitors of angiotensin-converting enzyme (ACEI) and angiotensin-receptors blockers (ARB) *versus* placebo or other classes of antihypertensive drugs for slowing the evolution of MA to proteinuria. However, it must be noted that many patients require three or more drugs to achieve the specified target levels of blood pressure control; even in those patients that failed to achieve the target levels, the treatment with ACEI was associated with a significant decrease in the incidence of cardiovascular events, phenomenon called "vasculoprotection".

The MICRO-HOPE Study [149] examined the effects of an ACEI (ramipril), administered for a 5 year follow-up period to a cohort of 3 557 microalbuminuric diabetic patients, on cardiovascular and renal outcomes. The primary endpoint (a composite of myocardial infarction, stroke or death from a cardiovascular cause) was reduced with 25% (p = 0.0004), compared to placebo; the secondary outcomes (total mortality and need for revascularization) were also significantly lowered, as well as the progression rate to overt nephropathy (16% reduction, p = 0.036). The most striking observation from this trial is that relatively large reductions in risk were achieved in the face of comparatively small reductions in blood pressure (the average reduction in blood pressure was 30/20 mmHg). This finding points towards possible direct effects of ACEI (as a class) on the heart and vasculature, in addition to their antihypertensive effects. It is also noteworthy, that the vasculoprotective effects of ramipril in HOPE study was even greater for diabetic patients, compared with non-diabetic high-risk population [150].

Apart from reducing incidence of cardiovascular events, the long-term aim is not slowing progression of albuminuria *per se*, although this could be useful as a surrogate marker, but primarily preservation of the renal function (and, perhaps structure), which, in order to be assessed, requires long-term studies of up to 6 to 8 years. Such a study [151], in microalbuminuric type 1 diabetic patients, showed that ACE treatment over 8 year period maintained an adequate GFR, whereas a clear-cut decline in GFR was reported in those who did not receive antihypertensive treatment. The better preservation of renal structure was also recently documented in these patients [152].

Two recent trials [153] aimed to assess the efficacy and safety of ARBs in preserving renal function and preventing cardiovascular events in type 2 diabetic patients. In the Irbesartan for Micro-Albuminuria in Type 2 Diabetes (IRMA 2) Study, 590 microalbuminuric type 2 diabetic patients were randomized to placebo or irbesartan (150 or 300 mg daily) for a 2 year follow-up period. The risk for progression from MA to macroproteinuria (overt nephropathy) was reduced with 68%, respectively 44% in the irbesartan treated groups (300 mg, respectively 150 mg daily); there was a reduction trend also in the cardiovascular events incidence rate (8.7 vs. 4.5%), but not statistically significant in view of the relatively small study size.

The Reduction in Endpoint in NIDDM with the Angiotensin II Antagonist Losartan (RENAAL) trial, an international multicentric study that enrolled over 1,500 type 2 diabetic microalbuminuric patients, aimed to verify the hypothesis that long-term treatment with ARB would increase the time to primary endpoint, defined as the doubling of serum creatinine, reaching ESRD or death. After a 3.4 year follow-up period the primary endpoint risk reduction was 22%, which means that one case of ESRD was prevented for every 16 treated patients. No significant reduction of cardiovascular mortality was observed. The time to doubling the serum creatinine was 198 days vs. 162 with placebo (25% risk reduction).

The mechanisms through ACEI improve the cardiovascular outcome in diabetic microalbuminuric patients were suggested by the findings of the HOPE study, which showed a significant reduction of 34% in the risk of development of type 2 diabetes in ramipril-treated patients without diabetes at the onset of the study, compared to placebo-treated group [150]. Furthermore, the ACEI perindopril was reported to reduce insulin resistance in obese non-diabetic subjects [154]. The improvement in the glucose metabolism associated with ACEI treatment might be caused by an increased blood flow through the microcirculation to adipose and skeletal muscle tissues and/or by an improved insulin action at the cellular level (post-receptor).

AGT II, acting via its specific type 1 receptor (AR1), interferes with insulin effect of phosphatidylinositol 3-kinase activation, probably through the competitive phosphorylation of the same substrates, the insulin receptor substrates (IRS) 1 and 2. Although the precise mechanism of inhibition of this major insulin signaling pathway is still unclear, it has been shown [155, 156] that AGT II inhibits the insulin-stimulated association between IRS1 and PI3-K in a proportion of 30 to 50% in a dose-dependent manner. This effect of AGT II is blocked almost completely by ACEI and partially by ARB. Another level where ACEI ameliorate insulin action is enhancing of GLUT4 glucose transporters translocation to the cell membrane. Even though the intimate mechanism of this effect is not completely understood, it was demonstrated that it is bradykinin-dependent [155, 157], at least in part, as well as the amelioration of the blood flow in the insulin-dependent tissues (adipose and skeletal muscle) microcirculation.

These findings are consistent with the data provided by the clinical studies, showing that ACEI, but not ARB treatment is associated with a reduction of the cardiovascular risk, because amelioration of the insulin resistance is followed by a better endothelial cells function and a decreased progression rate of atherosclerotic lesions.

In conclusion, ACEI should be a component of any therapeutic regime in diabetic and insulin resistant microalbuminuric patients (except intolerable cough is reported), in order to prevent the cardiovascular morbidity and mortality. ARBs, which have no effect on kinin metabolism, are effective for slowing the evolution of MA to overt proteinuria and chronic renal failure, but exert only a small, if any, vasculoprotective effect in microalbuminuric stage of diabetic renal disease. The association between ACEI and ARB (the "dual" RAS blockade) might be synergistic in the advanced stages of diabetic renal disease and reduce the cardiovascular risk associated with endothelial dysfunction as well as the cardiovascular morbidity, usually present in chronic renal failure.

STATINS

As previously discussed, hyperlipidemia and lipid glycoxidation process are important pathogenic mechanisms of endothelial dysfunction in diabetic patients with MA [158]. In present, the HMG-Coa reductase inhibitors, so-called "statins", are widely used in the treatment of hypercholesterolemia in type 2 diabetic patients and other insulin-resistant subjects, such as individuals with metabolic X syndrome; however, scant information is currently available about the effects of this therapy on endothelial functions in these patients.

Statins competitively inhibit HMG-CoA reductase, the enzyme that catalyzes the rate-limiting step in cholesterol biosynthesis [159]. The resultant reduction in hepatocyte cholesterol concentration triggers increased expression of hepatic LDL receptors, which will clear LDL from the circulation. Secondary, statins may inhibit hepatic synthesis of apolipoprotein B-100 and decrease the synthesis and secretion of triglyceride-rich lipoproteins [160].

The nature of the correlation between the extent of cholesterol reduction with statins and the degree of clinical benefit is controversial. In the Cholesterol And Recurrent Events (CARE) trial [161], as well as in the West Of Scotland Coronary Prevention Study (WOSCOPS) [162], the relative risk for an endpoint was progressively reduced with LDL levels declining up to a definite level (120 mg/dl, respectively 24%), but additional lowering of LDL did not produce additional risk reduction. These findings produced a debate on the vasculoprotective non-lipidic action mechanisms of the statins, involving the endothelial functions, vascular wall inflammation and immunomodulation.

Of particular importance, under these circumstances, appear to be the results from MRC / BHF Heart Protection Study [163], which showed a significant reduction of 27% (p = 0.0007) in the first cardiovascular event rate (coronary events, stroke and need for revascularization), among the 2426 diabetic patients whose pretreatment LDL cholesterol concentration was below 116mg/dl. These data provide direct evidence that statin therapy is beneficial in diabetic patients, even if they do not already have high LDL-cholesterol levels at baseline.

The effects of statins partially independent of cholesterol lowering (so-called "pleiotropic effects"), have been suggested also by the data from 4S and CARE studies, in which simvastatin and pravastatin reduced LDL to different degrees (35%, respectively 32%), with different effects on major coronary events (34%, respectively 24% reduction) (Table 15.17) [164].

Table 15.17

Clinical outcome studies using statins

(Adapted from: Maron DJ, *et al.*, *Circulation*, 2000, [164])

Study (n)	Prevention	Intervention	Baseline LDL (mg/dl)	% LDL reduction	On-trial LDL* (mg/dl)	% reduction in major coronary events	% reduction in total mortality	NNT
4S (4444)	secondary	Simvastatin 20–40 mg	188	35	120	34 (p < 0.0001)	30 (p = 0.003)	15
CARE (4159)	secondary	Pravastatin 40mg	139	32	95	24 (p = 0.003)	9 (p = NS)	33
LIPID (9014)	secondary	Pravastatin 40mg	150	25	113	24 (p < 0.0001)	22 (p < 0.0001)	28
WOSCOPS (6595)	primary	Pravastatin 40mg	192	26	142	31	22 (p = 0.051)	42
AFCAPS/ TexCAPS (6605)	primary	Lovastatin 20–40 mg	150	25	113	37 (p < 0.001)	0(NS)	24

*On-trial LDL values are calculated from published data.

Experimental data on cultured mesangial rat cell lines [165] treated with granulocyte / macrophage colony-stimulating factor showed that statins significantly reduced the production of interleukin IL-6 and macrophage chemotactic protein-1 (MCP-1), all inflammation-promoting factors involved in atherosclerosis progression. Recently, it was also demonstrated that lovastatin reduced *in vivo* the ability of leucocytes to migrate to the infection site by inhibiting chemokine production [166] and this effect was reversed by co-administration of mevalonate [167]. In the light of these observations, an anti-inflammatory action of statins, possibly mediated through inhibition of formation of non-lipidic mevalonate-derived products [167], appears to be relevant as a mechanism modulating the inflammatory process that accompanies endothelial cells dysfunction in the early stages of atherosclerosis.

Pleiotropic (non-lipidic) effects of statins affecting atherogenesis are necessarily targeted to preservation of normal endothelial functions, the most important being the nitric oxide production. The NO production by EC is influenced by biologic active molecules derived from the mevalonate pathway of cholesterol production (Figure 15.5, [167]), called isoprenoids (farnesyl-pyrophosphate and geranyl-geranyl-pyrophosphate). Isoprenoids are thought to play an important role in the post-translational modification of regulatory G proteins (Ras, Rab and Rho) [168], by covalently binding to these proteins; for example, geranyl-geranylation of GTP-binding protein Rho decreases endothelial cell NO-synthase expression by inhibiting the NF-kB transcriptional pathway. By inhibiting the formation of isoprenoids, statins upregulate eNOS and maintain NO-dependent vasodilatation.

Increasing evidence suggests that statins are able to downregulate IL-6 and MCP-1 transcription through the same mechanism [169] of interference with GTP-binding proteins/NF-kB transduction pathway. NF-kB, which is the key factor that promotes the transcription of both these cytokines [170], is activated, in inflammatory state, through GTP-binding proteins Ras-Rho that, in turn, require post-translational modification involving isoprenoids to be active.

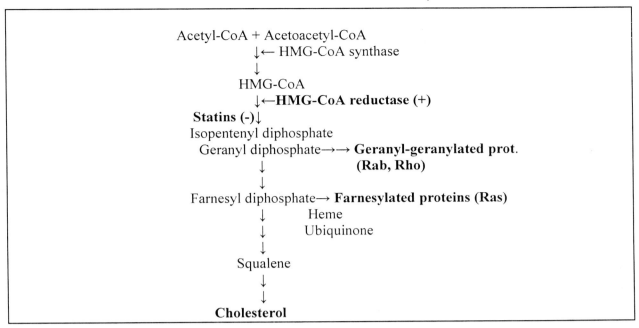

Figure 15.5

Cholesterol biosynthetic pathway, with mevalonate derivates and the action site of statins.
(Adapted from: Diomede L *et al., Arterioscl Thromb Vasc Biol*, 2001 [167]).

Another important topic concerning the beneficial role of statins in the atherosclerosis process is their possible immunomodulatory activity, which was revealed by two previously unknown immune effects of potential clinical relevance that have been recently reported. The first is that statins inhibit the expression of class II major histocompatibility antigens (MHC-II) on human macrophages, EC and smooth muscle cells, stimulated by interferon γ [171], possibly leading to a reduction of T cell proliferation and differentiation. This effect was demonstrated by mixed lymphocyte reaction on EC treated with statins [171].

The second immunosuppressive effect of statins is a selective blocking of LFA-1 (leucocyte function antigen 1, also known as CD11a/CD18), which, once expressed on the surface of leucocytes and activated, actions as an integrin and binds to intercellular adhesion molecule 1 (ICAM-1). In addition to its role in leucocyte recruitment and adhesion, LFA-1 seems to be also a potent co-stimulator of T cell proliferation.

Other equally important antiatherogenic effects of statins such as inhibiting oxidation-sensitive signaling pathways (LDLox dependent) or their angiogenetic effect, which are intervening later in the evolution of the atherogenic process, are beyond the scope of this chapter.

In conclusion, the above data about statin therapy in diabetic patients support a renewed emphasis on the control of cardiovascular "non-conventional" (inflammatory process, immune determination of atherosclerosis) as well as "classic" risk factors (hypertension, hypercholesterolemia) by an early intervention, for avoidance of the macrovascular events associated with diabetes mellitus.

The findings that statin therapy might be even more beneficial in diabetic than in non-diabetic patients for preventing cardiovascular events, and the benefit appears to be at least partially independent of cholesterol lowering, makes the decision about whether to initiate statin therapy be guided by an individual estimated risk of having a cardiovascular event in the future. MA is known to double this risk in the type 2 diabetes, so statins should be included in the majority of therapeutic regimens of this large category of patients.

REFERENCES

1. Mogensen CE, Christensen CK, Vittinghus. The stages in diabetic renal disease. With emphasis on

the stage of incipient diabetic nephropathy. *Diabetes*, **32:** 64–78, 1983.

2. Mogensen CE, Chachati A, Christensen CK. Microalbuminuria: an early marker for renal involvement in diabetes. *Uremia Invest*, **9:** 85–95, 1985–86.

3. Mogensen CE. Microalbuminuria as a predictor of clinical diabetic nephropathy. *Kidney Int*, **31:** 673–689, 1987.

4. Mogensen CE. Hyperfiltration, hypertension and diabetic nephropathy in IDDM patients. Based on the Golgi Lecture 1988. EASD meeting, Paris. *Diabetes Nutr and Metab*, **2:** 227–244, 1989.

5. Mogensen CE, Hansen KW, Osterby R, *et al.* Blood pressure elevation versus abnormal albuminuria in the genesis and prediction of renal disease and diabetes. *Diabetes Care*, **15:** 1192–1204, 1992.

6. Mogensen CE, Damsgaard EM, Froland A. GFR-loss, and cardiovascular damage in diabetes: a key role for abnormal albuminuria. *Acta Diabetol*, **29:** 201–213, 1992.

7. Parving H-H, Jensen HF, Mogensen CE, *et al.* Increased urinary albumin excretion rate in benign essential hypertension. *Lancet*, **1:** 1190–1192, 1974.

8. Campese VM, Bianchi S, Bigazzi R. Association between hyperlipidemia and microalbuminuria in essential hypertension. *Kidney Int*, **65 (Suppl. 71):** S10–S13, 1999.

9. Baenzinger JC. Reporting units for albumin/creatinine ratio. *Laboratory Med*, **31:** 597, 2000.

10. Viberti GC, Hill RD, Jarrett JR, *et al.* Microalbuminuria as a predictor of clinical nephropathy in insulin-dependent diabetes mellitus. *Lancet*, **1:** 1430–1432, 1982.

11. Mogensen CE. Microalbuminuria predicts clinical proteinuria and early mortality in maturity-onset diabetes. *N Engl J Med*, **310:** 356–60, 1984.

12. Dinneen SF, Gerstein HC. The association of microalbuminuria and mortality in non-insulin dependent diabetes mellitus. A systematic overview of the literature. *Arch Int Med*, **157:** 1413–1418, 1997.

13. Yudkin JS, Forrest RD, Jackson CA. Microalbuminuria as predictor of vascular disease in non-diabetic subjects. *Lancet*, **ii:** 530–533.

14. Damsgaard EM, Froland A, Jorgensen OD, *et al.* Microalbuminuria as predictor of increased mortality in elderly people. *BMJ*, **300:** 297–300, 1990.

15. Damsgaard EM, Froland A, Jorgensen OD, *et al.* Prognostic value of urinary albumin excretion rate and other risk factors in elderly diabetic patients and non-diabetic control subjects surviving the first 5 years after assessment. *Diabetologia*, **36:** 1030–1036, 1993.

16. Damsgaard EM, Mogensen CE. Microalbuminuria in elderly hyperglycaemic patients and controls. *Diabetic Med*, **3:** 430–435, 1986.

17. Vestbo E, Damsgaard EM, Mogensen CE. The relationship between microalbuminuria in first generation of diabetic and non-diabetic subjects and microalbuminuria and hypertension in the second generation (a population-based study). *Nephrol Dial Transplant*, **12,** Suppl.2: 32–36, 1997.

18. Vestbo E, Damsgaard EM, Froland A, *et al.* Urinary albumin excretion in a population-based cohort. *Diabetic Med*, **12:** 488–493, 1995.

19. Jager A, Kostense PJ, Nijpels G, *et al.* Microalbuminuria is strongly associated with NIDDM and hypertension but not with the insulin resistance syndrome: the Hoorn Study. *Diabetologia*, **41:** 694–700, 1998.

20. Mogensen CE. Microalbuminuria, blood pressure and diabetic renal disease: origin and development of ideas. In: Mogensen CE (ed). *The Kidney and Hypertension in Diabetes Mellitus*, Kluwer Academic Publishers, Dordrecht, The Netherlands, 2000, 655–706.

21. Turner RC, Millns H, Neil HA, *et al.*, for the United Kingdom Prospective Diabetes Study Group (UKPDS). Risk factors for coronary artery disease in non-insulin dependent diabetes mellitus. *BMJ*, **316:** 823–828, 1998.

22. Mogensen CE. Microalbuminuria in perspectives. In: Friedman EA and L'Esperance A (ed.) *Diabetic renal-retinal syndrome. Pathogenesis and management. Update 2002*, Kluwer Academic Publishers, Dordrecht/Boston/London, 2002, 105–120.

23. Rachmani R, Levi Z, Lidar M, *et al.* Considerations about the threshold value of microalbuminuria in patients with diabetes mellitus. Lessons from an 8 year follow-up study of 599 patients. *Diabetes Res Clin Pract*, **49:** 187–194, 2000.

24. Royal College of physicians of Edinburgh Diabetes Register Group. Near-normal urinary albumin concentrations predict progression to diabetic nephropathy in type 1 diabetes mellitus. *Diabetic Med.* **17:** 782–791, 2000.

25. Schultz CJ, Dalton NR, Neil HAW, *et al.* Risk of nephropathy can be detected before the onset of microalbuminuria during the early years after diagnosis of type 1 diabetes. *Diabetes Care*, **23:** 1811–1815, 2000.

26. Rostand SG, Kirk KA, Rutski EA, *et al.* Racial differences in the incidence of end stage renal disease. *N Engl J Med* **306:** 1276–1279, 1982.

27. Pugh JA, Stern MP, Haffner SM, *et al.* Excess incidence of treatment of end stage renal disease in Mexican Americans. *Am J Epidemiol*, **127:**135–144, 1988.

28. Haffner SM, Mitchell BD, Pugh JA, *et al*. Proteinuria in Mexican Americans and non-Hispanic Whites with NIDDM. *Diabetes Care*, **12**: 530–536, 1989.

29. Rostand SG. Diabetic renal disease in Blacks: inevitable or preventable? *N Engl J Med*, **321**: 1121–1122, 1989.

30. Seaquist ER, Goetz FC, Rich S, *et al*. Familial clustering of diabetic kidney disease: evidence for genetic susceptibility to diabetic nephropathy. *N Engl J Med*, **320**: 1161–1165, 1989.

31. Faronato PP, Maioli M, Tonolo G, *et al*. Clustering of albumin excretion rate abnormalities in Caucasian patients with NIDDM. *Diabetologia*, **40**: 816–823, 1997.

32. Canani LH, Gerchman F, Gross JL. Familial clustering of diabetic nephropathy in Brazilian type 2 diabetic patients. *Diabetes*, **48**: 909–913, 1999.

33. Pettitt DJ, Saad MF, Bennett PH, *et al*. Familial predisposition to renal disease in two generations of Pima Indians with type 2 (non-insulin dependent) diabetes mellitus, *Diabetologia*, **33**: 438–443, 1990.

34. Fogarty DG, Rich SS, Wantman M, *et al*. Albumin excretion in families with NIDDM is strongly influenced by a major gene: results of a segregation analysis. *Diabetes*, **47**, Suppl.1: A12 (abstr.), 1998.

35. Viberti GC, Keen H, Wiseman MJ. Raised arterial pressure in parents of proteinuric insulin dependent diabetics. *BMJ*, **295**: 515–517, 1987.

36. Krolewski AS, Canessa M, Warram JH, *et al*. Predisposition to hypertension and susceptibility to renal disease in insulin dependent diabetes mellitus. *N Engl J Med*, **318**: 140–145, 1988.

37. Takeda H, Ohta K, Hagiwara M, *et al*. Genetic predisposing factors in non insulin dependent diabetes with persistent albuminuria *J Exp Clin Med*, 17: 199–203, 1992.

38. Nelson RG, Pettitt DJ, de Courten MP, *et al*. Parental hypertension and proteinuria in Pima Indians with NIDDM. *Diabetologia*, **39**: 433–438, 1996.

39. Woods JW, Falk RJ, Pittman AW, *et al*. Increased red cell sodium-lithium countertransport in normotensive sons of hypertensive patients. *N Engl J Med*, **306**: 593–595, 1982.

40. Mangili M, Bending JJ, Scott G, *et al*. Increased sodium-lithium countertransport activity in red blood cells of patients with insulin dependent diabetes and nephropathy. *N Engl J Med*, **318**: 146–150, 1988.

41. Walker DJ, Tariq T, Viberti GC, *et al*. Sodium-lithium countertransport activity in red cells of patients with insulin dependent diabetes and nephropathy and their parents. *BMJ*, **301**: 635–638, 1990.

42. Kelleher C, Kingston SM, Barry DG, *et al*. Hypertension in diabetic clinic patients and their siblings. *Diabetologia*, **31**: 76–81, 1988.

43. Nelson RG, Pettitt DJ, Baird HR, *et al*. Prediabetic blood pressure predicts urinary albumin excretion after the onset of type 2 (non insulin dependent) diabetes mellitus in Pima Indians. *Diabetologia*, **36**: 998–1001, 1993.

44. Chowdury TA, Dyer PH, Barnett AH, *et al*. HLA and insulin (INS) genes in caucasians with type 1 diabetes and nephropathy. *Diabetologia*, **41**, Suppl.1: A296 (abstr.), 1998.

45. Mijovic C, Fletcher JA, Bradwell AR, *et al*. Phenotypes of the heavy chains of immunoglobulins in patients with diabetic microangiopathy: evidence for an immunogenetic predisposition. *BMJ*, **292**: 433–435, 1986.

46. Rigat B, Hubert C, Alhenc-Gelas F, *et al*. An insertion deletion polymorphism in angiotensin I converting enzyme gene accounting for half of the variance of serum enzyme levels. *J Clin Invest*, **86**: 410–415, 1990.

47. Cambien F, Costerousse O, Tiret L, *et al*. Plasma levels and gene polymorphism of angiotensin converting enzyme gene in relation with myocardial infarction. *Circulation*, **90**: 669–676, 1994.

48. Marre M, Jeunmaitre X, Gallois Y, *et al*. Contribution of genetic polymorphism in the renin-angiotensin system to the development of renal complications in insulin dependent diabetes. *J Clin Invest*, **99**:1585–1595, 1997.

49. Rogus JJ, Moczulski D, Freire MB, *et al*. Diabetic nephropathy is associated with AGT polymorphism T235: results of a family-based study. *Hypertension*, **31**: 627–631, 1998.

50. Doria A, Onuma T, Warram JH, *et al*. Synergistic effect of angiotensin II type 1 receptor genotype and poor glycaemic control on risk of nephropathy in IDDM. *Diabetologia*, **40**: 1293–1299, 1997.

51. Imperatore G, Hanson RL, Pettitt DJ, *et al*. The Pima Indians Gene Group: Sib-pair linkage analysis for susceptibility genes for microvascular complications among Pima Indians with type 2 diabetes. *Diabetes*, **47**: 821–830, 1998.

52. Moczulski DK, Burak V, Doria A, *et al*. The role of aldose reductase gene in the susceptibility to diabetic nephropathy in type II (non-insulin dependent) diabetes mellitus. *Diabetologia*, **42**: 94–97, 1999.

53. Zanchi A, Wantman M, Moczulski DK, *et al*. Genetic susceptibility to diabetic nephropathy in IDDM is related to polymorphism in the endothelial nitric oxide synthase (eNOS) gene. *Diabetes*, **47**, Suppl. 1: A52 (abstr.), 1998.

54. Fogarty RG, Moczulski DK, Makita Y, *et al.* Evidence for a susceptibility locus for diabetic nephropathy on chromosome 7q in Caucasian families with type 2 diabetes. *Diabetes,* **48, Suppl. 1:** A47 (abstr.), 1999.

55. Stamler J, Vaccaro O, Neaton JD, *et al.* Diabetes, other risk factors and 12 year cardiovascular mortality for men screened in Multiple Risk Factor Intervention Trial. *Diabetes Care,* **16:** 434–444, 1993.

56. Damsgaard EM, Froland A, Jorgensen OD, *et al.* Eight to nine year mortality in known non insulin dependent diabetics and controls. *Kidney Int,* **41:** 731–735, 1992.

57. Macleod JM, Lutale J, Marshall SM, *et al.* Albumin excretion and vascular deaths in NIDDM. *Diabetologia,* **38:** 610–616, 1995.

58. Gall M-A, Borch-Johnsen K, Hougaard P, *et al.* Microalbuminuria and poor glycemic control predict mortality in NIDDM. *Diabetes,* **44:** 1303–1309, 1995.

59. Thomas SM, Viberti GC. Microalbuminuria and cardiovascular disease. In: Mogensen CE (ed). *The Kidney and Hypertension in Diabetes Mellitus.* Kluwer Academic Publishers, Dordrecht, The Netherlands, 2000, 39–55.

60. Forsblom CM, Sane T, Groop OH, *et al.* Risk factors for mortality in type II (non-insulin dependent) diabetes mellitus: evidence of a role for neuropathy and a protective effect of HLA-DR4. *Diabetologia,* **41:**1253–1262, 1998.

61. Mattock MB, Barnes DJ, Viberti G, *et al.* Microalbuminuria and coronary heart disease in NIDDM: an incidence study. *Diabetes,* **47:**1786–1792, 1998.

62. Uusitupa MI, Niskanen KL, Siitonen O, *et al.* Ten-year cardiovascular mortality in relation to risk factors and abnormalities in lipoprotein composition in type 2 (non-insulin dependent) diabetic and non-diabetic subjects. *Diabetologia,* **36:**1175–1184, 1993.

63. Viberti GC, Hill RD, Jarrett RD, *et al.* Microalbuminuria as a predictor of clinical nephropathy in insulin dependent diabetes mellitus. *Lancet,* **1:**1430–1432, 1982.

64. Messent JW, Elliott TG, Hill RD, *et al.* Prognostic significance of microalbuminuria in insulin dependent diabetes mellitus: a twenty-three year follow-up study, *Kidney Int,* **41:** 836–9, 1992.

65. Rossing P, Hougaard P, Borch-Johnsen K, *et al.* Predictors of mortality in insulin dependent diabetes: 10 year observational follow-up study. *BMJ,* **313:** 779–784, 1996.

66. Earle KA, Mishra M, Morocutti A, *et al.* Microalbuminuria as a marker of silent myocardial ischemia in IDDM patients. *Diabetologia,* **39:** 854–856, 1996.

67. Sato L, Tarnow A, Parving H-H. Prevalence of left ventricular hypertrophy in diabetic patients with diabetic nephropathy. *Diabetologia,* **42, Suppl. 1:** 76–80, 1999.

68. Spring MW, Raptis AE, Chambers J, *et al.* Left ventricular structure and function are associated with microalbuminuria independently of blood pressure in type 2 diabetes. *Diabetes,* **46:** A0426 (abstr.), 1997.

69. Pedrinelli R, Gianfranco O, Carmassi F, *et al.* Microalbuminuria and endothelial dysfunction in essential hypertension. *Lancet,* **344:** 14–18, 1994.

70. Bigazzi R Bianchi S, Campese RM, *et al.* Prevalence of microalbumiunuria in a large population of patients with mild and moderate essential hypertension. *Nephron,* **61:** 94–97, 1992.

71. Hishiki S, Tochikubo O, Miyajima E, *et al.* Circadian variation of urinary microalbumin excretion and ambulatory blood pressure in patients with essential hypertension. *J Hypertens,* **16:** 2101–2108, 1998.

72. Bigazzi R, Bianchi S, Baldari D, *et al.* Microalbuminuria in salt-sensitive patients. A marker for renal and cardiovascular risk factors. *Hypertension,* **23:** 195–199, 1994.

73. Bigazzi R, Bianchi S, Nenci R, *et al.* Increased thickness of the carotid artery in patients with essential hypertension and microalbuminuria. *J Hum Hypertens,* **9:** 827–833, 1995.

74. Nilsson T, Svensson A, Lapidus L, *et al.* The relations of microalbuminuria to ambulatory blood pressure and myocardial wall thickness in a population. *J Intern Med,* **244:** 55–58, 1998.

75. Agewall S, Persson B, Samuelsson O, *et al.* Microalbuminuria in treated hypertensive men at high risk of coronary disease. The Risk Factor Intervention Study Group. *J Hypertens,* **11:** 461–469, 1993.

76. Erley CM, Risler T. Microalbuminuria in primary hypertension: is it a marker of glomerular damage? *Nephrol Dial Transplant,* **9:** 1713–1715, 1994.

77. Mann GF, Gerstein HC, Pogue J, *et al.* Renal insufficiency as a predictor of cardiovascular outcomes and the impact of ramipril: the HOPE randomized trial. *Ann Int Med,* **134:** 629–636, 2001.

78. Messent JW, Elliott TG, Hill RD, *et al.* Prognostic significance of microalbuminuria in insulin dependent diabetes mellitus: a twenty three year follow up study. *Kidney Int,* **41:** 836–839, 1992.

79. Rossing P, Hougaard P, Borch-Johnsen K, *et al.* Predictors of mortality in insulindependent diabetes: ten year observationai follow up study. *BMJ,* **313:** 779–784, 1996.

80. Agardh GH, Agardh E, Torffvit O. The association between retinopathy, nephropathy and long term metabolic control in type 1 diabetes mellitus: a 5 year follow up study of 442 adult patients in routine care. *Diab Res Clin Pract*, **35**: 113–121, 1997.

81. The Diabetes Control and Complications Trial Research. The effect of intensive treatment of diabetes on the development and progression of long term complications in insulin dependent diabetes mellitus. *N Engl J Med*, **329**: 977–986, 1993.

82. Bianchi S, Bigazzi R, Campese M, *et al*. Microalbuminuria in essential hypertension: significance, pathophysiology and therapeutic implications. *Am J Kidney Dis*, **34**: 973–995, 1999.

83. Rodicio J, Campo C, Ruilope L. Microalbuminuria in essential hypertension. *Kidney Int*, **54**: 551–554, 1998.

84. Agrawal B, Berger A, Wolf K, *et al*. Microalbuminuria screening by reagent strip predicts cardiovascular risk in hypertension. *J Hypertens*, **14**: 223–228, 1996.

85. Jensen JS, Feldt-Rasmussen B, Strandgaard S, *et al*. Arterial hypertension, microalbuminuria and risk of ischemic heart disease. *Hypertension*, **35**: 898–903, 2000.

86. Jager A, Kostense PJ, Ruhe HG, *et al*. Microalbuminuria and peripheral arterial disease are independent predictors of cardiovascular and all-cause mortality especially among hypertensive subjects: five-year follow-up of the Hoorn Study. *Arterioscl Thromb Vasc Biol*, **19**: 617–624, 1999.

87. Sethi AA, Nordestgaard BG, Agerholm-Larsen B *et al*. Angiotensinogen polymorphisms and elevated blood pressure in the general population. The Copenhagen City Heart Study. *Hypertension*, **37**: 875–881, 2001.

88. Parving H-H, Mogensen CE, Jensen HA, *et al*. Increased urinary albumin excretion rate in benign essential hypertension. *Lancet*, **1**: 1190–1192, 1974.

89. Lydakis C, Lip GY. Microalbuminuria and cardiovascular risk. *Q J Med*, **91**: 381–391, 1998.

90. Morimoto A, Uzu T, Fujii T, *et al*. Sodium sensitivity and cardiovascular events in patients with essential hypertension. *Lancet*, **350**: 1734–1737, 1997.

91. Meigs JB, D'Agostino RB, Nathan DM, *et al*. Longitudinal association of glycemia and microalbuminuria. *Diabetes Care*, **25**: 977–983.

92. Meigs JB, Nathan DM, Wilson PWF, *et al*. Metabolic risk factors worsen continuously across the spectrum of non-diabetic glucose tolerance: the Framingham Offspring Study. *Ann Intern Med*, **128**: 524–533, 1998.

93. Makimattila S, Virkamaki A, Groop P-H, *et al*. Chronic hyperglycaemia impairs endothelial function and insulin sensitivity via different mechanisms in insulin-dependent diabetes mellitus. *Circulation*, **94**: 1276–1282, 1996.

94. Calles-Escandon J, Cipolla M. Diabetes and endothelial dysfunction: a clinical perspective. *Endocrine Reviews*, **22**: 36–52, 2001.

95. De Mayer GR, Herman AG. Vascular endothelial dysfunction. *Progr Cardiovasc Dis*, **39**: 325–342, 1997.

96. Cohen RA. The role of nitric oxide and other endothelium-derived vasoactive substances in vascular disease. *Progr Cardiovasc Dis*, **38**: 105–128, 1995.

97. Brands MW, Fitzgerald SM. Acute endothelium-mediated vasodilatation is not impaired at the onset of diabetes. *Hypertension*, **32**: 541–547, 1998.

98. Huvers PC, De Leeuw PW, Houben AJ, *et al*. Endothelium-dependent vasodilatation, plasma markers of endothelial function and adrenergic vasoconstrictor responses in type 1 diabetes under near-normoglycaemic conditions. *Diabetes*, **48**: 2300–2307, 1999.

99. Clarkson P, Celermajer DS, Donald AE, *et al*. Impaired vascular reactivity in insulin dependent diabetes mellitus is related to disease duration and low density lipoprotein levels. *J Am Coll Cardiol*, **28**: 573–579, 1996.

100. Johnstone MT, Creager SJ, Scales KM, *et al*. Impaired endothelium-dependent vasodilatation in patients with insulin-dependent diabetes mellitus. Circulation, **88**: 2510–2516, 1993.

101. Cosentino F, Lutscher TF. Endothelial dysfunction in diabetes mellitus. *J Cardiovasc Pharmacol*, **32, Suppl. 3**: S54–S61, 1998.

102. Bloomgarten ZT. Endothelial dysfunction, neuropathy and the diabetic foot, diabetic mastopathy and the erectile dysfunction. *Diabetes Care*, **21**: 183–189, 1998.

103. Steinberg HO, Chaker H, Leaming R, *et al*. Obesity/insulin resistance is associated with endothelial dysfunction. Implications for the syndrome of insulin resistance. *J Clin Invest*, **97**: 2601–2610, 1996.

104. Caballero AE, Arora S, Saouaf R, *et al*. Microvascular and macrovascular reactivity is reduced in subjects at risk for type 2 diabetes. *Diabetes*, **48**: 1856–1862, 1999.

105. Ferri C, Bellini C, Desideri G, *et al*. Circulating endothelin-1 levels in obese patients with the metabolic syndrome. *Exp Clin Endocrinol Diab*, **105, Suppl. 2**: 38–40, 1997.

106.Calles-Escandon J, Ballor D, Harvey-Berino J, et al. Amelioration of the inhibition of fibrinolysis in elderly obese subjects by moderate energy intake restriction. *Am J Clin Nutr,* **64:** 7–11, 1996.

107.Fendri S, Roussel B, Lormeau B, et al. Insulin sensitivity, insulin action and fibrinolysis activity in non-diabetic and diabetic obese subjects. *Metabolism,* **47:** 1372–1375, 1998.

108.Serrano RM. Relationship between obesity and the increased risk of major complications in non-insulin dependent diabetes mellitus. *Eur J Clin Invest,* **28,** Suppl.2: 14–17, 1998.

109.Agewall S, Fagerberg B, Atvall S, et al. Microalbuminuria, insulin sensitivity and haemostatic factors in non-diabetic treated hypertensive men. Risk Factors Intervention Study Group. *J Intern Med,* **237:** 195–203, 1995.

110.Calles-Escandon J, Mirza SA, Sobel BE, et al. Induction of hyperinsulinemia combined with hyperglycemia and hypertriglyceridemia increases plasminogen activator inhibitor 1 in blood in normal human subjects. Diabetes, **47:** 290–293, 1998.

111.Cipolla MJ. Elevated glucose potentiates contraction of isolated rat resistance arteries and augments protein kinase-C induced intracellular calcium release. *Metabolism,* **48:** 1015–1022, 1999.

112.Cooper ME, Vranes D, Youssef S, et al. Increased renal expression of vascular endothelial growth factor (VEGF) and its receptor VEGFR-2 in experimental diabetes. *Diabetes,* **48:** 2229–2239, 1999.

113.Watts GF, Playford DA. Dyslipoproteinaemia and hyperoxidative stress in the pathogenesis of endothelial dysfunction in non-insulin dependent diabetes mellitus: a hypothesis. *Atherosclerosis,* **141:** 17–30, 1998.

114.Giugliano B, Ceriello A, Paolisso G. Oxidative stress and diabetic vascular complications. *Diabetes Care,* **19:** 257–267, 1996.

115.Cipolla MJ, Haker CT, Porter JM. Endothelial function and adrenergic reactivity in human type-2 diabetic resistance arteries. *J Vasc Surg,* **23:** 940–949, 1996.

116.Stehouwer CDA, Nauta JJP, Zeldenrust GC, et al. Urinary albumin excretion, cardiovascular disease and endothelial dysfunction in non insulin dependent diabetes mellitus. *Lancet,* **340:** 319–323, 1992.

117.Fioretto P, Stehouwer CDA, Mauer M, et al. Heterogenous nature of microalbuminuria in NIDDM: studies of endothelial function and renal structure. *Diabetologia,* **41:** 233–236, 1998.

118.Stehouwer CDA, Yudkin JS, Fioretto P, et al. How heterogenous is microalbuminuria in diabetes mellitus? The case for "benign" and "malignant"

microalbuminuria. *Nephrol Dial Transplant,* **13:** 2751–2754, 1998.

119.Stephenson JM, Fuller JH, Viberti G-C, et al. The EURODIAB IDDM Complications Study Group. Blood pressure, retinopathy and urinary albumin excretion in IDDM: The EURODIAB IDDM Complications Study. *Diabetologia,* **38:** 599–603, 1995.

120.Chavers BM, Mauer SM, Ramsay RC, et al. Relationships between glomerular and retinal lesions in IDDM patients. *Diabetes,* **43:** 441–446, 1994.

121.Forsblom CM, Groop PH, Ekstrand A, et al. Predictive value of microalbuminuria in patients with insulin dependent diabetes of long duration. *BMJ,* **305:** 1051–1053, 1992.

122.Parving H-H, Gall M-A, Skott P, et al. Prevalence and causes of microalbuminuria in non insulin dependent diabetic patients. *Kidney Int,* **41:** 758–762, 1992.

123.Fioretto P, Mauer M, Brocco E, et al. Patterns of renal injury in NIDDM patients with microalbuminuria. *Diabetologia,* **39:** 1569–1576, 1996.

124.Annuk M, Lind L, Linde T, et al. Impaired endothelium-dependent vasodilatation in renal failure in humans. *Nephrol Dial Transplant,* **16:** 302–306, 2001.

125.Ross R. Atherosclerosis: an inflammatory disease. *N Engl J Med,* **340:** 115–126, 1999.

126. Jager A, van Hinsbergh VWM, Kostense PJ, et al. Increased levels of soluble vascular cell adhesion molecule 1 are associated with risk of cardiovascular mortality in type 2 diabetes. The Hoorn Study. *Diabetes,* **49:** 485–491, 2000.

127.Bhagat K, Vallance P. Inflammatory cytokines impair endothelium-dependent dilation in human veins in vivo. *Circulation,* **96:** 3042–3047, 1997.

128.Stenvinkel P: Endothelial dysfunction and inflammation-is there a link? *Nephrol Dial Transplant,* **16:** 1968–1971, 2001.

129.Festa A, D'Agostino R, Howard G, et al. Chronic subclinical inflammation as part of the insulin resistance syndrome. The Insulin Resistance Atherosclerosis Study (IRAS). *Circulation,* **102:** 42–45, 2000.

130.Saydah SH, Eberhardt MS, Loria CM, et al. Age and the burden of death attributable to diabetes in the United States. *Am J Epidemiol,* **156:** 714–719, 2002.

131.Gaede P, Vedel P, Larsen N, et al. Multifactorial intervention and cardiovascular disease in patients with type 2 diabetes. *N Engl J Med,* **348:** 383–393, 2003.

132.Turner LC, Millins H, Neil HA, et al. Risk factors for coronary artery disease in non-insulin dependent diabetes mellitus: United Kingdom Prospective Diabetes Study (UKPDS:23). *BMJ*, **316:** 823–828, 1998.

133.Hanson L, Zanchetti A, Carruthes SG, *et al.* Effects of intensive blood pressure lowering and low dose aspirin in patients with hypertension: principal results of Hypertension Optimal Treatment (HOT) randomized trial. *Lancet,* **351:** 1755–1762, 1998.

134.Curb JD, Pressel SL, Cutler JA, *et al.* Effect of diuretic-based antihypertensive treatment on cardiovascular disease risk in older diabetic patients with isolated systolic hypertension. *JAMA,* **277:** 1356–1362, 1997.

135.Staessen JA, Fagard R, Thijs L, *et al.* Randomised double-blind comparison of placebo and active treatment for older patients with isolated systolic hypertension. *Lancet,* **350:** 757–764, 1997.

136.Lee M-K, Han DF, Lutterman JA, *et al.* Metabolic effects of troglitazone on fructose-induced insulinresistance in the rat. *Diabetes,* **43:** 1435–1439, 1994.

137.Miles PDG. TNF-α-induced insulin resistance in vivo and its prevention by troglitazone. *Diabetes,* **46:** 1678–1683, 1997.

138.Pasceri V, Wu HD, Willerson JT, *et al.* Modulation of vascular inflammation *in vitro* and *in vivo* by peroxisome proliferators-activated receptor-γ activators. *Circulation,* **101:** 235–238, 2000.

139. Jackson SM, Parhami F, Xi XP, *et al.* Peroxisome proliferators-activated receptor activators target human endothelial cells to inhibit leukocyte-endothelial cell interaction. *Arterioscl Thromb Vasc Biol,* **19:** 2094–2104, 1999.

140.Avena R, Mitchell ME, Nylen SE, *et al.* Insulin action enhancement normalizes brachial artery vasoactivity in patients with peripheral vascular disease and occult diabetes. *J Vasc Surg,* **28:** 1024–1031, 1998.

141.Tack CJ, Ong MK, Lutterman JA, *et al.* Insulin-induced vasodilatation and endothelial function in obesity/insulin resistance. Effects of troglitazone, *Diabetologia,* **41:** 569–576, 1998.

142.Nolan JJ, Ludvik B, Beerdsen P, *et al.* Improvement in glucose tolerance and insulin resistance in obese subjects treated with troglitazone. *N Engl J Med,* **331:** 1188–1193, 1994.

143.Ehrmann DA, Schmits FD. Troglitazone improves defects in insulin action, insulin secretion, ovarian steroidogenesis and fibrinolysis in women with ovarian polycystic syndrome. *J Clin Endocrinol Metab,* **82:** 2108–2116, 1997.

144.Ginsberg HN. Insulin resistance and cardiovascular disease. *J. Clin. Invest.,* **106:** 453–458, 2000.

145.Kumar S. Troglitazone, an insulin enhancer, improves metabolic control in NIDDM patients. Troglitazone Study Group. *Diabetologia,* **39:** 701–9, 1996.

146.Ibrahimi A. Evidence for a common mechanism of action for fatty acids and thiazolidinedione antidiabetic agents on gene expression in preadipose cells, *Mol Pharmacol,* **46:**1070–1076, 1994.

147.Braissant O, Foufelle F, Scott C, *et al.* Differential expression of peroxisome proliferators-activated receptors (PPARs): tissue distribution of PPAR-α, β and γ in the adult rat. *Endocrinology,* **137:** 354–366, 1996.

148.Sowers JR, Epstein M, Frohlich ED. Diabetes, hypertension and cardiovascular disease. An update. *Hypertension,* **37:** 1053–1059, 2001.

149.Effects of ramipril on cardiovascular and microvascular outcomes in people with diabetes mellitus: results of HOPE study and MICRO-HOPE substudy. *Lancet,* **355:** 253–259, 2000.

150.Warram JH, Scott LJ, Hanna LS, *et al.* Progression of microalbuminuria to proteinuria in type 1 diabetes. Non-linear relationship with hyperglycaemia. *Diabetes,* **49:** 94–100, 2000.

151.Mathiesen ER, Hommel E, Hansen HP, *et al.* Randomised controlled trial of long-term efficacy of captopril on preservation of kidney function in normotensive patients with insulin-dependent diabetes and microalbuminuria. *BMJ,* **319:** 24–25, 1999.

152.Rudberg S, Osterby R, Bangstad H-J, *et al.* Effect of angiotensin-converting enzyme inhibitor or beta-blocker on glomerular structural changes in young microalbuminuric patients with type 1 (insulin-dependent) diabetes mellitus. *Diabetologia,* **42:** 589–595, 1999.

153.Bloomgarden ZT. Angiotensin II receptor blockers and nephropathy trials. *Diabetes Care,* **24:** 1834–1838, 2001.

154.Fogari R, Zoppi A, Corradi L, *et al.* ACE inhibition but not angiotensin II antagonism reduced fibrinogen and insulin resistance in overweight hypertensive patients. *J Cardiovasc Pharmacol,* **32:** 616–620, 1998.

155.Folli F, Kahn CR, Hansen H, *et al.* Angiotensin II inhibits insulin signalling in aortic smooth muscle cell at multiple levels. *J Clin Invest,* **100:** 2158–2169, 1997.

156.Richey JM, Ader M, Moore D, *et al.* Angiotensin II induces insulin resistance independent of changes in interstitial insulin, *Am J Physiol,* **277:** E920–E926, 1999.

157.Henriksen EJ, Jacob S, Kinnick TR, *et al.* ACE inhibition and glucose transport in insulin-resistant muscle: roles of bradykinin and nitric oxide. *Am J Physiol,* **277**: R332–R336, 1999.

158. Watts GF, O'Brien SF, Silvester V, *et al.* Impaired endothelium dependent and independent dilatation of forearm resistance arteries in men with diet-treated non-insulin dependent diabetes: role of dyslipidemia, *Clin Sci*, **91**: 410–416, 1996.

159. Endo A, Tsujita Y, Kuroda M, *et al.* Inhibition of cholesterol synthesis *in vitro* and *in vivo* by ML-236A and ML 236B, competitive inhibitors of 3-hydroxy-3-methylglutaryl-coenzyme A reductase, *Eur J Biochem*, **77**: 31–36, 1977.

160. Grundy SM. Consensus statement: role of therapy with "statins" in patients with hypertriglyceridemia *Am. J. Cardiol.*, **81**, Suppl.4A: 1B–6B, 1998.

161. Sacks FM, Moye LA, Davis BR, *et al.* Relationships between plasma LDL concentrations during treatment with pravastatin and recurrent coronary events in the Cholesterol And Recurrent Events Trial. *Circulation,* **97**: 1446–1452, 1998.

162. West Of Scotland Coronary Prevention Study Group: Influence of pravastatin and plasma lipids on clinical events in the West Of Scotland Coronary Prevention Study (WOSCOPS). *Circulation,* **97**: 1440–1445, 1998.

163. Heart Protection Study Collaborative Group: MRC/BHF heart Protection Study of cholesterol-lowering with simvastatin in 5963 people with diabetes: a randomized placebo-controlled trial. *Lancet,* **361**: 2005–2016, 2003.

164. Maron DJ, Fazio S, MacRae FL. Current perspectives on statins, *Circulation,* **101**: 207–213, 2000.

165. Kim SI, Guijarro C, O'Donnell MP, *et al.* Human mesangial cell production of monocyte chemo-attractant protein-1: modulation by lovastatin. *Kidney Int,* **48**: 363–371, 1995.

166. Diomede L, Albani D, Fruscella P, *et al.* Cholesterol homeostasis and inflammation: relationship between sterol regulatory element binding protein-1 activation and leucocyte recruitment. *Eur Clin Invest,* **29**: 43–47, 1999.

167. Diomede L, Albani D, Sottocorno, M, *et al.* In vivo anti-inflammatory effect of statins is mediated by nonsterol mevalonate products. *Arterioscler Thromb Vasc Biol,* **21**: 1327–1332, 2001.

168. Palinski W, Tsimikas S. Immunomodulatory effects of statins: mechanisms and potential impact on arteriosclerosis. *J Am Soc Nephrol,* **13**: 1673–1681, 2002.

169. Kim SI, Kim HJ, Han DC, *et al.* Effects of lovastatin on GTP small binding proteins and on TGF-beta 1 and fibronectin expression. *Kidney Int,* **58**, Suppl. 77: 588–592, 2000.

170. Ueda A, Okuda K, Ohno S, *et al.* NFkB and Sp1 regulate transcription of human monocyte chemoattractant protein-1 gene. *J Immunol,* **153**: 2052–2063, 1994.

171. Kwak B, Mulhaupt F, Myit S, *et al.* Statins as a newly recognized type of immunomodulator. *Nat Med,* **6**: 1399–1402, 2000.

16

CARDIOVASCULAR RISK FACTORS IN TYPE 1 AND TYPE 2 DIABETES: COMMON CONVENTIONAL AND DIABETES-RELATED RISK VARIABLES?

Eckhard ZANDER, Wolfgang KERNER

Both in type 1 and type 2 diabetes macrovascular disease threatens the health and shortens life expectancy. In patients of both types of diabetes cardiovascular complications begin at earlier age than in the nondiabetic population and show a more rapid progression. In contrast to the nondiabetic population diabetes patients have not equally benefited from advances in reducing cardiovascular mortality. Besides the classical cardiovascular risk factors other non-conventional risk factors seem to explain the excess of cardiovascular mortality. In the present paper, we have reviewed the impact of conventional as well as non-conventional cardiovascular risk factors on cardiovascular disease morbidity and mortality in type 1 and type 2 diabetes. We have to take into consideration that both types of diabetes are different both in etiology and clinical presentation.

A risk factor represents an attribute or an exposure that is associated with increased probability of occurrence of a disease. Hyperglycemia is most likely a cardiovascular risk factor. HbA1c should be less than 7%. It is not completely resolved whether or not hyperinsulinemia associated with insulin resistance is atherogenic. The role of elevated cholesterol levels for cardiovascular disease in diabetes was shown in the Multiple Risk Factor data. Most consensus guidelines have established that LDL cholesterol should be brought to a value of less than 2.6 mmol/l (<100 mg/dl). Hypertension is of substantial importance for the reduced life expectancy in type 1 and type 2 diabetes and accelerates markedly the manifestation and progression of micro-and macroangiopathy. Clinical presentation of hypertension in both types of diabetes differs markedly. It is aimed to lower the blood pressure to <130/80 mmHg. Both in type 1 and type 2 diabetes smoking increases synergistically the micro- and macroangiopathy. Thrombosis due to hypercoagulability in atherosclerotic vessels increases cardiovascular morbidity. In both types of diabetes there is prospective evidence of hypertension, hyperlipoproteinemia and proteinuria including diabetes related variables for increased cardiovascular morbidity.

Macrovascular disease represents a major threat to the life of diabetes patients. Both type 1 and type 2 diabetes patients have an increased risk of cardiovascular disease in men and women [1].

Cardiovascular disease is the primary cause of mortality in type 2 diabetes patients, and the second one in type 1 diabetes [2, 3, 4]. Diabetes patients have at least a twofold to fourfold increased risk for having cardiovascular events compared with age-matched non-diabetic subjects [5]. Diabetes accelerates the atherosclerotic process [6, 7]. When compared with the nondiabetic population, both in type 1 and type 2 diabetes cardiovascular complications begin at an earlier age, showing a more rapid progression and leading more frequently to fatal events, like myocardial infarction, stroke and ischemic gangrene [8, 9, 10].

Indeed patients with type 2 diabetes have increased prevalence of traditional cardiovascular risk factors like hypertension, increased total and LDL cholesterol levels and smoking, even before manifestation of the disease. Beside other factors in type 1 diabetes, the aging process, high blood pressure, lipid abnormalities and nephropathy were found as coronary heart disease predictors [11]. Diabetes patients have not equally benefited from advances in reducing the coronary risk as the nondiabetic population have. The traditional risk factors do not fully explain the excess risk for cardiovascular disease in diabetes mellitus [12]. In addition to classical cardiovascular risk factors, still other non-conventional risk factors seem to explain the excess cardiovascular risk in diabetes.

Further, we have to take into consideration that type 1 and type 2 diabetes are different entities with a different natural history of the disease. Due to these differences the two entities are not easy to be compared.

In uncomplicated type 1 diabetes, the level of atherosclerotic risk factors does not show substantial abnormalities if the metabolic control is good. But, when microalbuminuria ensues blood pressure tends to increase and atherosclerotic plasma lipid abnormalities appear [13]. It is an open question whether or not the incidence of cardiovascular disease in type 1 diabetes patients who do not develop diabetic nephropathy is higher than in the general population [14].

In the present paper, we review the impact of conventional and various non-conventional cardiovascular risk factors on the manifestation and progression of cardiovascular disease (coronary heart disease, stroke, peripheral vascular disease) in type 1 and type 2 diabetes.

What is a risk factor?

A risk factor represents an attribute or exposure that is associated with increased probability of occurrence of a disease [14]. This is not necessarily a causal factor. Risk is used to indicate the likelihood of people who are exposed to certain factors (risk factors) to subsequently develop a particular disease. The absolute risk of a disease is identical with the incidence of the disease. The relative risk or risk ratio is the ratio of incidence in exposed persons to incidence in nonexposed persons. The attributable risk is defined as the difference between the incidence in the exposed and nonexposed. It is used to quantify the risk of disease in the exposed group that can be considered attributable to the exposure by removing the risk of disease that would have occurred anyway due to other causes.

HYPERGLYCEMIA

In observational studies, hyperglycemia is a cardiovascular risk factor [15, 16]. The role of hyperglycemia as an independent risk factor for the development of cardiovascular disease, however, was not fully supported by the UKPDS and other reports [17, 18]. Prospective observational studies have shown that cardiovascular risk increases with hyperglycemia and increased glycated hemoglobin [19, 20, 21]. In type 1 diabetes hyperglycemia accelerates the development of nephropathy, and increases *via* nephropathy the cardiovascular risk [22]. In type 2 diabetes the risk for cardiovascular disease was associated with hyperglycemia [23, 24], for stroke [25], and for total mortality [26]. UKPDS data have shown that there was no definite blood glucose level responsible for increased cardiovascular risk in diabetes patients [27]. In prospective population-based observational studies, the effect of hyperglycemia was less than that of conventional risk factors [15, 27].

But, hyperglycemia cannot be neglected as an important cardiovascular risk factor in both types of diabetes [18, 23, 29]. Nevertheless, the proof that optimal control of glycemia results in a reduction of CHD events remains to be shown by prospective studies.

In general, consensus guidelines have very much focused on HbA1c targets. HbA1c should probably be less than 7%.

Earlier and more intensive blood glucose control would probably reduce vascular events even further. Although the underlying pathophysiology remains to be elucidated, the factors thought to be involved include advanced glycation end-products (AGEs), oxidative stress, reductive stress, carbonyl stress, aldose reductase activity and protein kinase C activation [30, 31, 32].

Several recent papers have suggested that postprandial hyperglycemia is a better predictor for cardiovascular mortality than fasting blood glucose [33, 34]. The ADA commentaries stated that up to now, it is unclear whether excessive excursions of postprandial glucose have a significant impact on the development of diabetic microvascular or macrovascular complications independent of HbA1c levels. To address this fundamental question, studies must be designed to control fasting plasma glucose *versus* postprandial plasma glucose levels while aiming to achieve similar and acceptable HbA1c levels [35].

INSULIN RESISTANCE AND HYPERINSULINEMIA

It is well recognized that the cluster of risk factors in type 2 diabetes results in impaired sensitivity of various tissues (skeletal muscle, adipose tissue) to insulin. This cluster of risk factors is grouped around the unifying concept of insulin resistance syndrome [36, 37, 38, 39]. Hyperinsulinemia resulting from insulin resistance is frequently to be found in patients with type 2 diabetes and in subjects with impaired glucose tolerance. Hyperinsulinemia is frequently associated with obesity, arterial hypertension, lipid abnormalities and hypercoagulability [36, 40]. It seems unlikely that hyperinsulinemia of insulin resistance is atherogenic itself [38]. This issue is not completely resolved [41]. In order to elucidate the role of insulin resistance syndrome in the complex etiology of cardiovascular disease in diabetes, additional studies are needed in which insulin resistance has to be measured directly [38].

LIPID ABNORMALITIES AND CARDIOVASCULAR DISEASE IN DIABETES

Dyslipidemia (moderate to severe hypertriglyceridemia, low HDL cholesterol, normal to slightly elevated LDL cholesterol) is a major risk factor for coronary heart disease and cardiovascular disease in type 2 diabetes [42]. Most studies that have quantified the lipoproteins in diabetes have found that the major abnormality is hypertriglyceridemia [43, 44, 45]. Hypertriglyceridemia increases CHD risk through the accumulation of cholesterol-rich remnants and abnormal postprandial lipemia. It also shifts the low-density lipoprotein subfraction (LDL) towards the small dense particles, lowers HDL-cholesterol levels, and promotes abnormalities in major thrombotic and coagulation factors [46]. These abnormalities are already found in type 2 diabetes at the time of diagnosis [47]. Several data have shown that hypertriglyceridemia is an element of the insulin resistance syndrome [45]. Lowering of triglycerides with drugs like gemfibrozil, however, did not result in improved insulin sensitivity [48]. Further studies are needed to elucidate the role of elevated triglycerides in the pathogenesis of diabetic atherosclerotic disease [49].

The role of elevated cholesterol levels for coronary heart disease in diabetes was shown in the Multiple Risk Factor Intervention Trial data [50]. At any given serum cholesterol concentration those subjects with diabetes had an increased risk for coronary heart disease mortality that was two to four times greater than the risk in those without diabetes.

Randomized controlled trials have shown that lipid lowering therapy with statins or gemfibrozil resulted in the reduction of cardiovascular events and cardiovascular mortality in populations with predominantly non-diabetic patients [51, 52, 53, 54, 55]. In some of these studies significant effects were found in the subgroups of patients with diabetes [44]. Unfortunately, until now, no study has been published in which the effect of drug therapy of hyperlipidemia on cardiovascular endpoints is examined in a population of patients with diabetes.

Clinical presentation of hyperlipoproteinemia in patients with type 1 and type 2 diabetes is different. In contrast to type 2 diabetes, type 1 diabetes patients have normal lipid levels [56], but this is not the case in poorly controlled type 1 diabetes [57] and in type 1 diabetes patients with diabetic nephropathy [58], even in type 1 diabetes patients with incipient diabetic nephropathy [59]. When compared with non-nephropathic type 1 diabetes patients, nephropathic type 1 diabetes patients have a significantly increased cardiovascular morbidity and mortality [60].

Summing up, present evidence supports the necessity of rigorous treatment of hyper-lipoproteinemia in type 1 and type 2 diabetes patients. Throughout the world, most consensus guidelines have established that LDL cholesterol should be brought to a value of less than 2.6 mmol/l (<100 mg/dl), at least for patients with established atherosclerotic disease.

HYPERTENSION

Hypertension represents a major problem for health and quality of life of diabetes patients. Hypertension has substantial importance for reduced life expectancy of type 1 and type 2 diabetes patients. Arterial hypertension accelerates markedly the manifestation and progression of micro-and macrovascular complications both in type 1 and type 2 diabetes patients [4, 61, 62]. When compared with the non-diabetic population, diabetes patients have a twofold higher risk for development of hypertension [63, 64], and hypertensive diabetes patients have increased cardiovascular mortality [4, 62, 65, 66]. Both hypertension and diabetes mellitus are independent cardiovascular risk factors. They are frequently associated, and have a synergistic effect on the development of micro-and macrovascular diabetes complications, and even on the manifestation of diabetes mellitus itself [67, 68]. The causes of the higher risk for hypertension in patients with type 2 diabetes are unknown. Although hypertension is associated with insulin resistance and hyper-insulinism [36, 69], an elevated insulin level may not be an independent risk marker.

According to several studies, hypertension and particularly systolic blood pressure are dominant risk factors for coronary heart disease both in nondiabetic [70] and in diabetic subjects [71, 72]. Hypertension is the single most important risk factor for stroke in nondiabetic subjects [73] as well as in diabetic subjects [74, 75]. Hypertension is also a significant risk factor for amputation in type 2 diabetes [76].

Thus, type 2 diabetes patients are showing a cluster of cardiovascular risk factors with hypertension, lipid disorders and insulin resistance leading to increased cardiovascular mortality [77].

There are marked differences in the time courses of development of hypertension in patients with type 1 and type 2 diabetes. In patients with type 1 diabetes, blood pressure is typically normal at the onset of disease and during the following 5–10 years. Hypertension develops along with the presentation of microalbuminuria and nephropathy [78, 79, 80]. In patients with type 2 diabetes hypertension is present already at time of diagnosis of diabetes in a remarkable percentage of patients.

In diabetes patients with overt nephropathy cardiovascular mortality is increased. Hypertension and lipid disorders increase the cardiovascular risk both in nephropathic type 1 and in type 2 diabetes patients [81, 82].

Several controlled clinical trials have shown that rigorous blood pressure control markedly reduces cardiovascular morbidity and mortality and delays the development of end stage renal failure in diabetes [83, 84, 85]. Special benefits of aggressive blood pressure reduction with even greater reduction in cardiovascular mortality in type 2 diabetes patients have been observed in the SYSTEUR study [86]. Thus, available evidence suggests that blood pressure lowering drugs reduce both the risk of macrovascular and microvascular complications [87, 88, 89].

The National Kidney Foundation and the JNC-7 have urged physicians to lower the blood pressure of patients with both diabetes and hypertension to <130/80 mm Hg in its guidelines [90, 91].

SMOKING

There is substantial evidence that smoking increases synergistically with diabetes the morbidity and mortality in type 1 and type 2 diabetes patients [92, 93]. Smoking increases cardiovascular morbidity and total mortality in nondiabetic persons and also in patients suffering from type 1 and type 2 diabetes [94]. Smoking is a major avoidable risk factor for coronary heart disease, thus by cessation a decrease in cardiovascular morbidity and mortality in diabetes patients would be expected [95, 96].

HYPERCOAGULABILITY

In atherosclerotic vessels, vascular thrombosis significantly increases cardiovascular morbidity and mortality in diabetes patients. It is generally accepted that platelet dysfunction plays an important role in the pathogenesis of atherosclerosis in diabetes patients. Platelets from men and women with diabetes are often hypersensitive *in vitro* to platelet aggregating agents [97]. A major mechanism is increased production of thromboxane [98]. The HOT study has shown that a dosage of 75 mg aspirin was effective in reducing platelet aggregation [89]. Generally recommended dosages of aspirin are between 100 and 300 mg/day [99].

Summing up, all studies focused on diabetes and atherosclerosis have shown an increased risk for cardiovascular disease in diabetic men and women. There is an increased incidence of coronary heart disease and stroke in diabetes patients. However, the role of cardiovascular risk factors, increasing the risk in diabetes mellitus, in certain points has remained controversial. In order to implement cardiovascular interventions in diabetes patients, the strength of the associations between putative cardiovascular risk factors and cardiovascular end points in both types of diabetes needs to be elucidated.

In a cohort of 4743 diabetes patients, the WHO Multinational Study of Vascular Disease in Diabetes has prospectively studied the incidence of fatal and non-fatal cardiovascular disease outcomes for about 12 years [18]. The important findings are that blood pressure, serum cholesterol and proteinuria represent predictors for cardiovascular end points and for stroke in patients with type 1 and type 2 diabetes. Serum triglyceride concentrations were associated with death from cardiovascular disease in type 2 diabetes patients and in women with type 1 diabetes. Similar associations were detectable with the incidence of myocardial infarction and of stroke in patients with type 2 diabetes.

As shown in the WHO Multinational Study of Vascular Disease in Diabetes, the presence of retinopathy was related to cardiovascular disease death and incidence of myocardial infarction in both types of diabetes, and to stroke in type 2 diabetes [18].

In a recent cross–sectional study, comparing the risk factors for peripheral vascular disease in type 1 and type 2 diabetes, we found nearly identical associations in both types of diabetes, *i.e.* hypertension, coronary heart disease, nephropathy, neuropathy, foot ulceration and increased insulin requirement in type 1 diabetes, and for coronary heart disease, nephropathy, retinopathy, neuropathy, foot ulceration, increased insulin requirement and triglycerides in type 2 diabetes [100].

Almost identical CVD risk factors were also found for coronary heart disease, including the glucose-dependent microvascular complications such as nephropathy, neuropathy and proliferative retinopathy [101].

Current data show that the assessment of cardiovascular disease risk in both types of diabetes must include diabetes-related variables such as glucose control, nephropathy, neuropathy and retinopathy in addition to the classical risk factors as blood pressure, lipid disorders and smoking [18].

Recently, the ARIC Study provided evidence by a prospective study for the importance of several nontraditional risk factors for coronary heart disease in adults with type 2 diabetes, as albumin, fibrinogen, factor VIII, and von Willebrand factor and leukocyte account as being independently associated with coronary heart disease [102].

Thus, further compilation of diabetes related specific CVD risk tables could provide a significant contribution to a better prevention of cardiovascular disease in diabetes [103].

REFERENCES

1. Abbott RD, Donahue RP, Kannel WB, Wilson PW. The impact of diabetes on survival following myocardial infarction in men *vs.* women. Framingham Study. *JAMA*, **260**: 3456–3460, 1988.
2. Head JD, Fuller JH. International variations in mortality among diabetes patients: the WHO Multinational Study of Vascular Disease in Diabetics. *Diabetologia*, **33**: 477–481, 1990.

3. Krolewski AS, Kosinski EJ, Warram JH, Leland OS, Busick EJ, Asmal AC, Rand LI, Christlieb A, Bradley RF, Kahn CR. Magnitude and determinants of coronary artery disease in juvenile-onset, insulin-dependent diabetes mellitus. *Am J Cardiol*, **59**: 750–755, 1987.

4. Panzram G. Mortality and survival in type 2 (non-insulin-dependent) diabetes mellitus. *Diabetologia*, **30**: 123–134, 1987.

5. American Diabetes Association. Consensus Development Conference on the diagnosis of coronary heart disease in people with diabetes. *Diabetes Care*, **21**: 1551–1559, 1998.

6. Kannel WB, McGee DL. Diabetes and glucose tolerance as risk factors for cardiovascular disease: The Framingham Study. *Diabetes Care*, **2**: 120–126, 1979.

7. Krolewski AS, Warram JH, Rand LI, Kahn CR. Epidemiologic approach to etiology in type 1 diabetes and its complications. *N Engl J Med*, **329**: 977–986, 1993.

8. Brand FN, Abbott RD, Kannel WB. Diabetes, intermittent claudication, and risk of cardiovascular events. The Framingham Study. *Diabetes*, **38**: 504–509, 1989.

9. Fuller JH, Shipley MJ, Rose G, Jarrett RJ, Keen H. Coronary-heart-disease risk and impaired glucose tolerance. The Whitehall study. *Lancet*, **I** (8183): 1373–1376, 1980.

10. Manson JE, Colditz GA, Stampfer MJ, Willett WC, Krolewski AS, Rosner B, Arky RA, Speizer FE, Hennekens CH. A prospective study of maturity- onset diabetes mellitus and risk of coronary heart disease and stroke in women. *Arch Intern Med*, **151**: 1141–1147, 1991.

11. Forrest KYZ, Becker DJ, Kuller LH, Wolfson SK, Orchard TY. Are predictors of coronary heart disease and lower-extremity arterial disease in type 1 diabetes the same? A prospective study. *Atherosclerosis*, **148**: 159–169, 2000.

12. Damsgaard EM, Froland A, Mogensen CE. Over-mortality as related to age and gender in patients with established non-insulin-dependent diabetes mellitus. *J Diabetic Complications*, **11**: 77–82, 1997.

13. Deckert T, Poulsen JE, Larsen M. Prognosis of diabetes with diabetes onset before the age of thirty-one.1. Survival, causes of death, and complications. *Diabetologia*, **14**: 363–370, 1978.

14. Jarrett RJ. Risk factors for coronary heart disease in diabetes mellitus. *Diabetes*, **41** (Suppl 2): 1–3, 1992.

15. Laakso M. Hyperglycemia and cardiovascular disease in patients with type 2 diabetes. *Curr Opin Endocrinol Diabetes*, **7**: 197–202, 2000.

16. Stern M. Natural history of macrovascular disease in type 2 diabetes. Role of insulin resistance. *Diabetes Care*, **22 (Suppl 3)**: C2–C5, 1999.

17. Stratton IM, Adler AI, Neil HA, Matthews DR, Manley SE, Cull CA et al. (UKPDS 35). Associations of glycaemia with macrovascular and microvascular complications of type 2 diabetes (UKPDS 35): prospective observational study. *BMJ*, **321**: 405–412, 2000.

18. Fuller JH, Stevens LK, Wang SL, and the WHO Multinational Study Group. Risk factors for cardiovascular mortality and morbidity: The WHO multinational study of vascular disease in diabetes. *Diabetologia*, **44 (Suppl 2)**: S 54–S 64, 2001.

19. Hadden DR, Patterson CC, Atkinson AB, Kennedy L, Bell PM, McCance DR, Weaver JA. Macrovascular disease and hyperglycaemia: 10-year survival analysis in type 2 diabetes mellitus: the Belfast Diet Study. *Diabet Med*, **14**: 663–672, 1997.

20. Jarrett RJ, Mc Cartney P, Kenn H. The Bedford survey: ten year mortality rates in newly diagnosed diabetics, borderline diabetics and normoglycaemic controls and risk indices for coronary heart disease in borderline diabetics. *Diabetologia*, **22**: 79–84, 1982.

21. Klein R, Klein BE. Relation of glycaemic control to diabetic complications and health outcomes. *Diabetes Care*, **21 (Suppl 3)**: C39–C 43, 1998.

22. DCCT Research Group. Effect of intensive diabetes management on macrovascular events and risk factors in the Diabetes Control and Complications Trial. *Am J Cardiol*, **75**: 894–903, 1995.

23. Wei M, Gaskill SP, Haffner SM, Stern MP. Effects of diabetes and level of glycaemia on all-cause and cardiovascular mortality. The San Antonio Heart Study. *Diabetes Care,* **21**: 1167–1172, 1998.

24. Standl E, Balletshofer B, Dahl B, Weichenhain B, Stiegler H, Hormann A, Holle R. Predictors of 10-year macrovascular and overall mortality in patients with NIDDM: the Munich General Practitioner Project. *Diabetologia*, **39**: 1540–1545, 1996.

25. Lehto S, Ronnemaa T, Pyörälä K, Laakso M. Predictors of stroke in middle-aged patients with non-insulin-dependent diabetics. *Stroke,* **27**: 63–68, 1996.

26. Janka HU, Balleshofer B, Becker A, Gick MR, Hartmann J, Fung D, et al. Das metabolische Syndrom als potenter kardiovaskulärer Risikofaktor für vorzeitigen Tod bei Typ 2 Diabetikern. *Diab Stoffw*, **1**: 2–7, 1992.

27. UKPDS Group. Effect of intensive blood glucose control with metformin on complications in

overweight patients with type 2 diabetes (UKPDS 34). *Lancet,* **352:** 854–865, 1998.

28. Turner RC, Millns H, Neil HA, *et al* (UKPDS Group). Risk factors for coronary artery disease in non-insulin-dependent diabetes mellitus: United Kingdom Prospective Diabetes Study (UKPDS: 23). *BMJ,* **316:** 823–828, 1998.

29. Eckel RH. Natural history of macrovascular disease and classic risk factors for atherosclerosis. *Diabetes Care,* **22 (Suppl 3):** C21–C24, 1999.

30. Baynes JW, Thorpe SR. The role of oxidative stress in diabetic complications. *Curr Opin Endocrinol,* **3:** 277–284, 1997.

31. Lyons TJ, Jenkins AJ. Glycation, oxidation and lipoxidation in the development of complications of diabetes: a carbonyl stress hypothesis. *Diabetes Rev,* **5:** 365–391, 1997.

32. Ways DK, King G. Glucotoxicity: a role for protein kinase C activation. In: Betteridge DJ (ed).: *Current Perspectives,* Martin Dunitz, London, UK, 2000, 53–66.

33. DECODE – study group. Is fasting glucose sufficient to define diabetes? Epidemiological data from 20 European studies. The DECODE–study group. European Diabetes Epidemiology Group. Diabetes Epidemiology: Collaborative analysis of Diagnostic Criteria in Europe. *Diabetologia,* **42:** 647–654, 1999.

34. Shaw JE, Hodge AM, de Courten M, Chitson P, Zimmet PZ. Isolated post-challenge hyperglycemia confirmed as a risk factor for mortality. *Diabetologia,* **42:** 1050–1054, 1999.

35. American Diabetes Association. Postprandial blood glucose. *Diabetes Care,* **24:** 775–778, 2001.

36. Reaven GM. Role of insulin resistance in human disease. *Diabetes,* **37:** 1595–1607, 1988.

37. Adachi H, Hashimoto R, Tsuruta M, Jacobs DR, JR. Crow RS, Imaizumi T. Hyperinsulinemia and the development of ST-electrocardiographic abnormalities. An 11-year follow-up study. *Diabetes Care,* **20:** 1688–1692, 1997.

38. Depres JP, Lamarche B, Mauriege P, Cantin B, Dagenais GR, Moorjani S, Lupien PJ. Hyperinsulinemia as an independent risk factor for ischemic heart disease. *N Eng J Med,* **334:** 952–957, 1996.

39. Lehto S, Ronnemaa T, Pyörälä K, Laakso M. Cardiovascular risk factors clustering with endogenous hyperinsulinemia predict death from coronary heart disease in patients with type 2 diabetes. *Diabetologia,* **43:** 148–155, 2000.

40. European Arterial Risk Policy Group, IDF European Region. A strategy for arterial risk assessment and management in type 2 (non-insulin-dependent) diabetes mellitus. European Arterial Policy Group on behalf of the IDF European Region. *Diabet Med,* **14:** 611–621, 1997.

41. Stout RW. Insulin and atheroma: 20 year perspectives. *Diabetes Care,* **13:** 631–655, 1990.

42. Syvanne M, Taskinen MR. Lipids and lipoproteins as coronary risk factor in non-insulin-dependent diabetes mellitus. *Lancet,* **350 (Suppl 1):** S 20–S23, 1997.

43. Harris MI. Hypercholesterolemia in diabetes and glucose intolerance in the U.S. population. *Diabetes Care,* **14:** 366–374, 1991.

44. Dunn FL. Hyperlipidemia in diabetes mellitus. *Diabetes Metab Rev,* **6:** 47–61, 1990.

45. Steiner G. The dyslipoproteinemias of diabetes. *Atherosclerosis,* **110 (Suppl):** S 27–S33, 1994.

46. Betteridge DJ. Cardiovascular disease in diabetes: the scale of the challenge. *Medicographia,* **24:**9–14, 2002.

47. UK Prospective Diabetes Study Group. UK Prospective Diabetes Study 27: plasma lipids and lipoproteins at diagnosis of NIDDM by age and sex. *Diabetes Care,* **20:** 1683–1687, 1997.

48. Vuorinen-Markkolah, Yki-Jarvinen H, Taskinen MR. Lowering of triglycerides by gemfibrozil affects neither the glucoregulatory nor antilipolytic effects of insulin in type 2 (non-insulin-dependent) diabetic patients. *Diabetologia,* **36:** 161–169, 1993.

49. Steiner G. Risk factors for macrovascular disease in type 2 diabetes. Classic lipid abnormalities. *Diabetes Care,* **22(Suppl 3):** C6–C9, 1999.

50. Stamler J, Vaccaro O, Neaton JD. Diabetes, other risk factors, and 12-year cardiovascular mortality for men screened in the Multiple Risk Factor Intervention Trial. *Diabetes Care,* **16:** 434–444, 1993.

51. Goldberg RB, Mellies MJ, Sacks FM, Move LA, Howard BV, Howard WJ, Davis BR, Cole TG, Pfeffer MA, Braunwald E. Cardiovascular events and their reduction with pravastatin in diabetic and glucose-intolerant myocardial infarction survivors with average cholesterol levels: subgroup analyses in the cholesterol and recurrent events (CARE) trial. The CARE Investigators. *Circulation,* **98:** 2513–2519, 1998.

52. Manninen V, Tenkanen L, Koskinen P, Huttunen JK, Manttari M, Heinonen OP, Frick MH. Joint effects of serum triglyceride and LDL cholesterol and HDL cholesterol concentrations on coronary heart disease in the Helsinki Heart Study. Implications for treatment. *Circulation,* **85:** 37–45, 1992.

53. Pyörala K, Pedersen TR, Kjekshus J, Faergeman O, Olsson AG, Thorgeirsson G. Cholesterol lowering with simvastatin improves prognosis of diabetes patients with coronary heart disease. A subgroup analysis of the Scandinavian Simvastatin

Survival Study (4S). *Diabetes Care,* **20:** 614–620, 1997.

54. Tikkanen M, Laakso M, Ilmonen M, Helve E, Kaarsalo E, Kilkki E, Salveto J. Treatment of hypercholesterolemia and combined hyperlipidemia with simvastatin and gemfibrozil in patients with NIDDM. A multicenter comparison study. *Diabetes Care,* **21:** 477–481, 1998.

55. Downs JR, Clearfield M, Weis S, *et al.* Primary prevention of acute coronary events with lovastatin in men and women with average cholesterol levels: results of AFCAPS/Tex CAPS Air Force Texas Coronary Atherosclerosis Prevention Study. *JAMA,* **279**: 1615–1622, 1998.

56. Elkeles RS, Wu J, Hambley J. Hemoglobin A1, blood glucose, and high density lipoprotein cholesterol in insulin-requiring diabetes. *Lancet,* **II:** 547–549, 1978.

57. Lopes-Virella MF, Woltmann HJ, Mayfield RK, Loadholt CB, Colwell JA. Effect of metabolic control on lipid, lipoprotein, and apolipoprotein levels in 55 insulin-dependent diabetic patients. A longitudinal study. *Diabetes,* **32:** 20–25, 1983.

58. Jones SL, Close CE, Mattock MB, Jarrett RJ, Keen H, Viberti GC. Plasma lipid and coagulation factor concentrations in insulin-dependent diabetics with microalbuminuria. *BMJ,* **298:** 487–490, 1989.

59. Vannini G, Ciavarella A, Flammini M, Bargossi AM, Forlani G, Borgnino LC, Orsani G. Lipid abnormalities in insulin-dependent diabetic patients with albuminuria. *Diabetes Care,* **7:** 151–154, 1984.

60. Borch-Johnsen K, Andersen PK, Deckert T. The effect of proteinuria on relative mortality in type 1 (insulin-dependent) diabetes mellitus. *Diabetologia,* **28:** 590–596, 1985.

61. UKPDS-Group (UK Prospective Diabetes Study 38): Tight blood pressure control and risk of macrovascular and microvascular complications in type 2 diabetes. *BMJ,* **317:** 703–713, 1998.

62. Krolewski AS, Warram JH, Cupples A. Hypertension, orthostatic hypotension, and microvascular complications of diabetes. *J Chron Dis,* **38:** 319–326, 1985.

63. Kannel WB, McGee DL. Diabetes and cardiovascular risk factors. The Framingham Study. *Circ,* **1:** 8–13, 1979.

64. The Hypertension and Diabetes Study Group. Hypertension in newly presenting type 2 diabetic patients and the association with risk factors for cardiovascular and diabetic complications. *J Hypertens,* **11:** 309–317, 1993.

65. Morrish NJ, Stevens LK, Head J, *et al.* A prospective study on mortality among middle-aged diabetic patients (the London cohort of the WHO Multinational Study of Vascular Disease in Diabetics). II. Associated with risk factors. *Diabetologia,* **33:** 542–548, 1990.

66. Borch-Johnsen K, Nisson R, Nerup J. Blood pressure after 40 years of insulin–dependent diabetes. *Nephron,* **4:** 11–12, 1989.

67. Simonson DC. Etiology and prevalence of hypertension in diabetic patients. *Diabetes Care,* **11:** 821–827, 1988.

68. Gress TW, Nieto FJ, Shahar E, Wofford MR, Brancati FL. Hypertension and antihypertensive therapy as risk factors for type 2 diabetes mellitus. Atherosclerosis Risk in Communities Study. *N Engl J Med,* **342:** 905–912, 2000.

69. Ferrannini E, Natal A. Essential hypertension, metabolic disorders, and insulin resistance. *Am Heart J,* **121:** 1274–1282, 1991.

70. Ford ES, De Stefano F. Risk factors for mortality from all causes and from coronary heart disease among persons with diabetes: findings from the National Health and Nutrition Examination Survey. I Epidemiologic Follow-up Study. *Am J Epidemiol,* **133** : 1220–1230, 1991.

71. Stamler J, Vaccaro O, Neaton J, Wentworth D, for the Multiple Risk Factor Intervention Trial Research Group: Diabetes, other risk factors, and 12-yr cardiovascular mortality for men screened in the Multiple Risk Factor Intervention Trial. *Diabetes Care,* **16:** 434–444,1993.

72. Fitzgerald AP, Jarrett RJ. Are conventional risk factors for mortality relevant in type 2 diabetes? *Diabet Med,* **8:** 475–480, 1991.

73. Dunbabin DW, Sandercock PAG. Prevention stroke by modification of risk factors. *Stroke* **21(Suppl 12):** IV36–IV39, 1990.

74. Asplund K, Hagg F, Helmers C, Lithner F, Strand T, Wester PD. The natural history of stroke in diabetic patients. *Acta Med Scand,* **207:** 417–424, 1980.

75. Lavy S, Melamed E, Cahane E, Carmon A. Hypertension and diabetes as risk factors in stroke patients. *Stroke,* **4:** 751–759, 1973.

76. Lehto S, Rönnemaa T, Pyörälä K, Laakso M. Risk factors preventing lower extremity amputation in patients with NIDDM. *Diabetes Care,* **19:** 607–612, 1996.

77. The Hypertension and Diabetes Study Group. Hypertension in newly presenting type 2 diabetic patients and the association with risk factors for cardiovascular and diabetic complications. *J Hypertens,* **11:** 309–317, 1993.

78. Consensus Statement. Treatment of hypertension in diabetes. *Diabetes Care,* **16:** 1394–1401, 1993.

79. Hansen KW, Christensen CK, Andersen PH, Mau Pedersen M, Christiansen JS, Mogensen CE. Ambulatory blood pressure in microalbinuric type 1 diabetic patients. *Kidney Int,* **41:** 847–854, 1992.

80. Klein R. Hyperglycaemia and microvascular and macrovascular disease in diabetes. *Diabetes Care*, **18**: 258–268, 1995.
81. Mogensen CE. Microalbuminuria, blood pressure and diabetic renal disease: origin and development of ideas. *Diabetologia*, **42**: 263–285, 1999.
82. Gaede P, Vedel P, Parving HH, Pedersen O. Intensified multifactorial intervention in patients with type 2 diabetes mellitus and microalbuminuria: the STENO type 2 randomised study. *Lancet*, **I**: 617–622, 1999.
83. Lindholm LH. The outcome of STOP–hypertension 2 in relation to the 1999 WHO/ISH hypertension guidelines. *Blood Press Suppl*, **2**: 21–24, 2000.
84. Curb JD, Pressel MS, Cutler JA, Savage PJ, Applegate WB, Black H, Camel G, Davis BR, Frost PH, Gonzalez N, *et al.* Effect of diuretic-based antihypertensive treatment on cardiovascular disease risk in older diabetic patients with isolated hypertension. *JAMA*, **276**: 1886–1892.
85. Hansson L, Lindholm LH, Niskanen L, Lanke J, Hedner T, Niklason A, Luomanmaki K, Dahlhof B, de Faire U, Morlin C, *et al.* Effect of angiotensin-converting-enzyme inhibition compared with conventional therapy on cardiovascular morbidity and mortality in hypertension: the Captopril Prevention Project (CAPPP) randomized trial. *Lancet*, **353**: 611–616.
86. Tuomilehto J, Rastenyte D, Birkenhager WH, Thijs L, Antikainen R, Bulpitt CJ, Fletcher AE, Forette F, Goldhaber A, Palatini P, *et al.* for the Systolic Hypertension in Europe Trial Investigators. Effects of calcium channel blockers in older patients with diabetes and systolic hypertension. *N Engl J Med*, **340**: 677–684, 1999.
87. UK Prospective Diabetes Study Group. Tight blood pressure control and risk of macrovascular and microvascular complications in type 2 diabetes: UKPDS 38. *BMJ*, **317**: 706–713, 1998.
88. Estacio R, Raymond O, Jeffers B, Gifford N, Schrier R. Effect of blood pressure control on diabetic microvascular complications in patients with hypertension and type 2 diabetes. *Diabetes Care*, **23 (suppl 2)**: B54–B64, 2000.
89. Hannsson L, Zanchetti A, Carruthers A, *et al.* for the HOT Study Group. Effects of intensive blood pressure lowering and low-dose aspirin in patients with hypertension: principal results of the Hypertension Optimal Treatment (HOT) randomized trial. *Lancet*, **351**: 1755–1762, 1998.
90. Bakris GL, Williams M, Dworkin L, *et al.* Preserving renal function in adults with hypertension and diabetes. A consensus approach. *Am J Kidney Dis*, **36**: 646–661, 2000.
91. Chobanian AV, Bakris GL, Black HR, Cushmann WC, Green LA, Izzo JL, Jones DW, Materson BJ, Oparil S, Wright JT, Rotella EJ, and the National High Blood Pressure Education Program Coordinating Committee: The seventh Report of the Joint National Committee on Prevention, Detection and Evaluation and Treatment of High Blood Pressure. The JNC 7 Report. *JAMA,* **289**: 2534–2573, 2003.
92. Haire-Joshu D, Glassow RE, Tibbs TL. Smoking and diabetes. *Diabetes Care*, **22**: 1887–1898, 1999.
93. Mühlhauser I. Cigarette smoking and diabetes: an update. *Diabet Med*, **11**: 336–342, 1994.
94. Stamler J, Vaccaro O, Neaton JD, Wentworth D. Diabetes, other risk factors, and 12-yr cardiovascular mortality for men screened in the Multiple Risk Factor Intervention Trial. *Diabetes Care*, **16**: 434–444.
95. Dierkx RI, van de Hoek W, Hoekstra JB, Erkelens DW: Smoking in diabetes mellitus. *Neth J Med*, **48**: 150–162, 1996.
96. Canga N, DeIrala J, Vara E, Duaso MJ, Ferrer A, Martinez –Gonzalez MA. Intervention study for smoking cessation in diabetic patients. A randomized controlled trial in both clinical and primary care settings. *Diabetes Care*, **23**: 1455–1460, 2000.
97. ADA. Aspirin Therapy in Diabetes. *Diabetes Care*, **22** (suppl 1): S 60–S61, 1999.
98. Patrono C, Davi G. Antiplatelet agents in the prevention of diabetic vascular complications. *Diabetes Metab Rev*, **9**: 177–188, 1993.
99. European Arterial Risk Policy Group, International Diabetes Federation European Region. A strategy for arterial risk assessment and management in type 2 (non-insulin-dependent) diabetes mellitus. *Diabet Med*, **14**: 611–621, 1997.
100. Zander E, Heinke P, Reindel J, Kohnert KD, Kairies U, Braun J, Eckel L, Kerner W. Peripheral vascular disease in diabetes mellitus type 1 and type 2: Are there different risk factors? *VASA*, **31**: 249–254, 2002.
101. Zander E, Heinke P, Allwardt C, Gronwald S, Hahn JU, Schmidt J, Kerner W. Koronare Herzkrankheit und Diabetes mellitus: Unterscheiden sich die kardiovaskulären Risikofaktoren bei Typ 1 und Typ 2 Diabetes? *Diab Stoffw*, **11** (suppl 11): 97 (Abstract), 2002.
102. Saito I, Folsom AR, Brancati FL, Duncan BB, Chambless LE, McGovern PG. Nontraditional Risk Factors for Coronary Heart Disease Incidence among Persons with Diabetes: The Atherosclerosis Risk in Communities (ARIC) study. *Ann Intern Med*, **133**: 81–91, 2000.
103. Yudkin JS, Blauth C, Drury P, *et al.* Prevention and management of cardiovascular disease in patients with diabetes mellitus: An Evidence Base. *Diabetic Med*, **13**: 101–121, 1996.

17

IMPAIRED FASTING GLUCOSE AND IMPAIRED GLUCOSE TOLERANCE: DIFFERENCES IN PREVALENCE, METABOLIC CHARACTERISTICS AND ASSOCIATED RISK

Radu LICHIARDOPOL

The new classification of diabetes, released in 1997 by American Diabetes Association and in 1999 by the World Health Organization, identified Impaired Fasting Glycemia (IFG) and Impaired Glucose Tolerance (IGT) as fasting and respectively postprandial abnormalities of glucose regulation.

A number of epidemiological studies clearly demonstrated that IFG and IGT are not equivalent. Important differences in prevalence, phenotype, metabolic characteristics and associated risk exist between these two categories.

Most frequently these categories are expressed as an isolated increase of plasma glucose levels, either fasting (isolated IFG) or 2-h after oral glucose challenge (isolated IGT).

These distinct patterns of glucose intolerance are preserved during the progression to type 2 diabetes suggesting that they represent the expression of different pathophysiological mechanisms.

Therefore, the classification of glucose intolerance states should take into consideration the spectrum of glucose intolerance as the intermediary states between the two extremities: either isolated increase in fasting plasma glucose or post (prandial) oral glucose challenge.

Abbreviations List

ADA – American Diabetes Association
EGP – endogenous glucose production
FFA – free fatty acids
FPG – fasting plasma glucose
FPIS – first phase insulin secretion
HGP – hepatic glucose production
2-h PG – 2 hour plasma glucose after oral glucose challenge (75 g)
IFH – isolated fasting hyperglycemia

IGR – Impaired glucose regulation
I-IFG – isolated IFG (normal 2-h PG levels)
I-IGT – isolated IGT (normal FPG levels)
IMT – intima-media thickness
NGT – normal glucose tolerance
OGTT – oral glucose tolerance test (75 g)
PG – plasma glucose
WHO – World Health Organization

In 1997, the American Diabetes Association (ADA) Expert Committee [1] recommended that the diagnostic threshold for diabetes should be lowered to ≥ 7.0 mmol/l (126 mg/dl) fasting plasma glucose.

This recommendation was based on three different population studies showing that increasing fasting plasma glucose values ≥ 7 mmol/l (126 mg/dl) are associated with an increased risk for microvascular complications.

At the same time, the Expert Committee approved a new diagnostic category: Impaired Fasting Glucose (IFG), defined by fasting plasma glucose levels ≥ 6.1 mmol/l (110 mg/dl) but < 7.0 mmol/l (126 mg/dl).

This new category, based on fasting glucose levels, was created with the belief that it would be equivalent (in terms of microvascular and macrovascular complications risk) to Impaired Glucose Tolerance (IGT), defined by 2-h blood glucose levels between 140–199 mg/dl during a 75 g oral glucose tolerance test (OGTT).

ADA strongly recommended that fasting plasma glucose determination should be used in clinical and epidemiological studies and that 2-h plasma glucose need not be used.

The 1999 Report of a World Health Organization Consultation [2] on definition, diagnosis and classification of diabetes mellitus adopted the new diagnostic criteria for diabetes and impaired fasting glucose, but retained the former 2-h glucose diagnostic criteria for diabetes and IGT and suggested the use of fasting plasma glucose alone in epidemiological studies only when the use of OGTT is prevented.

Substantial discrepancies were subsequently demonstrated between IFG and IGT. It was found, in large epidemiological studies, that IFG and IGT are not equivalent: not only they do not identify the same group of individuals, but important differences in prevalence, associated cardiovascular risk and metabolic characteristics exist between these two categories.

PREVALENCE

A number of epidemiological studies analyzed whether fasting plasma glucose (FPG) value of 7.0 mmol/l (126 mg/dl) represents a value which had a similar diagnostic significance to a plasma glucose (PG) level of 11.1 mmol/l (200 mg/dl) 2-h post oral glucose load.

In a Polish study [3] using 75 g OGTT, from 1360 Caucasian subjects (759 women, 601 men) at increased risk for diabetes, with a mean age of 65.5 years and BMI of 28.2 kg/m^2 a number of 252 subjects with diabetes and 360 with Impaired Glucose Regulation (IGR) were identified by using combined criteria (ADA: fasting plasma glucose, WHO: 2-h post oral glucose load). From the total number of diabetic subjects, 220 had 2-h diabetic hyperglycemia (Table 17.1), and in this group 100 subjects had also increased FPG levels (40 had diabetic values and 60 had IFG values) whereas 120 subjects had normal FPG.

Table 17.1

Percentage of different phenotypes of plasma glucose response during OGGT in 252 newly detected diabetic subjects [3]

Phenotype	Plasma glucose levels (mg/dl)	Percentage (number of cases)
2-h DH	2-h PG ≥200; FPG < 126	**71%** (n = 180)
FDH	FPG ≥ 126; 2-h PG < 200	**13%** (n = 32)
CDH	FPG ≥ 126; 2-h PG ≥ 200	**16%** (n = 40)

2-h DH: 2-h diabetic hyperglycemia; FDH: Fasting diabetic hyperglycemia; CDH: combined diabetic hyperglycemia (Fasting + 2-h).

Therefore, using only FPG determination, as ADA recommended, in this group 47.6% of diabetic subjects (with 2-h diabetic hyperglycemia and normal FPG levels) would be found to be normal. Seventy-two subjects had diabetic levels of FPG, and 40 of them also had 2-h diabetic hyperglycemia while only 6 diabetic subjects (2.4%) had normal 2-h plasma glucose levels.

In the analyzed population, using only WHO diagnostic criteria, the prevalence of diabetes would be 16.2%, whereas using ADA criteria only the prevalence of diabetes would be 5.3%.

From a total of 360 subjects (Table 17.2) with impaired glucose regulation (IGR), 266 (74%) had IGT with normal FPG (postprandial nondiabetic hyperglycemia or isolated IGT), 44 subjects (12%) were found to have IFG with normal 2-h PG levels (fasting nondiabetic hyperglycemia or isolated IFG) and 50 subjects (14%) had IGT and IFG (mixed nondiabetic hyperglycemia). Therefore, using ADA criteria only, 74% of IGR subjects would be classified as having normal glucose tolerance.

Table 17.2

Percentage of different plasma glucose phenotypes during OGTT in 360 subjects with Impaired Glucose Regulation (IGR)

Phenotype	Plasma glucose levels (mg/dl)	Percentage (number of cases)
I–IGT	2-h PG: 140–199 FPG < 110	74% (n = 266)
I-IFG	FPG: 110–125 2-h PG < 140	12% (n = 44)
IFG/IGT	FPG: 110–125 2-h PG: 140–199	14% (n = 50)

I-IGT: Isolated IGT; I-IFG: Isolated IFG;

It can be observed that the same percentage of different phenotypes (defined by a predominant PG increase during OGTT: either fasting, 2-h post oral glucose load or a combination of the two) is present in both subgroups of diabetic and IGR subjects (Table 17.1 and 17.2).

This suggests that the pattern of glucose intolerance may be conserved during the natural history of the disease.

DECODE study (*Diabetes Epidemiology: Collaborative analysis of Diagnostic criteria in Europe*) reanalyzed European epidemiological data from 13 populations and three occupational based studies from eight European countries [4].

In this study 26,190 subjects (17,881 men, 8,309 women, age range: 17–92 years) were investigated by 75 g OGTT and WHO and ADA criteria concordance was analyzed. This study also evaluated, in individuals without known diabetes, the impact of the new (ADA) diagnostic criteria on the classification and prevalence of diabetes.

From a total of 1517 individuals, diagnosed with diabetes (previously unknown), 473 (31%) had 2-h diabetic hyperglycemia but nondiabetic (< 7.1 mmol/l or < 126 mg/dl) FPG levels. In this group, median FPG value was 6.0 mmol/l (108 mg/dl). In 613 (40.5%) individuals who had fasting diabetic hyperglycemia and 2-h nondiabetic glycemia, the median plasma glucose value 2-h post glucose load was 8.0 mmol/l (144 mg/dl). The remaining 431 (28.5%) newly diagnosed diabetics had mixed (fasting and 2-h post glucose) diabetic hyperglycemia.

According to these findings, at least in European populations, the majority of diabetic individuals manifest isolated diabetic hyperglycemia either fasting or 2-h post glucose challenge. The association between fasting and 2-h plasma glucose values was analyzed further in an extended DECODE study [5] in which epidemiological data from 20 European studies (17 population-based and 3 in occupational groups) were included. In this study 29,108 individuals (18,918 men, 10,190 women) without previously known diabetes were included, and all of them had a 75 g OGTT.

In total, 6,741 individuals (Table 17.3) disclosed IGR (impaired glucose regulation: I-IFG, I-IGT and IFG/IGT): 30% of them (n = 2,027) had nondiabetic fasting hyperglycemia (isolated IFG, having normal plasma glucose values 2-h post glucose load), 57% (n = 3,833) had 2-h nondiabetic hyperglycemia (isolated IGT, having normal FPG levels) and only 13% (n = 881) had mixed nondiabetic hyperglycemia (IFG + IGT).

It is therefore possible to affirm that glucose intolerance states, characterized by nondiabetic hyperglycemia (IGR), in the greatest percentage of cases, manifest as an isolated increase in plasma glucose levels: either fasting or post oral glucose load.

Table 17.3

DECODE study

Total number of cases with Impaired Glucose Regulation (IGR) diagnosed using both criteria: fasting and 2-h after 75 g oral glucose load. In this table, the IGR categories are presented as fasting (I-IFG), 2-h (I-IGT) or mixed (IFG/IGT) nondiabetic hyperglycemic states.

Phenotype	PG levels (mg/dl)	Percentage	No. of cases
I-IFG	FPG: 110–125 2-h : Normal	30%	2027
I-IGT	FPG: Normal 2-h : 140–199	57%	3833
IFG/IGT	FPG: 110–125 2-h : 140–199	13%	881
Total IGR cases	FPG: 110–125 or N 2-h : 140–199 or N	100%	6741

Table 17.4

DECODA Study

Total number of cases with Impaired Glucose Regulation (IGR) diagnosed using fasting and 2-h criteria.
IGR categories are presented as in Table 17.1. The data are similar to those reported in DECODE study (see Table 17.3)

Phenotype	PG levels (mg/dl)	Percentage	No. of cases
I-IFG	FPG: 110–125 2-h : Normal	20.2%	621
I-IGT	FPG: Normal 2-h : 140–199	64.4%	1984
IFG/IGT	FPG: 110–125 2-h : 140–199	15.4%	476
Total IGR cases	FPG: 110–125 or N 2-h : 140–199 or N	100%	3081

Table 17.5

Total number of cases with Impaired Glucose Regulation (IGR) diagnosed using fasting and 2-h criteria
in middle-aged Caucasian women [9]. IGR categories are presented as in Table 17.1.
The data are similar to those reported in DECODE and DECODA studies (see Tables 17.3 and 17.4).

Phenotype	PG levels (mg/dl)	Percentage	No. of cases
I-IFG	FPG: 110–125 2-h : Normal	25.8%	179
I-IGT	FPG: Normal 2-h : 140–199	54%	375
IFG/IGT	FPG: 110–125 2-h : 140–199	20.2%	140
Total IGR cases	FPG: 110–125 or N 2-h : 140–199 or N	100%	694

DECODA (*Diabetes Epidemiology: Collaborative analysis of Diagnostic criteria in Asia*) study [7] compared the prevalence of diabetes in Asian populations as diagnosed by fasting glucose values (ADA 1997 criteria) with prevalence as diagnosed by 2-h glucose values (WHO 1985 criteria).

From a total of 13,165 subjects, 3,081 were found with IGR (impaired glucose regulation). The great majority of cases (more than 84%) presented as isolated fasting or 2-h nondiabetic hyperglycemia, and only a minority (about 15%) was mixed (IFG+IGT) nondiabetic hyperglycemia (Table 17.4).

These data are similar to DECODE Study data (see Table 17.3).

Using both diagnostic criteria, 1,215 not previously known diabetics were diagnosed:

– 546 diabetic subjects (45%) had only 2-h plasma glucose (PG) diabetic levels; from these, 291 subjects (24%) had normal FPG and in the remaining 255 (21%) the FPG values were in the IFG range;

– 220 subjects (18%) had only fasting diabetic hyperglycemia: 101 (8%) with normal 2-h PG, 119 (10%) having 2-h PG values in the IGT range;

– 449 subjects (37%) had mixed diabetic hyperglycemia (fasting and 2-h PG in diabetes range).

An important part of the diabetic subjects had normal fasting (24%) or 2-h (8%) PG levels.

In Asian people, using only fasting criteria would miss (24% from diabetic and 60% from IGT subjects) an important percentage of people with glucose intolerance.

Similar data were reported in other small European studies [9, 10].

Comparing ADA and WHO diagnostic criteria in a group of 694 glucose intolerant middle-aged European women [9] it was found a poor concordance between the two criteria. Moreover, the two tests (fasting and 2-h PG) diagnosed two different groups with disturbed glucose metabolism. Using both diagnostic criteria (Table 17.5) the frequency of IGR categories was very similar to that reported in DECODE and DECODA studies.

PHENOTYPE DIFFERENCES BETWEEN IFG AND IGT

The DECODE study [5] investigated also the degree of concordance between a fasting plasma glucose value of 7.00 mmol/l (126 mg/dl) and a 2 h plasma glucose value of 11.1 mmol/l (200 mg/dl) by analyzing the ROC-curves of association between fasting and 2-h plasma glucose values.

It was found, in these European populations, that the cut-point value of fasting plasma glucose levels better associated to a 2-h plasma glucose of 11.1 mmol/l (200 mg/dl) was influenced by body weight and sex. In men, the optimal cut-point for this association was defined by a FPG level of 6.4 mmol/l (115 mg/dl) whereas in women this cut-point decreased to 5.8 mmol/l (104 mg/dl).

Only 54% of the people with a FPG > 5.5 mmol/l (99 mg/dl) will have glucose intolerance by the 2-h PG levels [5] whereas 100% of the people with a FPG ≥ 7.8 mmol/l (140 mg/dl) will have a 2-h PG > 11.1 mmol/l (200 mg/dl) [8]. In each age group (except in the fifth decade), women had significantly higher mean 2-h plasma glucose levels [6] than men, while the mean FPG levels were higher in men than in women between 30–69 years of age.

On the other hand, in obese people (BMI ≥ 30 kg/m^2), the "optimal FPG cut-point" was 6.6 mmol/l (119 mg/dl) and only 5.8 mmol/l (104 mg/dl) in normal weight people. FPG level associated to a 2-h PG diabetic level was greater in obese than in normoponderal people. The influence of body weight on this "optimal cut-point level" was similar in men and women.

During this data analysis it was also observed that a greater percentage of overweight individuals (BMI greater than 25 kg/m^2) and individuals below 65 years manifested more frequently isolated fasting hyperglycemia, while lean individuals had more frequently isolated post glucose load hyperglycemia.

Therefore, age and body weight were significantly associated with disagreement of ADA and WHO diagnostic criteria: in overweight middle-aged individuals diabetes was more frequently diagnosed by ADA (fasting only) criteria, whereas in lean, older individuals diabetes was more frequently diagnosed by WHO criteria.

The prevalence of isolated post load diabetic hyperglycemia (2-h plasma glucose ≥ 11.1 mmol/l and FPG < 7.0 mmol/l) or of isolated IGT increased more with age than isolated fasting diabetic hyperglycemia (FPG ≥ 7.0 mmol/l and 2-h plasma glucose < 11.1 mmol/l) or isolated IFG and this was more pronounced in women [6].

In the elderly population the increase in prevalence of diabetes and IGR resulted in principal from the increase in post load hyperglycemia than from the increase in fasting hyperglycemia.

In DECODE study, age and sex-specific prevalence of diabetes and IGR in 15,606 subjects with no prior history of diabetes and 1,325 subjects with known diabetes were analyzed [6].

It was observed that the mean values of plasma glucose increased with age but the increase was more pronounced in 2-h PG, especially after 50 years of age. The prevalence of IGT increased linearly with age whereas the prevalence of IFG tends to plateau in middle aged and decreases in older individuals.

IGT and diabetes defined by postload hyperglycemia was most prevalent in women, while the prevalence of IFG and diabetes defined by isolated fasting hyperglycemia was more prevalent in men.

Between diabetic individuals, those with fasting diabetic hyperglycemia and non diabetic 2-h post challenge PG values were most frequently middle aged, obese individuals, whereas aged, lean individuals had most frequently 2-h postchallenge diabetic hyperglycemia with non-diabetic FPG levels.

In a number of studies it was shown that ethnicity also may modulate the relationship between fasting and post glucose load glycemia.

A fasting PG level of 5.3–5.7 mmol/l (95–103 mg/dl) is the cut-point better associated to a 2-h PG level of 11.1 mmol/l (200 mg/dl) in Chinese, Brazilians and middle aged Caucasian women [11–13]. The corresponding FPG level is 6.4 mmol/l (115 mg/dl) in northern Europeans [14] and 7.1 mmol/l (128 mg/dl) respectively in South Asian people [15–16].

DIFFERENT PATHOPHYSIOLOGICAL MECHANISMS

It may be stated, as a general conclusion of these studies, that there is not a significant overlap between the categories of IFG and IGT. The majority of people with IGT do not have IFG, and the majority of people with IFG do not have IGT.

In DECODE and DECODA studies, in the category of Impaired Glucose Regulation (IGR) the majority of subjects (57%–64 %) had isolated IGT (isolated postprandial nondiabetic hyperglycemia with normal FPG levels), and only a minority (13%–15%) had mixed nondiabetic hyperglycemia (IFG+IGT). The percentage of subjects with nondiabetic fasting hyperglycemia (20%–30%) occupied an intermediary position (Table 17.3 and Table 17.4)

The fact that isolated increase of plasma glucose, either fasting or 2-h post oral glucose load, may co-exist with a different phenotype and that the people identified by one criteria may be different from people identified by the other, suggest that these abnormalities may represent different metabolic effects of a disturbed glucose homeostasis, possibly produced by distinct mechanisms that are differently influenced by age, sex and ethnicity.

Although a number of studies agree that IFG and IGT subjects are distinct phenotypes as reflecting the expression of different patho-physiological mechanisms, considerable controversy persists regarding the relative contribution of beta cell dysfunction and of insulin resistance in their pathogenesis.

Some studies show that IFG subjects are characterized by insulin resistance and hyperinsulinemia, whereas IGT subjects have reduced insulin response to glucose challenge [17–19]. Other studies report a reduced early insulin response in IFG and insulin resistance in IGT [20–22].

In the actual classification of Diabetes (WHO, 1999) IGT is a heterogeneous category including subjects with both normal and increased (in the IFG range) FPG levels.

If fasting and postprandial (2-h post oral glucose) hyperglycemia are due to different pathophysiological mechanisms, then it would be more appropriate to analyze separately IGT people with normal FPG levels (as isolated IGT or nondiabetic postprandial hyperglycemia) from IGT people with FPG levels in the IFG range (as mixed nondiabetic hyperglycemia or IFG+IGT)

and people with isolated IFG (nondiabetic fasting hyperglycemia, as having normal 2-h PG levels).

The majority of studies to date do not separate between these categories or when this is done the small number of individuals, in some of these categories, precludes statistical analysis.

On the other hand, there is a great variation between studies regarding the methods used to assess insulin action and secretion. In the majority of cases these are indirect estimates (surrogate indexes) of insulin action or secretion.

IFG is characterized by increased plasma glucose levels after an overnight fast.

It is generally accepted that the level of FPG is a function of endogenous glucose production [23], particularly the rate of gluconeogenesis.

Insulin modulates hepatic glucose production (HGP) by direct effect on liver enzyme activity and by indirect, peripheral, effect: reducing the free fatty acid supply to the liver [24] by inhibition of lipolysis, and by influencing the metabolic fate of intracellular glucose. A reduced insulin effect is accompanied by an increase in anaerobic glycolysis [25, 26] with an increased lactate production, a preferential gluconeogenetic substrate, leading to increased hepatic glucose production.

HGP is very sensitive to changes in portal insulin levels. In healthy subjects, a 5 µU/ml increase, above baseline, in portal insulin levels produced a 50% reduction in HGP, while a much greater increase in portal insulin levels was necessary to induce a similar decrease of HGP in diabetic subjects [27].

In newly diagnosed type 2 diabetes, isolated fasting hyperglycemia is more associated with insulin resistance, whereas in isolated postchallenge hyperglycemia the anomalies in insulin secretion are the most important determinant [28].

In a recent study [28], 181 newly diagnosed type 2 diabetic patients were separated in three subgroups according to fasting and 2-h (OGTT) PG levels: 54 subjects with fasting diabetic hyperglycemia (FDH), 65 subjects with 2-h diabetic hyperglycemia (2-h DH) and 62 subjects with combined (CH) diabetic hyperglycemia. The subjects with CH were more insulin resistant (HOMA) and had decreased insulin secretion as compared to FDH and 2-h DH subgroups of subjects.

Comparing FDH and 2-h DH subgroups it appeared that FDH was more associated with insulin resistance whereas in 2-h DH the anomalies in insulin secretion were the most important determinant.

In 297 subjects with IGR, in the same study population, the subgroup of subjects with isolated increase in FPG (IFG) was characterized more by insulin resistance, whereas in the subgroup of individuals with isolated increase in 2-h PG (isolated IGT) the defect in early insulin secretion was more important [29]. This again suggests that IFG and IGT are produced by different mechanisms and, during the natural history of diabetes the pathways leading to diabetes are different for IFG and IGT.

In 434 nondiabetic Pima Indians [30], a subgroup of 11 individuals with isolated IFG (I-IFG: normal 2-h PG levels) had similar impairments in insulin action as the subgroup (n = 98) of individuals with isolated IGT (I-IGT: normal FPG levels), but higher endogenous glucose production, whereas the subgroup with I-IGT had normal endogenous glucose production.

In the subgroup with I-IFG the increased basal endogenous glucose production was related to fasting plasma glucose levels.

There was a positive curvilinear relationship between basal endogenous glucose production and FPG levels even within the nondiabetic range.

The fasting plasma insulin levels were higher in I-IFG than in I-IGT group, but the difference was not significant after adjustment for age sex and percent body fat. It was presumed that high fasting insulin levels prevent an increase in basal endogenous glucose production (EGP) in I-IGT but not in I-IFG individuals.

While basal EGP was increased only in I-IFG and IFG/IGT and normal in I-IGT subgroup, reduced suppression of EGP under physiological levels of hyperinsulinemia (during hyperinsulinemic clamp) was observed in all three subgroups suggesting that hepatic insulin resistance is a common metabolic abnormality in all Pima Indians with IGR.

The reduced insulin action in all IGR subgroups was mainly due to a lower rate of nonoxidative glucose disposal, whereas oxidative glucose disposal was not different between IGR subgroup categories and normals.

Pima Indians with IGR had reduced first-phase insulin response to i.v. glucose. The reduction in first-phase insulin response was more pronounced in isolated IFG than in isolated IGT subgroup, and this was explained by the finding that first-phase insulin response was more closely related to the fasting than to the 2-h PG levels.

After adjustment for age and sex, individuals with I-IFG had significantly greater values for body weight, percent body fat and fat-free mass.

It was shown that liver fat accumulation (determined by proton spectroscopy) in obese nondiabetic women [31] with previous gestational diabetes as in normal weight or moderately overweight nondiabetic men [32] is associated more than any measure of body composition with features of insulin resistance syndrome.

Interindividual variation in hepatic insulin sensitivity may be related to variation in liver fat content. In a group of healthy nondiabetic men with high liver fat content [32] suppression of endogenous glucose production and of free fatty acids was significantly reduced as compared to a group of men with low liver fat content. The two groups had comparable values for age, BMI, waist to hip ratio, intraabdominal, subcutaneous and total fat.

In a prospective study of 216 Japanese-American nondiabetic men [33] followed for maximum 11 years, during age-related changes in fasting plasma glucose, fasting glucose was strongly associated with intraabdominal fat over time.

Therefore, it is possible to speculate that individuals with IFG characterized by features of insulin resistance syndrome may have increased hepatic insulin resistance. The combination of peripheral insulin resistance (reduced suppression of lipolysis) and hepatic insulin resistance could result in increased basal hepatic glucose production in IFG subjects.

In a recent study [34], insulin secretion and sensitivity were examined in 664 nondiabetic subjects: 13.6% (90 subjects) had isolated IFG (IFG with normal 2-h PG), 15.2% (101 subjects) had isolated IGT (IGT with normal FPG levels) and 16% (106 subjects) had IGT+IFG.

IFG was more prevalent in women and IGT was more prevalent in men.

FFA levels were significantly higher in IGT, as compared to IFG subjects. Isolated IFG and

IFG+IGT presented significantly higher levels of insulin resistance (HOMA) than isolated IGT groups.

The early insulin response, during OGTT, was reduced in all categories of glucose intolerance as compared to normal subjects. It was not a significant difference between IFG and IGT in early insulin response.

However, in factorial analysis, the "insulin resistance factor" was dominant in IFG and explained 28.4% of total variance whereas the "insulin secretion factor" was dominant and explained 31.1% of the variation in IGT.

The differences in insulin response were more pronounced during the second phase of insulin secretion.

Similar to normal subjects, the subjects with IFG reached the peak insulin level (during OGTT) after 60 minutes, whereas in the group of IGT subjects, the peak insulin level was attained after 90 minutes. When the incremental insulin levels during second phase insulin response were estimated taking into account the corresponding glucose values, a significant deficit for the second phase of insulin secretion in IGT, as compared to IFG subjects, was found. As a conclusion of this study, subjects with IGT presented a more severe deficit in early and late-phase insulin response as compared to IFG subjects.

In subjects with IGT, basal hepatic glucose output did not differ from normal subjects, but reduced suppression of basal endogenous glucose production after glucose ingestion is responsible for the increased rate of total systemic glucose appearance [35].

Hepatic insulin sensitivity was found to be normal during euglycemic clamp, but peripheral insulin sensitivity was markedly diminished [36] in IGT subjects. First-phase insulin secretion (FPIS) was significantly diminished and failure to suppress basal hepatic glucose output during postprandial state appeared to be due to decreased FPIS [36].

In IGT subjects, reduced early insulin release and reduced suppression of endogenous glucagon [35] were found to be significantly correlated to (reduced suppression of) endogenous glucose output during OGTT.

Tissue glucose uptake and hepatic glucose production have been measured during hyperglycemic clamp studies in normal human

subjects. Abolition of the FPIS by somatostatin with second phase insulin secretion replacement [37] was not accompanied by changes in peripheral glucose utilization whereas hepatic glucose production was dramatically increased, in spite of increased insulin and glucose levels. Replacement of both early and second phases of the insulin response leads to restoration of normal hepatic glucose production.

As compared to individuals with normal glucose tolerance, plasma glucose removal rates were similar [35] in individuals with IGT. However, these "normal rates" of glucose removal are inappropriate (high) when the concomitant increased plasma glucose and insulin levels are considered. This may express a state of peripheral insulin (and glucose) resistance [35].

Hyperglycemia observed post oral glucose challenge in IGT is the consequence of insufficient suppression of normal basal hepatic glucose production and of glucagon secretion in the postprandial state associated to an insufficient removal of the glucose load.

PROGRESSION TO DIABETES

In the Hoorn Study [38], a European population-based cohort of 1,342 men and women without known diabetes was followed for an average period of 6.4 years. A similar cumulative incidence of diabetes, either starting from isolated IFG (33%) or isolated IGT (34%), was found at the end of follow-up. The cumulative incidence of diabetes was double (64.5%) for combined IFG and IGT.

In the multiethnic population of Mauritius [39], from 3,229 nondiabetic subjects at baseline, 297 developed diabetes during a five-year mean follow-up. IGT was most frequent than IFG, but the percentage of people developing diabetes from IFG (22% from 148 subjects) or IGT (21% from 489 subjects) was almost equal and it was greater (38% from 118 subjects) when IFG and IGT were combined.

Other longitudinal studies had reported an excess cumulative incidence of diabetes from IGT than from IFG at baseline.

In an Italian study [40], an OGTT was done at baseline in a working population of 1,245 individuals aged 40–59 years and progression to diabetes was evaluated (on the basis of fasting plasma glucose only) 11.5 years later.

In the group of 50 subjects with isolated IGT at baseline 32.5% progressed to diabetes whereas from the group with isolated IFG (n = 25) only 9.1% progressed to diabetes till the end of the follow-up.

Similar data were reported in middle-aged [41] French men and in high-risk Chinese [42] subjects.

Different results were reported in other ethnic groups. In Hispanics and Pima Indians it was found that IFG was associated with a greater incidence of diabetes during longitudinal follow-up.

The incidence of diabetes during a longitudinal follow-up for up to 14 years [43] was compared in Hispanics (H) and Non Hispanic Whites (NHW) in the San Luis Valley Diabetes Study. The excess incidence of diabetes in H *versus* NHW occurred a decade earlier in males.

Starting from normal glucose tolerance (NGT) at baseline the annual incidence of diabetes was 5.1 *per* 1000, 30.3 *per* 1000 in those with IGT and 41.1 *per* 1000 in those with IFG at baseline.

There was an excess incidence of diabetes in H *versus* NHW with IFG (RR=1.7), but not in those with IGT (RR = 1.0).

These data suggest different pathways from NGT to diabetes in H and NHW.

In a group of 5,023 nondiabetic Pima Indians 31% of 93 subjects with isolated IFG, 20% of 537 subjects with isolated IGT and 41% of 126 subjects with combined IFG and IGT progressed to diabetes during a five-year follow-up [44].

The progression from normal glucose tolerance (NGT) and from IFG or IGT to diabetes was followed in the Baltimore Longitudinal Study of Aging [45, 46].

The ten-year cumulative incidence of progression from NGT to abnormal 2-h post glucose challenge plasma glucose levels (2-h PG) as defined by ADA 1997 and WHO 1999 criteria (≥ 7.8 mmol/l or 140 mg/dl) was four times greater (47.5%) than that of progression (13.5%) to abnormal fasting plasma glucose (FPG) levels (≥ 6.1 mmol/l or 110 mg/dl).

The ten-year cumulative incidence of progression from IFG or IGT (as defined by ADA 1997 and WHO 1999 criteria) at baseline to diabetes was 8.3% by increase (≥ 7.0 mmol/l or

126 mg/dl) in FPG only as compared to 37.4% for progression by increase in 2-h PG (≥ 11.1 mmol/l or 200 mg/dl) only.

The rate of progression was influenced by age (older subjects progressed more rapidly to abnormal 2-h PG), sex (men progressed faster than women), adiposity (subjects with obesity progressed more rapidly than lean subjects).

These data suggest than progression by increase in 2-h PG levels contributes more to diabetes incidence than progression by increase in FPG levels.

During the progression to diabetes two main phenotypes were observed:

– 2-h progressors. A more frequent phenotype characterized by development of IGT from NGT and progression to diabetes by increase in 2-h PG levels. In only a few cases this progression was accompanied by abnormal or diabetic FPG levels;

– Fasting progressors. A rarer phenotype consisting in the development of IFG from NGT and predominant progression to diabetes by increase in FPG levels; the increase in FPG levels was subsequently associated with IGT or diabetic 2-h PG levels.

These distinct phenotypes appear to be preserved during the natural history of diabetes; 42% NGT subjects, in whom glucose tolerance deteriorated during follow-up by developing abnormal FPG, did not associate abnormal 2-h PG and *vice-versa*.

If categories of FPG and 2-h PG are defined to include similar percentages of their respective distribution, their predictive value for diabetes is equivalent [46]. By using a lower level for diagnostic threshold of FPG the same sensitivity for predicting subsequent diabetes as for IGT can be obtained for IFG. For example in Pima Indians a FPG ≥ 5.7 mmol/l (≥ 103 mg/dl) is corresponding to a 2-h PG of ≥ 7.8 mmol/l (≥ 140 mg/dl), providing a similar prevalence of IGT and IFG and having the same sensitivity and specificity in predicting diabetes [47].

This level may differ (as stated before) in different ethnic groups.

In a subsidiary analysis of data from Baltimore Longitudinal Aging Study [46], the diagnostic thresholds for abnormal or diabetic FPG were set to lower levels (5.55 mmol/l or 100 mg/dl for the upper limit of "normal" and 6.1 mmol/l or

110 mg/dl for "diabetes") to obtain equal baseline prevalence for abnormal or diabetic 2-h PG and for abnormal or diabetic FPG.

Applying these new diagnostic thresholds the longitudinal probability of developing abnormal FPG or abnormal 2-h PG became roughly equal but was influenced in the same way by age, sex and adiposity.

This study [46] confirmed that fasting and postchallenge hyperglycemia represent distinct phenotypes and distinct pathways leading to diabetes.

Another important conclusion is that differences in the rate of progression to diabetes are influenced also by the (arbitrary) plasma glucose thresholds of diagnostic criteria.

IFG, IGT, CARDIOVASCULAR AND MORTALITY RISK

A metaregression analysis of available published data till 1996 [48] reviewed 20 prospective studies on the association between blood glucose levels and the cardiovascular risk.

A curvilinear relationship between cardiovascular events and blood glucose levels (fasting and post glucose challenge) with increasing risk even below the diabetic range of blood glucose levels was demonstrated. A relative risk of 1.33 was associated to a fasting plasma glucose level of 6.1 mmol/l (110 mg/dl) whereas a relative risk of 1.58 was associated with a 2-h plasma glucose level of 7.8 mmol/l (140 mg/dl).

The predictive value of 2-h glucose *versus* fasting glucose for an increased risk of coronary heart disease events (death or nonfatal myocardial infarction) was analyzed on five Finnish DECODE Study cohorts [49] including 6,766 subjects aged 30–89 years followed-up for 7–10 years. Standard 2-h 75 g OGTT was administred to all subjects according to WHO 1985.

The subjects with isolated 2-h postchallenge hyperglycemia (IGT or diabetes) were older than those with isolated fasting hyperglycemia (IFG or diabetes).

The subjects with IGT but normal fasting glucose had higher cholesterol levels than subjects with isolated IFG.

Survival in individuals with IFG was close to that in normoglycemic subjects and better than in individuals with IGT or diabetes.

In subjects without previous myocardial infarction, 2-h postchallenge glucose level was a stronger predictor of the risk for coronary heart disease events than fasting glucose [49].

In the DECODE study [50, 51] analysis of data from 13 prospective studies showed that the hazard ratio for all cause mortality increased with both fasting and 2-h plasma glucose levels. The association was stronger with 2-h than with fasting plasma glucose levels. The hazard ratio for all-cause mortality increased much more with increasing 2-h than with increasing fasting blood glucose levels. In the range of 2-h plasma glucose levels under 7.8 mmol/l (140 mg/dl) the hazard ratio increased with increasing fasting plasma glucose levels, but in the range of 2-h plasma glucose levels between 7.8–11.0 mmol/l (140–198 mg/dl) the hazard ratio for all-cause mortality was independent of fasting glucose levels.

The largest absolute number of excess deaths was observed in subjects with IGT, especially in those whose fasting glucose was normal.

After excluding the cases with known diabetes and after adjustment for the other cardiovascular risk factors, 44% of cases of cardiovascular death were associated with isolated IGT while no association was found with isolated IFG [51].

When analysis of the association between blood glucose levels and all-cause mortality was adjusted for other cardiovascular risk factors (total cholesterol, BMI, blood pressure and smoking) it was no more a relationship with fasting blood glucose levels below 7.0 mmol/l (126 mg/dl), but the association with 2-h blood glucose levels in the domain of IGT persisted.

Thus, the DECODE data found, in European population, a significant relationship between total mortality and 2-h blood glucose levels in the range of IGT but not with fasting blood glucose levels in the range of IFG. This relationship was independent of other cardiovascular risk factors. It appeared that 2-h plasma glucose level is a better predictor of death from all causes and from cardiovascular disease than FPG.

These data are concordant with data reported from other studies.

In the Funagata Diabetes Study [52, 53] 65% of the newly diagnosed diabetes had fasting glucose < 7.0 mmol/l (126 mg/dl) and 76% of the subjects with IGT had normal fasting glucose levels. In this study IGT was the most prevalent category of glucose intolerance. The subjects with IGT had increased risk for cardiovascular disease as high as subjects with diabetes, whereas no significant association was found between IFG and the risk for cardiovascular events.

In a group of 119 newly discovered diabetic patients in the RIAD Study [54] a significant increase in carotid intima-media thickness (IMT) was observed only in the subgroups with 2-h postchallenge hyperglycemia combined with either normal or impaired fasting glucose. By regression analysis, 2-h PG but not FPG was a significant determinant of IMT.

In the RIAD Study IMT of the common carotid artery was examined also in nondiabetic subjects [55] with isolated fasting hyperglycemia (IFH, n = 67), isolated postchallenge hyperglycemia (IPH, n = 82) and combined hyperglycemia (CH, n = 88). IMT was significantly increased in IPH group as compared to IFH and normoglycemic groups. IMT in IFH group was similar to IMT in normals.

Although hyperglycemia is a marker for premature death, the data presented support the conclusion that increased 2-h PG levels are more strongly associated with atherosclerosis, cardiovascular and total mortality than increased FPG levels.

Recently, a workshop convened by the International Diabetes Federation (IDF) [56] addressed these issues. The IFG/IGT consensus statement of IDF expert committee represents an important document for interpretation and understanding of the latest information of risk associated to IFG and IGT.

CONCLUSION

According to actual diagnostic thresholds (ADA 1997, WHO 1999), IGT is significantly more prevalent than IFG.

IFG and IGT may represent the expression of distinct pathophysiological mechanisms: IFG is associated with impaired suppression of endogenous glucose production in the fasting state, while IGT is associated with impaired suppression of endogenous glucose production after oral glucose challenge.

They express a different pattern of insulin secretion and sensitivity. IFG and IGT represent different phenotypic expressions and different pathways leading to diabetes that seems to be preserved during the course of its natural history.

The longitudinal probability to develop abnormal 2-h PG is significantly greater than to develop abnormal FPG. Progression to IGR and diabetes by increase in 2-h PG levels is the most frequent phenotype, but the differences in the rate of progression to diabetes are also influenced by the plasma glucose thresholds of diagnostic criteria.

It appears that IGT confer a greater risk for cardiovascular disease and mortality than IFG.

Taking into account that mechanisms leading to fasting and postchallenge (postprandial) hyperglycemia are different and the distinctive patterns of glucose intolerance categories may reflect the association in a different proportion of these mechanisms, a revision of the classification of hyperglycemia may be appropriate. In this classification, isolated fasting hyperglycemia should be separated from isolated postchallenge (postprandial) hyperglycemia.

REFERENCES

1. The Expert Committee on Diagnosis and Classification of Diabetes Mellitus. Report of the Expert Committee on the Diagnosis and Classification of Diabetes Mellitus. *Diabetes Care,* **20:** 1183–1197, 1997.
2. World Health Organization: Definition, Diagnosis and Classification of Diabetes Mellitus and its Complications. Report of a WHO Consultation. Part 1. Diagnosis and Classification of Diabetes Mellitus. Geneva, World Health Organization, 1999.
3. Drzewoski J, Czupryniak L: Concordance between fasting and 2–h post-glucose challenge criteria for the diagnosis of diabetes mellitus and glucose intolerance in high-risk individuals. *Diabetic Med,* **18:** 29–31, 2001.
4. DECODE Study Group on behalf of the European Diabetes Epidemiology Study Group: Will new diagnostic criteria for diabetes mellitus change phenotype of patients with diabetes? Reanalysis of European epidemiological data. *BMJ,* **317:** 371–375, 1998.

5. The DECODE Study group on behalf of the European Diabetes Epidemiology Group: Is fasting glucose sufficient to define diabetes? Epidemiological data from 20 European studies. *Diabetologia* , **42:** 647–654, 1999.

6. The DECODE Study group: Age and Sex-Specific Prevalences of Diabetes and Impaired Glucose Regulation in 13 European Cohorts. *Diabetes Care* , **26:** 61–69, 2003.

7. Qiao Q, Nakagami T, Tuomilehto J, Borch-Jonsen K, Balkau B, Iwamoto Y, Tajima N. The DECODA Study Group on Behalf of International Diabetes Epidemiology Group. Comparison of fasting and 2-h glucose criteria for diabetes in different Asian cohorts. *Diabetol ogia*, **43:** 1470–1475, 2000.

8. Shaw JE, Mc Carty D, Zimmet PZ, de Courten M. Type 2 Diabetes Worldwide According to the New Classification and Criteria. *Diabetes Care,* **23, Suppl 2:** B5–B10, 2000.

9. Larsson H, Berglund G, Lindgarde F, Ahren B. Comparison of ADA and WHO criteria for diagnosis of diabetes and glucose intolerance. *Diabetol ogia*, **41:** 1124–1125, 1998.

10. Schianca GPC, Rossi A, Sainaghi PP, Maduli E, Bartoli E. The Significance of Impaired Fasting Glucose Versus Impaired Glucose Tolerance. *Di abetes Care* , **25:** 1333–1337, 2003.

11. Larsson H, Ahren B, Lindgarde F, Berglund G. Fasting blood glucose in determining the prevalence of diabetes in a large homogenous population of Caucasian middle-aged women. *J Intern Med* , **237:** 537–541, 1995.

12. Borthiery AL, Malerbi DA, Franco LJ. The ROC curve in the evaluation of fasting capillary blood glucose as a screening test for diabetes and IGT. *Diabetes Care* , **17:** 1269–1272, 1994.

13. Ko GTC, Chan JCN, Lau E. Fasting plasma glucose as a screening test for diabetes and its relationship with cardiovascular risk factors in Hong Kong Chinese. *Diabetes Care,* **20:** 170–172, 1997.

14. Clements JP, French LR, Boen JR. A reassessment of fasting plasma glucose concentrations in population screening for diabetes mellitus in a community of northern European ancestry: The Wadena City Health Study. *Acta Diabetol* , **31:** 187–192, 1994.

15. Ramachandan A, Snehalatha C, Vijay V. Fasting plasma glucose in the diagnosis of diabetes mellitus: A study from Southern India. *Diabetic Med,* **10:** 811–813, 1993.

16. Cappuccio FP, Cook DG, Atkinson RW, Strazzulo P. Prevalence, detection and management of cardiovascular risk factors in different ethnic groups in south London. *Heart,* **78:** 555–563, 1997.

17. Tripathy D, Carlsson M, Almgren P, Isomaa B, Taskinen MR, Tuomi T, Groop LC. Insulin secretion and insulin sensitivity in relation to glucose tolerance: lessons from the Botnia Study. *Diabetes,* **49:** 975–980, 2000.

18. Guerrero-Romero F, Rodriguez-Moran M: Impaired glucose tolerance is a more advanced stage of alteration in the glucose metabolism than impaired fasting glucose. *J Diabetes Complications,* **15:** 34–37, 2001.

19. Weyer C, Bogardus C, Mott DM, Pratley RE: The natural history of insulin secretory dysfunction and insulin resistance in the pathogenesis of type 2 diabetes mellitus. *J Clin Invest,* **104:** 787–794, 1999.

20. Weyer C, Bogardus C, Pratley RE: Metabolic characteristics of individuals with impaired fasting glucose and/or impaired glucose tolerance. *Diabetes,* **48:** 2197–2203, 1999.

21. Davies MJ, Raymond NT, Day JL, Hales CN, Burden AC. Impaired glucose tolerance and fasting hyperglycemia have different characteristics. *Di abet Med,* **17:** 433–440, 2000.

22. Conget I, Fernandez Real JM, Costa A, Casamitjana R, Ricart W: Insulin secretion and insulin sensitivity in relation to glucose tolerance in a group of subjects at high risk for type 2 diabetes mellitus. *Med Clin,* **116:** 491–492, 2001.

23. DeFronzo RA, Bonadonna RC, Ferrannini E. Pathogenesis of NIDDM: a balanced overview. *Diab etes Care,* **15:** 358–368, 1992.

24. Bergman RN. Non-esterified fatty acids and the liver: why is insulin secreted into the portal vein? *Diabetol ogia,* **43:** 946–952, 2000.

25. Del Prato S, Gulli G, Bonadonna RC. Effect of hyperglycemia on glucose metabolism: regulatory role of basal plasma insulin levels. *Diabetes,* **41 (Suppl 1):** 188A (Abstract), 1992.

26. Del Prato S, Marchetti P, Bonadonna RC. Phasic Insulin Release and Metabolic Regulation in Type 2 Diabetes. *Diabetes,* **51 (Suppl 1):** S109-S116, 2002.

27. Groop LC, Bonadonna RC, Del Prato S, Ratheiser K, Zyck K, Ferrannini E, DeFronzo RA. Glucose and free-fatty acid metabolism in non-insulin dependent diabetes: evidence for multiple insulin resistance sites. *J Clin Invest,* **84:** 205–213, 1989.

28. Hanefeld M, Temelkova-Kurktschiev T, Henkel E, Fuecker K, Julius U, Koehler C. Newly Diagnosed Type 2 Diabetes with Isolated Fasting Hyperglycemia and Isolated Post-challenge Hyperglycemia is Different in Insulin Sensitivity and Secretion. *Diabetes,* **51 (Suppl.2):** A227 (Abstract), 2002.

29. Koehler C, Henkel E, Temelkova-Kurktschiev T, Fuecker K, Hanefeld M. Subjects with Isolated Impaired Fasting Glucose and Isolated Impaired Glucose Tolerance Exhibit Different Patterns of Insulin Secretion and Insulin Sensitivity. *Diabetes*, **51, Suppl 2:** A 939 (abstract), 2002.

30. Weyer C, Bogardus C, Pratley RE. Metabolic Characteristics of Individuals with Impaired Fasting Glucose and/or Impaired Glucose Tolerance. *Diabetes*, **48:** 2197–2203, 1999.

31. Tiikkainen M, Tamminen H, Hakkinen AM, Bergholm R, Vehrkavaara S, Halavaara J, Teramo K, Rissanen A, Yki-Jarvinen H: Liver-fat accumulation and insulin resistance in obese women with previous gestational diabetes. *Obes Res*, **10:** 859–869, 2002.

32. Seppala-Lindroos A, Vehkavaara S, Hakkinen AM, Goto T, Westerbacka J, Sovijarvi A, Halavaara J, Yki-Jarvinen H. Fat accumulation in the liver is associated with defects in insulin suppression of glucose production and serum free fatty acids independent of obesity in normal men. *J Clin Endocrinol Metab*, **87:** 3019–3022, 2002.

33. Tsai EC, Shofer JB, Boyko EJ, McNeely J, Leonetti DL, Fujimoto WY. Contrasting Influences of Fasting Glucose on Intra and Subcutaneous Abdominal Fat Change in Japanese-American Men. *Diabetes*, **51, Suppl 2:** A122 (abstract), 2002.

34. Hanefeld M, Koehler C, Fuecker K, Henkel E, Schaper F, Temelkova-Kurktschiev T. Insulin Secretion and Insulin Sensitivity Pattern is Different in Isolated Impaired Glucose Tolerance and Impaired Fasting Glucose: The Risk Factor in Impaired Glucose Tolerance for Atherosclerosis and Diabetes Study. *Diabetes Care*, **26:** 868–874, 2003.

35. Mitrakou A, Kelly D, Mokan M, Veneman T, Pangburn T, Reilly J, Gerich J. Role of reduced suppression of glucose production and diminished early insulin release in impaired glucose tolerance. *N Engl J Med*, **326:** 22–29, 1992.

36. Berrish TS, Hetherington CS, Alberti KGMM, Walker M. Peripheral and hepatic insulin sensitivity in subjects with impaired glucose tolerance. *Diabetologia*, **38:** 699–704, 1995.

37. Luzi L, DeFronzo RA. Effects of loss of first–phase insulin secretion on hepatic glucose production and tissue glucose disposal in humans. *Am J Physiol*, **257:** E241–E246, 1989.

38. de Vegt F, Dekker JM, Jager A, Hienkens E, Kostense PJ, Stehouwer CDA, Nijpels G, Bouter LM, Heine RJ. Relation of Impaired Fasting and Postload Glucose with Incident Type 2 Diabetes in a Dutch Population. The Hoorn Study. *JAMA*, **285:** 2109–2113, 2001.

39. Shaw JE, Zimmet PZ, de Courten M, Dowse GK, Chitson P, Gareeboo H, Hemraj F, Fareed D, Tuomilehto J, Alberti KGMM. Impaired Fasting Glucose or Impaired Glucose Tolerance. What best predicts future diabetes in Mauritius? *Diabetes Care*, **22:** 399–402, 1999.

40. Vaccaro O, Iovino V, Ruffa G, Rivellese AA, Imperatore G, Riccardi G. Risk of Diabetes in the New Diagnostic Category of Impaired Fasting Glucose. *Diabetes Care*, **22:** 1490–1493.

41. Charles MA, Fontbonne A, Thibult N, Warnet J, Rosselin GE, Eschwege E. Risk factors for NIDDM in white population. *Diabetes*, **40:** 796–799, 1991.

42. Chou P, Li CL, Wu GS, Tsai ST. Progression to Type 2 Diabetes among high-risk groups in Kin-Chen, Kinmen. Exploring the natural history of type 2 diabetes. *Diabetes Care*, **22:** 369–370, 1999.

43. Dabelea D, Scarbro S, Baron AE, Marshall JA, Baxter J, Hamman RF. No Excess Incidence of Type 2 Diabetes among Hispanics with Impaired Glucose tolerance *versus* Non-Hispanic Whites in the San Luis Valley Diabetes Study. *Diabetes*, **51, Suppl 2:** A 902 (abstract), 2002.

44. Gabir MM, Hanson RL, Dabelea D, Imperatore G, Roumain J, Bennett PH, Knowler WC. Plasma Glucose and Prediction of Macrovascular Disease and Mortality. Evaluation of 1997 American Diabetes Association and 1999 World Health Organization criteria for diagnosis of diabetes. *Diabetes Care*, **23:** 1113–1118, 2000.

45. Blake DR, Meigs JB, Muller DC, Nathan DM, Andres R. Cardiovascular Disease (CVD) Risk Profile among Subjects Progressing from Normal to Abnormal Glucose Homeostasis in the Baltimore Longitudinal Study of Aging (BLSA). *Diabetes*, **51, Suppl 2:** A889 (Abstract), 2002.

46. Meigs JB, Muller DC, Nathan DM, Blake DR, Andres R. The Natural History of Progression from Normal Glucose Tolerance to Type 2 Diabetes in the Baltimore Longitudinal Study of Aging. *Diabetes*, **52:** 1475–1484, 2003.

47. Gabir MM, Hanson RL, Dabelea D, Imperatore G, Roumain J, Bennett PH, Knowler WC. The 1997 American Diabetes Association and 1999 World Health Organization Criteria for Hyperglycemia in the Diagnosis and Prediction of Diabetes. *Diabetes Care*, **23:** 1108–1112, 2000.

48. Coutinho M, Gerstein HC, Wang Y, Yusuf S. The relationship between glucose and incident cardiovascular events. A metaregression analysis of published data from 20 studies of 95783

individuals followed for 12.4 years. *Diabetes Care,* **22:** 233–240, 1999.

49. Qiao Q, Pyörälä K, Pyörälä M, Nissinen A, Lindröm J, Tilvis R, Tuomilehto J. Two-hour glucose is better risk predictor for incident coronary heart disease and cardiovascular mortality than fasting glucose. *European Heart Journal,* **23:** 1267–1275, 2002.

50. The DECODE Study Group: Glucose tolerance and mortality: comparison of WHO and American Diabetes Association diagnostic criteria. *Lancet,* **354:** 617–621, 1999.

51. DECODE Study group. Glucose tolerance and cardiovascular mortality: comparison of fasting and 2-hour diagnostic criteria. *Arch Intern Med,* **161:** 397–405, 2001.

52. Sekikawa A, Tominaga M, Takahashi K, Eguchi H, Igarashi M, Ohnuma H, Sugiyama K, Manaka H, Sasaki H, Fukuyama H, Miyazawa K. Prevalence of diabetes and impaired glucose tolerance in Funagata Area, Japan. *Diabetes Care,* **16:** 570–574, 1993.

53. Tominaga M, Eguchi H, Manaka H, Igarashi K, Kato T, Sekikawa A. Impaired Glucose Tolerance Is a Risk Factor for Cardiovascular Disease, but Not Impaired Fasting Glucose. *Diabetes Care,* **22:** 920–924, 1999.

54. Hanefeld M, Koehler C, Henkel E, Fuecker K, Schaper F, Temelkova-Kurktschiev T. Post-challenge hyperglycemia relates more strongly than fasting hyperglycemia with carotid intima-media thickness: the RIAD Study. *Diabetic Med,* **17:** 835–840, 2000.

55. Temelkova-Kurkstchiev T, Henkel E, Schaper F, Koehler C, Siegert G, Hanefeld M: Prevalence and atherosclerosis risk in different types of non-diabetic hyperglycemia. Is mild hyperglycemia an underestimated evil? *Exp Clin Endocrinol Diabetes,* **108:** 93–99, 2000.

56. Unwin N, Shaw J, Zimmet P, Alberti KGMM: Impaired glucose tolerance and impaired fasting glycemia: the current status on definition and intervention. *Diabetic Med,* **19:** 708–723, 2002.

18

ENDOTHELIAL DYSFUNCTION, ATHEROSCLEROSIS AND ARTERIOSCLEROSIS IN DIABETIC PATIENTS WITH AND WITHOUT RENAL INVOLVEMENT

David GOLDSMITH, Andy SMITH, Karim BAKRI, Rashed BAKRI, Adrian COVIC

Macro- and microvascular diseases are the main causes of mortality in patients with type I and type II diabetes mellitus. There is now a worldwide epidemic of type II diabetes in both industrialised and poor nations, with predictable dire consequences. As well as taking action to stem the tide of growing obesity and sloth in society, now clearly seen even in childhood, there is an equally urgent need to look for reliable surrogates for eventual cardiovascular disease (or markers of susceptibility) so that targeted action can be taken to achieve prevention.

Endothelial function plays a key role in the pathogenesis of vascular disease in diabetic subjects. We shall explore the role of endothelial control on vascular smooth muscle tonus and how loss of endothelial functional integrity may arise from altered signal transduction, impaired release or increased destruction of endothelium-derived relaxing factors (EDRF) or decreased vascular muscle cell responsiveness to EDRF.

Vascular stiffness (measured directly as pulse wave velocity or, indirectly, as widened pulse pressure) has now been shown to be highly relevant for isolated systolic hypertension, most often seen in elderly subjects, but also seen in diabetics, especially with renal involvement (proteinuria to end-stage renal failure). Patients with stiffer vessels have more left ventricular hypertrophy and a poorer prognosis. The increase in vessel stiffening comes about in diabetic (and renal) patients through an increase of atherosclerosis and also, arteriosclerosis (medial thickening and calcification). Measures to reduce atherosclerosis and arteriosclerosis can now be taken in experimental and clinical settings and it is to be earnestly hoped that these can be translated into prevention and reversal of diabetic vasculopathy and the improved survival of diabetic subjects.

INTRODUCTION

The prevalence of diabetes mellitus has now attained epidemic proportions on a global scale. The explosion in type 2 diabetes (which now is the major issue) started in the post World War II years, initially in the industrialised countries, but now, in the early part of the 21st century, it is a worldwide phenomenon. Environmental stresses of abundant carbohydrate-rich food and an increasingly sedentary lifestyle, applied to a vulnerable genotype have produced increasing obesity, hypertension, gout, dyslipidaemia and diabetes. Shockingly, it is now possible to see type 2 diabetes in adolescents due to obesity and inactivity [1], not just in those with severe genetic predispositions, such as Indian-Asians, but in Caucasians too. Such children have clear-cut markers of atherosclerosis in early adolescence which augur very badly for the population [2].

It is now estimated that worldwide number of diabetics is approaching 200,000,000 and that this figure will increase by 50% in the next 25 years. This will impose a truly frightening burden on stretched health care systems and economies all around the world. Up to 25% of the population of the United Kingdom (approximately 55,000,000) is potentially at risk from these malign influences. For example, the leading cause of end-stage renal failure in most parts of the world is (type 2) diabetic nephropathy [3].

About 25% of type I diabetics will die from cardiovascular causes, but 75% of type 2 diabetics will succumb. There is a complex inter-relationship between atherosclerosis and diabetes, with overlap in hypertension, dyslipidaemia, thrombogenicity, inflammation and hyperuricaemia. If we start from the concept of insulin resistance conferring fundamental alterations to vascular and endothelial physiology, then we can see the attraction of the "common soil" hypothesis – namely that vascular risks clustering, type 2 diabetes and cardiovascular disease are multiple facets of the same underlying metabolic derangements [4].

One could convincingly argue that the development of type 2 diabetes in most cases is an example of failed primary prevention. However, such "prevention" will of necessity be a long-term relationship between patient and health care providers and involve education, application and motivation on both sides. There is presently depressingly little evidence of tangible progress, as obesity rates soar, dietary habits deteriorate and new diabetic patients arrive with increasing frequency [5].

In the likely absence of strong directed action to break the cycle of predispositions that conclude to diabetes, we may need to use surrogate markers of those most at risk, and target resources at this most vulnerable cohort. If there are reliable surrogate markers of increased vascular risk, these could be used to screen diabetic (and pre-diabetic) populations. However, despite of much effort, no genetic or vascular physiological parameter is currently suitable for this role.

In this chapter, we shall first discuss endothelial dysfunction, which plays a key role in the pathogenesis of diabetic vascular disease. Then, we shall discuss mechanisms, which underlie the acceleration of atherosclerosis in diabetes and finally, the important role played by increased vascular stiffening in the large arteries of diabetic patients. Endothelial dysfunction and increased large artery stiffness, once they can be robustly assessed without complex methods, hold promise as screening tools in the diabetic population to detect those at greatest risk of adverse cardiovascular outcomes.

ENDOTHELIAL DYSFUNCTION IN DIABETES

The endothelial cell layer is an "organ" of the most fundamental importance. Endothelial cell function can be assessed in different ways. For example, measurements (local or systemic spillover) of endothelial cell derived products can be made (endothelial secretory function – *e.g.*, thrombomodulin, von Willebrand factor, selectins, plasminogen activator inhibitor-1, homocysteine, endothelin, vascular endothelial growth factor). The vasoactive effects of endothelial stimuli can be quantified (endothelial vasomotor function) in several different ways. This latter aspect of endothelial reactivity will be the focus for this section. Endothelial vasomotor dysfunction is also recognised in old age, hypercholesterolaemia, smoking and renal failure.

Endothelial cells actively regulate basal vascular tone and vascular reactivity, in physiological and pathological settings. This is effected by endothelial cell layer response to mechanical forces and, also, to neuro-humoral mediators. The endothelial cell layer is capable of tonic and inducible release of several vaso-relaxing and vaso-constricting factors. Endothelium-derived vasorelaxing factors (EDRF) include nitric oxide (NO), prostacyclin and endothelium-derived hyperpolarising factor (see [6] for a detailed review). In health, the balance of release favours vasodilatation of muscular arteries and arterioles. Disturbance of endothelial vasomotor function consequently leads to vasoconstriction (in a relative or absolute sense).

In man, there are several competitive approaches to the measurement of endothelial vasomotor function. The differences in techniques employed and sometimes, the use of different vascular beds must go a long way to explain the lack of consensus that can be found in the many (mainly small) studies reported. Table 18.1 lists different techniques employed to assess endothelial vasomotor function (and "pre-atherosclerosis" markers).

Impaired responses to different endothelium-dependent agonists have been consistently described in several vascular beds of chemically-induced and genetic models of type 1 diabetes in animals. In human studies, most reports describe some abnormality in type 1 diabetic subjects, with or without diabetic or vascular complications; there are discrepant studies, perhaps reflecting covert differences in often small patient cohorts. The presence of clear-cut diabetic complications, typically microalbuminuria, has consistently seen reported abnormalities of endothelial vasorelaxation (see [6] for a detailed review).

Type 2 diabetics are more heterogeneous, and both animal model and human data are more discrepant. Clinical studies of type 2 diabetic patients are often confounded by the presence of multiple other cardiovascular risk factors, which may impinge on endothelial vasomotor reactivity. In particular, it is nearly impossible to locate type II diabetic subjects without any elevation of blood pressure or perturbation of lipid metabolism. It is not yet absolutely clear that type 2 diabetes *per se*, and not the constellation of shared vascular risks, disturbs endothelial vasomotor function. Part of this difficulty also lies in the fact that many of these studies are far too small to be reliable, and also that differences in patient characteristics and methodologies used make a meta-analysis impossible.

The reasons for endothelial dysfunction (impaired endothelium-dependent vasorelaxation) may involve several mechanisms. There are, may

Table 18.1

Tools to assess structure / function in pre-symptomatic vascular disease in man

DIRECT VASCULAR ASSESSMENT:
    Intracoronary Doppler wires, ultrasound, optical coherance tomography
    Venous plethysmography

CUTANEOUS ASSESSMENT:
    Laser Doppler flowmetry
    Nailfold capillary pressure measurements

INDIRECT VASCULAR ASSESSMENT:
    Vascular ultrasound – intima media thickness and plaque composition
    Thermal imaging of plaques
    Positron Emission Tomography (altered metabolism)
    Reactive Hyperaemia – Forearm Blood Flow by Ultrasound

BIOCHEMICAL MARKERS:
    Various secreted paracrine factors (*e.g.*, thrombomodulin, C-reactive protein, vWF)

PULSE WAVE CONTOUR ANALYSIS:
    Pulse wave analysis
    Pulse wave velocity
    Elastic incremental modulus (distensibility coefficient)

be, a decreased production, an enhanced inactivation, an impaired diffusion to the smooth muscle cells of the vessel media, an impaired responsiveness of the vessel wall smooth muscle cells to one or more of the EDRFs or enhanced generation of, or reactivity to, the endothelium-derived vasoconstricting factors. Depending on the model or type of diabetes studied, on the duration of diabetes, on the concurrent therapies in use, on the vascular bed studied it is possible to find evidence for all of these mechanisms. It may be naive to think that the same underlying fault can be responsible in every case. Endothelial cells from different vascular beds exhibit metabolic and structural differences and may be differentially affected by hyperglycaemia. Figure 18.1 shows some of the proposed mechanisms of endothelial dysfunction in diabetes.

Of necessity, most of the mechanistic studies have been done either *in vitro* or *in vivo,* in large conduit vessels, where vessel compliance is the target and separately, in small resistance arterioles, where local control of vessel bed perfusion is the issue. In the aorta, the current evidence tends to favour the elaboration of vasoconstrictor prostanoids and/or oxygen-derived free radicals (these may lead to premature destruction of NO and the formation of reactive species). Importantly and particularly in the context of diseased type 2 diabetics, abnormalities of endothelium-independent vasorelaxation can also be observed (*e.g.,* reduced vessel responsiveness to isosorbide dinitrate in type 2 diabetics with microalbuminuria).

Although the nature of the pathological link between high ambient glucose levels and diabetic complications is still not completely settled, it is accepted that hyperglycaemia induces repeated acute changes in intracellular metabolism, *e.g.,* activation of the polyol pathway, activation of diacylglycerol-protein kinase C, increased oxidative stress. Importantly, there are cumulative long-term changes in vessel structure and function due to the chemical alteration of macromolecule through formation of advanced glycation end-products (AGEs).

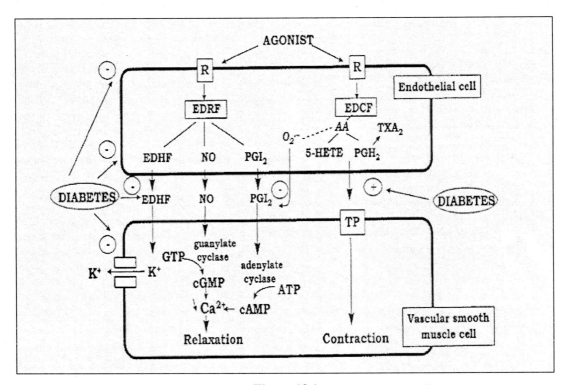

Figure 18.1
Mechanisms of endothelial dysfunction in diabetes.

Glycaemic control is a predictor of complications in type 1 and 2 diabetic patients, though the extent of the association is typically modest, especially in type 2 diabetics. Associations, in human studies, between elevation of glycated haemoglobin and extent of vasomotor abnormality are neither robust nor reliable.

In tissues that do not require insulin for cellular uptake of glucose (kidney, retina, nerves and blood vessels), hyperglycaemia activates the polyol pathway, resulting in the formation of sorbitol. Aldose reductase is the first and the rate-limiting step in the polyol pathway and reduces the aldehyde form of glucose to sorbitol. Several experimental and clinical studies have shown a link between increased polyol pathway activity and the occurrence of chronic diabetic complications. Chronic oral administration of aldose reductase inhibitors restored abnormal endothelium-dependent vasorelaxation, in several studies. Their use for the amelioration or prevention of diabetic neuropathy has to date been disappointing (see [6]).

Another glucose-mediated alteration in cellular metabolism that may account for abnormal endothelial function is the activation of protein kinase C. Hyperglycaemia leads to *de novo* synthesis of diacylglycerol, which leads to activation of the beta-isoform of protein kinase C. Protein kinase C inhibitors can also reverse the adverse vasomotor effects of elevated glucose, in several animal experimental models.

Glucose is known to bind non-enzymatically to free amino groups on proteins or lipids. Through a complex series of oxidative and non-oxidative reactions, AGEs are formed irreversibly and accumulate in tissues over time. Reactive carbonyl compounds can also behave similarly. AGEs, when bound to its receptor (RAGE), may trigger sustained cellular activation and oxidative stress. AGEs are known to quench NO. Taking all of the evidence together, it may be that AGE formation leads to structural and, consequentially, functional changes in the micro and macrovascular wall – in particular leading to cross-linking and increased vessel stiffening (see next section).

Oxidative stress, as an important pathogenetic element in the endothelial dysfunction of diabetes, is supported by considerable evidence (see [6]). Oxidative stress is defined as an increase in the steady-state levels of reactive oxidant species and may occur because of increased generation or because of decreased anti-oxidant capacity. Sources of increased reactive oxidant species, in diabetics, include auto-oxidation of glucose, AGE formation and AGE-binding to its receptors. Acute administration of scavengers of reactive oxidant species, such as superoxide dismutase with or without catalase, normalised the glucose-induced abnormal endothelium-dependent vasorelaxation, seen in several animal and experimental models. However, this effect is by no means universally seen across species, vascular beds and diabetic models.

ACE inhibitor used has been shown to ameliorate endothelial dysfunction in patients with diverse cardiovascular risks. The mechanism of action of ACE inhibitors is not known – but potential explanations include reduction of angiotensin-II induced NADH oxidase activity and hence, cellular production of superoxide anions. ACE inhibitors are known, also, to increase bradykinin levels and bradykinin is a potent vasodilator. Folate supplementation is known to reduce homocysteine levels (hyperhomocysteinaemia is seen at a very early stage of renal dysfunction and is also a feature of diabetes and familial hypercholesterolaemia).

Endothelial vasomotor dysfunction is often described in the context of impaired glucose tolerance and diabetes, in experimental and human settings. There are many reasons, at the cellular and metabolic level, why this should be so. Figure 18.2 shows the interaction between several intermediate steps and the induction of vascular changes. Manipulation, in man, of these complex vascular reactivity systems is however in its infancy and currently restricted to ACE inhibitors and possibly folate. It is of the utmost importance that future experimental and particularly human studies focus on highly clinically relevant models and with well-founded potential interventions.

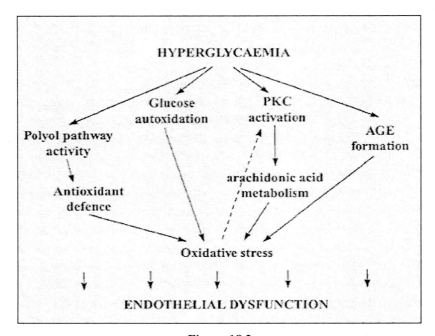

Figure 18.2

Effects of hyperglycaemia on metabolic pathways leading to endothelial dysfunction
and /or vessel structural changes.

ATHEROSCLEROSIS IN DIABETES

Diabetes is associated with a significantly higher incidence of coronary atheroma and with a 2–5 fold increased risk of fatal coronary events. It is now clear that the risk of a coronary event in diabetics is at the same level as is seen in non-diabetic with a prior myocardial infarction.

Atherosclerosis is a complex interplay between immune-mediated inflammation and lipid-storage disorder, leading to unstable atherosclerotic plaques, protruding into the lumen of blood vessels, leading either to rupture or to progressive luminal obliteration. The features of type 2 (in particular) diabetes, which contribute to this pathological maelstrom are well described – the initial disruption of the vascular endothelial cell layer function can be brought about by hyperglycaemia, altered lipoproteins, free fatty acids, derivates of glycation and oxidation and hypertension. Endothelial dysfunction is permissive of the deposition of lipid-rich particles in the vessel wall, where they are susceptible to oxidation and modification, promoting phagocytosis by macrophages, which then cause their phenotypic transformation into activated cells, in addition to

the cytokine, chemokine and growth factor influences and the migration and proliferation of fibroblasts and smooth muscle cells from the media into the intima [7]. The resulting vessel plaque may form a physical obstruction to blood flow, leading to chronic coronary insufficiency, or may rupture causing an acute coronary syndrome. The same conceptual issues are relevant to atherosclerosis in the carotid, renal arteries and peripheral vascular beds.

There are several mechanisms of increased vascular risk in diabetes. The first is the presence of platelet activation and hypercoagulability. Platelet activation can be demonstrated in the early stages of diabetes and insulin resistance. Diabetes, insulin resistance and hyperglycaemia are all pro-coagulant states. Enhanced expression of plasminogen activator inhibitor-1 (PAI-1) and down-regulation of anti-thrombin III activity, by non-enzymatic glycosylation, are just two reasons for hypercoagulability, independent of platelet activation [8].

Second, hypertension is nearly universal in diabetes, especially in type 2. Each 10 mm Hg rise in BP is associated with a 10% rise in the risk of death, MI, stroke or heart failure. Third, dyslipidaemia is a common feature in diabetes and insulin resistance. LDL-cholesterol levels are raised with the development of glyco-oxidised small dense LDL particles, which can enter in the damaged vessel wall, bind to exposed matrix proteins and caused macrophage activation. VLDL-cholesterol (*e.g.*, triglycerides and intermediate density lipoproteins) is also raised, and HDL-cholesterol significantly reduced [9]. Improved glycaemic control is associated with a reduction in the atherogenic lipid profile.

Of greatest recent topicality is the syndrome of chronic inflammation. Acute phase markers, such as serum – A component of amyloid, white cell count, and C-reactive protein are now linked with adverse cardiovascular outcome and may identify cohorts with a greater risk of future adverse events [10]. There are robust data showing elevated inflammatory markers in obese men and women [11]. The elevation of CRP in obese children, many years ahead of the development of advanced or symptomatic atherosclerosis, supports the idea that chronic inflammation is a promotor of accelerated vascular injury. It may be that adipocytes are the central players, releasing adipokines (leptin, resistin and adiponectin), as well as IL-6 and TNF-alpha. IL-6 is a key stimulus to hepatic synthesis of CRP. Table 18.2 lists the different ways in which inflammation might predispose to diabetes.

Patients with diabetes should arouse a very high index of suspicion for coronary artery disease, even if their symptoms are atypical. Autonomic neuropathy determines often "silences" chronic stable angina or even acute myocardial infarction. Stress echocardiography and electron-beam CT scanning of the cardiac vessels are promising screening tools to detect the presence of coronary disease.

Treatment of atherosclerosis (pre-clinical or clinical) should be aggressive and targeted. Blood pressure and blood glucose need intensively to be controlled in the acute and the chronic setting. Recently, it has been shown that intensive glucose control limits infarct size and reduces mortality in acute myocardial infarction and may also reduce progression in carotid intima-media thickness [12]. Antiaggregate therapy is essential – aspirin, clopidrogel and even both together. Two recent substudies of major hypertension trials (Hypertension Optimal Trial (HOT [13]) and UKPDS [14]) showed significant risk reduction in diabetic cohorts by aggressive BP reduction to 130/80 mm Hg. Two other recent studies (HOPE [15] and also LIFE [16]) have also shown overall greatest benefit on diabetic subjects. ACE inhibitors and angiotensin receptor blockers are now the first line therapy for hypertension in diabetes or, of course, micro-albuminuria at any BP level. The 4–S [17], the CARE and the Heart Protection Studies have all shown that diabetics have the most to gain from lipid-lowering therapy (predominantly with statin-based therapy). As triglycerides are also often raised, the use of fibrates is also justified in certain cases.

Diabetic patients have higher rates of complications and recurrences of stenoses in the context of coronary interventions. Mortality post-CABG is also greater in diabetics than in non-diabetics.

Table 18.2

Inflammation predisposing to diabetes: mechanisms

- Direct effect of cytokines on insulin-signalling cascade

- Proinflammatory cytokines induce lipolysis and hepatic de novo fatty acid synthesis

- Pro-inflammatory cytokine mediated endothelial cell dysfunction

- IL-6 mediated increased glucocorticoid receptor density and responsiveness

- Increased hepatic expression of Tanis (a novel gene whose protein product binds SAA and is dysregulated in insulin resistance states)

- Increased adiponectin release from adipocytes

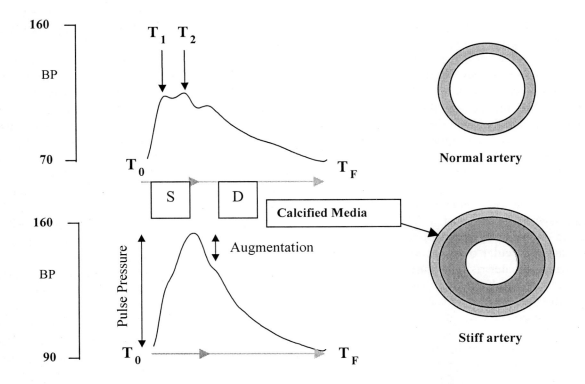

Figure 18.3

Augmentation index as a marker of arterial stiffness.

Typical pulse waveforms from normal (top) and stiffened (bottom) conduit arteries derived from percutaneous tonometry tracings. With reference to the normal artery: T_0 = time of start and T_F = time of finish of the cardiac cycle, T_1 = time to outgoing pressure peak and T_2 = time to peak of reflected wave. The peaks at T_1 and T_2 coincide in the stiffened artery leading to augmentation of the arterial pressure. The augmentation index is the augmentation divided by the pulse pressure × 100. S = systole and D = diastole.

The Bypass Angioplasty Revascularisation Investigation (BARI) reported an improved 5 years survival for surgical revascularisation compared to percutaneous coronary intervention [18]. One reason for this may be the increasingly routine use of internal mammary artery grafts, which are associated with marked extended patency rates compared to revascularisation using saphenous veins. Some of these results though need to be re-evaluated, as we know have drug-eluting stents, superstatins and adjunctive anti-platelet therapies (*e.g.*, glycoprotein IIb/IIIa receptor blockers) at our disposal.

ARTERIOSCLEROSIS IN DIABETES

Stiffening of the larger conduit arteries occurs with age, as a result of cyclic stress and strain effects and destruction of the medial and adventitial elastin fibres. The effect of loss of arterial compliance on the pulse waveform, leading to increased peripheral and central circulatory pulse pressure – PP – (simultaneously increasing cardiac afterload leading to LVH, and reducing coronary perfusion in diastole) is shown in Figure 18.3.

PP itself is determined by ventricular ejection (force / time) and by aortic cushioning function – the aorta is, of course, not only a conduit, but also a capacitance device for translating the "on-off" blood flow characteristics of the left ventricle into a smooth non-pulsatile blood flow pattern at capillary level. The degree to which the capacitance function can operate depends on arterial distensibility.

Aortic distensibility (elasticity) determines the degree of energy absorbed by the elastic aorta and its recoil in diastole – the aortic PP in health is modest and lower than peripheral arterial PP. Tempering the rise in aortic SBP protects the distal circulation against barotrauma and maintaining aortic DBP ensures adequate coronary perfusion – this constitutes perfectly aligned ventriculo-arterial coupling, as seen in young healthy adults. A stiffer, less healthy, aorta begins to fail in both of these tasks. As well as innate distensibility, there is another phenomenon that impinges on the pulse waveform characteristics – wave energy reflection. The energy propagated down the circulation eventually meets vessel branching points, where some of the anterograde energy is "reflected" and becomes retrograde. At some point down the aorta the incident and reflected energy waves summate. Where and when this happens depends on the speed of energy transfer along the aortic wall (pulse wave velocity – see below), on the degree of arterial luminal diameter mismatch (greater mismatch equates to greater reflection), and on the aortic length (closely correlated with subject height). In young healthy (tall) subjects energy summation takes place low in the abdominal aorta, in early diastole, helping to maintain coronary perfusion. Stiffer aortae, with greater pulse wave velocity, with constricted aortic branches and smaller subject height, all combine to cause greater reflection to occur in late systole (not as in diastole, as in the healthy state) and with energy summation happening closer to the aortic valve and coronary sinuses thereby prejudicing coronary perfusion.

PP is simple to measure, using familiar equipment, so it seems to be an attractive surrogate measure of aortic stiffness. However, because PP has its origins in both cardiac and aortic performance it is imperfect in this role. Wave reflections can be inferred from detailed computer-aided pulse wave contour analysis. Aortic pulse-wave velocity (PWV) is a direct measurement of arterial (aortic) stiffness. It is a directly-measured parameter derived from real-time measurement of the time taken for aortic mural energy waves (from cardiac contraction, aortic dilatation then recoil) to propagate down the aorta. PWV is greatly increased in hypertensive, diabetic and uraemic subjects, and in uraemic subjects it has a much better correlation with end-organ damage (LV mass) than does any measurement of peripheral BP. Increased arterial stiffness (increased pulse wave velocity) is, thus, mechanistically-linked with systolic hypertension, widened pulse pressure and left ventricular hypertrophy.

Importantly, both of these facets of arterial dysfunction (greater PWV and also increased wave energy reflection) contribute independently to the increased end-organ damage and premature mortality, seen in hypertension, diabetes and uraemia.

Large arterial structure is abnormal in diabetic patients, especially in those with chronic renal failure or on dialysis. All arteries are dilated, lengthened and tortuous, but with normal or even increased wall thickness. All portions of the arterial wall are involved in structural alterations, which have profound functional consequences. Proliferation of the intima, changes in the media (smooth muscle cell phenotypic alterations, elastic degeneration, reduplication, and cross-linking, and calcification) and adventitia (fibrosis) all conspire to "stiffened" arteries; this is most pronounced in the aorta and its major branches. All of these concepts are explained in greater detail in [19, 20].

In Aoun et al.'s study [21], one hundred and twenty-two diabetic patients were compared to 122 non-diabetic patients matched to the study group for sex, age, mean arterial pressure, number and localisation of the atherosclerotic alterations. Arterial stiffness was assessed by automatic measurement of the aortic pulse wave velocity (PWV) and by measuring the peripheral and carotid pulse pressure (PP) and reflected waves through analysis of the pulse wave, using the principle of applanation tonometry. Aortic PWV was significantly higher in the diabetic subgroup as well as PP at the peripheral and central levels for the same age and mean arterial pressure. In addition, renal failure was independently associated with an increased aortic PWV, but not PP, in the general population. Independent of the degree of renal failure, a fall in the glomerular filtration rate was also associated with increased aortic PWV. No interaction was noted between renal failure and diabetes mellitus. In conclusion, this study shows that diabetic patients have higher arterial stiffness compared to non-diabetic ones, having one or more cardiovascular risk factors, manifested by increased aortic PWV and PP. In addition, renal failure, irrespective of its degree and independent of diabetes mellitus, is associated with increased aortic PWV, but not with PP.

In a study to examine the implications of isolated office hypertension, Ribeiro *et al.* [22] tried to determine whether diabetes, smoking and dyslipidaemia were associated with greater than normal stiffness of aortic walls in subjects with white-coat hypertension. Arterial distensibility was assessed by automatic measurement of carotid-femoral PWV in 35 healthy normotensives, 46 white-coat hypertensives and 81 ambulatory hypertensives all matched for age, sex and body mass index. Nineteen normotensives (subgroup A), 28 WCH (subgroup A) and 37 ambulatory hypertensives (subgroup A) had only one or no other major cardiovascular risk factor, whereas 16 normo-tensives (subgroup B), 18 WCH (subgroup B) and 44 ambulatory hypertensives (subgroup B) had also some combination of non-insulin-dependent diabetes, smoking habit and dyslipidaemia. Both for the WCH and for ambulatory hypertensives diabetes and dyslipidaemia (subgroups B) were associated with higher PWV (11.6 ± 0.3 and 12.8 ± 0.3 m/s, respectively) than for subgroups A (9.3 ± 0.5 and 10.9 ± 0.6 m/s, respectively). In contrast, PWV for WCH in subgroup A (9.3 ± 0.5 m/s) did not differ from those for the normotensive subgroups A (9.2 ± 0.3 m/s) and B (9.6 ± 0.4 m/s). PWV was not correlated to levels of glycaemia, glycosylated haemoglobin and cholesterolaemia. These results suggest that, for ambulatory hypertensives and for WCH, both diabetes and dyslipidaemia are associated with an impairment of arterial distensibility, that can entail a greater than normal cardiovascular risk, which might dictate a more than usually stringent treatment of concomitant risk factors and possibly of high blood pressure.

The complex interplay between uraemia and diabetes, in respect of vascular stiffening and prognosis, was examined by Shoji *et al.* [23]. Aortic stiffness was compared between ESRD patients with and without diabetes, and the impact of aortic stiffness on cardiovascular mortality was examined in a prospective, observational cohort study. The cohort consisted of 265 ESRD patients on haemodialysis, including 50 diabetic patients studied between June 1992 and December 1998. At baseline, the diabetic ESRD patients had significantly higher aortic pulse wave velocity (PWV) than the nondiabetic patients. During a mean follow-up period of 63 months, 81 deaths,

including 36 cardiovascular deaths, were recorded. Kaplan-Meier analysis revealed higher all-cause or cardiovascular mortality rates in the diabetic compared with the nondiabetic patients and also, in those with higher aortic PWV than in those with lower aortic PWV. The effect of diabetes on cardiovascular death was significant in the Cox model, including age, years on hemodialysis, gender, smoking, C-reactive protein, haematocrit and body mass index as covariates. However, when aortic PWV was included as a covariate, the impact of diabetes was no longer significant, whereas aortic PWV was a significant predictor. In a model including 13 covariates, aortic PWV remained a significant predictor for cardiovascular and overall mortality, but not for non-cardiovascular death. These results demonstrate that the increased aortic stiffness of the ESRD patients with diabetes mellitus contributed to the higher all-cause and cardiovascular mortality rates.

While prevention is better than cure, especially in diabetic or uraemic subjects, there are several real and theoretical approaches to diminishing or even reversing the structural changes that have taken place in the great arteries. Of the various ways that arterial stiffening occurs, it should come as no surprise that the renin-angiotensin-aldosterone axis is very important. Recent evidence has emerged to suggest that ACEI can ameliorate some of the arteriosclerotic processes in uraemic large arteries, most likely by altering wave reflectance properties in the major/minor branching points in the distal circulation. Guerin *et al.*'s study of 150 HD patients, whose BP was monitored and treated vigorously for 51 months, showed that in some patients, despite successful BP lowering, the PWV increased [24]. The cohort of patients who had declines in *both PWV and BP* showed a marked survival advantage. The use of perindopril (but not nitrendipine or atenolol) was associated with a mortality risk ratio of 0.19 (CI 0.14–0.43). Reduction in arterial fibrosis by using ACEI and spironolactone has been reported. The thickening or fibrosis of the left ventricle in uraemia happens in parallel with similar mural changes in the large arteries, and both can regress. Nitrates also act to modulate reflected wave energy; eccentric dosing is necessary to prevent vascular tachyphylaxis. The majority of the effects of all these drugs is not on pulse-wave velocity, but more on reducing the extent and altering the timing of wave reflection, leading to reduced "late systolic" augmentation.

Asmar et al. [25] took 27 patients with mild to moderate essential hypertension and type 2 diabetes mellitus, and randomised them to once daily treatment with either telmisartan 40 mg or placebo, for three weeks and after a two-week washout period, crossed-over to the alternative treatment for a further three weeks. Carotid/femoral and carotid/radial PWV were measured non-invasively, using the automatic Complior device, and central parameters (central blood pressure, pulse contour analysis and augmentation index) were measured, using the SphygmoCor system, at the start and the end of each treatment period. Compared with placebo, treatment with telmisartan significantly reduced carotid/femoral PWV (mean adjusted treatment difference −0.95 m/s, 95% confidence intervals: −1.67, −0.23 m/s, p = 0.013), as well as peripheral and central diastolic, systolic and pulse pressure. In conclusion, the results of this study show that telmisartan is effective in reducing arterial stiffness in hypertensive patients with type 2 diabetes mellitus, and may potentially have beneficial effects on cardiovascular outcomes, beyond blood-pressure lowering effects in the patient group.

Finally, Ichihara et al. [26] studied the preventive effects of fluvastatin (20 mg daily versus placebo) on arterial PWV values in twenty-two patients with type 2 diabetes on haemodialysis with normal serum lipid levels. Their serum lipid levels, serum levels of C-reactive protein (CRP), arterial PWV and ankle-brachial indexes (ABI) were determined before, at 3 and 6 months after taking the medication to evaluate arterial stiffness. At the beginning of the follow-up, there were no differences in age, blood pressure, body mass index, serum haemoglobin A1c level, serum CRP level, serum lipid levels, PWV or ABI between the placebo- (n = 10) and the fluvastatin-treated patients (n = 12). After 6 months, the PWV and the serum oxidized low-density lipoprotein cholesterol (LDL-C) level increased significantly (from 1969 ± 140 to 2326 ± 190 cm/s and 70.4 ± 13.8 to 91.8 ± 15.5 U/l, respectively) in the placebo-treated patients. However, the fluvastatin group had a significantly reduced PWV (from 1991 ± 162 to 1709 ± 134 cm/s), oxidized LDL-C

serum levels (from 89.0 ± 9.6 to 73.0 ± 5.8 U/l) and CRP serum levels (from 0.97 ± 0.32 to 0.26 ± 0.16 mg/dl) compared with those in the placebo group. Long-term administration of fluvastatin prevents further worsening of arterial biomechanics in haemodialysis patients with type 2 diabetes mellitus, even in the presence of serum lipid levels in the normal range.

For many diabetic patients, vessel structural changes are too extreme to be reversed significantly. Prevention of some of the key processes that promote malign vascular changes must be a priority. Recent reports of agents that can reduce advanced glycation end (AGE) products, and more interesting, prevent collagen and elastin cross-linking in animal models and in man, are exciting [27–29].

Medial vascular calcification (an active regulated process [30]), typically seen in diabetic patients in large and small vessels, is associated with autonomic dysfunction, peripheral vascular disease and premature mortality from cardiovascular disease.

The role of renin-angiotensin-aldosterone genetic polymorphisms and the value of quenching excess oxidative stress and inflammation – to reduce endothelial damage – by use of vitamins, folic acid and endothelin-antagonists, urgently need more research. Much more information is also needed about the origins and time-course of these processes. So far, the vast majority of what we know is solely about haemodialysis patients. We must know at what stage in declining renal function these abnormalities begin. If one takes the analogy with left ventricular hypertrophy, these alterations may well start with near-normal renal function.

CONCLUSIONS

Old-age, diabetes and uraemia share a lot of cardiovascular risk factors and pathological mechanisms. These include abnormal autonomic function, deranged endothelial function, vessel dilatation and mural calcification, AGEs and oxidative stress. Increase in elastic artery stiffness is also common to all three. We will need to use of a variety of agents to counter raised BP, atherosclerosis, calcification and endothelial damage; the earlier these treatments can be employed the more likely they are to be beneficial.

For now, ACE inhibitors, ARBs, nitrates, statin-based lipid lowering therapy and the avoidance of promoting aggressive vascular calcification are the best remedies we currently have to ameliorate vascular functional decline. For many diabetic / renal patients – though this is a limited and only partly effective strategy – the anti-AGE / cross-chain linking agents may prove much more effective.

REFERENCES

1. Goran MI, Ball GD, Cruz ML. Obesity and risk of type 2 diabetes and cardiovascular disease in children and adolescents. *J Clin Endocrinol Metab,* **88:** 1417–1427, 2003.
2. Berenson GS, Srinivasan P, Bao W, Newmann WP, Tracy RE, Wattignay WA. Association between multiple cardiovascular risk factors and atherosclerosis in children and young adults. *N Engl J Med,* **338:** 1650–1656, 1998.
3. Lewis JB, Berl T, Bain RP, Rohde RD, Lewis EJ. Effect of intensive blood pressure control on the course of type 1 diabetic nephropathy. Collaborative Study Group [see comments]. *Am J Kidney Dis,* **34:** 809–817, 1999.
4. Shen BJ, Todaro JF, Niaura R, McCaffery JM, Zhang J, Spiro A, III, Ward KD. Are metabolic risk factors one unified syndrome? Modeling the structure of the metabolic syndrome X. *Am J Epidemiol,* **157:** 701–711, 2003.
5. Campbell I. The obesity epidemic: can we turn the tide? *Heart,* **89**(Suppl 2): ii22–24; 2003.
6. de Vriese AS, Verbeuren TJ, Van d, V, Lameire NH, Vanhoutte PM. Endothelial dysfunction in diabetes. *Br J Pharmacol,* **130:** 963–974, 2000.
7. Libby P, Ridker PM, Maseri A. Inflammation and atherosclerosis. *Circulation,* **105:** 1135–1143, 2002.
8. Beckman JA, Creager MA, Libby P. Diabetes and atherosclerosis: epidemiology, pathophysiology, and management. *JAMA,* **287:** 2570–2581, 2002.
9. Shoji T, Emoto M, Kawagishi T, Kimoto E, Yamada A, Tabata T, Ishimura E, Inaba M, Okuno Y, Nishizawa Y. Atherogenic lipoprotein changes in diabetic nephropathy. *Atherosclerosis,* **156:** 425–433, 2001.
10. Bell DS. Inflammation, insulin resistance, infection, diabetes, and atherosclerosis. *Endocr Pract,* **6:** 272–276, 2000.
11. Tamakoshi K, Yatsuya H, Kondo T, Hori Y, Ishikawa M, Zhang H, Murata C, Otsuka R, Zhu S, Toyoshima H. The metabolic syndrome is associated with elevated circulating C-reactive protein in healthy reference range, a systemic low-grade inflammatory state. *Int J Obes Relat Metab Disord,* **27:** 443–449, 2003.
12. Nathan DM, Lachin J, Cleary P, Orchard T, Brillon DJ, Backlund JY, O''Leary DH, Genuth S. Intensive diabetes therapy and carotid intima-media thickness in type 1 diabetes mellitus. *N Engl J Med,* **348:** 2294–2303, 2003.
13. Hansson L, Zanchetti A, Carruthers SG, Dahlof B, Elmfeldt D, Julius S, Menard J, Rahn KH, Wedel H, Westerling S. Effects of intensive blood-pressure lowering and low-dose aspirin in patients with hypertension: principal results of the Hypertension Optimal Treatment (HOT) randomised trial. HOT Study Group. *Lancet,* **351:** 1755–1762, 1998.
14. Efficacy of atenolol and captopril in reducing risk of macrovascular and microvascular complications in type 2 diabetes: UKPDS 39. UK Prospective Diabetes Study Group. *BMJ,* **317:** 713–720, 1998.
15. Yusuf S, Sleight P, Pogue J, *et al.* Effects of an Angiotensin-Converting-Enzyme Inhibitor, Ramipril, on Cardiovascular Events in High-Risk Patients. *N Engl J Med,* **342:** 145–153, 2000.
16. Lindholm LH, Ibsen H, Dahlof B, Devereux RB, Beevers G, de Faire U, Fyhrquist F, Julius S, Kjeldsen SE, Kristiansson K, Lederballe-Pedersen O, Nieminen MS, Omvik P, Oparil S, Wedel H, Aurup P, Edelman J, Snapinn S. Cardiovascular morbidity and mortality in patients with diabetes in the Losartan Intervention For Endpoint reduction in hypertension study (LIFE): a randomised trial against atenolol. *Lancet,* **359:** 1004–1010, 2002.
17. Pedersen TR. Coronary artery disease: the Scandinavian Simvastatin Survival Study experience. *Am J Cardiol,* **82:** 53T–56T, 1998.
18. Feit F, Brooks MM, Sopko G, Keller NM, Rosen A, Krone R, Berger PB, Shemin R, Attubato MJ, Williams DO, Frye R, Detre KM. Long-term clinical outcome in the Bypass Angioplasty Revascularization Investigation Registry: comparison with the randomized trial. BARI Investigators. *Circulation,* **101:** 2795–2802, 2000.
19. Goldsmith D, MacGinley R, Smith A, Covic A. How important and how treatable is vascular stiffness as a cardiovascular risk factor in renal failure? *Nephrol Dial Transplant,* **17:** 965–969, 2002.
20. Blacher J, Safar ME, Pannier B, Guerin AP, Marchais SJ, London GM. Prognostic significance of arterial stiffness measurements in end-stage renal disease patients. *Curr Opin Nephrol Hypertens,* **11:** 629–634, 2002.

21. Aoun S, Blacher J, Safar ME, Mourad JJ. Diabetes mellitus and renal failure: effects on large artery stiffness. *J Hum Hypertens*, **15:** 693–700, 2001.

22. Ribeiro L, Gama G, Santos A, Asmar R, Martins L, Polonia J. Arterial distensibility in subjects with white-coat hypertension with and without diabetes or dyslipidaemia: comparison with normotensives and sustained hypertensives. *Blood Press Monit,* **5:** 11–17, 2000.

23. Shoji T, Emoto M, Shinohara K, Kakiya R, Tsujimoto Y, Kishimoto H, Ishimura E, Tabata T, Nishizawa Y. Diabetes mellitus, aortic stiffness, and cardiovascular mortality in end-stage renal disease. *J Am Soc Nephrol*, **12:** 2117–2124, 2001.

24. London GM, Blacher J, Pannier B, Guerin AP, Marchais SJ, Safar ME. Arterial wave reflections and survival in end-stage renal failure. *Hypertension*, **38:** 434–438, 2001.

25. Asmar R. Effect of telmisartan on arterial distensibility and central blood pressure in patients with mild to moderate hypertension and Type 2 diabetes mellitus. *J Renin Angiotensin Aldosterone Syst* **2**(Suppl 2): S8–11, 2001.

26. Ichihara A, Hayashi M, Ryuzaki M, Handa M, Furukawa T, Saruta T. Fluvastatin prevents development of arterial stiffness in haemodialysis patients with type 2 diabetes mellitus. *Nephrol Dial Transplant*, **17:** 1513–1517, 2002.

27. Tamarat R, Silvestre JS, Huijberts M, Benessiano J, Ebrahimian TG, Duriez M, Wautier MP, Wautier JL, Levy BI. Blockade of advanced glycation end-product formation restores ischemia-induced angiogenesis in diabetic mice. *Proc Natl Acad Sci U S A,* **100**: 8555–8560, 2003.

28. Yang S, Litchfield JE, Baynes JW. AGE-breakers cleave model compounds, but do not break Maillard crosslinks in skin and tail collagen from diabetic rats. *Arch Biochem Biophys,* **412:** 42–46, 2003.

29. Candido R, Forbes JM, Thomas MC, Thallas V, Dean RG, Burns WC, Tikellis C, Ritchie RH, Twigg SM, Cooper ME, Burrell LM. A breaker of advanced glycation end-products attenuates diabetes-induced myocardial structural changes. *Circ Res*, **92:** 785–792, 2003.

30. Shanahan CM, Cary NR, Salisbury JR, Proudfoot D, Weissberg PL, Edmonds ME. Medial localization of mineralization-regulating proteins in association with Monckeberg's sclerosis: evidence for smooth muscle cell-mediated vascular calcification. *Circulation*, **100:** 2168–2176, 1999.

19

RENIN-ANGIOTENSIN-ALDOSTERONE SYSTEM AND DIABETES MELLITUS

Marius Marcian VINTILĂ, Monica Mariana BĂLUȚĂ, Vlad Damian VINTILĂ

The renin-angiotensin-aldosterone system (RAAS) is an important mechanism in the pathophysiology of hypertension and in the initiation and progression of atherosclerosis, leading to cardiovascular events. New evidence suggests that RAAS inhibition could also be helpful at preventing diabetes mellitus.

Diabetes increases the risk for atherosclerotic vascular disease. Both type 1 and type 2 diabetes are independent risk factors for the development of coronary artery disease and diabetic cardiomyopathy, which ultimately lead to heart failure irrespective of the initial event. The most common cause of death in diabetic patients is macrovascular disease, coronary disease being the predominant form.

In subjects with or without diabetes, endothelial dysfunction is one of the earliest abnormalities in vascular disease prior to overt atherosclerosis. Evidence from clinical trials suggest that breaking the chain of events by using agents such as ACE inhibitors can lead to improvements in endothelial dysfunction.

A substantial amount of data indicates that insulin resistance plays a major role in the development of glucose intolerance and diabetes. Angiotensin II (Ang II) negatively modulates insulin signaling by stimulating multiple serine phosphorylation events in the early components of the insulin-signaling cascade *in vitro*, therefore increasing insulin resistance.

The expression of angiotensin II-forming enzymes in adipose tissue is inversely correlated with insulin sensitivity. Some authors hypothesized that blockade of RAAS prevents diabetes by promoting the recruitment and differentiation of adipocytes. Increased formation of adipocytes would counteract the ectopic deposition of lipids in other tissues (muscle, liver, pancreas), thereby improving insulin sensitivity and preventing the development of type 2 diabetes.

Hypertension contributes to the development and progression of chronic complications of diabetes. In diabetes, hypertension is characterized by an upregulation of the RAAS and is associated with abnormal neurosympathetic autonomic function, with absence of nocturnal dipping of blood pressure or slowing of the heart rate, and endothelial dysfunction. These elements are also likely to play a role in the premature apoptosis of cardiac myocytes found in diabetes that, together with small and large vessel disease, are responsible for the characteristic cardiomyopathy.

The administration of converting enzyme inhibitors can slow the progression of renal damage in both diabetic and nondiabetic renal parenchymal disease. This effect appears to be an added action of converting enzyme inhibitors beyond their ability to lower systemic blood pressure, probably because they also selectively reduce renal glomerular pressure.

In the metabolic syndrome, modulation of the RAAS by ACE inhibition or by AT_1 receptor blockade acts on many targets, representing a first line intervention. It also reduces, at central and peripheral levels, the highly stimulated sympathetic drive, characteristic of most of these patients.

Aldosterone promotes vascular inflammation and perivascular fibrosis, synergizes with Ang II in inducing PAI-1 expression and has a significant pro-oxidative role in the pathogenesis of atherosclerosis. It promotes heart remodeling by myocyte hypertrophy and interstitial and perivascular fibrosis of the myocardium. Recent studies have examined the beneficial effect of aldosterone blockade in the prevention of recurrent heart failure and survival of patients with severe CHF (spironolactone – RALES) or in post myocardial infarction heart failure survivals (eplerenone – EPHESUS).

All over the world, diabetes is increasing in epidemic proportions. World Health Organization estimates that, while in the year 2000 the number of people with diabetes was about 177 million, by 2025, this will increase to at least 300 million. Primary prevention is the best method to limit this growth [1].

The renin-angiotensin-aldosterone system RAAS is an important mechanism in the pathophysiology of hypertension and in the initiation and progression of atherosclerosis, leading to cardiovascular events. New evidence suggests that RAAS inhibition could also be helpful in preventing diabetes mellitus [2].

The angiotensin converting enzyme ACE inhibitors and the angiotensin II receptor blockers ARB's are now widely used in the therapy of different conditions in which upregulation of RAAS induces detrimental effects. A number of clinical trials [4–7] reported that treatment with these drugs results in a marked reduction not only of diabetes-related cardiovascular complications, but also of new-onset diabetes. These actions may be mediated by antagonizing the direct effects of angiotensin II on inflammation, vascular endothelial function, hemostasis, risk of plaque ruptures and by determining improved blood flow to the pancreas [8], improved insulin sensitivity, a decrease in hepatic clearance of insulin and/or an effect on abdominal fat [9].

THE RENIN-ANGIOTENSIN-ALDOSTERONE SYSTEM

Angiotensinogen is the precursor of all angiotensin peptides and is synthesized by the liver. Renin is secreted into the lumen of renal afferent arterioles by juxtaglomerular cells. It cleaves four amino acids from angiotensinogen, thereby forming angiotensin I. In turn, angiotensin I is cleaved by ACE to form angiotensin II (Ang II), which plays an important homeostatic role through its endocrine and paracrine actions. One of these is the stimulation of aldosterone production in the zona glomerulosa of the adrenal cortex. Ang II and aldosterone are both involved in the pathophysiology of different complications generated by diabetes (Figure 19.1).

RENIN

Renin is a member of the aspartyl-proteinase family of enzymes and is synthesized as a pre-pro-protein in the juxtaglomerular apparatus of the kidney [10]. In the juxtaglomerular cells, it is stored in granules and released in response to specific stimuli, mainly drop of pressure in afferent arteriola. Renin is a double-domain enzyme, the N-terminal and C-terminal halves being similar [11]. Each domain contains a single aspartic acid residue, critical for its catalytic activity. In humans, the gene that encodes renin is located on the short arm of chromosome 1 (1q32–1q42).

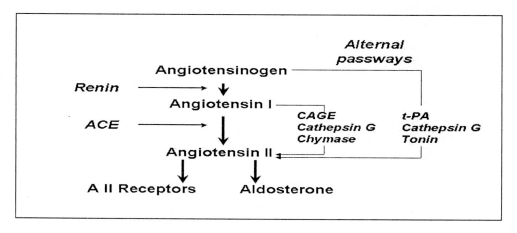

Figure 19.1

Renin-Angiotensin-Aldosterone System.

ANGIOTENSINOGEN

Angiotensinogen is the only known substrate for renin. Human angiotensinogen belongs to the serpin superfamily of proteins and is encoded by a gene on chromosome 1q42.3 near the renin gene [12]. Renin action on angiotensinogen is the first step of a catabolic cascade generating angiotensin peptides.

ANGIOTENSIN-CONVERTING ENZYME

The second step in the angiotensin peptides production is angiotensin-converting enzyme. ACE has a molecular weight considerably greater than that of renin, being a dipeptidyl-carboxyl-zinc-metallopeptidase usually bound to cell membranes [13]. In tissues that produce angiotensin II, it is also present in intracellular granules. In humans, two molecular forms of ACE are produced by separate promoter regions of a single gene located on chromosome 17q23. One is a germinal ACE and the second is a somatic or endothelial ACE, which consists of 1306 amino acids [14]. Somatic ACE molecule contains two homologous domains, with a functional active site each. The *in vivo* contribution of each active site to the release of Ang II and the inactivation of bradykinin (BK) is still unknown. It is probable that BK protection requires the inhibition of both active sites, while the selective inhibition of only one of the domains is sufficient to prevent the conversion of Ang I to Ang II. It might be suggested that the gene duplication of ACE in vertebrates may represent a means for regulating the cleavage of Ang I differently from that of BK [15].

ANGIOTENSIN RECEPTORS

In humans, the two primary forms of the angiotensin receptors are termed AT_1 and AT_2 [16]. They are encoded by a single gene on chromosome 3. The AT_1 receptor has seven transmembrane regions, with a disulfide bridge linking the first and fourth extracellular segments. The principal signaling mechanism involved in the AT_1 receptor operates through a G_q protein-mediated activation of phospholipase C [17]. The AT_2 receptor has a seven transmembrane domain structure too [18, 19].

ANGIOTENSIN PEPTIDES

The action of renin on angiotensinogen produces angiotensin I, a decapeptide that does not appear to be biologically active. But at least four peptides derived from angiotensin I have biologic activity [20, 21] (Figure 19.2).

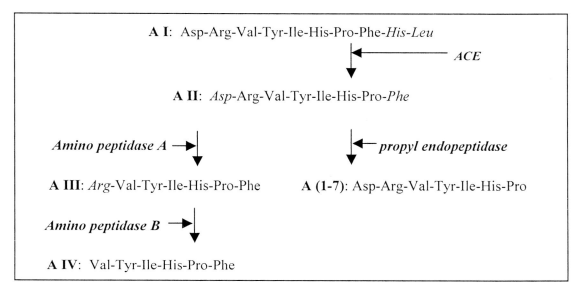

Figure 19.2
Angiotensin peptides.

Angiotensin II, formed by cleavage of the two carboxyl-terminal peptides by ACE [10] has full biologic activity. By further removing the N-terminal aspartic acid, *amino peptidase A* produces the heptapeptide angiotensin III (A III). The efficacy of A II and A III on renal blood flow and aldosterone secretion is equivalent, but A III has less pressor activity. *Amino peptidase B* cleaves an additional amino acid from A III to form angiotensin IV (angiotensin 3–8) [21]. A IV acting on a specific receptor activates endothelial plasminogen activator inhibitor-1 (PAI-1) production. That is why, by reducing A IV through a decrease of its precursors, ACE inhibitors promote fibrinolysis, one of their protective mechanisms. A IV may also be involved in the regulation of cerebral circulation and may produce vasodilation rather than vasoconstriction. A fourth biologically active compound is produced from angiotensin I by the action of a propyl endopeptidase to form angiotensin 1–7 [22], whose function in humans is unclear.

FUNCTIONS OF ANGIOTENSIN II

Angiotensin II is an octapeptide hormone that plays a central role in mediating the vasoactive, proliferative and inflammatory responses to arterial injury, as well as in promoting hypertension, cardiac remodeling and probably many other pathological processes, among which diabetes [2, 3].

The effects of the RAAS are systemic endocrine, or can be mediated by local paracrine actions [10, 23]. The endocrine part of the system consists initially in renin from the juxtaglomerular apparatus of the kidney and angiotensinogen from the liver. The levels of Ang I resulting from their interaction are dependent on the concentrations of each of these precursors. Endothelially expressed ACE activates plasma Ang I to Ang II.

Elements of the RAAS are present in various tissues, at least part of Ang II effects being mediated not by the circulating peptide, but by its local generation. In the heart, as well as in the fat cells Ang II may be generated by a nonrenin and/or nonACE system – the chymase system [24]. Interstitial angiotensin II modulates lipid and carbohydrate metabolism in a tissue specific fashion [25]. Now there is a lot of evidence suggesting that paracrine effects mediate many of the functions of angiotensin II.

The main physiologic function of Ang II, mediated by the AT_1 receptor, is to maintain normal blood pressure and extracellular volume and involves at least five mechanisms [10] :

1) constriction of vascular smooth muscle, thereby increasing blood pressure and reducing renal blood flow;

2) release of norepinephrine and epinephrine from the adrenal medulla;

3) augmentation of the sympathetic nervous system activity by increasing the central sympathetic outflow, thereby increasing norepinephrine discharge from sympathetic nerve terminals;

4) promotion of vasopressin release;

5) increasing aldosterone secretion.

In many respects, the action of angiotensin II through the AT_2 receptor antagonizes its effects through the AT_1 receptor. Thus, AT_2-mediated effects include vasodilatation, renal sodium loss, and apoptosis (thereby antagonizing the growth-promoting effects of AT_1 receptor activation). AT_2 receptors are highly expressed in fetal compared with adult tissues, unless the adult tissue is damaged [26].

Other functions of Ang II, mediated through the AT_1 receptor, include growth regulation of the heart, kidneys and vascular smooth muscle [27, 28]. Early studies demonstrated the role of Ang II in promoting cellular hypertrophy, characterized by increases in protein synthesis, cell size and polyploidy [29–31]. Ang II induced c-fos, c-jun and c-myc proto-oncogenes encoding transcription factors, that act in part as mediators of cell growth and differentiation.

However, Ang II serves a multiplicity of functions distinct from its ability to promote contraction or induce cellular hypertrophy.

Ang II induces tissue factor – the initiator of coagulation – and plasminogen type activator inhibitor-1 PAI-1, an inhibitor of fibrinolysis [32, 33]. This raised the possibility that Ang II could promote a procoagulant state. A significant improvement of the fibrinolytic balance was shown in patients after myocardial infarction with 14-day treatment with ramipril [34].

Angiotensin II is associated with elevated oxidative stress. Ang II stimulates the production of reactive oxygen species and activates a multitude of intracellular signals, including the mitogen-activated protein kinase, phosphatidylinositol 3-kinase/Akt and JAK/STAT pathways [35, 36]. Ang II decreases endothelium-dependent nitric oxide NO-mediated dilatation via superoxide production, by AT_1 receptor activation of NADPH oxidase. This may partly explain the impaired coronary flow regulation in heart diseases associated with an upregulated renin-angiotensin system [37].

Angiotensin II was also shown to induce JE/MCP-1, interleukin-6, and KC/gro chemokines, that are important in recruiting leukocytes at the sites of inflammation, thereby implicating Ang II as a proinflammatory molecule [38]. Ang II and aldosterone are also involved in regulating inflammatory and reparative processes that follow tissue injury [39, 40]. In this capacity, they stimulate cytokine production, inflammatory-cell adhesion, and chemotaxis; activate macrophages at sites of repair [41], and stimulate the growth of fibroblasts and the synthesis of type I and III fibrillar collagens, which govern the formation of scar tissue [42]. On the other hand, through these actions, Ang II augments vascular inflammation, induces endothelial dysfunction, and, in doing so, enhances the atherogenic process [43]. Recent studies have shown a high level of ACE activity in vulnerable plaques, so that plaque stabilization includes therapeutic RAAS antagonism to control the inflammatory processes in the vessel wall [44].

DIABETES AS A RISK FACTOR FOR CARDIOVASCULAR DISEASE. ASSOCIATION WITH OTHER RISK FACTORS AND CORRELATION WITH RAAS

Diabetes increases the risk for atherosclerotic vascular disease. Both type 1 and type 2 diabetes are independent risk factors for the development of coronary artery disease (CAD) and diabetic cardiomyopathy, which ultimately lead to heart failure irrespective of the initial event. This risk is greater in persons who have other known risk factors (such as dyslipidemia, hypertension, smoking, and obesity). Diabetes *per se*, as a risk factor for coronary disease, increases the risk of atherosclerotic events 2- to 4-fold, depending on gender and ethnic differences. Causation of accelerated atherosclerosis in diabetes is multifactorial and clearly begins years or even

decades prior to the diagnosis of type 2 diabetes. Atherosclerosis in diabetic patients is characterized by several factors, including an increase in rates of mortality following coronary events, in thrombosis and restenosis following invasive revascularization procedures, and in coronary event recurrence, and by the need for broad multitherapeutic intervention that goes well beyond maintenance of glycemic control [45, 47].

The most common cause of death in diabetic patients is macrovascular disease, with coronary disease being the predominant form [48]. Unlike microvascular disease, which occurs only in patients with diabetes mellitus, macrovascular disease resembles that in subjects without diabetes. However, subjects with diabetes have more rapidly progressive and extensive cardiovascular disease, with a greater incidence of multivessel disease and a greater number of affected vessel segments than in nondiabetic persons. Although the histopathology of atherosclerotic lesions in patients with diabetes appears similar if not identical compared with nondiabetic patients, the distribution of these lesions within the coronary circulation seems to be different. Patients with diabetes have a greater proportion of distal arterial disease, rendering invasive revascularization more difficult and less satisfactory, compared with nondiabetic patients. There is also an increased incidence of left main coronary artery disease or its equivalent, namely critical lesions at the proximal left anterior descending and circumflex branches of the left coronary artery.

The cardiovascular events associated with type 2 diabetes and the high incidence of other macrovascular complications, such as strokes and amputations, are a major cause of illness and an enormous economic burden. It is possible that these complications will even be prevented by early normalization of metabolic status. Treatment is aimed at lowering blood glucose levels to or near normal in all patients. Normalization of blood glucose has been demonstrated to be associated with a less atherogenic lipid profile [49].

ENDOTHELIAL DYSFUNCTION

In subjects with or without diabetes, endothelial dysfunction is one of the earliest abnormalities in vascular disease prior to overt atherosclerosis [50]. Evidence from clinical trials suggests that breaking the chain of events by using agents such as ACE inhibitors can lead to improvements in endothelial dysfunction [51].

Because macrovascular disease also occurs in nondiabetic subjects, diabetes is thought to accelerate the process by increasing endothelial cell dysfunction and by exacerbating dyslipidemia. The pathogenesis of endothelial cell dysfunction in diabetic arteries appears to involve RAAS upregulation and both insulin resistance and hyperglycemia. In the Heart Outcomes Prevention Evaluation (HOPE) trial [5], the ACE inhibitor arm was stopped early due to a consistent and significant benefit with ramipril; there was a 22% decline in the combined incidence of cardiovascular death, nonfatal MI and stroke. The findings from HOPE, together with the Trial on Reversing Endothelial Dysfunction (TREND), Brachial Artery ultrasound Normalization of Forearm Flow (BANFF), and Quinapril On Vascular ACE and Determinants of Ischemia (QUOVADIS) trials [52, 54] demonstrate that the endothelium is a vital regulator of vascular tone and smooth muscle cell proliferation, that can be effectively targeted with ACE inhibition.

There is also increasing evidence that angiotensin II is a major culprit in the vessel wall and the HOPE trial told us that it is important to inhibit RAAS to protect the vasculature. It seems that insulin resistant subjects, with or without diabetes, may have increased sensitivity to angiotensin II.

HYPERGLYCEMIA

The importance of hyperglycemia in the pathogenesis of diabetic macrovascular disease is suggested by the observation that carotid wall thickness is increased in persons with established diabetes but not in persons with impaired glucose tolerance [55]. The mechanisms by which hyperglycemia produces derangements in the macrovascular wall remain unclear, but they possibly include production of advanced glycosylation end-products AGE, enhancement of the polyol pathway and activation of protein-kinase C. Vascular endothelial cells express AGE-specific receptors (RAGE). This novel AGE-binding protein appears to be a member of the immunoglobulin superfamily, with three disulfide-bonded immunoglobulin homology units. RAGE

has been shown to mediate signal transduction *via* generation of ROS, activation of NFκB, and p21 ras. RAGE clearly plays a role in diabetic atherosclerosis. RAGE overexpression is associated with enhanced inflammatory reaction and this effect may contribute to plaque destabilization by inducing culprit metalloproteinase expression [56].

The United Kingdom Prospective Diabetes Study (UKPDS) identified hyperglycemia as an important risk factor for macrovascular disease in type 2 diabetes and numerous correlational studies show that hyperglycemia is a continuous risk factor for macrovascular disease [57].

The relative importance of hyperglycemia in type 1 patients is suggested by the 41% reduction in macrovascular disease (P = 0.06) observed in the intensive therapy group of the DCCT study [58].

HYPERINSULINEMIA AND INSULIN RESISTANCE

Angiotensin II negatively modulates insulin signaling by stimulating multiple serine phosphorylation events in the early components of the insulin-signaling cascade *in vitro* [59].

Ang II-induced insulin resistance cannot be attributed to impairment of early insulin-signaling steps only. Increased oxidative stress, possibly through impaired insulin signaling located downstream from phosphatidylinositol PI 3-kinase activation, is involved in Ang II-induced insulin resistance [60, 61].

A substantial amount of data indicates that insulin resistance plays a major role in the development of glucose intolerance and diabetes. Insulin resistance is a consistent finding in patients with type 2 diabetes, and resistance is present years before the onset of diabetes [62, 63]. Prospective studies provide evidence that insulin resistance predicts the onset of diabetes.

The mechanism by which the hyperinsulinemia contributes to cardiovascular disease is not well understood, and may not be simply explained by an association between insulin resistance and coexisting factors such as dyslipidemia. There are recent data that indicate the metabolic effects of insulin action are biochemically distinct from the mitogenic effects of the hormone.

DIABETES AND OBESITY

Obesity is the prime risk factor for the development of type 2 diabetes. Recent clinical trials revealed that blockade of the renin-angiotensin system, either by inhibiting the angiotensin-converting enzyme or by blocking the angiotensin type 1 receptor, may substantially lower the risk for type 2 diabetes [5, 7]. The mechanism underlying this effect is unknown. Angiotensin II markedly inhibits adipogenic differentiation of human adipocytes *via* the angiotensin type I receptor. The expression of angiotensin II-forming enzymes in adipose tissue is inversely correlated with insulin sensitivity. Some authors hypothesized that blockade of RAAS prevents diabetes by promoting the recruitment and differentiation of adipocytes. Increased formation of adipocytes would counteract the ectopic deposition of lipids in other tissues (muscle, liver, pancreas), thereby improving insulin sensitivity and preventing the development of type 2 diabetes [64].

The obesity seen in type 2 diabetes is central in distribution, with a large amount of abdominal or visceral fat. This is rich in highly metabolically active adipocytes, that are responsible for the formation and release of toxic substances (*e.g.*, tumor necrosis factor-α, PAI-1, interleukin-6, serum amyloid A, and asymmetric dimethylarginine, an endogenous nitric oxide synthase inhibitor). These mediators have a role in atherogenesis. Leptin and "resistin" are adipocyte hormones associated with insulin resistance and obesity [65]. High leptin levels are found in patients with obesity and type 2 diabetes, most likely as a consequence of a metabolic maladaptation. The novel cytokines "resistin" and "adiponectin" are closely linked to diabetes and obesity, and can be modified by peroxisome proliferator-activated receptor (PPARs) ligands.

Adipocyte-derived hormones may represent a mechanism linking insulin resistance to cardiovascular disease. The novel adipokine resistin exerts direct effects to activate endothelial cells by promoting endothelin-1 (ET-1) release, in part by inducing ET-1 promoter activity *via* the activator protein-1 (AP-1) site. Furthermore, resistin upregulates adhesion molecules and chemokines and downregulates tumor necrosis factor receptor-associated factor-3 (TRAF-3), an inhibitor of CD40 ligand signaling. In this fashion, resistin may be mechanistically linked to cardiovascular disease in the metabolic syndrome [66, 67].

Adiponectin has been suggested to play an important role in insulin sensitivity. Hypo-adiponectinemia is related to insulin resistance in essential hypertension and RAAS blockade increases adiponectin concentrations with improvement in insulin sensitivity [68].

DIABETES AND HYPERTENSION

Hypertension traditionally has been defined as a systolic blood pressure ≥ 140 mmHg and/or a diastolic blood pressure ≥ 90 mmHg [69, 70]. Most epidemiological studies have suggested that risk due to elevated blood pressure is a continuous function, so these cutoff levels are arbitrary. In the general population, the risk for target-organ damage appears to be the lowest when the systolic blood pressure is < 120 mmHg and the diastolic is < 80 mmHg [71, 72].

Hypertension contributes to the development and progression of chronic complications of diabetes. In diabetes, hypertension is characterized by an upregulation of the RAAS and is associated with abnormal neurosympathetic autonomic function, with absence of nocturnal dipping of blood pressure or slowing of the heart rate, and endothelial dysfunction. These elements are also likely to play a role in the premature apoptosis of cardiac myocytes found in diabetes, that together with small and large vessel disease are responsible for the characteristic cardiomyopathy.

In patients with type 1 diabetes, persistent hypertension is often a manifestation of diabetic nephropathy. In patients with type 2 diabetes, hypertension is often part of a syndrome that also includes glucose intolerance, insulin resistance, obesity, dyslipidemia, and coronary artery disease. Type 2 diabetes mellitus, hypertension, and obesity are commonly associated, and the frequency of this association may be greater than their occurrence in the general population suggesting a common etiology.

Control of hypertension has been demonstrated to reduce the rate of progression of diabetic nephropathy and reduce the cerebrovascular disease and cardiovascular disease. The primary goal of therapy for adults with diabetes according to WHO-ISH 1999 guideline should be to decrease blood pressure to < 130/85 mmHg or better below 130/80 as JNC 7 and ESH/ESC 2003 guidelines suggest [69, 71].

Insulin directly stimulates the calcium pump in insulin-sensitive tissues and promotes calcium loss from the cell [73]. Raising cytosolic calcium levels in an adipocyte can induce insulin resistance [74, 75]. If a cell is resistant to insulin, the insulin-induced calcium loss from cells would be decreased, and in vascular smooth muscle cells the resultant increase in intracellular calcium would enhance responsiveness to vasoconstrictors and increase blood pressure.

Other mechanisms proposed to explain the linkage between insulin resistance and hypertension are increased activity of the adrenergic nervous system [76] and increased renal sodium retention [77].

In addition to its involvement in primary hypertension, the renin-angiotensin system is a major factor in the most common cause of secondary hypertension due to diabetic nephropathy. It is known that RAAS activation and defective glucose control contribute to adverse renal outcomes. The local (intrarenal) renin-angiotensin system is activated to a variable degree in these subjects. This activation results in an elevation of hydraulic pressure in the glomeruli (so-called glomerular hypertension) secondary to the vasoconstrictor effect of angiotensin II on the efferent arteriole [78]. Chronic elevation of glomerular pressure leads to glomerular sclerosis and progressive loss of functioning nephron units.

The administration of converting enzyme inhibitors can slow the progression of renal damage in both diabetic and nondiabetic renal parenchymal disease [79, 80]. This effect appears to be an added action of converting enzyme inhibitors beyond their ability to lower systemic blood pressure, probably because they also selectively reduce renal glomerular pressure. Agents that only produce a decrease in systemic blood pressure equivalent to that accomplished by converting enzyme inhibitors do not afford the same degree of protection of renal function.

Current data suggest that in hypertensive patients with type 1 diabetes, ACE inhibitors can reduce the level of albuminuria and the rate of progression of renal disease to a greater degree than other antihypertensive agents that lower blood pressure by an equal amount. Other studies have shown that there is benefit in reducing the progression of microalbuminuria in normotensive patients with type 1 diabetes and in normotensive and hypertensive patients with type 2 diabetes.

Patients with diabetes mellitus seem to have a lower frequency of renal vascular hypertension, but the incidence of renal vascular disease is higher than in the nondiabetic population [81]. Most patients with renal vascular disease have either atherosclerotic plaques or fibromuscular disease, and in 10% of the cases, the lesion is in a segmental or branch artery.

Intensive treatment of hypertension in patients with newly diagnosed diabetes during an eight-year period, which decreased systolic and diastolic blood pressure by 10 and 5 mm Hg, respectively, significantly reduced both the absolute risk of stroke and the combined end point of diabetes-related death, death from vascular causes, and death from renal causes by 5 percent [82]. The Hypertension Optimal Treatment Study, which treated elevations in diastolic blood pressure for an average of 3.7 years, reported similar reductions in the risk of composite end points for macrovascular disease in subgroup analyses of patients with type 2 diabetes [83]. Treatment of systolic hypertension for 4.7 years in the Systolic Hypertension in the Elderly Program trial and 2 years in the Systolic Hypertension in Europe Trial reduced the absolute risk of cardiovascular events by 8 percent [84] and that of death from cardiovascular causes by 5 percent [85].

A provocative study, the Heart Outcomes Prevention Evaluation (HOPE) Trial, suggested that with essentially identical degrees of BP control, the inclusion of an ACE inhibitor (ramipril) might produce additional CV risk reduction as compared with placebo. In this study, ramipril was also associated with a reduced risk of developing type 2 diabetes in an otherwise high-risk but previously nondiabetic population [86].

Because of their efficacy as antihypertensive agents and the selective benefit they have in retarding progression of diabetic nephropathy, ACE inhibitors and ARB's are recommended as the primary treatment of all hypertensive diabetic patients with microalbuminuria or overt nephropathy. Because of the high proportion of patients who progress from microalbuminuria to overt nephropathy and subsequently to end stage renal disease, the use of ACE inhibitors is recommended for all type 1 patients with microalbuminuria, even if normotensive. The rate of progression from microalbuminuria to overt nephropathy and end stage renal disease in patients with type 2 diabetes is variable, but the use of ACE inhibitors in normotensive type 2 diabetics is useful because it is known that microalbuminuria is a risk factor for cardiovascular events. The effect of ACE inhibitors appears to be a class effect, so choice of agent may depend on cost and compliance issues.

More recently, similar studies have been performed with angiotensin receptor blocker (ARB) compounds. These agents have the additional advantage of relatively diminished cough, the latter being a common complication of the use of ACE inhibitors. Several studies that have assessed the nephroprotective and cardioprotective effects of angiotensin-II receptor antagonists have been completed. The results of the Reduction of Endpoints in NIDDM with the Angiotensin-II Antagonist Losartan (RENAAL), the Irbesartan Type 2 Diabetic Nephropathy Trial (IDNT), the Irbesartan in Patients with Type 2 Diabetes and Microalbuminuria Study (IRMA 2) and the Microalbuminuria Reduction with Valsartan Study (MARVAL) have shown that the angiotensin-II receptors blockers tested are protective of renal function in type 2 diabetics. The two latest agents have recently received FDA approval in patients with type 2 diabetes to reduce the progression of nephropathy [87–91]. The combination of angiotensin-II receptor blockers and ACE inhibitors may be more effective in reducing blood pressure and microalbuminuria. [92]

Lifestyle modifications such as weight loss, exercise, reduction of dietary sodium, smoking cessation and decreased alcohol consumption should be added to medication until blood pressure goals are reached.

DIABETES AND DYSLIPIDEMIA

Multiple modifiable risk factors for late complications in patients with type 2 diabetes, including hyperglycemia, hypertension, and dyslipidemia, increase the risk of a poor outcome [55]. Even if dyslipidemia and hypertension occur with great frequency in type 2 diabetic populations, there is still excess risk in diabetic subjects after adjusting for these other risk factors. Diabetes itself may confer 75% to 90% of the excess risk of coronary disease in these diabetic subjects and it enhances the deleterious effects of the other major cardiovascular risk factors. Subgroup analysis showed a large reduction in the absolute risk of cardiovascular events among diabetic patients with elevated serum total cholesterol concentrations who took statins for 5.4 years for secondary cardiovascular prevention [94–98].

Recent guidelines from the American Diabetes Association and other national guidelines recommend an intensified multifactorial treatment approach, although the effect of this approach has not been confirmed in long-term studies.

The Steno-2 Study compares the effect of a targeted, intensified, multifactorial intervention with that of conventional treatment on modifiable risk factors for cardiovascular disease in patients with type 2 diabetes and microalbuminuria. The results show that a focused, multifactorial intervention with continued patient education and motivation, strict targets and individualized risk assessment should be offered to patients with type 2 diabetes and microalbuminuria who are at increased risk for macrovascular and microvascular complications. Such patients may represent about one third of the population of patients with type 2 diabetes [99].

The direct impact of RAAS inhibition on diabetic dyslipidemia is not yet established. The main link could be the correction of cholesterol-induced endothelial dysfunction by associating ACE inhibitors or/and ARBs to antidyslipidemic therapy.

THE METABOLIC SYNDROME

The metabolic syndrome describes a high-risk population having 3 or more of the following clinical characteristics: abdominal obesity, atherogenic dyslipidemia (especially hypertriglyceridemia and low HDL), hypertension, and disturbed glucose and insulin metabolism (Table 19.1) [100].

Table 19.1

The diagnostic criteria suggested by the National Cholesterol Education Program (NCEP) for Metabolic Syndrome (3 of 5 Sufficient For Diagnosis)

1. Abdominal obesity	Waist >/=40" (male)
	Waist >/=35" (female)
2. Triglycerides	>150 mg/dL
3. HDL cholesterol	<40 mg/dL (males)
	<50 mg/dL (females)
4. Hypertension	>130/85 mm Hg
5. Impaired fasting glucose	>/=110 mg/dL

In the metabolic syndrome, modulation of the RAAS by ACE inhibition or by AT_1 receptor blockade acts on many targets, representing a first line intervention. As it was already shown, RAAS inhibition controls blood pressure, interferes endocrine and paracrine effect of visceral obesity and has favorable influences on insulin resistance. It also reduces, at central and peripheric levels, the highly stimulated sympathetic drive, characteristic of most of these patients.

Affected individuals can also exhibit prothrombotic and proinflammatory state associated with increased levels of C-reactive protein (CRP) leading to increased morbidity and mortality from atherosclerotic vascular disease. Data suggest that measurement of CRP adds clinically important prognostic information to the metabolic syndrome. Additive effects for CRP were also observed for patients with 4 or 5 characteristics of the metabolic syndrome. The use of different definitions of the metabolic syndrome had minimal impact on these findings [101].

The coagulation abnormalities are also complex and include factors predisposing to thrombosis, such as increased platelet activation and hyperaggregability and elevated procoagulants, such as fibrinogen and von Willebrand factor. Impaired fibrinolysis includes a high production and activity of PAI-1, together with low tissue plasminogen activity. PAI-1 levels are markedly elevated in atheroma specimens extracted from vessels of patients with long-standing type 2 diabetes [102–105]. It is known that PAI-1 is a risk factor for cardiovascular events and a risk factor to drive the development of other risk factors. At the molecular level, in humans, angiotensin and aldosterone drive PAI-1 production. It seems that PAI-1 also predicts the development of diabetes. A paper published in 2002 showed that C-reactive protein predicts the development of diabetes but in this work PAI-1 was a better predictor of the development of new onset diabetes in the studied population [59]. In an animal model, the PAI-1 expression in the injured tissue was prevented by an AT1 receptor blocker, which also protected from fibrosis.

DIABETIC CARDIOMYOPATHY

Diabetic patients show a prominent tendency to develop congestive heart failure early and with even relatively minor stimuli. In the Framingham Heart Study [106], diabetic men had twice the frequency of heart failure than did nondiabetic cohorts, whereas diabetic women had a 5-fold increased risk. This is likely a combination of extensive atherosclerotic disease of both epicardial and microvascular coronary arteries, coexistent hypertension and hyperglycemia, and possibly an autonomic neuropathy. The pathogenesis may involve formation of collagen acetylated glycation end-products [107, 108] and abnormalities in the handling of intracellular calcium [109].

In human subjects, diabetes has been shown to be associated with increased risk of apoptosis in myocytes, endothelial cells and fibroblasts, which may be related to increased RAAS upregulation. Enhanced tissue Ang II levels have been reported in diabetes and might lead to cardiac dysfunction through oxidative stress. Data suggest that local Ang II, acting *via* AT1 receptor-mediated NADPH oxidase activation, is involved in hyperglycemia-induced cardiomyocyte dysfunction, which also might play a role in diabetic cardiomyopathy [110, 111].

Diastolic filling abnormalities in type 2 diabetic subjects without clinical evidence of heart disease appear to be common and suggest the presence of early subclinical alterations in cardiac function.

The decrease in cardiac performance caused by progressive left ventricular systolic dysfunction evokes a series of neurohumoral changes that initially compensate, but ultimately further compromise the heart. Catecholamine release, *via* activation of the sympathetic nervous system, represents an attempt to maintain cardiac output, but later increase myocardial oxygen consumption and eventually lead to further cardiac dysfunction. In addition, increases in angiotensin II level through activation of the RAAS can result in myocardial necrosis and apoptosis as a consequence of vasoconstriction or a direct effect on cardiac myocytes [112]. Several studies have linked these effector hormones with mortality and poor prognosis in patients with severe chronic heart failure CHF [113].

The results of the CONSENSUS trial proved that ACE inhibitors significantly reduce both morbidity and mortality in patients with severe CHF [114].

In addition to vasodilatation, the mechanism by which ACE inhibitors reduce morbidity and mortality seems to relate to suppression of neurohumoral factors (*i.e.*, angiotensin II, norepinephrine). This hypothesis is supported by the finding that enalapril further improved survival compared with the combination of hydralazine and isosorbide dinitrate in the Second Veterans Administration Cooperative Vasodilator-Heart Failure Trial II (V-HeFT II).

In severe CHF refractory to conventional therapy, high doses of loop diuretics are used to overcome diuretic resistance [115]. However, this is commonly associated with marked increases in circulating renin levels, which promotes a sodium retentive state, both through a proximal tubular action of angiotensin II [116] and a distal tubular action of aldosterone. Association of an ACE inhibitor limits the development of diuretic resistance.

In the Studies of Left Ventricular Dysfunction (SOLVD) Trials and Registry, diabetes was found to be an independent risk factor for mortality and morbidity in both symptomatic and asymptomatic heart failure [117]. A retrospective analysis on patients enrolled in the SOLVD trials show that enalapril reduces the risk to develop diabetes mellitus in patients with left ventricular dysfunction. With an absolute risk reduction of 16.5%, it is necessary to treat 6 patients with left ventricular dysfunction with enalapril for 2.9 years to prevent one new case of diabetes. This beneficial effect is even more striking in patients with impaired fasting plasma glucose [118].

ALDOSTERONE – THE LAST LINK

The last link to bind the diabetic patient to cardiologist, in terms of RAAS involvement is aldosterone [119]. Identification of aldosterone receptors not only in the kidney, but throughout the body, including vasculature and heart led to a sticking amount of research. Important effects of aldosterone on the cardiovascular system were discovered. Aldosterone promotes vascular inflammation and perivascular fibrosis, synergizes with Ang II in inducing PAI-1 expression and has a significant pro-oxidative role in the pathogenesis of atherosclerosis. It promotes heart remodeling by myocyte hypertrophy and interstitial and perivascular fibrosis of the myocardium [120, 121].

In diabetic patients, as it was already discussed elsewhere in this paper, there is an important overstimulation of the RAAS, leading not only to high levels of Ang II and low levels of BK, but also to an increased aldosterone activity. New data suggest that age-related alterations in telomere length could influence age-dependent expression of genes leading to hypertension and hyperaldosteronism, most commonly encountered in individuals with diabetes mellitus.

Recent studies have examined the effect of aldosterone blockade in the prevention of recurrent heart failure and survival of patients with severe CHF (spironolactone – RALES) or in post myocardial infarction heart failure survivals (eplerenone – EPHESUS).

RALES, Randomized Aldactone Evaluation Study, was the first clinical trial to examine the effect of spironolactone on morbidity and mortality [122]. Patients with NYHA class III-IV CHF and ejection fractions < 35% were randomized to receive either a low dose of spironolactone (25 mg/d) or placebo. Patients continued to receive their pre-existing drug regimens, including an ACE inhibitor and a loop diuretic, with or without digitalis. Ten percent of placebo-treated and 11% of spironolactone-treated patients also received a β-blocker. The Data and Safety Monitoring Board recommended early termination of the trial after only 24 months, when an interim analysis revealed that mortality was significantly reduced by spironolactone. Patients treated with spironolactone had a 30% reduction in the risk of death from all causes (P < 0.001) and a 31% reduction in the risk of death from cardiac causes. Spironolactone also had a positive effect on morbidity, with a significant improvement in NYHA functional class compared to placebo (P < 0.001).

EPHESUS (Eplerenone Postacute Myocardial Infarction Heart Failure Efficacy and Survival Study) evaluates successfully the role of aldosterone antagonism early in the course of heart failure[123, 124]. At a mean dose of 43 mg once daily, eplerenone reduced total mortality by 15%, cardio-vascular mortality/cardiovascular hospitalizations by 13%, cardiovascular mortality by 17%, sudden cardiac death by 21%, total mortality/total hospitalization by 8%, and episodes of hospitalization for heart failure by 23%. These effects were relatively consistent across a number of predefined subsets.

COULD RAAS INHIBITION PROVIDE DIABETES PRIMARY PREVENTION?

The mechanisms by which ACE inhibition exerts its protective effect against diabetes are not completely understood. ACE inhibitors not only block the conversion of angiotensin I to angiotensin II, but also increase bradykinin levels through inhibition of kinase II-mediated degradation. In animals, it was described improved insulin sensitivity with some angiotensin converting enzyme inhibitors through an increase in endogenous kinins. The higher kinin level leads to increased production of prostaglandins and nitric oxide, which improve muscle sensitivity to insulin and exercise induced glucose metabolism, resulting in enhanced insulin-mediated glucose uptake. Furthermore, the peripheral vasodilatory actions of ACE inhibitors (through diverse mechanisms, including prostaglandin and nitric oxide) lead to an improvement in skeletal muscle blood flow, the primary target of insulin action and an important determinant of glucose uptake. Clinical evidence supporting this effect has been recently provided by analyzing retrospectively a subgroup of obese, hypertensive, and dyslipidemic patients who have shown improved insulin sensitivity with enalapril in SOLVD Study. A similar effect has been reported with captopril. Finally, ACE inhibitors inhibit the vasoconstrictive effect of angiotensin II in the pancreas and increase islet blood flow [8], which could improve insulin release by β-cells. These experimental and clinical studies suggest that ACE inhibition increases insulin sensitivity, skeletal muscle glucose transport and pancreatic blood flow, which probably all contribute to the prevention of diabetes mellitus.

To resume, the principal mechanisms experimentally proved to ameliorate glucose metabolism through RAAS modulation, either by ACE inhibition or by AT1 receptor antagonism are:

1. enhancement of glucose uptake by improvement of skeletal muscle blood flow;

2. enhancement of insulin production by increase in pancreatic islet blood flow;

3. reduction in A II-induced sympathetic drive, with consecutive glycemia reduction;

4. diminution in lipolysis and FFA release, inducing an increase in energetic glucose consumption;

5. adiponectin-induced promotion of adipocyte recruitment and differentiation, counteracting the ectopic deposition of lipids;

6. reduction in intracellular AT 1 receptor signaling, with less protein-kinase Cα induced phosphorylation of Insulin Receptor Signal-1 (IRS-1), upregulation of insulin receptor and reduction in insulin resistance.

All these data suggest that ACE inhibitors may lower the risk of developing diabetes, but the final proof comes from large clinical trials. In the HOPE study, significantly fewer patients in the ramipril group than in the placebo group had a new diagnosis of diabetes (102 *vs.*155; relative risk 0.66; P < 0.001), or complications related to diabetes (299 *vs.* 354; relative risk 0.84; P = 0.03) [5]. Angiotensin II AT_1 receptor blockers showed the same effect. In the LIFE study losartan compared to atenolol in 9193 patients over 4.8 years reduced new-onset diabetes (241 *vs.* 319; relative risk reduction 25%; P = 0.001) [7].

Another problem is appropriate RAAS inhibition regimens used to treat diabetic patients with cardiovascular diseases, to prevent disease progression and to interrupt the chain of events that leads from risk factors to end-stage cardiac disease [125].

REFFERENCES

1. King H, Aubert RE, Herman WH. Global burden of diabetes, 1995–2025: prevalence, numerical estimates, and projections. *Diabetes Care,* **21:** 1414–1431, 1998.
2. Ruiz-Ortega M, Lorenzo O, Ruperez M, Esteban V, Suzuki Y, Mezzano S, Plaza JJ, Egido J. Role of the renin-angiotensin system in vascular diseases: expanding the field. *Hypertension,* **38:** 1382–1387, 2001.
3. Taubman MB. Angiotensin II A Vasoactive Hormone With Ever-Increasing Biological Roles. *Circulation Research,* **92:** 9, 2003.
4. Vermes E, Ducharme A, Bourassa GM, Lessard M, White M, Tardif JC. Enalapril Reduces the Incidence of Diabetes in Patients With Chronic Heart Failure. Insight From the Studies Of Left Ventricular Dysfunction (SOLVD). *Circulation,* **107:** 1291, 2003.
5. Yusuf S, Sleight P, Pogue J, *et al.* for the Heart Outcomes Prevention Evaluation Study Investigators. Effects of an angiotensin-converting enzyme inhibitor, ramipril, on cardiovascular events in high-risk patients. *N Engl J Med ,* **342:** 145–153, 2000.
6. Hansson L, Lindholm LH, Niskanen L *et al.* Effect of angiotensin-converting-enzyme inhibition compared with conventional therapy on cardiovascular morbidity and mortality in hypertension: the Captopril Prevention Project (CAPP) randomised trial. *Lancet,* **353:** 611–616, 1999.
7. Dahlöf B, Devereux RB, Kjeldsen SE, *et al.* Cardiovascular morbidity and mortality in the Losartan Intervention For Endpoint reduction in hypertension study (LIFE): a randomised trial against atenolol. *Lancet,* **359:** 995–1003, 2002.
8. Carlsson PO, Berne C, Jansson L. Angiotensin II and the endocrine pancreas: effects on islet blood flow and insulin secretion in rats. *Diabetologia,* **41:** 127–133, 1998.
9. Engeli S, Gorzelniak K, Kreutz R, Runkel N, Distler A, Sharma AM. Co-expression of renin-angiotensin system genes in human adipose tissue. *J Hypertens,* **17:** 555–560, 1999.
10. Williams GH, Dluhy RG. Diseases of the adrenal cortex. In Braunwald E, Fauci AS, Kasper D, *et al.* (eds). Harrison's Principles of Internal Medicine, 15th ed. New York, McGraw-Hill, 2001, pp 2084–2105.
11. Baxter JD, Dunkin K, Chu W, *et al.* Molecular biology of human renin gene. *Recent Prog Horm Res,* **47:** 211–257, 1991.
12. Gaillard-Sanchez I, Mattei MG, Clauser E, *et al.* Assignment by in situ hybridization of angiotensinogen to chromosome band 1q42: the same region as human renin gene. *Hum Genet,* **84:** 341–343, 1990.
13. Bernstein KE, Shai SY, Howard T, *et al.* Structure and regulated expression of angiotensin-converting enzyme and the receptor for angiotensin II. *Am J Kidney Dis,* **21(4 suppl 1):** 53–57, 1993.
14. Corvol P, Michaud A, Soubrier F, *et al.* Recent advances in knowledge of the structure and function of the angiotensin I converting enzyme. *J Hypertens,* **13:** S3–S10, 1995.
15. Georgiadis D, Beau F, Czarny B, Cotton J, Yiotakis A, Dive V. Roles of the Two Active Sites of Somatic Angiotensin-Converting Enzyme in the Cleavage of Angiotensin I and Bradykinin. Insights From Selective Inhibitors. *Circ Res,* **93:**148, 2003.
16. Timmermans PB, Wong PC, Chiu AT, *et al.* Angiotensin II receptors and angiotensin II receptor antagonists. *Pharmacol Rev,* **45:** 205–251, 1993.
17. Shibata T, Suzuki C, Ohnishi J, *et al.* Identification of regions in the human angiotensin II receptor type 1 responsible for Gi and Gq coupling by mutagenesis study. *Biochem Biophys Res Commun,* **218:** 383–389, 1996.
18. Tsuzuki S, Ichiki T, Nakakubo H, *et al.* Molecular cloning and expression of the gene encoding human angiotensin II type 2 receptor. *Biochem Biophys Res Commun,* **200:** 1449–1454, 1994.
19. Nahmias C, Strosberg AD. The angiotensin AT2 receptor: searching for signal-transduction pathways and physiological function. *Trends Pharmacol Sci,* **16:** 223–225, 1995.
20. Wright JW, Harding JW. Brain angiotensin receptor subtypes AT1, AT2, and AT4 and their functions. *Regul Pept,* **59:** 269–295, 1995.
21. Hall KL, Venkateswaran S, Hanesworth JM, *et al.* Characterization of a functional angiotensin IV receptor on coronary microvascular endothelial cells. *Regul Pept,* **58:** 107–115, 1995.
22. Benter IF, Ferrario CM, Morris M, *et al.* Antihypertensive actions of angiotensin (1–7) in spontaneously hypertensive rats. *Am J Physiol,* **269:** H313–H319, 1995.
23. Paul M, Wagner J, Dzau VJ. Gene expression of the renin-angiotensin system in human tissues: quantitative analysis by the polymerase chain reaction. *J Clin Invest,* **91:** 2058–2064, 1993.

24. Harp JB, DiGirolamo M. Components of the renin-angiotensin system in adipose tissue: changes with maturation and adipose mass enlargement. *J Gerontol A Biol Sci Med Sci,* **50:** 270–276, 1995.

25. Boschmann M, Jordan J, Adams F, Christensen NJ, Tank J, Franke G, Stoffels M, Sharma AM, Luft FC, Klaus S. Tissue-Specific Response to Interstitial Angiotensin II in Humans. *Hypertension,* **41:** 37, 2003.

26. Inagami T, *et al.* Molecular biology of angiotensin II receptors: an overview. *J Hypertens,* **12:** S83–S94, 1994.

27. Tian Y, Balla T, Baukal AJ, *et al.* Growth responses to angiotensin II in bovine adrenal glomerulosa cells. *Am J Physiol,* **268:** E135–E144, 1995.

28. Cox BE, Word RA, Rosenfeld CR. Angiotensin II receptor characteristics and subtype expression in uterine arteries and myometrium during pregnancy. *Endocrinology,* **81:** 49–58, 1996.

29. Geisterfer AA, Peach MJ, Owens GK. Angiotensin II induces hypertrophy, not hyperplasia, of cultured rat aortic smooth muscle cells. *Circ Res,* **62:** 749–756, 1988.

30. Berk BC, Vekshtein V, Gordon HM, Tsuda T. Angiotensin II-stimulated protein synthesis in cultured vascular smooth muscle cells. *Hypertension,* **13:** 305–314, 1989.

31. Naftilan AJ. The role of angiotensin II in vascular smooth muscle cell growth. *J Cardiovasc Pharmacol,* **20(suppl 1):** S37–S40, 1992.

32. Vaughan DE, Lazos SA, Tong K. Angiotensin II regulates the expression of plasminogen activator inhibitor-1 in cultured endothelial cells: a potential link between the renin-angiotensin system and thrombosis. *J Clin Invest,* **95:** 995–1001, 1995.

33. Brown NJ, Agirbasli MA, Williams GH, *et al.* Effect of activation and inhibition of the renin-angiotensin system on plasma PAI-1. *Hypertension,* **32:** 965–971, 1998.

34. Vaughan DE, Rouleau J-L, Ridker PM *et al.* Effects of ramipril on plasma fibrinolytic balance in patients with acute myocardial infarction. *Circulation,* **96:** 442–447, 1997.

35. Berk BC, Corson MA. Angiotensin II signal transduction in vascular smooth muscle: role of tyrosine kinases. *Circ Res,* **80:** 607–616, 1997.

36. Griendling KK, Ushio-Fukai M, Lassegue B, Alexander RW. Angiotensin II signaling in vascular smooth muscle: new concepts. *Hypertension,* **29:** 366–373, 1997.

37. Zhang C, Hein T W, Wang W, Kuo L. Divergent Roles of Angiotensin II AT1 and AT2 Receptors in Modulating Coronary Microvascular Function. *Circ Res,* **92:** 322, 2003.

38. Phillips MI, Kagiyama S. Angiotensin II as a pro-inflammatory mediator. *Curr Opin Investig Drugs,* **3:** 569–577, 2002.

39. Weber KT. Hormones and fibrosis: a case for lost reciprocal regulation. *News Physiol Sci,* **9:** 123–8, 1994.

40. Weber KT, Swamynathan SK, Guntaka RV, Sun Y. Angiotensin II and extracellular matrix homeostasis. *Int J Biochem Cell Biol,* **31:** 395–403, 1999.

41. Dzau VJ. Mechanisms of protective effects of ACE inhibition on coronary artery disease. *Eur Heart J,* **19:** J2–J6, 1998.

42. Weber KT. Angiotensin II and connective tissue: homeostasis and reciprocal regulation. *Regul Pept,* **82:** 1–17, 1999.

43. Brasier AR, Recinos A 3rd, Eledrisi MS. Vascular Inflammation and the Renin-Angiotensin System. *Arterioscler Thromb Vasc Biol,* **22:** 1257, 2002.

44. Scholkens BA, Landgraf W. ACE inhibition and atherogenesis. *Internist,* **42:** 1219–1225, 2001.

45. Haffner SM, Lehto S, Ronnemaa T, *et al.* Mortality from coronary heart disease in subjects with type 2 diabetes and in nondiabetic subjects with and without prior myocardial infarction. *N Engl J Med,* **339:** 229–234, 1998.

46. The BARI Investigators. Influence of diabetes on 5-year mortality and morbidity in a randomized trial comparing CABG and PTCA in patients with multivessel disease. The Bypass Angioplasty Revascularization Investigation (BARI). *Circulation,* **96:** 1761–1769, 1997.

47. Islam MA, Blankenship JC, Balog C, *et al,* for the EPISTENT Investigators. Effect of abciximab on angiographic complications during percutaneous coronary stenting in the Evaluation of Platelet IIb/IIIa Inhibition in Stenting Trial (EPISTENT). *Am J Cardiol,* **90:** 916–921, 2002.

48. Bohannon NJV. Coronary artery disease and diabetes. *Postgrad Med,* **105:** 66–80, 1999.

49. GarberAJ. Cardiovascular Complications of Diabetes: Prevention and Management. *Clin Cornerstone,* **5(2):** 22–37, 2003.

50. Ross R. Atherosclerosis: an inflammatory disease. *N Engl J Med,* **340:** 115–126, 1999.

51. Johnstone MT, Craeger SJ, Scales KM, *et al.* Impaired endothelium dependent vasodilatation in patients with insulin-dependant diabetes mellitus. *Circulation,* **88:** 2510–2516, 1993.

52. Mancini GBH, Henry GC, Macaya C, *et al.* Angiotensin-converting enzyme inhibition with quinapril improves endothelial vasomotor dysfunction in patients with coronary artery disease. The TREND (trial on reversing endothelial dysfunction) study. *Circulation,* **94:** 258–265, 1996.

53. Anderson TJ, Elstein E, Haber H, *et al.* Comparative study of ACE-inhibition, angiotensin II antagonism, and calcium channel blockade on flow mediated vasodilation in patients with coronary disease (BANFF study). *J Am Coll Cardiol,* **35:** 60–66, 2000.

54. Oosterga M, Voors AA, Veeger JGM, *et al.* Beneficial effects of quinapril on ischemia in coronary bypass surgery patients: one-year clinical follow-up of the QUO VADIS study. *Circulation,* 99: 2486–2491, 1999.

55. Wagenknecht LE, Zaccaro D, Espeland MA, Karter AJ, O'Leary DH, Haffner SM. Diabetes and Progression of Carotid Atherosclerosis. The Insulin Resistance Atherosclerosis Study. *Arterioscler Thromb Vasc Biol,* 23: 1035, 2003.

56. Cipollone F, Iezzi A, Fazia M, Zucchelli M, Pini B, Cuccurullo C, De Cesare D, *et al.* The Receptor RAGE as a Progression Factor Amplifying Arachidonate-Dependent Inflammatory and Proteolytic Response in Human Atherosclerotic Plaques. Role of Glycemic Control. *Circulation,* 108: 1070, 2003.

57. Gerstein HC. Is glucose a continuous risk factor for cardiovascular mortality? *Diabetes Care,* 22: 659–660, 1999.

58. The effect of intensive treatment of diabetes on the development and progression of long-term complications in insulin-dependent diabetes mellitus: the Diabetes Control and Complications Trial Research Group. *N Engl J Med,* 329: 977–986, 1993.

59. Haffner SM, Hanley AJG. Do Increased Proinsulin Concentrations Explain the Excess Risk of Coronary Heart Disease in Diabetic and Prediabetic Subjects? *Circulation,* 105: 2008, 2002.

60. Folli F, Saad MJA, Velloso L, Hansen H, Caradente O, Feener EP, Kahn CR. Crosstalk between insulin and angiotensin II signaling systems. *Exp Clin Endocrinol Diabetes,* 107: 133–139, 1999.

61. Ogihara T, Asano T, Ando K, Chiba Y, Sakoda H, *et al.* Angiotensin II–Induced Insulin Resistance Is Associated With Enhanced Insulin Signaling. *Hypertension,* 40: 872, 2002.

62. Bloomgarden ZT. American Association of Clinical Endocrinologists (AACE) Consensus Conference on the Insulin Resistance Syndrome: 25–26 August 2002, Washington, DC. *Diabetes Care,* 26(4): 1297–1303, 2003.

63. Hanefeld M, Koehler C, Fuecker K, Henkel E, Schaper F, Temelkova-Kurktschiev T. Insulin Secretion and Insulin Sensitivity Pattern Is Different in Isolated Impaired Glucose Tolerance and Impaired Fasting Glucose: The Risk Factor in Impaired Glucose Tolerance for Atherosclerosis and Diabetes Study. *Diabetes Care,* 26(3): 868 – 874, 2003.

64. Hong Y, Pedersen NL, Brismar K, de Faire U. Genetic and environmental architecture of the features of the insulin-resistance syndrome. *Am J Hum Genet,* 60: 143–152, 1997.

65. Jansson PA, Pellmé F, Hammarstedt A, Sandqvist M, *et al.* A novel cellular marker of insulin resistance and early atherosclerosis in humans is related to impaired fat cell differentiation and low adiponectin. *FASEB J,* 17: 1434–1440, 2003.

66. Sharma A, Janke J, Gorzelniak K, Engeli S, Luft F. Angiotensin Blockade Prevents Type 2 Diabetes by Formation of Fat Cells. *Hypertension,* 40: 609, 2002.

67. Verma S, Li SH, Wang CH, Fedak PWM, Li RK, Weisel RD, Mickle DAG. Resistin Promotes Endothelial Cell Activation. Further Evidence of Adipokine-Endothelial Interaction. *Circulation,* 108: 736, 2003.

68. Furuhashi M, Ura N, Higashiura K, *et al.* Blockade of the Renin-Angiotensin System Increases Adiponectin Concentrations in Patients With Essential Hypertension. *Hypertension,* 42: 76, 2003.

69. 1999 World Health Organization – International Society of Hypertension Guidelines for the Management of Hypertension. *J Hypertens,* 17: 151–183, 1999.

70. 2003 European Society of Hypertension – European Society of Cardiology Guidelines for the management of arterial hypertension. *J Hypertens,* 21: 1011–1053, 2003.

71. The Seventh Report of the Joint National Committee on Prevention, Detection, Evaluation, and Treatment of High Blood Pressure: the JNC 7 Report. *JAMA,* 289: 2560–2572, 2003.

72. Kottke TE, Stroebel EJ, Hoffman RS. JNC 7 – It's more than High Blood Pressure. *JAMA,* 289: 2573–2575, 2003.

73. Levy J, Gavin JR III, Hammerman MR, *et al.* Ca^{2+} + Mg^{2+} ATPase activity in kidney basolateral membrane in non insulin dependent diabetic rats: effect of insulin. *Diabetes,* 35: 899–905, 1986.

74. Draznin B, Lewis D, Houlder N, *et al.* Mechanism of insulin resistance induced by sustained levels of cytosolic free calcium in rat adipocytes. *Endocrinology,* 125: 2341–2349, 1989.

75. Draznin B, Sussman KE, Eckel RH, *et al.* Possible role of cytosolic free calcium concentrations in mediating insulin resistance of obesity and hyperinsulinemia. *J Clin Invest,* 28: 1848–1852, 1988.

76. Anderson EA, Hoffman RP, Balon TW, *et al.* Hyperinsulinemia produces both sympathetic neural activation and vasodilation in normal humans. *J Clin Invest,* 84: 2246–2252, 1991.

77. DeFronzo RA, Cooke CR, Adres R, *et al.* The effect of insulin on renal handling of sodium, potassium, calcium and phosphate in man. *J Clin Invest,* 55: 845–855, 1975.

78. Hollenberg NK, Raij L. Angiotensin-converting enzyme inhibition and renal protection: an assessment of implications for therapy. *Arch Intern Med,* 153: 2426–2435, 1993.

79. Lewis EJ, Hunsicker LG, Bain RP, *et al.* The effect of angiotensin-converting enzyme inhibition in diabetic nephropathy. The Collaborative Study Group. *N Engl J Med,* **329:** 456–462, 1993.

80. Maschio C, Alberti D, Janin G, *et al.* Effect of the angiotensin-converting-enzyme inhibitor benazepril on the progression of chronic renal insufficiency. The Angiotensin-Converting-Enzyme Inhibition in Progressive Renal Insufficiency Study Group. *N Engl J Med,* **334:** 939–945, 1996.

81. Albers FJ. Clinical characteristics of atherosclerotic renovascular disease. *Am J Kidney Dis,* **24:** 636–641, 1994.

82. UK Prospective Diabetes Study (UKPDS) Group. Tight blood pressure control and risk of macrovascular and microvascular complications in type 2 diabetes: UKPDS 38. *BMJ,* **317:** 703–713, 1998. [Erratum, *BMJ,* **318:** 29, 1999]

83. Hansson L, Zanchetti A, Carruthers SG, *et al.* Effects of intensive blood-pressure lowering and low-dose aspirin in patients with hypertension: principal results of the Hypertension Optimal Treatment (HOT) randomised trial. *Lancet,* **351:** 1755–1762, 1998.

84. Staessen JA, Fagard R, Thijs L, *et al.* Randomised double-blind comparison of placebo and active treatment for older patients with isolated systolic hypertension. *Lancet,* **350:** 757–764, 1997.

85. Curb JD, Pressel SL, Cutler JA, *et al.* Effect of diuretic-based antihypertensive treatment on cardiovascular disease risk in older diabetic patients with isolated systolic hypertension. *JAMA,* **276:** 1886–1892, 1996. [Erratum, *JAMA,* **277:** 1356, 1997]

86. The Heart Outcome Prevention Evaluation Study Investigators. Effects of ramipril on cardiovascular and microvascular outcomes in people with diabetes; results of the HOPE study and the MICRO-HOPE substudy. *Lancet,* **355:** 253–259, 2000.

87. Brenner BM, Cooper ME, deZeeuw D, *et al.* Effects of losartan on renal and cardiovascular outcomes in patients with type 2 diabetes and nephropathy. *N Engl J Med,* **345:** 861–869, 2001.

88. Rodby RA, Rohde RD, Clarke WR, *et al.* The irbesartan type II diabetic nephropathy trial: study design and baseline patient characteristics. *Nephrol Dial Transplant,* **15:** 487–497, 2000.

89. Parving HH, Lehnert H, Brochner-Mortensen J, *et al.* The effect of irbesartan on the development of diabetic nephropathy in patients with type 2 diabetes. *N Engl J Med,* **345:** 870–878, 2001.

90. Viberti G, Wheeldon NM. MicroAlbuminuria Reduction with VALsartan (MARVAL) Study Investigators. Microalbuminuria reduction with valsartan in patients with type 2 diabetes mellitus: a blood pressure-independent effect. *Circulation,* **106(6):** 672–8, 2002.

91. Mogensen CE, Neldam S, Tikkanen I, *et al,* for the CALM Study Group. Randomised controlled trial of dual blockade of renin-angiotensin system in patients with hypertension, microalbuminuria, and non-insulin dependent diabetes: The Candesartan and Lisinopril Micro-albuminuria (CALM) study. *BMJ,* **321:** 1440–1444, 2000.

92. Sowers JR. Hypertension in type 2 diabetes: update on therapy. *Cardiovasc Rev Rep,* **23:** 41–46, 2002.

93. Stamler J, Vaccaro O, Neaton JD, Wentworth D. Diabetes, other risk factors, and 12-yr cardiovascular mortality for men screened in the Multiple Risk Factor Intervention Trial. *Diabetes Care,* **16:** 434–444, 1993.

94. Pyörälä K, Pedersen TR, Kjekshus J, Færgeman O, Olsson AG, Thorgeirsson G. Cholesterol lowering with simvastatin improves prognosis of diabetic patients with coronary heart disease: a subgroup analysis of the Scandinavian Simvastatin Survival Study (4S). *Diabetes Care,* **20:** 614–620, 1997. [Erratum, *Diabetes Care,* **20:** 1048, 1997.]

95. Sacks FM, Pfeffer MA, Moye LA, *et al.* The effect of pravastatin on coronary events after myocardial infarction in patients with average cholesterol levels. *N Engl J Med,* **335:** 1001–1009, 1996.

96. The Long-Term Intervention with Pravastatin in Ischaemic Disease (LIPID) Study Group. Prevention of cardiovascular events and death with pravastatin in patients with coronary heart disease and a broad range of initial cholesterol levels. *N Engl J Med,* **339:** 1349–1357, 1998.

97. Heart Protection Study Collaborative Group. MRC/BHF Heart Protection Study of cholesterol lowering with simvastatin in 20 536 high-risk individuals: a randomised placebo-controlled trial. *Lancet,* **360:** 7–22, 2002.

98. Sever PS, Dahlof B, Poulter NR, *et al,* for the ASCOT investigators. Prevention of coronary and stroke events with atorvastatin in hypertensive patients who have average or lower-than-average cholesterol concentrations, in the Anglo-Scandinavian Cardiac Outcomes Trial – Lipid Lowering Arm (ASCOT-LLA): a multicenter randomized controlled trial. *Lancet,* **361:** 1149–1158, 2003.

99. Gaede P, Vedel P, Larsen N, Jensen GVH, Parving HH, Pedersen O. Multifactorial Intervention and Cardiovascular Disease in Patients with Type 2 Diabetes. *N Engl J Med,* **348:** 383–393, 2003.

100. Grundy SM. The National Cholesterol Education Program (NCEP)-The National Cholesterol Guidelines in 2001, Adult Treatment Panel (ATP) III. Approach to lipoprotein management in 2001 National Cholesterol Guidelines. *Am J Cardiol,* **90:** 11i–21i, 2002.

101. Ridker PM, Buring JE, Cook N, Rifai N. C-Reactive Protein, the Metabolic Syndrome, and Risk of Incident Cardiovascular Events. An 8-Year Follow-Up of 14719 Initially Healthy American Women. *Circulation,* **107:** 391, 2003.

102. Juhan-Vague I, Alessi MC, Morange PE. Hypofibrinolysis and increased PAI-1 are linked to atherothrombosis via insulin resistance and obesity. *Ann Med,* **32(suppl 1):** 78–84, 2000.

103. Fujii S, Goto D, Zaman T, *et al.* Diminished fibrinolysis and thrombosis: clinical implications for accelerated atherosclerosis. *J Atheroscler Thromb,* **5:** 76–81, 1998.

104. Sobel BE. The potential influence of insulin and plasminogen activator inhibitor type 1 on the formation of vulnerable atherosclerotic plaques associated with type 2 diabetes. *Proc Assoc Am Physicians,* **111:** 313–318, 1999.

105. Festa A, D'Agostino R Jr, Mykkanen L, *et al.* Relative contribution of insulin and its precursors to fibrinogen and PAI-1 in a large population with different states of glucose tolerance. The Insulin Resistance Atherosclerosis Study (IRAS). *Arterioscler Thromb Vasc Biol,* **19:** 562–568, 1999.

106. Kannel WB, Hjortland M, Castelli WP. Role of diabetes in congestive heart failure: the Framingham Study. *Am J Cardiol,* **34:** 29–34, 1974.

107. Vlassara H. Recent progress in advanced glycosylation end-products and diabetic complications. *Diabetes,* **46:** S19–S25, 1997.

108. Brownlee M. Glycation and diabetic complications. *Diabetes,* **43:** 836–841, 1994.

109. Frustaci A, Kajstura J, Chimenti C, *et al.* Myocardial cell death in human diabetes. *Circ Res,* **8:** 1123–1132, 2000.

110. Tan LB, Jalil JE, Pick R, *et al.* Cardiac myocyte necrosis induced by angiotensin II. *Circ Res,* **69:** 1185–1195, 1991.

111. Privratsky J, Wold L, Sowers J, Quinn M, Ren J. AT1 Blockade Prevents Glucose-Induced Cardiac Dysfunction in Ventricular Myocytes. Role of the AT1 Receptor and NADPH Oxidase. *Hypertension,* **42:** 206, 2003.

112. Swedberg K, Eneroth P, Kjekshus J, *et al.* Hormones regulating cardiovascular function in patients with severe congestive heart failure and their relation to mortality. *Circulation,* **82:** 1730–1736, 1990.

113. Swedberg K, Eneroth P, Kjekshus J, *et al,* for the CONSENSUS Trial Study Group. Effects of enalapril and neuroendocrine activation on prognosis in severe congestive heart failure (Follow-up of the CONSENSUS trial). *Am J Cardiol,* **66:** 40D–45D, 1990.

114. The CONSENSUS Trial Study Group. Effects of enalapril on mortality in severe congestive heart failure: results of the Cooperative North Scandinavian Enalapril Survival Study (CONSENSUS). *N Engl J Med,* **316:** 1429–1435, 1987.

115. Gerlag PG, Van Meyel JJ. High-dose furosemide in the treatment of refractory congestive heart failure. *Arch Intern Med,* **148:** 286–291, 1988.

116. Cogan MG. Angiotensin II: a powerful controller of sodium transport in the early proximal tubule. *Hypertension,* **15:** 451–458, 1990.

117. Shindler DM, Kostis JB, Yusuf S, Quinones MA, Pitt B, Stewart D, Pinkett T, Ghali JK, Wilson AC. Diabetes mellitus, a predictor of morbidity and mortality in the Studies of Left Ventricular Dysfunction (SOLVD) Trials and Registry. *Am J Cardiol,* **77:** 1017–1020, 1996.

118. Vermes E, Ducharme A, Bourassa GM, Lessard M, White M, Tardif JC. Enalapril Reduces the Incidence of Diabetes in Patients With Chronic Heart Failure. Insight From the Studies Of Left Ventricular Dysfunction (SOLVD). *Circulation,* **107:** 1291, 2003.

119. Delcayre C, Silvestre JS, Garnier A, *et al.* Cardiac aldosterone production and ventricular remodeling. *Kidney Int,* **57:** 1346–1351, 2000.

120. Weber KT, Gerling IC, Kiani MF, Guntaka RV, Sun Y, Ahokas RA, Postlethwaite AE, Warrington KJ. Aldosteronism in heart failure: a proinflammatory / fibrogenic cardiac phenotype. Search for biomarkers and potential drug targets. *Curr Drug Targets,* **4(6):** 505–16, 2003.

121. Brown NJ, Kim KS, Chen YQ, *et al.* Synergistic effect of adrenal steroids and angiotensin II on plasminogen activator inhibitor-1 production. *J Clin Endocrinol Metab,* **85:** 336–344, 2000.

122. Pitt B, Zannad F, Remme W, *et al,* for the RALES Investigators. The effect of spironolactone on morbidity and mortality in patients with severe heart failure. *N Engl J Med,* **341:** 709–717, 1999.

123. Stier C Jr, Koenig S, Lee D, Chawla M, Frishman W. Aldosterone and Aldosterone Antagonism in Cardiovascular Disease: Focus on Eplerenone (Inspra). *Heart Dis,* **5(2):** 102–118, 2003.

124. Salam AM. Selective aldosterone blockade with eplerenone in patients with congestive heart failure. *Expert Opin Investig Drugs,* **12(8):** 1423–7, 2003.

125. Ghosh J, Weissm M, Kay R, Frishman W. Diabetes Mellitus and Coronary Artery Disease. Therapeutic Considerations. *Heart Dis,* **5(2):** 119–128, 2003.

20

THE INVOLVEMENT OF AUTONOMIC NEUROPATHY IN CARDIOVASCULAR FUNCTION IN DIABETES MELLITUS

Ioana Maria BRUCKNER, Mihaela Victoria VLĂICULESCU, Anca Maria NEGRILĂ

Neuropathy is well defined as a distinct entity in the diabetic patient. Although in the past clinicians focused on peripheral sensitive diabetic neuropathy, in the latest years autonomic diabetic neuropathy has become an item more and more tackled in literature, as a frequent and severe complication of diabetes mellitus.

Alteration of sympathetic/ parasympathetic balance within the framework of diabetic neuropathy is associated with great morbidity and an unfavorable outcome, therefore early diagnosis and therapeutic intervention become compulsory.

Because cardiac autonomic neuropathy (CAN) associated symptoms are sometimes diverse and insensitive, and due to its important prognostic implications, sensible and specific diagnostic means are necessary.

The use of Ewing's battery of tests in current clinical practice allows early detection of CAN, also in asymptomatic stages. Other diagnostic means, as ECG and blood pressure monitoring or echocardiography, can be helpful, but their contribution to diagnosis is disputed for the time being.

Many prospective studies have demonstrated a high mortality among patients with CAN. The most important predictors are reduced heart rate variability (HRV) and the lengthening of QT interval (expression of ventricular repolarization changes). At the same time we must consider that the out of balance autonomic function could be due to ischemic heart disease, heart failure or other conditions, rising even more the risk of death.

Reaching a good metabolic control seems to be the most efficient method to prevent and to slow CAN progression. Some specific therapeutic means are used for the particular presentation of CAN.

Abbreviations List

ABPM – ambulatory blood pressure monitoring
AGE – advanced glycosylation end-product
BRS – baroreflex sensitivity
CAN – cardiac autonomic neuropathy
DAN – diabetic autonomic neuropathy
DM – diabetes mellitus
ECG – electrocardiogram
GLA – gamma linoleic acid

HRV – heart rate variability
GLA – gamma linoleic acid
ISA – intrinsic sympathetic activity
MIBG – metaiodobenzylguanidine
NO – nitric oxide
QTc – corrected QT
QTd – QT dispersion
PCK – proteinkinase C
SMI – silent myocardial ischemia

DIABETIC AUTONOMIC NEUROPATHY

INTRODUCTION, EPIDEMIOLOGY

Diabetic autonomic neuropathy (DAN) is one of the least recognized and understood complications of diabetes, which has come into the focus in recent years. Because of its association with adverse outcomes and its impact on the quality of life, cardiac autonomic neuropathy (CAN) is clinically one of the most important forms of diabetic autonomic neuropathy.

CAN is associated with a poor prognosis and may result in an increased incidence of silent myocardial infarction and ischemia, exercise intolerance, severe postural hypotension and enhanced intraoperative instability. Hence, early detection aimed at the prevention of advanced symptomatic stages of this complication is essential.

Although the impact of CAN is increasingly recognized, only little and contradictory information exists about its frequency in representative diabetic populations, the reported prevalence of CAN varying considerably among authors. The clinic-based DiaCAN Study has reported prevalence rates of definite CAN of 16.8% among 647 unselected type 1 diabetic patients and 22.1% in 524 type 2 diabetic patients attending clinics or outpatient diabetes centers. In 130 newly diagnosed type 1 diabetic patients the prevalence of definite CAN, reported by Ziegler *et al.* [1], was 9.2%. According to this study, CAN is not necessarily a late complication of diabetes. Nevertheless, other studies reported a prevalence as high as 90% of CAN in potential recipients of a pancreas transplant. Such variance of the prevalence depends on numerous factors such as whether the study was carried out in the community, clinics or tertiary referral centers or the type and number of the tests performed. Therefore, further studies to assess the real prevalence of autonomic dysfunction in the diabetic populations are needed.

PATHOGENESIS OF DIABETIC AUTONOMIC NEUROPATHY – A BRIEF REVIEW

Diabetic neuropathy implies a multifactorial and usually multifocal impairment of peripheral and autonomic nerves by a metabolic insult combined with neurovascular insufficiency.

The *metabolic* theory implies a complex chain of events involving glucose-induced activation of the polyol pathway, leading to accumulation of sorbitol and fructose in nerves, damaging them by an incompletely known mechanism. This is accompanied by myoinositol depletion, impaired protein kinase C (PKC) activity and reduced nerve Na/K-ATP-ase activity. All these can cause direct neural damage and decreased nerve blood flow. It has been demonstrated that impaired activity of Na/K-ATP-ase or increased activity of PKC leads to the up-regulation of the inflammatory cytokines interleukin-1β and tumor necrosis factor-α gene expression in mononuclear cells. Cytokines, in turn, can modulate the activity of Na/K-ATP-ase, closing the "circle".

Deficiencies of dihomo-γ-linoleic acid as well as the consequent decrease in prostanoid synthesis and reduced availability of N-acetyl-L-carnitine have also been implied in the development of neuropathy [2].

An activated polyol pathway may also disturb normal nerve function by oxidizing the NADPH/NADP+ and reducing the NADH/NAD+ redox couples, which leads to increased oxidative stress with increased free radical production, followed by vascular endothelium damage and reduced nitric oxide bioavailability.

High surrounding glucose levels will also result in protein glycation, followed by reactive oxygen species oxidation. This generates advanced glycosylation end-products (AGEs). Reactive oxygen species will further enhance AGEs formation, which, in turn, will accelerate AGEs formation, process known as autooxidative glycosylation.

Hormones are other factors contributing to cardiovascular complications, especially increased levels of insulin, an antiatherogenic factor, which loses its effects in insulin-resistant states. This, along with IFG I, IFG II and GH promote the proliferation of smooth muscle cells. A matter of debate is the role of angiotensin due to its properties, as treatment with its inhibitors was shown to lower the risk of nephropathy and, as a consequence, of cardiovascular complications.

The *vascular* hypothesis relies on studies suggesting that absolute or relative ischemia may exist in the nerves because of altered function of the endoneurial or epineurial blood vessels. Investigations on biopsy material from patients with neuropathy show graded structural changes in nerve microvasculature including basement membrane thickening, pericyte degeneration and endothelial cells hyperplasia [3]. There are also a number of functional disturbances like endothelial dysfunction, platelet activation, altered fibrinolysis and reduction in the expression of endothelial nitric oxide synthesis that have been demonstrated in the microvasculature of the nerves of diabetic patients [4].

Nitric oxide (NO) has been suggested as the potential bridge between the metabolic and the vascular theories. One of the actions of the cytokines mentioned above is the increase in activity of inducible nitric oxide synthesis. Excess nitric oxide production may result in formation of peroxynitrite and damage endothelium and neurons by a process referred to as nitrosative stress [5].

The autoimmune damage of the nerves by antibodies against nerve growth factors, sympathetic and parasympathetic ganglia, phospholipids and the reduction in neurohormonal growth factors may also be involved in the pathogenesis of DAN.

Nevertheless, we must emphasize that all the above-mentioned pathogenic mechanisms are better sustained by clinical studies for peripheral neuropathy. Pathological data and studies of autonomic tissue are limited and have not yet been adequately quantified.

PHYSIOPATHOLOGIC CONSIDERATIONS AND CLINICAL FEATURES OF CARDIOVASCULAR AUTONOMIC NEUROPATHY

Considering the presence or absence of clinical features, CAN can be divided into two:

1. *subclinical neuropathy*, which can be diagnosed only by tests, such as the classical Ewing battery, which is also called cardiovascular autonomic dysfunction;

2. *clinical neuropathy*, which presents typical symptoms and signs.

The clinical manifestations of CAN are often hard to recognize if you do not bear them in mind. It is said, "Awareness is the first step in

recognition". According to that, we tried to summarize the main clinical features of cardiovascular autonomic neuropathy:

– reduced heart rate variability, fixed heart rate;

– increased resting heart rate, sinus tachycardia;

– postural hypotension with systolic blood pressure fall $\geq$ 30 mmHg;

– increased mortality and predisposition to sudden death;

– increased prevalence of silent myocardial ischemia/infarction;

– reduced circadian variation of heart rate and blood pressure;

– hypersensitivity to α- and β-adrenergic agonists due to autonomic denervation;

– inadequate increase in heart rate and blood pressure with exercise;

– impaired left ventricular diastolic function / ejection fraction;

– intraoperative cardiovascular instability;

– QTc interval prolongation, increased QT dispersion.

HEART RATE CHANGES IN CAN

It has long been recognized that resting tachycardia and fixed heart rate are characteristic findings in diabetic patients with advanced CAN. The pathogenetic mechanism of these features has been elucidated by Ewing *et al.* in the early 1980s when they admitted that the parasympathetic involvement is the first event and the more severe one as compared to the sympathetic impairment. Others consider that both sympathetic and parasympathetic impairments occur early but with different degrees of intensity [6]. As soon as relative parasympathetic "failure" occurs, heart rate increases substantially, resting heart rates of 90–100 beats/min and occasionally heart rate increments up to 130 beats/min being observed in association with CAN. In time, heart rate may decline with increasing severity of sympathetic damage and therefore does not provide a reliable diagnostic criterion for CAN. This also happens to the patients with heart failure, in whom tachycardia is a compensatory hemodynamic response. Following the complete loss of autonomic control, heart rate stabilizes at a fixed level and remains unchanged consequently [7].

Resting tachycardia is not a benign phenomenon. It was demonstrated that it contributes to the progression of atherosclerosis by decreasing elasticity and distensibility of the vascular wall in the elastic arteries. In addition, animal studies have reported vascular degenerative changes, like increased coronary calcification, induced by tachycardia in arterial sites exposed to shear stress [8].

The above-mentioned hypothesis was also verified by epidemiological data. It seems that resting tachycardia clusters with other cardiovascular risk factors, especially those that are more common in the insulin resistance syndrome, like hypercholesterolemia, hypertriglyceridemia and the reduction of HDL-cholesterol levels. The follow-up analysis in the Framingham Study [9] also demonstrated a correlation between tachycardia at rest and cardiovascular mortality. Therefore, tachycardia must be considered an important cardiovascular risk factor.

The hallmark and earliest indicator of subclinical and symptomatic CAN is reduced heart rate variability (HRV) which can be detected using various noninvasive autonomic reflex tests. A fixed heart rate, defined as unresponsiveness to moderate exercise, stress or sleep indicates almost complete cardiac denervation.

The evaluation of heart rate variability is an important step in the management of diabetic patients, because a low and inflexible HRV seems to be associated with poor cardiovascular prognosis [10].

Recently, as a component of autonomic dysfunction, the neuropathic postural tachycardia syndrome has been described, characterized by chronic orthostatic symptoms along with a severe increase in heart rate occurring in orthostatism, but it does not involve orthostatic hypotension. Several lines of evidence indicate that this disorder may result from the sympathetic denervation of legs [11, 12].

POSTURAL HYPOTENSION

Postural hypotension is recognized as the clinical hallmark of CAN in diabetic patients, the relationship between postural hypotension and autonomic dysfunction being first suggested by Rundles in 1945 [13].

Although there is much debate regarding the diagnostic criteria, it is generally agreed that postural hypotension in diabetic patients is defined as a decrease in systolic blood pressure upon standing up of 30 mmHg or more.

From the clinical point of view, postural hypotension is characterized by weakness, fainting, dizziness, visual impairment and even syncope following the transition to the standing up posture. In some cases this complication may become disabling, but the blood pressure fall may also be asymptomatic. In their evolution, patients with diabetes have a great variability of the severity of postural hypotension; the cause of this fluctuation is unknown.

The pathophysiology of orthostatic hypotension is complex. The plasma norepinephrine response to standing up is variable. Thus, the majority of patients have a blunted response, which has been described as **hypoadrenergic postural hypotension**. This results in insufficient elevation of peripheral vascular resistance and limited changes in cardiac output; stroke volume is of secondary importance only.

There are also individuals who, in turn, may show a normal or even increased adrenergic response to standing up, which has been termed **hyperadrenergic postural hypotension** [14]. This pattern is not attributed to sympathetic neuropathy, but to intravascular volume depletion, associated with a substantially lower total red blood cells mass. This is often related to diabetic nephropathy and decreased erythropoietin secretion as a manifestation of renal autonomic denervation [15].

The renin system seems also involved in the pathogenesis of orthostatic hypotension. Several studies demonstrated the significant attenuation of the increase in plasma renin activity after standing up in patients with CAN. However, the underlying causes of these changes have not yet been elucidated. In addition to the role of sodium retention and reduced adrenergic activity, the importance of nephropathy is also debated.

It is important to emphasize that orthostatic symptoms can be easily misjudged as hypoglycemia, and the differentiation of severe orthostatic hypotension from syncope induced by insulin through severe hypoglycemia can be occasionally difficult.

Postural hypotension can be influenced by many factors. Fluid retention from any cause, for example, can alleviate the orthostatic blood pressure fall. Thus, improvement of this symptom can reflect a deterioration of renal function or a progression in ventricular dysfunction. On the other hand, postural hypotension can be aggravated by a number of drugs including vasodilators, diuretics, phenothiazines, tricyclic antidepressants, and in particular insulin. The diurnal variation of blood pressure is partially dependent on the timing of insulin administration. There are two ways by which insulin mediates hypotension: it increases capillary permeability, producing a mild intravascular depletion and directly stimulates endothelial release of NO [16].

DENERVATION HYPERSENSITIVITY

Diabetic patients with CAN may show an increased vascular sensitivity to infusions of alpha- adrenergic and beta-adrenergic agonists. This is attributed to denervation hypersensitivity like an up-regulation phenomenon, because of sympathetic nerve degeneration. As a result, infusions of alpha-adrenergic agonists in diabetic patients with CAN lead to an increase in arterial pressure after significantly lower doses than in healthy subjects.

EXERCISE INTOLERANCE

In diabetic patients with asymptomatic CAN and without evidence of heart disease, exercise capacity, evaluated as the greatest tolerable workload and maximal oxygen uptake, is diminished. The responses to exercise of the heart rate, blood pressure, cardiac stroke volume and splanchnic vascular resistance are also diminished. Thus, CAN contributes to impaired exercise tolerance.

In addition to that, a decrease in exercise capacity and blood pressure response to exercise appears in patients with postural hypotension. It should also be noted that decreased ejection fraction, systolic dysfunction and diastolic filling impairment limit exercise tolerance. Because patients with autonomic neuropathy may also have difficulties with thermoregulation, they should be advised to avoid physical exercise in extreme temperatures and to pay attention to adequate hydration.

Therefore, autonomic testing is a very useful method to identify patients with potentially poor exercise performance. In addition to that, a graded exercise ECG test may be helpful to prevent

unwanted events when they are introduced to exercise training programs.

SILENT MYOCARDIAL INFARCTION AND ISCHEMIA

The poor cardiovascular prognosis of autonomic neuropathy is partially attributable to undetected silent ischemia and myocardial infarction. Many diabetic patients with severe coronary stenoses are symptoms-free; however, the presence and severity of symptoms do not predict the outcome.

The incidence of silent myocardial ischemia (SMI) has been reported as approximately 2 to 4 % in the symptom-free general population and 30 to 50 % in patients with coronary artery disease [17].

Several clinical studies have examined the possible relationship between CAN and SMI but the literature data are contradictory [18]. Many scientific data suggest that the poor cardiovascular prognosis related to CAN in previous studies was probably associated with undetected SMI in many patients [19]. Nevertheless, the risk linked to CAN appears to be mostly independent of SMI and seems to be highest when CAN is associated with SMI, the majority of studies showing that in asymptomatic diabetic patients CAN is a better predictor of major cardiac events than SMI. That is the reason why CAN should be searched for in the largest possible number of diabetic patients, and, in those with cardiovascular risk factors, SMI should also be assessed.

The absence of ischemic pain seems to be due primarily to the impairment of sympathetic afferent fibers, due to dysautonomy or ischemia, the sympathetic innervation of the heart being highly sensitive to ischemia. This was confirmed by metaiodobenzylguanidine (MIBG) scintigraphy and thallium scintigraphy performed on patients with SMI [20] and implies the decrease of the diabetic individual sensitivity to regional ischemia by interruption of pain transmission. Studies performed by dynamic contrast-enhanced magnetic resonance perfusion imaging during baseline conditions and after Dipyridamole-induced vasodilatation concluded that diabetic patients with CAN have an additional decreased myocardial perfusion reserve capacity when challenged with a vasodilator. This could be due to defective myocardial sympathetic vasodilatation or to a lack of ability to maintain blood pressure during vasodilatation [21] and may contribute to the great incidence of SMI in these patients.

The absence of ischemic pain has a negative impact on cardiovascular outcomes in diabetic patients because it implies the loss of a limiting factor that would otherwise restrict physical activity, increasing the risk of acute myocardial infarction and sudden cardiac death. Cardiovascular dysautonomy is also implied in the delay of perception of angina as it was confirmed by ECG Holter monitoring, by inducing a longer latency period between the onset of ST segment depression, marker of ischemia, and the perception of angina [22]. Painless or atypical infarction also carries an increased risk for the patient, delaying the prompt diagnosis and appropriate medical treatment. According to this, chest pain in any location in a patient with diabetes should be considered to be of myocardial origin until proved otherwise; but, of equal importance, unexplained fatigue, confusion, peripheral edema, nausea and vomiting, diaphoresis, arrhythmias, dyspnea or sudden hyperglycemic crises as ketoacidosis of unknown origin, should alert the physician to the possibility of a silent myocardial infarction. In addition to all that, we must also take into account that, due to the underlying alteration of circadian autonomic tone, acute coronary syndromes in diabetic subjects are characterized by the presence of a marked attenuation of the "classical" morning peak [23, 20].

As mentioned before, the data regarding the consistent association between CAN and the presence of SMI and their causality relation are contradictory. It has recently been argued that the increased incidence of coronary artery disease in diabetes reflects mainly accelerated coronary atherosclerosis and that there is no convincing clinical and epidemiological evidence for a major role of CAN in the lack of ischemic pain. Nevertheless, there are authors who report that autonomic dysfunction may be involved in the pathogenesis of atherosclerosis. This would have important implications in our understanding of the pathogenesis of coronary atherosclerosis in diabetic patients. A direct effect of autonomic dysfunction on atherosclerosis is certainly possible as sympathetic denervation may cause dedifferentiation of vascular smooth cells and

transition to a secretory phenotype [24]. This phenotype is associated with extracellular matrix production and migration of the cells to the intima, features characteristic for atherosclerosis. H. Colhoun et al. [25] demonstrated that reduced HRV, a characteristic feature of CAN, is associated with increased coronary calcification, and that this association was not secondary to ischemia. Edmonds et al. [26] also attributed Monckeberg's sclerosis, the calcification of arterial tunica media, to the neuropathic impairment of the sympathetic system.

Given the complex mechanisms of silent myocardial ischemia even in the absence of diabetes, further studies are needed to clarify the exact role of CAN in this context.

INTRAOPERATIVE CARDIOVASCULAR INSTABILITY

Perioperative cardiovascular morbidity and mortality is 2 to 3 fold increased in patients with diabetes. This seems to be related to abnormal blood pressure and heart rate responses to general anesthesia produced mainly by the incomplete compensation between the vasodilation effect of anesthesia and the impaired autonomic response of vasoconstriction and tachycardia. Therefore, in patients undergoing general anesthesia there is a greater decline in heart rate and blood pressure during induction of anesthesia accompanied by a lesser degree of increase following tracheal intubation and extubation, as compared to nondiabetic subjects. However, some patients may show important hypertensive reactions during induction of anesthesia.

The imbalance between the anesthesia-induced vasodilatation and the abnormal autonomic response can also favor the development of more severe intraoperative hypothermia. This may lead to failure to maintain a normal body temperature during the intervention and can be accompanied by other complications like impaired wound healing and altered drug metabolism.

There are also authors [27] who report that diabetic patients require more often intraoperative blood pressure support by vasopressor drugs and there are many more cardiorespiratory arrests during or right after anesthesia in diabetics than in non-diabetic persons. All these data suggest that preoperative screening of cardiac autonomic function provides useful information for identifying patients who are at risk of intraoperative cardiovascular lability and complications.

DISTURBANCES OF THE PHYSIOLOGICAL CIRCADIAN RHYTHM OF BLOOD PRESSURE

It is well known that blood pressure is not an invariable biological parameter. During 24 hours, blood pressure follows a physiologic pattern with moderate nocturnal falls in both systolic and diastolic blood pressure compared with the daytime values. A 10–15% reduction of blood pressure below mean daytime values is considered normal ("dipper" pattern). The circadian blood pressure curves are best offered by 24-hour ambulatory blood pressure monitoring (ABPM).

It is shown by an increasing number of studies that diabetic patients with CAN are characterized by a "non-dipper" pattern of blood pressure values, that is defined by a day to night fall in either systolic or diastolic blood pressure of less than 10%. This seems to be due to a lower daytime sympathetic as well as a lower nocturnal parasympathetic activity along with an attenuation of the diurnal variability of sympathetic / parasympathetic activity ratio. Consequently, the diabetic patients with autonomic dysfunction seem to have a relative dominance of nocturnal sympathetic activity, thought to be responsible for the loss of the nocturnal blood pressure fall.

Edmonds et al. have reported the presence of a strong correlation between orthostatic hypotension and the loss of physiologic diurnal blood pressure variability [26]. They recommend that when a non-dipper pattern of circadian blood pressure is found, postural hypotension should also be looked for and, conversely, the presence of orthostatic hypotension justifies the performance of an ABPM to determine the pattern of the circadian blood pressure variability.

The blunted circadian variation in ambulatory blood pressure imposes a constant pressure load leading to unfavorable effects expressed by an increased severity of target-organ damage, including increased left ventricular mass, impaired left ventricular diastolic function, signs of renal damage and retinal changes. It should be stressed that this also applies for normotensive patients [28]. There are also some interesting studies [29, 30], which reported no correlations between the non-dipper status and cardiovascular events or left ventricular hypertrophy, probably related to the lack of reproducibility due to the reduced number of patients included. This assumption is confirmed by another study which showed a positive relation between target organ damage and the absence of the blood pressure circadian variability only when the non-dipping status was well characterized by multiple ABPMs.

Studies performed in our departments, sustaining data from literature, showed that there is a significant association between the presence of CAN and the development of left ventricular hypertrophy and ventricular diastolic dysfunction in normotensive subjects who are free of a clinically detectable heart disease. We believe that the main determinant of this association is the constant 24-hour pressional load induced by a non-dipper pattern of the blood pressure variability that exerts on "target-organs" relatively similar effects as those of hypertension [31].

A non-dipper pattern is a good predictor of diabetic nephropathy and retinopathy too. Even since 1994 V. Spallone et al., trying to evaluate the relationship between autonomic neuropathy, nephropathy and 24-h blood pressure profile in insulin-dependent diabetes mellitus, found that CAN is associated with reduced nocturnal falls in blood pressure and increased urinary albumin excretion. At that time, they suggested a pathogenetic role of autonomic neuropathy in the development of nephropathy through changes in nocturnal glomerular function and may be through increased kidney vulnerability to hemodynamic forces [32]. Many authors have underlined the correlation between the loss of nocturnal decline in blood pressure and the development of permanent microalbuminuria in normotensive diabetic patients [33]. Microalbuminuria is a well-established independent cardiovascular risk factor [34, 35]. Thus, any marker of a disturbed blood pressure regulation pattern could be useful in the early detection of these patients, in order to favorably influence of cardiovascular outcome and to prevent the progress of diabetic nephropathy.

We must also emphasize the importance of the pulse pressure, a parameter offered by ABPM analysis, representing the fluctuation of blood pressure between systolic and diastolic values. It is now recognized that pulse pressure is a more convenient factor appreciating the pressional load than the values of blood pressure recorded by sphygmomanometer. Our studies performed in hypertensive patients compared to normotensive subjects with autonomic dysfunction demonstrated insignificant differences in values of pulse pressure between the two groups [31]. This suggests that the non-dipper pattern of the circadian blood pressure variability may be equal or even more harmful than arterial hypertension itself for the "target-organs". In addition, pulse pressure becomes an important index of cardiovascular risk, target-organ damage and cardiovascular prognosis.

LEFT VENTRICULAR DYSFUNCTION

Cardiovascular autonomic neuropathy may be associated with abnormalities in left ventricular systolic and particularly diastolic function. This association was found even in the absence of a clinically detectable cardiac disease.

The first detectable abnormality is the impairment of diastolic function, echocardiographic studies showing a significant correlation between CAN presence and reduced peak diastolic filling rate, delayed isovolumetric relaxation and augmented atrial contribution to diastolic filling [38]. It seems that the degree of left ventricular dysfunction correlates well with the severity of autonomic dysfunction.

The impairment of diastolic function is followed by the development of systolic dysfunction. Characteristic changes include the prolongation of the pre-ejection period and the shortening of left ventricular ejection time. These changes are associated with a worsening of ejection fraction to appropriately increase with exercise, contributing to the exercise intolerance of these patients.

However, it is difficult to judge whether autonomic neuropathy is an independent contributor to all these abnormalities because there are several other factors that can be implicated in the pathogenesis of "diabetic myocardial disease", such as the microangiopathic or metabolic changes as well as the interstitial myocardial fibrosis.

INCREASED MORTALITY RISK AND PREDISPOSITION TO SUDDEN DEATH

The increased mortality risk associated with diabetic autonomic neuropathy is a well-established issue. Only 25–50% of the people with diabetes who have symptomatic CAN survive ten years, suggesting that autonomic failure is, as already emphasized before, a major cause of adverse outcome, with abnormal heart rate variability being associated with more than five-fold increase in mortality in type 1 diabetic patients [37]. According to data from consistent studies [38], a correlation between sudden cardiac death and the presence of markers of abnormalities in ventricular repolarization such as QT interval length and, respectively, dispersion was identified, that may be involved in the genesis of ventricular tachyarrhythmia.

QT interval length is influenced by the autonomic tone, QT prolongation being regarded because of an imbalanced distribution of sympathetic and parasympathetic activity in the heart with a positive correlation with the severity of CAN [39]. The same mechanism is responsible for an impaired QT heart-rate dependence and a reversed day-night pattern.

In recent years, QT dispersion (QTd) has been proposed as a sensitive marker for arrhythmic risk, predicting mortality in type 1 diabetes [40].

Even if there are some authors that deny the implication of QT interval abnormalities in the genesis of malign ventricular arrhythmia, the prolongation of QT interval still remains a specific marker of autonomic neuropathy and we must keep in mind, for diabetic patients with CAN, to avoid therapeutic agents that might influence the length of QT interval such as class I-A antiarrhythmics, erythromycin, phenothiazines, tricyclic antidepressants a.s.o.

Concerning the antiarrhythmic drugs, it should be reminded that autonomic neuropathy has a major influence on their efficacy. For example, digitalis exerts its effects by vagal fibers; therefore, a reduction in its antiarrhythmic efficacy should be expected in patients with parasympathetic impairment. Similarly, patients with a major sympathetic dysfunction will not respond adequately to beta-blockers, depriving them from their antianginal and heart rate reducing effects.

There are also many other factors potentially implicated in the genesis of fatal cardiac arrhythmia and sudden death. Attenuated heart rate variability and reduced baroreflex sensitivity (BRS) are faithful predictors of sudden death from cardiac causes. In addition to these, the potential role of prolonged ventricular late potentials detected by signal-averaged ECG in the etiology of ventricular tachyarrhythmia and sudden death in diabetic patients with CAN was emphasized. The increased risk of autonomic cardiorespiratory arrest is another characteristic feature of CAN. Although the exact mechanism is still unknown, it seems that reduced sensitivity to hypoxia and the loss of hypoxia-activated reflexes resulting from damage of afferent pathways or the respiratory center itself results from autonomic neuropathy [5]. A reduced bronchial smooth muscle tone by parasympathetic impairment has also been found, that may constitute the link between CAN and obstructive sleep apnea that was recently described and contributes to hypoxia. Silent myocardial ischemia, impaired diastolic or systolic ventricular performance, alteration of the circadian rhythm of heart rate and blood pressure are other factors that can be implicated in sudden death prediction too.

However, we should not forget that sudden death in diabetics can also result from a reduced awareness of hypoglycemia with impaired counter-regulation and increased prevalence of severe unrecognized hypoglycemia. These are characteristic features of CAN and are often implied in cases of death occurring in a good general condition and without any warning sign ("dead in bed" syndrome). Remarkably, it was found that hypoglycemia in patients with type 2 diabetes could be occasionally accompanied by increased QT dispersion [41].

DIAGNOSTIC METHODS

Symptom-based diagnosis of diabetic cardiovascular autonomic neuropathy (CAN) proves to have low sensitivity; therefore, diagnosis by means of objective cardiovascular tests is indicated. In time, a great variety of parameters has been used, but part of them was abandoned because of their inaccuracy, invasiveness and potential side effects. Diabetic autonomic neuropathy (DAN) presence and severity may be detected by performing a set of standard, non-invasive, relatively simple and non-time consuming cardiovascular tests, based on the assumption that abnormalities of cardiovascular reflexes are an indicator of the diffuse involvement of the neural autonomic system.

During the Conference of San Antonio [42], several clarifications have been brought in respect to diagnosing and categorizing CAN.

1. Symptoms specific to diabetic neuropathy do not exclusively suffice for diagnosis.

2. Use of standard, non-invasive, quantitative, combined tests is necessary; in their assessment one should consider age, pathological and therapeutic connections.

3. Additional evidence should be brought to establish whether these tests are relevant or not for monitoring patients.

In 1985, Ewing [43] chose a set of five cardiovascular tests, which describe the neural autonomous system adequately, meet the scientific standards and are simple enough to be used during current clinical practice. These tests consist of measuring the response of heart rate to certain stimuli (deep inspiration, Valsalva maneuver, standing up) and of blood pressure to standing up and hand gripping, respectively.

CHANGES OF HEART RATE DURING BREATHING

Respiratory arrhythmia (*i.e.*, increase of heart rate while breathing in and decrease thereof while breathing out) is a physiological phenomenon under parasympathetic control and diminishes while getting older. The maximum amplitude of this arrhythmia corresponds to a respiratory rate of 6 *per* minute.

Patients suffering from DAN have low or no respiratory arrhythmia.

Technique: ECG is performed for one minute while the patient breathes by 6 breaths *per* minute.

Results are expressed as:

– beat-by-beat variability (*i.e.*, the difference between the highest and the lowest heart rate, which normally equals or exceeds 15 *per* minute and pathologically is less than 10 *per* minute);

– E/I ratio (*i.e.*, time elapsed between two heartbeats measured during expiration (E) divided by the time elapsed between two heartbeats during inspiration (I)).

An alternative technique consists of assessing the E/I ratio during a single deep inspiration.

CHANGE OF HEART RATE WHEN STANDING UP

The physiological reaction to changing from a lying down to a standing up position is biphasic and under both sympathetic and parasympathetic control (the first phase consists of an increase in heart rate, reaching its maximum level on the 5th beat after standing up; the second phase consists of a decrease in heart rate, reaching its minimum level on the 30th beat after standing up).

Technique: ECG is performed while the patient is lying down and then continued while the patient is standing up by himself until the 30th heart beat, at least.

The ratio between the shortest and longest period elapsed between two heartbeats, namely the RR interval before the 30th heart beat and, respectively, the RR interval before the 15th heart beat (30:15 ratio), which normally equals or exceeds 1.04, may decrease under 1 for patients suffering from CAN.

CHANGE OF HEART RATE DURING VALSALVA MANEUVER (VALSALVA QUOTIENT)

The Valsalva maneuver (enforced exhalation with glottal stop) determines sympathetic and parasympathetic changes in heart rate and blood pressure. Under normal conditions blood pressure and heart rate decrease, and after removing the constraint blood pressure increases over the initial value while heart rhythm is slowing. In the case of patients suffering from CAN, these changes in blood pressure and heart rate are not influenced by age. Blood pressure decreases during the maneuver, but the going back to normal is slower, without rebound, while heart rate is not influenced.

Technique: the patient breathes out by means of a device attached to a manometer at a pressure of 40 mm Hg for 15 seconds. Meanwhile, ECG is performed. Valsalva ratio is obtained by dividing the longest period between two heartbeats (on the 20th beat after starting the maneuver, approximately) by the shortest (during the entire maneuver). A mean is calculated based on 3 consecutive Valsalva maneuvers.

The normal value of the ratio equals or exceeds 1.21; a value of 1.20 or under is pathological.

The disadvantage is that this method may determine vitreous hemorrhage or retinal detachment in the case of patients suffering from proliferative retinopathy and may also interfere with heart deficiency, in which case the heart rate does not change significantly, regardless of autonomic neuropathy being present or not.

CHANGE OF BLOOD PRESSURE WHEN CHANGING THE POSITION FROM LYING DOWN TO STANDING UP

Upon standing up, blood shifts to the lower extremities, leading to a decrease of blood pressure. As a normal reaction, the sympathetic system rapidly intervenes and brings blood pressure back to normal mainly by constraining peripheral and splanchnic blood vessels more than by increasing the heart rate.

Weakening of sympathetic reflexes (during advanced stages of CAN) leads to postural hypotension, namely a decrease by more than 30 mmHg of systolic blood pressure measured one minute after getting in upright position.

BLOOD PRESSURE RESPONSE TO HAND GRIPPING

During this maneuver, peripheral vessels resistance does not change, but blood pressure increases. Consequently, heart blood volume and blood pressure increase. Heart rate growth is slower and blood pressure growth is more temperate in the case of patients suffering from CAN.

Technique: A handgrip dynamometer is pressed to the limit for a couple of seconds, then by 30% of initial force for another 3–5 minutes. Blood pressure is measured every minute.

The results are expressed by the increase of diastolic blood pressure right after releasing handgrip by at least 16 mmHg in excess of the previous value.

331

In order to reduce the time necessary for CAN investigation, the following sequence of 4 tests is recommended: heart rate response to Valsalva maneuver, heart rate reaction to deep breathing, blood pressure response to hand gripping, heart rate and then blood pressure response to getting in an upright position. These tests can be carried out in 15–20 minutes, and the interpretation of the results may be performed with computer help.

Ewing's set of tests is also useful for evaluating CAN severity. Each test is granted 0, 1 or 2 points for normal, borderline and pathological, respectively. Summing up these points leads to a scoring directly correlated to the severity of CAN.

Some tests may not be applied to certain patients. Thus, the elderly have frequently additional diseases at the same time, which diminish the accuracy of cardiovascular tests (HTA, clinical lung diseases, myocardial ischemia, etc) and frequently use medication interfering with the neural autonomic system. Sinus rhythm and absence of extrasystoles are essential conditions that some patients do not fulfill. Changes in blood pressure during Valsalva maneuver and handgrip can trigger brain hemorrhage and complications of proliferative retinopathy and must be avoided in the case of high-risk patients, as mentioned. In order to obtain accurate results, any medication that has an influence over the autonomic status, heart rate and blood pressure should be stopped for 24–48 hours, if possible.

An easier algorithm begins with determining beat-by-beat variability (the most sensitive test) and 30:15 ratio. If these tests lead to normal results, there is no point in continuing the investigations. If at least one result of these tests is abnormal, the next step is to perform the Valsalva maneuver and the handgrip test. The third step is to investigate whether postural hypotension occurs. Bellavere (1985) considers that beat-by-beat variability test can make the diagnosis of CAN even if other changes are absent, as the other tests only contribute to evaluating its severity.

Other non-invasive tests for autonomic dysfunction diagnosis are under study, as well:

– Squatting test – getting from squatting to standing up position amplifies diastolic blood pressure response and may be used as early diagnosis test, especially for young people;

– Cold water pressure test – one of CAN characteristics is that blood pressure takes more time to return to normal after exposure to cold water;

– Cough-test – cough induces a cholinergic response, leading to acceleration of heart rate. Its advantages are that it is easy to perform, reproducible, is less risky than the Valsalva maneuver and correlates very well with lying down to standing up test;

– Brain stress test is less standardized;

– Effort test; both blood pressure and heart rate have delayed responses in the case of patients suffering from CAN;

– Tilting test;

– Sitting down to standing up test.

Another category of tests includes investigations with significant contribution to CAN diagnosis, but costly, technically difficult and time consuming (MIBG and C-HED scan, ECG and blood pressure Holter). I-131-metaiodobenzyl-guanidine (MIBG) is a norepinephrine analogue, which serves as a direct evidence for sympathetic activity. MIBG scan identifies areas with high density of postsynaptic ends, which actively uptake this tracer.

Diabetic patients show less MIBG myocardial uptake than non-diabetic ones, differentiated by location (more intense to the base than to the apex); given these uptake irregularities, a qualitative analysis of the images is necessary in order to interpret data obtained.

MIBG scan is more sensitive than Ewing clinical tests. Uptake deficiencies are more frequent and larger for diabetic patients ($13 \pm 15\%$ *versus* $2 \pm 2\%$; $p < 0.0001$) and heart/lung uptake ratio is lower (1.22 ± 0.18 *versus* 2 ± 0.28; $p<0.005$). The latter is an indicator of the global sympathetic cardiac function. MIGB scan must be associated with perfusion scan, due to the fact that tracer uptake depends on the local blood flow.

MIBG uptake deficiencies relate inversely proportional to the markers of sympathetic modulation like the area under the curve of the low frequency band and the total power of HRV in the spectral analysis of heart rate.

Certain authors have demonstrated that using a newer tracer, namely C11-hydroxiephedrine (C-HED) leads to identifying 40% more patients suffering from CAN (*i.e.*, with early CAN) than clinical cardiovascular tests. Almost all patients suffering from clinical CAN show global and local HED uptake irregularities. This is correlated with a poor coronary blood flow, coronary flow reserve and LV diastolic dysfunction.

Ambulatory blood pressure monitoring (ABPM) contributes to white coat hypertension recognition, indicates the hypertensive charge during 24 hours, blood pressure decrease by night (dipper/non-dipper pattern) and helps in establishing the optimum medicating timetable.

Left ventricle hypertrophy is attested as an independent indicator of mortality and morbidity and represents an adapting reaction of the left ventricle to an increase in wall stress. It depends on high blood pressure duration and blood pressure circadian variability. Unfortunately, blood pressure Holter is not a reproducible method as regards dipper/non-dipper pattern. Therefore, there are some authors considering that the non-dipper profile diagnosed based on a single Holter record does not identify the patients with more severe heart dysfunction.

Among the parameters offered by the integrated analysis of the 24-hour blood pressure recordings, mean ABPM values seems to be better correlated with clinically relevant cardiovascular events than casual blood pressure readings. This hypothesis is sustained by many trials, such as a subgroup- analysis of elderly hypertensive participants of the Syst-Eur (Systolic Hypertension in Europe) Trial [44], which showed that every 10 mmHg increase in mean systolic blood pressure recorded during the night period was associated with a 31 % increase in cardiovascular risk.

Performing **Holter ECG** is a widely used method to identify silent ischemia, arrhythmia, QT and HRV. O'Sullivan [45] showed, based on 24-hour ECG ambulatory Holter-monitoring recordings, that silent ischemia occurs in 64.7% of diabetic patients with autonomic neuropathy, whereas its incidence in diabetics without neuropathy is as low as 4.1 % [39]. Valensi *et al.* [19] also showed that the prevalence of silent myocardial ischemia in diabetic patients with no cardiac history and with a normal 12-lead ECG was high (almost 30%). Significant coronary stenoses are found in coronarography in approximately one-third of the patients with SMI. Therefore, all efforts should be made for diagnosing SMI.

One of the QT determining factors is the neural autonomic system. QT prolongation, present within CAN, is a sudden death risk marker. QT dispersion, an indicator of heterogeneity in recovery of excitability with non-uniform repolarization, has been proposed as another factor, which identifies patients who are at risk for sudden death from specifically re-entry arrhythmia. QTd is statistically related to the duration of QTc (corrected QT interval) but increased QTd and increased QTc identify different groups of patients with different risk of cardiac events. Thus, prospective evaluation is necessary to determine the predictive value of these tests. It should be stressed, however, that there are also many other factors that can interfere with the QT interval profile, such as ischemia or disturbances of serum electrolytes or recent myocardial infarction, heart failure and hypertrophic cardiomyopathy, suggesting that all these factors should always be taken into account.

Many authors reported the poor prognosis associated to HRV decrease. **Spectrum analysis of heart rate** in the ECG record shows 3 peaks:
 – VLF (very low frequency) 0–0.04 Hz;
 – LF (low frequency) ≈ 0.1 Hz – expresses the maximum level of sympathetic activity;
 – HF (high frequency) – indicates parasympathetic influence.

Low frequency to high frequency ratio is a general indicator of autonomic function; further to the spectral analysis of heart rate, simultaneous sympathetic and parasympathetic dysfunctions were demonstrated during early stages of CAN, but different in intensity [5].

In the last few years, there was a trend toward the use of **baroreflex sensitivity assessment**. Its clinical importance was proved by the ATRAMI Study (Autonomic Tone and Reflexes After Myocardial Infarction) [46], which provided clinical evidence for a significant prognostic value of baroreflex sensitivity in patients with a recent myocardial infarction, independently of left ventricular ejection fraction and ventricular arrhythmia.

THERAPEUTICAL APPROACH

There are many ways to counteract cardiovascular autonomic neuropathy. This implies an etiologic treatment, a pathogenic one and a direct modulation of autonomic system.

ETIOLOGIC TREATMENT

After 5 years of monitoring patients with IDDM within DCCT [47, 48], it was noted that 8.7% of the patients under conventional insulin treatment as compared to 4.3% of those under intensive insulin treatment developed HRV abnormalities. This fact underlines the importance of a good metabolic control in the prevention of chronic diabetic complications.

In non-insulin depending diabetic patients suffering an acute myocardial infarction, the intensive treatment with insulin has shown a 28% reduction of 1-year mortality, comparing with those patients receiving a conventional treatment. This favorable effect can be attributed to the benefic influences of insulin on endothelial properties, platelet aggregation, lipidic status, systolic ventricular function and, last but not least, on autonomic tone [49].

PATHOGENETIC TREATMENT

Assuming the different pathogenetic mechanisms, specific treatment measures have been undertaken for the management of cardiovascular autonomic neuropathy.

1. *The Polyol pathway* might be influenced by aldose-reductase inhibitors. This assumption has been confirmed by two clinical trials with tolrestat, which showed favorable influence on CAN, but at the risk of an inadmissible level of liver toxicity. Therefore, tolrestat has been put off sale. Another aldose-reductase inhibitor, namely epalrestat, proved its effectiveness in improving HRV after 3 years of treatment (150 mg three times a day); no significant favorable results were obtained after 1 and, respectively, 2 years of medication [50].

2. *Formation of glycosylation end-products* involved in CAN pathogenesis might be prevented by aminoguanidine, which acts as a competitive inhibitor of AGEs. Further studies are needed to demonstrate its specific benefits on CAN.

3. *Abnormalities of essential fatty acids and prostanoids metabolism* may be theoretically neutralized by γ linoleic acid. There is no sufficient evidence for the moment supporting this hypothesis [51].

4. Under the assumption that CAN is determined by *ischemia,* vasodilators, as well as drugs diminishing endothelial dysfunction and oxidative stress seem to be valuable.

Accordingly, there are studies involving alpha-lipoic acid like DEKAN (Deutsche Kardiale Autonome Neuropathie), which showed improvement in heart rate variability indexes, without correspondence in symptoms, with a daily oral dose of 800mg. These effects may be due to some metabolic actions: it increases glucose uptake and it is also a potent scavenger for hydroxyl free radicals, by improving the nerve perfusion and lowering the oxidative stress. To a certain extent, it alleviates neurogenic pain [52, 53, 54].

Quinapril [55] is shown to stimulate parasympathetic activity (measured by changes in HRV and frequency domain indices) in patients suffering from CAN; malign heart arrhythmia risk decreased starting with the 3rd month of treatment.

5. *Deprivation of neural growth factors* has been demonstrated by experiments on animals suffering from CAN; no evidence has been found yet to sustain the therapeutic effect of substituting such factors [56].

Influencing directly the neural autonomic system

We can modulate autonomic tonus by means of a large variety of drugs. For example, some of them lead to HRV increase, such as ACE inhibitors, selective beta-blockers without intrinsic sympathetic activity (ISA), digoxin and verapamil. Other drugs induce HRV decrease and should be avoided (class Ic antiarrhythmic drugs, beta-blockers with ISA, clonidine, tricyclic antidepressant drugs).

This interference with the neural autonomic system constitutes an additional argument in favor of using ACE inhibitors, selective beta-blockers, calcium channel blockers in patients suffering from diabetes mellitus (DM) and CAN, a combination frequently associated with high blood pressure and coronary artery disease.

Diabetic patients seem to benefit from selective beta-blockers to an even higher extent than non-diabetic patients do. This could be related to the high risk of arrhythmia and the high mortality rate after myocardial infarction in patients with CAN, and is correlated with the extended myocardial ischemia, a typical finding in diabetic patients.

There are reports regarding administration of vitamin E, a well-known antioxidant, as a therapeutic agent. The clinical data support its rather beneficial effects on sympathetic modulation expressed by RR interval, total power, high frequency and low frequency component of HRV [57].

Postural hypotension treatment is difficult as it hardens reaching the target blood pressure, which is lower for diabetic patients as compared to non-diabetic subjects. The treatment involves the increase of venous return through basic measures and pharmaceutical means.

Some examples of *basic measures* are as follows:

– wearing elastic stockings;

– using an elasticised garment reaching from the metatarsus to the costal margin);

– using foldable chairs on a regular basis;

– performing easy physical exercise;

– keeping a head-up bed position;

– sitting on the bed edge before standing up;

– crossing the legs;

– squatting;

– increasing daily salt ingestion by 2–6 g if not prohibited;

– avoiding psychotropic, diuretic and vasodilator drugs;

– changing insulin administration timetable if proven to be the cause of postural hypotension (by its vasodilation properties).

Pharmaceutical treatment is relatively effective, but has many adverse effects, some of them significant.

Midodrine, an alpha1- adrenergic agonist, leads to blood pressure increase by arteries and veins constriction, an advantage being that it does not act directly on the heart and central neural system. The maximum dosage is 10 mg three to four times a day.

Fludrocortisone, a mineralocorticoid, induces systolic and diastolic blood pressure increase due to salt and water retention, but also by means of a vasoconstrictor effect on partly denervated vessels. These effects are doubled by vascular distensibility decrease due to the increase of water content within vessels wall. The inconvenience thereof consists of high blood pressure presence in the lying down position, chronic heart failure and ankle swelling, as well as hypokalemia. The treatment starts with 0.1 mg per day, adjustable according to clinical symptoms (average dosage is 0.2–0.3 mg *per* day). Based on the observation that there are individuals with autonomic neuropathy who are anemic and have a decreased red-cell mass, Cazzola *et al.* [58] suggested that CAN may have a role in the regulation of red-cell volume. The reasonable cause probably is the decreased erythropoietin secretion as a manifestation of renal autonomic denervation. Recently, *erythropoietin* proved its short-term effectiveness in the case of patients with CAN and a low hematocrit. Further studies are needed to asses the long-term effects of this treatment. Until then erythropoietin should not be prescribed as a first line therapeutic agent, and should be prescribed to patients nonresponding to midodrine and fludrocortisone.

Non-steroid anti-inflammatory drugs, dihydro-ergotamine, coffeine and clonidine have also been recommended.

Diabetic neuropathy is an early complication, although the symptom-based diagnosis is more belated. Cardiac autonomic neuropathy (including the asymptomatic one) correlates with a high mortality, and is involved in the pathogenesis of diabetic nephropathy and cardiovascular diseases.

The standardized Ewing set of tests is the most useful mean for diagnosis. Some other clinical tests and paraclinical investigations become more and more accepted.

The treatment relies mainly on an etiologic basis, but today there are more and more attempts to influence the evolution of CAN by pathogenic interventions.

REFERENCES

1. Ziegler D. Diabetic cardiovascular autonomic neuropathy: Prognosis, diagnosis and treatment. *Diabetes Metab Rev*, **10**: 339–383, 1994.
2. Zochodne DW, Ho LT. Normal blood flow but lower oxygen tension in diabetes of young rats: microenvironment and the influence of sympathectomy. *Can J Pharmacol*, **70**: 651, 1993.
3. Cameron N, Eaton S, Cotter M, Tesfaye S. Vascular factors and metabolic interactions in the pathogenesis of diabetic neuropathy. *Diabetologia*, **44**: 1973–1988, 2001.
4. Tuck RR, Schmelzer JD, Low PA. Endoneurial blood flow and oxygen tension in the sciatic nerve of rats with experimental diabetic neuropathy. *Brain*, **107**: 935, 1984.

5. Vinik A, Mitchell B, Maser R, Freeman R. Diabetic autonomic neuropathy. *Diabetes Care*, **26**: 1553–1562, 2003.

6. Kempler P. Pathomorphology and pathomechanism of neuropathies. In: Kempler P (ed). *Neuropathies. Pathomechanism, clinic diagnosis, therapy.* Springer Scientific Publisher, 2002, 21–41.

7. Mangoni AA, Mircoli L, Giannattasio C, Ferrari AU, Mancia G. Heart rate-dependence of arterial distensibility in vivo. *J Hypertens*, **14**: 897–902, 1996.

8. Beer PA, Glagor S, Zarin CK. Retarding effect of lowered heart rate on coronary atherosclerosis. *Science*, **226**: 18–182, 1984.

9. Gilman MW, Kannel WB, D'Agostino RB. Influence of heart rate on mortality among persons with hypertension. The Framingham Study. *Am Heart J*, **125**: 1148–1154; 1993

10. Dekker JM, Schrouten EG, Klootwijk P, Pool J, Swenne CA, Kromhout D. Heart rate variability from short ECG recordings predicts mortality from all causes in middle – aged and elderly men: The Zutphen Study. *Am J Epidemiol*, **145**: 899–908, 1997.

11. Braune S, Wrocklage C, Schulte-Monting J, Schnitzer R, Lucking CH. Diagnosis of tachycardia syndromes associated with orthostatic symptoms. *Clin Auton Res*, **9**: 97–101, 1999.

12. Jacob G, Costa F, Shannon J, Robertson RM, Wathen M, Stein M, Braggioni I, Black B, Robertson D. The neuropathic postural tachycardia syndrome. *N Engl J Med*, **343**: 1008–1014, 2000.

13. Rundles PW. Diabetic neuropathy, general review report of 125 cases. *Medicine*, **24**: 111–116, 1945.

14. Cryer PE, Silverberg AB, Santiago JV. Plasma catecholamines in diabetes: the syndromes of hypoadrenergic and hyperadrenergic postural hypotension. *Am J Med*, **64**: 407–414, 1978.

15. Braggioni I, Garcia F, Inagami T, Haile V. Hyporeninemic normoaldosteronism in severe autonomic failure. *J Clin Metab*, **76**: 580–586, 1993.

16. Vinik AI, Erbas T. Recognition and treating diabetic autonomic neuropathy. *Cleveland Clinic Journal of Medecine*, **68**: 345–349, 2001.

17. Deedmania PC, Carbajal EV. Silent myocardial ischemia. A clinical perspective. *Arch Intern Med*, **151**: 2373–2381, 1991.

18. Koistinen MJ, Airaksinen KEJ, Huikuri KV, Pirttiaho H, Linnaluoto MK, Ikaheimo MJ, Takkunen JT. Asymptomatic coronary artery disease in diabetes: associated with autonomic neuropathy? *Acta Diabetol*, **28**: 199–202, 1992.

19. Valensi J, Sachs RN, Harfouche B, Lormeau B, Paries J, Cosson E, Paycha F, Lentenegger M, Attali JR. Predictive value of cardiac autonomic neuropathy in diabetic patients with or without silent myocardial ischemia. *Diabetes Care* **24**: 339–343, 2001.

20. Kostinen MJ, Airaksinen KE, Huikuri HV, Linnaluoto MM, Heikkila J. No difference in cardiac innervation of diabetic patients with painful and asymptomatic coronary artery disease. *Diabetes Care*, **19**: 231–233, 1996.

21. Taskiran M, Fritz-Hansen T, Verner R, Larsson HBW, Hilsted J. Decreased myocardial perfusion reserve in diabetic autonomic neuropathy. *Diabetes,* **51**: 3306–3310, 2002.

22. Marchant B, Umachandran V, Stevenson R, Kopelman PG, Timmis AD. Silent myocardial ischemia: Role of subclinical neuropathy in patients with and without diabetes. *J Am Coll Cardiol*, **22**: 1433–1437, 1992.

23. Rana J, Mukamal KJ, Morgan JP, Muller JE, Mittleman MA. Circadian variation in the onset of myocardial infarction. *Diabetes*, **52**: 1464–1468, 2003.

24. Dimitriadou V, Aubineau P, Taxi J, Seylaz J. Ultrastructural changes in the cerebral artery wall induced by long-term sympathetic denervation. *Blood Vessels*, **25**: 122–143, 1988.

25. Colhoun H, Francis DP, Rubens MB, Underwood R, Fuller JH. The association of heart-rate variability with cardiovascular risk factors and coronary artery calcification. *Diabetes Care*, **24**: 1108–1114, 2001.

26. Edmonds ME, Watkins PJ. Clinical presentation of diabetic autonomic failure. In: Bannister R (ed). *Autonomic failure. A textbook of clinical disorders of the autonomic nervous system.* Oxford University Press, Oxford, 1998, 632–653.

27. Burgos LG, Ebert EJ, Aviddao C, Turner LA, *et al.* Increased intraoperative cardiovascular morbidity in diabetics with autonomic neuropathy. *Anaesthesiology*, **70**: 591–597, 1989.

28. Roman MJ, Pickering TG, Schwartz JE, Cavallini MC, Pini R, Devereux RB. Is the absence of diurnal-nocturnal fall in blood pressure (non)dipping associated with cardiovascular target organ damage? *J Hypertens*, **15**: 969–978, 1997.

29. Mochijuchi J, Okutani N, Donfei Y, Iwasaki H, Tagusagawa H, Kohno I, *et al.* Limited reproducibility of circadian variation in blood pressure: dippers and nondippers. *Am J Hypertens*, **11**: 403–409, 1998.

30. Manning G, Rushton L, Donelly R and Millar Craig MW. Variability of diurnal changes in ambulatory blood pressure and nocturnal dipping

status in untreated hypertensive and normotensive subjects. *Am J Hypertens*, **13**: 1035–1038, 2000.

31. Vlaiculescu M, Homentcovschi C, Gurghean A, Dodan R, Muraru M, Bruckner I. The lack of blood pressure circadian variability – more harmful than arterial hypertension for the target organ? – Oral communication – The Annals of the Romanian Federation of Diabetes, Nutrition and Metabolic Diseases, Cluj-Napoca, 2002.

32. Spallone V, Gambardella S, Maiello M, Barini A, Frontoni S, Menzinger G. Relationship between autonomic neuropathy, 24h blood pressure profile and nephropathy in normotensive IDDM patients. *Diabetes Care*, **6**: 578–584, 1994.

33. Sundkvist G, Lilja B. Autonomic neuropathy predicts deterioration in glomerular filtration rate in patients with IDDM. *Diabetes Care*, **16**: 773–779, 1993.

34. Mogensen CE, Keane W, Bennett P, Jerums G, Parving H, Passa P, *et al*. Prevention of diabetic renal disease with special reference to microalbuminuria. *Lancet*, **346**: 1080–4, 1995.

35. Mogensen CE. Systemic blood pressure and glomerular leakage with particular reference to diabetes and hypertension. *J Intern Med*, **235**: 297–316, 1994.

36. Oh JK, Appleton CP, Hatle LK, Nishimura RA, Seward JB, Tajik AJ. The invasive assessment of left ventricular diastolic function with two-dimensional and Doppler echocardiography. *J Am Soc Echocardiogr*, **10**: 246–270, 1997.

37. Levitt NS, Stransberry KB, Wynchack S, Vinik AI. The natural progression of autonomic neuropathy and autonomic tests in a cohort of people with IDDM. *Diabetes Care*, **19**: 751–754, 1996.

38. Kahn JK, Hisson JC, Vinik AI. QT interval prolongation and sudden death in diabetic autonomic neuropathy. *J Clin Endocrinology and Metabolism*, 751–754, 1987.

39. Kempler P. Cardiac autonomic neuropathy: is it a cardiovascular risk factor in type 2 diabetes? In: Hancu N (ed*). Cardiavascular risk in type 2 diabetes mellitus. Assessment and control.* Springer–Verlag, Berlin, Heidelberg, 2003, 181–189.

40. Veglio M, Giunti S, Stevens L, Fuller J, Perin P. The EURODIAB IDDM Complications Study Group: Prevalence of QT Interval Dispersion in Type I Diabetes and its Relation with Cardiac Ischemia. *Diabetes Care*, **25**: 702–707, 2002.

41. Landstedt-Hallin L, Englund A, Adamson U, Lins PE. Increased QT dispersion during hypoglycemia in patients with type 2 diabetes mellitus. *J Intern Med*, **246**: 299–307, 1999.

42. American Diabetes Association and American Academy of Neurology. Report and recommeandations of the San Antonio Conference on diabetic neuropathy (Consensus Statement). *Diabetes*, **37**: 1000–1004, 1988.

43. Ewing DJ, Marty CN, Young RJ, Clarke BF. The value of cardiovascular autonomic function tests: 10 Years experiences in diabetes. *Diabetes Care*, **8**: 491–498, 1985.

44. Birkenhager WH, Staessen JA, Gasowski J, de Leenw PW. Effects of antihypertensive treatment on endpoints in the diabetic patients randomised in the Systolic Hypertention in Europe (Syst-Eur) Trial. *J Nephrol*, **13**: 232–237, 2000.

45. O'Sullivan JJ, Conroy RM, Mc Donald K, Mc Kenna TJ, Maurer BJ. Silent ischemia in diabetic men with autonomic neuropathy. *Br Heart J*, **66**: 313–315, 1991.

46. La Rovere MT, Bigger JT Jr. Marcus FI, Mortara A, Schwartz PJ. Baroreflex sensitivity and heart rate variability in prediction of total cardiac mortality after myocardial infarction. ATRAMI (Autonomic Tone and Reflexes After Myocardial Infarction) investigators. *Lancet*, **351**: 478–484, 1998.

47. The Diabetes Control and Complications Trials Complications Group. The effect of intensive treatment of diabetes on the development and progression of long-term complications in insulin - dependent diabetes mellitus. *N Engl J Med*, **329**: 977–986, 1993.

48. The DCCT Research Group: The effect of intensive diabetes therapy on measures of autonomic nervous system function in the Diabetes Control and Complications Trial (DCCT). *Diabetologia*, **41**: 416–23, 1998.

49. Malmberg K-Prospective randomised study of intensive insulin treatment on long term survival after acute myocardial infarction in patients with diabetes (DIGAMI*). Br Med J*, **314**: 1512, 1997.

50. Ikeda T, Iwata K, Tanaka Y. Long term effect of epalrestat on cardiac autonomic neuropathy in subjects with non-insulin dependent diabetes mellitus. *Diabetes Res Clin Pract*, **43**: 193–198, 1999.

51. Keen H.,Payan J., Allawi J.*et al*. Treatment of diabetic neuropathy with gamma-linolenic acid. *Diabetes Care*, **16**: 8–15, 1993.

52. Ziegler DH, Schats F, Conrad FA, Gries H, *et al*. Effects of treatment with the antioxidant alpha-lipoic acid on cardiac autonomic neuropathy in NIDDM patients. A 4 month randomized controlled multicenter trial (DEKAN Study). Deutche kardiale autonome neuropathie. *Diabetes Care*, **20(3)**: 369–73, 1997.

53. Ziegler D, Gries FA. Alpha-lipoic acid in treatment of peripheral and cardiac autonomic neuropathy. *Diabetes*, **46:** S62–S66, 1997.

54. Ziegler D, Hanefeld M, Ruhnau KJ, Hasche H, Lobish M, Schutte K, Kerum G, Malessa R. Treatment of symptomatic polyneuropathy with the antioxidant alpha-lipoic acid: a 7-month multicenter randomized controlled trial (ALADIN III Study). ALADIN Study Group. Alpha Lipoic Acid in Diabetic Neuropathy, *Diabetes Care*, **22:** 1296–1301, 1999.

55. Kontopoulos AG, Athyros VG, Didangelos TP, Papageorgiou AA, Avramidis MJ, Mayroudi MC, Karamitsos DT. Effect of chronic quinapril administration on heart rate variability in patients with diabetic autonomic neuropathy. *Diabetes Care,* **20:** 355–61, 1997.

56. Apfel SC, Adornato BT, Dyck P J, *et al.* Results of a double-blind, placebo-controlled trial of recombinant human nerve growth factor in diabetic neuropathy. *Am Neurol,* **40:** T194, 1996.

57. Manzella D, Barbieri M, Ragno E, Paolisso G. Chronic administration of pharmacologic doses of vitamin E improves the cardiac autonomic nervous system in patients with type 2 diabetes. *Am J of Clinical Nutrition,* **73:** 1052–1057, 2001.

58. Cazzola M, Mercuriali F, Brugnara C. Use of Recombinant Human Erythropoietin outside the setting of uremia. *Blood*, **89:** 4248–4267, 1997.

21

SCREENING FOR SUBCLINICAL COMPLICATIONS IN YOUNG TYPE 1 DIABETIC PATIENTS: EXPERIENCE ACQUIRED IN BRUSSELS

Harry DORCHY

Clinical studies conducted since the 1970s by the pediatric diabetology group of the Free University of Brussels have demonstrated that screening for subclinical retinopathy, neuropathy, and nephropathy should be started at puberty and at least 3 years after the diabetes diagnosis with the goal of detecting early abnormalities responsible for subclinical disorders that can be reversed by improved metabolic control, thus preventing the occurrence of irreversible potentially incapacitating lesions. A 1974 retinal fluorescein angiography study showed that the development of microaneurysms, which are irreversible lesions, could be preceded by fluorescein leakage due to disruption of the blood-retinal barrier. Risk factors for early retinopathy include: duration of diabetes, age at diagnosis (with younger children having longer times to retinopathy), puberty and sex (with onset one year earlier in girls than in boys), long-term bad metabolic control over several years, high cholesterol levels and excessive body mass index (BMI). On the other hand, rapid improvement of diabetic control may worsen diabetic retinopathy (1985). Minimal EEG abnormalities were found in relationship with frequent and severe hypoglycemic comas and/or convulsions, and retinopathy (1979). Desynchronization of action potentials in distal nerve fibers preceded conduction velocity slowing (1981). A single high glycated hemoglobin value was associated with peroneal motor nerve conduction slowing (1985), which was not observed in the femoral nerve (1987). Sympathetic skin response (1996) and statistical analysis of heart rate variability (2001) could have some interest for the diagnosis of early diabetic autonomic neuropathy. Early microproteinuria is of mixed origin, being both glomerular (microalbumin) and tubular (β2-microglobulin). Exercise testing to exhaustion did not provide additional information more than the basal excretion testing did (1976). Microtransferrinuria (1984) and urinary acid glycosaminoglycans output (2001) could also be predictive markers of glomerular dysfunction. Physical training reduced exercise-related proteinuria by half (1988). High levels of serum lipoprotein (a) were not associated with the presence of subclinical complications (1996). On the other hand, ultra sensitive C-reactive protein could be an interesting indicator for the risk of developing early complications (2002). Poor metabolic control was associated with higher levels of triglycerides, total cholesterol, LDL cholesterol, and apolipoprotein B (1990). Decreased glutathione peroxidase, glutathione reductase, and vitamin C levels, denoting moderate oxidative stress, were found (1996), although there was no evidence of increased LDL cholesterol peroxidation (1998). Erythrocytes exhibited increased glycolytic activity, and neutrophils decreased migration, in relationship with metabolic control (1992). The degree of metabolic control influenced serum triiodothyronine levels (1985), magnesium concentrations (1999) and infection by *Helicobacter pylori* (1997). Insulin therapy could activate the complement pathway if intermediate and long-acting insulin preparations without protamine sulphate are used (1992), and provoke higher BMI in adolescents on 4 insulin injections (1988). Well-being was inversely related to glycated hemoglobin levels (1997).

INTRODUCTION

ROLE OF GLYCEMIC CONTROL

The principal aims of therapeutic management of the child, adolescent and adult with type 1 diabetes are to allow good quality of life [1, 2] and to avoid long-term complications (retinopathy, neuropathy, nephropathy, etc.) by maintaining blood glucose concentrations close to the normal range [3–5], even if it is possible that some complications – namely nephropathy – could be influenced by genetic factors [6–8].

Repeated determinations of glycated hemoglobin levels (HbA1c) provide a good criterion of overall control. They must be under 7% [4], (the upper normal limit is about 6%) which is possible, in our experience, even in diabetic children and adolescents [9–12]. The number of daily insulin injections, 2 or 4, by itself does not necessarily give better results, but the 4-injection regimen allows greater freedom, taking into account that the proper insulin adjustment is difficult before adolescence. Successful glycemic control in young patients depends mainly on the quality and intensity of diabetes education. Any dogmatism must be avoided. Details on our way of treating diabetic children and adolescents have been published elsewhere [13–18]. The mean HbA1c levels of our diabetic children and adolescents are among the lowest in a comparison of major studies of glycemic control in diabetic children [19], and in the international comparisons by the Hvidøre Study Group on Childhood Diabetes [20–23]. In unselected patients, we obtain a mean HbA1c of approximately 140 percent of normal mean being 100%, *i.e.* about 7 percent if the normal mean is 5% [9–11].

SUBCLINICAL COMPLICATIONS

Clinical studies conducted since the 1970s by our team [9, 24] have demonstrated that screening for subclinical retinopathy, neuropathy, and nephropathy should be started at puberty and three years after diagnosis (Figure 21.1), as also shown by the Berlin group [25], with the goal of detecting early abnormalities responsible for functional disorders that can be reversed by improved metabolic control, thus preventing the occurrence of potentially irreversible incapacitating

lesions [26–28]. This motivates both the patient and the multidisciplinary diabetes team in order to obtain good HbA1c levels.

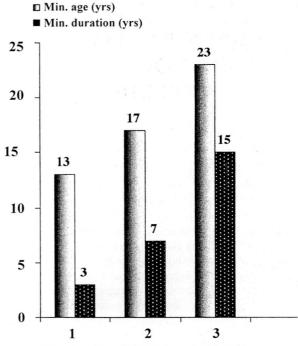

Figure 21.1

In 90 young diabetics who underwent tests for early retinopathy (fluorescein angiography), neuropathy (nerve conduction velocities), nephropathy (microalbuminuria), the youngest patients with one, two, or three subclinical complications were 13, 17, and 23 years of age, respectively, and corresponding minimal disease durations were 3, 7, and 15 years (from ref. 9).

EFFECT OF PUBERTY

Diabetic complications are very rare before puberty, except if metabolic control is very bad as shown in cases of Mauriac syndrome [29]. The years of insufficient glycemic control before puberty influence the development of microvascular complications [30, 31]. Prepubertal diabetes duration remains a significant predictor of retinopathy in young adults. The effect of time on the risk of retinopathy and microalbuminuria is not uniform, with an increasing delay in the onset of complications in those with longer prepubertal duration [32]. We have shown earlier in a longitudinal study that the younger the child was when he or she became diabetic, the longer the retinopathy-free period [33]. Moreover, girls acquired their first retinal lesions one year earlier than boys, although age at onset of diabetes did not differ between boys and girls [34], maybe because puberty appears earlier in girls than in boys. Hormonal changes could be involved in the development of complications [35]. Insulin resistance during puberty, related to BMI and adiposity among others, could be a factor favoring complications [36].

PERSONAL EXPERIENCE

The purpose of this paper is to briefly summarize our clinical studies, begun more than 30 years ago, on the screening for subclinical complications in young type 1 diabetic people. It is not an extensive review of the scientific literature. Of course, the cited articles have a bibliography brought up to date from the moment of their publication.

Only few general or review papers on complications in diabetic children have been published during the latest years [37–44]. Recommended screening procedures for diabetic complications in children have been published by the International Society for Pediatric and Adolescent Diabetes (ISPAD) [45].

RETINOPATHY

CONTRIBUTION OF FLUORESCEIN ANGIOGRAPHY

Used for the first time by Novotny and Alvis in 1961 [46], the retinal fluorescein angiography is a considerable progress. This allows detection of early abnormalities that are undetectable by regular ophthalmoscopy; it enables the study of the vascular walls and the perturbations of the dynamic circulation. The principle of the angiofluororetinography is simple. After intravenous injection of fluorescein (10 ml of a 10% sodium solution), the retina is lit up by an electronic flash [47–49] crossing a blue filter, giving an intense light, the wavelength being more or less 4,900 Å, which corresponds to the absorption band of fluorescein. A photograph is taken at the same time behind a yellow filter that only allows the passage of the light emitted by the fluorescein, eliminating all interferences. The photographic sequence entails one per second for 10 or 15 seconds. Two complementary photographs are taken 15 to 30 minutes after the fluorescein injection. In

practice, for many ophthalmologists the method for obtaining the best photographs remains unclear, and subsequent interpretation of these pictures is difficult. Paradoxically, fluorescein angiography (a sensitive method) is prescribed most often for patients who already show retinal lesions by normal ophthalmoscopy (a less sensitive method) so that the initial abnormalities of diabetic retinopathy may not be seen for several years [37, 48, 49].

Among 114 diabetics whose disease was diagnosed before the age of 14, with duration of diabetes ranging from 1 month to 19 years (mean: 6 years), retinopathy was diagnosed in 21 patients (18%) by regular ophthalmoscopy with green filter, whereas fluorescein angiography evidenced abnormalities in 39 patients (34%) [49]. Compared with regular ophthalmoscopy, fluorescein angiography doubles the diagnosis of incipient retinopathy.

CHARACTERIZATION OF EARLY STAGES OF DIABETIC RETINOPATHY: FLUORESCEIN LEAKS

Since 1994, the late Daniel Toussaint and myself have shown that microaneurysms could be preceded by a functional abnormality characterized by the appearance of fluorescein leaks secondary to an increased permeability of the pigment epithelium and retinal capillaries [28, 47–54] (Figure 21.2 and Figure 21.3a). These leakages are different from those seen later in the disease in the (pre)proliferative stage (Figure 21.3b). Even though our first studies were published in French (not in English) [47, 48], in 1978, Arnall Patz, from the Wilner Ophthalmological Institute of the John Hopkins Hospital, in fairness, wrote in the New England Journal of Medicine that: "Drs. Dorchy and Toussaint have pioneered in the use of fluorescein angiography in the study of diabetic retinopathy and have defined early changes observed in patients with juvenile-onset diabetes... Their observations of capillary leakage as a result of vascular incompetence before specific morphologic lesions occur represent an important contribution" [55]. However, nearly three decades after our first publication [47], it is difficult to persuade some diabetologists or ophthalmologists of the importance of fluorescein leaks as an incipient functional abnormality.

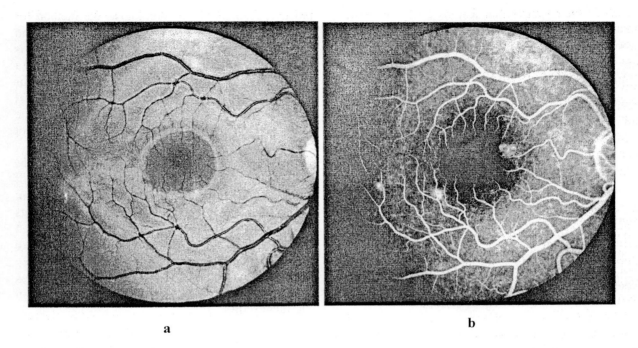

a   b

Figure 21.2

Whereas the red-free photograph was apparently normal (a), the fluorescein angiogram demonstrated fluorescein leakage with no other lesions characteristic of diabetic retinopathy (b) (courtesy of Professor C. Verougstraete, ophthalmology).

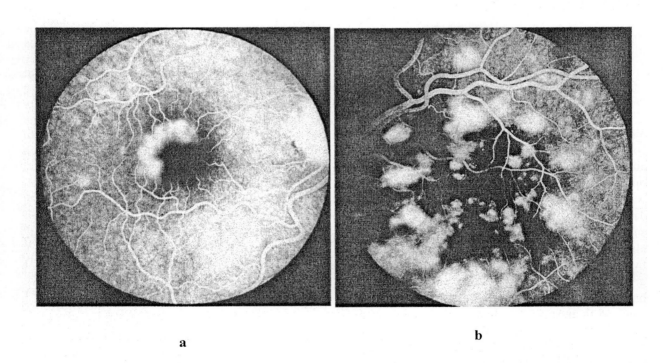

a   b

Figure 21.3

Comparison between fluorescein leaks in early retinopathy (fundoscopy, not shown here, was normal) (a), and myriad of fluorescein leaks presaging proliferative retinopathy in a patient with very poor metabolic control, (b) (courtesy of Professor C. Verougstraete, ophthalmology).

In 1991, we published a longitudinal study of 161 type 1 diabetic children and adolescents, which investigated, by fluorescein angiography, the nature of the initial vascular changes in childhood diabetes, their frequency, and their occurrence [56]. The criteria for inclusion were to have at least one normal angiogram no more than 3 years before the occurrence of the first observed angiographic changes or to have one normal eye. The different types of significant retinal abnormalities, isolated or not, as well as the mean duration of diabetes and age, are shown in Table 21.1. Although capillary nonperfusion was rarely an initial lesion, occurring after a longer duration of diabetes and at a later age than the other abnormalities, no significant difference could be found between the various types of lesions for either the patient's age at onset or the duration of diabetes. The type of initial abnormality was also unrelated to sex, age at onset of diabetes, or long-term glycemic control evaluated by mean values of glycated hemoglobin from either the onset of follow-up or from 1977 onwards, when the method became available.

Retinopathy was not found in children <12 years of age and was detected only after 3 years of diabetes. However, we published the case of a boy with Mauriac syndrome who had become diabetic at 19 months of age and showed retinopathy at 11 years of age [29]. The longest retinopathy-free period was 16 years, which confirms our previous cross-sectional and longitudinal study [34] (Figure 21.4). The mean interval between the onset of retinopathy in the two eyes was 1.2 years with a maximum of 6 years. The conclusion of this study was that if microaneurysms, isolated or associated with other abnormalities, are the most frequently observed lesion (65% of the eyes), leakages were seen in 52% of the eyes, and in the absence of other lesions, in 18% of cases.

We also observed in a 14-years-old adolescent a rare manifestation of capillary permeability involving the optic disc capillaries, resulting in transient leakage at the level of the optic nerves (Figure 21.5), consecutive to rapid improvement in the degree of control as shown by Daneman *et al.* [58].

Table 21.1

Frequency, mean duration of diabetes, age at occurrence, and types of significant abnormalities
in 118 eyes of 69 young diabetic patients
with incipient retinopathy (from ref. 56)

Type of abnormality	Eyes (%)	Eyes with single type of abnormality (%)	Mean duration of diabetes (yr)	Mean age (yr)
Microaneurysms	65	31	8.1	16.6
Leakage	52	18	8.3	16.5
Hemorrhages	25	8	7.6	15.9
Areas of capillary non-perfusion	11	0	9.2	18
Capillary remodeling	6	1	9	16.4
All abnormalities	100	58	8.2	16.4

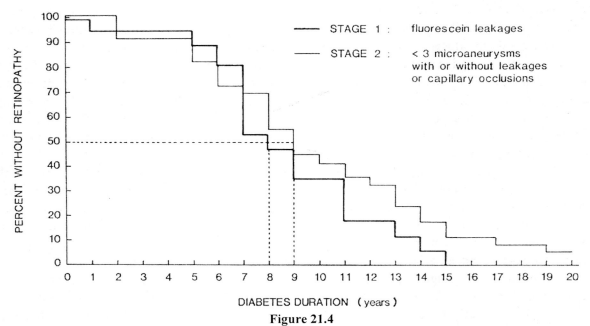

Figure 21.4
Median diabetes duration among patients who developed retinopathy at stages 1 or 2 at any time during the study (from ref. 34).

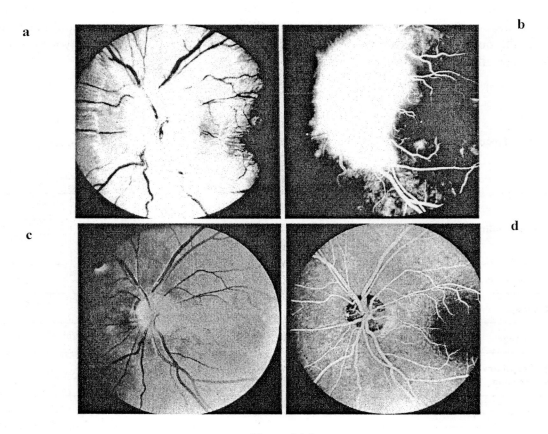

Figure 21.5
Left eye showing severe papilledema, through a green filter (a), and 20 seconds after fluorescein injection (b). In (c) and (d), same subject after 10 days of steroid therapy (from ref. 57).

CLASSIFICATION OF DIABETIC RETINOPATHY

Since 1979 [49], we proposed a new classification of diabetic retinopathy (Figure 21.6) taking into account the existence of early fluorescein leaks, which have been quantified by Cunha-Vaz *et al.* using fluorophotometry [59]. Haut *et al.* [60], reviewing the literature, consider that only fluorescein angiography can take into consideration the functional evaluation of the retinal circulation with unquestionable pathogenic correlation and adapted treatment; edematous diabetic retinopathy corresponds to capillary dilatation and ischemic diabetic retinopathy corresponds to capillary occlusion. Macular diseases are classified according to these same criteria.

Comparative data from literature on the use of fluorescein angiography in diabetic children and adolescents have been recently published by Salardi *et al.* [61].

Several reasons can explain why the initial leakages pass unnoticed by several authors: 1) angiofluorographies should be carried out before the appearance of detectable lesions by ophthalmoscopy or by fundus photography; 2) the dose of fluorescein must be sufficient; 3) angiofluorographic investigation demands meticulousness as well as the subsequent quality of the photographic development and impression at a magnification of 13×13 cm; 4) the number of exposures must be numerous, including late-phase photographs. Even if digital retinal imaging is very fashionable, until now its accuracy has proved unsatisfactory.

The ISPAD recommendations [45] for diabetic retinopathy screening are: "Early retinopathy is asymptomatic but may be detected by sensitive methods (*e.g.*, fundus photography or fluorescein angiography) in a large proportion of young people with diabetes duration of more than 10 years. Fluorescein angiography is not performed in many pediatric centers but is a sensitive method of detecting early functional vascular abnormalities of the retina which are potentially reversible by improvements in metabolic control".

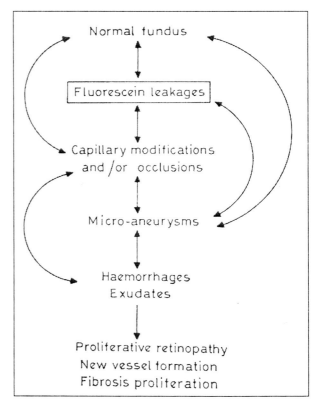

Figure 21.6
Proposed classification of diabetic retinopathy
(from ref. 49).

MECHANISMS OF INCREASED VASCULAR PERMEABILITY

Whereas some of the mechanisms that lead to proliferation in the late stages of retinopathy have been explained, the early processes, which launch the onset of the disease, are still obscure. In 1994, Wardle [62] reviewed the factors involved in increased vascular permeability in diabetics, namely hyperglycemia leading to increased production of diacylglycerol and thence protein kinase C, non-enzymatic glycation generating free radicals and lipid peroxides, sorbitol formation, loss of endothelial cell surface heparan sulphates, and the activation of arachidonate derivatives that affect endothelial cell contractibility. Schmetterer and Wolzt [63] have analyzed other mechanisms: C-peptide could prevent increased retinal blood flow; impaired blood rheology contributes to altered retinal blood flow; the altered endothelin-1 system could be linked to perturbations in the retinal response to hypoxia; vascular endothelial growth factor (VEGF) contributes to the retinal perfusion abnormalities; the exact role of the angiotensin-renin system in the regulation of retinal blood flow is still not clear; recently, it has been shown that not only vascular cells, but also Müller cells of the retina are affected, and express endothelin as well as nitric oxide, etc.

The blood-retinal barrier (BRB) acts at two levels: pigmentary epithelium (external barrier) and endothelial cells of the retinal capillaries. These two cell types are united by tight junctions that prevent the passage of substances (including fluorescein) in the intercellular spaces. Tight junctions are comprised of at least seven proteins. Occludin is a 65-kDa protein specific to cells that contain tight junctions, and is thought to span across the plasma membrane, conferring the cell-to-cell interaction of tight junctions. Antonetti et al. [64] have suggested that VEGF decreases retinal endothelial cell occluding content, which accounts for at least some of the loss of BRB integrity and the increased vascular permeability.

FACTORS RELATED TO DIABETIC RETINOPATHY

We conducted several studies to determine the relationship between some clinical and biological factors and diabetic retinopathy. Ancient studies have been summarized elsewhere [53, 65]. Residual endogenous insulin secretion, measured by C-peptide immunoreactivity, was significantly higher in patients without retinal abnormalities. In this group, however, the duration of diabetes was shorter.

The effect of *duration of diabetes* has been found constantly since our first study in 1977 [34, 48, 49, 56].

The effect of *age at onset*, before or after puberty, plays an important role. In patients whose diabetes started before age 11 (*i.e.*, before puberty) mean duration of diabetes before occurrence of retinopathy in the first affected eye was 8.5 years, whereas in patients whose diabetes began later, it was 5.2 years (p <0.001) [24, 33]. Moreover, there was a linear negative correlation between the

duration of diabetes free of retinopathy, and the age at onset of diabetes (r = − 0.72; p < 0.001). In the patients who became diabetic before puberty, the "good" control subgroup (mean age at onset of diabetes = 5.5 years) had their first retinal abnormality after a mean duration of diabetes of 11.7 years while in the "poor" control subgroup (mean age at onset of diabetes = 6.9 years), this duration was only 7.6 years (p < 0.001).

In our studies of 1977 and 1979 [48, 49], insufficient or poor long-term *metabolic control*, evaluated according to clinical estimates, increased the frequency of retinopathy. However, in 1977, Malone *et al.* [66] did not observe a relationship between frequency of retinopathy and the degree of control, because of bad control criteria [67]. After the introduction of glycated hemoglobin as an objective marker of glycemic control, we found no relationship between diabetic retinopathy and total glycated hemoglobin repeatedly measured during a test period of one year [68]. Correlations between retinopathy and glycated hemoglobin appear when measured during several years [34, 69, 70].

We did not find any relationship between the prevalence of retinopathy and the presence of *HLA-DR3 and/or DR4 antigens* [34, 69].

In 1999, we illustrated the *major role of metabolic control* in diabetic retinopathy with the case report of two homozygous twins becoming diabetic at age 8 years [5]. They share the HLA-DQ genotype, which is associated with the highest risk of type 1 diabetes in Belgium: A1*0301-B1*0302 / A1*0501-B1*0201. Their personal medical history, blood pressure, lipoprotein levels, and way of life were very similar, except that one brother had always been very compliant, which resulted in good metabolic control of his diabetes (hemoglobin A1c always <115% of normal values, the upper limit being 100%). His brother, in contrast, had shown, since shortly after the onset of diabetes, a poor metabolic control (hemoglobin A1c from 130% to 150% of normal values). The twin with poor metabolic control had the first signs of retinopathy, as determined by fluorescein angiography, at age 17, three years before his brother, and had a higher level of severity of retinopathy than his brother all through the follow-up. He had a major proliferative retinopathy with bilateral rubeosis at age 31, after 23 years of diabetes (Figure 21.7a); at the same time, his brother only showed moderate background retinopathy (Figure 21.7b).

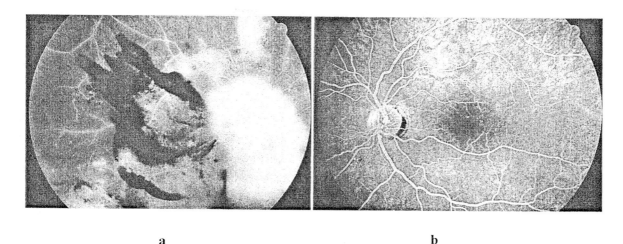

a   b

Figure 21.7

Fluorescein angiogram (a), of twin with poor metabolic control at age 31 (after 23 years of diabetes), showing major proliferative retinopathy with vitreous hemorrhage. In (b), fluorescein angiogram of twin with good metabolic control at same age and same duration of diabetes showing mild background retinopathy (from ref. 5).

At age 32, the twin with poor metabolic control had a slightly reduced peroneal motor nerve conduction velocity. Neither of the 2 brothers had abnormal microalbuminuria. In conclusion, by suppressing the differential genetic influence on diabetic retinopathy evolution and reducing to a minimum external and personal differences, this naturally occurring twin study points out the major importance of the metabolic control on the development of diabetic retinopathy.

In 1991, we published a longitudinal study [56], begun in the 1970s [48], in order to detect the initial retinal abnormalities at fluorescein angiography in 161 type 1 diabetic children and adolescents. Sixty-nine of them developed an incipient retinopathy. In the year 2000, 32 subjects (15 females and 17 males), among these 69 patients who developed incipient retinopathy, were always treated by our team [71]. Their mean age was 33 years and their mean diabetes duration was 26 years. Some potential risk factors (glycated hemoglobin, total cholesterol, blood pressure, BMI, insulin dose, frequency of home blood glucose monitoring and of clinic attendance, smoking tobacco, presence of other complications), measured during the whole follow-up, were analyzed in relationship with the evolution of retinopathy to the proliferative stage, using fluorescein angiography. Proliferative retinopathy was diagnosed in 6 patients (19%),

3 males and 3 females. Its occurrence was significantly related to poor glycemic control during the preceding years, cumulated glycated hemoglobin being 143% vs. 120% (100% is the upper normal limit) (p = 0.049), to cumulated cholesterol levels above 200 mg/dl (p = 0.014), to a higher BMI, 27 kg/m^2 vs. 22 (p = 0.035), and to the presence of other complications (p = 0.029). In conclusion, our data suggest that the risk factors for developing proliferative retinopathy are long-term bad metabolic control, which is well known, and an *elevated BMI*, which is novel, as noticed by Zhang *et al.* [72]. They confirm the importance of maintaining a glycated hemoglobin level always < 120% of the upper normal limit, as we have shown in homozygous diabetic twins [5].

In an as-yet unpublished longitudinal study, we tried to determine the risk factors associated with the progression of non-proliferative diabetic retinopathy, in extension of our previous longitudinal study on the first microangiographic abnormalities in diabetic children [56]. Appearance of retinopathy was significantly correlated with cumulated glycated hemoglobin levels >125% of the upper normal limit, cumulated mean cholesterol level >220 mg/dl, and BMI >27 kg/m^2. Worsening of retinopathy, observed in a period of 3 years, was significantly correlated with raised glycated hemoglobin levels.

The results prove the deleterious effect of bad glycemic control during 3 years.

NEUROPATHY

ELECTRO-ENCEPHALOGRAM (EEG)

In 1979, we published a study on EEG in diabetic children [73]. Abnormal EEG patterns were found in 15 of 61 patients (25%). Among the abnormal EEG patterns, 6 were diffuse (non-rhythmic slowing) and 9 were paroxysmal (spike-and-wave in 5, spikes in 1, sharp waves in 1, bursts of delta waves in 2). A significant positive correlation was found between minor EEG abnormalities and long-term degree of diabetic control according to clinical estimates, but no definite increase was noted in relation to the duration of diabetes. Eighty *per* cent of the patients having more than 5 severe hypoglycemic attacks showed evidence of abnormal EEG, suggesting that hypoglycemic coma or convulsions are closely related to EEG abnormalities (minor hypoglycemic episodes had no effect on the EEG). With the sensitive technique of fluorescein angiography, we demonstrated a clear correlation between incipient retinal angiopathy and EEG abnormalities, perhaps because both retinal and brain capillaries have tight junctions that become leaky in the presence of chronic hyperglycemia. In conclusion, the factors that most positively relate to pathologic electrocerebral activity in diabetic children are frequent and severe hypoglycemic attacks, comas and/or convulsions, and vascular changes in the retina. In 1995, Hauser *et al.* [74] demonstrated that the level of HbA1c influences the EEG and that improvement of glucose metabolism is an important factor in avoiding EEG abnormalities in young diabetic patients. In 1996, Bjorgaas *et al.* [75], in a controlled blind study, have shown that episodes of severe hypoglycemia may affect slightly the fronto-central function in some diabetic children. Putative mechanisms of cerebral abnormalities in diabetes have been reviewed by Biessels *et al.* [76].

AFFERENT NERVE ACTION POTENTIAL AND CEREBRAL SOMATOSENSORY EVOKED POTENTIALS

Clinical neuropathy is rare in children and adolescents with satisfactory glycemic control. Sensitive tests can detect subclinical neurological abnormalities, the natural history of these being unclear [45].

In 1981, in a pilot study, we measured the afferent conduction of nerve impulses from digits to the cortical sensory area [77]. The recording of the afferent nerve impulse volley at different levels of the peripheral and central nervous system (CNS) is particularly rewarding in the precise determination of mild, subclinical abnormalities. The cerebral somatosensory evoked potential affords ultimately critical data allowing an evaluation of the propagation of the same volley in the CNS, namely the spinal cord and intracerebral pathway. In diabetic patients without clinical neuropathy, subclinical neuropathy, characterized by desynchronization of action potentials in the median nerve, precedes conduction velocity (CV) slowing. A reduction of the maximal CV is not the sole feature indicating a dysfunction of the peripheral nerve. Additional evidence of a pathological process can be demonstrated by late components of the nerve action potential (NAP) (Figure 21.8). Late components result from small-demyelinated segments of the nerve, not sufficiently important to slow maximal CV (Figure 21.9). In the patient illustrated in Figure 21.8b, the 13.3-ms latency of the last deflection points to an additional delay. A demyelinated segment of 3.7 cm, corresponding to approximately 18 internodes, either clustered or randomly distributed along the nerve, should be postulated to account for such an abnormality. There is a distal predominance of these abnormalities. By contrast, the central CV is normal.

If the recording of the afferent nerve impulse volley at different levels is particularly sensitive in the determination of subclinical alterations, it cannot be proposed as a routine diagnostic tool. Indeed, this technique is time-consuming, unpleasant for the patient and requires sophisticated electronic equipment. Less invasive methods, but less sensitive, can be used to evidence peripheral sensory nerve dysfunction [78].

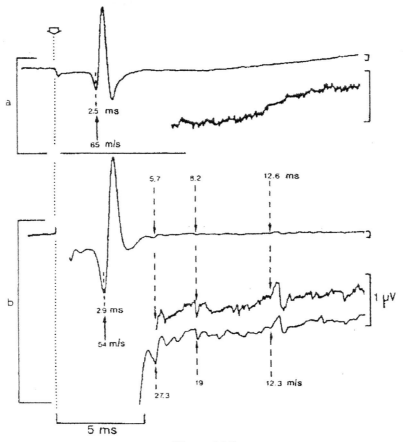

Figure 21.8

In a, sensory NAP recorded at the wrist in a normal subject aged 14 at 2 different magnifications. In b, sensory NAP recorded at the wrist in a diabetic patient aged 14. Dotted lines indicate the onset of 3 late components. Two separate runs are illustrated to demonstrate the consistency of these abnormal responses (from ref. 77).

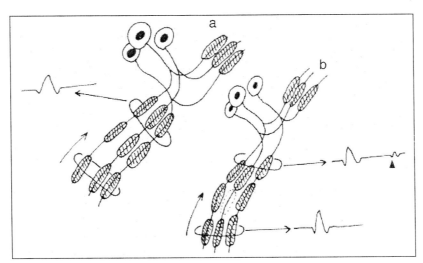

Figure 21.9

Theoretical drawing of a sensory myelinated nerve consisting of 3 nerve fibers.

In (a): normal nerve with triphasic NAP. In (b): diabetic nerve; the middle fiber presents a demyelinated node. The delay of the nerve fiber action potential at this site accounts for the late deflection (arrow) of the compound response recorded proximally to the lesion (from ref. 77).

PERONEAL AND FEMORAL MOTOR NERVE CONDUCTION VELOCITY

In 1985, we published a study in which we have investigated incipient diabetic motor neuropathy [79]. Peroneal motor nerve conduction velocity (PMNCV) was measured in 61 diabetic children and adolescents (age range: 7–22 yr; diabetes duration: 1–15 yr) whose type 1 diabetes became clinically apparent before the age of 14 years. They had no neurological symptoms. PMNCV in diabetic patients (48.3±5.6 m/s) was significantly lower than in controls (56.5±5.5 m/s), 23 diabetics (36%) having a value higher than 2 SD below the mean for normal subjects. Moreover, late components, indicating low CV in some fibers, were detected in 5 patients with normal CV. This attests a subclinical neuropathy even in those patients in whom PMNCV is normal. It must be emphasized that the PMNCV is in fact the CV in the fasted fibers and thus, when normal, gives no clue to the function of the nerve trunk considered as a whole. There was a highly significant negative correlation between PMNCV and HbA1 levels concomitant with PMNCV measurement (r = –0.43; p < 0.001) or mean annual HbA1 concentrations preceding PMNCV (r = –0.42; p <0.001). The relationship between PMNCV and the clinical score of diabetic control since the onset of the disease was also significant. Age, duration of diabetes and HLR-DR antigens were unrelated to PMNCV. EEG abnormalities and retinopathy, whose pathogenesis is different, were not necessarily associated with subclinical neuropathy. Being easy and sensitive, PMNCV determination provides the pediatric diabetologist and the patient himself with an important motivation to improve diabetic control.

In order to compare the prevalence of diabetic neuropathy in proximal and distal peripheral nerves, femoral and peroneal motor conduction was also evaluated in 61 diabetic children, adolescents and young adults (age range: 6–24 years; diabetes duration: 1–17 years) whose type 1 diabetes had become clinically apparent before the age of 14 years [80]. They had no neurological symptoms. Femoral motor nerve conduction velocity (FMNCV) in diabetic patients (63.8±10.4 m/sec) was not significantly different from FMNCV in control subjects (65.6±7.1 m/sec). However, 13% of the patients have a value more than 2 SD below the mean for normals. By contrast, PMNCV in diabetic patients (50.2± ±6.9 m/sec) was significantly lower than in controls (54.1±3.5 m/sec), 31% of the patients having a value more than 2 SD below the mean for normals, which confirms our previous study [79]. Peroneal nerve abnormality was negatively correlated with HbA1 levels, while femoral nerve abnormality was positively correlated with the presence of retinopathy. This discrepancy is not fully understood. Age and duration of diabetes were unrelated to femoral or peroneal motor nerve conduction velocity. Our data emphasize the occurrence of subclinical proximal neuropathy in diabetic children and adolescents. However, for a routine diagnostic tool PMNCV determination must be chosen. Moreover, very recently, Carrington et al. [81] have concluded that PMNCV is the best predictor for foot ulceration.

SYMPATHETIC SKIN RESPONSE

The sympathetic skin response (SSR) is a transient reflex change in the electrical potential of the skin that can be elicited by a variety of stimuli. The SSR is generated by the sweat glands, and can be measured with surface electrodes connected to a standard electromyogram instrument. During our study on the evolution of subclinical complications [70], the SSR test was performed on 108 diabetic subjects with a mean age of 21 years (range: 8–37 years) and a mean duration of diabetes of 14 years (range: 6–31 years) [24]. A palmar electrode was used to record the SSR, with a stimulating electrode placed at the level of the supra-orbital nerve. Abnormal palmar amplitude is <500 μV. Slowing of palmar amplitude was detected in 16 patients, i.e. 15%, while prevalence of subclinical retinopathy, motor-sensory neuropathy, and nephropathy was, respectively, 49%, 45%, and 11%. As a multiplicity of factors may intrude upon the measurement of this highly complex neurological reflex, the use of SSR testing could not to be a reliable and consistent index of the autonomic dysfunction [82].

HEART RATE VARIABILITY: STATISTICAL AND SPECTRAL ANALYSIS

Since the 1970s, a lot of tests have been proposed for the diagnosis of diabetic autonomic neuropathy, namely 5 simple non-invasive cardiovascular reflex tests (Valsalva maneuver, heart rate response to deep breathing, heart rate response to standing up, blood pressure response to standing up, blood pressure response to sustained handgrip) [83]. In 2001, we carried out a preliminary study in order to determine whether the double, statistical and spectral, analysis of the heart rate variability (HRV), a refined testing, could be used to detect cardiac autonomic neuropathy (CAN) in young adult diabetic patients, who already present ocular, renal or neurological complications [84]. The study included 8 type 1 diabetic patients with a median age of 29 years, and median illness duration of 18 years. Retinopathy (fluorescein angiography) was diagnosed in 7 of them, peripheral neuropathy (conduction velocities in sensory and motor nerves) in 5, and nephropathy (microalbuminuria) in 3. Five-time domain and 3 frequency domain HRV indices were determined from 24-h Holter recordings and then compared to reference values. In the 8 patients, CAN was assessed at different degrees of severity (Figure 21.10). Abnormalities were characterized by a slowing in activity of both vagal and sympathetic nervous system, with a sympathetic-vagal balance in favor of the sympathetic nervous system. The severity of CAN was associated with increasing age and diabetes duration, as well as with the number and severity of the other complications. The statistical and spectral analysis of HRV seems to be an efficient tool in the evaluation of cardiac autonomic function. As it has been demonstrated that diabetic complications may appear from puberty and after 3 years of illness duration, it would be useful to apply this method in young diabetic patients from adolescence [85, 86].

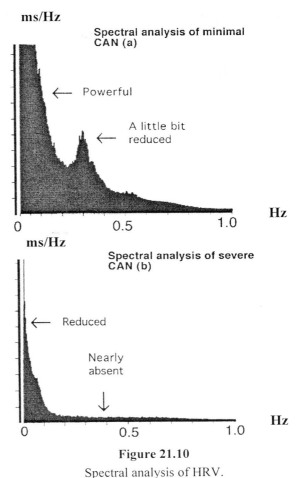

Figure 21.10

Spectral analysis of HRV.

Illustration of the sympathetic-vagal imbalance. (a) – minimal CAN. (b) – severe CAN.

NEPHROPATHY

GLOMERULAR HYPERFILTRATION

Diabetic nephropathy and end-stage renal failure have been a major cause of mortality amongst young adults with type 1 diabetes. In the 1970s, the cumulative incidence of nephropathy, defined as persistent proteinuria, was about 40% after 40 years of type 1 diabetes [87]. The incidence increases sharply 10 years after onset of diabetes but it is low after 35 years. In recent decades, a decrease in clinical nephropathy in some countries probably reflects improvements in diabetes management and glycemic control [45].

In patients with type 1 diabetes, micro-albuminuria (MA), defined as an albumin excretion rate between 20–200 µg/min, precedes persistent proteinuria and is an accepted early sign of nephropathy and glomerular damage [88]. However, MA can be preceded by glomerular hyperfiltration. Glomerular hyperfiltration in diabetes mellitus was first described by a Belgian man, P. Cambier [89]. Soper *et al.* [90] have shown that poor glycemic control directly correlates with hyperfiltration and renal hyperperfusion in early type 1 diabetes. In our experience, glomerular filtration rate, determined by ^{51}Cr-EDTA at the onset of diabetes, is >145 ml/min/1.73 m in 75% of diabetic children under 15 years of age [91]. Later, there is normalization when good HbA1c is obtained.

MARKERS OF EARLY GLOMERULAR AND TUBULAR DYSFUNCTION DURING EXERCISE

In 1975, Mogensen and Vittinghus [92] proposed a light physical exercise stress test (100W) to elicit and screen for the early presence of albuminuria in diabetic adults. In 1976, in a preliminary study [93], our group did not find exercise until exhaustion to be a stimulating effect on proteinuria in diabetic children under 16 years of age. In order to verify our previous results on a greater number of young patients, we determined whether protein excretion during intense physical exercise is an earlier sign of renal dysfunction in diabetic adolescents than the basal measurements [94]. Urinary creatinine, total proteins, albumin, and β2-microglobulin were studied before, immediately after, and 30 minutes after exercise until exhaustion on a bicycle ergometer in a group of 21 adolescent diabetic boys (Albustix negative) and in a comparable control group. The controls, as well as the diabetic subjects, ranged from 13 to 25 years of age, and the duration of diabetes varied from 3 to 14 years. Among the 21 diabetic subjects, 11 had an incipient retinopathy diagnosed by fluorescein angiography. Urinary output of creatinine was similar in diabetic and in nondiabetic groups, and did not vary during exercise. At rest, the urinary output of total proteins, albumin, and β2-microglobulin was significantly higher in diabetic subjects than in controls (Figure 21.11). These data suggest that the subclinical proteinuria of diabetes is of mixed origin, being both glomerular and tubular. An exercise test leading to exhaustion did not give

any additional information other than the basal excretion. There was no difference between diabetic subjects with early retinal vascular changes and those free from all retinopathy (Figure 21.11). From these results, it may be concluded that exhaustive physical exercise does not provoke, in diabetic patients, an enhanced dysfunction of the kidney, while moderate loads induce a slight increase in postexercise proteinuria in diabetic patients, which is not observed in a healthy population [95].

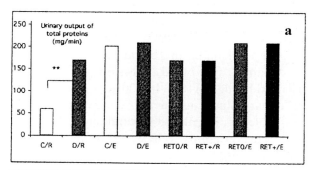

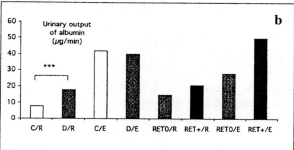

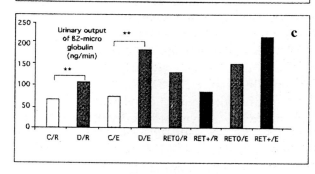

Figure 21.11

Urinary output of total proteins (a), albumin (b), and β2-microglobulin (c) in controls (C) and in diabetic subjects (D), at rest (R) and after exercise until exhaustion (E). At rest, the urinary output of total proteins, albumin, and β2-microglobulin was significantly higher in diabetic subjects than in controls. There was no difference between diabetic patients with subclinical retinopathy (RET+) and those free from all retinopathy (RET0) (from ref. 94).

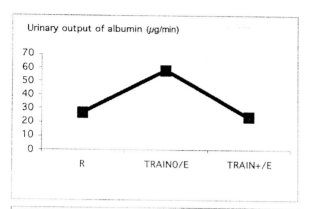

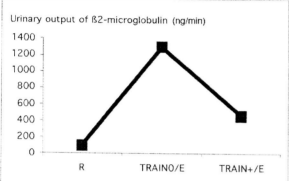

Figure 21.12

Urinary excretion of albumin and β2-microglobulin at rest (R) and 15 minutes after physical exercise (E), before (TRAIN0) and after training (TRAIN+) on a regular basis, six hours per day during 15 days, in 21 adolescents (from ref. 96).

We also investigated the potential benefit of exercise training on the renal handling of plasma proteins in a young diabetic population (11 to 18 years old; diabetes duration: 1–13 years) who participated in a 15-day sport camp with a daily exercise period of about 6h of various physical activities [96]. Under the influence of training, both albumin and β2-microglobulin excretion were reduced by half for the same load of exercise (Figure 21.12). Whether this effect is beneficial for diabetic adolescents remains an open question.

URINARY EXCRETION OF TRANSFERRIN AND ACID GLYCOSAMINOGLYCANS

It has been proposed that the determination of urinary transferrin is more sensitive than the determination of albumin for early detection of glomerular dysfunction [97]. Earlier (in a pilot study published in 1984) we had shown that urinary transferrin excretion is higher than normal even in patients with normal MA [98]. Transferrin is a protein very similar to albumin in molecular weight (mw) (90,000 *vs*. 69,000) and shape, but with a higher isoelectric point. In general, proteins with high isoelectric points are filtered more easily through the glomerular barrier. Abnormal transferrin or MA excretion was unrelated to incipient retinopathy diagnosed by fluorescein angiography or subclinical neuropathy revealed by slowing of peroneal motor nerve conduction velocity. On the other hand, urinary excretion of α2-HS-glycoprotein (mw: 49,000) and immunoglobulin G (mw: 160,000) was normal.

Recently we tried to confirm, with a better methodology, whether increased urinary transferrin excretion (UTE) could be found in patients with normal urinary albumin, in a larger population [99]. The study included 105 patients (64 boys, 41 girls). The median age was 16 years (5–42) and the median duration of diabetes was 8 years (1–32). They had a mean HbA1c level of 7.4% (upper normal limit: 6.1%). Blood pressure was normal (< 14/9 cm Hg). Urine was collected overnight and kept at 4°C until albumin and transferrin determination (1–2 days). Albumin was determined by immunoturbidimetry and transferrin by nephelometry. Normal values were measured in 27 healthy subjects: albumin < 31 mg/g creatinine; UTE < 0.002 mg/g creatinine. Slightly elevated MA was found in 7 patients (6.7%) and a higher UTE in 4 patients (3.8%), after a minimum duration of diabetes of 6 years. Only 2 subjects (1.9%) had concomitantly increased MA and UTE. Taken together, there was no correlation between urine albumin and UTE (p = 0.77). The conclusion was that, in this unselected population of young diabetic subjects with a variable degree of glycemic control, the prevalence of abnormal MA or UTE is low. There is no relationship between urine albumin and UTE. UTE contributes less than MA as a marker of early renal dysfunction in young diabetic patients. It is interesting to note that the prevalence of subclinical nephropathy is lower than that observed 10 years ago [9].

Acid glycosaminoglycans (GAG) are incorporated within the glomerular membrane. Their negative charges prevent the transfer of macromolecules through the membrane. In adult diabetic patients, it has been shown that the synthesis of GAG is reduced, which could contribute to impairment in the glomerular anionic filtration barrier. Therefore we tried to answer the following question: would GAG excretion be an earlier marker of glomerular dysfunction than microalbuminuria [100]? The study included 101 patients (60 boys, 41 girls). Their mean age was 17 years and the mean duration of diabetes was 8 years. They had a mean HbA1c level of 7.4% (upper normal limit: 6.1%). Urine was collected overnight and kept at 4°C until albumin and GAG determination (1–2 days). Albumin was determined by an immunological technique (nephelometry) while GAG was assayed by an ELISA system using the diethyl ethylene blue method (colorimetry). Normal values are: albumin <20 μg·min^{-1}; GAG < 25 μg·min^{-1}. Slightly elevated microalbuminuria (mean: 35 μg.min^{-1}) was diagnosed in 5 patients (5%) and a higher GAG excretion rate (mean: 47 μg.min^{-1}) in 6 other patients (6%). Taken together, there was no correlation between albumin and GAG urine excretion (p = 0.16). In conclusion, in this unselected population of young diabetic subjects with a variable degree of glycemic control, the prevalence of abnormal microalbumin or GAG urine excretion is low. There is no relationship between albumin and GAG excretion. The independent predictive value of GAG as an early marker of glomerular dysfunction should be confirmed in a prospective study.

In the literature, other markers of both glomerular and tubular dysfunction have been studied: 1) glomerular: fibronectin, laminin P1, type IV collagen, etc.; 2) tubular: retinal binding protein, α1 microglobulin, Tamm-Horshall protein, N-acetyl-β-D-glucosaminidase, etc. [101]. There is not yet consensus as to which will emerge as being widely accepted for use. Kordonouri et al. [102] have confirmed our findings from 1982 [94], i.e. that in diabetic children and adolescents both glomerular and tubular dysfunction may be present. Therefore, the sole measurement of MA is not satisfactory, even if it is proposed in the ISPAD guidelines [45]. Schultz et al. [103] have suggested that a rise in albumin-to-creatinine ratio within the normal range may be a risk marker for diabetic nephropathy. HbA1c is a determinant of risk for MA, but pubertal factors have a greater effect on rates of progression of urine albumin excretion during adolescence. It has been shown that, in patients with microalbuminuria, the risk of progression to overt proteinuria can be reduced by improving glycemic control, only if the HbA1c is maintained below 8.5%. Moreover, below that value, the risk declines as the level of HbA1c decreases [104]. Diabetic nephropathy is limited to a subset of patients with long-standing poorly controlled diabetes and an apparent hereditary predisposition. Sodium-hydrogen exchange appears to detect a subset of diabetic patients prone to develop renal damage [105]. Several observational follow-up studies have found that the D allele of the insertion / deletion polymorphism of the ACE gene is associated with an increased risk of renal function loss, even during ACE inhibition [106]. Losartan could have similar renoprotective effects in diabetic patients with ACE II and DD genotypes.

PREDICTIVE MARKERS FOR DIABETIC TRIOPATHY

LIPOPROTEIN (a)

Ten years ago, the role of lipoprotein (Lp) (a) as a genetically determined marker to predict complications in diabetic adults was controversial [107]. This protein is composed of apolipoprotein (a) covalently linked to apoprotein B-100. The homology of structure of Lp(a) to plasminogen was evoked to provide a link between the clotting and lipoprotein system. In 1993, Coupe et al. [108] have shown that only pubertal and postpubertal young diabetic patients had higher serum Lp(a) levels than control subjects. In 1996, we published a study [109] on an eventual relationship between Lp(a) and three main complications (retinopathy, neuropathy, nephropathy) diagnosed with sensitive methods even at a subclinical level in 106 young type 1 diabetic patients, between 1 and 30 years of age. The patients were subdivided according to puberty and to the presence or not of subclinical complications (no complications [n = 32]; retinopathy at fluorescein angiography [n = 28]; neuropathy diagnosed by reduced peroneal motor nerve conduction velocity [n = 30]; nephropathy determined by the presence of microalbuminuria [n = 15]). Lp(a) concentrations were not significantly increased in the whole group of diabetic patients. There was no difference between girls and boys, or between the prepubertal children and the others. There were no significant correlations between the markers of metabolic control (HbA1c or fructosamine) and Lp(a). Nevertheless, if the diabetic patients were divided into two groups according to the levels of HbA1c (<7.6 or ≥7.6%), Lp(a) tends to be higher in the poorly controlled, but not to any significant degree. On the other hand, significant increases of total cholesterol, triglycerides, low-density lipoprotein cholesterol (LDL-c) and apolipoprotein B levels were observed in poorly controlled patients. Lp(a) concentrations were significantly lower in patients with subclinical neuropathy or nephropathy than in patients without these complications, but not in patients with retinopathy versus no retinopathy. These results were confirmed by categorical analysis (i.e. Lp(a) ≤ 30 vs. > 30 mg/dl). In conclusion, Lp(a) levels are not significantly increased in poorly controlled young type 1 diabetic patients. High levels of Lp(a), in young diabetic patients, are not markers for subclinical complications (retinopathy, neuropathy and nephropathy). On the contrary, low Lp(a) levels were found in subjects with subclinical neuropathy or nephropathy. Recently Hernandez et al. [110] have observed that LDL cholesterol (positively) and triglycerides (negatively) were independently related to Lp(a) concentration in diabetic patients, whatever the Lp(a) phenotype. These results indicate that Lp(a) concentrations depend on lipid profiles and suggest that treatment of diabetic dyslipidemia may also affect Lp(a) concentrations. In a review of the literature published in 2003 [111], it is stated that the contribution of Lp(a) to the enhanced risk of vascular disease in the diabetic population is not yet clearly defined.

Ultra sensitive CRP

Observations support the theory that chronic low-degree inflammation is involved in the initiation or progression of atherosclerosis. A feature of inflammatory activity is the increase in plasma concentration of acute-phase proteins produced by the liver such as the C-reactive protein (CRP). Ridker et al. [112] have conducted a prospective study among 28,263 apparently healthy post-menopausal women over a mean follow-up period of 3 years to assess the risk of cardiovascular events associated with the base-line levels of 12 markers of inflammation and also homocysteine and lipids. The conclusion is that the addition of the measurements of ultra

sensitive CRP (US-CRP) and of total cholesterol and HDL-cholesterol, is the best method to identify persons at high risk for future cardiovascular events. Little information exists in young type 1 diabetic patients. In type 1 diabetic patients, Sckalkwijk et al. [113], have found a correlation between C-reactive protein and markers of endothelial dysfunction suggesting a relation between activation of the endothelium and chronic inflammation. There are no data in diabetic children and adolescents on a possible relationship between US-CRP and complications.

Therefore, we initiated a study in order to investigate the impact of the diabetic state (HbA1c, blood lipids, subclinical complications, etc.) on the levels of US-CRP. US-CRP was determined in 126 young type 1 diabetic patients (55 girls and 71 boys), excluding the youngest that are certainly free of subclinical complications, and in 52 healthy controls [114]. The patients were divided into 2 groups according to the presence of subclinical complications: retinopathy (fluorescein angiography); neuropathy (conduction velocities); nephropathy (microalbuminuria). 81 subjects (group A) were free of complications (mean age ± SD: 16 ± 6 years; diabetes duration: 7 ± 4 years); 45 had at least 1 subclinical complication (mean age ± SD: 27 ± 7 years; diabetes duration: 19 ± 8 years). US-CRP was measured by a nephelometric assay. Blood lipids and HbA1c (HPLC) were also determined. Circulating levels of US-CRP were significantly higher in patients than in controls (2.6 ± 4 mg/l vs. 0.6 ± 0.6; $p < 0.001$). This difference persisted when comparing normal subjects with those of group A (2.0 ± 3.1; $p < 0.01$) and of group B (3.6 ± 5.1; $p < 0.001$) (Figure 21.13). Group B patients also had significantly higher levels of lipids (except for HDL-cholesterol) than those of group A (Figure 21.13). US-CRP levels were significantly correlated to diabetes duration (in group A only), total cholesterol (TC), TC/HDL-C ratio, LDL-C, triglycerides (TG), but not with HDL-C, HbA1c, or blood glucose. The multivariate regression analysis showed that US-CRP concentration and the TC/HDL-C ratio interact independently on the risk for subclinical complications. In conclusion, mean plasma concentration of US-CRP increased nearly 3-fold in diabetic patients without subclinical complications and 5-fold in those with subclinical complications in parallel with higher levels of TC, LDL-C and TG. US-CRP seems to be an interesting indicator of the risk for developing early complications.

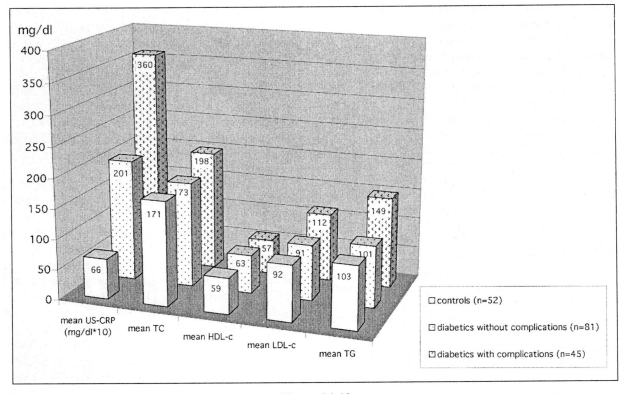

Figure 21.13

Mean values of US-CRP, TC, HDL-c, LDL-c, TG in controls and in diabetic patients without
or with subclinical complications.

OTHER SUBCLINICAL COMPLICATIONS

(Apo)LIPOPROTEINS ABNORMALITIES

Many studies have demonstrated that the atherosclerotic process begins in childhood in association with high blood cholesterol levels [115]. Lipid levels show a strong familial aggregation that has both a genetic and environmental component. In the 1980s, data on lipoprotein abnormalities and their relationship with glycemic control were controversial. To clarify this question, we began a study [116] in which plasma levels of triglycerides (TG), total cholesterol (TC), HDL- and LDL-cholesterols, apolipoproteins (Apo) A1 and B were measured in 120 young patients aged from 4 to 32 years (mean ± 1 SD: 17 ± 6 years) whose diabetes had been present for a mean period of 10 ± 6 years (range: less than one year to 25 years). The results

obtained were analyzed in relation to total glycated hemoglobin (N: 6.8 ± 0.6%) and plasma fructosamine (N: 1.9 ± 0.2 mmol/l) levels. The patients were divided into 3 groups according to their HbA1 level: group 1: <9%; group 2: 9% ≤ HbA1< 11%; group 3: ≥11 %. The most significant increases of TG, TC, LDL-C and ApoB levels were observed in group 3, *i.e.* in patients whose diabetes was the most poorly controlled (HbA1: 12.9 ± 1.3%; fructosamine: 4.6 ± 0.9 mmol/l). These parameters were significantly correlated with HbA1 (p < 0.01) and even more significantly with fructosamine (p < 0.001). No significant difference in HDL-C and ApoA1 levels was found in the 3 groups of patients. HDL2-C or HDL3-C were unrelated to metabolic control [117]. Thus, TG, TC, LDL-C and ApoB are increased in young diabetics whose HbA1 and fructosamine levels exceed reference values by more than 5 standard deviations. Consequently, blood glucose should be maximized and dietary counseling should be provided, namely in Belgium where the fat intake is too high, and the polyunsaturated-to-saturated fat ratio too low at 0.45 [18]. An Australian group has shown that a modest increase in the monounsaturated fat content of an adolescent diet has the potential to improve glycemic control and lipid profile [118]. Evidence that postprandial lipoproteins are themselves atherogenic is expanding and with this new information, new emphasis must be placed on measures to normalize both fasting and postprandial apo B-containing lipoprotein abnormities in order to prevent the vascular complications of diabetes [119]. Of course, hyperlipidemia is in part genetically determined and it has been demonstrated that both mean parental total cholesterol and HbA1c were significant determinants of the child's total cholesterol [120].

OXIDATIVE STRESS

Endothelial dysfunction, a forerunner of diabetic angiopathy, is present early in the course of childhood diabetes. The mechanisms of such endothelial dysfunction are not clear, but oxidative stress has been proposed as one of the putative mechanisms of vascular injury in diabetes. It results from the balance between the different antioxidant defenses, non-enzymatic (vitamins C, E or A, free radical scavengers) and enzymes (red cell superoxide dismutase [SOD], red cell glutathione peroxidase [GPX], glutathione reductase [GRD]), and the free radical production [121]. Recent studies have pointed out the key role of superoxide production in the endothelial cells at the mitochondrial level during hyperglycemia in the activation of the pathways involved in the pathogenesis of diabetic complications. These include increased polyol pathway flux, increased advanced glycation end-product formation, activation of protein kinase C, and increased hexosamine pathway flux [122]. Superoxide overproduction is accompanied by increased nitric oxide generation, which in turn damages DNA. This leads to activation of the nuclear enzyme poly(ADP-ribose) polymerase, which depletes the intracellular content of its substrate NAD, slowing the rate of glycolysis, electron transport, and ATP formation.

In a first study [123–125], some biological parameters involved in cell defense against oxygen radicals (plasma vitamins C and E, GPX, GRD and SOD) were measured in single blood samples from 119 diabetic infants, adolescents and young adults. Data were studied in relation to residual insulin secretion determined by C peptide, level of metabolic control appreciated by glycated hemoglobin, lipid abnormalities and subclinical complications (retinopathy by fluorescein angiography, neuropathy by peroneal motor nerve conduction velocity and nephropathy by microalbuminuria). There was no change in antioxidant parameters with residual insulin secretion. Patients with poor glycemic control and high plasma lipids had higher levels of plasma vitamin E. Patients with subclinical nephropathy had lower plasma vitamin C levels and those with neuropathy showed lower GPX activity. Plasma vitamin C concentrations and GRD activities were negatively correlated with the age of the patients and with duration of diabetes. We concluded that higher transport capacity of vitamin E probably explains the elevated levels of vitamin E observed in patients with high lipid levels. The lower levels of vitamin C in the presence of nephropathy may be due to an increased renal excretion of this vitamin, as also shown by Hirsch et al. [126]. The lower GPX activity associated with subclinical neuropathy confirms the animal studies having demonstrated that oxidative stress can reduce Na^+-K^+-ATPase activity [127]. The reduction of GPX, GRD activities and vitamin C levels confirms the existence of an oxidative stress in young type 1 diabetic subjects. Another pediatric study has shown that systemic oxidative stress is present upon early onset of diabetes and is increased by early adulthood [128].

As oxidized LDL and autoantibodies to oxidized LDL seem to play an important role in the atherogenic process, and as studies in young type 1 diabetic patients are scarce, it was decided to evaluate autoantibodies against oxidized LDL (o-LAB) and antioxidant status in relationship with levels of HbA1c and lipids, and with the presence of subclinical complications (retinopathy by fluorescein angiography, neuropathy by peroneal motor nerve conduction velocity and nephropathy by microalbuminuria) [129]. The study included 110 young type 1 diabetic patients, with a median age of 15 years and a median diabetes duration of 5 years. The mean ± SEM of HbA1c levels was 7.1 ± 0.2 % (upper normal limit: 6.1 %). Subclinical complications were detected in 26 patients. Total antioxidant status (TAS), vitamin A or E were not decreased in the patients and no significant differences were noted between the different subgroups of patients classified according to their subclinical complications. HbA1c levels were not related to antioxidants. Autoantibodies against LDL-lipoproteins decreased with age and diabetes duration, as reported in healthy non-diabetic subjects. The decrease of o-LAB could be associated with the onset of the atherosclerotic process if we consider that o-LAB antibodies are an accompanying immunological expression of lipid peroxidation. The titers of circulating o-LAB antibodies reflect the balance between the amount of antibodies generated and released into the circulation and the consumption of these antibodies. In conclusion, in diabetic patients with a more or less good diabetic control, increased lipid peroxidation or reduced lipid antioxidant defense could not be demonstrated, even for the patients with subclinical complications. Recently, Varvarovska *et al.* [130] have shown reduced plasma antioxidant capacity in diabetic children, but their mean HbA1c level was high: 9.2 % (upper normal limit: 5.8 %).

To fight against the oxidative stress, antioxidant drugs, in particular vitamins C and E, have failed to demonstrate any effect [122]. In the latest few years, lipoic acid has been found to reduce neuropathic symptoms [127]. Statins, ACE inhibitors, and angiotensin 1 inhibitors can also reduce intracellular oxidative stress generation. Finally, the best way to avoid increased superoxide production is to maintain blood glucose values close to the normal range.

METABOLIC DISRUPTIONS IN RED AND WHITE CELLS

Metabolic and structural modifications of the red blood cell may play a role in the pathogenesis of diabetic microangiopathy. Impaired deformability of the diabetic erythrocyte affecting the blood flow at the capillary level, increased glycation of membrane proteins and hemoglobin, decreased intra-erythrocytic adenosine triphosphate (ATP) level have been implicated as causative factors in the development of vascular complications. Ditzel [131] pointed out the importance of the alterations of oxygen delivery to the tissues in the disease: in the acidotic patient, the acidosis and hypophosphatemia interfere with the red cell 2,3 diphosphoglycerate (2,3 DPG) generation. The resulting increase in hemoglobin-oxygen affinity together with an excessive formation of glycated hemoglobin could be, in part, responsible for tissue hypoxia. Data concerning diabetic red cell glycolysis activity, ATP and 2,3 DPG levels are rather fragmentary and mainly focused on adult diabetes. Therefore, we published in 1992 a paper the aim of which being to study this metabolic pathway in red cells from type 1 diabetic children and adolescents [132]. Erythrocytes from young type 1 diabetic patients (n = 11), incubated in their plasma in anaerobic conditions, exhibited higher glucose consumption than cells from controls (n = 11). This increased metabolic activity is believed to reflect erythrocyte alterations dependent on the degree of metabolic control, as glucose consumption was significantly correlated to glycated hemoglobin (HbA1) and to glucose levels ($p < 0.05$ and $p < 0.01$, respectively). Red cell hexokinase (HK) and pyruvate kinase (PK) activities were similar in both groups whereas phosphofructokinase (PFK) activity was slightly higher in patients' cells ($p < 0.05$). No difference was found between patients and controls for red cell ATP and 2,3 DPG levels. However, the concentrations of these glycolytic products seem also closely related to the glucose homeostasis in diabetes. Indeed, within the diabetic group, ATP levels showed a negative relationship with glucose level ($p < 0.05$) and 2,3 DPG a positive relationship with HbA1 ($p < 0.05$). In conclusion, higher glycolytic activity is present in young diabetic red cells. This activity as well as ATP and 2,3 DPG levels are related to the degree of short- or long-term diabetic control. These findings stress the importance of a careful metabolic control to avoid hematological disturbances.

In the literature, some diabetic patients have been shown to present disturbances to one or more functions of their polymorphonuclear neutrophils (PMN). Abnormalities of adherence, chemotaxis, phagocytosis, nitroblue tetrazolium (NBT) reduction, superoxide anion formation, chemiluminescence and bacterial killing have all been described, and may play a role in the decreased host resistance to infections, which is observed in poorly controlled diabetic patients. The published data are, however, equivocal; for instance, the PMN dysfunction has been attributed to serum and / or cellular abnormalities. These discrepancies may be due to at least 2 factors: 1) the variability of the methods used; 2) the variable and sometimes poorly defined clinical status of the patients under consideration. The aims of our work [133] were to compare PMN functions in type 1 diabetic children with controls and to determine the role of glycation. Twenty unselected young type 1 diabetic patients aged between 13 and 25 years, with a diabetes duration of 2–16 years, were involved in the study. The following PMN functions were analyzed: random and induced migration, *Staphylococcus aureus* and baker's yeast phagocytosis, staphylococcus aureus killing, spontaneous and stimulated NBT reduction, myeloperoxidase score. The effect of the glycation of normal serum on baker's yeast was measured. No significant difference between patients and controls was observed in the PMN functions studied. When diabetic serum was used in the tests, random and induced PMN migrations correlated negatively with the HbA1 level. However, there was a positive correlation between baker's yeast phagocytosis and HbA1 level. The nature of the relevant glycated proteins, which stimulate phagocytosis, is unknown. In conclusion, the PMN dysfunction, which occurs in type 1 diabetes, is a result of both inhibiting and stimulating phenomena and is related to glycated hemoglobin levels.

LOW T_3 SYNDROME

As type 1 diabetes is frequently associated with thyroid autoimmunity [134], in 1985 we published a study on thyroid function (thyroid stimulating hormone, TSH; triiodothyronine, T_3; reverse T_3, rT_3; thyroxine, T_4; free T_4, FT_4) in relationship with the presence of thyroid antibodies (antithyroglobulin and antithyroid microsomes antibodies) as well as with the degree of metabolic control (HbA1c; upper normal limit: 6.5%) [135]. The serum levels of thyroid hormones and TSH were compared in 64 type I diabetic children and adolescents (13.8 ± 4.2 years; diabetes duration: 5.6 ± 3.9 years) without ketosis and in 28 age matched normal subjects (13.9 ± 4.9 years). In diabetic children, HbA1c

was 8.1 ± 2.5%. Only T_3 levels were significantly different in the diabetic patients (2.38 ± ± 0.41 nmol/l) than in the controls (2.64 ± ± 0.52 nmol/l) ($p < 0.01$) confirming the existence of the 'low T_3 syndrome' in diabetic children as already described in diabetic adults with poor metabolic control. A negative correlation was found between T_3 and blood glucose as well as glycated hemoglobin suggesting that short-term hyperglycemia could regulate T_3 concentration. Low T_3 level is secondary to an impaired peripheral T_3 production from T_4. This conversion is catalyzed by the enzyme T_{4-5} deiodinase; the activity of this enzyme has been shown to be reduced by hyperglycemia in diabetic rats. Thyroid function was not different in diabetic children with or without thyroid antibodies. We conclude that serum T_3 level is influenced by the degree of metabolic control and that thyroid function in diabetic children should be assessed by the measurement of the serum concentration of T_4, FT_4 and TSH. The negative correlation between HbA1c and T_3 has been confirmed by Radetti *et al.* [136].

Recently, Kordonouri *et al.* [137] found that 10% of diabetic patients, with a median age of 13 years, had elevated titers of antibodies to thyroperoxidase – anti-TPO – (more in girls than in boys), and 6% had antibodies to thyroglobulin. Because 50% of children with diabetes and significant titers of anti-TPO develop thyroid problems within 3–4 years, examinations of thyroid antibodies should be performed yearly.

MAGNESIUM AND HbA1c

Pediatric studies on magnesium depletion in type 1 diabetic patients are scarce, and there are no data on erythrocyte magnesium content (EMC), which is important since 99% of total magnesium (Mg) is intracellular. Moreover, in the pediatric studies there are no data on the relationships between hypomagnesemia and HbA1c levels or subclinical complications. Therefore, we have carried out a study in order to answer these questions [138].

Serum Mg levels, EMC, magnesuria, and HbA1c were determined in 118 type 1 diabetic subjects (105 boys and 83 girls) aged 19 ± 8 years (mean ± SD) with a diabetes duration of 11 ± ± 8 years, and in 96 controls. Mg was measured by colorimetric calmagite kits and HbA1c using a HPLC method. We searched for subclinical retinopathy (fluorescein angiography), neuropathy (conduction velocities in the limbs), nephropathy (microalbuminuria and $\beta2$-microglobulinuria) in patients aged >12 years with a diabetes duration >3 years.

The mean ± SD Mg serum concentration was 1.8 ± 0.2 mg/dl in the diabetic population and 2.0 ± 0.2 mg/dl in the controls ($p < 0.001$). The mean EMC was 5.0 ± 0.5 mg/dl in the patients, vs. 5.3 ± 0.2 mg/dl in the controls ($p < 0.001$). In 14% of the patients, serum Mg levels were less than -2 SD below the normal mean, while 6% of the diabetic subjects had EMC less than -2 SD below the normal mean. In diabetic patients, serum Mg levels were positively correlated with EMC ($r = 0.19$; $p < 0.01$) and negatively with age ($r = -0.24$; $p < 0.01$), duration of diabetes ($r = -0.19$; $p < 0.05$), HbA1c ($r = -0.16$; $p < 0.05$). EMC levels were negatively correlated to magnesuria ($r = -0.31$; $p < 0.05$), which is related to microalbuminuria ($r = 0,24$; $p < 0.05$) and $\beta2$-microglobulinuria ($r = 0.26$; $p < 0.05$). In the 74 diabetic patients with one or more subclinical complications, serum Mg levels were significantly lower than in the patients without complications (1.8 ± 0.2 mg/dl vs. 1.9 ± 0.2 mg/dl; $p < 0.01$). It has been shown that low plasma magnesium concentration was associated with development and progression of retinopathy [139].

In conclusion, lower serum Mg levels and EMC are found in type 1 young diabetic patients. Hypomagnesemia is related to age, duration of diabetes, bad glycemic control, and presence of subclinical complications. An increased renal magnesium clearance during hyperglycemia has been shown [140]. Mg depletion should be searched for, even in the pediatric population and supplementation with Mg should be considered.

HELICOBACTER PYLORI (HP) AND HbA1c

Many studies have been published to elucidate the prevalence of HP infection in childhood [141]. The prevalence of HP in children living in developed countries is low (15–25%) compared to the prevalence in children living in developing countries (40–60%). In 1996, Oldenburg et al. [142] have found that the age-adjusted seroprevalence of HP (IgG and IgA) in type 1 and type 2 diabetic patients was higher than in control subjects in several age groups.

In a preliminary study summarized in 1997 [143], we studied the prevalence of HP-seropositivity in 278 diabetic children with a mean age of 18 years and a mean duration of diabetes of 10 years, 69% being European Caucasians (EC) and 31% mainly Moghrabin Caucasians (MC). Anti-HP IgG (Elisa Cobas Core) were detected in 18% of the patients (32% in the MC group and 11% in the EC group). The age of seropositive children was lower in the MC group than in the EC group. Less than half of seropositive subjects have abdominal complaints. We have also evidenced that HP-positive diabetic children, adolescents and young adults had higher HbA1c levels than our total diabetic population (139% vs. 120% of normal values, the upper normal limit being 100%). In 43 out of the 49 seropositive patients, it was possible to verify the presence of HP in the stomach by a ^{13}C-urea breath test and an upper gastrointestinal endoscopy with biopsies for histology and HP-culture. An active infection has been proved in 81% of the seropositive subjects. In conclusion, HP-positive patients have a significantly higher HbA1c level than HP-negative ones. One third of young MC is HP-seropositive, mainly before the age of 18 years, which is 3 times more than in EC, probably due to a lower mean socio-economic status. In a Turkish study, anti-HP IgG was positive in 56% of diabetic children and in 31% of controls [144].

In another study we examined the relationships between HbA1c levels and eradication of HP infection. [145]. A total of 47 patients (age: 18 ± 6 years; diabetes duration: 9 ± 5 years) with HP infection, proved by histology, culture and ^{13}C-urea breath test (UBT), were included in the study during a 6 month period after a bi-therapy based on a bacterial antibiogram. HP eradication was checked with UBT 2 months after the end of treatment. HbA1c levels, measured by an HPLC method at diagnosis, 2 and 6 months after treatment, were expressed as % of normal values, the upper normal limit being 100%. Eradication of HP infection was obtained in 32/47 patients (68%). Age and diabetes duration were not significantly different in the eradicated and non-eradicated groups, nor was the ratio immigrants/non-immigrants. HbA1c levels were significantly higher in HP-non eradicated patients than in HP-eradicated subjects at diagnosis (147% *vs.* 136%), 2 months after treatment (147% *vs.* 137%), and 6 months after treatment (145% *vs.* 135%). However, treatment of HP infection, whether successful or not, did not modify HbA1c levels after 2 and 6 months. In conclusion, eradication of HP infection is less efficient in type 1 diabetic subjects with the poorest glycemic control, and eradication of HP has no influence on HbA1c levels during the following 6 months. Similarly, in type 1 diabetic adults, de Luis *et al.* [146] did not observe improvement in HbA1c levels 6 months after treatment for HP infection. Ojetti *et al.* [147] have reported that 38% of type 1 diabetic patients, compared with 5% in controls, were re-infected with HP 1 year after successful eradication. Better metabolic control in diabetic patients in whom HP has been eradicated compared with re-infected subjects was observed.

COMPLICATIONS RELATED TO TREATMENT

COMPLEMENT ACTIVATION BY ZINC INSULINS

Nearly 20 years ago, we determined the effect of the switch-over from porcine (Actrapid MC and Monotard MC to semi-synthetic human insulins (Actrapid HM and Protaphane HM) in a prospective study comparing complement evaluation (CH50, C3, C3d/C3, C4) as well as other immunological factors (insulin antibodies, autoantibodies, etc.), metabolic control (HbA1, lipids, etc.) and clinical data (insulin dose/kg, number of hypoglycemic episodes, etc.) [148]. Forty-six type 1 diabetic children and adolescents (mean age ± SD: 14.3 ± 3.8 years) participated in the trial. The duration of diabetes ranged from 1.0 to 16.9 years (mean ± SD: 7.3 ± 3.7). The study protocol consisted of a 9-month period during which, at monthly intervals, the subjects were assessed clinically and blood samples taken for measurement of biological data. After 3 months,

porcine insulins were switched to human insulins. The main results were as follows:

1) The insulin dose/kg was increased after the switchover (porcine insulin: 0.90 ± 0.03 U/kg; human insulin: 0.98 ± 0.03 U/kg; p <0.001). This can perhaps be explained by the different bioavailabilities of Monotard MC and Protaphane HM.

2) The objective degree of metabolic control (HbA1), as well as the HDL-cholesterol level and the apolipoproteins A1/B ratio, were not statistically different before and after the switchover.

3) IgG insulin antibody binding was not statistically different on transfer from porcine insulin to semi-synthetic insulin.

4) Mean level of total IgE and IgE specific insulin antibodies, determined before and after the switchover, were not different.

5) Autoantibodies and antinuclear factor were unchanged.

6) The prevalence of immune complexes was decreased by half (p < 0.05) after 6 months on human insulin.

7) The patients treated by porcine insulins had an increased complement activity (CH50) (p < 0.001) and an increased C3 activation (p < 0.001) as compared to controls while mean C4 remained unchanged. Moreover, there was an increased mean value of C3 breakdown product C3d and of the catabolic index C3d/C3 (p < 0.001). After the switchover to human insulins, CH50, C3 and C3d/C3 ratio decreased to the values observed in healthy controls.

In conclusion, the main feature of this prospective study was the demonstration of an abnormal *in vivo* complement metabolism in diabetic children and adolescents treated with porcine insulins Actrapid MC and Monotard MC, and its correction using semisynthetic human insulins Actrapid HM and Protaphane HM.

The prospective study was prolonged until 2 years in 45 diabetic children and adolescents in order to follow the evolution of the insulin antibodies [149]. IgG insulin antibodies were detected in 21 children out of 45 (47%) at a mean level of 0.96 mU/ml (0.77–1.15). A significant and important decrease of both the number of patients having insulin antibodies and the level of insulin antibodies was observed 18 months after the switchover. After 24 months, IgG insulin antibodies were only present in 5 patients (11%) at a mean level reduced by half (0.53 mU/ml; p <0.05). Four patients out of the five (80%) had HLA-DR3/4 antigens while this phenotype was only prevalent in 26% of the initial patient cohort. The prevalence of autoantibodies and of antinuclear factors showed no significant variations. The practical implication of these findings was that the use of human insulins could be of interest even in patients previously treated by porcine insulins because of the decrease of insulin antibodies.

In order to understand the abnormal *in vivo* complement metabolism in type 1 diabetic children treated with monocomponent porcine insulin Monotard MC and its correction after switchover to human insulin Protaphane HM [148], we have investigated the ability of different kinds of insulin preparations to induce complement activation *in vitro* [150]. Freshly collected serum samples from healthy blood donors were incubated with commercial rapid and intermediate or long-acting (by protamine sulphate [PS] or zinc) insulin preparations for 2 hours at 37 degrees C. The C3d content of the supernatants was measured by turbidimetry as a marker of C3 complement fraction consumption. Only long-acting preparations of insulins without protamine sulphate were associated with highly significant increased levels of C3d, whatever the source of insulin, animal or human. Moreover, addition of exogenous protamine sulphate was able to inhibit the C3 conversion. This effect was dose-dependent and peaked at the concentration of commercial NPH insulin preparations. The mechanism by which protamine sulphate inhibits complement activation *in vitro* could be related to its ability to interfere with the physical nature of the solid surfaces presented by the insulin crystals. Indeed, insulin crystals were rapidly cleared (< 5 min) in the incubated serum when small doses of protamine sulphate were added. The complement activating capacity of long-acting insulin without protamine was dose dependent, equivalent to the known complement activator

Zymosan, and abolished in the presence of EDTA (Figure 21.14). In conclusion, the study has documented the ability of some protracted insulin preparations to activate the complement system *in vitro* if they lack protamine sulphate. On the other hand, short-acting and NPH insulins are not complement activators. The practical conclusion is to avoid the use of zinc insulins, which are complement activators. Moreover, NPH and zinc insulins differ in their ability to form stable mixtures with neutral insulin solutions, since only NPH insulin can be mixed with regular insulin without changing the specific course of effect of regular insulin, and the variability of resorption from the subcutaneous deposit is higher for zinc insulins than for NPH.

[LysB28, ProB29]-human insulin analogue is not a complement activator *in vitro* [151].

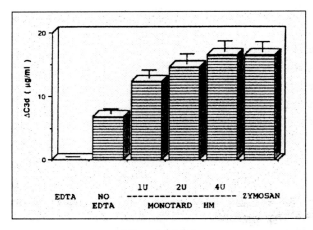

Figure 21.14

In vitro C3d generation performed at 37°C for 2 hours, in the presence of 3 doses of Monotard HM insulin (1, 2, and 4 units), EDTA and Zymosan. Mean increments of C3d from basal serum levels (before incubation) are expressed as μg/ml (± SEM) (from ref. 150).

OVERWEIGHT IN ADOLESCENTS ON 4 DAILY INSULIN INJECTIONS

In a preliminary study published more than 15 years ago, when the basal-bolus regimen was made easier due to the invention of the pen injector (NovoPen), we have evaluated the use of the NovoPen and in 23 type 1 diabetic adolescents and young adults between 14 and 28 years of age [152]. All patients were diabetic before age 15 and the duration of diabetes varied from 5 to 23 years. All patients were previously treated with a conventional regimen of Actrapid HM and Monotard HM or Protaphane HM twice daily (0.98 ± 0.24 U/kg/day). The patients used NovoPen to inject Actrapid HM in a bolus regimen with Ultratard HM as basal insulin, administered before bedtime. The mean duration of the NovoPen experience was 8.1 months. During the first 4 months after transfer to NovoPen, the total daily dosage of insulin was higher than 1 U/kg; afterwards the insulin needs to be decreased to 0.8 U/kg (at 12 months). On the other hand, the weight/height ratio increased significantly from the 4th month. After one year, the mean increase was 14%. The mean level of HbA1c was unchanged after the transfer to NovoPen. The patients' self-evaluation of the therapy was documented by asking them to fill in a questionnaire: 91% of the patients considered the use of NovoPen more pleasant than the previous injection therapy, and 87% reported a greater freedom regarding diet.

Later in more large studies we confirmed that HbA1c levels were unrelated to the number of insulin injections [9–11]. We observed that after the age of 13 years, BMI was significantly higher in girls and in adolescents on four daily injections, because of greater dietary freedom [11]. The Hvidøre Study Group on Childhood Diabetes has confirmed our findings showing that the increase in daily insulin injections was not associated with changes in the average HbA1c levels of the participating centers [20–23], and that adolescent girls, but to a lesser extent also boys, on 4 or more injections had significantly higher BMI than girls on twice-daily insulin [20]. The adjustment of insulin dosage is more complicated in the basal-bolus regimen because dose alteration cannot be done only according to sliding scales based on the glycemia immediately preceding the insulin injection. Insulin dose alteration must be retrospective according to previous experiences,

prospective according to physical activity and programmed meals, with only a "touch" of compensatory adaptation according to the present glucose level [9–18]. The proper use of this system gives more freedom for sports and meals, but young patients rarely succeed in following it. On the other hand, the proper use of the two-injection regimen, in countries where the meal schedule allows correct allocation of diet, may lead to "intensive conventional therapy" and good metabolic control.

WELL-BEING INDICES AND HbA1c

Therapeutic constraints should not decrease the quality of life and well-being of patients. Therefore, we carried out a study in order to evaluate by a questionnaire the well-being of our autonomous diabetic adolescents and young adults in relationship with their HbA1c levels and other characteristics [1]. A total of 100 unselected subjects (73 men and 44 women), with a mean age of 21 years (14–38) and mean diabetes duration of 12 years (0–26), were included in the study over a 3-month period. Mean age at onset of diabetes was 10 years. Twenty-five percent of the patients were of Moroccan origin. All the patients were autonomous for self-management and treatment. Their socioeconomic status was not different from that of the normal population. The mean annual HbA1c level in the 100 diabetic patients was 7.3 (4.7–11.7). Well-being was measured using a questionnaire developed by a working group of the World Health Organization, International Diabetes Federation and St Vincent Declaration [153]. The questionnaire included 4 subscales labeled depression, anxiety, energy and positive well-being. The measurement of all 4 subscales involved 22 items and allowed an estimation of general well-being. General well-being in women was not as good as in men due to a greater tendency toward depression. Well-being was better in patients with a professional activity than in the others. Patient's age, duration of diabetes, number of insulin injections, frequency of home blood glucose monitoring, presence of 1 or 2 subclinical complications, had no effect on well-being. On the other hand, well-being was negatively correlated with the HbA1c levels: the higher the HbA1c, the higher the anxiety and the depression, and the lower the energy and the positive well-being (Figure 21.15). In conclusion, well-being was mainly associated with HbA1c levels; it improved with better glycemic control.

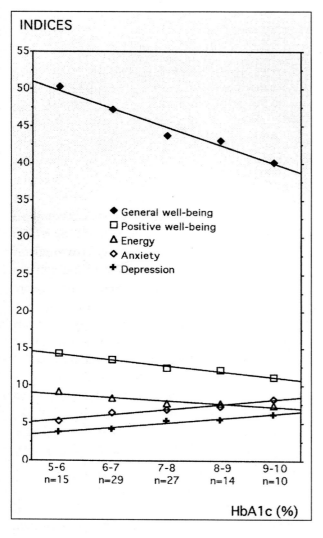

Figure 21.15

Well-being is negatively correlated with HbA1c levels: higher HbA1c leads to higher anxiety and depression, and lower energy and positive well-being (from ref. 1).

CONCLUSION

Successful treatment is reflected in good HbA1c associated with less severe hypoglycemic events, a better quality of life, lack of long-term complications and is not necessarily exportable without adjustment to the local way of life and the socio-economic status. No dogmatism! Only the objective result is important.

Our "recipes" have been summarized [9–11, 15, 18, 154]:

– Critical mass of patients; friendly contacts and personalized long-term follow-up until adulthood, at the age where clinical complications are possible which gives the so-called pediatric diabetologist more motivation to require good control.

– High frequency of home blood glucose monitoring, of HbA1c measurements and of long-term consultations; screening for subclinical complications by sensitive methods from puberty in order to increase the motivation of both the patient and the doctor (see below).

– Two daily insulin injections in children <15 years: easy and effective; an individualized mixture of insulins in a syringe gives better results, in terms of HbA1c, than the use of premixed insulins with a pen injector; the proportion of carbohydrates of the mid-morning snack must be more important than that for breakfast.

– Basal-bolus regimen in adolescents: increased flexibility in daily life and dietary freedom, but more complicated; no simplistic sliding scales; insulin dose alteration must be triple: 1) retrospective, according to numerous previous experiments, in order to enjoy more freedom for meals, sports, etc.; 2) prospective according to programmed changes in meals and sports; 3) with only a "touch" of compensatory adaptation according to the present glycemia. This needs psychological maturity, otherwise the multiple injection system leads to anarchy and obesity, mainly in adolescent girls.

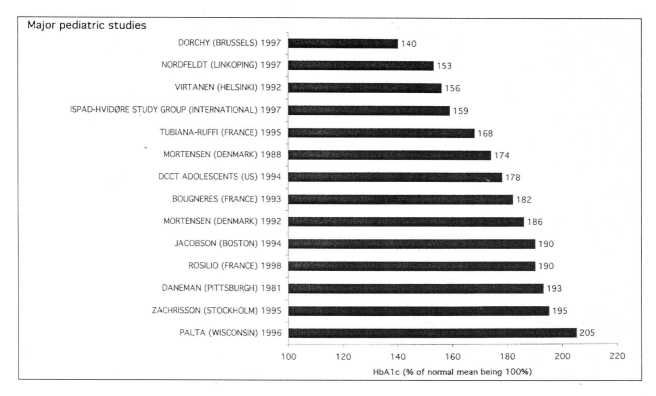

Figure 21.16

Comparison of glycated hemoglobin levels in major pediatric studies.

HbA1c is expressed in % of normal mean being 100% (from ref. 19).

– Fast-acting analogs in the basal-prandial regimen: no systematic replacement of rapid-acting insulins if the time period between 2 injections exceeds 3 or 4 hours; in our experience, the fast-acting analogs are recommended under well defined circumstances; 1) to correct hyperglycemia rapidly; 2) to allow to eat something between the main meals; 3) to allow a snack at 4 o'clock if the period between lunch and dinner exceeds 6–8 h, *i.e.* the length of action of the rapid-acting insulins; 4) if the patient sleeps in, in order to avoid the cumulation of the activities of the rapid-acting insulins injected before late breakfast and before lunch, the analog can replace the rapid-acting insulin before breakfast; 5) if dinner is near bedtime, in order to avoid the cumulation of the activities of the rapid-acting insulin injected before dinner, and of the intermediate-acting insulin injected at bedtime, the analog can replace the rapid-acting insulin before late dinner, reducing the risk of nocturnal hypoglycemia.

In 1998, Rosilio *et al.* [19] summarized the main pediatric studies on glycemic control since 1981 (Figure 21.16), showing that the best results, in terms of HbA1c, were obtained by our team in Brussels [11], with 2 or 4 insulin injections. The classic twice-daily insulin regimen is appropriate for Belgian children and adolescents until the end of the secondary school, according to Belgian customs, namely those concerning the meal timetable. In the most recent publications [155–159] on HbA1c in relation with the use of multiple injection regimen or of insulin pumps, the results are poorer than what we published 10 years ago with 2 (children) or 4 injections (adolescents) [9, 11].

The motivation of both the patient and the doctor is fundamental in order to obtain for life good glycemic control. After age 13 and 3 years of diabetes, we perform every year: retinal fluorescein angiography, measurements of motor and sensitive conduction velocities (which is different from a painful electromyography), and dosage of microalbuminuria and ß2-microglobulinuria. The majority of my colleagues use only the dosage of microalbuminuria and the observation of the eye fundus at regular ophthalmoscopy. It is important to be able to say to the patient, for example, "You have no complaint, but, as you can see on this photograph, there are 2 leakages of fluorescein in your left eye; it is reversible if you improve your HbA1c; otherwise, that will become an irreversible lesion leading later to overt complications". The same message for the slowing of conduction velocity or the presence of abnormal microalbuminuria. For many ophthalmologists, the most important operational outcome for retinal screening is the detection of severe lesions that must be treated by laser therapy in order to avoid blindness and, therefore, they do not understand why use fluorescein angiography if fundus at regular ophthalmoscopy or through digital non-mydriatic retinal imaging is normal [160]. Tele-ophthalmology *via* stereoscopic digital imaging has even been proposed [161]. A virtual doctor for a real diabetic patient...

At the onset of diabetes, we look for eventual EEG abnormalities; therefore, in the case of convulsions during severe hypoglycemia we are able to exclude epilepsy. Every year, we check for lipoproteins abnormalities, US-CRP raise, autoimmune disorders (namely thyroid antibodies and antigliadin (IgG and IgA) antibodies plus possibly anti-endomysial (IgA antibodies), serum and erythrocyte magnesium content, anti-HP IgG, complement consumption, as well as other classical measurements (urea, creatinine, etc.). Of course we search for hypertension, lipodystrophies, necrobiosis lipoidica diabeticorum, etc. We have never met impaired growth, except in cases of Mauriac syndrome [29], or limited joint mobility [162], probably because of the good mean HbA1c of our patients. Diabetes-related foot problems usually occur in older people with neuropathy and vascular complications [45].

The most important message to give to diabetic children, adolescents and young adults is that potentially disabling complications are not due to diabetes *per se* (if true, they should be ineluctable), but to long-term hyperglycemia and are therefore avoidable. We have a marker to claim that complications are not developing: to

obtain a glycated hemoglobin level under 7% [4]. The Hvidøre studies [20–23], performed in developed countries without financial restrictions, have shown that treatment of childhood diabetes is in general inadequate, and that levels of HbA1c are very different. Diabetes treatment teams should individually explore the reasons for failure without any prejudice or bias [9, 11, 15, 18]. Education and multidisciplinary team concepts for pediatric and adolescent diabetes mellitus [163–165], as well as educational vacation camps [166], must be evaluated objectively. Quality of care and patient well-being should be compared across diabetology teams with the goal of optimizing both these parameters [167].

REFERENCES

1. Dorchy H, Olinger S. Bien-être des diabétiques insulino-dépendants. Evaluation chez 100 adolescents et adultes jeunes en fonction de leur contrôle métabolique. *Presse Méd*, **26**: 1420–1424, 1997.

2. Hoey H, Aanstoot HJ, Chiarelli F, Daneman D, Danne T, Dorchy H, Fitzgerald M, Garandeau P, Greene S, Holl RW, Hougaard P, Kaprio E, Kocova M, Lynggaard H, Martul P, Matsuura N, McGee HM, Mortensen HB, Robertson K, Schoenle E, Søvik O, Swift P, Tsou RM, Vanelli M, Åman J, for the Hvidøre Study Group on Childhood Diabetes. Good metabolic control is associated with better quality of life in 2,101 adolescents with type 1 diabetes. *Diabetes Care*, **24**: 1923–1928, 2001.

3. Pirart J. Diabète et complications dégénératives. Présentation d'une étude prospective sur 4.400 cas observés entre 1947 et 1973. *Diabète Métab*, **3**: 97–107, 173–182, 245–256, 1977.

4. The Diabetes Control and Complications Trial Research Group. The effect of intensive treatment of diabetes on the development and progression of long-term complications in insulin-dependent diabetes mellitus. *N Engl J Med*, **29**: 977–986, 1993.

5. Verougstraete C, Libert J, Dorchy H. Discordant diabetic retinopathy in homozygous twins: the importance of good metabolic control. *J Pediatr*, **134**: 658, 1999.

6. Alcolado J. Genetics of diabetic complications. *Lancet*, **351**: 230–231, 1998.

7. Kao Y, Donaghue KC, Chan A, Bennetts BH, Knight J, Silink M. Paraoxonase gene cluster is a genetic marker for early microvascular complications in type 1 diabetes. *Diabet Med*, **19:** 212–215, 2002.

8. Mogensen CE. Genetics and diabetic renal disease: still a black hole. *Diabetes Care*, **26:** 1631–1632, 2003.

9. Dorchy H. Quel contrôle glycémique peut être obtenu chez des jeunes diabétiques sans sécrétion résiduelle d'insuline endogène? Quelle est la fréquence des hypoglycémies sévères et des complications subcliniques? *Arch Pédiatr*, **1:** 970–981, 1994.

10. Dorchy H. Dorchy's recipes explaining the "intriguing efficacy of Belgian conventional therapy". *Diabetes Care*, **17:** 458–460, 1994.

11. Dorchy H, Roggemans MP, Willems D. Glycated hemoglobin and related factors in diabetic children and adolescents under 18 years of age: a Belgian experience. *Diabetes Care*, **20:** 2–6, 1997.

12. Dorchy H, Roggemans MP, Willems D. Hémoglobine glyquée chez des jeunes diabétiques de moins de 18 ans non sélectionnés. Comparaison de 2 méthodes de dosage par HPLC. *Rev Méd Brux*, **18:** 59–63, 1997.

13. Czernichow P, Dorchy H. Traitement et insulinothérapie. In: Czernichow P, Dorchy H, (eds). *Diabétologie pédiatrique*, Doin, Paris, 1989, 445–496.

14. Dorchy H. Traitement du diabète de type I chez l'enfant et l'adolescent. *Rev Praticien* (Paris), **46:** 577–586, 1996.

15. Dorchy H. Insulin regimens and insulin adjustments in diabetic children, adolescents and young adults : personal experience. *Diabetes Metab,* (Paris) **26:** 500–507, 2000.

16. Dorchy H. Choix des insulines et adaptation des doses chez les enfants et adolescents diabétiques: expérience personnelle. *Rev Méd Brux*, **21:** 19–27, 2000.

17. Dorchy H. Sport et diabète de type 1: experience personnelle. *Rev Méd Brux*, 23: A211–A217, 2002.

18. Dorchy H. Dietary management for children and adolescents with diabetes mellitus: personal experience and recommendations. *J Pediatr Endocrinol Metab*, **16:** 131–148, 2003.

19. Rosilio M, Cotton JB, Wielliczko MC, Gendrault B, Carel JC, Couvaras O, Ser N, Bougnères PF, Gillet P, Soskin S, Garandeau P, Stuckens C, Le Luyer B, Jos J, Bony-Trifunovic H, Bertrand AM, Leturcq F, Lafuma A. Factors associated with glycemic control: a cross sectional nationwide study in 2,579 French children with type 1 diabetes. *Diabetes Care*, **21:** 1146–1153, 1998.

20. Mortensen H, Hougaard P, The Hvidøre Study Group On Childhood Diabetes. Comparison of metabolic control in a cross-sectional study of 2,873 children and adolescents with IDDM from 18 countries. *Diabetes Care*, **20:** 714–720, 1997.

21. Mortensen HB, Robertson KJ, Aanstoot H-J, Danne T, Holl RW, Hougaard P, Atchinson JA, Chiarelli F, Daneman D, Dinesen B, Dorchy H, Garandeau P, Greene S, Hoey H, Kaprio EA, Kocova M, Lynggaard H, Martul P, Matsuura N, Schoenle EJ, Søvik O, Swift P, Tsou RM, Vanelli M, Åman J, for the Hvidøre Study Group on Childhood Diabetes. Insulin management and metabolic control of type 1 diabetes mellitus in childhood and adolescence in 18 countries. *Diabet Med*, **15:** 752–759, 1998.

22. Danne T , Mortensen HB, Hougaard P, Lynggaard H, Aanstoot H-J, Chiarelli F , Daneman D, Dinesen B, Dorchy H, Garandeau P, Greene S, Hoey H, Holl RW, Kaprio EA, Kocova M, Martul P, Matsuura N, Robertson KJ, Schoenle EJ, Søvik O, Swift PGF, Tsou RM, Vanelli M, Aman J, for The Hvidøre Study Group on Childhood Diabetes. Persistent differences among centers over 3 years in glycemic control and hypoglycemia in a study of 3,805 children and adolescents with type 1 diabetes from the Hvidøre Study Group. *Diabetes Care*, **24:** 1342–1347, 2001.

23. Holl RW, Swift PGF, Mortensen HB, Lynggaard H, Hougaard P, Aanstoot H-J, Chiarelli F, Daneman D, Danne T, Dorchy H, Garandeau P, Greene S, Hoey H, Kaprio EA, Kocova M, Martul P, Matsuura N, Robertson KJ, Schoenle EJ, Søvik O, Tsou RM, Vanelli M, Aman J, for The Hvidøre Study Group on Childhood Diabetes. Insulin injection regimens and metabolic control in an international survey of adolescents with type 1 diabetes over 3 years: results from the Hvidøre study group. *Eur J Pediatr*, **162:** 22–29, 2003.

24. Dorchy H. Dépistage des complications subcliniques chez les jeunes diabétiques: l'expérience bruxelloise. *Ann Pédiatr* (Paris) **45:** 585–606, 1998.

25. Danne T, Kordounouri O, Hovener G, Weber B. Diabetic angiopathy in children. *Diabetic Med*, **14:** 1012–1025, 1997.

26. Dorchy H, Toussaint D. Reversal of complications of diabetes mellitus with improved metabolic control. *J Pediatr*, **100:** 337–338, 1982.

27. Dorchy H, Loeb H. Functional abnormalities precede structural lesions in diabetic children and adolescents. *Transplantation Proc*, **18:** 1494–1495, 1986.

28. Dorchy H. Characterization of the early stages of diabetic retinopathy: importance of the breakdown

of the blood-retinal barrier. *Diabetes Care*, **16**: 1213–1214, 1993.

29. Dorchy H, Van Vliet G, Toussaint D, Ketelbant-Balasse P, Loeb H. Mauriac syndrome: three cases with angiofluorescein study. *Diabète Métab*, **5**: 195–200, 1979.

30. Goldstein DE, Blinder KJ, Ide CH, Wilson RJ, Wiedmeyer HM, Little RR, England JD, Eddy M, Hewett JE. Anderson RR. Glycemic control and development of retinopathy in youth-onset insulin-dependent diabetes mellitus. *Ophthalmology*, **100**: 1125–1132, 1993.

31. Donaghue KC, Fung ATW, Hing S, Fairchild J, King J, Chan A, Howard NJ, Silink M. The effect of prepubertal diabetes duration on diabetes. Microvascular complications in early and late adolescence. *Diabetes Care*, **20**: 77–80, 1997.

32. Donaghue KC, Fairchild JM, Craig ME, Chan AK, Hing S, Cutler LR, Howard NJ, Silink M. Do all prepubertal years of diabetes duration contribute equally to diabetes complications? *Diabetes Care*, **26**: 1224–1229, 2003.

33. Dorchy H, Veroustraete C, Verstappen A, De Schepper J, Haentjens M, Toussaint D. Longitudinal study on the first microangiographic abnormalities in childhood diabetes. Types of lesions and risk factors. *Hormone Res*, **35**: 54, 1991.

34. Dorchy H, De Schepper J, Haentjens M, De Maertelaer V, Verougstraete C, Loeb H. The course of incipient diabetic retinopathy in youth -as revealed by fluorescein angiography. *Pediatr Adolesc Endocrinol*, **18**: 101–106,.1989.

35. Williamson JR, Rowold E, Chang K, Marvel J, Tomlinson M, Sherman WR, Ackerman KE, Berger RA, Kilo C. Sex steroid dependency of diabetes-induced changes in polyol metabolism, vascular permeability, and collagen cross-linking. *Diabetes*, **35**: 20–27, 1986.

36. Moran A, Jacobs DR, Steinberger J, Hong CP, Prineas R, Luepker R, Sinaiko AR. Insulin resistance during puberty. Results from clamp studies in 357 children. *Diabetes*, **48**: 2039–2044, 1999.

37. Weber B. Rétinopathie diabétique. In: Czernichow P, Dorchy H (eds). *Diabétologie pédiatrique*. Doin, Paris, 1989, 259–282.

38. Dorchy H. Complications neurologiques. In: Czernichow P, Dorchy H (eds). *Diabétologie pédiatrique*. Doin, Paris, 1989, 307–325.

39. Drummond KN. Rein et diabète. In: Czernichow P, Dorchy H, (eds). *Diabétologie pédiatrique*. Doin, Paris, 1989, 283–306.

40. Couper J. Microvascular complications of insulin-dependent diabetes: risk factors, screening and intervention. *J Paediatr Child Health*, **32**: 7–9, 1996.

41. Sochett E, Daneman D. Early diabetes-related complications in children and adolescents with type 1 diabetes. Implications for screening and intervention. *Endocrinol Metab Clin North Am*, **28**: 865–882, 1999.

42. Brink S. Complications of pediatric and adolescent type 1 diabetes mellitus. *Current Diabetes Reports*, **1**: 47–55, 2001.

43. Chiarelli F, Mohn A, Tumini S, Trotta D, Verrotti A. Screening for vascular complications in children and adolescents with type 1 diabetes mellitus. *Horm Res*, **57** (suppl 1): 113–116, 2002.

44. Chiarelli F, Mohn A. Angiopathy in children with diabetes. In: Brink S, Serban V (eds). *Pediatric and Adolescent Diabetes*. Brumar, Timişoara, 2003, 299–324.

45. ISPAD (International Society for Pediatric and Adolescent Diabetes) - Consensus guidelines 2000, Swift PGE ed. Zeist, Netherlands: *Publ Medforum* 2000; 95–101.

46. Novotny HR, Alvis DL. A method of photographing fluorescence in circulating blood in the human retina. *Circulation*, **24**: 82–86, 1961.

47. Toussaint D, Dorchy H. Exploration angiofluorescéinique de la rétinopathie diabétique infantile: étude préliminaire. *Bull Soc Belge Ophtalmol*, **168**: 783–800, 1974.

48. Dorchy H, Toussaint D, Devroede M, Ernould C, Loeb H. Diagnostic de la rétinopathie diabétique infantile par angiographie fluorescéinique. Description des lésions initiales. *Nouv Presse Méd*, **6**: 345–347, 1977.

49. Dorchy H, Toussaint D, Vanderschueren-Lodeweyckx M, Vandenbussche E, Devroede M, Loeb H. Leakage of fluorescein: first sign of juvenile diabetic retinopathy. *Acta Pædiatr Scand*, suppl. **277**: 47–53, 1979.

50. Dorchy H, Toussaint D. Fluorescein leakage: first sign of juvenile diabetic retinopathy. *Lancet*, **1**: 1200, 1978.

51. Dorchy H. Toussaint D. Mise en evidence d'un trouble précoce de la perméabilité des capillaries rétiniens diabétiques par angiographies fluorescéinique. In: *Journées de diabétologie de l'Hôtel-Dieu*, Flammarion Médecine-Sciences, Paris, 1979, 35–45.

52. Dorchy H, Toussaint D. Rupture précoce de la barrière hémato-rétinienne chez les jeunes diabétiques. Trouble fonctionnel initial de la rétinopathie dans le diabète de type 1 chez l'enfant et l'adolescent. *Rev Méd Brux*, **5**: 319–331, 1984.

53. Dorchy H, Toussaint D. Early breakdown of the blood-retinal barrier in diabetic children: incipient

functional abnormality in diabetic retinopathy. *Diabetes in the Young (Bulletin of ISGD)*, **12**: 18–46, 1985.

54. Dorchy H. Early diabetic retinopathy. *Diabetologia*, **30**: 274, 1987.

55. Patz A. Retinal vascular diseases (reply to a letter). *N Engl J Med*, **299**: 1017–1018, 1978.

56. Veroustraete C, Toussaint D, De Schepper J, Haentjens M, Dorchy H. First microangiographic abnormalities in childhood diabetes-types of lesions. *Graefe's Arch Clin Exp Ophthalmol*, **229**: 24–32, 1991.

57. Dorchy H, Toussaint D, Verougstraete C, Lemiere B. Transient acute disc swelling associated with improved metabolic control in an adolescent with type 1 diabetes: role of dexamethazone therapy. *Eur J Pediatr*, **143**: 187–190, 1985.

58. Daneman D, Drash A, Lobes LA, Becker DJ, Baker LM, Travis LB. Progressive retinopathy with improved control in diabetic dwarfism (Mauriac's syndrome). *Diabetes Care*, **4**: 360–365, 1981.

59. Cunha-Vaz JG, Fonseca JR, Abreu JF, Ruas MA. Detection of early retinal changes in diabetes by vitreous fluorophotometry. *Diabetes*, **28**: 16–19, 1979.

60. Haut J, Redor JY, Abboud E, van Effenterre G, Moulin F. Classification of diabetic retinopathy. *Ophthalmologica*, **195**: 145–155, 1987.

61. Salardi S, Rubbi F, Puglioli R, Brancaleoni A, Bacchi-Reggiani L, Ragni L, Cacciari E. Diabetic retinopathy in childhood: long-term follow-up by fluorescein angiography beginning in the first months of disease. *J Pediatr Endocrinol Metab*, **14**: 507–515, 2001.

62. Wardle EN. Vascular permeability in diabetics and implication for therapy. *Diabetes Res Clin Pract*, **23**: 135–139, 1994.

63. Schmetterer L, Wolzt M. Ocular blood flow and associated functional deviations in diabetic retinopathy. *Diabetologia*, **42**: 387–405, 1999.

64. Antonetti DA, Barber AJ, Khin S, Lieth E, Tarbell JM, Gardner TW. Vascular permeability in experimental diabetes is associated with reduced endothelial occluding content. Vascular endothelial growth factor decreases occluding in retinal endothelial cells. *Diabetes*, **47**: 1953–1959, 1998.

65. Dorchy H, Toussaint D, Haumont D, Loeb H. Relationship between some clinical and biological factors and incipient diabetic retinopathy diagnosed by fluorescein angiography. *Am J Ophthalmol*, **96**: 108–110, 1983.

66. Malone JI, Van Cader TC, Edwards WC. Diabetic vascular changes in diabetes. *Diabetes*, **26**: 673–679, 1977.

67. Dorchy H, Loeb H. More on "diabetic control"! What is it? *J Pediatr*, **90**: 502–503, 1977.

68. Dorchy H, Despontin M, Haumont D, Toussaint D, De Vroede M, Loeb H. Hémoglobine glycosylée et estimation clinique du degré de contrôle du diabète. Relations avec la glycémie, la cholestérolémie, la triglycéridémie, la durée du diabète et la rétinopathie. Etude de 85 enfants et adolescents diabétiques. *Ann Pédiatr*, **29**: 319–326, 1982.

69. Verougstraete C, Haentjens M, Dorchy H. Analyse de la micro-angiopathie des jeunes diabétiques par l'angiographie rétinienne. Relations avec la durée du diabète, l'HbA1, les antigènes HLA-DR et la neuropathie. *J Fr Ophtalmol*, **9**: 665–666, 1986.

70. Dorchy H, Roggemans MP, Willems D. Quel contrôle glycémique peut être obtenu chez des jeunes diabétiques et quelle est la fréquence des complications subcliniques? Avec 4 ans de recul supplémentaire. *Arch Pédiatr*, **3**: 294–296, 1996.

71. Dorchy H, Claes C, Verougstraete C. Risk factors of developing proliferative retinopathy in type 1 diabetic patients. Role of BMI. *Diabetes Care*, **25**: 798–799, 2002.

72. Zangh L, Krentowski G, Albert A, Lefebvre P. Risk of developing retinopathy in Diabetes Control and Complications Trial type 1 diabetic patients with good or poor metabolic control. *Diabetes Care*, **24**: 1275–1279, 2001.

73. Haumont D, Dorchy H, Pelc S. EEG abnormalities in diabetic children. Influence of hypoglycemia and vascular complications. *Clin Pédiatr*, **18**: 750–753, 1979.

74. Hauser E, Strohmayer C, Seidl R, Birnbacher R, Lischka A, Schober E. Quantitative EEG in young diabetics. *J Child Neurol*, **10**: 330–334, 1995.

75. Bjorgaas M, Sand T, Gimse R. Quantitative EEG in type 1 diabetic children with and without episodes of severe hypoglycemia: a controlled, blind study. *Acta Neurol Scand*, **93**: 398–402, 1996.

76. Biessels GJ, Kappelle AC, Bravenboer B, Erkelens DW, Gispen WH. Cerebral function in diabetes mellitus. *Diabetologia*, **37**: 643–650, 1994.

77. Noël P, Dorchy H, Loeb H. Neurophysiological evaluation of subclinical neuropathy in juvenile diabetes. *Pediatr Adolesc Endocrinol*, **9**: 130–139, 1981.

78. Barkai L, Kempler P, Vamosi I, Lukacs K, Marton A, Keresztes K. Peripheral sensory nerve dysfunction in children and adolescents with type 1 diabetes mellitus. *Diabet Med*, **15**: 128–133, 1998.

79. Dorchy H, Noël P, Krüger M, De Maertelaer V, Dupont D, Toussaint D, Pelc S. Peroneal motor nerve conduction velocity in diabetic children and adolescents. Relationship to metabolic control,

HLA-DR antigens, retinopathy, and EEG. *Eur J Pediatr*, **144**: 310–315, 1985.

80. Krüger M, Brunko E, Dorchy H, Noël P. Femoral versus peroneal neuropathy in diabetic children and adolescents. Relationships to clinical status, metabolic control and retinopathy. *Diabète Métab*, **13**: 110–115, 1987.

81. Carrington AL, Shaw JE, Van Schie CH, Abbott CA, Vileikyte L, Boulton AJ. Can motor nerve conduction velocity predict foot problems in diabetic subjects over a 6-year outcome period? *Diabetes Care*, **25**: 2010–2015, 2002.

82. Bril V, Ngo M. Limits of the sympathetic skin response in patients with diabetic polyneuropathy. *Muscle Nerve*, **23**: 1427–1430, 2000.

83. Vinik AI, Maser RE, Mitchell BD, Freeman R. Diabetic autonomic neuropathy. *Diabetes Care*, **26**: 1553–1579, 2003.

84. Kandel K, Rondia G, Dorchy H. Cardiac autonomic neuropathy in type 1 diabetic patients: diagnosis by statistic and spectral analysis of heart rate variability. *J Pediatr Endocrinol Metab*, **14** (suppl 3): 1072, 2001.

85. Massin MM, Derkenne B, Tallsund M, Rocour-Brumioul D, Ernould C, Lebrethon M-C, Bourguignon J-P. Cardiac autonomic dysfunction in diabetic children. *Diabetes Care*, **22**: 1845–1850, 1999.

86. Riihimaa PH, Suominen K, Jantti V, Knip M, Tapanainen P, Tolonen U. Cardiovascular autonomic reactivity is decreased in adolescents with type 1 diabetes. *Diabet Med*, **19**: 932–938, 2002.

87. Anderson AR, Sandahl CJ, Andersen JK, Kreiner S, Deckert T. Diabetic nephropathy in type 1 insulin-dependent diabetes: an epidemiological study. *Diabetologia*, **25**: 496–501, 1983.

88. Arun CS, Stoddart J, Mackin P, MacLeod JM, New JP, Marshall SM. Significance of microalbuminuria in long-duration type 1 diabetes. *Diabetes Care*, **26**: 2144–2149, 2003.

89. Cambier P. Application de la théorie de Rehberg à l'étude clinique des affections rénales et du diabète. *Ann Méd*, **35**: 273–299, 1934.

90. Soper CPR, Barron JL, Hyer SL. Long-term glycaemic control directly correlates with glomerular filtration rate in early type 1 diabetes mellitus before the onset of microalbuminuria. *Diabet Med*, **15**: 1010–1014, 1998.

91. Dorchy H. Néphropathie diabétique: évolution naturelle, diagnostic précoce, prévention. *CR Soc Belge Pédiatr*, **24**(4): 11–20, 1992

92. Mogensen CE, Vittinghus E. Urinary albumin excretion during exercise in juvenile diabetes. A provocation test for early abnormalities. *Scand J Clin Lab Invest*, **35**: 295–300, 1975.

93. Poortmans J, Dewancker A, Dorchy H. Urinary excretion of total protein, albumin and ß2-microglobulin during exercise in adolescent diabetics. *Biomedicine Express*, **25**: 273–274, 1976.

94. Poortmans J, Dorchy H, Toussaint D. Urinary excretion of total proteins, albumin, and ß2-microglobulin during rest and exercise in diabetic adolescents with and without retinopathy. *Diabetes Care*, **5**: 617–623, 1982.

95. Poortmans JR, Dorchy H. Exercise, kidney responses and diabetes. In: Kawamori R, Vranic M, Horton ES, Kubota M (eds). *Glucose fluxes, exercise and diabetes*, Smith-Gordon, Great Britain, 1995, 85–90.

96. Poortmans JR, Waterlot B, Dorchy H. Training effect on postexercise microproteinuria in type I diabetic adolescents. *Pediatr Adolesc Endocrinol*, **17**: 166–172, 1988.

97. Bernard AM, Ouled A., Goemare-Vanneste J, Antione JL, Lauwerys RR, Lambert A, Vandeleene B. Microtransferrinuria is a more sensitive indicator of early glomerular damage in diabetes than micro-albuminuria. *Clin Chem*, **34**: 1920–1921, 1988.

98. Poortmans J, Dorchy H, De Maertelaer V. Subclinical proteinuria in type 1 diabetic children and adolescents: relationship to duration of diabetes, metabolic control, HLA-DR type, retinopathy and neuropathy. *Diabetic Nephropathy*, **3**: 123–126, 1984.

99. Carlier L, Willems D, Dorchy H. Would increased urine transferring excretion be a predictive marker of early glomerular dysfunction in type 1 young diabetic patients? *J Pediatr Endocrinol Metab*, **14**(suppl 3): 1072, 2001.

100. Poortmans JR, Dorchy H. Would acid aminoglycans be a predictive marker of early glomerular dysfunction in type 1 young diabetic patients? *J Pediatr Endocrinol Metab*, **14**(suppl 3): 1072, 2001.

101. Hong CY, Chia KS. Markers of diabetic nephropathy. *J Diabetes Complications*, **12**: 43–60, 1998.

102. Kordonouri O, Kahl A, Jörres A, Hopfenmüller W, Danne T. The prevalence of incipient tubular dysfunction, but not glomerular dysfunction, is increased in patients with diabetes onset in childhood. *J Diabetes Complications*, **13**: 320–324, 1999.

103. Schultz CJ, Neil HAW, Dalton RN, Dunger DB. Risk of nephropathy can be detected before the onset of microalbuminuria during the early years after diagnosis of type 1 diabetes. *Diabetes Care*, **23**: 1811–1815, 2000.

104. Warram JH, Scott LJ, Hanna LS, Wantman M, Cohen SE, Laffel LMB, Ryan L, Krolewski AS. Progression of microalbuminuria to proteinuria in type 1 diabetes. Nonlinear relationship with hyperglycemia. *Diabetes*, **49**: 94–100, 2000.

105. Koren W, Koldanov R, Pronin VS, Postnov IY, Peleg E, Rosenthal T, Berezin M, Postnov YV. Enhanced erythrocyte Na+/H+ exchange predicts diabetic nephropathy in patients with IDDM. *Diabetologia*, **41**: 201–205, 1998.

106. Andersen S, Tarnow L, Cambien F, Rossing P, Juhl T, Deinum J, Parving HH. Long-term renoprotective effects of losartan in diabetic nephropathy. *Diabetes Care*, **26**: 1501–1506, 2003.

107. Haffner SM. Lipoprotein (a) and diabetes: an update. *Diabetes Care*, **16**: 835–840, 1993.

108. Couper JJ, Bates DJ, Cocciolone R, Magarey AM, Boulton TJC, Penfold JL, Ryall RG. Association of lipoprotein (a) with puberty in IDDM. *Diabetes Care*, **16**: 869–873, 1993.

109. Willems D, Dorchy H, Dufrasne D. Serum lipoprotein (a) in type 1 diabetic children and adolescents: relationships with HbA1c and subclinical complications. *Eur J Pediatr*, **155**: 175–178, 1996.

110. Hernandez C, Chacon P, Garcia-Pascual L, Simo R. Differential influence of LDL cholesterol and triglycerides on lipoprotein(a) concentrations in diabetic patients. *Diabetes Care*, **24**: 350–355, 2001.

111. Koschinsky ML, Marcovina SM. The relationship between lipoprotein(a) and the complications of diabetes mellitus. *Acta Diabetol*, **40**: 65–76, 2003.

112. Ridker PM, Hennekens CH, Buring JE, Rifai N. C-reactive protein and other markers of inflammation in the prediction of cardiovascular disease in women. *N Engl J Med*, **342**: 836–843, 2000.

113. Schalkwijk CG, Poland DC, van Dijk W, Kok A, Emeis JJ, Drager AM, Doni A, van Hinsbergh VW, Stehouwer CD. Plasma concentration of C-reactive protein is increased in type I diabetic patients without clinical macroangiopathy and correlates with markers of endothelial dysfunction: evidence for chronic inflammation. *Diabetologia*, **42**: 351–357, 1999.

114. Dorchy H, Coulon B, Willems D. Increased levels of ultra sensitive CRP in young type 1 diabetic patients with or without subclinical complications. *J Pediatr Endocrinol Metab*, **15**(suppl 4): 1063, 2002.

115. American Diabetes Association. Management of dyslipidemia in children with diabetes. *Diabetes Care*, **26**: 2194–2197, 2003.

116. Willems D, Dorchy H. Taux des lipoprotéines et des apolipoprotéines chez les jeunes diabétiques insulinodépendants. Relations avec l'hémoglobine glycosylée et la fructosamine. *Presse Méd*, **19**: 17–20, 1990.

117. Willems D, Dorchy H. Sous-fractions du HDL-cholestérol chez les jeunes diabétiques insulinodépendants. *Presse Méd*, **20**: 86, 1991.

118. Donaghue KC, Pena MM, Chan AKF, Blades BL, King J, Storlein LH, Silink M. Beneficial effects of increasing monounsaturated fat intake in adolescents with type 1 diabetes. Diabetes Res *Clin Pract*, **48**: 193–199, 2000.

119. Tomkin GH, Owens D. Abnormalities in apo B-containing lipoproteins in diabetes and atherosclerosis. *Diabetes Metab Res Rev*, **17**: 27–43, 2001.

120. Abraha A, Schultz C, Konopelska-Bahu T, James T, Watts A, Stratton IM, Matthews DR, Dunger DB. Glycaemic control and familial factors determine hyperlipidaemia in early childhood diabetes. Oxford Regional Prospective Study of Childhood Diabetes. *Diabet Med*, **16**: 598–604, 1999.

121. West IC. Radicals and oxidative stress in diabetes. *Diabet Med*, **17**: 171–180, 2000.

122. Ceriello A. New insights on oxidative stress and diabetic complications may lead to a "causal" antioxidant therapy. *Diabetes Care*, **26**: 1589–1596, 2003

123. Ndahimana J, Dorchy H, Vertongen F. Activité anti-oxydante érythrocytaire et plasmatique dans le diabète de type 1. *Presse Méd*, **25**: 188–192, 1996.

124. Dorchy H, Ndahimana J, Vertongen F. Erythrocyte and plasma antioxidant activity and subclinical complications in young diabetic patients. *Diabetes Care*, **19**: 1165, 1996.

125. Dorchy H. Lower plasma vitamin C levels in young type I diabetic patients with microalbuminuria. *J Diabetes Complications*, **13**: 119, 1999.

126. Hirsch IB, Atchley DH, Tsai E, Labbé RF, Chait A. Ascorbic acid clearance in diabetic nephropathy. *J Diabetes Complications*, **12**: 259–263, 1998.

127. Sytze van Dam P. Oxidative stress and diabetic neuropathy: pathophysiological mechanisms and treatment perspectives. *Diabetes Metab Res Rev*, **18**: 176–184, 2002.

128. Dominguez C, Ruiz E, Gussinye M, Carrascoa A. Oxidative stress at onset and in early stages of type 1 diabetes in children and adolescents. *Diabetes Care*, **21**: 1736–1742, 1998.

129. Willems D, Dorchy H, Dufrasne D. Serum antioxidant status and oxidized LDL in well-

controlled young type 1 diabetic patients with and without subclinical complications. *Atherosclerosis*, **137** (suppl): S61–S64, 1998.

130. Varvarovska J, Racek J, Stozicky F, Soucek J, Trefil L, Pomahacova R. Parameters of oxidative stress in children with type 1 diabetes mellitus and their relatives. *J Diabetes Complications*, **17**: 7–10, 2003.

131. Ditzel J. Oxygen transport impairment in diabetes. *Diabetes*, **25**: 832–838, 1976.

132. Cauchie P, Vertongen F, Bosson D, Dorchy H. Erythrocyte metabolic alterations in type I diabetes: relationship to metabolic control. *Ann Biol Clin*, **50**: 9–13, 1992.

133. Dorchy H, Cantinieaux B, De Maertelaer V, Hariga C, Mascart F, Fondu P. Granulocyte functions in non-acidotic juvenile diabetes: evidence of a stimulating effect of plasma protein glycosylation. *Diabetes in the Young (Bulletin of ISGD)*, **28**: 11–14, 1992.

134. Dorchy H, Lemiere B, Toussaint D, Gausset P. Anticorps anti-cellules des îlots de Langerhans et spécifiques d'organes chez les jeunes diabétiques. Relations avec l'âge, le début et la durée du diabète, la sécrétion résiduelle d'insuline endogène et la rétinopathie. *Nouv Presse Méd*, **10**: 2795–2798, 1981.

135. Dorchy H. Bourdoux P, Lemiere B. Subclinical thyroid hormone abnormalities in type 1 diabetic children and adolescents. Relationships to metabolic control. *Acta Pædiatr Scand*, **74**: 386–389, 1985.

136. Radetti G, Paganini C, Gentili L, Barbin F, Pasquino B, Zachmann M. Altered adrenal and thyroid function in children with insulin-dependent diabetes mellitus. *Acta Diabetol*, **31**: 138–140, 1994.

137. Kordonouri O, Deiss D, Dänne T, Dorow A, Bassir C, Grüters-Kieslich A. Predictivity of thyroid autoantibodies for the development of thyroid disorders in children and adolescents with type 1 diabetes. *Diabet Med*, **19**: 518–521, 2002.

138. Dorchy H, Declercq S, Willems D. Decreased magnesium levels in serum and erythrocytes of young type 1 diabetic subjects. Relationships with glycated hemoglobin levels (HbA1c) and subclinical complications. *Diabetes Res Clin Pract*, **44**: S27, 1999.

139. De Valk HW, Hardus P, Van Rijn H, Ekelens D. Plasma magnesium concentration and progression of retinopathy. *Diabetes Care*, **22**: 864–865, 1999.

140. Djurhuus MS, Skott P, Vaag A, Hother-Nielsen O, Andersen P, Parving HH, Klitgaard NA. Hyperglycaemia enhances renal magnesium excretion in type 1 diabetic patients. *Scand J Clin Lab Invest*, **60**: 403–409, 2000.

141. Megraud F, Brassens-Rabbé MP, Denis F, Belbouri A, Hoa DQ. Seroepidemiology of Campylobacter pylori infection in various populations. *J Clin Microbiol*, **27**: 1870–1873, 1989.

142. Oldenburg B, Diepersloot RJA, Hoekstra JBL. High seroprevalence of Helicobacter pylori in diabetes mellitus patients. *Dig Dis Sc*, **41**: 458–461, 1996.

143. Scaillon M, Bontems P, Dorchy H, Cadranel S. Infection à Helicobacter Pylori chez les jeunes diabétiques: prevalence chez les caucasiens européens et maghrébins résidant en Belgique. *CR Soc Belge Pédiatr (Mini Acta)*, **29**: 112, 1997.

144. Arslan D, Kendirci M, Kurtoglu S, Kula M. Helicobacter pylori infection in children with insulin dependent diabetes mellitus. *J Pediatr Endocrinol Metab*, **13**: 553–556, 2000.

145. Scaillon M, Dorchy H, Cadranel S. Relationship between glycated haemoglobin (HbA1c) and eradication of Helicobacter pylori (HP) infection in young type 1 diabetic patients. *Diabetes Res Clin Pract*, **44**: S28, 1999.

146. de Luis DA, Cordero JM, Caballero C, Boixeda D, Aller R, Canton R, de la Calle H. Effect of the treatment of Helicobacter pylori infection on gastric emptying and its influence on the glycaemic control in type 1 diabetes mellitus. *Diabetes Res Clin Pract*, **52**: 1–9, 2001.

147. Ojetti V, Pitocco D, Bartolozzi F, Danese S, Migneco A, Lupascu A, Pola P, Ghirlanda G, Gasbarrini G, Gasbarrini A. High rate of Helicobacter pylori re-infection in patients affected by type 1 diabetes. *Diabetes Care*, **25**: 1485, 2002.

148. Dorchy H, Duchateau J. D'Hooge D. Normalization of complement activation and consumption in diabetic children and adolescents after switch-over from porcine to semisynthetic human insulin. *Diabète Métab*, **14**: 415–421, 1988.

149. Dorchy H, Duchateau J, Bosson D, D'Hooge D. Transfer from porcine insulins to semisynthetic human insulins decreases insulin antibodies and circulating immune complexes in diabetic children and adolescents? A two year follow-up. *Diabète Métab*, **15**: 107–110, 1989.

150. Duchateau J, Schreyen H. Dorchy H. Intermediate and long-acting preparations without protamine sulphate are complement activators in vitro. *Diabète Métab*, **18**: 272–276, 1992.

151. Duchateau J, Schreyen H. Dorchy H. Lack of in vitro complement activation by the human insulin analogue LYS (B28) PRO (B29). *Diabète Métab*, **20**: 562–563, 1994.

152. Dorchy H. Le stylo-injecteur d'insuline chez le jeune diabétique: liberté et prise pondérale excessive. *Pédiatrie*, **43**: 697–702, 1988.

153. Bradley C, Gamsu DS for the Psychological Well-being Working Group of the WHO/IDF St Vincent

Declaration Action Programme for Diabetes. Guidelines for encouraging psychological well-being, *Diabet Med*, **11**: 510–516, 1994.

154. Dorchy H. Improving outcomes for young people with diabetes. *Diabet Med*, **19**: 702–703, 2002.

155. Levine BS, Anderson BJ, Butler DA, Antisdel JE, Brackett J, Laffel LM. Predictors of glycemic control and short-term adverse outcomes in youth with type 1 diabetes. *J Pediatr*, **139**: 174–176, 2001.

156. Dabadghao P, Vidmar S, Cameron FJ. Deteriorating diabetic control through adolescence-do the origins lie in childhood? *Diabet Med*, **18**: 889–94, 2001.

157. Litton J, Rice A, Friedman N, Oden J, Lee MM, Freemark M. Insulin pump therapy in toddlers and preschool children with type 1 diabetes mellitus. *J Pediatr*, **141**: 490–495, 2002.

158. Barton DM, Baskar V, Kamalakannan D, Buch HN, Gone K, Wilson E, Anderson J, Abdu TA. An assessment of care of paediatric and adolescent patients with diabetes in a large district general hospital. *Diabet Med*, **20**: 394–398, 2003.

159. Weintrob N, Benzaquen H, Galatzer A, Shalitin S, Lazar L, Fayman G, Lilos P, Dickerman Z, Phillip M. Comparison of continuous subcutaneous insulin infusion and multiple daily injection regimens in children with type 1 diabetes: a randomized open crossover trial. *Pediatrics*, **112**: 559–564, 2003.

160. Cavallerano AA, Cavallerano JD, Katalinic P, Tolson AM, Aiello LP, Aiello LM, Joslin Vision Network Clinical Team. Use of Joslin Vision Network digital-video nonmydriatic retinal imaging to assess diabetic retinopathy in a clinical program. *Retina*, **23**: 215–223, 2003.

161. Tennant MT, Rudnisky CJ, Hinz BJ, MacDonald IM, Greve MD. Tele-ophthalmology *via* stereoscopic digital imaging: a pilot project. *Diabetes Technol Ther*, **2**: 583–587, 2000.

162. Infante JR, Rosenbloom AL, Silverstein JH, Garzarella L, Pollock BH. Changes in frequency and severity of limited joint mobility in children with type 1 diabetes mellitus between 1976-78 and 1998. *J Pediatr*, **138**: 33–37, 2001.

163. Laron Z, Galatzer A, Amir S, Gil R, Karp M, Mimouni M. A multidisciplinary, comprehensive, ambulatory treatment scheme for diabetes mellitus in children. *Diabetes Care*, **4**: 342–348, 1979.

164. Lemiere B, Goethals D, Dorchy H, Loeb H. Medico-social profile of a pediatric Diabetology unit. *Pediatr Adolesc Endocrinol*, **10**: 192–197, 1982.

165. Brink SJ, Miller M, Moltz K. Education and multidisciplinary team care concepts for pediatric and adolescent diabetes mellitus. *J Pediatr Adolesc Endocrinol*, **15**: 1113–1130, 2002.

166. Dorchy H, Ernould C. Les colonies de vacances pour enfants et adolescents diabétiques. *Diabète Métab (Paris)*, **16**: 513–521, 1990.

167. Dorchy H. (R)évolution de la diabétologie pédiatrique et optimisation du traitement. *Ann Pédiatr (Paris)*, **45**: 521–529, 1998.

22

COMPLICATIONS OF TYPE 1 DIABETES MELLITUS IN CHILDREN AND TEENAGERS

Stuart J. BRINK

The complications of type 1 diabetes mellitus are usually subclinical throughout most of the pediatric and adolescent years but begin to surface after longer duration and worse metabolic control. There is no "grace" period for the beginnings of such complications although there seems to be an accelerated phase of appearance around the time of puberty. Duration of diabetes and long-standing glycemic control, age and pubertal status all are critical factors associated with the development of the microvascular and eventually macrovascular problems of diabetes. Genetic factors accessible *via* analysis of family history as well as lipid, blood pressure and smoking exposure are also important factors in the appearance and severity of such problems. The DCCT proved the importance of improved glycemic control and especially the longevity of such interventions even when control is not sustained for at least 6 years after the end of the DCCT itself. The key outcomes of the DCCT, retinopathy, nephropathy and neuropathy, all showed a significant decreased risk when treatment included individualized and targeted glucose and A1c values. The main mechanism for achieving such risk reductions involved utilization of a multidisciplinary same-philosophy-of-care approach by nurses, dietician, psychologists and therapists as well as physicians working in a coordinated fashion with a goal of specific glycemic targets/outcomes. Other pediatric and adolescent-based natural history and intervention studies in Paris, France, Brussels, Belgium, Oslo, Norway, Sydney, Australia and Leicester, England all support the findings of the DCCT vis-à-vis youngsters with type 1 diabetes mellitus. With education and supportive therapy, microangiopathic complications can be reduced. Metabolic control counts.

INTRODUCTION

Modern treatment of type 1 diabetes mellitus in children and teenagers requires knowledge of the physiology of nutrition and of insulin treatment. Division of the effects of insulin into basal and bolus concepts allows more physiologic attention to the different characteristics required for modern treatment. Balancing patient and family needs against the rigors of multiple injections is a difficult chore but increasingly accomplished coupled with frequent blood glucose monitoring. Such monitoring allows the variabilities of food absorption, gut motility, food-to-food interactions as well as the variabilities in insulin preparations and absorption characteristics and kinetics to be known and used as part of the treatment itself. Even under ideal conditions in clinical research centers, however, current treatment is far from adequate compared to what was accomplished by the millions of beta cells in a functioning pancreas. Nevertheless, new insulin analogs and insulin pump concepts allow more patients to be successful in their self-treatment endeavors than ever before.

Attempts to mimic normal pancreatic function continue to evolve and all such intensified treatment programs are based upon frequent capillary blood glucose monitoring and pattern analysis by the patient and/or parent. Short term therapeutic goals include avoiding hypoglycemia and hyperglycemia extremes. This is especially true for avoiding diabetic ketoacidosis as well as avoiding the most severe types of hypoglycemia (that requiring assistance of others as well as avoiding unconsciousness or hypoglycemia-induced seizures). Other short term treatment goals include avoiding the extreme variability of day-to-day glucose values. All this is accomplished by paying attention not only to activity and illness but also to daily optimized nutrient provision and insulin delivery while using frequent blood glucose monitoring for pattern identification and adjustment.

Most pediatric endocrinologists and pediatric diabetologists believe that modern treatment also allows the reduction or avoidance of the most severe long term complications seen in the past with type 1 diabetes. Not only can early blindness and cataract formation be avoided almost completely but growth and pubertal abnormalities

should also be assigned to the dustbin of medical history when reasonable application of current insulin and monitoring tools are available and applied around the world. Where severe complications continue, it behooves the clinicians caring for such patients to investigate the causes of such problems. If there is systematic lack of education, then this should be corrected. If there is a lack of reasonable self-care supplies (strips, reliable insulin, syringes) then this too must be addressed. Often these are political and socioeconomic problems but sometimes the will to access and utilize new medical information must also be addressed with appropriately trained and updated medical care teams specializing in diabetes.

Carbohydrate counting and meal planning are key to provision of such care since insulin alone is insufficient to improve specific glycemic control. Blood glucose monitoring identifies problem areas and allows for frequent adjustments compensating for insulin deficiency, growth needs and activity changes each day. Ongoing education with a focus on a multidisciplinary cooperative team effort allows these treatment choices to be used and adapted to the individual and tailored for the specifics of the society in which the child or adolescent resides [1]. Key theoretical and practical research carried out over the past twenty years in many parts of the world support such treatment concepts. Recent research suggests that even those with the worst existing levels of education and motivation benefit greatly from application of a behavioral approach to improving compliance and providing information aimed at improved glycemia [2, 4]. With the incidence of type 1 diabetes increasing, it is critical that such complications be prevented if possible, identified early if unavoidable and treated appropriately and aggressively.

AUTOIMMUNOPATHIES ASSOCIATED WITH TYPE 1 DIABETES MELLITUS: THYROID, CELIAC, ADRENAL

Type 1 diabetes mellitus is associated with other autoimmunopathies (thyroid disease, celiac disease, vitiligo and adrenal insufficiency) [4]. Such disorders are not caused by having diabetes or by poorly controlled diabetes but most likely reflect the common genetic predisposition with such autoimmune disease and the autoimmune type of type 1 diabetes mellitus. HLA studies, when available and less expensive in the future, hold the promise of identifying subgroups of patients who may be at higher risk for such concomitant autoimmunopathies. For now, however, on clinical grounds it is not usually possible to identify which individual patients are most susceptible to such risks and therefore screening recommendations have been developed.

Thyroid dysfunction including euthyroid goiters, Hashimoto's thyroiditis and compensated as well as full-fledged hypothyroidism as well as hyperthyroidism are all more commonly seen in patients with type 1 diabetes mellitus. Thyroid dysfunction is associated with significant morbidity but not usually mortality whether or not it co-exists with diabetes. The impact of thyroid abnormalities on growth and development is particularly pertinent when dealing with children and adolescents. In the adult years, however, bone mineralization as well as abnormalities of lipids and cardiac function are associated with undiagnosed and untreated thyroid problems. As a consequence of such known risks, recommendations from the ADA [5] as well as ISPAD [6] include routine screening for thyroid disease. Hashimoto's thyroiditis with positive thyroid autoantibodies (thyroglobulin and/or thyroid microsomal antibodies) occurs in 20–40% of young people with type 1 diabetes. A palpable or enlarged thyroid gland (goiter) may be present in 10–20% [4]. This author suggests, at a minimum, that this be done at diagnosis and at least annually with T4, sensitive TSH and thyroid antibodies. Most goiters usually are not very large and usually not noted by patients or family members; often the patient is clinically euthyroid. Development of an obvious goiter, abnormal growth velocity or unexplained weight gain coupled with any other classical symptoms of hypo- or hyperthyroidism should warrant immediate thyroid function and antibody testing. When evaluating hyperlipidemia, consideration of thyroid function should also occur since treatment of underlying subtle hypothyroidism may also "cure" the abnormal lipid levels. Synthetic thyroid hormone replacement is appropriate for the treatment of compensated or more total

hypothyroidism while anti-thyroid medications such as propylthiouracil or methimazole are available for hyperthyroidism; radioiodine can also safely be used in children and adolescents although not commonly recommended as frequently as in adult patients. Usually there is no concomitant change in metabolic control with either hypothyroidism or hyperthyroidism. Most thyroid disorders do not produce obvious glucose control abnormalities nor do treatments change glucose control appreciably in this author's experience. It is reasonable to also screen other family members with thyroid antibodies and perhaps a sensitive TSH assay since thyroid disorders are frequently found in numerous relatives as a result of inherited genetic predisposition.

Celiac disease is increased in frequency (approximately 2–8%) [6] in association with type 1 diabetes presumably related to HLA B8-DR3 commonality between the two conditions with prevalence from 10–50 times higher than in the general pediatric and adolescent population. Certain ethnic groups, specifically southern Mediterranean (i.e. Italy) [7], may be at higher risk than other populations. With current screening techniques using very sensitive transglutaminase assays, subclinical celiac disease may be detected at diagnosis or with annual antibody screening blood testing. Often such youngsters are completely asymptomatic or only have nonspecific symptoms such as vague abdominal complaints (flatulence, dyspepsia, diarrhea, nonspecific abdominal pains), increased hypoglycemia, slowed growth velocities and/or delayed puberty. Iron deficiency anemia may result. Jejunal biopsy shows villous atrophy and avoidance of gluten in the meal-plan usually eliminates even subtle symptoms of celiac disease as well as causes the positive antibodies (gliadin, endomysial or transglutaminase) to become negative as long as gluten is avoided [8]. It is reasonable if celiac disease is diagnosed, to also then test other members of the nuclear family since they are at higher risk for also having asymptomatic celiac disease.

Adrenal insufficiency can be screened with available adrenal autoantibodies and may occur in 2–4% of youngsters with type 1 diabetes [4, 9]. It should be suspected if there is a sudden decrease in insulin requirements or if there is unexpected hypoglycemia or when hypoglycemia occurs without other explanations, increasing in frequency or intensity. Abnormalities of growth rate, progressive weight loss, unexplained tiredness or increasing skin pigmentation should also prompt testing of adrenal antibodies and cortisol as well as ACTH levels. Definitive testing involves measurement of serum electrolytes (hyponatremia and usually but not always hyperkalemia), blood cortisol (low) and ACTH (high) levels as well as positive antibodies if such are available. When available, ACTH stimulation testing can confirm lack of appropriate increase in serum cortisol levels by 30–60 minutes after the ACTH is given. Successful treatment with replacement doses of adrenal glucocorticoids is confirmed with prompt return to health, weight gains, loss of lassitude and return to normal skin pigmentation as the ACTH levels normalize. Some Addisonian patients require mineralocorticoid replacement with 9-α-fludrocortisone as well.

Polyendocrine autoimmunopathy syndrome [4, 9] with type 1 diabetes can include not only thyroid and adrenal disorders but also vitiligo, alopecia, hypoparathyroidism, pernicious anemia with positive gastroparietal antibodies and hypophysitis. Exactly how commonly these other entities occur is not well known in children and adolescents but all such entities are certainly less common than thyroid disease and celiac disease. Clinical concern and treatment should be based upon an increased awareness of the possibility of such abnormalities coupled with appropriate history and physical findings, confirmatory tests when available and therapeutic response to treatment when prescribed. Family history may also provide a clue to such diagnoses.

GROWTH AND GONADAL/PUBERTY PROBLEMS

With reasonable glucose control, it is now rare to have major growth problems or abnormalities of puberty. However, in individual patients where glucose control is particularly problematic or in parts of the world where glucose control remains elusive, such problems may be frequent. Reasons for poor growth [10, 11], delayed puberty and menometrorrhagia [12, 13] should be investigated since other causes may also exist related or unrelated to diabetes. Thyroid disorders and celiac disease are especially important because of their increased frequency in type 1 diabetes patients and because both can be specifically treated with our current understanding of their pathophysiology.

Puberty should be staged and documented according to Tanner stages. Growth should be assessed and plotted at least quarterly on standardized country and sex-specific charts to document normalcy and adequate growth progress. This allows early identification of abnormalities [14] and appropriate investigation as to causality and treatment. The importance of a detailed family history when investigating growth and pubertal disorders cannot be overemphasized since familial patterns may be more important than glycemic control. Classical Mauriac syndrome (growth failure, fatty hepatomegaly, delayed puberty associated with chronic inadequate insulin) [15] now is quite rare with reasonable metabolic control as long as sufficient insulin is available to avoid chronic ketosis. Mauriac syndrome may be more commonly seen in those parts of the world where insulin is not always available but can occur in the developed world when insulin is not faithfully administered or major psychosocial problems cause chronic insulin omission. Sexual and physical abuse is often an underlying factor when recurrent ketoacidosis and severe growth failure occur related to chronic hyperglycemia.

LIMITED JOINT MOBILITY (LJM)

Limited joint mobility [16, 17] is most likely a biochemical marker of tissue advanced glycation end-products (AGEs) associated with chronic hyperglycemia [18]. The importance of limited joint mobility may be its ability, in concrete fashion, to show the patient and family something that is abnormal and is caused by high sugar levels. While there may be different genetic susceptibilities for LJM, these may be the same generalized susceptibilities that select those at higher risk for renal or cardiovascular compromise. In our own LJM studies, LJM presence was associated with complication risks as high as 400–600% compared to those without LJM [16]. Limited joint mobility should be assessed clinically at least annually by placing the hands in a 'prayer position'. This author has developed a 5 stage system that stratifies risk (Brink-Starkman LJM stages: stage 0 = no stiffness or contractures; stage 1 = stiffness of fingers only; stage 2 = stiffness and contractures only of the fifth fingers bilaterally; stage 3 = stiffness and contractures of more than just the fifth fingers bilaterally; stage 4 = stiffness and contractures of the fingers plus the wrists; stage 5 = spine, neck and other joints also involved) [16].

OSTEOPENIA

Osteopenia prevalence, incidence and frequency in childhood and adolescent type 1 diabetes are unknown. Conflicting research studies have been published describing abnormalities in vitamin D and its metabolites as well as parathyroid hormone but there is documentation of increased urinary losses of calcium in those with type 1 diabetes [19]. Known decreases in type 1 diabetes related to IGF-1 levels may also be contributing factors for osteopenia and lower bone density measurements [20]. There is no increase in incidence of fractures in youngsters with diabetes whether or not they are in adequate or inadequate glucose control. In a prospective study utilizing a cohort of teenage and post-teenage young adult women with type 1 diabetes compared to age-matched controls, significant bone density abnormalities were not present in the teenagers but were present in the young adult women despite no differences found in IGF-1 and IGF-binding protein 3 levels as well as in osteocalcin and N-telopeptide levels [21].

DCCT AND OTHER STUDIES

The Diabetes Control and Complications Trial (DCCT) [22] continues to be the premier large, prospective and randomized multi-centered research trial evaluating long term microangiopathic complications associated with type 1 diabetes mellitus. 1441 patients participated in 29 centers in the United States of America and Canada as part of the DCCT and proved the importance of glycemic control to decrease retinopathy, nephropathy and neuropathy. Analysis of the results from the cohort of teenagers who participated in the DCCT was presented separately from those of the entire DCCT study participants

but did not change the study outcome [23]. By the conclusion of the DCCT, the adolescent cohort were young adults but there is no other large, multicentered, prospective and randomly designed treatment study involving younger children to address the issue of importance of glycemic control vis-à-vis long term microangiopathies let alone those macrovascular complications that take even longer to become clinically apparent. Earlier studies by Pirart [24] showed similar importance of improved control but with less scientifically rigid study design. The adolescent cohort of the DCCT – compared to the adults in the same study – had more difficulty controlling blood glucose levels (higher A1c) and were more likely to have severe hypoglycemia during the study. However, similar differences between the intensive vs conventional treatment groups occurred in the adolescent cohort compared to the adult cohort when analyzed by hemoglobin A1c levels obtained and intention to treat.

The DCCT conclusively and overwhelming proved the glucose hypothesis: elevated blood glucose levels are significantly associated with retinopathy as well as neuropathy and nephropathy even with follow-up of less than 10 years duration in an otherwise young and healthy population of adolescents and young adults with type 1 diabetes mellitus. Primary prevention of retinopathy was reduced by 76% and secondary progression of retinopathy was reduced by 54%. The development of proliferative or severe nonproliferative retinopathy was reduced by 47%, microalbuminuria reduction of 39%, frank albuminuria reduction by 54% and clinical neuropathy by 60% [22]. This occurred in association with targeted glycemic goals utilizing capillary blood glucose self-monitoring and improving and sustaining the improvement of hemoglobin A1c values. The chief adverse event associated with intensive therapy was a two to three fold increase in severe hypoglycemia but no increase in deaths or motor vehicle accidents nor any change in intellectual capacity or any other psychosocial adverse events was documented. These goals were achieved either through multi-dose insulin algorithms or insulin pump treatment and supported by a multidisciplinary diabetes team of nurse educators, nutritionists, diabetologists and psychosocial support staff [25]. It is the opinion of this author that the nurse educators and dieticians working together with a common philosophy of empowerment helped teach, support and focus the efforts of our patients during the DCCT [26]. The DCCT (Figure 22.1) results provide a gold standard to improve glycemic control for all with diabetes while always stressing the importance of minimizing and preventing severe episodes of hypoglycemia. Using an intent-to-treat analysis four years after the conclusion of the DCCT, treatment benefits persist (Figure 22.2) [27]. This benefit is also sustained at six years after the conclusion of the DCCT as well [28]. Studies at other centers show that not only can such control be achieved in children and adolescents but also the amount of hypoglycemia that occurred in the DCCT cohort can be reduced significantly [29, 30, 31].

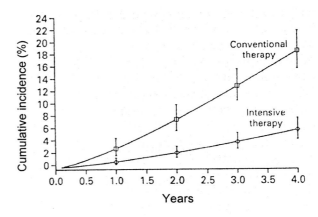

Figure 22.2

Four year follow-up of DCCT (with permission of Dr David Nathan on behalf of the DCCT Research Group).

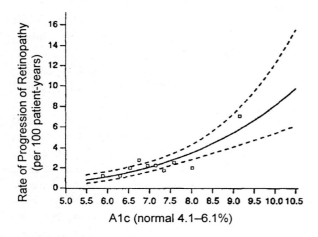

Figure 22.1

DCCT Retinopathy Rates (with permission of Dr David Nathan on behalf of the DCCT Research Group).

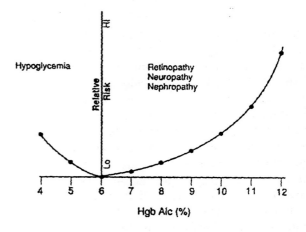

Figure 22.3

J curve: Hypoglycemia *vs.* Complications Risk *v.s.* A1c Achieved (with permission of Dr Richard Dickey, Hickory NC).

The most important antecedents for the development of long-term microvascular complications in children and adolescents are (1) longer duration of diabetes, (2) poor glycemic control and (3) others in the family with similar microangiopathic (*i.e.* hyperlipidemia, hypertension, angina and myocardial infarction) risks [9]. Pubertal factors, presumably hormonally medicated such as gonadal steroids and growth hormone, accelerate the progression of microvascular complications [6]. The DCCT demonstrated that **any** improvement in glycemic control helps reduce these same risks with the greatest improvement occurring in those with the highest A1c levels and thus the largest starting risk.

Smoking [32] and hyperlipidemia [33] as well as any degree of higher blood pressure [6, 34] are also other key risk factors for microangiopathies. From the diagnosis of type 1 diabetes and at all points in its treatment, the aim of therapy should be the best possible metabolic control while avoiding recurrent and severe episodes of hypoglycemia (see Figure 22.3) [35]. *Any* level of sustained improvement in glycemic control is associated with risk reduction [36, 37]. The DCCT found that for every 10% improvement in hemoglobin A1c (*e.g.* 9% down to 8.1%) a 44% risk reduction occurred. The DCCT also did not demonstrate any specific hemoglobin A1c threshold below which diabetes complications will not occur [36]. Other studies suggest that the rate of complications changes more dramatically above hemoglobin A1c levels around 8–8.5% (using a DCCT reference standard assay) [38, 39] but the different interpretations of these studies remain controversial. While most diabetes associated complications do not become clinically apparent before adulthood [40], those youngsters in the worst glycemic control for the longest periods of time may have clinically apparent abnormalities of growth and puberty as well as limited joint mobility, retinopathy, neuropathy, hypertension and proteinuria [41].

RETINOPATHY

Past surveys demonstrated a 5–10% chance of becoming legally blind in people with diabetes but the earliest ability to detect minor microaneurisms is rarely seen before five years duration of type 1 diabetes. Using fundus photography, retinopathy reaches a prevalence of 50% by the tenth year of duration of type 1 diabetes. However, clinically significant retinopathy is virtually nonexistent before puberty. This has led to speculation that the increases in sex steroids as well as the growth hormone axis (increased growth hormone and decreased insulin-like growth factors) or some combination facilitate or contribute in association with increased burden of glycemia on the retinal and other microcirculations. As a result of such studies large organizations such as ISPAD (International Society for Pediatric and Adolescent Diabetes) Consensus Guidelines and the Guidelines of the American Diabetes Association recommend direct ophthalmoscopy at least annually after five years duration of diabetes and/or the onset of puberty [5, 6]. Stereo fundus photography and/or fluorescein angiography are more expensive and require special equipment and trained technologists but are also very sensitive methods for detecting early retinal abnormalities [42].

Earlier research [43] suggested the years prior to puberty were not very important in the development of type 1 diabetes complications but more recent studies from Brussels [44], Berlin [45], Leicester [46] and Sydney [47] all suggest that this is not so. Duration of diabetes as well as degree of long-term glycemic control are most important in determining risks of retinopathy as well as renal and neurologic complications. Familial susceptibilities to such damage also may be important to elucidate.

Enhancement of retinal visualization with ophthalmic eye drops may be helpful but, with training and practice, many pediatric diabetologists become quite skilled at visualization in a completely darkened room with a cooperative patient. A skilled ophthalmologist knowledgeable in retinal pathology and detection should be consulted with any abnormal symptoms (e.g. floaters, persistent blurry vision) or physical signs (e.g. hemorrhage, exudates, cataracts, new retinal blood vessel formation) and for routine annual examination at puberty or after five years duration of diabetes. Any rapid improvement in glycemic control especially with hemoglobin A1c levels above 10% can be associated with significant deterioration of retinopathy. This would likely occur in anyone who is pregnant and quickly decides to take better care of themselves in an effort to decrease miscarriage and prematurity. This would also occur in any patients with poor glycemic control who decide to intensify their treatment and succeed. Under such circumstances, immediate ophthalmologic referral is important not only to document pre-existing retinopathy but also to allow sequential follow-up and assessment of subtle changes that may require laser therapy [48, 49].

Background or nonproliferative diabetic retinopathy (NPDR) is often the earliest abnormality detected. NPDR appears as small red dots through the ophthalmoscope. Dot hemorrhages and microaneurisms appear similar to each other and may require expert ophthalmoscopy, fundus photography or angiography to be able to tell them apart or document their severity particularly in the outer portions of the retina not easily seen by a non-ophthalmologist. Protein or lipid exudates are also seen in NPDR and there are several protocols [50] designed to document such findings as well as the changes via sequential examinations. Most of the time, there are no visual symptoms associated with NPDR. However, if the macula is edematous, then vision can be compromised. As retinopathy progresses and retinal hypoxia is associated with neovascularization, new blood vessels can form in response to nonperfusion or hypoxic retinal damage. This can include dilated or irregular blood vessels and also intraretinal microvascular abnormalities (IRMA). Proliferative retinopathy (PDR) involves new blood vessel formation to a greater extent than preproliferative retinopathy and carries the risk of spontaneous hemorrhage. If scar tissue forms on or around the retina or fibrous traction occurs as hemorrhages resolve, retinal detachment can occur with sudden blindness and the need for emergency operative repair. High risk retinal findings include new vessel formation around the disk (NVD), NVD associated with preretinal or vitreous hemorrhage or extensive formation of new vessels elsewhere (NVE) in the retina. Diabetic macular edema involving the central portion of the retina often produces dramatic decrease in visual acuity when the fovea is involved [51, 52, 53]. Focal or panretinal photocoagulation was demonstrated by the Early Treatment Diabetic Retinopathy Study (ETDRS) and the Diabetic Retinopathy Study (DRS) Research Group [54, 55] and saves vision.

If macular edema, preretinal or vitreous hemorrhage or new vessels are seen or if there are any new findings of background, preproliferative or proliferative retinopathy, urgent ophthalmologic consultation should be arranged for consideration of laser treatment.

NEPHROPATHY

Many previous epidemiological studies [56, 57] have demonstrated that up to 30–40% of patients with type 1 diabetes develop end-stage retinal failure and require dialysis or kidney transplantation. Not only is glycemic control critical in the development of diabetic nephropathy [58], but smoking, hyperlipidemia and hypertension seem to be independent co-factors increasing the risk of nephropathy [59] as already referenced above. Genetic predisposition [60, 61] also adds risk. Knowledge of such risk makes obtaining a family history of cardiovascular diseases and hypertension extremely important to identify patients at higher risk who should be considered for earlier treatment for minimal hypertension or advancing microalbuminuria with medications like ACE inhibitors [62, 63, 64]. Danish pediatric cross sectional studies [65] have confirmed such findings. Predictors of microalbuminuria were defined in Pittsburgh [66] and confirmed that,

even with the normal level, stratification of albumin excretion was able to predict those more likely to show progression over time towards increased protein losses [67]. Other research looking for pathophysiologic mechanisms suggests involvement of the sodium-lithium countertransport system [68, 69]. In recent years, there is also an impression, documented in Sweden [70], of a declining incidence of nephropathy that may well be related to gradual improvement in overall glycemic control in the past decade or two.

With diabetic nephropathy and its associated end-stage renal failure such a major cause of mortality among young adults with type 1 diabetes, ways to screen for incipient renal involvement are very important. Focusing on improved glycemic control is as important as identifying ways to reduce other risk factors [71]. Screening with timed urine samples using very sensitive "microalbumin" assays is a mainstay coupled with assessment of lipids and blood pressure. It is generally acknowledged that elevated urinary albumin excretion predicts later diabetic nephropathy while elevated blood pressure may be associated not only with familial hypertension predisposition but also with subtle diabetic kidney disease. With increasing amounts of microalbuminuria or microalbuminuria identifying populations at risk, premature cardiovascular death occurs [72]. Beginning at puberty or five years after diagnosis of type 1 diabetes mellitus, urinary protein should be screened using either a random microalbumin/creatinine ratio, timed overnight microalbumin assay / albumin excretion rate assessment or 24 hour timed urinary microalbumin / albumin excretion rate measurement. There is no convincing evidence that one or the other is any better but there are wide day-to-day variations particularly associated with intercurrent viral illness or stresses as well as changes in day-to-day-activity intensity. Pediatric and adolescent normative data is now available that suggests that children and adolescents without diabetes rarely excrete albumin on such timed collections higher than 7.2–7.6 µg/minute [6]. Persistent microalbuminuria should be diagnosed only after two or three consecutive urine specimens consistently show such abnormalities and glomerulonephritis, urinary tract infection, menstrual bleeding or vaginal discharge and strenuous exercise are excluded from the differential diagnosis. This author prefers overnight timed urine collections to avoid some of the problems of 24 hour collections. Overnight timed collections are not affected by posture or exercise and can be done in the convenience of the home for improved facility of collection. Timed microalbumin overnight results < 95th percentile for age are approximately < 7–20 µg/min corrected for body surface area. There may be minor differences for increased male muscle mass compared to female muscle mass in mid-late puberty or later age that are likely more important for researchers than for clinicians. Recent dipstick methods (*e.g.* Micral-Test ®) may also be used for screening purposes.

Reducing total protein, especially animal-source protein, to less than 20% of calorie contribution has also been shown to reduce microalbuminuria but it is unknown if this has any long term benefits or merely reduces protein urinary loss [73]. This author has had great difficulty moving the total protein contribution to the meal plan to less than 20% given the style of foods available in the USA despite coordinated nutrition, nursing and physician recommendations when microalbuminuria and/or hypertension or even if treatment is already prescribed with ACE inhibitors. Short of a full vegetarian meal plan, this approach may be theoretically beneficial but is extremely difficult to sustain.

Blood pressure readings should be assessed at least annually and compared to age and sex matched normative standards. Particular attention to blood pressure readings in those with intermittent or persistent microalbuminuria or proteinuria and those in whom there is a positive family history of hypertension, kidney, stroke or heart problems. Home blood pressure monitoring or ambulatory 24 hour home monitoring of blood pressure may be helpful to determine when and if antihypertensive treatment should be instituted. This author prefers single nightly doses of ACE inhibitors (*e.g.* lisinopril) since such a dose schedule may be easier to remember, side effects (*e.g.* coughing and tiredness) may be minimized and documented decreases in microalbuminuria as well as blood pressure readings have been demonstrated. If lipid abnormalities are also present, lipid-lowering statin medications can be

used at the same time without any increase in side effects. Improvement in glycemic control remains the mainstay of reducing microalbuminuria [22] but antihypertensive treatment and reducing all the other possible risk factors should not be minimized. If progression of microalbuminuria produces frank proteinuria, uncontrolled hypertension or overt evidence of early renal failure, involvement of knowledgeable nephrologists is warranted. Recent research may provide new diagnostic and therapeutic agents that allow identification of underlying high risk contribution to atherosclerotic plaque formation and perhaps target specific perturbations of diabetic vasculature (*i.e.* RAGE: receptor for advanced glycation end-products) and therefore bypass part of the need for improved glycemic control by "blocking" the effects of chronic hyperglycemia [74].

NEUROPATHY

Diabetic neuropathy results in significant morbidity of the peripheral and/or autonomic nervous systems [75]. Pathophysiologically, such end-organ disease may reflect a combination of metabolic and vascular assaults on the nervous tissue compared to retinopathy and nephropathy which are likely direct insults to the microvascular circulation. Hyperglycemia is associated with increases in sorbitol accumulation and direct toxic effects on the nerve as well as abnormalities of myoinositol, phosphoinositide and Na^+/K^+ ATPase activity [76]. The vascular hypothesis of neuropathy suggests that local ischemia also commonly occurs [77].

Occasionally, teenagers present with severe painful neuritis or with problematic gastroparesis. Often – but not exclusively – this type of dramatic neuropathy presents in the cohort of extremely long duration poor glycemic control. Subtle and subclinical diabetic neuropathy can be detected in adolescents [78, 79] if appropriate techniques are utilized. In those who are smokers, such neuropathies may also occur earlier and with more intensity. The DCCT proved the association of neuropathy with glycemic control [22]. Long term follow-up in the Oslo Study [80] confirmed that hemoglobin A1c, a surrogate marker for longitudinal glycemic control, was associated with near normal nerve function if < 8.4% over 18 years in a young adult cohort.

Peripheral neuropathy most commonly presents in a typical "glove and stocking" distribution involving pain, hyperaesthesia and/or loss of sensation to pinprick or plastic filament testing. Reflexes can be absent or reduced in the lower extremities and vibratory sensation decreased or absent. Amyotrophy is less common and at times can be unilateral. Any such changes should be distinguished from other neurologic abnormalities (*e.g.* tumors compressing nerves). Pressure neuropathies most commonly involve the median nerve and are associated with carpal tunnel syndrome while limited joint mobility is painless and usually asymptomatic.

Autonomic neuropathy [81] can include gastroparesis, bloating with decreased appetite, constipation, diarrhea if the gastrointestinal system is involved, postural hypotension or QT abnormalities [82] as well as resting tachycardia if the cardiac system is involved, urinary retention and impotence if the genitourinary system is involved, sweating abnormalities and absent or abnormal pupillary responses.

Delayed gastric emptying and hypoglycemia unawareness syndrome may be two of the most common subclinical autonomic neuropathies in the pediatric or adolescent age group. Both have enormous clinical implications. Delayed food absorption can wreck havoc with insulin decision causing both hyperglycemia as well as hypoglycemia from mismatched insulin-food choices.

In the DCCT, hypoglycemia was increased three-fold in the intensively treated cohort [29] but other study groups achieving tight glycemic control do not also report so much hypoglycemia [30, 31]. With hypoglycemic problems often a major barrier to improving overall glycemic control [83], strategies to decrease episodes of hypoglycemia are being sought. While hypoglycemia, per se, is not a direct neuropathic complication, hypoglycemia unawareness may at least in part be an autonomic neuropathy. Hypoglycemia of increasing frequency changes counter-regulatory hormone response to hypoglycemia and sets up a vicious circle of worsening recognition, less physiologic response, worse ability to metabolically self-correct and, therefore, more severe and more frequent hypoglycemia. Hypoglycemia fears also set up large barriers toward improved control. If such hypoglycemia is unrecognized and does not cause any symptoms, then nocturnal hypoglycemia will not likely awaken a child, adolescent or adult. What might be mild episodes of symptomatic hypoglycemia can quickly escalate into recurring episodes of unconsciousness and/or hypoglycemic convulsions [84, 85, 86, 87]. With the advent of near-continuous glucose monitoring, and the documentation of the incredible frequency of unrecognized hypoglycemia, it is possible that this type of hypoglycemia unawareness is much more common than previously recognized [88]. Abnormalities of cardiac conduction, although rare, may be related to the syndrome of unexplained sudden death [89].

Tests for neuropathy are often not standardized but start with a detailed neurologic examination including vibratory sensation, deep tendon reflexes and filament sensory testing. Others including nerve conduction studies as well as cardiovascular reflex testing are often relegated to research studies since they involve large expenditures of time, equipment and tester proficiency to be reliable. A detailed history and systems review (numbness and tingling, pains, cramping, weakness; bloating, constipation and diarrhea; bladder distension; impotence; irregular heartbeat or fainting) may point out the need for more specific testing. Treatment with aldose reductase inhibitors to interfere with sorbitol accumulation has not demonstrated clinical utility and most other treatments (*e.g.* vitamin and mineral supplementation) for either nonspecific, not very efficacious or merely designed for symptomatic relief, lessening of anxiety or depression. Improved control, as in the DCCT, has been demonstrated to be of benefit if the neuropathy is not far advanced [90].

NECROBIOSIS LIPOIDICA DIABETICORUM

Necrobiosis lipoidica diabeticorum usually occurs in young adolescent or young adult females with diabetes and consists of indurated plaques. Most often these occur on the anterior shins and usually are bilateral. They consist of round or oval reddened areas without tenderness. Sometimes these areas coalesce with very thin skin. There can be some central atrophic areas in a pinkish base, often but not always associated with some ulceration and secondary infection. Pathogenesis is unclear although there seems to be some local inflammatory response as well as abnormalities of the microcirculation. Anecdotally, steroids applied as creams or ointments superficially and/or locally injected sometimes have been helpful as have local vitamin E oils but without adequate long term prospective studies. Low dose aspirin to decrease platelet adhesion have also been recommended but treatments are all empiric, symptomatic and with poor results. Common sense prevention of skin breakdown and local infection is important with appropriate hygienic dressing. Association with glycemic control has been difficult to prove [91].

CONCLUSION

It is believed that the complications of diabetes can be minimized and/or prevented with reasonable control of chronic hyperglycemia following the treatment protocols similar to those of the DCCT. While such complications often do not appear clinically in the pediatric and adolescent ages, the underlying mechanisms responsible for the development of complications of type 1 diabetes are already at work. Metabolic control matters. Our job as care providers for youngsters with type 1 diabetes should be to offer education, support and encouragement for the best possible glycemic control while avoiding frequent or severe episodes of hypoglycemia. This can be done with modern treatment options, involved families, home monitoring and ongoing educational and psychosocial diabetes team strategies.

REFERENCES

1. Brink SJ, Moltz KC, Miller M. Education and multidisciplinary team care concepts for pediatric and adolescent diabetes mellitus. *J Pediatr Endocr Metab*, **15:** 113–1130, 2002.
2. Anderson BJ. Who benefits from intensive therapy in type 1 diabetes? *Diabetes Care*, **26:** 2204–5, 2003.
3. Wysocki T, Harris MA, Wilkinson K, Sadler M, Mauras N, White NH. Self-management competence as a predictor of outcomes of intensive therapy or usual care in youth with type 1 diabetes. *Diabetes Care*, **26:** 2043–2047, 2003.
4. Brink SJ. Thyroid dysfunction in youngsters with IDDM. *J Pediatr Endocrin*, **1:** 181–184, 1985.
5. American Diabetes Association. Standards of Medical Care for Patients with Diabetes Mellitus. *Diabetes Care*, **24:** (S1)S33–S43, 2003.
6. Swift PGF, ed. *ISPAD Guidelines 2000*. Zeist, Netherlands: Medial Forum International; 2000.
7. Pocecco M, Ventura A. Coeliac disease and insulin dependent diabetes mellitus: a causal association? *Acta Paediatr*, **84:** 1432–1434, 1995.
8. Carlsson A, Axelsson IE, Borulf SK, Bredberg AC, Lindberg BA, Sjoberg KG, Ivarsson S-A. Prevalence of IgA-antiendomysium and IgA-antigliadin autoantibodies at diagnosis of insulin-dependent diabetes mellitus in Swedish children and adolescents. *Pediatrics*, **103:** 1248–1252, 1999.
9. Silink M, ed. *APEG Hand book on Childhood and Adolescent Diabetes: The Management of Insulin-Dependent (Type 1) Diabetes Mellitus (IDDM)*. Parramatta NSW, Australia: Australasian Paediatric Endocrine Group, 1996.
10. Brown M, Ahmed ML, Clayton K, Dunger DB. Growth during childhood and final height in type 1 diabetes. *Diabetic Med*, **11:** 182–187, 1994.
11. Clarke WL, Vance ML, Rogol AD. Growth and the child with diabetes mellitus. *Diabetes Care*, **16:** 101–106, 1993.
12. Kjaer K, Hagen C, Sando SH. Epidemiology of menarche and menstrual disturbances in an unselected group of women with insulin-dependent diabetes mellitus compared to controls. *J Clin Endocrin Metab*, **75:** 524–529, 1992.
13. Adcock CJ, Perry LA, Lindsell AM. Menstrual irregularities are more common in adolescents with type 1 diabetes: association with poor glycemic control and weight gain. *Diabetic Med*, **11:** 465–470, 1994.
14. Batch JA. Growth and puberty. In: Werther GA and Court JM, eds. *Diabetes and the Adolescent*. Melbourne, Australia: Miranova Publishers, 1998: 93–112.
15. Mauriac P. Hepatomegalies de l'enfance avec troubles de la croissance et du metabolism des glucides. *Paris Med*, **2:** 525–528, 1934.
16. Brink SJ. Limited joint mobility (LJM). In: Brink SJ, ed. *Pediatric and Adolescent Diabetes Mellitus*. Chicago: Year Book Medical Publishers, 1987: 305–312.
17. Rosenbloom AL. Skeletal and joint manifestation of childhood diabetes. *Pediatr Clin North Am*, **31:** 569–489, 1984.
18. Brownlee M. Glycation and diabetic complications. *Diabetes*, **43:** 836–884, 1994.

19. Becker DJ. Complications of IDDM in childhood and adolescence. In: Lifshitz F. *Pediatric Endocrinology. Third Edition.* New York, Marcel Dekker, 1996, p. 585.

20. Yakar S, Rosen CJ, Beamer WG, Ackert-Bicknell CL, Wu Y, Liu JL, Ooi G, Setse J, Frystyk J, Boisclair YR, LeRoith D. Circulating levels of IGF-1 directly regulate bone growth and density. *J Clin Invest,* **110:** 771–781, 2002.

21. Liu EY, Wactawski-Wende J, Donahue RP, Dmochowski J, Hovey KM, Quattrin T. Does low bone mineral density start in post-teenage years in women with type 1 diabetes? *Diabetes Care,* **26:** 2365–2369, 2003.

22. DCCT Research Group. The effect of intensive treatment of diabetes on the development and progression of long-term complications in insulin-dependent diabetes mellitus. *New Engl J Med,* **329:** 977–986, 1993.

23. DCCT Research Group. Effect of intensive diabetes treatment on the development and progression of long-term complications in adolescents with insulin-dependent diabetes mellitus. *J Pediatr,* **125:** 177–188, 1994.

24. Pirart J. Diabetes mellitus and its degenerative complications: a prospective study of 4400 patients observed between 1947 and 1973. *Diabetes Care,* **1:** 168–88, 1978.

25. Ahern JA, Wesche J. Strand T, Grove N, Brenneman A, Tamborlane W for the DCCT Research Group. The impact of the trial coordinator in the Diabetes Control and Complications Trial (DCCT). *Diabetes Educ,* **19:** 509–512, 1993.

26. Brink SJ. How to apply the DCCT experience to children and adolescents. *Ann Med,* **29:** 419–424, 1997.

27. DCCT/Epidemiology of Diabetes Interventions and Complications Research Group. Retinopathy and nephropathy in patients with type 1 diabetes four years after a trial of intensive therapy. *New Engl J Med,* **342:** 381–389, 2000.

28. DCCT/Epidemiology of Diabetes Interventions and Complications Research Group. Effect of intensive therapy on the microvascular complications of type 1 diabetes mellitus. *J Amer Med Assoc,* **287:** 2563–2569, 2002.

29. DCCT Research Group. Hypoglycemia in the Diabetes Control and Complications Trial. *Diabetes,* **46:** 271–286, 1997.

30. Nordfeldt S and Ludvigsson J. Severe hypoglycemia in children with IDDM. A prospective population study, 19921994. *Diabetes Care,* **20:** 497–503, 1997.

31. Dorchy H. What glycemic control can be achieved in young diabetics without residual secretion of endogenous insulin? What is the frequency of severe hypoglycemia and subclinical complications? *Arch Pediatrie,* **1:** 970–981, 1994.

32. Couper JJ. Staples AJ, Cocciolone R, Nairn J, Badcock N, Henning P. Relationship of smoking and albumin excretion in children with IDDM. *Diabetic Med,* **11:** 666–669, 1994.

33. Kordonouri O, Danne T, Hopfenmuller W, Enders I, Hovener G, Weber B. Lipid profiles and blood pressure: are they risk factors for the development of early background retinopathy and incipient nephropathy in children with insulin-dependent diabetes mellitus? *Acta Paediatr,* **104:** 1079–1084, 1996.

34. Chase HP, Garg SK, Jackson WE, Thomas MA, Harris S, Marshal G, Crews MJ. Blood pressure and retinopathy in type 1 diabetes. *Ophthalmology,* **97:** 155–159, 1990.

35. Brink SJ and Moltz K. The message of the DCCT for children and adolescents. *Diabetes Spectrum* 1997; 248–267.

36. DCCT Research Group. The relationship of glycemic exposure (HbA1c) to the risk of development and progression of retinopathy in the Diabetes Control and Complications Trial. *Diabetes,* **44:** 968–983, 1995.

37. Zhang LY, Krzentowski G, Albert A, Lefebvre PJ. Risk of developing retinopathy in Diabetes Control and Complications Trial for type 1 diabetic patients with good or poor metabolic control. *Diabetes Care,* **24:** 1275–1279, 2001.

38. Danne T, Weber B, Harman R, Enders I, Burger W, Hovener G. Long term glycemic control has a nonlinear association to the frequency of background retinopathy in adolescents with diabetes. Follow-up of the Berlin Retinopathy Study. *Diabetes Care,* **17:** 1390–1396, 1994.

39. Warram JH, Manson JE, Krolewski AS. Glycated hemoglobin and the risk of retinopathy in insulin-dependent diabetes mellitus. *New Engl J Med,* **332:** 1305–1306, 1995.

40. Brink SJ. Pubertal and post-pubertal diabetes. In: Brink SJ, ed. *Pediatric and Adolescent Diabetes Mellitus,* Chicago: Year Book Medical Publishers, 1987, 89–137.

41. Santiago JV, ed. *Medical Management of Insulin-Dependent (Type 1) Diabetes. Second Edition.* Alexandria, VA, USA: American Diabetes Association, 1994.

42. DCCT Research Group. Color photography *vs.* fluorescein angiography in the detection of diabetic retinopathy in the Diabetes Control and Complications Trial. *Arch Ophthalmol,* **107:** 236–243, 1989.

43. Kostraba JN, Dorman JS, Orchard TJ, Becker DJ, Yuskashi O, Ellis D, Drash AL. Contribution of

diabetes duration before puberty to the development of microvascular complications in IDDM subjects. *Diabetes Care*, **12**: 686–693, 1989.

44. Dorchy H. What level of HbA1c can be achieved in young patients beyond the honeymoon period? *Diabetes Care*, **16**: 1311–1313, 1993.

45. Burger W, Hovener G, Dusterhus R, Hartman R, Weber B. Prevalence and development of retinopathy in children and adolescents with type 1 (insulin-dependent) diabetes mellitus. A longitudinal study. *Diabetologia*, **29**: 17–22, 1986.

46. McNally PG, Raymond NT, Swift PGF, Hearnshaw JR, Burden AC. Does the prepubertal duration of diabetes influence the onset of microvascular complications? *Diabetes Med*, **10**: 906–916, 1993.

47. Donaghue KC, King J, Fung ATW, Chan A, Hing S, Howard NJ, Fairchild J, Silink M. The effect of prepubertal diabetes duration on diabetes microvascular complications in early and late adolescence. *Diabetes Care*, **20**: 77–80, 1997.

48. Daneman D, Drash AL, Lobes LA, Becker DJ, Baker LM, Travis LB. Progressive retinopathy with improved control in diabetic dwarfism (Mauriac syndrome) *Diabetes Care*, **4**: 360–365, 1981.

49. Dahl-Jorgensen K, Brinchmann-Hansen O, Hansen KF, Sandvik L, Aagenaes O. Rapid tightening of blood glucose control leads to transient deterioration in retinopathy in insulin dependent diabetes mellitus – the Oslo Study. *BMJ*, **290**: 811–815, 1985.

50. Donaghue K. Retinopathy. In: Werther GA and Court JM, eds. *Diabetes and the Adolescent*, Melbourne, Australia: Miranova Publishers, 1998, 157–173.

51. Klein R, Klein BEK, Moss SE, Davis MD, DeMets DL. The Wisconsin epidemiology study of diabetic retinopathy. II. Prevalence and risk of diabetic retinopathy when age at diagnosis is less than 30 yr. *Arch Ophthalmol*, **102**: 520–526, 1984.

52. Krolewski AS, Warram JH, Rand LI, Kahn CR. Epidemiologic approach to the etiology of type 1 diabetes mellitus and its complications. *New Engl J Med*, **317**: 1390–1398, 1987.

53. Kostraba JN, Klein R, Dorman JS, Becker DJ, Drash AL, Maser RE. The Epidemiology of Diabetes Complications Study IV. Correlates of diabetic background and proliferative retinopathy. *Am J Epidemiol*, **133**: 381–391, 1991.

54. Early Treatment Diabetic Retinopathy Study Research Group. Treatment techniques and clinical guidelines for photocoagulation of diabetic macular edema. *Ophthalmology*, **94**: 761–774, 1987.

55. Diabetic Retinopathy Study Research Group. Photocoagulation treatment of proliferative diabetic retinopathy: clinical application of Diabetic Retinopathy Study (DRS) Findings. *Ophthalmology*, **88**: 583–600, 1981.

56. Andersen AR, Christiansen JS, Anderson JK, Kreiner S, Deckert T. Diabetic nephropathy in type 1 (insulin-dependent) diabetes: an epidemiological study. *Diabetologia*, **25**: 496–501, 1983.

57. Mogensen CE. Natural history of renal functional abnormalities in human diabetes mellitus: from normoalbuminuria to incipient and overt nephropathy. *Contemp Issues Nephrol*, **20**: 19–49, 1989.

58. Couper JJ. Jones TW, Donaghue KC, Clarke CF, Thomsett MJ and Silink M. The Diabetes Control and Complications Trial. Implications for children and adolescents. Australasian Paediatric Endocrine Group. *Med J Austr*, **162**: 369–372, 1995.

59. Cruickshanks KJ, Orchard TJ, Becker DJ. The cardiovascular risk profile of adolescents with insulin-dependent diabetes mellitus. *Diabetes Care*, **8**: 118–124, 1985.

60. Seaquist E, Goetz F, Rich S, Barbosa J. Familial clustering of diabetic kidney disease. *New Engl J Med*, **320**: 1161–1165, 1989.

61. Krolewski AS, Canessa M, Warram JH. Predisposition to hypertension and susceptibility to renal disease in insulin dependent diabetes mellitus. *New Engl J Med*, **318**: 140–145, 1988.

62. Laffel LM, McGill JB, Gans DJ. The beneficial effect of angiotensin converting enzyme inhibition with captopril on diabetic nephropathy in normotensive IDDM patients with microalbuminuria. North American Microalbuminuria Study Group. *Am J Med*, **99**: 497–504, 1995.

63. Cook JJ, Balfe JW, Spino M, Sachet E, Daneman D. Angiotensin converting enzyme inhibitor therapy decreases microalbuminuria in normotensive children with IDDM. *J Pediatr*, **117**: 39–45, 1990.

64. Rudberg S, Aperia A, Freyschuss U, Persson B. Enalapril reduces microalbuminuria in young, normotensive type 1 (insulin-dependent) diabetic patients irrespective of a hypotensive effect. *Diabetologia*, **33**: 470–476, 1990.

65. Mortensen HB, Marinelli K, Norgaard K. A nationwide cross-sectional study of urinary albumin excretion rate, arterial blood pressure and blood glucose control in Danish children with type 1 diabetes mellitus. *Diabetic Med*, **7**: 887–897, 1990.

66. Coonrad BS, Ellis D, Becker DJ, Bunker CH, Kelsey SF, Lloyd CE, Drash AL, Kuller LH, Orchard TJ. Predictors of microalbuminuria in individuals with IDDM: Pittsburgh Epidemiology

of Diabetes Complications Study. *Diabetes Care*, **16:** 1376–1383, 1993.

67. Schultz CJ, Neil HAW, Dalton RN, Dunger DB on behalf of the Oxford Regional Prospective Study Group. Risk of nephropathy can be detected before the onset of microalbuminuria during the early years after diagnosis of type 1 diabetes. *Diabetes Care*, **23:** 1811–1815, 2000.

68. Houtman PN, Campbell FM, Shah V, Grant DB, Dunger DB and Dillon MJ. Sodium-lithium countertransport in children with diabetes and their families. *Arch Dis Child*, **72:** 133–136, 1995.

69. Chiarelli F, Casani A, Tumini S, Kordonouri O, Danne T. Diabetic nephropathy in childhood and adolescence. *Diabetes Nutr Metab*, **12:** 144–153, 1999.

70. Bojestig M, Arnqvist HJ, Hermansson G, Karlberg BE, Ludvigsson J. Declining incidence of nephropathy in insulin dependent diabetes mellitus. *New Engl J Med*, **330:** 15–18, 1994.

71. Cooper ME, Allen TJ, Couper J. Nephropathy and hypertension. In: Werther GA and Court JM, eds. *Diabetes and the Adolescent.* Melbourne, Australia: Miranova Publishers; 1998, 139–156.

72. Allen KV, Walker JD. Microalbuminuria and mortality in long-duration type 1 diabetes. *Diabetes Care*, **26:** 2389–2391, 2003.

73. Brodsky IG, Robins DC, Hiser E. Effects of low protein diet on protein metabolism in insulin dependent diabetes mellitus patients with early nephropathy. *J Clin Endocrin Metab*, **75:** 351–357, 1992.

74. Cipollone F, Iezzi A, Fazia M, Zucchelli M, Pini B, Cuccurullo C, De Cesare D, De Blasis G, Muraro R, Bei R, Chiarelli F, Schmidt AM, Cuccurullo F, Mezzetti A. The receptor RAGE as a progression factor amplifying arachidonate-dependent inflammatory and proteolytic response in human atherosclerotic plaques. Role of glycemic control. *Circulation*, **108:** 2254–2262, 2003.

75. Clarke C. Neuropathy. In: Werther GA and Court JM, eds. *Diabetes and the Adolescent.* Melbourne, Australia: Miranova Publishers, 1998, 175–189.

76. Greene DA, Lattimer SA, Sima AF. Sorbitol, phosphoinositides and sodium-potassium ATPase in the pathogenesis of diabetic complications. *New Engl J Med*, **316:** 599–606, 1987.

77. Young RJ, Macintyre CC, Martyn CN, Prescott RJ, Ewing DJ, Smith AF, Viberti G, Clarke BF. Progression of subclinical polyneuropathy in young patients with type 1 (insulin-dependent) diabetes: association with glycaemic control and microangiopathy (microvascular complications). *Diabetologia*, **29:** 156–161, 1986.

78. Barkai L, Madacsy L, Kassay L. Investigation of subclinical signs of autonomic neuropathy in the early stages of childhood diabetes. *Horm Res*, **34:** 54–59, 1990.

79. Becker DJ, Greene DA, Aono SA, Aono M, D'Antonio J, Orchard T, Drash AL. Assessment of subclinical autonomic and peripheral neuropathy in childhood insulin-dependent diabetes mellitus. *Pediatr Adol Endocrin*, **17:** 173–178, 1988.

80. Larsen JR, Sjoholm H, Hanssen KF, Sandvik L, Berg TJ, Dahl-Jorgensen K. Optimal blood glucose control during 18 years preserves peripheral nerve function in patients with 30 years duration of type 1 diabetes. *Diabetes Care*, **26:** 2400–2404, 2003.

81. Verrotti A, Chiarelli F, Blasetti A, Morgese G. Autonomic neuropathy in diabetic children. *J Paediatr Child Health*, **31:** 545–548, 1995.

82. Barkai L, Madacsy L. Cardiovascular autonomic dysfunction in diabetes mellitus. *Arch Dis Child*, **73:** 515–518, 1995.

83. Brink SJ. Hypoglycaemia in children and adolescents with type 1 diabetes mellitus. *Diab Nutr Metab*, **12:** 108–121, 1999.

84. Amiel SA, Tamborlane WV, Sacca L, Sherwin RS. Hypoglycemia and glucose counterregulation in normal and insulin-dependent diabetic subjects. *Diabetes Metab Rev*, **4:** 71–89, 1988.

85. Cryer PE. Iatrogenic hypoglycemia as a cause of hypoglycemia-associated autonomic failure in IDDM: a vicious cycle. *Diabetes*, **4:** 255–260, 1992.

86. Cryer PE, Fisher JN, Shamoon H. Hypoglycemia. *Diabetes Care*, **17:** 734–75, 1994.

87. White NH, Skor DA, Cryer PE, Bier DM, Levandoski L, Santiago JV. Identification of type 1 diabetic patients at increased risk for hypoglycemia during intensive therapy. *New Engl J Med*, **308:** 485–491, 1983.

88. Gibson LC, Halvorson MJ, Carpenter S, Kaufman FR. Short-term use of the Minimed continuous monitoring system to determine patterns of glycemia in pediatric patients with type 1 DM. *Diabetes*, **6(S1):** 1664, 2000.

89. Sovik O. Dead-in-bed syndrome in young diabetic patients. *Diabetes Care*, **22:** B40–B42, 1999.

90. White N, Waltman S, Krupi T, Santiago J. Reversal of neuropathic and gastrointestinal complications related to diabetes mellitus in adolescents with improved metabolic control. *J Pediatr*, **99:** 41–45, 1981.

91. Kelly WF, Nicholas J, Adams J, Mahmood R. Necrobiosis lipoidica diabeticorum: association with background retinopathy, smoking and proteinuria. A case control study. *Diabetic Med*, **10:** 725–728, 1993.

23

AN EVIDENCE BASED APPROACH TO THE MANAGEMENT OF CARDIOVASCULAR DISEASES IN DIABETES MELLITUS

Umair MALLICK, Maria DOROBANȚU, Billy IQBAL, Dan CHEȚA

Diabetes mellitus and its cardiovascular complications are an important cause of morbidity and mortality worldwide. With the recent advancements in diagnostic, investigative and treatment techniques in the light of growing epidemiological and clinical evidence, international experts have developed guidelines to improve management and outcomes of patients with cardiovascular diseases. The interplay of multiple risk factors in different population groups in the developed world, as well as in countries with economies in transition, needs to be better understood. There is a growing need for defining effective key public health strategies for prevention and management of rising clinical and economic burden of diabetes and cardiovascular diseases.

This chapter is aimed towards readers with a basic knowledge of medicine. A summary of fundamental concepts in epidemiology, pathophysiology and principals of evidence based management in patients with diabetes and cardiovascular diseases is given. Many of these issues are already discussed in other chapters, in details. However, we attempt to address these issues using an approach that integrates principals of evidence-based medicine. For further information regarding detailed medical management of patients with diabetes and cardiovascular diseases, we recommend readers to consult the existing international and national guidelines.

INTRODUCTION

The prevalence of diabetes mellitus has shown a dramatic increase over the latest 50 years all across the globe. It is estimated that approximately 156 million individuals are currently diagnosed with diabetes and this number is expected to increase to an alarming 300 million in 2025 [1]. Only in the United States over 15 million people are known diabetics and approximately one third of these still remain undiagnosed [2]. The most prevalent form of diabetes is type 2 diabetes (formerly known as non-insulin dependent diabetes mellitus) and accounts for 90–95% of all diabetics. The remaining 5–10% have type 1 diabetes (formerly known as insulin-dependent diabetes mellitus). Patients with diabetes are at high risk of developing cardiovascular diseases (CVD). There is an increasing evidence that cardiovascular complications of diabetes mellitus are the most common cause of death and disability in these patients. It is well established that atherosclerosis is the main underlying pathophysiological mechanism that results in the development of cardiovascular complications, in association with poor glycaemic control. Diabetics with cardiovascular disease have a poorer prognosis when compared to their non-diabetic counterparts. Despite recent advancements in screening, detection and emerging evidence to guide therapy and improve outcomes in these patients, diabetes remains a constantly growing clinical and public health threat worldwide. Higher prevalence of cardiovascular complications possesses an increasing clinical and economic burden.

Using data from recently published clinical trials and current updated expert guidelines, an evidence-based approach to the management of cardiovascular complications in diabetes is justified. In this chapter, we aim to describe an overview of an evidence based approach towards management of important cardiovascular complications in diabetes and also review scope of CVD in diabetic patients taking the readers through epidemiological aspects of cardiovascular complications as a consequence of diabetes. With a better understanding of molecular mechanisms, recent research has highlighted potential novel biological risk markers in cardiovascular diseases frequently found in association with diabetes. It is crucial to recognise this concept in our appreciation of treatment strategies aiming at the prevention of cardiovascular events during long-term follow-up, which will be discussed in this chapter. We also explain recent advances in the pathophysiology of diabetic vascular disease to provide a thorough understanding of biological, clinical and epidemiological aspects of cardiovascular complications in diabetes. There is a growing awareness about the risk assessment for primary and secondary prevention of coronary artery disease (CAD). We describe, in brief, an overview of recently developed evidence based models to estimate risk of cardiovascular events that may guide us towards a better control of risk factors. Overall, the primary goal of this chapter is to introduce readers key notions of the currently existing evidence regarding the growing burden of diabetes and its vascular complications and their management. It is beyond scope of this chapter to give in depth management of CVD and diabetes, which is discussed in details in other chapters in this book.

RISK FACTORS AND DIABETES

Both type 1 and type 2 diabetes are independent risk factors for cardiovascular disease in men and women. Several risk factors including inappropriate lifestyle, physical inactivity, obesity and smoking contribute towards development of cardiovascular diseases, as well as diabetes in a similar fashion. Conventional risk factors for CVD, such as hypertension and elevated low-density lipoprotein cholesterol, remain principal determinants of cardiovascular disease in diabetics in addition to impaired glucose tolerance, insulin resistance, albuminuria, inflammatory processes and subclinical atherosclerosis. Early detection of cardiovascular disease and its risk factors, and their better control can delay the onset of cardiovascular complications in diabetics. Clustering of risk factors, that leads to enhancement of atherosclerotic processes in diabetics, affects the macro- and microvasculature resulting in a wide range of vascular disorders. These disorders can be broadly grouped into macrovascular complications, affecting medium sized vessels and microvascular complications that include small vessels of kidneys, eyes and other microvasculature.

CARDIOVASCULAR COMPLICATIONS IN DIABETES

Diabetes is a major risk factor for atherosclerosis, and its effect is so pronounced that the inherent protection conferred by the female gender is largely eliminated in diabetic women with cardiovascular event rate, being similar in both diabetic men and women [3]. Macrovascular complications of diabetes primarily refer to coronary artery disease, cerebrovascular disease and peripheral arterial disease and microvascular complications, including diabetic nephropathy, retinopathy and neuropathy.

MACROVASCULAR DISEASE

Macrovascular disease is the leading cause of death in patients with diabetes, accounting for 65% of all deaths in diabetic people, of which 80% is due to coronary artery disease and 15% to cerebrovascular disease [3]. In the UK Prospective Diabetes Study, the mortality rate due to macrovascular complications was 70 times higher than of microvascular complications [4].

Coronary artery disease

Diabetes is a strong risk factor and accelerates the natural course and development of atherosclerotic lesions in the coronary arteries. It is associated with a 2-fold increased risk in men and a 4-fold increased risk in women for developing coronary artery disease [5]. The risk of myocardial infarction in patients with diabetes and no history of coronary artery disease was found to be similar to that of non-diabetic individuals who have previously had a myocardial infarction [6]. Therefore, the Adult Treatment Panel of the National Cholesterol Education Program established diabetes as a "coronary artery disease" risk equivalent, implicating aggressive treatment of cardiovascular risk factors in diabetic individuals [7]. Diabetes also worsens outcomes in acute coronary syndromes. Diabetic patients with unstable angina are more likely to develop myocardial infarction, and diabetic patients with a myocardial infarction have a worse prognosis compared to their non-diabetic counterparts [8]. In the OASIS (Organization to Assess Strategies for

Ischemic Syndromes) registry, observing the outcomes of patients with unstable angina, diabetes independently increased mortality by 57% [9]. The FINMONICA Myocardial Infarction Register showed that after a myocardial infarction, diabetes increased the 1-month mortality rates by 58% in men and 160% in women, and 1-year mortality rates were increased by 38% in men and 86% in women [10]. A Swedish study found that over 50% of diabetic patients die 5 years after a myocardial infarction – that was greater than double the rate found in non-diabetic patients [11]. The SHOCK (SHould we emergently revascularize Occluded Coronaries for cardiogenic shocK?) registry, examining the role of diabetes in cardiogenic shock complicating myocardial infarction, showed diabetes to increase mortality by 36% [12]. In addition, diabetes is a recognized risk factor for poor outcome after both percutaneous and surgical revascularization procedures.

Cerebrovascular disease

Diabetes adversely affects the cerebrovascular arterial circulation and increases the risk of stroke. Analysis of panoramic radiographs for routine dental treatment revealed over a 5-fold excess prevalence of calcified carotid atheromas in patients with diabetes [13]. In the Multiple Risk Factor Intervention Trial (MRFIT), a 12-year follow-up study of 347,978 men aged 35–57 years, the risk of stroke was 3 times higher in diabetic patients [14]. Diabetes particularly increases the incidence of stroke in younger patients – an average diabetic stroke patient was found to be 3.2 years younger than an average non-diabetic stroke patient [15]. The Baltimore-Washington Cooperative Young Stroke Study [16], examining young white and black adults aged 18–44 years, found greater than a 10-fold increased risk of stroke in young diabetic patients, ranging as high as 23-fold in young white men with diabetes. Diabetes doubles the rate of first recurrent stroke [17] and trebles the rate of stroke-related dementia [18]. Patients with diabetes have a slower recovery from stroke, and mortality is increased independent of stroke severity. It has been identified as the strongest risk factor for stroke-related mortality, greater than hypertension, hypercholesterolaemia and smoking, with an increased mortality rate of almost 4-fold in men and 6-fold in women with diabetes [19].

Peripheral arterial disease

Diabetes increases the incidence and severity of peripheral arterial disease of 2- to 4-fold [20]. Data from the Framingham Study found men with diabetes to have a two-fold excess of carotid bruits and women with diabetes to have a two-fold excess of femoral bruits [21]. Diabetes is associated with non-palpable pedal pulses and lower ankle-brachial pressure indices. In the Hoorn Study, there was a 3-fold excess prevalence of an abnormal ankle-brachial pressure index (defined as less than 0.9) in diabetic individuals. Moreover, the prevalence of any peripheral arterial disease in diabetics was more than double that found in non-diabetics [22]. Diabetic patients are more frequently symptomatic, with the frequency of intermittent claudication being increased by more than 3-fold in men and 8-fold in women [23]. In the US, 50–70% of all non-traumatic lower-extremity amputations can be attributed to diabetes, being the leading cause for all non-traumatic amputations [24].

MICROVASCULAR DISEASE

Microangiopathy, an important long term complication of diabetes, is a specific but generalized disorder of the small blood vessels. Clinical manifestations of this disorder result from involvement of eyes, kidney and vasa vasorum of peripheral nerves. Unlike macrovascular complications, the incidence and progression of microvascular disease correlate highly with the level of glycaemia. Mechanisms of development of these complications are still not clear. Poor glycaemic control and duration of illness are considered to be major susceptibility factors.

Diabetic Nephropathy

Diabetes significantly affects the kidneys, causing glomerulopathy, arteriolar hyalinosis and tubulo-interstitial lesions, often referred to collectively as diabetic nephropathy. It is characterized by proteinuria > 300 mg/24h,

hypertension and a progressive decline in renal function. At its extreme, diabetic nephropathy results in end-stage renal disease, requiring dialysis or transplantation. However, the early stage of the disease is characterized by low, but abnormal, levels of proteinuria. This is known as "microalbuminuria" and is defined as proteinuria of 30–300mg/24h, being highly predictive of overt diabetic nephropathy, especially in type 1 diabetes. Diabetes is the leading cause of end-stage renal disease in the US. It accounts for approximately one-third of all patients with end-stage renal disease [25]. Approximately 35% of patients with type 1 diabetes of 18 years duration will show signs of diabetic renal involvement. Approximately one third of patients starting renal dialysis have type 2 diabetes [26]. Diabetic nephropathy dramatically increases the prevalence of coronary artery disease. For patients with type 1 diabetes, the presence of diabetic nephropathy (proteinuria > 300mg/24h) increases the risk of cardiovascular mortality almost 10-fold [27]. For patients with diabetes who are on renal dialysis, the annual mortality rates are greater than 20% [26].

Diabetic Retinopathy

Diabetic retinopathy is a progressive disease, resulting from a combination of microvascular leakage and microvascular occlusion in the retinal circulation. It is the commonest cause of blindness in people aged 30–69 years. Compared to non-diabetics, the risk of blindness is increased to 20-fold in diabetic individuals. One fifth of patients diagnosed with type 2 diabetes have retinopathy at time of diagnosis. In type 1 diabetes, vision-threatening retinopathy almost never occurs in the first 5 years after diagnosis or before puberty. However, after 15 years, almost all patients with type 1 diabetes, and two-thirds of patients with type 2 diabetes have background retinopathy.

Diabetic Neuropathy

Diabetic neuropathies can present in many ways, but the commonest form is a diffuse distal progressive polyneuropathy (in a glove and stocking distribution). It mainly affects the feet, predominantly sensory, often asymptomatic, and affects 40–50% of all patients with diabetes.

THE PATHOPHYSIOLOGY OF DIABETES AND CARDIOVASCULAR DISEASE

ATHEROSCLEROSIS IN DIABETES

Atherosclerosis is considered an inflammatory process, with associated fibrosis and lipid deposition. In sites predisposed to atherosclerosis, one of the earliest changes is the movement of monocytes, leaving the arterial wall. Monocytes adhere to the endothelial cells and squeeze between them to the subendothelial space, where they become tissue macrophages. Such endothelial cells overlying atherosclerotic plaques show increased expression of cell adhesion molecules. Macrophages express low-affinity scavenger receptors, which take up oxidized low-density lipids (LDL), transforming them into foam cells. Foam cells and the endothelial cells, together, release growth factors, cytokines and chemo-attractant molecules, which stimulate the proliferation and migration of vascular smooth muscle cells into the atherosclerotic lesion and their subsequent production of collagen and extracellular matrix. This results in the development of fatty streaks or plaques, on the luminal surface of the arterial wall. Erosion or rupture of such lesions, with exposure of underlying collagen, is a potent stimulus for thrombus formation, leading to acute vascular occlusion and clinical sequels.

The impact of diabetes on endothelial cell, vascular smooth muscle cell and platelet function and its effect on the coagulation cascade leads to an accelerated course of atherosclerosis and an increased thrombotic tendency, accounting for the increased cardiovascular morbidity and mortality. The effect of diabetes on each of the above and alterations in signalling cascades and molecular mechanisms will now be discussed.

ENDOTHELIAL CELL DYSFUNCTION IN DIABETES

Endothelial cells line the inner surface of all blood vessels, providing a metabolically active interface between the circulating blood and the vessel wall. Their position allows them to modulate blood flow, coagulation, thrombosis and leucocyte diapedesis [28]. The endothelial glucose concentration mirrors that in the extracellular environment. These cells produce important vasoactive substances contributing to vascular structure and function. These include nitric oxide (NO), reactive oxygen species (ROS), endothelins, prostaglandins and angiontensin-II (AT-II). Amongst them, NO plays a crucial role in mediating vascular smooth muscle relaxation [29]. It also inhibits platelet activation, attenuates the inflammatory response by decreasing the adhesion and migration of inflammatory cells and decreases vascular smooth muscle cell migration and proliferation [30, 31]. NO is produced constitutively in endothelial cells by nitric oxide synthase (eNOS), by oxidation of N-terminus of L-arginine. It acts in a paracrine fashion, mediating its vasodilator effect by activating guanylate cyclase and subsequent production of cyclic GMP, in neighbouring vascular smooth muscle cells [32]. In diabetes, the metabolic derangements including hyperglycaemia, excess free fatty acid production, advanced glycation end-products and insulin resistance all contribute to a decreased bioavailability of NO, achieved through a number of different mechanisms. Studies have shown that hyper-glycaemia decreases endothelium-derived NO production [33, 34].

Hyperglycaemia increases the production of ROS, especially of the superoxide anion (SO_2^-), *via* the mitochondrial electron transport chain in both endothelial cells and vascular smooth muscle cells [35]. ROS can activate protein kinase C (PKC) and increase the formation of AGEs (as discussed later), which may further lead to ROS production [36]. This increased oxidative stress decreases the bioavailability of NO by a number of mechanisms.

PKC is a family of at least a dozen kinases implicated in the cardiovascular complications of diabetes [37]. Although several isoforms are present in THE vascular tissue, studies have shown preferential activation of the β-isoform (PKC_β) in animal models of diabetes [38–40]. PKC is an important signalling enzyme contributing to endothelial dysfunction in diabetes. Impaired endothelium-dependent vasodilatation in rabbit aorta due to hyperglycaemia is reversed by

PKC inhibition [33]. PKC inhibition, by administering PKC_β inhibitors, in healthy adults with diabetes has shown to prevent the abnormal endothelium-dependent vasodilatation due to hyperglycaemia [41]. Hyperglycaemia leads to increased formation of diacylglycerol (DAG) from glycolytic intermediates, which is a major endogenous cofactor for PKC activation [42]. PKC may be activated directly by SO_2^- and free fatty acids (FFAs) [43, 44]. Thus, diabetes leads to a greater PKC activation, and this has a number of effects on the vascular function, promoting atherosclerosis through a series of mechanisms. In summary, these include an increased production of ROS, decreased NOS activation, an enhanced expression of endothelin-1 (a potent vasoconstrictor) and of pro-inflammatory cytokines, as well as an increased thrombotic tendency due to an increased expression of tissue-factor (TF) gene in endothelial cells [33, 37, 44–46]. This also involves an increased expression of growth factors and their receptors in the endothelial cells, vascular smooth muscle cells, platelets and monocytes-macrophages. These include platelet derived growth factor-β (PDGF-β) receptor and transforming growth factor-β (TGF-β) that results in an increased extracellular matrix production in atherosclerotic lesions [47–49].

In diabetes, the hyperglycaemia leads to non-enzymatic glycation of many molecules. These include haemoglobin, many other proteins and even lipids. The production of ROS leads to the formation of reactive carbonyl groups on glucose molecules. This allows glucose to form covalent links between a whole spectrum of molecules, leading to the formation of aldinine or Schiff bases, which then undergo slow chemical reactions to yield glycated products. Such advanced glycation end-products (AGEs) are increased in diabetes [50]. AGEs affect cellular function by activating the receptor for AGEs (RAGE) found in cells throughout the body [51]. RAGE activation can further increase ROS production [52] and increase the activation of transcription factor κB (TF-κB) and activator protein-1 which results in up-regulation of genes encoding leucocyte cell adhesion molecules (LCAM), leucocyte-attracting chemokines and pro-inflammatory cytokines, such as IL-1 and tumor necrosis factor (TNF), platelet derived

growth factor (PDGF) and IGF-1 all of which being implicated in atherosclerosis [53–55]. Glycation of LDLs increases their susceptibility to oxidative modifications, increasing the levels of oxidized LDLs, crucial for atherosclerosis [56].

In diabetes, decreased uptake of free fatty acids (FFAs) by striated muscle and increased release by adipose tissue leads to an elevated FFAs level [57, 58]. As a result, the liver increases its production of very low-density lipids (VLDLs). Further, the activity of lipoprotein lipase, the enzyme responsible for catabolizing triglyceride-rich lipoproteins, is also decreased in diabetes. Thus, increased hepatic synthesis of VLDLs and decreased clearance of triglyceride-rich particles leads to the characteristic hypertriglyceridaemia in diabetes [59, 60]. This provides a substrate for cholesterol ester transfer protein, which promotes the transfer of cholesterol from high-density lipids (HDL) to LDL. This modification of LDL yields a smaller, more dense and atherogenic LDL. Both increased LDL and decreased HDL levels are associated with endothelial dysfunction [61]. Increased FFAs levels, in addition to leading to a more atherogenic environment, increase the production of ROS and activation of PKC [45], as discussed above. Infusion of FFAs in animals and humans has shown a decreased endothelium-dependent vasodilatation [62]. Co-administration of ascorbic acid attenuates this response, implicating oxidative stress in mediating this abnormality [63].

VASCULAR SMOOTH MUSCLE DYSFUNCTION IN DIABETICS

The changes in vascular smooth muscle function and signal transduction in diabetes are similar to those in endothelial cells. The impaired vasodilatation caused by decreased endothelial production of NO is augmented by the decreased vasodilator response of vascular smooth muscle cells (VSMCs) to NO in diabetic patients [64]. In addition to decreased NO production, the endothelial production of vasoconstrictor prostanoids, endothelin and angiotensin II is increased in diabetes [65, 66]. *In vitro* studies have shown that hyperglycaemia increases the expression of cyclo-oxygenase-2 (COX-2) mRNA in human aortic endothelial cells [36]. Endothelin-1 activates endothelin-A receptors on adjacent VSMCs to cause vasoconstriction. By increasing renal salt and water retention, endothelin-1 can indirectly stimulate the renin-angiotensin system, thereby inducing vascular smooth muscle hypertrophy [67].

Hyperglycaemia increases the production of ROS and AGEs and activates PKC in VSMCs, as it does in endothelial cells [45]. Diabetes increases the migration of VSMCs into atherosclerotic lesions, where they replicate and lay down a complex extracellular matrix. As a source of collagen, VSMCs confer stability to the atherosclerotic lesions, decreasing the likelihood of plaque rupture and subsequent thrombosis. In diabetes, the increased cytokine production by endothelial cells decreases the production of collagen by VSMCs [68]. In addition, the breakdown of collagen is increased due to increased matrix metalloproteinase activity [69]. Advanced atherosclerotic lesions in diabetic individuals have been shown to contain fewer VSMCs as a result of increased apoptosis [70]. Inducers of VSMC apoptosis include oxidized LDL, ROS and pro-inflammatory cytokines, such as IL-1 and TNF [71], all of which being increased in diabetes. As a result of decreased collagen content and fewer VSMCs in atherosclerotic lesions, diabetes increases the propensity for plaque instability, rupture and subsequent thrombosis.

IMPAIRED PLATELET FUNCTION AND ABNORMAL COAGULATION IN DIABETES

Most acute coronary events occur with less than one-third narrowing of the vessel lumen [72]. Therefore, thrombosis subsequent to endothelial injury and plaque rupture remains a key to cardiovascular morbidity and mortality. In addition to modulating vascular function, platelets play a crucial role in thrombus formation. In diabetes, changes in platelet structure and function contribute to the progression of atherosclerosis and an enhanced thrombotic potential. Like endothelial cells, glucose entry into platelets is independent of insulin, and the intra-platelet glucose concentration mirrors that in the extra-cellular environment. Similar to its effect in endothelial cells and VSMCs, hyperglycaemia increases the production of ROS and the activation of PKC, leading to a decreased production of platelet-derived NO [73].

In diabetes, platelets exhibit increased sensitivity to aggregating agents including ADP, thrombin, epinephrine and collagen. This enhanced platelet sensitivity has been shown to result from increased glycosylation of LDLs [74]. Intra-platelet magnesium concentration is an important predictor of platelet thrombosis, and correlates positively with blood glucose levels [75, 76]. Increased calcium and decreased magnesium levels may be associated with enhanced platelet aggregation in diabetes [77]. Intra-platelet calcium concentration is crucial for platelet function, regulating platelet shape change, secretion, aggregation and thromboxane formation. Most platelet aggregants initiate aggregation by activating PLC-mediated signalling pathway, resulting in increased intra-platelet calcium concentration [78]. Platelets from diabetic patients have been shown to have higher calcium content than those from in non-diabetic patients [79, 80]. Presence of higher plasma levels of platelet release products, such as β-thromboglobulin, platelet factor 4 and thromboxane B_2 in diabetics demonstrates the platelet hyperactivity in diabetes [81].

In diabetes, there is increased expression of GpIb and GpIIb/IIIa on the platelet membrane leading to increased vWF- and fibrin-platelet interaction [80]. The levels of plasminogen activator inhibitor-1 (PAI-1) are elevated [82], which inhibits the formation of plasmin from plasminogen, resulting in decreased fibrinolytic activity [81, 83]. The expression of tissue factor, fibrinogen, factor VII, factor XI, factor XII, kallikrein and vWF is increased [81], and the levels of endogenous anticoagulants such as anti-thrombin III and protein C are decreased in diabetes [84]. Taken together, the abnormalities in platelet function and coagulation yield an enhanced thrombotic potential in diabetes, increasing the likelihood of thrombus formation and vascular occlusion after plaque rupture or erosion.

MANAGEMENT OF RISK FACTORS AND ATHEROSCLEROSIS IN DIABETICS

Methods of risk assessment and management of risk factors have been discussed in depth in other chapters of this book. However, we would like to reinforce the fact that due to the important role of established risk factors in the development of atherosclerotic cardiovascular complications, an aggressive approach towards management of atherosclerosis in diabetics is warranted. Please see Tables 23.1 and 23.2, indicating goals for risk factor management and guide to comprehensive risk reduction for patients with vascular diseases. In an individual several risk factors may co-exist. Risk assessment is target-driven, intensive intervention directed at multiple risk factors reduces the risk of cardiovascular events, as well as microvascular events by 50% in patients with type 2 diabetes [85]. Use of effective strategies for a better control of hypertension, dyslipidaemia together with an emphasis on lifestyle modifications including weight management, exercise and diet in association with targeting metabolic disturbances illustrates a clustered approach towards management of the risk factors. The interaction of diabetes mellitus and other risk factors for cardiovascular disease (Figure 23.1) is most evident in the data from the Multiple Risk Factor Intervention Trial (MRFIT) [86]. The trial involved approximately 350,000 nondiabetic and 5000 diabetic men aged between 35 and 57 years free of myocardial infarction at baseline. The subjects were initially screened during the recruitment phase and then followed for 6 years for mortality. Data showed that in both groups, major risk factors such as smoking, hypercholesterolemia and hypertension have additive effects on risk. Diabetics appeared to have two to three times the risk of dying of a cardiovascular event regardless of number of risk factors present. Even without any of these risk factors, risk in a diabetic patient is equivalent to a nondiabetic with two of the three factors. Considering that hypertension and dyslipidaemia are found in approximately 50% of adult diabetics, it is evident that an individual with NIDDM generally has five to 10 times the risk of a healthy, nondiabetic individual. Based on presence or absence of diabetes as well as other risk factors, recent guidelines for prevention of coronary heart disease recommend use of risk assessment charts to estimate absolute risk of developing coronary artery disease [87]. These guidelines are compiled by panels of experts who make recommendations on appropriate use of medications and interventions based on evidence from randomized clinical trials.

Table 23.1

Goals for Risk Factor Management in Patients with Diabetes

Risk Factor	Goal of Therapy	Recommendation body*
Cigarette smoking	Complete cessation	ADA
Blood pressure	<130/85 mm Hg <130/80 mm Hg	JNC VI (NHLBI) ADA
LDL cholesterol	<100 mg/dL	ATP III (NHLBI), ADA
Triglycerides 200–499 mg/dL	Non-HDL cholesterol <130 mg/dL	ATP III (NHLBI)
HDL cholesterol <40 mg/dL	Raise HDL (no set goal)	ATP III (NHLBI)
Prothrombotic state	Low-dose aspirin therapy (patients with CHD and other high-risk patients)	ADA
Glucose	Hemoglobin A1c <7%	ADA
Overweight and obesity BMI >25 kg/m²)	Lose 10% of body weight in 1 year	OEI (NHLBI)
Physical inactivity	Exercise prescription dependent on patient status	ADA
Adverse nutrition		ADA, AHA, and NHLBI's ATP III, OEI, and JNC VI

* JNC VI indicates the 6th report of the Joint National Committee on Prevention, Evaluation, and Treatment of High Blood Pressure; NHLBI, National Heart, Lung, and Blood Institute; ATP III, National Cholesterol Education Program Adult Treatment Panel III; HDL, high-density lipoprotein; and OEI, Obesity Education Initiative Expert Panel on Identification, Evaluation, and Treatment of Overweight and Obesity in Adults. See Ref. [135].

Table 23.2

Guide to comprehensive risk reduction for patients with coronary and other vascular disease who have diabetes [136]

Risk Intervention	Recommendations
Smoking Goal: complete cessation	Strongly encourage patient and family to stop smoking Provide counseling, nicotine replacement, and formal cessation programs as appropriate
Blood pressure control Goal: ≤135/85 mm Hg	Initiate lifestyle modification–weight control, physical activity, alcohol moderation, and moderate sodium restriction–in all patients with blood pressure >135 mm Hg systolic or 85 mm Hg diastolic Add blood pressure medication, individualized to other patient requirements and characteristics (*i.e.* age, race, need for drugs with specific benefits) if blood pressure is not <140 mm Hg systolic or < 90 mm Hg diastolic in 3 months or if initial blood pressure is >160 mm Hg systolic or >100 mm Hg diastolic

Lipid management Primary goal: LDL ≤100 mg/dL	Start AHA Step II Diet in all patients: ≤30% fat, <7% saturated fat, <200 mg/d cholesterol
	Assess fasting lipid profile. Immediately start cholesterol-lowering drugs when baseline LDL >130 mg/dL

Secondary goals: HDL >35 mg/dL TG<200 mg/dL	LDL<100 mg/dL No drug therapy	LDL 100 to 129 mg/dL Consider adding drug therapy to diet, as follows LDL≥130 mg/dL Add drug therapy to diet, as follows	HDL<35 mg/dL Emphasize weight management and physical activity Advise smoking cessation
		↘ ↙ Suggested drug therapy	
		TG<200mg/dL TG 200 to 400 mg/dL TG>400mg/dL	
		Statin Resin Statin Fibrate Consider combined drug therapy (statin+fibrate)	

Glucose control Goal: near normal fasting glucose Goal: HbA1c≤1% above normal	First-step therapy: weight reduction and exercise Second-step therapy: oral hypoglycaemic agents (sulfonylureas and/or metformin; ancillary: acarbose, glitazone) Third-step therapy: insulin therapy
Physical activity: Goal: minimum goal 30 minutes 3 to 4 times *per* week	Assess risk, preferably with exercise test, to guide prescription Encourage minimum of 30 to 60 minutes of moderate-intensity activity 3 or 4 times weekly (walking, jogging, cycling, or other aerobic activity) supplemented by an increase in daily lifestyle activities (eg, walking breaks at work, using stairs, gardening, household work) Maximum benefit 5 to 6 hours a week Advise medically supervised programs for moderate- to high-risk patients
Weight management	Start intensive dietary therapy and appropriate physical activity, as outlined above, in patients whose BMI is ≥25 kg/m^2 Particularly emphasize need for weight loss in patients with hypertension, elevated triglycerides, or elevated glucose levels
Antiplatelet agents/ anticoagulants	Start aspirin 80 to 325 mg/d if not contraindicated Manage warfarin to international normalized ratio 2 to 3.5 for post-MI patients not able to take aspirin
ACE inhibitors in post-MI patients	Start early post-MI in stable high-risk patients (anterior MI, previous MI, Killip class II [S3 gallop, rales, radiographic congestive heart failure]) Continue indefinitely for all with LV dysfunction (ejection fraction ≤40%) or symptoms of failure Use as needed to manage blood pressure or symptoms in all other patients
β-Blockers	Start in high-risk post-MI patients (arrhythmia, LV dysfunction, inducible ischemia) at 5 to 28 days. Continue 6 months minimum. Observe usual contraindications. Appropriate use of β-blockers not contraindicated in patients with diabetes Use as needed to manage angina, rhythm, or blood pressure in all other patients
Estrogen	Observational studies (but not clinical trials) suggest benefit. Limited data in diabetic women Individualize recommendation consistent with other health risks

TG indicates triglycerides; MI, myocardial infarction; and LV, left ventricular.

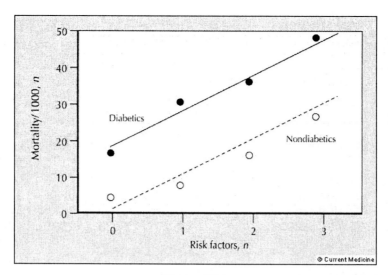

Figure 23.1

Interaction of diabetes mellitus and risk factors for CVD.

The interaction of diabetes mellitus and other risk factors for cardiovascular disease (CVD). (From www.incirculation.net, adapted from the American Diabetes Association American Diabetes Association, Consensus statement. *Diabetes Care*, **12**: 573–579, 1989, and from Braunwald's Atlas of Heart Diseases).

Diabetes is under diagnosed in various parts of the world. However, principals for detection of subclinical diabetes have not been fully established despite the fact that diabetics are recognised as high-risk group of individuals. Use of screening tests is recommended when these could be used rapidly, are inexpensive, can be applied on wide scales and that could lead to change in management and improvement in outcomes. Due to non-availability of data from clinical trials and cost-effectiveness issues, screening of diabetic patients for cardiovascular disease using non invasive or invasive testing has not been recommended. Further clinical trials are mandatory to guide decision making in this high risk population [88].

GLYCAEMIC CONTROL

Studies have shown that adequate glycaemic control and improvement in insulin sensitivity are mainstay of pharmacological treatments in the management of atherosclerosis and vascular complications. A "tight" glucose control decreases the microvascular complication rate. Please see Table 23.3 showing relationship between improved glycaemic control and risk of cardiovascular disease in diabetics. In the Diabetes Control and Complication Trial [89], involving patients with type 1 diabetes, intensive insulin therapy was associated with a reduced risk of developing microalbumiuria by 39%, albuminuria by 54%, retinopathy by 76%, and clinical neuropathy by 60%. Similarly, in the UK Prospective Diabetes Study [4], involving patients with type 2 diabetes, a 1% means reduction in HbA1c was associated with a reduction in total mortality by 21%, myocardial infarction by 14% and total microvascular complications by 37%. Use of biguanide metformin and thiazolidinedione class of hypoglycaemic agents improves insulin sensitivity. Later are known to bind peroxisome proliferator–activated receptor (PPAR), a nuclear receptor expressed on monocyte/macrophages of atherosclerotic lesions [90] and participates in the regulation of adipose differentiation [91], also inhibits matrix metalloproteinase-9 in human macrophages [90] and improves endothelial function in patients with type 2 diabetes [92, 93]. Studies evaluating role of these agents are ongoing.

Table 23.3

Relationship Between Improved Glycaemic Control and Risk of Cardiovascular Disease in Patients with Diabetes

Trial Risk	No. of Patients	Duration, y	Glycemic Control	Outcome	Rate	% Relative
Kuusisto 1997	1059	7.2	HbA1c ≥10.7% vs. <10.7%	CHD death	NA	1.4
San Antonio Heart Study, 1998	875	7.5	FPG 8 to 11.5 mmol/L vs. <8 mmol/L	CV death	6.3 vs. 2.8	2.9
UKPDS 1998	3055	7.9	HbA1c >7.5% vs. <6.2%	Fatal MI	NA	1.72
					Any MI/angina	1.52

HbA1c indicates glycosylated hemoglobin; FPG, fasting plasma glucose; CHD, coronary heart disease; CV, cardiovascular; MI, Myocardial infarction; and NA, not applicable. See Ref. [131, 137].

DRUGS FOR PRIMARY AND SECONDARY PREVENTION OF CARDIOVASCULAR COMPLICATIONS IN DIABETICS

Aspirin, in a daily dose of 75–150mg, is recommended in all patients with type II diabetes [94]. Unless contraindicated aspirin should be given as secondary prevention for cardiovascular events in type II diabetes [95]. According to Antiplatelet Trialists' Collaboration in a meta-analysis of 145 trials of antiplatelet agents, 4502 diabetic subjects were included. In majority of these trials aspirin was used. Analysis of this subgroup showed that incidence of cardiovascular events (i.e. cardiovascular death, myocardial infarction, and stroke) was reduced from 22.3% to 18.5% by the antiplatelet agents [96]. A recent meta-analysis of four controlled trials of Aspirin concluded that aspirin, for primary prevention, is safe and worthwhile with coronary event risk of ≥ 1.5% per year; safe but of limited value at 1% per year; and unsafe at coronary event rate of 0.5% per year with coronary heart disease [97]. Use of angiotensin converting enzyme inhibitors (ACE-inhibitors) and morerecently angiotensin II receptor blockers (ARBs) has proved to significantly reduce cardiovascular

events and mortality in patients at high risk for cardiovascular disease on the basis of diabetes and prevalent cardiovascular risk factors. A controlled multicenter trial GISSI 3 compared treatment with lisinopril plus nitrates with only nitrates started within 24 hours immediately after an acute myocardial infarction [98]. More than 19,000 patients and 2790 patients with diabetes were enrolled. Outcomes at 6-week and 6-month mortality rates in the two groups showed that lisinopril reduced mortality by 30% at 6 weeks. This effect was statistically significant and was still evident after 6 months (Figure 23.2). In carotid artery stenosis, indications for carotid revascularization are the same for both diabetic and non-diabetic patients.

In summary, presence of risk factors in an individual has significant impact on absolute risk of developing CHD event (Table 23.4). Meticulous efforts are needed to increase patient awareness of classical cardiovascular risk factors, to ensure smoking cessation, control of blood pressure, blood lipids, blood glucose and body weight [93]. Patients at high risk of atherosclerotic cardiovascular disease should be assessed using appropriate investigating techniques, and evidence based pharmacological interventions should be used. Table 23.5 gives a summary of diagnostic methods to detect clinical and subclinical cardiovascular disease in the diabetic patient.

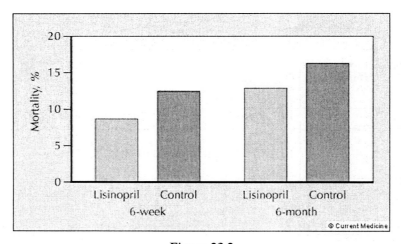

Figure 23.2

ACE inhibitors reduce cardiovascular mortality in diabetes.

Angiotensin-converting enzyme (ACE) inhibitors reduce cardiovascular mortality in diabetes. (From www.incirculation.net, adapted from Zuanetti *et al.* and from Braunwald's Atlas of Heart Diseases)

Table 23.4

Examples showing the impact of a single risk factor, multiple risk factors and clinically established coronary heart disease on the absolute risk of developing a coronary heart disease event over 10 years [101].

Sex	Age (years)	Plasma cholesterol (mmol/1)	Systolic blood pressure (mmHg)	Smoking	Clinical CHD	Minimum estimate of the 10-year risk
Male		7	120	"	"	10%
Male	50	6	140	+	"	20%
Male	50	7	120	"	+	>20%
Male	50	6	140	+	+	>40%

CHD, Coronary Heart Disease

Table 23.5

Detection of Clinical and Subclinical Cardiovascular Disease in the Diabetic Patient [136]

Stress testing for coronary heart disease
Consult AHA guidelines for exercise treadmill testing
Special considerations for exercise testing in diabetic patients
Blood pressure and heart rate responses often blunted (due to elevated resting heart rate)
Painless ST-segment depression common in diabetic patients
Diagnostic specificity of ST-segment depression often reduced (due to previous silent myocardial infarction, conduction abnormalities, and increases in LV mass)
Exercise or pharmacological stress 201Tl (or 99Tc) perfusion scintigraphy favourable alternative for exercise testing in diabetic patients
Ambulatory ECG monitoring for silent ischemia: may be helpful in some diabetic patients, but not recommended routinely
Noninvasive evaluation of cardiac function
Echocardiography (with Doppler) and radionuclide ventriculography
Special considerations for diabetic patients
Diastolic dysfunction common in asymptomatic diabetic patients
Diastolic dysfunction often precedes systolic dysfunction
LV wall motion abnormalities: suggests diabetic cardiomyopathy

Table 23.5

(continued)

Evaluation of autonomic dysfunction
Bedside evaluation of autonomic dysfunction
Two or more of the following tests are abnormal
– Resting heart rate (supine) 100 bpm
– Excess diastolic blood pressure response to hand-grip exercise
– Abnormal expiratory/inspiratory RR-interval ratio
– Postural hypotension
Significance of autonomic dysfunction in diabetic patients
– Carries poor prognosis (50% mortality in 5 years)
– Sudden death common; consider electrophysiological study for syncope workup
– Enhanced complications after elective surgical procedures
– Increased danger with general anesthesia
Detection of subclinical cardiovascular disease
History: Assess carefully for claudication, angina, dyspnea on exertion, cerebrovascular disease
Physical exam: routine cardiovascular examination; assess for carotid and femoral artery bruits; evaluate peripheral artery pulses; ratio of ankle-to-brachial artery systolic blood pressure (marker of subclinical peripheral vascular disease)
Laboratory: check for microalbuminuria
ECG: LV hypertrophy strong predictor of CHD morbidity and mortality
Electron beam CT: coronary calcium score highly correlated with total coronary atherosclerosis burden (role in risk assessment currently under investigation)
Carotid ultrasound: detects subclinical carotid atherosclerosis (role in risk assessment currently under investigation)
LV indicates left ventricular.

MANAGEMENT OF CORONARY ARTERY DISEASE IN DIABETICS: WHAT IS THE EVIDENCE?

CAD accounts for 75% of all deaths in diabetics, and approximately 20% – 25% of patients with non ST segment elevation myocardial infarction or unstable angina (NSTEMI/UA) are diabetics [99]. The main underlying mechanism in acute coronary syndromes (ACS) involves dislodging of atherosclerotic plaque that is known to be more common in diabetics. Evidence suggests that on coronary angiograms diabetics have greater proportion of ulcerated plaques (94% vs 60%, and intracoronary thrombi (94% vs 55%,) than non-diabetics [100]. In addition to increased prevalence of co-morbidities including autonomic dysfunction, patients with diabetes have a higher threshold for perception of angina and an increased LV dysfunction [99]. In Table 23.6 we give priorities of coronary heart disease prevention in clinical practice as recommended by European Society of Cardiology (ESC) Second Joint Task Force Guidelines on coronary prevention [101]. Expert guidelines for management of ACS categorize patients with ACS in high risk group in the presence of diabetes in addition to the presence of other markers of high risk including troponin elevation, ST segment depression, haemodynamic and arrhythmic instability [99, 102]. Diabetes is recognized as an important factor in risk stratification of patients with coronary artery disease (CAD), being a marker of acute and long term risk. A summary of recommendations from the American College of Cardiology (ACC) and American Heart Association (AHA) guidelines for the management of diabetic patients with ACS according to the level of evidence is given in Table 23.7. Please refer to Tables 23.8 and 23.9 for definitions of class and levels of evidence as used in the ACC/AHA guidelines for the management of non ST elevation ACS, respectively. Due to a higher long term risk of mortality in diabetics ACC/AHA and the ESC for the management of ACS recommend long term use of evidence based therapy including aspirin, beta blockers, statins and angiotensin converting enzyme inhibitors (ACE-inhibitors), and an aggressive risk management with a tight glucose control and an adequate blood pressure management in all patients with established CAD [99, 102]. Clopidogrel has shown clear short and long term improvement in clinical outcomes in the patients with ACS without ST segment elevation as shown in CURE (Clopidogrel in Unstable Angina to Prevent Recurrent Events) trial [103].

Table 23.6

Priorities of coronary heart disease prevention in clinical practice [99]

1. Patients with established coronary heart disease or other artherosclerotic disease
2. Healthy individuals who are at high risk of developing coronary heart disease or other atherosclerotic disease, because of a combination of risk factors – including smoking, raised blood pressure, lipids (raised total cholesterol, and LDL-cholesterol, low HDL-cholesterol and raised triglycerides) raised blood glucose, family history of premature coronary disease – or who have severe hypercholesterolaemia, or other forms of dyslipidaemia, hypertension or diabetes
3. Close relatives of patients with early-onset coronary heart disease or other atherosclerotic disease healthy individuals at particularly high risk
4. Other individuals met in connection with ordinary clinical practice

HDL, High Density Lipids
LDL, Low Density Lipids

Table 23.7

Recommendations for the management of diabetic patients with ACS according to level of evidence

(Adapted from ACC/AHA Guideline update for the management of non- ST elevation ACS -2002) [99]

Class I recommendations	Level of evidence	Class II recommendations	Level of evidence
Diabetes is an independent risk factor in patients with UA/NSTEMI.	A	PCI for diabetic patients with 1-vessel disease and inducible ischemia.	B
Medical treatment in the acute phase and decisions on whether to perform stress testing and angiography and revascularization should be similar in diabetic and nondiabetic patients.	C	Abciximab for diabetics treated with coronary stenting.	B
Attention should be directed toward tight glucose control.	B		
For patients with multi-vessel disease, CABG with use of the internal mammary arteries is preferred over PCI in patients being treated for diabetes.	B		

For definitions of classes and levels of evidence according to ACC/AHA guidelines please see Table 23.8
UA/NSTEMI – Unstable Angina/Non ST Elevation Myocardial Infarction
PCI – Percutaneous Coronary Intervention
CABG – Coronary Artery Bypass Grafting

Table 23.8

Definition of customary classifications used for recommendations by ACC/AHA Guidelines for the management of non ST elevation ACS 2002 [99]

Class I	Conditions for which there is evidence and/or general agreement that a given procedure or treatment is useful and effective
Class II	Conditions for which there is conflicting evidence and/or a divergence of opinion about the usefulness/efficacy of a procedure or treatment
	Class IIa Weight of evidence/opinion is in favour of usefulness/efficacy
	Class IIb Usefulness/efficacy is less well established by evidence/opinion
Class III	Conditions for which there is evidence and/or general agreement that the procedure/treatment is not useful/effective and in some cases may be harmful

Table 23.9

Definition of levels of evidence indicating weight of evidence used for recommendations by ACC/AHA Guidelines for the management of non ST elevation ACS 2002 [99]

Level of evidence	Definition
A	The weight of the evidence was ranked highest (A) if the data were derived from multiple randomized clinical trials that involved large numbers of patients.
B	Intermediate if the data were derived from a limited number of randomized trials that involved small numbers of patients or from careful analyses of nonrandomized studies or observational registries.
C	A lower rank (C) was given when expert consensus was the primary basis for the recommendation.

Beta blockers and diuretics should be used with caution in patients with diabetes during an acute coronary event due to effects on glucose tolerance and electrolyte imbalance, as hypokalaemia caused by diuretics may inhibit insulin release. Despite concerns about the effects of β-blockers on hypoglycaemia awareness, data have established that these drugs are beneficial. According to analysis of 2723 patients with type 2 diabetes and established CAD from BIP (Bezafibrate Infarction Prevention) study, 33% of the patients (n = 911) received the β-blocker propranolol. Over 5 years, the β-blocker-treated patients had a 44% lower mortality, most of which was due to a decrease in cardiovascular deaths [104].

Use of ACE inhibitors is recommended in patients with LV dysfunction and also in all diabetics with an ST elevation ACS as post discharge therapy in the absence of any contraindications. Other chapters in this book cover stepwise management of ACS in details.

Large amount of data exists regarding revascularization in diabetic patients with ACS. Data from recent randomized clinical trials (BARI, EAST, CASS, NHLBI and Duke University registries) show complex outcomes in patients with diabetes undergoing coronary revascularization [105–111]. The US guidelines recommend coronary artery bypass grafting (CABG) in patients with and without ST elevation ACS with multi-vessel disease, using internal mammary artery (evidence level B) and PCI in diabetics with mono-vessel disease (evidence level C) [99]. Diabetic patients undergoing coronary artery stenting seem to have better outcomes as compared to those undergoing percutaneous transluminal coronary angioplasty (PTCA) and reduced restenosis rates of 63% *vs.* 36% in diabetics *vs.* non diabetics undergoing balloon PTCA at 6 months compared with 25% and 27% undergoing stents (P = NS) [112]. In addition, benefits of drug eluting stents as compared to bare metal stents have been shown to be significant in the diabetic patients with coronary artery disease. Similar effects were seen when diabetics were compared with non-diabetics in these studies.

Glycoprotein IIb/IIIa inhibitors have emerged as an important anti-thrombotic therapy in high risk patients with ACS. In a meta-analysis of six randomized trials it was demonstrated that diabetic patients with ACS derive particular benefit from GPIIb/IIIa inhibitors [113]. Among 6,458 patients, this antiplatelet treatment was associated with a significant mortality reduction at 30 days from 6.2% to 4.6% (relative risk 0.74; 95% CI: 0.59 – 0.02). Among 1,279 diabetic patients undergoing PCI during index hospitalization, the use of GPIIb/IIIa inhibitors was associated with a mortality reduction at 30 days from 4.0 to 1.2% (ARR: 2.8%, relative risk 0.30: 95% CI 0.14 – 0.69). It should be stressed that in patients with an ST segment elevation myocardial infarction (STEMI) diabetic retinopathy is not a contraindication to thrombolytic therapy.

The unfavorable outcome in diabetic patients is related to metabolic factors causing an increased oxygen consumption of free fatty acids during acute myocardial ischaemia. An association between glycaemia with microvascular and macrovascular complications was observed in a prospective observational study of 4,585 diabetic patients (UKPDS) [4]. Data revealed that each 1% reduction in updated haemoglobin A1c was associated with a 21% diabetes related mortality reduction, and a 14% reduction in the incidence of myocardial infarction during 10 year follow-up. Strict attention to the glycaemic control by use of insulin glucose infusion followed by multiple-dose insulin treatment has been shown to reduce long-term mortality [114, 115]. The DIGAMI (Diabetes mellitus, Insulin Glucose infusion in Acute Myocardial Infarction) investigators demonstrated that long-term metabolic control will improve prognosis of myocardial infarction patients with previously diagnosed diabetes mellitus, or an abnormal blood glucose concentration during the acute phase. Patients enrolled in the DIGAMI trial (N = 620) were randomized to receive a 24 h insulin-glucose infusion, followed by subcutaneous insulin four times daily for at least three months, or control therapy. Control patients were treated according to standard practice, and did not receive any insulin unless clinically indicated. Long-term metabolic control was associated with a 35% reduced incidence of all-cause death during one year follow-up (odds ratio 0.65, and 95% CI 0.44 to 0.95). One year mortality among hospital survivors was 43% reduced (odds ratio 0.57, and 95% CI 0.35 to 0.94). Insulin infusion and long-term insulin treatment should therefore be part of routine management of diabetic patients after acute coronary syndromes. Several ongoing trials are investigating the role of glucose-insulin and potassium infusion as myocardial protective agent in acute ischaemic state in patients with ST segment elevation MI.

MANAGEMENT
OF HYPERTENSION IN DIABETICS

Hypertension (>140/90 mmHg) is more commonly associated with type 2 diabetes (70%) as compared to type 1, resulting in an increased risk of cardiovascular and renal complications [116]. When blood pressure is lowered in the diabetic patients (both type 1 and 2) with hypertension, there is a significant decrease in cardiovascular morbidity and mortality as compared to the non-diabetic hypertensives (Table 23.10). The HOT (Hypertension Optimal Treatment) study investigators compared the effects of different levels of hypertension treatment on the development of cardiovascular events. The study enrolled 18,790 patients including 1501 diabetics from 26 countries. Three different target levels of diastolic blood pressure were achieved using felodipine and additional agents. A remarkable reduction of 50% in the cardiovascular end points was seen when diastolic blood pressure was titrated beyond < 90 mmHg to < 80 mmHg [117]. Table 23.11 summarises trials that showed a relationship between blood pressure lowering and the risk of cardiovascular disease in patients with diabetes.

Table 23.10

Major cardiovascular events in patients with diabetes mellitus in relation to target blood pressure groups [99]

Blood pressure, mm Hg	Events, *n*	Events/1000 patients year	*P* for trend	Comparison	Relative Risk (95% CI)
≤ 90 (*n* = 501)	45	24.4		90 *vs.* 85	1.32 (0.84–2.06)
≤ 85 (*n* = 501)	34	18.6		85 *vs.* 80	1.56 (0.91–2.67)
≤ 80 (*n* = 499)	22	11.9	0.005	90 *vs.* 80	2.06 (1.24–3.44)

Table 23.11

Relationship Between Blood Pressure Lowering and Risk of Cardiovascular Disease in Patients with Diabetes [131]

| Trial | No. of Patients | Duration, y | Blood Pressure Control | | | Outcome | Risk Reduction, % |
			Less Tight	Tight	Initial Therapy		
SHEP, 1996	583	5	155/72*	143/68*	Chlorthalidone	Stroke CV events CHD	NS 34 56
Syst-Eur, 1999	492	2	162/82	153/78	Nitrendipine	Stroke CV events	69 62
HOT, 1998	1501	3	144/85*	140/81*	Felodipine	CV events MI Stroke CV mortality	51 50 NS 67
UKPDS, 1999	1148	8.4	154/87	144/82	Captopril or atenolol	Diabetes-related end points Deaths Strokes Microvascular end points	34 37 44 37
HOPE, Micro-HOPE 2000	3577	4.5	Changes in systolic (2.4 mm Hg) and diastolic (1.0 mm Hg)		Ramipril vs. placebo	CV events CV mortality MI Stroke Total mortality New-onset diabetes	25 37 22 33 24 34
CAPP, 2001	572	7	155/89 vs. 153/88		Captopril vs. diuretics or β-blockers	Fatal +NFMI+ stroke +CV deaths	41
IDNT, 2001	1715	2.6	≤135/85		Irbesartan vs. Amlodipine or placebo	Doubling of serum creatinine + end-stage renal disease + death from any cause	23 (vs. amlodipine) 20 (vs. placebo)
IRMA, 2001	590	2	144/83 143/83 141/83		Irbesartan 150 mg or 300 mg vs. placebo	Onset of diabetic nephropathy	35 (100 mg) 65 (300 mg)
RENAAL, 2001	1513	3.4	152/82 vs. 153/82		Losartan vs. placebo in addition to conventional therapy	Doubling of serum creatinine End-stage renal disease Death	25 28 NS
LIFE, 2002	1195	4.8	146/79 vs. 148/79		Losartan vs. atenolol	CV events Total mortality in diabetics New-onset diabetes	22 25 25

SHEP indicates Systolic Hypertension in the Elderly Program; Syst-Eur, Systolic, hypertension in Europe; HOT, Hypertension Optimal Treatment; CAPP, Captopril Prevention Program; IDNT, Irbesartan Diabetic Nephropathy Trial; IRMA, IRbesarlan MicroAlbuminuria in type 2 diabetes; REENAL, Reduction in End points in NIDDM with Angiotensin II Antagonist Losartan; CVD, cardiovascular disease; CHD, coronary heart disease; CV, cardiovascular; MI, myocardial infarction; NFMI, nonfatal myocardial infarction; and NS, not significant.

*Blood pressure in diabetic+nondiabetic population because blood pressure is not reported for diabetic patients alone. Data derived from Sowers JR, Haffner S. Treatment of cardiovascular renal risk factors in the diabetic hypertensives. *Hypertension*, **40:** 781–788, 2002 [137].

Hypertensive patients frequently exhibit a condition known as 'metabolic syndrome' associating insulin resistance (with the concomitant hyperinsulinaemia), central obesity and characteristic dyslipidaemia (high plasma triglycerides and low high-density lipoprotein cholesterol) [118, 119]. These patients are prone to develop type 2 diabetes [120].

Prevalence of microalbuminuria, left ventricular hypertrophy (LVH), and electrocardiographic signs of myocardial ischaemia are twice as common at the initial diagnosis of diabetes, when hypertension is present. Similarly, hyporeninemic hypoaldosteronism manifesting with hyperkalaemia is more commonly found in the diabetics with hypertension.

TREATMENT CONSIDERATIONS IN DIABETIC HYPERTENSIVES

Goals for treatment in hypertension in diabetics according to the recent European Hypertension Society guidelines and their position statement on anti-hypertensive therapy in diabetics are given in Tables 23.12 and 23.13 respectively. High doses of diuretics or beta-blockers may induce insulin resistance in the diabetics. Diabetic neuropathy may add to the postural hypotension and impotence that frequently complicate anti-hypertensive therapy. Autonomic nervous system involvement in diabetics should be carefully evaluated by measuring orthostatic changes in blood pressure. According to recent European and British guidelines for the management of hypertension threshold for treatment for diabetics is >140/90 mmHg with an optimal BP target of 130/80 mmHg [121, 122]. Hypertension in patients with type 1 diabetes often indicates the presence of nephropathy. Target blood pressure is aimed even lower (125/75 mm Hg) when there is proteinuria of >1 g/24 h in these patients [116].

Table 23.12

Position statement: Goals of Treatment in hypertension in diabetics

(Adapted from European Hypertension Society Guidelines 2003) [121]

- The primary goal of treatment of the patient with high blood pressure is to achieve the maximum reduction in the long-term total risk of cardiovascular morbidity and mortality. This requires treatment of all the reversible risk factors identified, including smoking, dyslipidaemia or diabetes, and the appropriate management of associated clinical conditions, as well as treatment of the raised blood pressure *per se*.
- On the basis of current evidence from trials, it can be recommended that blood pressure, both systolic and diastolic, be intensively lowered at least below 140/90 mmHg and to definitely lower values, if tolerated, in all hypertensive patients, and below 130/80 mmHg in diabetics, keeping in mind, however, that systolic values below 140 mmHg may be difficult to achieve, particularly in the elderly.

Table 23.13

Position statement: antihypertensive therapy in diabetics

(Adapted from European Hypertension Society Guidelines, 2003) [121]

- Non-pharmacological measures (particularly weight loss and reduction in salt intake) should be encouraged in all patients with type 2 diabetes, independently of the existing high blood pressure.
These measures may suffice to normalize blood pressure in patients with high normal or grade 1 hypertension, and can be expected to facilitate blood pressure control by antihypertensive agents.
- The goal blood pressure during behavioural or pharmacological therapy is below 130/ 80 mmHg.
- To reach this goal, most often combination therapy will be required.
- It is recommended that all effective and well tolerated antihypertensive agents are used, generally, in combination.
- Available evidence indicates that renoprotection benefits from the regular inclusion in these combinations of an ACE inhibitor in type 1 diabetes and of an angiotensin receptor antagonist in type 2 diabetes.
- In type 2 diabetic patients with high normal blood pressure, who may sometimes achieve blood pressure goal by monotherapy, the first drug to be tested should be a blocker of the renin–angiotensin system.
- The finding of microalbuminuria in type 1 or 2 diabetics is an indication for antihypertensive treatment, especially by a blocker of the renin–angiotensin system, irrespective of the blood pressure values.

TREATMENT OPTIONS IN HYPERTENSIVE PATIENTS WITH TYPE 1 DIABETES

ACE inhibitors are recommended as first line therapy. Dosage should be titrated to the maximum dose recommended or tolerated. However, use of Angiotensin II antagonists is recommended if intolerance to ACE inhibitors develops such as cough. Thiazide diuretics, calcium antagonists, cardioselective beta-blockers or alpha blockers can also be considered. Type 1 diabetic subjects with persistent microalbuminuria or proteinuria and 'normal' blood pressures may also benefit from ACE-inhibition titrated to the recommended maximum dose.

HYPERTENSION IN TYPE 2 DIABETES

In type 2 diabetes, a rapid decline in renal function is seen in patients with established nephropathy due to hypertension. Threshold for intervention with antihypertensive therapy is >130/80 mmHg. For optimal control systolic blood pressure should be targeted to be below 130 mmHg and diastolic blood pressure below 80 mmHg [121].

Evidence suggests that patients with type 2 diabetes with established nephropathy, deterioration in the renal function is more rapid in the presence of hypertension, and ACE inhibitors delay progression from microalbuminuria to overt nephropathy. Due to the presence of other cardiovascular risk factors in patients with type 2 diabetes, such as obesity, multi-factorial approach should be adapted in the treatment strategies, in addition to simple blood pressure lowering. Aspirin should be offered to all patients with type 2 diabetes [122]. ACE inhibitors, dihydropyridine calcium antagonists, low dose thiazide diuretics or beta-blockers using the criteria for non-diabetic patients, are recommended for patients with type 2 diabetes without nephropathy.

Recent evidence with angiotensin II receptor antagonists has shown a significant reduction of cardiovascular events, cardiovascular death and total mortality in diabetics when losartan was compared with atenolol [122]. If renal endpoints are also considered, the benefits of angiotensin II receptor antagonists become more evident. Another trial [123] showed a reduction in renal dysfunction and failure by the use of irbesartan rather than amlodipine, and similarly, LIFE (Losartan Intervention For Endpoint reduction in hypertension) trial [124] showed significant reduction in the incidence of new proteinuria by losartan as compared to atenolol. European Society of Hypertension guidelines from 2003 recommend use of angiotensin II receptor antagonists for renoprotection in patients with type 2 diabetes [121].

MANAGEMENT OF DYSLIPIDAEMIA IN DIABETICS

Patients with type 2 diabetes are likely to have dyslipidaemia characterized by high triglycerides, small LDL particles and low HDL cholesterol serum levels, known as lipid atherogenic triad. Evidence suggests that lowering cholesterol levels can significantly reduce cardiovascular events in diabetic patients with CAD. A large pool of data is available from high quality randomized clinical trials showing benefits of statins (3-Hydroxy 3-Methylglutaryl Coenzyme-A reductase inhibitors) in patients with diabetes with or without established CAD (Table 23.14). Larger studies like Scandinavian Simvastatin Survival Study (4S) [125] and Cholesterol and Recurrent Events (CARE) [126] trials have demonstrated clear reduction of 55% and 24% in cardiovascular events in patients with diabetes with CAD and elevated LDL cholesterol levels, as compared to non-diabetics. The recently completed Heart Protection Study enrolled 20,536 high risk individuals, including patients with coronary disease and diabetes mellitus, with total cholesterol levels >135 mg/dl (3.5 mmol/l) [127]. During long-term follow-up, individuals randomised to simvastatin had a 13% lower mortality than those receiving placebo (hazard ratio 0.87, and 95% CI 0.81 to 0.94). The incidence of major cardiovascular events was 24% reduced (hazard ratio 0.76, and 95% CI 0.72 to 0.81). These data suggest that statin treatment should be extended to patients with cholesterol levels below 5 mmol/l (190 mg/dl).

Table 23.14

Relationship Between Lipid Lowering With Statins and Risk of Cardiovascular Disease in Patients with Diabetes

Trial (Diabetic Subgroups)	No. of Patients	Event Rate, %		Risk Reduction %	Outcome
		Placebo	Statin		
Primary prevention					
AFCAPS, 1998	155	8.4	4.8	43	Fatal +NFMI, sudden death
Secondary prevention					
4S, 1999	202	45	22	51	Fatal CHD +NFMI
CARE, 1996	602	37	29	22	Fatal CHD +NFMI + revascularization
LIPID, 1998	782	23	19	17	Fatal CHD +NFMI
Primary and secondary prevention HPS, 2002	5986			24	Fatal + NFMI, strokes, and revascularization

NFMI indicates nonfatal myocardial infarction; CHD, coronary heart disease. See ref. [131,137].
AFCAPS, The Air Force/Texas Coronary Atherosclerosis Prevention Study; 4S, Scandinavian Simvastatin Survival Study; CARE, Cholesterol and Recurrent Events; LIPID, Long-term Intervention with Pravastatin in Ischemic Disease (LIPID) Study; HPS, Heart Protection Study

LDL lowering is now recognized as the first priority in the control of diabetic dyslipidaemia [128]. The combination of low-dose statin with nicotinic acid or fibrates for combined hyper-lipidaemia is a safe approach when performed with appropriate monitoring and after careful patient education [129]. Similarly, statin treatment should be implemented in the majority of type 2 diabetic patients with LDL >100 mg/dl. However, since beneficial effect of statins in the large Phase III trials was only seen after long-term (5 to 6 years) use, the cost-effectiveness of treatment of patients with a limited life-expectancy can therefore be questioned [130].

MANAGEMENT OF PERIPHERAL ARTERIAL DISEASE IN DIABETICS

PAD is a clinical marker of atherosclerosis requiring an aggressive approach towards management of risk factors. Principals of management in diabetic patients involve prevention of cardiovascular events and improvement of functional status of patients using pharmacological or revascularization and rehabilitative measures.

Progressive worsening claudication and critical limb ischaemia are the main indications for peripheral revascularization, performed using endovascular or open surgical techniques. These procedures include percutaneous transluminal angioplasties with or without stenting and surgical grafting. Data suggest no significant differences between outcomes for peripheral revascularization between diabetics and non diabetics. It has been reported that graft patency rates are comparable between diabetic and non diabetic population. However, due to the presence of critical limb ischaemia and foot infection, rates of limb loss were observed more frequently in diabetics. Similarly, increased preoperative cardiovascular event rates have been seen in the diabetics [130].

MANAGEMENT OF CEREBROVASCULAR DISEASE

Diabetes increases stroke related mortality, doubles the rate of recurrent stroke and trebles the rate of stroke related dementia [131]. According to a nine year follow up report from ARIC study involving 13,700 individuals aged 45 to 64 years, there was a similar risk of stroke (RR 1.05; 95% CI 0.61 to 1.79; P = 0.87), but a lower risk of CHD events and mortality from CVD in diabetic patients without MI *vs.* nondiabetic patients with MI (95% CI, 1.22 to 2.72; P = 0.003) [132].

COST ISSUES, DIABETES AND PREVENTION OF COMPLICATIONS

According to estimates only in the US in the year 2002 direct medical and indirect costs (due to work loss, disability and premature mortality) due to diabetes were around 132 billion US Dollars [133]. Cardiovascular disease is the most costly complication of diabetes, accounting for more than $17.6 billion of the $91.8 billion annual direct medical costs for diabetes in 2002. Statistics from the American Diabetes Association indicate that chronic complications of diabetes are responsible for six million days of hospital bed use per year with an average length of hospital stay of about 9 days. In 2002 diabetes-related hospitalizations totaled 16.9 million days and accounted for a loss of nearly 88 million disability days. In the United Kingdom the costs of diabetes have also reached alarming figures representing 9% of total healthcare costs translating into a total of approximately 4–6 billion £ (Great Britain Pounds) *per annum* [134]. Over 80% of these costs relate to the long term complications.

Cost-effectiveness of a primary prevention program is mainly influenced by prevalence of disease and clinical outcomes as a consequence of the illness. Primary prevention is aimed at individuals without any manifestations of the disease and is based on risk factor modification. Screening of individuals for risk factors can be costly as many people may have to be screened in order to identify one person with the risk factor and many people with the risk factor may have to be treated for one person to benefit. On the other hand, secondary prevention involves individuals with evidence of an illness (*i.e.* high risk population). This group of individuals has high risk of recurrent events due to complications and contains a bigger prevalence of individuals with modifiable risk factors. Cost-effectiveness ratios produced by this group are more favourable as compared to those in the primary prevention group mainly due to that fact that fewer people must be screened and treated to benefit one person with the risk factor and also screening is more efficient in these individuals. However, further data from high quality clinical trials are needed to refine estimates of the costs and benefits of these programs so that informed policy choices can be made for this high risk population.

CONCLUSIVE REMARKS

Cardiovascular diseases are frequent complications in patients with diabetes mellitus. Enough data is available to warrant and to guide a better control of risk factors in patients with high risk of developing cardiovascular diseases. Due to a high risk of mortality, patients with diabetes developing cardiovascular complications should be aggressively managed. A better risk factor management in patients with evidence of atherosclerosis and diabetes can significantly reduce mortality. Lipid lowering therapy, tight glycaemic control and more recently use of novel therapies to improve insulin sensitivity is mainstay of management of these patients. Large amount of data from clinical trials and registries is pooled into expert guidelines for the management of cardiovascular conditions. These guidelines provide a thorough and stepwise management of patients with cardiovascular conditions in acute hospital settings, as well as in community care. In order to reduce this ever-increasing clinical and economic burden of cardiovascular complications in patients with diabetes, use of expert guidelines for primary and secondary prevention as well as management of cardiovascular diseases in routine practice should be strongly recommended. Further efforts are needed to focus on developing strategies for dissemination and implementations of guidelines in practice.

REFERENCES

1. King H, Aubert RE, Herman WH. Global burden of diabetes, 1995–2025: prevalence, numerical estimates, and projections. *Diabetes Care*, **21**(9): 1414–1431, 1998.

2. Diabetes Statistics. National Diabetes Information Clearinghouse. Bethesda, Md: National Institute of Diabetes and Digestive and Kidney Diseases, *NIH publication*, 99–3296, 1999.

3. National Diabetes Data Group, Diabetes in America, 2nd Edition. Bethesda: NIH, 1995.

4. Stratton IM, Adler AI, Neil HA, Matthews DR, Manley SE, Cull CA, Hadden D, Turner RC, Holman RR. Association of glycaemia with macrovascular and microvascular complications of type 2 diabetes (UKPDS 35): prospective observational study. *Brit Med J*, **321**(7258): 405–412, 2000.

5. Clinical Guidelines on the Identification, Evaluation, and Treatment of Overweight and Obesity in Adults: the Evidence Report. Bethesda, Md: National Institute of Health, National Heart, Lung, and Blood Institute, 1998.

6. Haffner SM, Lehto S, Ronnemaa T, Pyorala K, Laakso M. Mortality from coronary heart disease in subjects with type 2 diabetes and in nondiabetic subjects with and without prior myocardial infarction. *N Engl J Med*, **339**(4): 229–234, 1998.

7. Expert Panel on Detection, Evaluation, and Treatment of High Blood Cholesterol in Adults. Executive Summary of the Third Report of the National Cholesterol Education Program (NCEP) Expert Panel on Detection, Evaluation, and Treatment of High Blood Cholesterol in Adults (Adult Treatment Panel III). *JAMA,* **285**(19): 2486–2497, 2001.

8. Kjaergaard SC, Hansen HH, Fog L, Bulow I, Christensen PD. In-hospital outcome for diabetic patients with acute myocardial infarction in the thrombolytic era. *Scand Cardiovasc J*, **33**(3): 166–170, 1999.

9. Malmberg K, Yusuf S, Gerstein HC, Brown J, Zhao F, Hunt D, Piegas L, Calvin J, Keltai M, Budaj A. Impact of diabetes on long-term prognosis in patients with unstable angina and non-Q-wave myocardial infarction: results of the OASIS (Organization to Assess Strategies for Ischemic Syndromes) Registry. *Circulation*, **102**(9): 1014–1019, 2000.

10. Miettinen H, Lehto S, Salomaa V, Mahonen M, Niemela M, Haffner SM, Pyorala K, Tuomilehto J. Impact of diabetes on mortality after the first myocardial infarction. The FINMONICA Myocardial Infarction Register Study Group. *Diabetes Care*, **21**(1): 69–75, 1998.

11. Herlitz J, Karlson BW, Lindqvist J, Sjolin M. Rate and mode of death during five years of follow-up among patients with acute chest pain with and without a history of diabetes mellitus. *Diabet Med*, **15**(4): 308–314, 1998.

12. Shindler DM, Palmeri ST, Antonelli TA, Sleeper LA, Boland J, Cocke TP, Hochman JS. Diabetes mellitus in cardiogenic shock complicating acute myocardial infarction: a report from the SHOCK Trial Registry. Should we emergently revascularize Occluded Coronaries for cardiogenic shock? *J Am Coll Cardiol*, **36**(3 Suppl A): 1097–1103, 2000.

13. Friedlander AH, Maeder LA. The prevalence of calcified carotid artery atheromas on the panoramic radiographs of patients with type 2 diabetes mellitus. *Oral Surg Oral Med Oral Pathol Oral Radiol Endod,* **89**(4): 420–424, 2000.

14. Stamler J, Vaccaro O, Neaton JD, Wentworth D. Diabetes, other risk factors, and 12-yr cardiovascular mortality for men screened in the Multiple Risk Factor Intervention Trial. *Diabetes Care*, **16**(2): 434–444, 1993.

15. Jorgensen H, Nakayama H, Raaschou HO, Olsen TS. Stroke in patients with diabetes. The Copenhagen Stroke Study. *Stroke*, **25**(10): 1977–1984, 1994.

16. Rohr J, Kittner S, Feeser B, Hebel JR, Whyte MG, Weinstein A, Kanarak N, Buchholz D, Earley C, Johnson C, Macko R, Price T, Sloan M, Stern B, Wityk R, Wozniak M, Sherwin R. Traditional risk factors and ischemic stroke in young adults: the Baltimore-Washington Cooperative Young Stroke Study. *Arch Neurol*, **53**(7): 603–607, 1996.

17. Hankey GJ, Jamrozik K, Broadhurst RJ, Forbes S, Burvill PW, Anderson CS, Stewart-Wynne EG. Long-term risk of first recurrent stroke in the Perth Community Stroke Study. *Stroke*, **29**(12): 2491–2500, 1998.

18. Luchsinger JA, Tang MX, Stern Y, Shea S, Mayeux R. Diabetes mellitus and risk of Alzheimer's disease and dementia with stroke in a multiethnic cohort. *Am J Epidemiol*, **154**(7): 635–641, 2001.

19. Tuomilehto J, Rastenyte D, Jousilahti P, Sarti C, Vartiainen E. Diabetes mellitus as a risk factor for death from stroke. Prospective study of the middle-aged Finnish population. *Stroke,* **27**: 210–215, 1996.

20. Newman AB, Siscovick DS, Manolio TA, Polak J, Fried LP, Borhani NO, Wolfson SK. Ankle-arm index as a marker of atherosclerosis in the Cardiovascular Health Study. Cardiovascular Heart Study (CHS) Collaborative Research Group. *Circulation*, **88**: 837–845, 1993.

21. Abbott RD, Brand FN, Kannel WB. Epidemiology of some peripheral arterial findings in diabetic men and women: experiences from the Framingham Study. *Am J Med,* **88**: 376–381, 1990.

22. Beks PJ, Mackaay AJ, de Neeling JN, de Vries H, Bouter LM, Heine RJ. Peripheral arterial disease in relation to glycaemic level in an elderly Caucasian

population: the Hoorn study. *Diabetologia*, **38**: 86–96, 1995.

23. Kannel WB, McGee DL. Update on some epidemiologic features of intermittent claudication: the Framingham Study. *J Am Geriatr Soc*, **33**: 13–18, 1985.

24. Diabetes-related amputations of lower extremities in the Medicare population–Minnesota, 1993–1995. MMWR *Morb Mortal Wkly Rep,* **47**: 649–652, 1998.

25. Shumway JT, Gambert SR. Diabetic nephropathy-pathophysiology and management. *Int Urol Nephrol,* **34**: 257–264, 2002.

26. US Renal Data System. USRDS 1994 Annual Data Report. Bethesda Md: *National Institute of Health, National Heart, Lung, and Blood Institute*, 1994.

27. Borch-Johnsen K, Kreiner S. Proteinuria: value as predictor of cardiovascular mortality in insulin dependent diabetes mellitus. *Br Med J (Clin Res Ed),* **294**: 1651–1654, 1987.

28. Cines DB, Pollak ES, Buck CA, Loscalzo J, Zimmerman GA, McEver RP, Pober JS, Wick TM, Konkle BA, Schwartz BS, Barnathan ES, McCrae KR, Hug BA, Schmidt AM, Stern DM. Endothelial cells in physiology and in the pathophysiology of vascular disorders. *Blood,* **91**: 3527–3561, 1998.

29. Verma S, Anderson TJ. The ten most commonly asked questions about endothelial function in cardiology. *Cardiol Rev*, **9**: 250–252, 2001.

30. Sarkar R, Meinberg EG, Stanley JC, Gordon D, Webb RC. Nitric oxide reversibly inhibits the migration of cultured vascular smooth muscle cells. *Circ Res*, **78**: 225–230, 1996.

31. Kubes P, Suzuki M, Granger DN. Nitric oxide: an endogenous modulator of leukocyte adhesion. *Proc Natl Acad Sci USA*, **88**: 4651–4655, 1991.

32. Moncada S, Higgs A. The L-arginine-nitric oxide pathway. *N Engl J Med*, **329**: 2002–2012, 1993.

33. Tesfamariam B, Brown ML, Cohen RA. Elevated glucose impairs endothelium-dependent relaxation by activating protein kinase C. *J Clin Invest*, **87**: 1643–1648, 1991.

34. Williams SB, Goldfine AB, Timimi FK, Ting HH, Roddy MA, Simonson DC, Creager MA. Acute hyperglycemia attenuates endothelium-dependent vasodilation in humans *in vivo. Circulation*, **97**: 1695–1701, 1998.

35. Nishikawa T, Edelstein D, Du XL, Yamagishi S, Matsumura T, Kaneda Y, Yorek MA, Beebe D, Oates PJ, Hammes HP, Giardino I, Brownlee M. Normalizing mitochondrial superoxide production blocks three pathways of hyperglycaemic damage. *Nature,* **404**: 787–790, 2000.

36. Cosentino F, Eto M, De Paolis P, van der Loo B, Bachschmid M, Ullrich V, Kouroedov A, Delli Gatti C, Joch H, Volpe M, Luscher TF. High glucose causes upregulation of cyclooxygenase-2 and alters prostanoid profile in human endothelial cells: role of protein kinase C and reactive oxygen species. *Circulation*, **107**: 1017–1023, 2003.

37. Koya D, King GL. Protein kinase C activation and the development of diabetic complications. *Diabetes*, **47**: 859–866, 1998.

38. Nagpala PG, Malik AB, Vuong PT, Lum H. Protein kinase C beta 1 overexpression augments phorbol ester-induced increase in endothelial permeability. *J Cell Physiol*, **166**: 249–255, 1996.

39. Kunisaki M, Bursell SE, Umeda F, Nawata H, King GL. Normalization of diacylglycerol-protein kinase C activation by vitamin E in aorta of diabetic rats and cultured rat smooth muscle cells exposed to elevated glucose levels. *Diabetes*, **43**: 1372–1377, 1994.

40. Inoguchi T, Battan R, Handler E, Sportsman JR, Heath W, King GL. Preferential elevation of protein kinase C isoform beta II and diacylglycerol levels in the aorta and heart of diabetic rats: differential reversibility to glycemic control by islet cell transplantation. *Proc Natl Acad Sci USA*, **89**: 11059–11063, 1992.

41. Beckman JA, Goldfine AB, Gordon MB, Garrett LA, Creager MA. Inhibition of protein kinase Cbeta prevents impaired endothelium-dependent vasodilatation caused by hyperglycemia in humans. *Circ Res*, **90**: 107–111, 2002.

42. Xia P, Inoguchi T, Kern TS, Engerman RL, Oates PJ, King GL. Characterization of the mechanism for the chronic activation of diacylglycerol-protein kinase C pathway in diabetes and hyper-galactosemia. *Diabetes,* **43**: 1122–1129, 1994.

43. Inoguchi T, Li P, Umeda F, Yu HY, Kakimoto M, Imamura M, Aoki T, Etoh T, Hashimoto T, Naruse M, Sano H, Utsumi H, Nawata H. High glucose level and free fatty acid stimulate reactive oxygen species production through protein kinase C-dependent activation of NAD(P)H oxidase in cultured vascular cells. *Diabetes,* **49**: 1939–1945, 2000.

44. Dimitriadis E, Griffin M, Owens D, Johnson A, Collins P, Tomkin GH. Oxidation of low-density lipoprotein in NIDDM: its relationship to fatty acid composition. *Diabetologia,* **38**: 1300–1306, 1995.

45. Takagi C, Bursell SE, Lin YW, Takagi H, Duh E, Jiang Z, Clermont AC, King GL. Regulation of retinal hemodynamics in diabetic rats by increased expression and action of endothelin-1. *Invest Ophthalmol Vis Sci*, **37**: 2504–2518, 1996.

46. Hink U, Li H, Mollnau H, Oelze M, Matheis E, Hartmann M, Skatchkov M, Thaiss F, Stahl RA, Warnholtz A, Meinertz T, Griendling K, Harrison DG, Forstermann U, Munzel T. Mechanisms

underlying endothelial dysfunction in diabetes mellitus. *Circ Res*, **88**: E14–E22, 2001.

47. Kawano M, Koshikawa T, Kanzaki T, Morisaki N, Saito Y, Yoshida S. Diabetes mellitus induces accelerated growth of aortic smooth muscle cells: association with overexpression of PDGF beta-receptors. *Eur J Clin Invest*, **23**: 84–90, 1993.

48. Inaba T, Ishibashi S, Gotoda T, Kawamura M, Morino N, Nojima Y, Kawakami M, Yazaki Y, Yamada N. Enhanced expression of platelet-derived growth factor-beta receptor by high glucose. Involvement of platelet-derived growth factor in diabetic angiopathy. *Diabetes*, **45**: 507–512, 1996.

49. Nabel EG, Shum L, Pompili VJ, Yang ZY, San H, Shu HB, Liptay S, Gold L, Gordon D, Derynck R *et al*. Direct transfer of transforming growth factor beta 1 gene into arteries stimulates fibrocellular hyperplasia. *Proc Natl Acad Sci USA*, **90**: 10759–10763, 1993.

50. Brownlee M, Cerami A, Vlassara H. Advanced glycosylation end-products in tissue and the biochemical basis of diabetic complications. *N Engl J Med*, **318**: 1315–1321, 1988.

51. Schmidt AM, Yan SD, Wautier JL, Stern D. Activation of receptor for advanced glycation end-products: a mechanism for chronic vascular dysfunction in diabetic vasculopathy and atherosclerosis. *Circ Res*, **84**: 489–497, 1999.

52. Schmidt AM, Stern D. Atherosclerosis and diabetes: the RAGE connection. *Curr Atheroscler Rep*, **2**: 430–436, 2000.

53. Kirstein M, Brett J, Radoff S, Ogawa S, Stern D, Vlassara H. Advanced protein glycosylation induces transendothelial human monocyte chemotaxis and secretion of platelet-derived growth factor: role in vascular disease of diabetes and aging. *Proc Natl Acad Sci USA*, **87**: 9010–9014, 1990.

54. Vlassara H, Brownlee M, Manogue KR, Dinarello CA, Pasagian A. Cachectin/TNF and IL-1 induced by glucose-modified proteins: role in normal tissue remodelling. *Science*, **240**: 1546–1548, 1988.

55. Kirstein M, Aston C, Hintz R, Vlassara H. Receptor-specific induction of insulin-like growth factor I in human monocytes by advanced glycosylation end-product-modified proteins. *J Clin Invest*, **90**: 439–446, 1992.

56. Bowie A, Owens D, Collins P, Johnson A, Tomkin GH. Glycosylated low density lipoprotein is more sensitive to oxidation: implications for the diabetic patient? *Atherosclerosis*, **102**: 63–67, 1993.

57. Boden G. Free fatty acids, insulin resistance, and type 2 diabetes mellitus. *Proc Assoc Am Physicians*, **111**: 241–248, 1999.

58. Kelley DE, Simoneau JA. Impaired free fatty acid utilization by skeletal muscle in non-insulin-dependent diabetes mellitus. *J Clin Invest*, **94**: 2349–2356, 1994.

59. Sniderman AD, Scantlebury T, Cianflone K. Hypertriglyceridemic hyperapob: the unappreciated atherogenic dyslipoproteinemia in type 2 diabetes mellitus. *Ann Intern Med*, **135**: 447–459, 2001.

60. Cummings MH, Watts GF, Umpleby AM, Hennessy TR, Naoumova R, Slavin BM, Thompson GR, Sonksen PH. Increased hepatic secretion of very-low-density lipoprotein apolipoprotein B-100 in NIDDM. *Diabetologia*, **38**: 959–967, 1995.

61. de Man FH, Weverling-Rijnsburger AW, van der Laarse A, Smelt AH, Jukema JW, Blauw GJ. Not acute but chronic hypertriglyceridemia is associated with impaired endothelium-dependent vasodilatation: reversal after lipid-lowering therapy by atorvastatin. *Arterioscler Thromb Vasc Biol*, **20**: 744–750, 2000.

62. Steinberg HO, Tarshoby M, Monestel R, Hook G, Cronin J, Johnson A, Bayazeed B, Baron AD. Elevated circulating free fatty acid levels impair endothelium-dependent vasodilatation. *J Clin Invest*, **100**: 1230–1239, 1997.

63. Pleiner J, Schaller G, Mittermayer F, Bayerle-Eder M, Roden M, Wolzt M. FFA-induced endothelial dysfunction can be corrected by vitamin C. *J Clin Endocrinol Metab*, **87**: 2913–2917, 2002.

64. Williams SB, Cusco JA, Roddy MA, Johnstone MT, Creager MA. Impaired nitric oxide-mediated vasodilatation in patients with non-insulin-dependent diabetes mellitus. *J Am Coll Cardiol*, **27**: 567–574, 1996.

65. De Vriese AS, Verbeuren TJ, Van de Voorde J, Lameire NH, Vanhoutte PM. Endothelial dysfunction in diabetes. *Br J Pharmacol*, **130**: 963–974, 2000.

66. Luft FC. Proinflammatory effects of angiotensin II and endothelin: targets for progression of cardiovascular and renal diseases. *Curr Opin Nephrol Hypertens*, **11**: 59–66, 2002.

67. Hopfner RL, Gopalakrishnan V. Endothelin: emerging role in diabetic vascular complications. *Diabetologia*, **42**: 1383–1394, 1999.

68. Hussain MJ, Peakman M, Gallati H, Lo SS, Hawa M, Viberti GC, Watkins PJ, Leslie RD, Vergani D. Elevated serum levels of macrophage-derived cytokines precede and accompany the onset of IDDM. *Diabetologia*, **39**: 60–69, 1996.

69. Uemura S, Matsushita H, Li W, Glassford AJ, Asagami T, Lee KH, Harrison DG, Tsao PS. Diabetes mellitus enhances vascular matrix metalloproteinase activity: role of oxidative stress. *Circ Res*, **88**: 1291–1298, 2001.

70. Fukumoto H, Naito Z, Asano G, Aramaki T. Immunohistochemical and morphometric evaluations of coronary atherosclerotic plaques associated with myocardial infarction and diabetes mellitus. *J Atheroscler Thromb*, 5: 29–35, 1998.

71. Geng YJ. Molecular signal transduction in vascular cell apoptosis. *Cell Res*, 11: 253–264, 2001.

72. Ross R. Atherosclerosis – an inflammatory disease. *N Engl J Med*, 340: 115–126, 1999.

73. Assert R, Scherk G, Bumbure A, Pirags V, Schatz H, Pfeiffer AF. Regulation of protein kinase C by short term hyperglycaemia in human platelets *in vivo* and *in vitro*. *Diabetologia*, 44: 188–195, 2001.

74. Vinik AI, Erbas T, Park TS, Nolan R, Pittenger GL. Platelet dysfunction in type 2 diabetes. *Diabetes Care*, 24: 1476–1485, 2001.

75. Shechter M, Merz CN, Paul-Labrador MJ, Kaul S. Blood glucose and platelet-dependent thrombosis in patients with coronary artery disease. *J Am Coll Cardiol*, 35: 300–307, 2000.

76. Shechter M, Bairey Merz CN, Paul-Labrador MJ, Shah PK, Kaul S. Plasma apolipoprotein B levels predict platelet-dependent thrombosis in patients with coronary artery disease. *Cardiology*, 92: 151–155, 1999.

77. Paolisso G, Barbagallo M. Hypertension, diabetes mellitus, and insulin resistance: the role of intracellular magnesium. *Am J Hypertens*, 10: 346–355, 1997.

78. Tchobroutsky G. Relation of diabetic control to development of microvascular complications. *Diabetologia*, 15: 143–152, 1978.

79. Pellegatta F, Folli F, Ronchi P, Caspani L, Galli L, Vicari AM. Deranged platelet calcium homeostasis in poorly controlled IDDM patients. *Diabetes Care*, 16: 178–183, 1993.

80. Tschope D, Rosen P, Gries FA. Increase in the cytosolic concentration of calcium in platelets of diabetics type II. *Thromb Res*, 62: 421–428, 1991.

81. Carr ME. Diabetes mellitus: a hypercoagulable state. *J Diabetes Complications*, 15: 44–54, 2001.

82. Juhan-Vague I, Roul C, Alessi MC, Ardissone JP, Heim M, Vague P. Increased plasminogen activator inhibitor activity in non insulin dependent diabetic patients-relationship with plasma insulin. *Thromb Haemost*, 61: 370–373, 1989.

83. Nordt TK, Bode C. Impaired endogenous fibrinolysis in diabetes mellitus: mechanisms and therapeutic approaches. *Semin Thromb Hemost*, 26: 495–501, 2000.

84. Ceriello A, Giugliano D, Quatraro A, Marchi E, Barbanti M, Lefebvre P. Evidence for a hyperglycaemia-dependent decrease of antithrombin III thrombin complex formation in humans. *Diabetologia*, 33: 163–167, 1990.

85. Gaede P, Vedel P, Larsen N, *et al*. Multifactorial intervention and cardiovascular disease in patients with type 2 diabetes. *N Engl J Med*, 348: 383–393, 2003.

86. Stamler J, Wentworth D, Neaton J, *et al*. Diabetes and risk of coronary, cardiovascular, and all causes mortality: findings for 356,000 men screened by the Multiple Risk Factor Intervention Trial (MRFIT). *Circulation,* 70: (suppl 2) 161, 1984.

87. Wood D, *et al*. Recommendations of the Second Joint Task Force of the European and other Society on Coronary Prevention. *Eur Heart J*, 19: 1434–1503, 1998.

88. Writing Group III: Risk Assessment in Persons With Diabetes. Prevention Conference VI Diabetes and Cardiovascular Disease. *Circulation*, 105: 144–152, 2002.

89. The Diabetes Control and Complications Trial Research Group. The effect of intensive treatment of diabetes on the development and progression of long-term complications in insulin-dependent diabetes mellitus. *N Engl J Med*, 329: 977–986, 1993.

90. Marx N, Sukhova G, Murphy C, *et al*. Macrophages in human atheroma contains PPARgamma: differentiation–dependent peroxisomal proliferators–activated receptor gamma (PPARgamma) expression and reduction of MMP-9 activity through PPARgamma activation in mononuclear phagocytes in vitro. *Am J Pathol*, 153: 17–23, 1998.

91. Putsch J. Peroxisome proliferator–activated receptors in vascular biology and atherosclerosis: emerging insights for evolving paradigms. *Curr Atheroscler Rep*, 2: 327–335, 2000.

92. Watanabe Y, Sunayama S, Shimada K, *et al*. Troglitazone improves endothelial dysfunction in patients with insulin resistance. *J Atheroscler Thromb*, 7: 159–163, 2000.

93. Marx N, Mackman N, Schonbeck U, *et al*. PPARalpha activators inhibit tissue factor expression and activity in human monocytes. *Circulation*, 103: 213–219, 2001.

94. Burden AC, McNally TG, Feehally J, Wallis J. Increased incidence of end staged renal failure from Diabetes mellitus in an Asian ethnic group in the United Kingdom. *Diab Med*, 9: 641–645, 1992.

95. Nelson RG, Bennett PH, Beck GJ, Tan M, *et al*. Development and progression of renal disease in Pima-Indians with NIDDM. Diabetic Renal Disease Group. *N Engl J Med*, 335: 1636–1642, 1996.

96. Antiplatelet Trialist's randomised trials of antiplatelet therapy. Prevention of death,

myocardial infarction and stroke by prolonged antiplatelet therapy in various categories of patients. *BMJ,* **308:** 81–106, 1994.

97. Samuganthan TS, Ghahramani P, Jackson PR, Wallis EJ, *et al.* Aspirin for primary prevention of coronary heart disease: Safety and absolute benefit related to coronary risk derived from meta-analysis of randomised trials. *Heart,* **85:** 265–271, 2001.

98. Zuanetti G, Latini R, Maggioni AP, *et al.* Effect of ACE Inhibitor lisinopril on mortality in diabetic patients with acute myocardial infarction: data from GISSI 3 study. *Circulation,* **96:** 4239–4245, 1997.

99. Braunwald E *et al.* ACC/AHA Guidelines update for the management of patients with unstable angina and non-ST-segment elevation myocardial infarction. A report of American College of Cardiology/ American Heart Association Task Force on Practice Guidelines (Committee on the management of patients with unstable angina). *J Am Coll Cardiol,* **36:** 970–1062, 2002.

100. Silva JA, Escobar A, Collins TJ, Ramee SR, White CJ. Unstable angina: a comparison of angioscopic findings between diabetic and nondiabetic patients. *Circulation,* **92:** 1731–1736, 1995.

101. Wood D, De Backer G, Faergeman O, Graham I, Mancia G, Pyörälä K. Prevention of coronary heart disease in clinical practice. Recommendations of the Second Joint Task Force of European and other Societies on Coronary Prevention. *Eur Heart J,* **19:** 1434–1503, 1998.

102. Bertrand ME Chair, Simoons ML, Fox KA, Wallentin LC, Hamm CW, McFadden E, De Feyter PJ, Specchia G, Ruzyllo W. Management of acute coronary syndromes: acute coronary syndromes without persistent ST segment elevation. Recommendations of the Task Force of the European Society of Cardiology. *Eur Heart J,* **23:** 1809–1840, 2002.

103. Yusuf S, Zhao F, Mehta SR, Chrolavicius S, Tognoni G, Fox KK. Effects of clopidogrel in addition to aspirin in patients with acute coronary syndromes without ST-segment elevation. *N Engl J Med,* **345:** 494–502, 2001.

104. Jonas M, Reicher-Reiss H, Boyko V, *et al.* Usefulness of beta-blocker therapy in patients with non-insulin-dependent diabetes mellitus and coronary artery disease: Bezafibrate Infarction Prevention (BIP) Study Group. *Am J Cardiol,* **77:** 1273–1277, 1996.

105. Weintraub WS, Stein B, Kosinski A, *et al.* Outcome of coronary bypass surgery versus coronary angioplasty in diabetic patients with multivessel coronary artery disease. *J Am Coll Cardiol,* **31:** 10–19, 1998.

106. Detre KM, Guo P, Holubkov R, *et al.* Coronary revascularization in diabetic patients, a comparison of the randomized and observational components of the Bypass Angioplasty Revascularization Investigation (BARI). *Circulation,* **99:** 633–640, 1999.

107. Influence of diabetes on 5-year mortality and morbidity in a randomized trial comparing CABG and PTCA in patients with multivessel disease: the Bypass Angioplasty Revascularization Investigation (BARI). *Circulation,* **96:** 1761–1769, 1997.

108. Kip KE, Faxon DP, Detre KM, Yeh W, Kelsey SF, Currier JW. Coronary angioplasty in diabetic patients: the National Heart, Lung, and Blood Institute Percutaneous Transluminal Coronary Angioplasty Registry. *Circulation,* **94:** 1818–1825, 1996.

109. King SB III, Kosinski A, Guyton RA, Lembo NJ, Weintraub WS. Eight year mortality in the Emory Angioplasty vs Surgery Trial (EAST). *J Am Coll Cardiol,* **35:** 1116–1121, 2000.

110. Kuntz RE. Importance of considering atherosclerosis progression when choosing a coronary revascularization strategy: the diabetes-percutaneous transluminal coronary angioplasty dilemma. *Circulation,* **99:** 847–851, 1999.

111. Barsness GW, Peterson ED, Ohman EM, *et al.* Relationship between diabetes mellitus and long-term survival after coronary bypass and angioplasty. *Circulation,* **96:** 2551–2556, 1997.

112. Levine GN, Jacobs AK, Keeler GP, *et al.* Impact of diabetes mellitus on percutaneous revascularization (CAVEAT-I) CAVEAT-I Investigators. Coronary Angioplasty Versus Excisional Atherectomy Trial. *Am J Cardiol,* **79:** 748–755, 1997.

113. Roffi M, Chew DP, Mukherjee D, *et al.* Platelet glycoprotein inhibitors reduce mortality in diabetic patients with non-ST segment elevation acute coronary syndromes. *Circulation,* **104:** 2767–2771, 2001.

114. Malmberg K. Prospective randomised study of intensive insulin treatment on long-term survival after acute myocardial infarction in patients with diabetes mellitus. DIGAMI (Diabetes Mellitus, Insulin Glucose Infusion in Acute Myocardial Infarction) Study Group. *Br Med J,* **314:** 1512–1515, 1997.

115. Malmberg K, Ryden L, Efendic S, *et al.* Randomized trial of insulin-glucose infusion followed by subcutaneous insulin treatment in diabetic patients with acute myocardial infarction (DIGAMI study): effects on mortality at 1 year. *J Am Coll Cardiol,* **26:** 57–65, 1995.

116. Ramsay LE, Williams B, Johnston GD, MacGregor GA, Poston L, Potter JF, Poulter NR, Russel G. Guidelines for management of hypertension: report

of the third working party of the British Hypertension Society. *J Hum Hypertens*, **13**: 569–592, 1999.

117. Hansson L, Zanchett A, Carruthers SG, *et al*. Effects of intensive blood-pressure lowering and low-dose aspirin in patients with hypertension: principal results of the Hypertension Optimal Treatment (HOT) randomized trial. *Lancet*, **351**: 1755–1762, 1998.

118. Reaven G. Metabolic syndrome: pathophysiology and implications for management of cardiovascular disease. *Circulation*, **106**: 286–288, 2002.

119. Reaven GM, Lithell H, Landsberg L. Hypertension and associated atherosclerosis in hypertension: results of the Plaque Hypertension Lipid Lowering Italian Study (PHYLLIS). *J Hypertens*, **21**(suppl 4): S346, 2003.

120. Haffner SM. The prediabetic problem: development of non-insulindependent diabetes mellitus and related abnormalities. *J Diabet Complic*, **11**: 69–76, 1997.

121. European Society of Hypertension–European Society of Cardiology Guidelines Committee. 2003 European Society of Hypertension–European Society of Cardiology guidelines for the management of arterial hypertension. *Journal of Hypertension*, **21**: 1011–1053, 2003.

122. Williams B, Poulter NR, Brown MJ, Davis M, McInnes GT, Potter JF, Sever PS, McG Thom S; the BHS guidelines working party, for the British Hypertension Society. British Hypertension Society guidelines for hypertension management 2004 (BHS-IV): Summary. *Brit Med J*, **328**: 634–640, 2004.

123. Lewis EJ, Hunsicker LG, Clarke WR, Berl T, Pohl MA, Lewis JB, *et al*. Renoprotective effect of the angiotensin-receptor antagonist irbesartan in patients with nephropathy due to type 2 diabetes. *N Engl J Med*, **345**: 851–860, 2001.

124. Lindholm LH, *et al*. Cardiovascular morbidity and mortality in patients with diabetes in the Losartan Intervention For Endpoint reduction in hypertension study (LIFE): a randomised trial against atenolol. *Lancet*, **359**: 1004–1010, 2002.

125. Pyorala K, Pedersen TR, Kjekshus J, *et al*. Cholesterol lowering with simvastatin improves prognosis of diabetic patients with coronary heart disease: a subgroup analysis of the Scandinavian Simvastatin Survival Study (4S). *Diabetes Care*, **20**: 614–620, 1997.

126. Goldberg RB, Mellies MJ, Sacks FM, *et al*. Cardiovascular events and their reduction with pravastatin in diabetic and glucose-intolerant myocardial infarction survivors with average cholesterol levels: subgroup analyses in the cholesterol and recurrent events (CARE) trial. The Care Investigators. *Circulation*, **98**: 2513–2519, 1998.

127. Heart Protection Study Collaborative Group. MRC/BHF Heart Protection Study of cholesterol lowering with simvastatin in 20,536 high-risk individuals: a randomised placebo-controlled trial. *Lancet*, **360**: 7–22, 2002.

128. American Diabetes Association. Management of dyslipidemia in adults with diabetes (Position Statement). *Diabetes Care*, **22**: S56–S59, 1999.

129. Tikkanen MJ. Statins: within-group comparisons, statin escape and combination therapy. *Curr Opin Lipidol*, **7**: 385–388, 1996.

130. Van Hout BA, Simoons ML. Cost-effectiveness of HMG coenzyme reductase inhibitors; whom to treat? *Eur Heart J*, **22**: 751–761, 2001.

131. Lüscher TF, Creager MA. Clinical cardiology: new frontiers. diabetes and vascular disease pathophysiology, clinical consequences, and medical therapy: Part II. *Circulation*, **108**: 1655–1661, 2003.

132. Lee CD, Folsom AR, Pankow JS. Brancati FL; Atherosclerosis Risk in Communities (ARIC) Study Investigators. Cardiovascular Events in Diabetic and Nondiabetic Adults With or Without History of Myocardial Infarction. *Circulation*, **109**: 855–860, 2004.

133. American Diabetes Association. National Diabetes Fact Sheet. http://www.diabetes.org/diabetes-statistics/national-diabetes-fact-sheet.jsp, accessed in March 2004.

134. Currie CJ, *et al*. NHS acute sector expenditure for diabetes: the present, future, and excess in-patient cost of care. *Diabetic Medicine*, **14**: 686–692, 1997.

135. Grundy SM, Garber A, Goldberg R, Havas S, Holman R, Lamendola C, Howard WJ, Savage P, Sowers J, Vega GL. Writing Group IV: Lifestyle and medical management of risk factors. Prevention Conference VI, Diabetes and Cardiovascular Disease. *Circulation*, **105**: e153–e158, 2002.

136. Grundy SM, Benjamin IJ, Burke GL, Chait A, Eckel RH, Howard BV, Mitch W, Smith SC, Jr, Sowers JR. AHA Scientific Statement Diabetes and Cardiovascular Disease. A Statement for Healthcare Professionals From the American Heart Association. *Circulation*, **100**: 1134–1146, 1999.

137. Sowers JR, Haffner S. Treatment of cardiovascular and renal risk factors in the diabetic hypertensive. *Hypertension*, **40**: 781–788, 2002.

24

PRACTICAL APPROACH TO THE MULTIFACTORIAL RISK IN TYPE 2 DIABETES

Nicolae HÂNCU, Anca CERGHIZAN, Cornelia BALA

Type 2 diabetes is clearly associated with an increase in cardiovascular risk and cardiovascular disease.

The risk is multifactorial, including at least five "bad companions": hyperglycemia, hypertension, dyslipidemia, obesity and smoking. The prothrombotic state can also be added.

To achieve a reduction of cardiovascular morbidity and mortality, the global approach to cardiovascular risk is needed, by obtaining the control of all these five factors.

The global approach means the following steps: 1) the identification and evaluation of each risk factor, 2) the evaluation of global cardiovascular risk, 3) the intervention for each risk factor.

The implementation of global approach to cardiovascular risk in type 2 diabetes is a huge task for practitioners implying a high effort. But this is worth doing because the significant benefits have been demonstrated.

OVERVIEW
OF CARDIOVASCULAR RISK

FROM THE GENERAL POPULATION TO PEOPLE WITH TYPE 2 DIABETES

Global cardiovascular risk represents the action and consequences of all risk factors which simultaneously or sequentially act on the body, leading to atherogenesis/atherosclerosis with their clinical or subclinical entities: coronary heart disease, cerebrovascular disease, peripheral arteriopathy, aortic aneurism [1].

Type 2 diabetes carries a heavy burden of cardiovascular disease, being recently considered by some authorities as *a cardiovascular disease* [2]. Hence *preventing this complication of diabetes is undoubtedly one of the biggest therapeutic challenges for the new millenium.*

There is growing evidence that through the control of multiple risk factors these tremendous complications could be reduced. This is a complex but achievable and affordable task [3].

Risk factors and the global risk

The concept of global risk has emerged from the well-known investigations: the Framingham Study [4], the Multiple Risk Factors Intervention Trial – MRFIT [5] and the Münster Heart Study – PROCAM [6]. It was clearly showed that the development of coronary heart disease is mainly caused by two or more risk factors, which have a multiplicative effect, the global risk being greater than would be expected from a simple addition of each risk [7].

The true sense of risk factors is mainly referred to coronary heart disease although, for practical reasons, it has been extrapolated to other atherosclerotic cardiovascular diseases or macrovascular diseases.

Cardiovascular risk factors can be characterized as: modifiable or non-modifiable risk (Table 24.1): as causal, conditional, predisposing or plaque burden risk (Table 24.2): as absolute, relative or attributable risk (Table 24.3).

Table 24.1

Lifestyle and characteristics associated with increased risk of future coronary heart disease events (from [8] with kind permission)

Lifestyle	Biochemical or physiological characteristics (modifiable)	Personal characteristics (non-modifiable)
Diet high in saturated fat, cholesterol and calories Cigarette smoking Excess alcohol consumption Physical inactivity	Elevated blood pressure Elevated plasma total cholesterol (LDL-cholesterol) Low plasma HDL-cholesterol Elevated plasma triglycerides Hyperglycemia/Diabetes Obesity Thrombogenic factors	Age Sex Family history of CHD or other atherosclerotic vascular disease at early age (in men < 55 years, in women < 65 years) Personal history of CHD or other atherosclerotic vascular disease

Table 24.2

Categories of risk factors according to mechanism emerge (from [1] with kind permission)

Category	Risk factors
Causal or major	• Cigarette smoking • High blood pressure • Elevated serum cholesterol or LDL cholesterol • Low HDL cholesterol • High plasma glucose

Table 24.2

(continued)

Category	Risk factors
Conditional	Elevated levels of: • Serum triglycerides • Lipoprotein (a) • Small, dense LDL particles • Homocysteine • Coagulation factors (fibrinogen, PAI-1)
Predisposing	• Obesity • Physical inactivity • Family history of premature CHD • Male sex • Possibly behavioral, socio-economic and ethnic factors • Insulin resistance
Plaque burden	• Age • Intimal medial thickness of the carotid arteries (measured by sonography) • Coronary calcium scores (measured by electron-beam computerized tomography – EBCT) • Subclinical ischemia (during exercise testing)

Table 24.3

Absolute, relative and attributable risk (from [1] with kind permission)

Absolute risk (AR)	Definition	The probability of developing CHD over a finite period
	Stratification of probability	Low risk: low probability of CHD High risk: high probability of CHD
	Stratification according to period of developing CHD	Short-term: $\leq$ 10 years Long-term: > 10 years or over a lifetime
	Importance	AR should provide a guide to intensify the management in case of: High short-term risk High long-term risk
Relative risk (RR)	Definition	RR is the ratio of two levels of absolute risk (AR): RR= AR of the subject / AR of a baseline population
	Importance	RR has advantage in risk assessment and risk reduction strategy
Attributable risk (ATR)	Definition	ATR is the difference in absolute risk between the considered subject and that of a control group
	Importance	ATR is low in young adulthood and high in older age group

Primary and secondary prevention

The concept of risk factors is related to the primary and the secondary prevention of coronary heart disease and other atherosclerotic diseases. In Table 24.4 are described the main characteristics of the two preventive strategies.

Table 24.4

The concept of primary and secondary prevention (from [1] with kind permission)

Primary prevention (PP)	Definition	All actions to modify risk factors or their development in order to delay or prevent new-onset coronary heart disease
	Importance	PP has to be considered for high risk persons both in short and long term
	Short-term, high risk prevention	The likelihood to develop a major coronary event is similar to that of patients with established coronary heart disease The patients focused are those with coronary heart disease risk equivalents (see below)
	CHD risk equivalents	Are considered for the patients without CHD but having at least one of the followings: 1. Abdominal aortic aneurism 2. Ischemia of the extremities 3. Substantial carotid atherosclerosis documented by clinical cerebral symptoms (transient ischemic attacks or stroke), sonography or angiography 4. Type 2 diabetes mellitus 5. Absolute risk > 20% in 10 years
	Recommendations	For persons with CHD equivalents the strategy used for secondary prevention is recommended
	Long-term high risk prevention	Focuses the persons either with multiple marginal risk factors or by a single categorical risk factor All persons in this category deserve attention Long-term prevention represents a certain progress in preventive cardiology
Secondary prevention (SP)	Definition	SP means therapy to reduce recurrent CHD events and decrease coronary mortality in patients with established CHD
	Recommendations for	1. Control of risk factors 2. Direct protection of coronary arteries from plaque eruption

Peculiarity of cardiovascular risk in type 2 diabetes

Cardiovascular risk in people with type 2 diabetes is similar to that of the general population but also has many and important peculiarities.

• All risk factors are considered potential determinants of macrovascular disease in type 2 diabetes. They are important even when atherosclerotic disease had already appeared, because they contribute to disease progression [8–11].

• The causal or major risk factors (Table 24.5) act also as independent determinants of cardiovascular disease. Very often they are clustered as in the metabolic syndrome [12]. Two reports from AHA (American Heart Association) and NHLBI (National Heart, Lung and Blood Institute) have defined the metabolic syndrome and the significance of diabetes mellitus. It has been shown that: 1) the metabolic syndrome is a predictor of diabetes; 2) diabetes increases the cardiovascular risk of the metabolic syndrome; 3) risk assessment should be a compulsory part of the practical approach; 4) for the management of insulin resistance and hyperglycemia, metformin, thiazolidinediones or their combination are recommended [13, 14].

Table 24.5

The five determinants of the Metabolic X Syndrome according to the ATP III [15]. Its diagnosis is made when any three of the five determinants are identified*

The determinants	Suggestive values

1. Abdominal obesity:
  waist circumferences
  – Men
  – Women
	
	> 102 cm
	> 88 cm

2. Plasma triglycerides	≥ 150 mg/dl [1.7 mmol/dl]

3. HDL cholesterol
  – Men
  – Women
	
	< 40 mg/dl [1.03 mmol/dl]
	< 50 mg/dl [1.29 mmol/dl]

4. Blood pressure	≥ 130/ ≥ 85 mmHg
5. Fasting glucose	≥ 110 mg/dl [6.1 mmol/dl]

* According to the WHO Report [98], the definition of the metabolic X syndrome is suggested when glucose intolerance (IGT or IGF) or diabetes mellitus and/or insulin resistance is associated with two or more of other components as follows: raised blood pressure, raised plasma triglycerides and/or low HDL cholesterol, central obesity, microalbuminuria.

The five determinants of the Metabolic X Syndrome according to the ATP III [15]. The diagnosis is made when any three of the five determinants are identified

• The predisposing factors (Table 24.2) also influence the development of macrovascular disease in type 2 diabetes [2]. Conversely, macrovascular disease and hyperglycemia can be prevented and controlled by controlling some of the predisposing factors [16].

• Conventional cardiovascular risk factors have the same impact in diabetics as in non-diabetic individuals [8, 5, 17]. However, in diabetes, at any given risk factor levels, there is a much higher risk of an atherosclerotic cardiovascular event than in non-diabetic people [8, 5].

• Type 2 diabetes is associated with more significant cardiovascular risk factors than type 1 diabetes [8].

• Premenopausal women with diabetes are not protected from cardiovascular disease: both women and men with diabetes are seen as having similar cardiovascular risks [18].

• The cardiovascular risk factors in type 2 diabetes have a distinct spectrum in different manifestations of macrovascular disease as shown in Table 24.6.

• The analysis of baseline risk factors and their predictive power to cardiac end points in UKPDS have shown that [19]:

– Patients without evidence of atherosclerotic disease at diagnosis of type 2 diabetes had a quintet of modifiable risk factors: increased LDL cholesterol, decreased HDL cholesterol, hypertension, hyperglycemia, smoking and age as a non-modifiable risk factor. They have a different position in the model for coronary heart disease, non-fatal or fatal myocardial infarction and fatal myocardial infarction (Table 24.7).

– Coronary risk factors in the general population change their importance once type 2 diabetes has developed. Abdominal obesity, sedentarism and hyperinsulinism were not found to be major risk factors in type 2 diabetes. Plasma triglycerides level was not found to be an independent risk factor, possibly because of the great variability of this lipid parameter. But postprandial triglycerides values may have an additional atherogenic role to the fasting levels [20].

– The variation of these risk factors and subsequent modification of coronary risk is shown in Table 24.8 according to the UKPDS data [20].

Table 24.6

The spectrum of risk in macrovascular disease of type 2 diabetes (from [1] with kind permission)

Risk factor	Coronary heart disease	Stroke	Amputation
Hyperglycemia	+	++	+++
Hemoglobin A1c	+	++	+++
Total cholesterol	++	+	+
HDL cholesterol	+++	++	(+)
Total triglycerides	+++	++	(+)
Hypertension	(+)	++	(+)
Duration of diabetes	+	+	+++
Medial arterial calcification	+++	+	+++

Table 24.7

Risk factors for coronary heart disease in UKPDS: stepwise selection adjusted for age and sex in 2693 persons with type 2 diabetes with depended variable as time to first event (from [1] with kind permission)

Position in model	Coronary artery disease	Non-fatal or fatal myocardial infarction	Fatal myocardial infarction
First	LDL cholesterol	LDL cholesterol	Diastolic blood pressure (BP)
Second	HDL cholesterol	Diastolic BP	LDL cholesterol

Table 24.7

(continued)

Position in model	Coronary artery disease	Non-fatal or fatal myocardial infarction	Fatal myocardial infarction
Third	Hemoglobin A1c	Smoking	Hemoglobin A1c
Fourth	Systolic BP	HDL cholesterol	–
Fifth	Smoking	Hemoglobin A1c	–

Table 24.8

Variation of the main risk factors and modification of coronary risk; compiled from UKPDS data
(from [1] with kind permission)

Risk factors	Variation	Coronary risk
LDL cholesterol	↓ 40 mg/dl (1 mmol/l)	↓ 36%
HDL cholesterol	↑ 4 mg/dl (0.1 mmol/l)	↓ 15%
Hemoglobin A1c	↑ 1%	↑ 11%
Systolic blood pressure	↑ 10 mmHg	↑ 15%

• The importance of cardiovascular risk factors in type 2 diabetes has also emerged from impressive interventional trials, where hyperglycemia, hypertension and dyslipidemia have been focused.

– Intensive glycemic control, as achieved in UKPDS with either sulphonylurea or insulin, reduced significantly only the microvascular but not the macrovascular complications [21, 22, 23]. However, in obese people with type 2 diabetes, well controlled with metformin, a significant reduction of macrovascular complication was demonstrated [24].

– Another important conclusion comes from UKPDS [25, 26] where it was demonstrated that the tight control of blood pressure leads to a significant reduction of both microvascular and macrovascular disease. A similar conclusion has been drawn from HOPE, microHOPE and HOT studies [27, 28].

– The post-hoc analysis of the diabetic subgroups from 4S and CARE studies has shown that secondary prevention in diabetic patients treated with simvastatin or pravastatin is effective [29, 30, 31, 32]. Moreover, the cardiovascular effect of LDL reduction by statins was greater (4S) or as great (CARE) as in the general population [33]. Heart Protection Study, which included 20536 high-risk individuals, from which 5963 subjects with diabetes, clearly showed that treatment with 40 mg Simvastatin daily decreases the rate of major vascular events (major coronary events, strokes, and revascularisations) by about one-quarter, irrespective of the initial cholesterol concentrations. The reduction was statistically significant in all subgroups, including the subgroup of people with diabetes [34]. The proportional reduction in risk was also about a quarter among various subcategories of diabetic patients studied, including: those with different duration, type, or control of diabetes; those aged over 65 years at entry or with hypertension; and those with total cholesterol below 5.0 mmol/l (193 mg/dl) [35]. In the more recent ASCOT Study, treatment with Atorvastatin 10 mg in hypertensive patients with average or lower than average cholesterol concentrations, produced a 36% reduction in fatal and nonfatal myocardial infarction, but the subgroup with diabetes benefited less than that without diabetes (explained by a low number of events in the diabetic patients) [36]. The results of Collaborative Atorvastatin Diabetes Study (CARDS) have been recently published [37]. It has been demonstrated that atorvastatin 10 mg daily is safe and efficacious in reducing the risk of first cardiovascular event, including stroke, in patients with type 2 diabetes without high LDL-cholesterol. Despite the fact that these results are directly applicable to most patients with type 2 diabetes, there is a serious care gap in the use of lipid-lowering drugs for that group of persons [38].

These results emphasize the role of the control of dyslipidemia in type 2 diabetes persons [39].

– In addition, we must mention the beneficial effects of aspirin on macrovascular disease both in primary and secondary prevention [40, 41, 17].

• Important data comes from post-myocardial infarction surveys. Haffner [33], based on two prospective studies [42, 43], concluded that patients with type 2 diabetes without preexisting myocardial infarction have a risk of developing myocardial infarction similar to non-diabetic patients with previous myocardial infarction. In addition the pre-hospital mortality is higher in patients with diabetes than in non-diabetic patients. It can be concluded that in people with type 2 diabetes, the treatment of cardiovascular risk factors must be as aggressive as in patients with established coronary heart disease [33]. Another important demonstration of the role of diabetes in the occurrence of myocardial infarction have recently come from the INTERHEART study [44], which included 11 119 cases of myocardial infarction and 13 648 controls from 52 countries. In this study, the first three clinical risk factors for myocardial infarction were current smoking, psychosocial factors (depression, general stress, low locus of control and major life events), and **diabetes** (odd ratio 2.87, 2.67 and 2.37, respectively).

• All these facts clearly suggest that:

– The prevention of macrovascular disease in type 2 diabetes could be achieved by controlling the cardiovascular risk [45–50].

– This can be accomplished only with a multifactorial intervention strategy, which must focus at least five *bad companions* in diabetes: hyperglycemia, hypertension, dyslipidemia, obesity and smoking.

– The interventions should be as aggressive and intensive as for patients with macrovascular disease and that all patients with type 2 diabetes

must be considered as candidates for secondary prevention irrespective of their cardiovascular status. In the new AHA guidelines on primary prevention of coronary heart disease, people with type 2 diabetes are included in the group of *coronary heart disease risk equivalents*. For them, secondary prevention is suggested [51, 52].

• Until recently, there was no intensive multifactorial intervention trial in type 2 diabetes to demonstrate the benefits on macrovascular disease endpoints and related mortality [53], this having been shown only for microvascular complications [54]. The results of Steno-2 Study, published in January 2003, demonstrated that a targeted, intensified, multifactorial intervention in people with type 2 diabetes and microalbuminuria, reduces the risk of cardiovascular and microvascular events by about 50 percent [55]. The ADDITION study (Anglo-Danish-Dutch Study of Intensive Treatment In People with Screen Detected Diabetes in Primary Care) [56], which began in 2000 and the ACCORD study (Action to Control Cardiovascular Risk in Diabetes) [19] have the same main objectives.

• In addition there are many other factors both traditional and novel which are not included in Table 24.1. Only a part of them are shown in Table 24.9. Not all factors presented here are validated by clinical trials. As a consequence not all of them are mentioned in clinical guidelines. Until the large-scale studies define which factors are valid, more important or even specific for diabetes, practitioners should extrapolate the data from the general population to people with diabetes.

Table 24.9

Traditional and so called novel cardiovascular risk factors for people with diabetes (from [1] with kind permission)

Traditional risk factors	**So called novel risk factors**
Poor glycemic control	Increased Lp(a)
Dyslipidemia	Increased IDL
• ▲ total cholesterol	Increased small dense LDL
• ▲ LDL cholesterol	Glycated and oxidized lipoproteins and
• ▼ HDL cholesterol	albumin
• ▲ triglycerides	Immune response to modified lipoprotein
Hypertension	Increased cholesterol ester transfer
Abdominal obesity	protein
Insulinresistance / hyperinsulinism	Low level of paraoxonase (PON) and
Physical inactivity	certain PON genotypes

Table 24.9

(continued)

Traditional risk factors	So called novel risk factors
Hypercaloric / hyperlipidic intake Smoking Increasing age Personal and familial history of atherosclerosis Long duration of diabetes Microalbuminuria Hemostatic factors • impaired fibrinolytic activity: fibrinogen, PAI-1*, tPA activity* • FPA, TAT, f VII* • platelets, leucokytes and erythrocytes abnormalities • plasma viscosity	Hyperhomocysteinemia Markers of inflammation • increased white blood cell count • increased C-reactive protein Infections with • Chlamydia pneumoniae • Helicobacter pylori Periodontal disease Markers of endothelial dysfunction • increased von Willebrand factor • increased trombomodulin • increased adhesion molecules Medial artery calcification Postprandial state Depression Erectile dysfunction

*PAI-1: plasminogen activator inhibitor 1; tPA: tissue plasminogen activator; FPA: fibrinopeptide A; TAT: thrombin – antithrombin; fVII: coagulation factor VII.

PRACTICAL APPROACH TO THE CONTROL OF RISK IN PEOPLE WITH TYPE 2 DIABETES

In daily practice, a stepwise implementation for controlling the global cardiovascular risk is needed as shown in Table 24.10.

Table 24.10

The stepwise control of cardiovascular risk in persons with type 2 diabetes (from [1] with kind permission)

Actions	Focus on
Step1: IDENTIFICATION	Cardiovascular risk factors (as much as possible) Cardiovascular disease as: • Coronary heart disease (CHD) • CHD equivalents: aortic aneurism, ischemia of the extremities, carotid atherosclerosis
Step 2: INTERPRETATION	Global cardiovascular risk: scores and stratification high, medium, low Type of prevention: • Primary: short term high risk, long term high risk • Secondary Objectives to be achieved for each factor and disease
Step 3: INTERVENTION	For all identified risk factors and disease with appropriate clinical management, that is: • Lifestyle optimization: diet, physical exercise, alcohol reduction • Drugs • Therapeutical education • Current monitoring • Global evaluation

These actions are in line with the new proposals from the American Heart Association regarding … *the pathway from risk assessment to risk reduction* [57] where three steps are involved:

• measurements of risk factors,

• interpretation of risk-related data with an estimation of risk in both absolute and relative terms,

• intervention to minimize the actual risk or to prevent the development of other risks.

In the light of these considerations we will focus on the practical aspects of identification and evaluation of cardiovascular risk and disease in people with type 2 diabetes.

IDENTIFICATION AND EVALUATION OF CARDIOVASCULAR RISK AND DISEASE IN TYPE 2 DIABETES

IDENTIFICATION AND EVALUATION OF THE MAIN RISK FACTORS

Identification and evaluation of the main cardiovascular risk factors in patients with type 2 diabetes is strongly and unanimously recommended in all principal international guidelines [2, 7, 8, 58–73].

The identification and evaluation of risk factors in persons with type 2 diabetes should be made according to Grundy's recommendations (1999) [2, 12] as summarized in Table 24.11.

The depression and erectile dysfunction must also be considered as risk factors in the clinical practice [74, 75, 21].

In Table 24.12 a summary of the levels of main cardiovascular risk factors is presented. Few of them have to be adapted to ADA's recommendations [65].

The identification and evaluation of cardiovascular risk factors require a few comments:

• The assessment of major (causal) and predisposing risk factors is compulsory, while the evaluation of conditional factors should be optional.

• The glycemic status should be evaluated with HbA1c, fasting and postprandial glycemia [76], as shown in Table 24.13. Both will be correlated with the macro- or microvascular risk as it has been recommended by recent guidelines.

• The assessment of waist circumference will easily offer a clinical marker of insulin resistance. For the screening of the metabolic syndrome in patients with diabetes an initial and very simple step has been suggested, by identifying the persons with hypertensive waist, that is: enlarged waist ($\geq$ 88 cm for women and $\geq$ 102 cm for men) and high blood pressure (> 130/85 mmHg) [77].

• Regarding the conditional risk factors (Lp(a), LDL type B, apoprotein B, homocysteine, fibrinogen, PAI-1) their role in risk stratification is not yet sufficiently known. In addition, their measurements are not yet widespread recommended in daily practice [51].

Table 24.11

The priority of identification and evaluation of cardiovascular risk factors in type 2 diabetes
(from [1] with kind permission)

Compulsory assessment		Optional assessment
Causal or major RF	Predisposing RF	Conditional RF
Cigarette smoking Blood pressure Lipids and lipoproteins Albuminuria Glycemic control	Body fat: BMI Fat distribution: waist circumference (insulin- resistance as clinical marker) Physical activity Family history	Lipoprotein (a) Small LDL particles (LDL – B) Apoprotein B Homocysteine Fibrinogen Plasminogen activator inhibitor 1

Table 24.12

The levels of main cardiovascular risk factors suggested to be assessed in type 2 diabetes mellitus by the European Arterial Risk Policy Group on behalf of the International Diabetes Federation (from [1] with kind permission)*

Risk factor	Low risk	Moderate risk	High risk
Total serum cholesterol mmol/l	< 5.2	5.2 – 6.5	> 6.5
mg/dl	< 200	200 – 250	> 250
LDL cholesterol mmol/l	< 3.0	3.0 – 4.0	> 4.0
mg/dl	< 115	115 – 154	> 154
HDL cholesterol mmol/l	> 1.2	1.0 – 1.2	< 1.0
mg/dl	> 46	38 – 46	< 38

Table 24.12

(continued)

Risk factor	Low risk	Moderate risk	High risk
Serum triglycerides mmol/l	< 2.3	2.3 – 4.0	> 4.0
mg/dl	< 204	204 – 354	> 354
Blood pressure (mmHg)	< 140/90	140/90 –160/95	> 160/95
Glycated haemoglobin (%Hb)[a]	< 6.5	6.5 – 8.5	> 8.5
Body mass index (kg/m^2)	< 25.0	25.0 – 30.0	> 30.0
Raised albumin excretion[b]:	–	–	–
– albumin, mg/l	< 15	–	> 15
– albumin: creatinine ratio mg/mmol	< 2.5[c] / 3.5[d]	–	> 2.5[c] / 3.5[d]
Smoking (cigarettes/day)	Not smoking	1 – 10	> 10
Ethnic group	Europid	–	Non Europid
Personal or family history of arterial disease	None	Family history of MI/stroke	Previous MI/ stroke /PVD

[a] HbA1c: assumes a DCCT standardized assay (normal < 6.1%)
[b] Early morning urine sample
[c] Men
[d] Women
MI, myocardial infarction
PVD, peripheral vascular disease

* According to the ADA's recommendations [65], the low risk category should include:
  - LDL cholesterol < 100 mg/dl (< 2.6 mmol/l) (B – evidence level)
  - Triglycerides < 150 mg/dl (< 1.7 mmol/l) (C – evidence level)
  - HDL cholesterol – in men: > 45 mg/dl (> 1.15 mmol/l) (C – level evidence)
                        – in women: > 55 mg/dl (> 1.7 mmol/l) (C – level evidence)
  - Blood pressure < 130/0 mmHg (A – level evidence)
  - Waist: in men <94 cm; in women < 80 cm

Table 24.13

The blood glucose control assessment (from [59] with kind permission)

	Low risk	Arterial risk	Macrovascular risk
HbA1c (DCCT standardized) % Hb	≤ 6.5	> 6.5	> 7.5
Venous plasma glucose			
Fasting/pre-prandial			
mmol/l	≤ 6.0	> 6.0	≥ 7.0
mg/dl	< 110	≥ 110	> 125
Self-monitored blood glucose			
Fasting/pre-prandial			
mmol/l	≤ 5.5	> 5.5	> 6.0
mg/dl	< 100	≥ 100	≥ 110
Post-prandial (peak)			
mmol/l	< 7.5	≥ 7.5	> 9.0
mg/dl	< 135	≥ 135	> 160

SCREENING AND DIAGNOSIS OF MACROVASCULAR DISEASE

Screening and diagnosis of macrovascular disease should be part of the global evaluation of each person with type 2 diabetes.

The objectives of cardiovascular investigations in people with type 2 diabetes are as follows:
- The early detection of clinical and sub-clinical coronary heart disease or cardiomyopathy, cerebrovascular disease and peripheral arteriopathy [78, 79].

• To establish the coronary heart disease risk equivalents (see also Table 24.4): abdominal aortic aneurism, ischemia of the extremities, carotid atherosclerosis [52, 2].

• Their complete diagnosis.

It is beyond the scope of this chapter to detail the diagnosis of cardiovascular disease, which will follow the current guidelines.

ASSESSMENT OF GLOBAL CARDIOVASCULAR RISK IN PEOPLE WITH TYPE 2 DIABETES: TOOLS AND RULES

Based on the large prospective studies (Framingham, PROCAM), charts and scores have been developed to estimate the absolute risk for a coronary event in the next 10 years.

Three tools are recommended: the Coronary Chart developed by the Second Joint Task Force of European and other Societies on Coronary Prevention [8] thereafter to be referred to as Euro'98, Risk Stratification Chart for diabetic subjects with or without microalbuminuria [80] (UK'99) and the New Framingham Risk Scores [51, 52, 81, 82].

Very recently, two new methods to estimate the risk were developed: the charts of the Third Joint Task Force of European and other Societies on Cardiovascular Disease Prevention in Clinical Practice [83] to be referred as Euro'2003 and the UKPDS Risk Engine [84, 85], developed from the data of the United Kingdom Prospective Diabetes Study (UKPDS).

CORONARY CHART "EURO'98"

This chart is based on a risk function derived from the Framingham Study [8]. It is based on five risk factors: total cholesterol level, systolic blood pressure, age, sex and smoking status. The absolute 10 years risk of developing coronary heart disease (angina, non-fatal myocardial infarction or coronary death) can be estimated in the general population or in people with diabetes (Plate 24.1).

Coronary risk chart for primary CHD prevention in diabetes mellitus (from 8 with kind permission).

RISK STRATIFICATION CHARTS "UK'99"

This chart [80] is also based on the Framingham equations. It can estimate the 10 years absolute risk of coronary heart events for non-diabetic and diabetic people, with or without microalbuminuria. The risk has been calculated for men and women according to age (30–70 years), systolic blood pressure, total to high density lipoprotein cholesterol ratio and smoking status. The coronary absolute risk predicted refers to angina, myocardial infarction and coronary death [80]. The charts are shown in Plate 24.2. The number of patients required to treat for 10 years to prevent one coronary heart disease event are also outlined. The calculations reveal that interventions reduce the risk of a coronary risk event by 25% [80].

For a busy practitioner it is wise to count the number of different risk factors. Two additional risk factors in a patient with diabetes aged above 50 years can give a 40% risk of cardiovascular event in 10 years.

THE NEW FRAMINGHAM RISK SCORES

The new Framingham risk scores [51, 52, 81, 82] estimate both absolute risk and relative risk. However, the ATP III [15] do suggest to use in practice the absolute coronary risk, according to the data presented in Figure 24.1.

The first step is to calculate the points for each major risk factor: age, total and HDL cholesterol, systolic blood pressure, diabetes and smoking status. The score is obtained by adding up the points separately for men and women (Figure 24.1). This corresponds to the absolute risk for developing, in 10 years, either total coronary heart disease (all forms of clinical coronary heart disease) or hard coronary heart disease (myocardial infarction and coronary death).

Estimate of 10-Year Risk for Men — Framingham Point Scores

Age	Points
20-34	-9
35-39	-4
40-44	0
45-49	3
50-54	6
55-59	8
60-64	10
65-69	11
70-74	12
75-79	13

Total cholesterol	Points				
Age	20-39	40-49	50-59	60-69	70-79
< 160	0	0	0	0	0
160-199	4	3	2	1	0
200-239	7	5	3	1	0
240-279	9	6	4	2	1
≥ 280	11	8	5	3	1

	Points				
Age	20-39	40-49	50-59	60-69	70-79
Nonsmoker	0	0	0	0	0
Smoker	8	5	3	1	1

HDL (mg/ dl)	Points
≥ 60	-1
50-59	0
40-49	1
< 40	2

Systolic BP (mmHg)	If Untreated	Treated
< 120	0	0
120-129	0	1
130-139	1	2
140-159	1	2
≥ 160	2	3

Point Total	10-Year Risk (%)
< 0	< 1
0	1
1	1
2	1
3	1
4	1
5	2
6	2
7	3
8	4
9	5
10	6
11	8
12	10
13	12
14	16
15	20
16	25
≥ 17	≥ 30

10-Year Risk___%

Estimate of 10-Year Risk for Women — Framingham Point Scores

Age	Points
20-34	-7
35-39	-3
40-44	0
45-49	3
50-54	6
55-59	8
60-64	10
65-69	12
70-74	14
75-79	16

Total cholesterol	Points				
Age	20-39	40-49	50-59	60-69	70-79
< 160	0	0	0	0	0
160-199	4	3	2	1	1
200-239	8	6	4	2	1
240-279	11	8	5	3	2
≥ 280	13	10	7	4	2

	Points				
Age	20-39	40-49	50-59	60-69	70-79
Nonsmoker	0	0	0	0	0
Smoker	9	7	4	2	1

HDL (mg/ dl)	Points
≥ 60	-1
50-59	0
40-49	1
< 40	2

Systolic BP (mmHg)	If Untreated	Treated
< 120	0	0
120-129	1	3
130-139	2	4
140-159	3	5
≥ 160	4	6

Point Total	10-Year Risk (%)
< 9	< 1
9	1
10	1
11	1
12	1
13	2
14	2
15	3
16	4
17	5
18	6
19	8
20	11
21	14
22	17
23	22
24	27
≥ 25	≥ 30

10-Year Risk___%

Figure 24.1

The new Framingham Risk Scores (from [15] with kind permission).

Risk assessment for determining the 10-year risk for developing CHD is carried out using Framingham risk scoring (for men and for women). The risk factors included in the Framingham calculation of 10-year risk are: age, total cholesterol, HDL cholesterol, systolic blood pressure, treatment for hypertension and cigarette smoking. The first step is to calculate the number of points for each risk factor. For initial assessment, values for total cholesterol and HDL cholesterol are required. Because of a larger data base, Framingham estimates are more robust for total cholesterol than for LDL cholesterol. Note, however, that LDL cholesterol level remains the primary target of therapy. Total cholesterol and HDL cholesterol values should be the average of at least two measurements obtained from lipoprotein analysis. The blood pressure value used is that obtained at the time of assessment, regardless of whether the person is on antihypertensive therapy. However, if the person is on antihypertensive treatment, an extra point is added beyond points for the blood pressure reading because treated hypertension carries residual risk. The average of several blood pressure measurements, as recommended by the Joint National Committee (JNC), is needed for an accurate measure of baseline blood pressure. The designation "smoker" means any cigarette smoking in the past month. The total risk score sums the points for each risk factor. The 10-year risk for myocardial infarction and coronary death (hard CHD) is estimated from total points, and the person is categorized according absolute 10-year risk as indicated.

EURO'2003 CHARTS FOR FATAL CVD (CARDIOVASCULAR DISEASE)

This chart is based on the SCORE (Systematic Coronary Risk Evaluation) system, derived from a large dataset of prospective European studies and predicts any kind of fatal atherosclerotic endpoints (myocardial infarction, ischaemic stroke and peripheral arterial disease) over a ten-year period [83].

In SCORE the following risk factors are considered: gender, age, smoking, systolic blood pressure and total cholesterol. Since the chart predicts fatal events the threshold for being at high risk is defined as $\geq 5\%$, instead of the previous $\geq 20\%$ in charts using a composite coronary endpoint. Euro'2003 includes two risk charts: one for the high-risk regions of Europe and the other for the low risk regions (Plate 24.3a and 3b).

UKPDS RISK ENGINE

UKPDS Risk Engine [84, 85] is a model for predicting the absolute risk of coronary heart disease (CHD) and of first stroke in male and female with type 2 diabetes, and it is the first diabetes-specific model available at the moment. The equations are based on data from 4549 newly-diagnosed type 2 diabetic patients enrolled in the UK Prospective Diabetes Study. The first model estimates the absolute risk of CHD and incorporates glycemia, systolic blood pressure and lipid levels as risk factors, in addition to age, sex, ethnic group, smoking status and time since diagnosis of diabetes [82]. The second model estimates the risk of first stroke, the variables included are duration of diabetes, age, sex, smoking, systolic blood pressure, total cholesterol to HDL cholesterol ratio and presence of atrial fibrillation [85]. Both models are incorporated in the UKPDS Risk engine software, which is available at the website http://www.dtu.ox.ac.uk/riskengine/.

FUNCTIONS, LIMITS AND INTERPRETATION OF RESULTS

The main functions and the potential uses of these tools [8, 51, 52, 80–85] are:

- To assess the global cardiovascular risk in terms of absolute and relative risk,
- To help us to tailor a plan for intervention and to predict and evaluate its effect,
- To educate and to motivate patients,
- To motivate physicians in order to become more involved in cardiovascular risk control.

Before using these tools, practitioners should be informed about their limits [8, 51, 52, 80–85]:

- All these tools can be used only for people without atherosclerotic cardiovascular disease,
- They overestimate the risk in young people and underestimate it in the case of clustering risk factors with people displaying the metabolic syndrome,
- For certain reasons a few risk factors are not used in the tools: obesity, familial history, physical inactivity, LDL cholesterol, triglycerides, and fibrinogen. Nevertheless they remain an important target for intervention.

To interpret the values provided by this estimation, a few rules have to be taken into consideration:

- People with an absolute coronary risk $\geq 20\%$ (or total CVD risk $\geq 5\%$) have the likelihood of developing a coronary event similar to those with established coronary heart disease. They have to be submitted for short-term high-risk primary prevention [47].
- If the absolute risk is $< 20\%$ but the relative risk is moderate or high (Figure 24.1) a young person should be considered a candidate for long-term high-risk action because in time, a moderate or high relative risk will become a high absolute risk [40].
- All those with coronary heart disease equivalents (Table 24.4) must be considered as having a high absolute risk ($\geq 20\%$). Recommendations used for secondary prevention should be applied.
- People with type 2 diabetes represent a coronary heart disease equivalent and must be treated appropriately [52]. However, it is recognized that the absolute risk of these persons is underestimated by Framingham Scores [81]. That is why the risk estimated by means of this tool should be elevated to a higher risk category

[86]. Alternatively, estimates of individual risk could be abandoned and all people with diabetes could be treated with statins and other effective agents, as suggested by a recent review on the prediction of risk in people with diabetes [87]. The new model from the UKPDS Risk Engine can offer supplementary information regarding the absolute risk of coronary events and stroke in this category of patients [84, 85].

TARGETING OBJECTIVES AND PLANNING INTERVENTIONS

The link between the assessment of cardiovascular risk and intervention should be the interpretations of the results and finally the targeting of objectives and planning of the interventions. The clinical judgment has an important role in these actions.

After data collection, the following parameters have to be interpreted:

• Levels of individual risk factors and cardiovascular status and how are they modified versus optimal or reasonable standards,

• Absolute risk,

• Patient education and his or her desire, willingness and possibilities to change.

This interpretation would further allow establishing [1]:

• The realistic and individualized objectives for each risk factor, which have to be agreed by the persons,

• The priorities of the objectives, which are to be approached,

• The methods of intervention,

• The stepwise implementation of these methods.

The clinical management is the most important part of the intervention. It must be adapted to each focused factor and encompasses four programs:

• **T**herapeutical program: lifestyle optimization and pharmacotherapy,

• **E**ducation or more precisely *therapeutical education* as a specific part of a global education program to be applied for people with type 2 diabetes [88],

• **M**onitoring program that is a regular control of the patient's specific parameters,

• **E**valuation: an annual full review of the person.

The acronym of these actions is THEME, a suggestive term for practitioners [89].

INTERVENTIONS FOR THE GLOBAL CONTROL OF CARDIOVASCULAR RISK

SECONDARY PREVENTION

These recommendations represent the secondary prevention of atherosclerotic cardiovascular disease. In Table 24.14 the strategies proposed by the Second Joint Task Force of European and other Societies on Coronary Prevention [8] for the general population are shown.

Table 24.14

Lifestyle and therapeutic goals for patients with CHD, or other atherosclerotic disease, and for healthy high-risk individuals (from [8] with kind permission)

Patients with CHD or other atherosclerotic disease	Healthy high-risk individuals. Absolute CHD risk ≥20% over 10 years, or will exceed 20% if projected to age 60
1	2
Lifestyle Stop smoking, make healthy food choices, be physically active and achieve ideal weight.	
Other risk factors Blood pressure <140/90 mmHg, Total cholesterol <5.0 mmol/l (190 mg/dl) LDL cholesterol <3.0 mmol/l (115 mg/dl) When these risk factor goals are not achieved by lifestyle, blood pressure and cholesterol lowering drug therapies should be used.	

Table 24.14

(continued)

1	2
Other prophylactic drug therapies	
Aspirin (at least 75 mg) for all coronary patients, those with cerebral atherosclerosis and peripheral atherosclerotic disease. β-blockers in patients following myocardial infarction. ACE inhibitors in those with symptoms or signs of heart failure at the time of myocardial infarction, or with chronic LV systolic dysfunction (ejection fraction <40%). Anticoagulants in selected coronary patients.	Aspirin (75 mg) in treated hypertensive patients and in men at particularly high CHD risk.
Screen close relatives	
Screen close relatives of patients with premature (men <55 yrs, women <65 yrs) CHD	Screen close relatives if familial hypercholesterolaemia or other inherited dyslipidaemia is suspected.

Table 24.15

Primary prevention in coronary asymptomatic patients at high short-term risk (CHD risk equivalents)
(from [52] with kind permission)

Patient selection (CHD risk equivalents)
  Symptomatic peripheral arterial disease
  Abdominal aortic aneurysm
  Symptomatic carotid artery disease
  Type 2 diabetes[*]
  Multiple risk factors (Framingham risk for hard CHD >20% / 10 years)[**]
Smoking goal: complete cessation
Blood pressure goal: ≤149/90 mmHg (≤130/85 mmHg in type 2 diabetes)[*]
Primary lipid goal: LDL cholesterol ≤100 mg/dl[***]
Glucose goal: near normal glucose and near normal hemoglobin A1c(<7%)
Antiplatelet therapy: aspirin 80 mg/dl if not contraindicated
Life habits: NCEP/AHA step II diet, weight loss in overweight patients (goal body mass index 21–25 kg/m^2), moderate-intensity exercise (30 – 60 minutes) 3 or 4 times weekly

[*]Includes Americans of white, Hispanic, black, and South Asian origin. May not include Americans of East Asian origin.

[**]Accuracy of absolute risk enhanced by substitution of noninvasive estimates of coronary plaque burden for age as a risk factor.

[***]Most patients with baseline LDL cholesterol levels > 130 mg/dl will require cholesterol-lowering drugs to achieve the target of therapy. When on-treatment serum LDL cholesterol is in the range of 100 to 129 mg/dl, several therapeutic option are available: to increase the drug dose (or to combine with another cholesterol-lowering drug) to achieve an LDL cholesterol <100 mg/dl, to add another lipid-lowering drug to improve triglyceride and HDL cholesterol levels, or to aggressively modify other risk factors. Clinical judgments is required whether to start (or to increase the dose of) cholesterol-lowering drugs in patients > 65 years old.

* The newest ADA's recommendations: < 130/80 mmHg.

Table 24.16

Long-term primary prevention in the clinical setting (from [52] with kind permission)

All categorical risk factors should be treated professionally
Smoking goal: smoking cessation
Blood pressure goal: <140/90 mmHg*
Serum cholesterol and lipid goals
Desirable LDL cholesterol: <130 mg/dl
Very high LDL cholesterol (≥ 190 mg/dl)
Most patients will require cholesterol-lowering drugs
Two or more risk factors* (absolute risk <20%/10 years for hard CHD)
LDL cholesterol goal: <130 mg/dl
Zero to 1 risk factor*:
Acceptable LDL cholesterol: 130 to 159 mg/dl
Elevated triglycerides (>200 mg/dl) or low HDL cholesterol (<35 mg/dl)
Emphasize weight reduction and increase physical activity
Consider nicotinic acid or fibric acid only after LDL cholesterol goal of <130 mg/dl is achieved (limited clinical trial evidence of efficacy)
Life habits: NCEP/AHA step I diet, weight loss in overweight patients (goal: body mass index 21 – 25 kg/m^2), moderate-intensity exercise (30 – 60 minutes) 3 or 4 time weekly
* Includes risk factors other than LDL cholesterol >160 mg/dl. Ie. cigarette smoking, hypertension, low HDL cholesterol (<35 mg/dl), family history of premature CHD, age (men ≥ 45 years; women >55 years or postmenopausal)

* The newest ADA's recommendations: < 130/80 mmHg.

Lifestyle and therapeutic goals for patients with CHD, or other atherosclerotic disease, and for healthy high-risk individuals (from 8 with kind permission)

For the people with diabetes and cardiovascular disease, American Heart Association has proposed the following prophylactic measures [2]:

- Smoking cessation
- Blood pressure control
- Glucose control
- Regular physical activity
- Weight management
- Antiplatelet agents
- ACE inhibitors in post MI patients
- β blockers
- Estrogens

PRIMARY PREVENTION

According to the concept of primary prevention of coronary heart disease and other atherosclerotic cardiovascular disease [52] the

strategies for general population are shown in Table 24.15 and 24.16.

The greatest part of the measures used for secondary prevention can also be used for primary prevention in people with diabetes [2].

SOME PRACTICAL ASPECTS OF CLINICAL MANAGEMENT RELATED TO THE GLOBAL CARDIOVASCULAR RISK IN TYPE 2 DIABETES

In this chapter we only want to underline some practical aspects regarding: 1) lifestyle optimization, 2) glycemic control, 3) the management of hypertension and microalbuminuria, 4) weight management, 5) lipids control and 6) the anti – aggregant treatment. These will be based on the quality of evidence proposed in the recent ADA's recommendations for clinical practice [65].

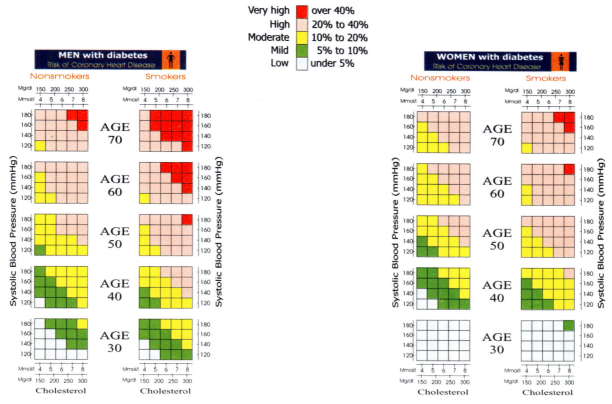

Plate 24.1

Coronary risk chart for primary CHD prevention in diabetes mellitus (from [8] with kind permission). Ten-year risk level.

How to use the Coronary Risk Chart for Primary Prevention.

The chart is for estimating coronary heart disease (CHD) risk for individuals who have not developed symptomatic CHD or other atherosclerotic disease. Patients with CHD are already at high risk and require intensive lifestyle intervention and, as necessary, drug therapies to achieve risk factor goals.

- To estimate a person's absolute 10 year risk of a CHD event, find the table for their gender, smoking status and age. Within the table, find the cell nearest to their systolic blood pressure (mmHg) and total cholesterol (mmol/l or mg/dl).
- The effect of lifetime exposure to risk factors can be seen by following the table upwards. This can be used when advising younger people.
- High risk individuals are defined as those whose 10 year CHD risk exceeds 20% or will exceed 20% if projected to age 60
- CHD risk is higher than indicated in the chart for those with familial hyperlipidemia, those with a family history of premature cardiovascular disease, those with low HDL cholesterol (these tables assume HDL cholesterol to be 1.0 mmol/l or 39 mg/dl in men and 1.1 mmol/l or 43 mg/dl in women), those with raised triglyceride levels > 2.0 mmol/l or 180 mg/dl, as the person approaches the next age category.
- To find a person's relative risk, compare their risk category with that for other people of the same age. The absolute risk shown here may not apply to all populations, especially those with a low CHD incidence. Relative risk is likely to apply to most populations.
- The effect of changing cholesterol, smoking status or blood pressure can be read from the chart.

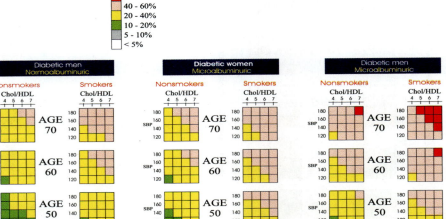

Plate 24.2

Ten-year risk of CHD diabetic men and women without and microalbuminuria (from [80] with kind permission).

Risk tables diabetic patients (J.S. Yudkin & N. Chaturvedi).

In order to read a person's risk, identify the chart relating to the person's gender, age and smoking status. Within the chart, find the cell nearest to the person's level of total: high density lipoprotein cholesterol ratio and systolic blood pressure. Compare the cell tone with the key and read the risk level. For south Asian subjects, people with symptomatic or asymptomatic cardiovascular disease, a family history of coronary disease at an early age, central obesity, or left ventricular hypertrophy, the risk level will be greater than that indicated in the chart by around one category. The risk will be higher at lower levels, or if concentrations of triglyceride exceed 2.2 mmol/l. Chol/HDL= total cholesterol: high density lipoprotein cholesterol ratio. SBP = Systolic Blood Pressure in mmHg.

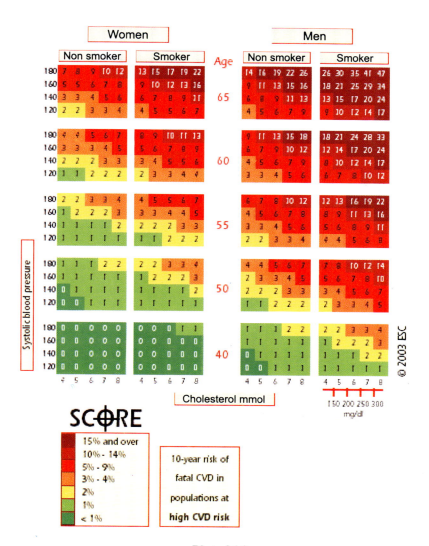

Plate 24.3a

Ten years of fatal CVD in high risk regions of Europe by gender, age, systolic blood pressure, total cholesterol and smoking status (from [83] with kind permission).

• The high risk chart should be used in all the countries of Europe other than Belgium, France, Greece, Italy, Luxembourg, Spain, Switzerland and Portugal.

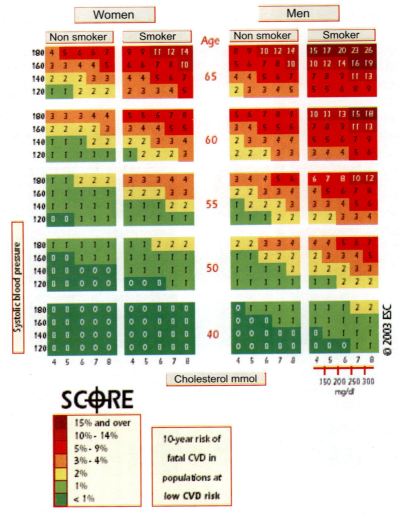

Plate 24.3b

Ten years of fatal CVD in low risk regions of Europe by gender, age, systolic blood pressure, total cholesterol and smoking status (from [83] with kind permission).

• The low risk chart should be used in Belgium, France, Greece, Italy, Spain, Switzerland and Portugal; the high risk chart should be used in all other countries of Europe.

• To estimate a person's total ten year risk of CVD death, find the table for their gender, smoking status and age. Within the table find the cell nearest to the person's systolic blood pressure (mmHg) and total cholesterol (mmol/l or mg/dl).

• The effect of lifetime exposure to risk factors can be seen by following the table upwards. This can be used when advising young people.

• Low risk individuals should be offered advice to maintain their low risk status. Those who are at 5% risk or higher or will reach this level in middle age should be given maximal attention.

• To define a person's relative risk, compare their risk category with that of a non-smoking person of the same age and gender, blood pressure <140/90 mmHg and total cholesterol < 5mmol/l (190 mg/dl).

• The cart can be used to give some indications of the effect of changes from one category to another, for example when the subject stops smoking or reduces other risk factors.

Qualifiers:

Note that total CVD risk may be higher than indicated in the chart:

– as the person approaches the next age category

– in asymptomatic subjects with pre-clinical evidence of atherosclerosis (*e.g.* CT scan, ultrasonography)

– in subjects with strong family history of premature CVD

– in subjects with low HDL cholesterol levels, with raised triglyceride level, with impaired glucose tolerance, and with raised levels of C-reactive protein, fibrinogen, homocysteine, apolipoprotein B or Lp(a)

– in obese or sedentary subjects.

Accordingly, three levels of evidence have been defined [65]:

• A-level of evidence based on large well-designed clinical trials or well-done meta-analysis,

• B-level of evidence that comes from well-conducted cohort studies,

• C-level of evidence from poorly controlled or uncontrolled studies.

A separate category of recommendations is based on expert opinion (E-level) in which there is yet no evidence from clinical trials, in which clinical trials may be unpractical, or in which there is conflicting evidence [65].

The clinical judgment should also be added to the evidences in order to treat individuals with certain peculiarities and needs.

Lifestyle optimization

• Lifestyle optimization is a compulsory objective. According to IDF recommendations [59] a four-point plan should be implemented: 1) a balanced diet, 2) physical exercise, 3) seeking good medical advice and taking control of your life and 4) social events. The first two points are strongly related to cardiovascular risk and ample evidence was provided (A, B and C levels) [65, 73] supporting their importance. The therapeutic education is the best method to accomplish these objectives.

• Smoking cessation is extremely important and must be maintained. This can be achieved with intensive therapeutic education [88].

Glycemic control

• According to the international guidelines [58] the management of hyperglycemia should be based on four steps [58]: 1) lifestyle optimization, 2) oral monotherapy, 3) oral combined therapy and 4) insulin therapy (Figure 24.2). Achievement of metabolic control is a step-by-step process. If the glycemic objectives are not achieved, the next step has to be initiated [58].

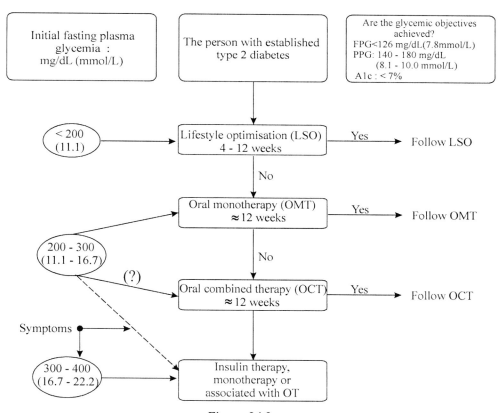

Figure 24.2

Step strategy suggested for glycemic control in type 2 diabetes (from [1] with kind permission).

The initiation and duration of each step is determined by fasting glycemic values, glycemic related symptoms, global risk, achievement of glycemic objectives based on existing evidence and clinical judgment.

• Regarding insulin therapy in type 2 diabetes mellitus, it has the following indications [58]: failure to achieve glycemic control despite maximum doses of combinations of blood glucose lowering agents, decompensation due to intercurrent events, perioperative management, pregnancy and lactation, failure of vital organs, allergy or other serious reactions to oral drugs, marked hyperglycemia at the time of presentation and acute myocardial infarction. It should be mentioned that in every patient who needs prandial insulin, the use of a rapidly-acting insulin analogue should be prescribed [58], while as basal insulin, glargine would be preferred [90].

• There are some evidence (A, B and C level) regarding the possibilities to achieve the treatment targets and also to reduce the cardiovascular risk by controlling glycemia [65].

Management of hypertension and microalbuminuria

• The goal of treatment is systolic blood pressure < 130 mmHg (B-level of evidence) and diastolic blood pressure < 80 mmHg (A-level of evidence) [72, 91].

• Patients with a blood pressure of 130–139/80–89 mmHg should be given lifestyle optimization therapy alone for a maximum of 3 months. If targets are not achieved, the pharmacotherapy should be initiated (A-level of evidence) [72]. A reduction of blood pressure can be achieved by reduction of sodium intake and modest weight loss (A-level of evidence).

• If the initial levels of blood pressure are ≥ 140/90 mmHg, drug therapy should be prescribed in addition to lifestyle optimization (A-level of evidence) [72, 91].

• The drugs of choice are: ACE-inhibitors (particularly if microalbuminuria is present and/or in the presence of heart failure), calcium channel blockers, β_2-blockers (particularly in the presence of chronic coronary artery disease), α_1-blockers (particularly if dyslipidemia is present) and thiazide diuretics. As diuretic, indapamide can also be recommended [58]. If ACE inhibitors are not tolerated, angiotensin-receptor blockers (ARBs) may be used [72]. In patients with type 2 diabetes, hypertension, macroalbuminuria (>300 mg/day), nephropathy, or renal insufficiency, an ARB should be strongly considered [72]. The use of α_1-blockers was recently reconsidered as a result of the ALLHAT Study where they were associated with a higher incidence of heart failure [92]. It seems reasonable to use these as second-line agents when preferred classes have been ineffective or when other specific indications, such as benign prostatic hypertrophy (BPH), are present [72].

• The rational combinations suggested would be [58]: ACE-inhibitors + low-dose thiazides or calcium channel blockers, calcium channel blockers or α_1-blockers + β_2-blockers and/or diuretics, with the same comments for the use of alpha-blockers.

• ACE-inhibitors seem to have additional benefits on cardiovascular events, metabolic abnormalities and microalbuminuria mainly in patients over the age of 55 with or without hypertension but with another cardiovascular risk factor (A-level of evidence) [72, 93, 94, 95].

• In individuals with microalbuminuria, reduction of protein intake to $0.8–1.0$ $g \cdot kg^{-1} \cdot wt^{-1}$ per day may slow the progression of nephropathy (C-level evidence) [73].

• Very recent data shows that the risk of cardiovascular disease is continuous and beginning at 115/75 mmHg it doubles at each increment of 20/10 mmHg [96, 97]. These findings could have an impact on the management of high blood pressure in the near future.

• In the recent American guidelines for the management of hypertension [96] values of blood pressure of 120–139/80–89 mmHg are considered as prehypertension and lifestyle changes are recommended to prevent cardiovascular disease.

Weight management

This must be a priority of any strategy. Practitioners should not forget the benefits that could be achieved by moderate weight loss and its maintenance (A and B evidence level) [65, 73]. The role of weight control in persons with type 2 diabetes has been pointed out by the ADA Position Statement [98]. For all overweight and obese people the objective of weight control is the long-term weight loss on the order of 5–7% of starting weight. Moderate weight loss improves glycemic control, reduces cardiovascular risk and can prevent the development of diabetes mellitus in those with prediabetes.

Lipid control

The *lipid objectives* for adults with diabetes are as follows [66]:
- LDL cholesterol < 100 mg/dl (2.6 mmol/l) (B-level of evidence)
- HDL cholesterol – in men: > 45 mg/dl (1.15 mmol/l)

         – in women: > 55 mg/dl (1.40 mmol/l) (C–level of evidence)
- Triglycerides < 150 mg/dl (1,7 mmol/l) (C-level of evidence).

Because diabetes mellitus is considered a coronary risk equivalent, the lipid objective is LDL cholesterol < 100 mg/dl (< 2.6 mmol/l) as lowering LDL cholesterol is associated with reduction in cardiovascular events (A-level of evidence), it represents the first priority of therapy [66, 67].

The same LDL-cholesterol targets (< 100 mg/dl) in patients with "coronary risk equivalents" (including those with diabetes) were established by National Cholesterol Education Program (NCEP)/Adult Treatment Panel (ATP) III in 2001 [15]. Very recently, the importance of diabetes as coronary heart disease equivalent has been reinforced by the new NCEP Report [99]. The Report includes the persons with diabetes in the high risk category. When the risk is very high the recommended LDL-cholesterol goal should be < 70 mg/dl. Moreover, when the high-risk patient has high triglycerides or low-HDL cholesterol, the combination of fenofibrate or nicotinic acid (slow released form) with statin can be used.

The following *order of priorities for treatment* of dyslipidemia in adult with type 2 diabetes should be considered [66, 62]:
- For LDL cholesterol lowering:
– If the level is 100–129 mg/dl (2.6–3.3 mmol/l) lifestyle optimization should aggressively be given, or treatment with statins must be prescribed, mainly in the presence of atherosclerotic cardiovascular disease. If HDL cholesterol is < 40 mg/dl, fenofibrate can be used [66].
– If the initial level is ≥ 130 mg/dl (3.3 mmol/l) statins and lifestyle modification treatment should concomitantly be used.
– According to an expert opinion statins should be initiated if the absolute coronary risk is ≥ 15%.

- For HDL cholesterol rising, the lifestyle optimization and glycemic control may be useful. Statins modestly raise HDL. A greater increase is achieved with fibrates.
- For triglyceride lowering, the first priority is to achieve glycemic control. Fibrates (gemfibrozil, fenofibrate) are used in patients with high levels (≥ 400 mg/dl) of triglycerides. Statins at high doses are moderately effective in this respect.
- For combined hyperlipidemia the first choice is to improve glycemic control plus high dose statins. As second choice fibrates should be added to statins. The drugs for the third choice are resins plus fibrates or statins plus nicotinic acid. The association of hypolipidemic drugs can develops secondary effects such as myositis or deterioration of glycemic control. They must be monitored carefully [66].

Anti–aggregation treatment

Acetylsalicylic acid should be used for both primary and secondary prevention according to ADA's [100] and AHA's recommendations (see also Tables 24.14 and 24.15). In terms of "evidence" the following recommendations should be considered [65]:
- Therapy with aspirin (75–325 mg/day) in all adult patients with diabetes and macrovascular disease (A–level evidence).
- As primary prevention, aspirin (75–325 mg/day) is indicated in patients ≥ 40 years of age, with diabetes and one or more other cardiovascular risk factors.

BENEFITS AND COSTS

Steno-2 Study, the first multifactorial intervention trial on cardiovascular risk in persons with type 2 diabetes, showed a 50 % reduction of cardiovascular events (and of microvascular complications), demonstrating that the multifactorial strategy is beneficial [54, 55]. Other trials having the same objective are ongoing. The benefits of such interventions can be evaluated by measuring the mortality and morbidity, macro- and microvascular complications of diabetes, metabolic and hypertensive control and endpoints related to visits to outpatient clinics and hospital admission [56].

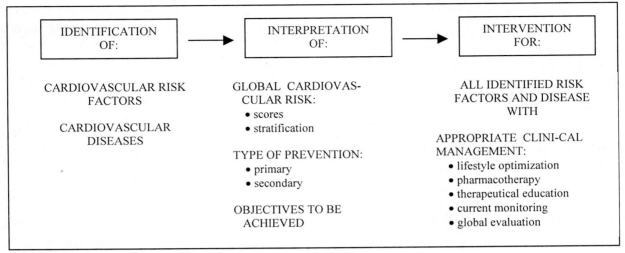

Figure 24.3

The suggested stepwise approach of the global cardiovascular risk in persons with type 2 diabetes
(from [1] with kind permission).

All large interventions which have focused on one or two factors in people with type 2 diabetes were cost-effective. This cannot yet be said regarding an intensive multifactorial strategy. However, the cost-effectiveness data from UKPDS [16, 23] regarding the intensive glycemic or blood pressure control and also from lipid – lowering trials [56] could allow to think that global interventions are also justified from the economic point of view in people with type 2 diabetes. In addition, the results from DIGAMI study [102, 103, 104] clearly showed that intensive insulin treatment after acute myocardial infarction in persons with diabetes along with its favorable endpoints is also cost-effective.

CONCLUDING REMARKS

Type 2 diabetes has a high prevalence of cardiovascular events, which are determined by multiple risk factors. This global cardiovascular risk can be stepwise approached as is suggested in Figure 24.3.

All steps are important and all of them must be carefully accomplished. The practical approach of the global cardiovascular risk is a dynamic and flexible process.

The model of multiple cardiovascular risk factor intervention ought to be implemented in daily practice as much as possible. This offers a unique opportunity [53] to reduce the devastating cardiovascular morbidity and mortality in people with type 2 diabetes.

REFERENCES

1. Hâncu N, Cerghizan Anca. Global Approach to Cardiovascular Risk in Type 2 Diabetic Persons. In: Hâncu N (ed) *Cardiovascular Risk in Type 2 Diabetes Mellitus*, Springer-Verlag Berlin, Heidelberg, New-York, 2003, 240–276.
2. Grundy SM, Benjamin IJ, Burke GL, Chait A, Eckel RH, Howard BV, Mitch W, Smith SC, Sowers JR. Diabetes and cardiovascular disease. A statement for health care professionals from the American Heart Association. *Circulation*, **100:** 1134–1146, 1999.
3. Savage PJ, Narayan Venkat KM. Reducing cardiovascular complications of type 2 diabetes. *Diabetes Care,* **22:** 1769–1770, 1999.
4. Kannel WB. Contributions of the Framingham Study to the conquest of coronary artery disease. *American Journal of Cardiology*, **62:** 1109–1112, 1988.
5. Stamler J, Vaccaro O, Neaton JR, Wentworth D for the Multiple Risk Factor Intervention Trial Research Group. *Diabetes Care*, **16:** 434–444, 1998.
6. Assman G, Cullen P, Schulte H. The Münster Heart Study (Procam). Results of follow-up at 8 years. *European Heart Journal* **19** (Suppl. A):A2–A11, 1998.

7. International Task Force for Prevention of Coronary Heart Disease. Coronary Heart Disease: reducing the risk. The scientific background for primary and secondary prevention of coronary heart disease. A worldwide view. *Nutr Metab Cardiovasc Dis*, **8**: 205–271, 1998.

8. Wood D, De Backer G, Faergeman O, Graham I, Mancia G, Pyörälä K. Prevention of coronary heart disease in clinical practice. Recommendations of the Second Joint Task Force of European and other Societies on Coronary Prevention. *European Heart Journal*, **19**: 1434–1503, 1998.

9. Garber AJ. Diabetes and vascular disease. *Diabetes, Obesity and Metabolism*, **2** (Suppl. 2):S1–S5, 2000

10. Brown WV. Risk factors for vascular disease in patients with diabetes. *Diabetes, Obesity and Metabolism*, **2** (Suppl. 2):S11–S18, 2000.

11. Gavin J, Kagan S. Vascular disease prevention in patients with diabetes. *Diabetes, Obesity and Metabolism*, **2** (Suppl. 2):S25–S36, 2000.

12. Grundy SM. Small LDL atherogenic dyslipidemia and the metabolic syndrome. *Circulation*, **95**: 1–4, 1997.

13. Grundy SM, Brewer HB, Cleeman JI, Smith SC, Lenfant C; for the Conference Participants. Definition of Metabolic Syndrome. Report of the National Heart, Lung, and Blood Institute/ American Heart Association Conference on Scientific Issues Related to Definition. *Circulation*, **109**: 433–438, 2004.

14. Grundy SM, Hansen B, Smith SC, Cleeman JI, Kahn RA; for the Conference Participants. Clinical Management of Metabolic Syndrome. Report of the National Heart, Lung, and Blood Institute/ American Heart Association Conference on Scientific Issues Related to Management. *Circulation*, **109**: 551–556, 2004.

15. Expert Panel on Third Report of the National Cholesterol Education Program (NCEP). Detection, evaluation and treatment of high blood cholesterol in adults (Adult Treatment Panel III). *NIH Publication* No 01–3670, 2001.

16. UK Prospective Diabetes Study (UKPDS). Intensive blood-glucose control with sulphonylureas or insulin compared with conventional treatment and risk of complications in patients with type 2 diabetes (UKPDS 33) *Lancet*, **352**: 837–853, 1998.

17. Standl E. Cardiovascular risk in type 2 diabetes. *Diabetes, Obesity and Metabolism*, **1** (Suppl. 2):S24–S36, 1999.

18. Laakso M, Lehto S. Epidemiology of macrovascular disease in diabetes. *Diabetes Reviews*, **5**: 294–315, 1997.

19. Lorber D. Complicating matters. *Practical Diabetology*, **19**: 35, 2000.

20. Turner RC, Millns H, Neil HAW, Stratton IM, Manley SE, Matthews DR, Holman PR for the UKPDS Group. Risk factors for coronary artery disease in non-insulin dependent diabetes mellitus: United Kingdom prospective diabetes study (UKPDS: 23). *British Medical Journal*, **316**: 823–828, 1998

21. Talbot F, Nouwen A. A review of the relationship between depression and diabetes in adults. *Diabetes Care*, **23**: 1556–1562, 2000.

22. Mommier L. The role of blood glucose - lowering drugs in the light of the UKPDS. *Diabetes, Obesity and Metabolism*, **1** (Suppl. 2): S14–S23, 1999.

23. Turner RC. The U.K. Prospective Diabetes Study. *Diabetes Care*, **21** (Suppl. 3): C35–C38, 1998.

24. UK Prospective Diabetes Study (UKPDS) Group. Effect of intensive blood control with metformin on complications in overweight patients with type 2 diabetes (UKPDS 34). *Lancet*, **352**: 854–865, 1998.

25. Mogensen CE. Combined high blood pressure and glucose in type 2 diabetes: double jeopardy. *British Medical Journal*, **317**: 693–694, 1998.

26. UK Prospective Diabetes Study Group. Tight blood pressure control and risk of macrovascular and microvascular complications in type 2 diabetes (UKPDS 38). *British Medical Journal*, **317**: 703–713, 1998.

27. Hansson L, Zanchetti A, Capruthers SG *et al.* for the HOT Study Group. Effects of intensive blood pressure lowering and low-dose aspirin in the patients with hypertension: principal results of the Hypertension Optimal Treatment (HOT) randomised trial. *Lancet*, **351**: 1755–1762, 1998.

28. Heart Outcomes Prevention Evaluation (HOPE) Study Investigators. Effects of ramipril on CV and microvascular outcomes in people with diabetes mellitus: results of HOPE study and MICRO-HOPE substudy. *Lancet*, **355**: 252–259, 2000.

29. Garber AJ. Implications of cardiovascular risk in patients with type 2 diabetes who have abnormal lipid profiles: is lower enough? *Diabetes, Obesity and Metabolism*, **2**: 263–270, 2000.

30. Haffner SM. The Scandinavian Simvastatin Survival Study (4S) subgroup analysis of diabetic subjects: implications for the prevention of coronary heart disease. *Diabetes Care*, **20**: 469–471, 1997.

31. Sacks FM, Pfeffer MA, Moye LA. *et al* for the Cholesterol and Recurrent Events Trial Investigators. The effects of pravastatin on coronary events after myocardial infarction in patients with average cholesterol levels: Cholesterol and Recurrent Events Trial

Investigators. *New England Journal of Medicine,* **335:** 1001–1009, 1996

32. Steiner G. Lipid intervention trials in diabetes. *Diabetes Care,* **23,** (Suppl. 2):B49–B53, 2000.

33. Haffner SM. Patients with type 2 diabetes: the case for primary prevention. *Amer J Med,* **107** (2A): 435–455, 2000.

34. Heart Protection Study Collaborative Group. MRC/BHF Heart Protection Study of cholesterol lowering with simvastatin in 20 536 high-risk individuals: a randomised placebo-controlled trial. *Lancet,* **360:** 7–22, 2002.

35. Heart Protection Study Collaborative Group. MRC/BHF Heart Protection Study of cholesterol-lowering with simvastatin in 5963 people with diabetes: a randomised placebo-controlled trial. *Lancet,* **361:** 2006–2016, 2003.

36. Sever PS et al for the ASCOT Investigators. Prevention of coronary and stroke events with atorvastatin in hypertensive patients who have average and lower than average cholesterol concentrations, in the Anglo-Scandinavian Cardiac Outcomes Trial- Lipid Lowering Arm (ASCOT-LLA): a multicentre randomised controlled trial. *Lancet,* **361:** 1149–1158, 2003.

37. Colhoum HM, Betteridge JD, Durrington PN, Hitman GA, Neil HAW, Livinstone SJ, Thomason MJ, Mackness MI, CharltonMenys V, Fuller JH, on behalf of CARDS investigators. Primary prevention of cardiovascular disease with atorvastatin in type 2 diabetes in the Collaborative Atorvastatin Diabetes Study (CARDS):multicentre randomized placebo-controlled trial. *Lancet,* **364:** 685–696, 2004.

38. Leiter LA, Betteridge DJ and AUDIT Investigators. The AUDIT Study: a worldwide survey of physicians attitudes about diabetic dyslipidemia. *Diabetes,* **53 (suppl 2):** A285, 2004.

39. Cullen P *et al.* Dyslipidemia and cardiovascular risk in diabetes. *Diabetes, Obesity and Metabolism,* **1:** 189–198, 1999.

40. Pozzili P, Leslie RDG. Aspirin and diabetes. *Practical Diabetes International,* **16:** 265–261, 1999.

41. Colwell JA. Aspirin in diabetes. *Diabetes Care,* **20:** 1767–1771, 1997.

42. Haffner SM, Lehto S, Rőnnemaa T, Pyőrälä K, Laakso M. Mortality from coronary heart disease in subjects with type 2 diabetes and in non-diabetic subjects with and without prior myocardial infarction. *New England Journal of Medicine,* **339:** 229–234, 1998.

43. Miettinen H, Lehto S, Salomaa VV, *et al.* Impact of diabetes on mortality after the first myocardial infarction. *Diabetes Care,* **21:**69–75, 1998.

44. Yusuf S, Hawken S, Dans T, Avezum A, Lanas F, McQueen M, Budaj A, Pais P, Varigas J, Lisheng L, on behalf of the INTERHEART Study Investigators. Effect of potentially modifiable risk factors associated with myocardial infarction in 52 countries (the INTERHEART study): case-control study. *Lancet,* **364:** 937–952, 2004

45. Cockram C *et al.* Diabetes and cardiovascular disease. International Diabetes Federation, 2001.

46. Heinig RE. What should the role of ACE inhibitors be in the treatment of diabetes? Lessons from HOPE and MICRO-HOPE. *Diabetes, Obesity and Metabolism,* **4** (Suppl. 1): S19–S26, 2002.

47. Reaven GM. Multiple CHD risk factors in type 2 diabetes: beyond hyperglycemia. *Diabetes, Obesity and Metabolism,* **4** (Suppl. 1): S13–S18, 2002.

48. Garber AJ. Attenuating CV risk factors in patients with diabetes: clinical evidence to clinical practice. *Diabetes, Obesity and Metabolism,* **4** (Suppl. 1): S5–S12, 2002.

49. Hâncu N, De Leiva A. La hiperglicemia como factor de riesgo cardiovascular. *Cardiovascular risk factors,* **10:** 262–270, 2001.

50. Hâncu N, De Leiva A. Enfermedad cardiovascular en la diabetes mellitus: impacto sanitario y patogenia. *Cardiovascular Risk Factor,* **10:** 251–262, 2001.

51. Grundy SM et al from AHA Task Force on risk reduction. Primary prevention of coronary heart disease: guidance from Framingham. *Circulation,* **97:** 1876–1887, 1998.

52. Grundy SM. Primary prevention of coronary heart disease – integrating risk assessment with intervention. *Circulation,* **100:** 988–998, 1999.

53. Cockroft JR, Wilkkinson IB, Yki-Järvinen H. Multiple risk factor intervention in type 2 diabetes: an opportunity not to be missed. *Diabetes, Obesity and Metabolism,* **3:** 1–8, 2001.

54. Gaede P, Vedel P, Parving HH, Pedersen O. Intensified multifactorial intervention in patients with type 2 diabetes mellitus and microalbuminuria: the Steno type 2 randomized study. *Lancet,* **353:** 617–622, 1999.

55. Gæde P and others. Multifactorial Intervention and Cardiovascular Disease in Patients with Type 2 Diabetes. *New England Journal of Medicine,* **348:** 383–393, 2003.

56. Lawritzen T, Griffin S, Borch-Johnsen K et al for the ADDITION Study Group. The ADDITION Study: proposed trial of the cost-effectiveness of an intensive multifactorial intervention on morbidity and mortality among people with type 2 diabetes detected by screening. *International Journal of Obesity,* (**Suppl.3**): S6–S11, 2000.

57. Greenland P, Grundy S, Pasternak RC, Lenfant C. Problems on the pathway from risk assessment to risk reduction. *Circulation*, **97**: 1761–1762, 1998.

58. Boulton AJ *et al.* Recommendations for the management of patients with type 2 diabetes mellitus in the Central, Eastern and Southern European Region – Consensus statement. *Int J Postgrad Training Med*, **8**: 3–26, 2000.

59. European Diabetes Policy Group. A desktop guide to type 2 diabetes mellitus. International Diabetes Federation – European Region, 1998–1999.

60. International Diabetes Federation – European Region. Hypertension in people with type 2 diabetes – knowledge-based diabetes specific guidelines. International Diabetes Federation (European Region), 1997.

61. World Health Organization – International Society of Hypertension. Guidelines for the management of hypertension. *Journal of Hypertension*, **17**: 151–183, 1999.

62. Henry RR, Saudek CD from International Consensus Group. Managing dyslipidemia in patients with diabetes in the primary care settings – recommendations of an International Consensus Group. The John Hopkins University School of Medicine, Office of CME, 2000.

63. European Arterial Risk Policy Group on behalf of the International Diabetes Federation (European Region). A strategy for arterial risk assessment and management in type 2 (non-insulin-dependent) diabetes mellitus. *Diabetic Medicine*, **14**: 611–621, 1997.

64. Gotto AM *et al.* from ILIB (International Lipid Information Bureau). The ILIB Lipid Handbook for Clinical Practice. ILIB, New York, 2000.

65. American Diabetes Association. Position statement: Standards of medical care for patients with diabetes mellitus. *Diabetes Care*, **27** (Suppl. 1): S15–S35, 2004.

66. American Diabetes Association. Position statement: Management of dyslipidemia in adults with diabetes. *Diabetes Care*, **27** (Suppl. 1): S68–71, 2004.

67. Scheen AJ, Lefebvre PJ. Management of the obese diabetic patient. *Diabetes Reviews*, **7**: 77–93, 1999.

68. Maggio CA, Pi-Sunyer FX. The prevention and treatment of obesity – application to type 2 diabetes. *Diabetes Care*, **20**: 1744–1766, 1997.

69. Williams G. Obesity and type 2 diabetes: a conflict of interests? *International Journal of Obesity*, **23** (Suppl. 7)**:** 32–35, 1999.

70. Betteridge J. Diabetic dyslipidemia. *Diabetes, Obesity and Metabolism*, **2** (Suppl. 1): S31–S36, 2000.

71. Hansson L. The impact of antihypertensive therapy in type 2 diabetes. *Diabetes, Obesity and Metabolism*, **2** (Suppl.1): S37–S41, 2000.

72. American Diabetes Association. Position statement: Treatment of hypertension in adults with diabetes. *Diabetes Care*, **27** (Suppl. 1): S65–67, 2004.

73. American Diabetes Association. Position statement: Evidence-based nutrition principles and recommendations for the treatment and prevention of diabetes and related complications. *Diabetes Care*, **26** (Suppl. 1): S51–S61, 2003.

74. Vinik A, Richardson D. Erectile dysfunction in diabetes. *Diabetes Reviews*, **6**:16–33, 1998

75. Shabsigh R. *et al.* Erectile dysfunction and depression: a dynamic association. *Sexual Dysfunction*, **1**: 42–45, 1999.

76. Kelley DE. Approaches to preventing mealtime hyperglycaemic excursions. *Diabetes, Obesity and Metabolism*, **4**: 11–18, 2002.

77. Hâncu ND *et al.* „Hypertensive waist" as a cardiovascular risk factor in newly diagnosed type 2 diabetes persons. *Diabetologia*, **47**, suppl 1: A419, 2004.

78. Horvit PK, Garber AJ. Diabetes and cerebrovascular disease. *Clinical Diabetes*, **15**: 253–256, 1997.

79. Cooper Stephanie, Caldwell JH. Coronary artery disease in people with diabetes: diagnostic and risk factor evaluation. *Clinical Diabetes*, **17**: 58–70, 1999.

80. Yudkin JS, Chaturvedi N. Developing risk stratification charts for diabetic and nondiabetic subjects. *Diabetic Medicine*, **16**: 219–227, 1999.

81. Wilson PWF, D'Agostino RB, Levy D, Belanger AM, Silbershatz H, Kannel WB. Prediction of coronary heart disease using risk factor categories. *Circulation*, **97**: 1837–1847, 1998.

82. Grundy SM, Pasternak R, Greenland P, Smith S, Fuster U. Assessment of cardiovascular risk by use of multiple-risk-factor assessment equations. A statement for health care professionals from the American Heart Association and the American College of Cardiology. *Journal of American College of Cardiology*, **34**: 1348–1359, 1999.

83. Third Joint Task Force of European and other Societies on Cardiovascular Disease Prevention in Clinical Practice. European guidelines on cardiovascular disease prevention in clinical practice. Executive summary. *European Heart Journal*, **24**: 1601–1610, 2003.

84. Stevens RJ, Kothari V, Adler AI, Stratton IM, Holman RR on behalf of the United Kingdom Prospective Diabetes Study (UKPDS) Group. The UKPDS risk engine: a model for the risk of

coronary heart disease in Type II diabetes (UKPDS 56). *Clinical Science*, **101**: 671–679, 2001.

85. Kothari V, Stevens RJ, Adler AI, Stratton IM, Manley SE, Neil A, Holman RR for the UK Prospective Diabetes Study Group. UKPDS 60. Risk of stroke in type 2 diabetes estimated by the UK Prospective Diabetes Study risk engine. *Stroke*, **33**: 776–1781, 2002.

86. Game FL, Jones AF. Coronary heart disease risk assessment in diabetes mellitus – a comparison of PROCAM and Framingham risk assessment functions. *Diabetic Medicine*, **18**: 355–359, 2001.

87. Winocour PH, Fisher M. Prediction of cardiovascular risk in people with diabetes. *Diabetic Medicine*, **20**: 515–527, 2003.

88. Golay A, Assal JP. Cardiovascular risk in diabetes and therapeutic patient education. *Int J Metab*, **2**: 47, 1999.

89. Hâncu N (1999) Abordarea în practică a dislipidemiilor: necesități, posibilități, bariere. In: Dabelea Dana (Ed) *Actualități în lipidologie*. Editura Mirton, Timișoara, 1999, 184–189.

90. Herbst KL, Hirsch IB. Insulin strategies for primary care providers. *Clin Diab*, **20**: 11–17, 2002.

91. Guidelines Committee. European Society of Hypertension-European Society of Cardiology guidelines for the management of arterial hypertension. *Journal of Hypertension*, **21**(6): 1011–1053, 2003.

92. ALLHAT Collaborative Research Group. Validation of Heart Failure Events in the Antihypertensive and Lipid Lowering Treatment to Prevent Heart Attack Trial (ALLHAT) Participants Assigned to Doxazosin and Chlorthalidone. *Curr Control Trials Cardiovasc Med*, **3**, 2002.

93. Gerstein HC. Cardiovascular and metabolic benefits of ACE inhibition. *Diabetes Care*, **2**: 882–883, 2000.

94. Heart Outcomes Prevention Evaluation (HOPE) Study Investigators. Effects of an angiotensin-converting-enzyme inhibitor, ramipril, on cardiovascular events in high risk patients. *New England Journal of Medicine*, **342**: 145–153, 2000.

95. Mathiensen ER. Effects of ACE inhibition on cardiovascular outcomes in people with diabetes mellitus. The findings of the HOPE study. *International Diabetes Monitor*, **12**: 1–4, 2000.

96. Aram V. Chobanian, George L. Bakris, Henry R. Black, William C. Cushman, Lee A. Green, Joseph L. Izzo, Jr, Daniel W. Jones, Barry J. Materson, Suzanne Oparil, Jackson T. Wright, Jr, and Edward J. Roccella. The Seventh Report of the Joint National Committee on Prevention, Detection, Evaluation, and Treatment of High Blood Pressure: The JNC 7 Report. *JAMA*, **289**: 2560–2571, 2003.

97. Prospective Studies Collaboration. Age-specific relevance of usual blood pressure to vascular mortality: a meta-analysis of individual data for one million adults in 61 prospective studies. *Lancet*, **360**: 1903–1913, 2002.

98. American Diabetes Association. Position Statement: Weight Management Through Lifestyle Modification for the Prevention and Management of Type 2 Diabetes: Rationale and Strategies: A statement of the American Diabetes Association, the North American Association for the Study of Obesity, and the American Society for Clinical Nutrition *Diabetes Care*, **27**: 2067–2073, 2004.

99. Grundy SM, Cleeman JI, Merz CN, *et al.* Implications of recent clinical trials for the National Cholesterol Education Program Adult Treatment Panel III guidelines. *Circulation*, **110**: 227–239, 2004.

100. American Diabetes Association. Position statement: Aspirin therapy in diabetes. *Diabetes Care*, **27** (Suppl. 1): S72–S73, 2004.

101. World Health Organization. Definition, diagnosis and classification of diabetes mellitus and its complications. Part 1: diagnosis and classification of diabetes mellitus. WHO, Dept of Noncommunicable DiCare Surveillance. Geneva, 1999.

102. Almbrad B *et al.* Cost effectiveness of intense insulin treatment after acute myocardial infarction in patient with diabetes mellitus: results from DIGAMI study. *European Heart Journal*, **21**: 733–739, 2000.

103. Yudkin JS. Managing the diabetic patient with acute myocardial infarction. *Diabetic Medicine*, **15**: 276–281, 1998.

104. Malmberg K for the DIGAMI (Diabetes mellitus Insulin Glucose infusion in Acute Myocardial Infarction) study group. Prospective randomized study of intensive insulin treatment of long term survival after acute myocardial infarction in patients with diabetes mellitus. *British Medical Journal*, **314**: 1512–1515, 2000.

25

HYPERTENSION IN DIABETES MELLITUS

Gheorghe S. BĂCANU, Viorel ŞERBAN, Romulus TIMAR, Adrian VLAD, Laura DIACONU

The prevalence of hypertension in diabetic patients is 1.5 to 3 times greater compared to general population. The high prevalence of hypertension in type 2 diabetes, up to 60–80%, is explained by the common risk factors the two diseases share: insulin resistance and android obesity. The prevalence of hypertension in type 1 diabetes mellitus is lower, up to 10–30%, and its existence suggests the presence of diabetic nephropathy.

Regarding the cardiovascular risk, diabetes mellitus is currently considered to be equivalent to the presence of coronary heart disease, while its association with hypertension further increases this risk. MRFIT study has demonstrated that diabetic subjects who are also hypertensive have a three-fold increase in cardiovascular mortality compared with their nondiabetic counterparts. Furthermore, the combination of hypertension with hyperglycemia facilitates the development and progression of diabetic nephropathy and retinopathy. Therefore, in diabetic patients it is mandatory to consider equally important both a good glycemic control and the normalization of blood pressure values. Dyslipidemia and obesity are also frequent comorbidities of diabetes mellitus and require careful treatment in order to decrease the cardiovascular risk.

There is extensive evidence that the aggressive treatment of hypertension in diabetes is important for reducing both cardiovascular and microvascular complications; however, the ideal strategy for treating hypertension in persons with diabetes is less clear.

This chapter focuses on the particularities of hypertension in diabetic patients and aims to provide to clinicians an evidence based guide for the management of hypertension in diabetes mellitus.

Abbreviations List

AGEs – Advanced Glycation End-products
AASK – African-American Study of Kidney Disease
ABCD study – Appropriate Blood Pressure Control in Diabetes study
ACE – Angiotensin Converting Enzyme
ACEI – Angiotensin Converting Enzyme Inhibitor
ALLHAT – Antihypertensive and Lipid Lowering Treatment to Prevent Heart Attacks Trial
ARB – Angiotensin II Receptor Blocker
AT 1 receptors – Angiotensin type 1 receptors
AT 2 receptors – Angiotensin type 2 receptors
AT II – Angiotensin II
BB – Beta-blocker
CALM – Candesartan and Lisinopril Microalbuminuria study
CAPPP – Captopril Prevention Project
CCB – Calcium Channel Blocker
DCCB – Dihydropyridine CCB
FACET – Fosinopril *versus* Amlodipine Cardiovascular Events Trial
HOPE study – Heart Outcomes Prevention Evaluation study
HOT study – Hypertension Optimal Treatment study

HYVET – Hypertension in the Very Elderly Trial
IDNT – Irbesartan Diabetic Nephropathy Trial
IRMA 2 – Microalbuminuria in Hypertensive Patient with Type 2 Diabetes Mellitus
JNC – Joint National Committee on Prevention, Detection, Evaluation and Treatment of High Blood Pressure
LIFE – Losartan Intervention for End point reduction in Hypertension Trial
non-DCCB– non -Dihydropyridine CCB
NORDIL – Nordic Diltiazem Study
RAS – Renin Angiotensin System
RENAAL study – Reduction of Endpoints in NIDDM with the Angiotensin II Antagonist Losartan study
SHEP study – Systolic Hypertension in Elderly patients study
STOP-2 – Swedish Trial in Old Patients with Hypertension
Syst-Eur – Systolic Hypertension in Europe Trial
UKPDS – United Kingdom Prospective Diabetes Study
Val-HeFT – Valsartan in Heart Failure Trial
WHO -; World Health Organization

THE IMPORTANCE OF THE ASSOCIATION OF HYPERTENSION WITH DIABETES MELLITUS

Arterial hypertension is more frequent in diabetic subjects than in general population. Hypertension can develop in the course of type 1 or 2 diabetes or can be present from the diagnosis of type 2 diabetes.

Regarding the cardiovascular risk, diabetes mellitus is currently considered to be equivalent to the presence of coronary heart disease, while its association with hypertension further increases this risk. MRFIT study [1] has demonstrated that diabetic subjects who are also hypertensive have a three fold increase in cardiovascular mortality compared with their nondiabetic counterparts. Furthermore, the combination of hypertension with hyperglycemia facilitates the development and progression of diabetic nephropathy and retinopathy. Therefore, in diabetic patients it is mandatory to consider equally important both a good glycemic control and the normalization of blood pressure values. Dyslipidemia and obesity are also frequent comorbidities of diabetes mellitus and require careful treatment in order to decrease the cardiovascular risk [1].

DEFINITION AND CLASSIFICATION OF HYPERTENSION

DEFINITION AND CLASSIFICATION OF HYPERTENSION IN GENERAL POPULATION

Due to the linear relationship between hypertension and cardiovascular risk, and also because there is much arbitrary in establishing normal range for blood pressure values, various expert groups and committees have given different definitions of hypertension. In order to reduce confusion and give practitioners a reference basis, WHO has decided in 1999 to adopt the definition and classification of hypertension established at the 6th Report of Joint National Committee on Prevention, Detection, Evaluation and Treatment of Arterial Hypertension from the USA [2]. According to JNC 6, hypertension is defined as an increase, usually permanent, of systolic blood pressure to 140 mm Hg or greater and/or of diastolic blood pressure to 90 mm Hg or greater, in a subject not taking antihypertensive medication.

The latest JNC Report, JNC 7, from 2003 [3] introduces a new category, named *prehypertension*, while grades 2 and 3 hypertension from the previous classification have been merged. JNC 7 classification is presented in Table 25.1.

Table 25.1

Classification of Blood Pressure for adults (JNC 7–2003)

Category	Systolic Blood Pressure (mmHg)	Diastolic Blood Pressure (mmHg)
Normal	< 120	< 80
Prehypertension	120–139	80–89
Stage 1 Hypertension	140–159	90–99
Stage 2 Hypertension	≥160	≥100

The introduction of prehypertension as a stage of hypertension aims to underline the importance and the role of measures for health education that aim to reduce blood pressure values and to prevent the development of high blood pressure in general population.

DEFINITION OF HYPERTENSION IN DIABETIC PATIENTS

Data from clinical trials enrolling diabetic patients have demonstrated a continuous increase in cardiovascular risk once blood pressure is greater than 140/80 mm Hg, and have also shown evident clinical benefits if blood pressure values are reduced below 130/80 mm Hg. Furthermore, studies on diabetic patients have shown that diabetic retinopathy and nephropathy have an accelerated progression when diastolic blood pressure is greater than 70 mm Hg [4, 5]. That is why, in our opinion, it is more appropriate to define hypertension in diabetic subjects as values above 130 mm Hg for the systolic pressure and above 80 mm Hg for the diastolic value, comparatively with 140/90 mm Hg for the general population. In elderly diabetics with systolic hypertension, the reduction of systolic blood pressure under 140 mm Hg has proved to be beneficial [5, 6]. These are the reasons for considering the new JNC 7 classification of hypertension [3] more adequate and more correlated with the cardiovascular risk in diabetic patients.

STRATIFICATION OF CARDIOVASCULAR RISK

The relationship between blood pressure and the risk for cardiovascular events is continuous and independent of other risk factors. The higher the blood pressure of, the greater the risk of myocardial infarction, heart failure, stroke and renal impairment. In subjects aged between 40 and 70 years, every 20 mm Hg increase in systolic blood pressure or 10 mm Hg increase in diastolic blood pressure is accompanied by a doubling of cardiovascular risk. On the other hand, the association of high blood pressure with other risk factors, such as diabetes mellitus, smoking, hypercholesterolemia, further increases cardiovascular morbidity and mortality [7].

Consequently, a correct therapeutic decision must take into account not only blood pressure values but also the presence of other risk factors, target organ involvement, other cardiovascular or renal conditions, concomitant diseases, diabetes mellitus, and also other patient-related factors (psychosocial and economic) [2, 3, 7].

Factors that contribute to the increase of absolute risk for developing major cardiovascular events in hypertensive patients are: age (above 55 years in men and above 65 years in women), smoking, diabetes mellitus, hypercholesterolemia, and family history of early cardiovascular disease. Additionally, the following conditions also increase the absolute cardiovascular risk: the presence of target organ disease (left ventricular hypertrophy; proteinuria and/or slight increase in plasmatic creatinine between 1.2–2 mg/dL; carotid, iliac or femoral atheromatous plaques on ultrasound or on radiographic examination, focal or diffuse narrowing of the retinal arteries), and other associated clinical conditions represented by: cerebrovascular disease (ischemic and hemorrhagic stroke, transitory ischemic attack), cardiac disease (myocardial infarction, angina pectoris, congestive heart failure), renal disease (diabetic nephropathy, renal failure), vascular disease (dissecting aneurysm, symptomatic peripheral arterial disease), advanced hypertensive retinopathy (with hemorrhages, exudates, papillary edema) [8].

Based on the presence of the above-mentioned factors, four categories of cardiovascular risk are defined: low, moderate, high and very high, each category representing an interval of absolute risk for developing major cardiovascular events. Within each interval, the individual risk is determined by the severity and the number of risk factors present [9] (Table 25.2).

Table 25.2

Risk stratification for prognosis in hypertensive patients

Other risk factors and history of disease	SBP = 140–159 mmHg DBP = 90–99 mmHg	SBP=160–179 mmHg DBP = 100–109 mmHg	SBP ≥ 180 mmHg DBP ≥ 110 mmHg
No other risk factor	Low* <15%	Medium 15–20%	High 20–30%
1–2 risk factors	Medium 15–20%	Medium 15–20%	Very high > 30%
3 or more risk factors or hypertensive end-organ disease or diabetes mellitus	High 20–30%	High 20–30%	Very high >30%
Associated conditions	Very high >30%	Very high risk >30%	Very high risk >30%
* risk for major cardiovascular events in 10 years SBP= systolic blood pressure, DBP= diastolic blood pressure			

Patients with diabetes mellitus belong to the high or very high risk group, as follows: patients with grade 1 or 2 hypertension (according to JNC 6–WHO 1999 [6]), with no associated clinical conditions, are classified in the high risk group, while those diabetic patients with grade 3 hypertension or those with associated clinical conditions regardless of blood pressure values belong to the very high risk group.

Diabetic patients from the high-risk group have a 20 to 30% probability to develop a major cardiovascular event within the following 10 years, whereas in those from the very high-risk group this probability exceeds 30%.

EPIDEMIOLOGY OF HYPERTENSION IN DIABETIC PATIENTS

The prevalence of hypertension in diabetics is 1.5 to 3 times greater compared to general population [10, 11]. The occurrence and evolution of hypertension differ significantly in type 1 compared to type 2 diabetes mellitus.

Hypertension is found in 10 to 30% of patients with type 1 diabetes, and its existence suggests the presence of diabetic nephropathy. In these patients, hypertension is characterized by high values of both systolic and diastolic blood pressure. Blood pressure is usually normal at diagnosis and remains so in the first 5 to 10 years of disease. Approximately 50% of type 1 diabetes patients with diabetes duration over 30 years present high blood pressure; this subgroup consists mainly of patients who have developed diabetic nephropathy. Type 1 diabetes patients, with a disease duration of 30 years or more who do not have diabetic nephropathy seldom present hypertension [6, 7, 12].

On the opposite, in type 2 diabetes patients, the prevalence of hypertension at diagnosis or shortly after is high. In UKPDS [13, 14, 15], 32% of the men and 45% of the women with recently diagnosed type 2 diabetes were also hypertensive. Hypertension often precedes type 2 diabetes and can be present in subjects with impaired glucose tolerance or with impaired fasting glucose. Blood pressure increase is usually correlated with the presence of obesity and advanced age of the patient.

In type 2 diabetes, isolated systolic hypertension can also occur and is frequently attributed to macrovascular disease and to the reduction of elastic properties of the arteries. Furthermore, systolic blood pressure increases with age, thus contributing to the high prevalence of hypertension in type 2 diabetic patients.

The evolution of diabetic nephropathy and the contribution of impaired renal function to the development of hypertension in type 2 diabetes mellitus are not well precised. However, in type 2 diabetic patients and microalbuminuria, the prevalence of hypertension is approximately 70% [12].

The high prevalence of hypertension in type 2 diabetes, up to 60–80%, is explained by the common risk factors the two diseases share: insulin resistance and abdominal (android) obesity.

PATHOPHYSIOLOGY

The pathophysiological mechanisms that underlay the association of hypertension with diabetes mellitus are not completely identified; however it seems that they involve a complex interaction between genetic factors predisposing for hypertension and metabolic abnormalities present in diabetes mellitus [12].

In type 1 diabetes, hypertension usually develops secondary to diabetic nephropathy, while in type 2 diabetes, it is most often essential.

Essential hypertension associated with diabetes has generally the same pathogenic mechanisms as those encountered in non-diabetic subjects, with insulin resistance and hyperinsulinemia playing an important role.

An extremely important factor in the development of hypertension in diabetics is insulin resistance; however, it is not yet clear whether insulin resistance *per se* or the resultant hyperinsulinemia lead to raised blood pressure values in diabetic patients. Furthermore, the association of hypertension to diabetes worsens insulin resistance [16, 17].

Although there are rare situations when hyperinsulinemia and/or insulin resistance are not associated with hypertension, *i.e.*, insulinoma, polycystic ovary disease, excessive obesity, recent data from the European Group for the Study of Insulin Resistance have suggested that blood pressure values are higher in subjects with insulin resistance than in control group, regardless of age, gender or body mass index. The relationship between hypertension and insulin resistance is stronger in normal weight subjects than in obese ones. Hypertensive, type 2 diabetes patients with normal weight have a higher insulin resistance compared with normotensive patients. In obese type 2 diabetes patients, no significant differences regarding insulin resistance have been demonstrated between normotensive and hypertensive individuals. The correlation between hypertension and insulin resistance may vary with the degree of adipose excess; however, a threshold for obesity probably exists that, if exceeded, this relationship disappears [17].

There is a tight relationship between non-dipper type hypertension and insulin resistance. Non-dipper hypertension is characterized by the absence of nocturnal decrease of blood pressure. Studies performed have shown that non-dipper hypertensive patients have a higher fasting insulinemia and more severe insulin resistance compared with dipper hypertensive patients [17].

There are several pathways through which insulin resistance and hyperinsulinemia may lead to hypertension. Firstly, in diabetes mellitus there is a selective tissular insulin resistance. In the kidney, insulin acts directly on sodium reabsorption, by stimulating Na^+/H^+ pump or Na^+/K^+ ATP-ase from the renal tubuli. In type 2 diabetes mellitus, because of the insulin resistance, insulinemia is increased during the entire day and this could play a role in the initiation and maintenance of high sodium levels. Secondly, hyperinsulinemia with subsequent stimulation of carbohydrate metabolism leads to sympathetic nervous system stimulation and to an increase of circulating norepinephrine, which may result in vasoconstriction. In obese subjects, the activation of sympathetic nervous system is also determined by leptin. This activation results in an increased release of free fatty acids from the adipose tissue, that will determine a reduction in hepatic clearance of insulin, will alter the uptake and utilization of glucose in the muscle and, through the inhibition of NO synthesis, is associated with an increase in vascular reactivity to pressor stimuli. The combined effects of volemic expansion and vasoconstriction will, in

turn, lead to an increase in systolic blood pressure [18, 19].

Insulin also exerts several actions on the metabolism of intracellular electrolytes. There is evidence that insulin determines a rise in intracellular calcium concentration through voltage-dependant calcium channels, and also through a mechanism mediated by protein kinase C. Furthermore, hyperglycemia *per se* leads to increased intracellular calcium both in the myocardium and in the smooth muscle cells from the arterial wall, determining an increased vascular tonus and thus contributing to increased peripheral vascular resistance. Furthermore, high intracellular calcium stimulates Na^+/H^+ antiporter, which, at the kidney level, increases sodium reabsorption in contort distal tubuli, while at the smooth muscle level results in high intracellular sodium and pH. The rise of intracellular pH stimulates protein synthesis that will eventually result in arterial wall hypertrophy. Insulin determines vascular smooth muscle proliferation both *in vitro*, in human arterial cell cultures, and *in vivo*, in aorta from rats. This insulin action is mediated through a direct effect on vascular smooth muscle cell, increased expression of IGF-1 at this level, stimulation of endogenous angiotensinogen synthesis that will determine the local rise of angiotensin II, potentiation of mitogen effect of PDGF (platelet derived growth factor) and increased expression of α1 receptors. Hypertrophy of the vascular wall may lead to increased peripheral vascular resistance and thus determine hypertension [20, 21].

Hypertension in diabetic patients is characterized by plasma expansion, abnormalities in angiotensin-renin system, increased peripheral vascular resistance, and decreased activity of plasmatic renin.

Experimental and clinical data are indicative that hypertension in diabetes mellitus is volume-dependent, the main mechanism involved being hyperglycemia that raises extracellular osmolality and produces an expansion of plasma volume and an increase in total body sodium with approximately 10% compared with non-diabetics.

The role of angiotensin-renin system has been extensively studied, the activity of plasmatic renin being normal or low in most hypertensive diabetic patients. Low-renin-activity hypertension of diabetic patients involves several mechanisms:

raised extracellular volume, impaired renin secretion or synthesis from juxtaglomerular apparatus, decreased prostacyclin secretion, impaired transformation of prorenin in renin. On the other hand, the decreased activity of plasmatic renin or the decreased sensitivity to intrarenal action of angiotensin II leads to renal vasodilatation, contributing to the development of nephropathy [18].

Hyperglycemia, impaired volemia and autonomic nervous system dysfunction may determine in diabetic subjects a raised vascular reactivity to vasopressor stimuli (norepinephrine, angiotensin II), favoring the development of hypertension. Vascular hyperactivity may precede hypertension and may be independent of blood pressure values. Increased vascular tonus may partially result from the alteration of vasodilatation mechanisms. Several clinical and experimental data support the role of insulin in the regulation of vascular tonus through direct interaction both with the endothelium and with vascular smooth muscle cell, with nitric oxide and Na^+/K^+ ATP-ase as vasodilating effectors. In type 2 diabetes, NO-dependent vasodilatation is impaired either because of decreased NO synthesis, or of increased NO inactivation, or secondary of a reduced reactivity of vascular smooth muscle cells to NO; the latter mechanism might also involve advanced end-glycation products. Supplementarily, there is a decrease in prostacyclin synthesis (with vasodilating properties), while endothelin 1 (vasoconstrictor and mitogen for vascular smooth muscle cell) is increased [21].

Secondary hypertension associated with diabetes is due in most cases to diabetic nephropathy, but it may also be the consequence of renal artery stenosis (usually atherosclerotic) or of an associated chronic pyelonephritis.

A tight relationship exists between hypertension and diabetic nephropathy, which is why renal mechanisms are of paramount importance in the pathogenesis of hypertension. The most common mechanism involves the hydrosaline retention and impairment of water excretion capacity, leading to hypervolemia and high blood pressure values; hypertension itself accelerates the deterioration of renal function in diabetic patients, creating a vicious cycle.

There is a genetic susceptibility for hypertension and nephropathy in diabetic patients, represented by the family history of high blood pressure and the increase in Na^+/Li^+ antiporter activity. It seems that the increase in Na^+/Li^+ antiporter reflects the raised activity of membrane Na^+/H^+ pump that will produce high intracellular sodium concentration, followed by an increased sensitivity of the arterial wall to various pressor stimuli [21].

DIAGNOSIS

Given the frequent association of hypertension with diabetes mellitus, it is mandatory that all diabetic patients are investigated for hypertension; conversely, all hypertensive patients, especially if obese, should be investigated for diabetes [22, 23].

The diagnosis of hypertension in diabetic patients is based on multiple measurements of blood pressure, in standard conditions and is established if blood pressure is greater than 130/80 mmHg in at least three different determinations, separated by one week interval [6, 12, 22].

Blood pressure is measured at the office, using the classical method, with mercury sphygmomanometer, twice at each visit, with at least 5-minute interval between determinations [23]. The values thus obtained, with strict observation of measuring conditions, are at the basis of all hypertension classifications and are used for correct staging of the patients and for monitoring the results of therapy. Blood pressure should be measured in both arms, in clino- and orthostatic position, to evidentiate eventual orthostatic hypotension, a consequence of diabetic autonomic neuropathy. According to JNC 6 [2], orthostatic hypotension is defined as a reduction in standing position in systolic blood pressure more than 30 mm Hg or in diastolic blood pressure of more than 15 mm Hg, (according to JNC 7 [3] a decrease of both values of blood pressure with more than 10 mm Hg) associated with symptoms such as giddiness, syncope.

In certain situations, continuous, 24-hours ambulatory non-invasive monitoring of blood pressure is required, most effective and most accurate being automatic ambulatory blood pressure monitoring. In diabetic patients, this method presents several advantages: allows a correct diagnosis, avoiding "white-coat" hypertension, permits a more accurate evaluation of blood pressure variation over 24 hours and the identification of the lack of nocturnal variability of blood pressure (non-dipper hypertension) that relates closely to the cardiovascular risk, allows a better assessment of efficacy of different hypotensor drugs, especially regarding their duration of action and their effect on nocturnal variations of blood pressure [24].

CLINICAL EXAMINATION OF HYPERTENSIVE DIABETIC PATIENTS

The assessment of hypertensive diabetic patients must review the following aspects:

— eventual concomitant medication that may influence blood glucose or blood pressure: non-steroidal anti-inflammatory drugs, amphetamines, sympathicomimetic drugs (nasal decongestives, anorexigens), oral contraceptives, steroid hormones, etc;

— the identification of secondary forms of hypertension, some of them surgically treatable: chronic renal or renovascular diseases, aortic coarctation, pheochromocytoma, Cushing syndrome, primary hyperaldosteronism, thyroid and parathyroid conditions, etc;

— target organ diseases: cardiac (left ventricular hypertrophy, angina pectoris or myocardial infarction, coronary revascularization, heart failure), renal (chronic renal conditions), cerebral (stroke, transitory ischemic attack), retinal (retinopathy);

— family history of diabetes mellitus, hypertension, cardiovascular disease, renal disease, etc;

— personal history of cardiovascular or cerebrovascular disease, diabetic nephropathy, diabetic retinopathy, etc;

— duration of hypertension and blood pressure values;

— duration of diabetes and quality of glycemic control;

— results of previous hypotensor and antidiabetic therapy, as well as possible side effects of these medications;

— presence of other cardiovascular risk factors: obesity, dyslipidemia, smoking;

— lifestyle characteristics: diet, sodium intake, alcohol intake, smoking, physical activity;

— psychosocial and environmental factors that may influence blood pressure or glycemic control.

Physical examination should include:

— at least two determinations of blood pressure, both in clinostatism and in standing position, in both arms; the efficacy of blood-pressure lowering medication is controlled by measuring blood pressure in the arm with the highest value;

— measurement of height, weight, BMI and waist-to-hip ratio;

— complete system and organ examination;

— funduscopic examination for detection of hypertensive and/or diabetic retinopathy;

— neurological examination;

— identification of physical signs indicative of secondary hypertension: palpable lumbar masses (in polycystic kidney), abdominal and lumbar murmurs (renovascular disease), absent pulse at the femoral arteries (aortic coarctation), abdominal obesity with vergetures (Cushing syndrome), tachycardia with paroxysmic headache, sweating (pheochromocytoma).

The following investigations are recommended: chest X-ray, electrocardiogram, cardiac ultrasound, hemoglobin, hematocrit, blood electrolytes, blood glucose, glycemic profile, glycated hemoglobin, serum lipids (total cholesterol, HDL cholesterol, LDL cholesterol, triglycerides), urea, creatinine, uric acid, creatinine clearance, complete urinalysis, proteinuria, albuminuria. Serum lipids, fasting glycemia, glycated hemoglobin, blood electrolytes, and creatinine must be measured before initiating blood pressure-lowering therapy and 6–12 weeks thereafter in order to assess the impact of the medication on carbohydrate, lipid, hydroelectrolytic metabolism, and renal function. The moment and frequency of these investigations depend on the severity of target organ involvement and on the effect of chosen therapy [22, 25, 26].

MANAGEMENT OF ARTERIAL HYPERTENSION IN THE DIABETIC PATIENT

TREATMENT GOALS

The main goals of blood pressure-lowering therapy are:
– reduction of blood pressure values to the normal range;
– decrease of hypertension-associated morbidity and mortality, including the prevention and treatment of target organ disease;
– the control of other modifiable cardiovascular risk factors that may influence the disease evolution [27].

These aims can be achieved in most cases using nonpharmacological and pharmacological measures in association. Epidemiological data showed that blood pressure values over 120/70 mmHg are associated with an increased rate of cardiovascular events and mortality in diabetic patients. Therefore, in these patients a target value of less than 130/80 mmHg is recommended [6, 12].

Two large trials, UKPDS [13, 14] and HOT [28] have followed the benefits of achieving a good blood pressure control in hypertensive diabetic subjects and have demonstrated the existence of a direct and continuous relationship between cardiovascular risk and blood pressure, but without evidentiation of an inferior threshold. In UKPDS [13, 14] each 10 mmHg reduction of mean systolic blood pressure has been associated with a reduction with 12% of all diabetic complications, with 15% of diabetes related mortality, with 11% of myocardial infarction, and with 13% of microvascular complications. Similarly, in the HOT study, optimal results have been obtained in the group with a mean diastolic pressure of 80 mmHg [28].

In patients with renal failure and proteinuria, recommended target values for blood pressure are even lower, of less than 125/75 mmHg [6].

It is very important that these therapeutic goals to be achieved with as few drug side effects as possible and with preservation of patients' quality of life.

THERAPEUTIC STRATEGY

Patients with diabetes should be treated to a diastolic blood pressure of less than 80 mmHg and to a systolic blood pressure less than 130 mmHg. The strategy is presented below [2, 3, 5, 6, 12, 29, 30]:
– Patients with a systolic blood pressure between 130 and 139 mmHg or a diastolic blood pressure between 80 and 89 mmHg should be given lifestyle/behavioral therapy alone for a maximum of 3 months and then, if targets are not achieved, should also be treated pharmacologically.
– Patients with systolic blood pressure between 140 and 159 mmHg or diastolic blood pressure between 90 and 99 mmHg should receive drug therapy (monotherapy) in addition to lifestyle/behavioral therapy.
– Patients with systolic blood pressure of 160 mmHg or over or DBP equal or greater than 100 mmHg should receive drug therapy, two-drug combination.
– Most patients with hypertension will require two or more antihypertensive medications to achieve target blood pressure.
– Initial drug therapy may be from any drug class currently indicated for the treatment of hypertension. However, some drug classes (ACEIs, ARBs, BBs, and diuretics) have been repeatedly shown to be particularly beneficial in reducing cardiovascular events during the treatment of uncomplicated hypertension and are therefore preferred agents for initial therapy.
– In patients with type 1 diabetes, with or without hypertension, with any degree of albuminuria, ACEIs proved to be effective in delaying the progression of nephropathy.
– In patients with type 2 diabetes, hypertension and microalbuminuria, ACEIs and ARBs have been shown to delay the progression to macroalbuminuria. In those with type 2 diabetes, hypertension, macroalbuminuria (>300 mg/day), nephropathy, or renal insufficiency, an ARB should be strongly considered.
– In patients with a recent myocardial infarction, the addition of BB is considered to reduce mortality. In patients with microalbuminuria or overt nephropathy, in whom ACEIs or ARBs are not well tolerated, a non-DCCB or a BB should be considered.
– In elderly hypertensive patients, blood pressure should be lowered gradually to avoid complications.
– The most effective therapy prescribed by the most careful clinician will control hypertension only if patients are motivated. Motivation improves when patients have positive experiences with, and trust in, the clinician.

An algorithm for the treatment of hypertension is presented in Figure 25.1.

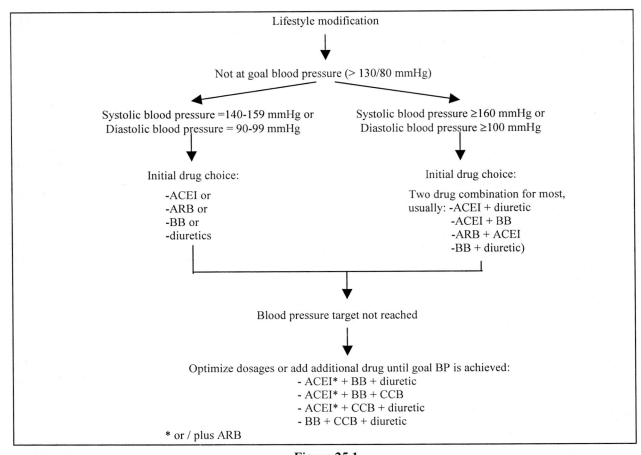

Figure 25.1

Algorithm for treatment of hypertension.

BEHAVIORAL TREATMENTS OF HYPERTENSION

Reductions in daily sodium intake to 10–20 mmol (230–460 mg) per day have resulted in decreases in systolic blood pressure of 10–12 mmHg. The results from controlled trials in essential hypertension have shown that moderate sodium restriction (from a daily intake of 200 mmol [4,600 mg] to 100 mmol [2,300 mg] of sodium per day) is accompanied by a reduction of 5 mmHg for systolic and 2–3 mmHg for diastolic blood pressure [31, 32]. Even when pharmacological agents are used, there is often a better response when there is concomitant salt restriction caused by the aforementioned volume component of hypertension that is almost always present. The efficacy of these measures in diabetic individuals is not known [33, 34]. Weight reduction can reduce blood pressure independent of sodium intake and can also improve blood glucose and lipid levels. The loss of 1 kg body weight has resulted in decreases

in mean arterial blood pressure of approximately 1 mmHg [12, 35, 36]. The role of very low calories diets and pharmacological agents that induce weight loss in the management of hypertension in diabetic patients has not been adequately studied. Some appetite suppressants, both prescription and over-the-counter, may induce rises in blood pressure levels and therefore must be used with care [37].

Moderately intense physical activity, such as 30–45 min of brisk walking most days of the week, has been shown to lower blood pressure [38]. Smoking cessation and moderation of alcohol intake are mandatory.

A number of epidemiological studies suggest an inverse relationship between calcium, magnesium, and potassium intake [39] and blood pressure level. There are no randomized clinical trials on magnesium supplementation in diabetic subjects with hypertension.

The impact of lifestyle modifications is presented in Table 25.3 [2].

Table 25.3

Lifestyle modifications to manage hypertension

Modification	Recommendation	Approximate systolic blood pressure reduction (range)
Weight reduction	Maintain normal body weight (body mass index 18.5–24.9 kg/m^2).	5–20 mmHg/10 kg weight loss
Diet	Consume a diet rich in fruits, vegetables, and low-fat dairy products with a reduced content of saturated and total fat.	8–14 mmHg
Dietary sodium reduction	Reduce dietary sodium intake to no more than 100 mmol *per* day (2.4 g sodium or 6 g sodium chloride).	2–8 mmHg
Physical activity	Engage in regular aerobic physical activity such as brisk walking (at least 30 min *per* day, most days of the week).	4–9 mmHg
Moderation of alcohol consumption	Limit consumption to no more than 2 drinks (1 oz or 30 mL ethanol; *e.g.*, 24 oz beer, 10 oz wine, or 3 oz 80-proof whiskey) *per* day in most men and to no more than 1 drink *per* day in women and lighter weight persons.	2–4 mmHg

CHARACTERISTICS OF THE IDEAL ANTIHYPERTENSIVE DRUG [40]

– Efficient as monotherapy in more than 50% of all patients
– Blood pressure control during all activities for 24 hours
– Once-a-day dosing with high trough-to-peak ratio
– Hemodynamically logical and effective: reduces systemic vascular resistance, improves arterial compliance, preserves cardiac output and maintains perfusion to all vital organs
– Favorable biochemical effects, metabolic effects and risk factor profile
– Reduces structural, vascular smooth muscle and cardiac hypertrophy
– Reduces all end-organ damage
– Low incidence of side effects
– Good compliance with drug regimen
– Reasonable cost

RENIN ANGIOTENSIN SYSTEM INHIBITORS

Any initial treatment for uncomplicated hypertension should not simply lower elevated blood pressure, but also specifically address the pathophysiology of hypertension, and prevent or reverse its complications.

Activation of the RAS plays an important role in the pathogenesis of hypertension, atherosclerosis, heart failure, and diabetic nephropathy. Hypertensive patients with a high plasma renin activity are at a higher risk for myocardial infarction and death. Locally produced AT II in the tissue plays an important role in the cardiovascular and renal pathological changes in diabetes and hypertension [41].

Most of the physiologic effects of AT II, the active component of RAS, are mediated through the activation of AT1 receptors. These effects include vasoconstriction, proximal tubular sodium reabsorption, secretion of aldosterone from the adrenal glands, activation of the sympathetic nervous system, and cell proliferation. AT2 receptors, which are present in abundance during the fetal life, are expressed only in a few organs, including the heart, the adrenal gland, and the kidney, during adulthood. The number of these receptors increases during certain disease states. Their function is not completely understood. AT II induces vasodilatation, mediated by bradykinin, nitric oxide, and cyclic GMP through the activation of its type 2 receptors [41].

AT II causes vasoconstriction, vascular myocyte hypertrophy that enhances the vasoconstrictive response to vasopressors, plasma volume expansion (through increasing aldosterone and antidiuretic hormone and through hemodynamic renal effects) and activates the sympathetic nervous system.

Also, AT II is involved in atherosclerosis through up-regulation of vascular cell adhesion molecule proteins production, stimulation of leukocytes chemotaxis, macrophages activation, enhance of superoxide anion formation, which promotes production of oxidized LDL cholesterol, increase of platelet adhesiveness and plasminogen activator inhibitor type 1, stimulation of vascular myocyte migration from medial to intimal vascular layer and increase of tissue collagen deposition in vascular wall. AT II within the cardiac wall promotes left ventricular hypertrophy and congestive heart failure through cardiac myocyte hypertrophy and fibroblast proliferation. At renal level AT II promotes sodium retention, shifts pressure natriuresis toward higher blood pressure, increases transforming growth factor-β [42]. It is evident that AT II has a negative impact on micro- and macroangiopathy through additional mechanisms rather than through merely elevating blood pressure, and seems logical that a drug that reduces or eliminates the effects of AT II should be effective in hypertension treatment.

Angiotensin Converting Enzyme Inhibitors

When first discovered, the ACEIs antihypertensive effect was believed to result primarily from the blockade of the converting enzyme within the pulmonary circulation to eliminate AT II. However, it was subsequently demonstrated that though there is an initial fall in plasma angiotensin II when an ACEI is given to hypertensive patients, this effect lasts only several weeks. By 6 months, the plasma angiotensin II level returns to normal while the blood pressure remains controlled [43]. The antihypertensive effect of ACEIs results from the transient reduction of angiotensin II and the accumulation of bradykinin since the converting enzyme is also kinase II, the enzyme responsible for degradation of bradykinin [42]. Inhibition of circulatory and tissular angiotensinogen converting enzyme decreases the production of AT II and its vasoconstrictive, proliferative and prothrombotic effects. Also, increase in bradykinin levels associated with the use of ACEIs increases PGI 2 release, NO and tissue-plasminogen activator production and has vasodilatator, antiproliferative and fibrinolytic effects and might be responsible for the improvement in insulin sensitivity [44]. The elevation of bradykinin levels may also contribute to the occurrence of the side effects of ACEIs, such as cough and angioedema.

Several long-term randomized controlled trials (Table 25.4) have demonstrated the beneficial effects of ACEIs in lowering elevated blood pressure, reducing cardiovascular morbidity and mortality, total mortality and microvascular complications in diabetic patients. Some of these studies have suggested that ACEIs may have additional beneficial effects independent of lowering blood pressure.

Table 25.4

Large studies evaluating ACE inhibitors in patients with diabetes mellitus

Trial	Population with Diabetes (%)	Intervention	Follow-up (years)	Blood Pressure (BP) effects	Main Results
UKPDS [13,14] 1998	1148 (100)	Target BP: 144/82 *vs.* 154/87 mmHg Captopril *vs.* atenolol	9	Similar reduction of BP with both drugs	Captopril treatment not superior; reduction in diabetes related events (24%), death (32%) and acute myocardial infarction (21%) in tight BP control group
ABCD [51] 1998	470 (100)	Enalapril *vs.* nisoldipine	5	Similar reduction of BP with both drugs	Fatal and nonfatal acute myocardial infarction: 25 cases in nisoldipine group *vs.* 5 cases in enalapril group
FACET [52] 1998	380 (100)	Fosinopril *vs.* amlodipine	3	Systolic BP significantly higher with fosinopril	Fosinopril treatment superior; decrease in major cardiovascular events (51%) with fosinopril

Table 25.4

(continued)

Trial	Population with Diabetes (%)	Intervention	Follow-up (years)	Blood Pressure (BP) effects	Main Results
CAPPP [48] 1999	572 (5.2)	Captopril *vs.* β-blocker or diuretic	6	Baseline BP greater in Captopril group; similar reduction with both drugs	Captopril treatment superior in cohort with diabetes; decrease in primary outcome (40%), acute myocardial infarction (65%), cardiovascular events (33%) in captopril group
HOPE [45], 2000	3578 (38.5)	Ramipril *vs.* placebo	4.5	In ramipril group BP was lower with 2.4 /1 mm Hg	Ramipril treatment superior; decrease in primary outcome (25%), acute myocardial infarction (22%), stroke (33%), total mortality (16%), overt nephropathy (24%)
ALLHAT [49] 2003	12063 (36)	Chlortalidone vs. lisinopril vs. amlodipine	4.9	Systolic BP significantly higher in amlodipine and lisinopril group	No differences in non fatal myocardial infarction, coronary heart disease deaths and total mortality; Congestive heart failure more frequent in lisinopril and amlodipine groups; borderline elevated risk for combined cardiovascular disease with lisinopril vs. diuretic

Cardiovascular protective effects of ACEIs

The HOPE study [45] investigated the effects of ACE inhibition on the development and progression of atherosclerotic process [46]. In this study, 9297 patients with established atherosclerotic disease or diabetes with at least one other cardiovascular risk factor, *i.e.*, hypertension, hypercholesterolemia, smoking, or microalbuminuria, were randomized to treatment with ramipril *versus* placebo. At the beginning of the study 38% of participants had diabetes, and 47% had mildly elevated blood pressure. After a 4.5-year follow-up period, in the ramipril-treated group was reported a 22% reduction in the primary outcome (combined incidence of myocardial infarction, stroke, or death from cardiovascular disease), incidence of myocardial infarction was reduced by 22%, stroke by 33%, all-cause mortality by 24%, microvascular complications by 16% and overt nephropathy by 24%, despite only modest reduction of blood pressure (−3/2 mmHg). Mean systolic blood pressure in the ramipril-treated group was 136 mm Hg, whereas it was 139 mm Hg in the placebo-treated group. The lower cardiovascular risk in the ramipril group persisted after adjustment for blood pressure differences, therefore, it has been suggested that part of the cardioprotective properties of ACE inhibition are independent of their antihypertensive effects. The HOPE trial also demonstrated that ramipril use results in a 34% reduction in the development of new cases of diabetes [45].

The results of comparative trials of ACEIs, BBs, CCBs and diuretics are discordant. The UKPDS [13, 14] and STOP-2 [47] found that ACEIs were equivalent to BB and diuretics, while in CAPPP [48], ACEIs were superior in hypertensive diabetics. The ALLHAT trial [49] compared ACEIs, CCBs and thiazide diuretics. Blood pressure control was slightly but significantly different between groups; systolic blood pressure was better decreased in the diuretic group, while diastolic blood pressure was better decreased in the CCB group. In a prespecified subgroup analysis of 12,063 patients with type 2 diabetes, no significant differences were seen between the groups regarding the primary outcomes of nonfatal acute myocardial infarction plus CHD death or all-cause mortality. However, the risk for heart failure was the lowest in the diuretic group. In addition, the ACEI group had a borderline elevated risk for combined cardiovascular disease compared to the diuretic group [46]. The conclusion of this study, that diuretics are superior to ACEIs and CCBs, seems excessive because the study included a large number of African Americans, which have poorer response to ACEIs; systolic blood pressure was significantly higher in ACEI and CCB treated groups and the antihypertensive therapeutic combinations were inappropriate for ACEI [50].

The ABCD trial [51] demonstrated that ACE inhibition may be superior to calcium-channel blockade in the reduction of CVD events in patients with diabetes. Similar outcomes were shown by the FACET [52], which compared the effects of fosinopril with amlodipine on serum lipid levels and glycemic control in 380 patients with type 2 diabetes and hypertension. The FACET [52] results indicated that despite similar metabolism of both medications, an ACEI, fosinopril, significantly lowered the risk the combined outcome of stroke, myocardial infarction, and hospitalization for congestive heart failure, compared to CCB-amlodipine therapy. It should be noticed that patients treated with both fosinopril and amlodipine had the fewest cardiovascular events [53].

In the ACEI group, the risk of acute myocardial infarction was significantly decreased in the ABCD [51] and the CAPPP [48] trial was nonsignificantly lower in the FACET [52], and was nonsignificantly higher in the UKPDS [14] compared to the alternative treatment. For the outcome of stroke, no significant differences were evident among treatments in any of the trials. In the ACEI group, the risk of combined cardiovascular events was significantly decreased in the ABCD trial, the CAPPP and the FACET, and was nonsignificantly increased in the UKPDS [14] compared with the alternative treatment; the risk of all-cause mortality was significantly decreased in the CAPPP [48], was

nonsignificantly lower in the ABCD trial and the FACET, and was nonsignificantly higher in the UKPDS. Meta-analysis [53] of the ABCD, CAPPP and FACET trials showed a significant advantage of ACEIs over alternative treatment modalities in reducing acute myocardial infarction (63% reduction), cardiovascular events (51% reduction), and all-cause mortality (62% reduction). These findings were not observed in the UKPDS, which compared captopril with atenolol. The ACEIs did not appear to be superior to other agents for the outcome of stroke in any of the trials [53].

The greater benefit of ACEIs in major cardiovascular events was not explained by differences in blood pressure control, metabolic control, or other measured risk factors [53]. This indicates that other mechanisms linked to ACE inhibition may have played an additional role in the prevention of major clinical events. One of the possible mechanisms of such CVD protection is improvement of insulin sensitivity by ACEIs. The HOPE trial also demonstrated that ramipril use results in a 34% reduction in the development of new cases of diabetes. Similarly, the CAPPP showed a reduction of 11% in the new cases of diabetes with the use of an ACEI [48]. These results suggest possible benefits from the ACEIs beyond their antihypertensive effect. Improving insulin resistance as demonstrated in other animal and human studies could be, in part, responsible for these observations [54]. It has been suggested that endogenous AT II, through its effects on insulin signaling, is involved in insulin resistance [55]. Bradykinin type 2 receptor-deficient mice had higher insulin levels and lower insulin sensitivity than normal mice when both groups were treated with captopril [56]. This finding suggests a possible role for bradykinin in reducing insulin resistance during treatment with ACEIs [41]. Other metabolic favorable effects of ACEIs include reduction of low-density lipoprotein particle oxidation [57], improvement of hypercoagulation [58], attenuation of oxidative stress [59], and enhancement of endothelial nitric oxide function [60]. ACEIs may also enhance endothelial integrity by decreasing expression of vascular cell adhesion molecules [61], and normalizing vascular permeability [62].

Renoprotective effects of ACEIs in type 1 diabetic patients

Several randomized, placebo-controlled studies have enrolled type 1 and type 2 diabetic patients with microalbuminuria or macroalbuminuria to evaluate the benefit of ACEI therapy. These studies have shown significant reductions in the urinary albumin excretion rate with the use of different ACEIs. A large placebo controlled trial using captopril [63] showed a significant decrease in the progression of diabetic nephropathy in proteinuric (urinary albumin excretion rate > 0.500mg/24 h) hypertensive type 1 diabetic patients. Captopril treatment was associated with a 48% reduction in the incidence of doubling of serum creatinine and a 50% reduction in the incidence of end-stage renal disease or death. The differences in systolic and diastolic blood pressure levels between the two groups (placebo and captopril) studied were small, suggesting that ACEIs have a renal protective effect independent of their antihypertensive effect. This is the only randomized, placebo-controlled trial of ACEI therapy in proteinuric hypertensive type 1 diabetic patients that assessed hard renal outcomes [41].

There are studies showing that in patients with microalbuminuria (urinary albumin excretion rate of 30–300 mg/24 h) and hypertension, ACEIs decrease the progression to overt proteinuria (urinary albumin excretion rate >300 mg/24 h) [64, 65]. Also, in studies of type 1 patients with microalbuminuria without a clinical diagnosis of hypertension, several small clinical trials suggest that ACEIs may be beneficial in delaying the progression of nephropathy [66, 67]. A recent meta-analysis [86] of data obtained for 698 patients enrolled in several small trials has shown a statistically significant decrease in progression to macroalbuminuria [12].

Renoprotective effect of ACEIs in type 2 diabetic patients

There is little evidence that the use of ACEIs as prophylactic treatment in type 1 or type 2 diabetic patients without microalbuminuria can prevent the development of diabetic nephropathy, although there was a nonsignificant decrease in the development of microalbuminuria in type 2 diabetic patients in the MICRO-HOPE study [45].

In the MICRO-HOPE study [45], ramipril compared with placebo reduced the relative risk of developing overt proteinuria from microalbuminuria by 24% (p < 0.027) and the risk for combined microvascular outcome of overt nephropathy, dialysis or laser therapy by 16%. Transition from normo- to macroalbuminuria was also significantly decreased when enalapril was compared with placebo in a group (n = 194) of normotensive normoalbuminuric type 2 diabetic patients [69]; only 6.5% of patients treated with the ACEI developed proteinuria compared with 19% of those receiving placebo. Comparison between the effect of ACEIs and other therapies on creatinine clearance and proteinuria has been performed in several small studies with follow-up periods lasting from 3 to 5 years. A greater reduction in proteinuria was obtained with ACEIs in the absence of significant differences in glomerular filtration rate [70].

Some limited evidence showed that ACEIs may have hypertension-independent renoprotective effects in patients with diabetes: some short-term trials [71–73] and the placebo-controlled study of Ravid *et al.* [74] that showed renoprotective effects after 7 years of treatment with enalapril in normotensive microalbuminuric type 2 diabetic patients. Other studies have reported similar degrees of renal protection when nifedipine [75], amlodipine [76], nitrendipine [77], atenolol [69], or nisoldipine [78] were compared with an ACEI. Development of microalbuminuria or overt proteinuria did not differ in patients receiving captopril or atenolol in the UKPDS study [14], or in those receiving either enalapril or nisoldipine in the ABCD [51] studies. So far, there are no long-term trials comparing angiotensin II receptor blockers with ACEIs in patients with diabetes. Early data on renal outcomes appear to be equivalent [79] and effects on intermediate end points such as blood pressure control seem to be similar, although angiotensin II receptor blockers may be slightly better tolerated [46].

Diabetic retinopathy and ACEIs

In the UKPDS [13, 14], there was a significant reduction of 34% in the number of patients requiring photocoagulation and showing deterioration of the retinopathy by two or more steps and a 47% reduction in the risk of decreasing vision in both eyes was associated with tight blood pressure control. This benefit was achieved with either the ACE inhibitor or the beta-blocker, suggesting that the reduction in blood pressure, rather than ACE inhibition itself, may be of primary importance.

ACEI therapy has been associated with lower levels of vascular endothelial growth factor in patients with proliferative diabetic retinopathy [80], and animal models suggest a strong potential benefit for ACE inhibition as a treatment for diabetic retinopathy [81]. Although conclusive proof of a specific and independent benefit for ACE inhibition in treating diabetic retinopathy has not been demonstrated, clinical trials are now under way to further elucidate these issues. In the meantime, ACE inhibition in appropriate patients with diabetic retinopathy is of value in reducing the risk of renal disease and lowering blood pressure, which have been associated with progression of diabetic retinopathy [82].

Conclusions

ACEIs are useful in the management of hypertension in diabetic patients with or without diabetic nephropathy. They are also effective in decreasing cardiovascular mortality and morbidity in patients with congestive heart failure and post myocardial infarction [12]. The UKPDS [13, 14] showed similar beneficial effects of the ACE inhibitor captopril and the β-blocker atenolol on diabetes-related mortality and microvascular and cardiovascular complications in patients with type 2 diabetes. Data from recent trials [45, 51, 52] support the view that, compared with the alternative agents tested, ACEIs appear to provide a special advantage in addition to blood pressure control. The question of whether atenolol is equivalent to captopril remains open. Because many studies demonstrated the benefits of ACEIs on multiple adverse outcomes in patients with diabetes, including macrovascular and microvascular complications, in patients with either mild or more severe hypertension and in type 1 and type 2 diabetes, the established practice of choosing an ACEI as the first–line agent in most patients with diabetes is reasonable [83]. In Table 25.5 are presented some of the ACEIs frequently used in clinical practice.

Table 25.5

Angiotensin converting enzyme inhibitors

Drug	Daily dose (mg)	Observations
Benazepril*	10–40	Contraindications: pregnancy, bilateral renal artery stenosis or renal artery stenosis of the unique kidney, hypersensitivity to this drug
Captopril*	12.5–150	
Cilazapril	2.5–5	
Enalapril*	2.5–40	
Fosinopril	10–40	Adverse effects: cough, angioedema, hypotension, decline of renal function in patients with renal impairment
Lisinopril*	5–40	
Perindopril*	4–8	
Quinapril*	10–40	
Ramipril*	2.5–10	Cautions: monitor serum creatinine and K^+ levels, adjust dosage in patients with serum creatinine ≥ 221 mmol/l (2.5mg/dL) for drugs marked with *
Trandolapril*	2–4	

Angiotensin II AT 1 receptor blockers

AT 1 receptors are responsible for the majority of cardiovascular action of AT II and are subject to genetic polymorphism. So far, three genetic types of AT 1 receptors (A, B, C) have been identified. The homozygote type CC is most frequently associated with left ventricular hypertrophy and with the risk for myocardial infarction. AT 1 receptor blockers prevent the binding of AT II, generated both in the classic pathway of ACE and in the non-ACE alternate pathway, and consecutively lowers blood pressure through vasodilatation, decrease in sympathetic activity, decreased aldosterone synthesis, decrease retention of sodium and water. They determine an increase in circulating AT II and stimulate AT 2 receptors (if they are expressed). Lack of AT 2 receptor blocking permits the maintenance of favorable effects of AT II mediated through these receptors: vasodilatation with increased coronary blood flow, a better myocardial oxygenation, myocardial protection during ischemic events and antiproliferative effects. ARBs do not interfere with bradykinin and substance P catabolism, therefore avoiding ACEIs side effects (cough, bronchospasm) [84].

Currently, there is a large range of AT 1 receptor blockers, known as sartans: losartan, irbesartan, candesartan, valsartan, telmisartan, eprosartan, and olmesartan (Table 25.6).

Table 25.6

Angiotensin II receptor AT 1 blockers

Drug	Daily dose (mg)	Observations
Irbesartan	150–300	Effective in controling blood pressure, renal and cardiovascular protective effects
Losartan	50–100	
Valsartan	80–320	Should be strongly considered in the presence of diabetic nephropathy in type 2 diabetes
Candesartan	8–35	
Telmisartan	40–80	Cautions: monitor of renal function and serum K^+ levels,
Eprosartan	400–800	Contraindications: pregnancy, hypersensitivity to these drugs
Olmesartan	20–40	

All ARBs have duration of action of approximately 24 hours, which allows the administration once daily. The selectivity for AT 1 receptors compared to AT 2 receptors is extremely important. This selectivity is over 20,000 for valsartan, over 10,000 for candesartan, over 8,000 for irbesartan, over 3,000 for telmisartan and over 1,000 for eprosartan and losartan.

ARBs reduce systolic and diastolic blood pressure in a dose-dependent manner. The blood pressure lowering is maintained 24 hours in case of single dose administration. The trough-to-peak ratio (T/P) is between 60 and 100%. Monotherapy with ARBs achieves blood pressure control in over 50% of subjects with grade 1 and grade 2 hypertension. When associated with other blood pressure lowering agents, target values are reached in over 80% of the patients [84, 85].

Sartans can be associated with BBs, CCBs, ACEIs, diuretics. The association with ACEIs is extremely useful, decreasing both circulating AT II and its action on AT 1 receptors.

ARBs do not interfere with carbohydrate and lipid metabolism. Side effects during sartan therapy are rare and side effect-related treatment drop-out rate is low.

Renoprotective effects of ARBs

Several studies in type 2 diabetic patients with hypertension have shown that ARBs reduce albuminuria, can even restaurate normoalbuminuria and retard development and progression of nephropathy (Table 25.7).

Table 25.7

Studies evaluating ARBs in hypertensive diabetic patients

Trial	n	Follow-up (years)	Intervention	Renal outcomes	Cardiovascular outcomes
RENAAL [86]	1513	3.4	Losartan vs. placebo	Doubling of serum creatinine: ↓25% ESRD: ↓ 28% Proteinuria: ↓ 35%	Mortality and morbidity from cardiovascular causes, all-cause mortality were similar Rate of first hospitalization for heart failure ↓ 32% with losartan
IDNT [87]	1715	2.6	Irbesartan 300mg vs. amlodipine 10mg vs. placebo	Doubling of serum creatinine: Irbesartan vs. placebo ↓ 33%, Irbesartan vs. amlodipine ↓ 37% ESRD: irbesartan vs. both placebo or amlodipine ↓ 23%	Mortality and morbidity from cardiovascular causes, all-cause mortality were similar
IRMA 2 [88]	590	2	Irbesartan 300 mg vs. placebo	Progression to overt nephropathy: 300mg irbesartan 5.2%, 150mg irbesartan 9.7%, placebo 14.9% Restoration of normoalbuminuria: 34%	Not studied
CALM [91]	199	0.5	Candesartan vs. lisinopril vs. combination	UAER: candesartan ↓ 44%, lisinopril ↓ 39%, combination ↓ 50%	Not studied
LIFE [93]	1195	4	Losartan vs. atenolol	Not studied	Mortality from cardiovascular causes, stroke, miocardial infarction ↓ 24.5 % with losartan
ESRD = end-stage renal disease, UAER = urinary albumin excretion					

The RENAAL study [86] examined the effect of losartan when added to conventional antihypertensive therapy in 1,513 diabetic type 2 subjects with diabetic nephropathy. Mean follow-up was 3.4 years. Patients in the losartan group had a 16% risk reduction in the composite primary end point (doubling of serum creatinine, end-stage renal disease, or death, a 25% risk reduction in the doubling of serum creatinine, and a 28% reduction in end-stage renal disease. Proteinuria was reduced by 35%. The benefits exceeded those attributable to changes in blood pressure.

In IDNT [87], the effect of irbesartan added to conventional therapy was compared with amlodipine and placebo also added to conventional therapy in 1,715 hypertensive diabetic type 2 patients with overt nephropathy treated for a mean duration of 2.6 years. Treatment with irbesartan (300 mg) was associated with a reduction of the risk of the primary composite end point (doubling of serum creatinine, development of end-stage renal disease or death) of 20% compared with the placebo group and 23% compared with the amlodipine group. The risk of doubling serum creatinine was 33% lower compared with the placebo group and 37% compared with the amlodipine group (10 mg). The relative risk of end-stage renal disease was 23% lower in the irbesartan group than in the placebo or amlodipine groups. These differences were not explained by the blood pressure reduction achieved. There were no significant differences in the rates of death or cardiovascular composite outcomes.

IRMA 2 investigators [88] examined the effect of irbesartan *vs.* placebo on the development of diabetic nephropathy in 590 type 2 hypertensive diabetic subjects with microalbuminuria. Follow-up was for 2 years. They found that in 5.2% of the 300-mg irbesartan and in 9.7% of the 150-mg irbesartan group, the primary outcome (time to onset of diabetic nephropathy, defined by persistent albuminuria, with a urinary albumin excretion rate >200 μg/min and >30% higher than baseline) was achieved, compared with 14.9% of the placebo group. It was reported a dose-dependent beneficial effect of irbesartan on the level of microalbuminuria and a more frequent restoration of normoalbuminuria in the 300 mg irbesartan group. Although both doses of irbesartan produced comparable reductions in

blood pressure, only the 300 mg dose was renoprotective. They concluded that irbesartan had a renoprotective effect independent of any blood pressure-lowering effect.

In these three studies, systolic blood pressure remained above goal blood pressure suggested by guidelines (< 130/80 mmHg for IRMA 2 and < 125/75 mmHg for RENAAL and IDNT). This confirms the difficulty of controlling blood pressure in diabetic patients. Benefit was thus obtained in the absence of strict blood pressure control. Renal protection in type 2 diabetes by a similar degree of blood pressure control independent of the type of therapy remains unexplored. Interestingly, the positive data of the RENAAL study [86] was obtained while approximately 90% of patients were receiving a calcium channel blocker (two thirds a dihydropyridine calcium antagonist) in addition to losartan and other antihypertensive agents. These data indicate that in the presence of renal damage and proteinuria, the combination of an ARB and a calcium channel blocker is totally safe. However, the IDNT data suggest that calcium channel blocker use without concurrent angiotensin II blockade with an ARB does not afford renoprotection [70].

ACEIs and/or ARBs in hypertensive type 2 diabetic patients

So far there are no long-term trials comparing angiotensin II receptor blockers with ACEIs in patients with diabetes. Early data on renal outcomes appear to be equivalent [79] and effects on intermediate end points such as blood pressure control seem to be similar, although angiotensin II receptor blockers may be slightly better tolerated [46]. In most patients, renal function continues to decline at an accelerated rate (>5 mL/min/year) despite treatment with either an ACEI (type 1 diabetes) or an ARB (type 2 diabetes), and end-stage renal disease is not prevented [89]. Possible reasons for this include insufficient blood pressure lowering and incomplete RAS blockade [90].

Several small studies have shown the benefits of combining lower doses of ACEIs and ARBs. In the CALM study, dual blockade of the RAS using candesartan and lisinopril for 6 months found that the combination of both agents reduced blood pressure and urinary albumin levels to a greater extent than either medication alone [91]. However, published studies of ACEI plus ARB combinations have important shortcomings, including small numbers of study subjects, short-term follow-up (1 to 6 months), mixed renal diseases, lack of control of sodium intake, variable doses of both classes of agents, low doses of ACEI or ARB, variation in proteinuria measurements, and lack of safety data reporting [90].

Cardiovascular protective effects of ARBs

Long-term data on cardiovascular outcomes using this class of drugs are limited (Table 25.7). The RENAAL [86] study compared the effects of losartan vs. placebo when added to conventional antihypertensive therapy in hypertensive type 2 diabetic patients. There were no differences between the two groups for all-cause mortality and the composite of mortality and morbidity from cardiovascular causes. Rate of first hospitalization for heart failure was 32% lower on losartan. In the IDNT [87] study there were no significant differences in the rates of death or cardiovascular composite outcomes, between the groups treated with irbesartan, amlodipine or placebo in addition to conventional antihypertensive therapy. The addition of valsartan to chronic ACEI treatment in patients with heart failure in the Val-HeFT [92] study did not reduce mortality but was associated with a 27.5% reduction in hospitalization. This effect was largely related to the significant reduction in morbidity and mortality associated with the use of valsartan in those who could not tolerate ACEIs; once these patients were removed from the analysis, the reduction in hospitalization seen with valsartan was not significant anymore [41].

LIFE study [93] has demonstrated a 25% reduction of risk for composite end point (represented by cardiovascular mortality, myocardial infarction, and stroke) in the subgroup of patients with DM and a 38% reduction of general mortality risk.

All these studies confirm that ARBs are first line agents for the treatment of hypertension in diabetic patients.

BETA-BLOCKERS

BBs have been convincingly shown to reduce total and cardiovascular morbidity and mortality of hypertensive diabetic patients. In diabetic patients, after myocardial infarction, these agents confer a twice as high protective effect when compared to non-diabetic patients [94]. However, most paradoxically, β-blocking agents are used less frequently in diabetes probably because of concern about possible adverse metabolic effects, hypoglycemia unawareness or less nephroprotective effects of β1 -selective BBs.

Unlike diuretics, CCBs and ACEIs, there are no prospective, randomized, placebo-controlled mortality trials in hypertensives involving diabetics who received BBs. In the STOP-2 study [47] that involved 719 hypertensive elderly diabetics, conventional therapy (a mixture of diuretics and BBs given as first line therapy), did not differ from ACEIs or CCBs in preventing cardiovascular events. In the UKPDS [14] the ACEI was not superior to the BB in reducing either primary or secondary clinical end-points. The blood pressure at base-line and after 9 years of follow-up was the same in both drugs groups. Although no significant differences existed between the two drugs, the trends of all 7 primary endpoints (i.e., any diabetes end point, deaths related to diabetes, all cause mortality, myocardial infarction, stroke, peripheral vascular disease and microvascular disease) favored the BB. Also, a large majority of the secondary end points showed trends favoring the BB. β-1 blockade was at least as "reno-protective" as ACE-inhibition in the UKPDS [14] study. At baseline, 20% of patients assigned to atenolol and 16% of those assigned to captopril had albuminuria (>50 mg/L); after 9 years, the proportions were 26% and 31% respectively, and there was no difference in the plasma creatinine concentration (or in those who had more than a two-fold increase in plasma creatinine concentration between the atenolol and captopril groups). Non-compliance was slightly worse on atenolol due to cold feet (4%) and bronchospasm (6%).

The LIFE study [93] involved 1195 diabetics with hypertension and left ventricular hypertrophy by ECG, mean age 67 years, who were randomized to atenolol or losartan and followed up for a mean of 4.7 years. Blood pressure control was similar with both agents. In contrast to the UKPDS [14] study, atenolol came out second best. The primary endpoint was 24% less frequent in the losartan group; all-cause mortality was 39% less frequent in the losartan group; there were no significant differences in the frequency of non-fatal and fatal stroke and myocardial infarction in the two drug groups, though the trends favored losartan. Losartan was better tolerated than atenolol. ECG-left ventricular hypertrophy was reversed more effectively by losartan. The change in serum-creatinine over 4 years was similar in both groups.

It is apparent that studies favoring BBs (including UKPDS) involve younger, middle-aged hypertensives with a mean age in the low 50s with a relatively compliant vascular system as evidenced by mean pulse-pressures ranging between 59–65 mmHg. By contrast, the studies generally unfavorable to BBs as first-line therapy (including the LIFE study) involve elderly hypertensives with a mean age around 70 years, with a relatively non-compliant, stiff vascular system as evidenced by mean pulse-pressures ranging between 76–97 mmHg [95]. Evidence also indicates that β1 receptor responses of the heart decline with age. Thus, first line BB therapy would be ideally suited to younger/middle aged hypertensives, say less than 60–65 years old, where β1 receptor activity has not been downgraded and the vascular system is relatively compliant and elastic. In the elderly hypertensive, BBs are relatively ineffective in reversing left ventricular hypertrophy and reducing the frequency of heart attacks. Initiating BB therapy in the elderly hypertensive should be on the back of low dose diuretic therapy which does improve vascular compliance, reverses left ventricular hypertrophy and reduces the frequency of cardiovascular events, including heart attacks. If, however, an elderly hypertensive has a history of myocardial infarction, a BB should be considered as first-line therapy [95].

Effects of β-blockers on blood glucose

β2 receptors appear to play an important role in the stimulated hepatic glucose production in humans. Adverse effects of blockade of β2 receptors on glucose metabolism have been recognized and repeatedly described. In contrast to unselective BB, β1 selective blockers appear to be without relevant influence on glucose metabolism. However, in some studies, adverse effects of β1 selective blockers have been described. A validity of this conclusion is brought into question by significant weight gain in the BB treated groups

during the study period [14]. In such circumstances, it is impossible to demonstrate any specific metabolic effect of an antihypertensive drug, as even small changes in body weight may markedly affect glucose tolerance and insulin sensitivity. It is of note that the impressive benefits of BB therapy of patients were observed despite simultaneous gain in body weight [14].

β-blockers and hypoglycemia unawareness

Theoretically, BBs could diminish the adrenergic counterreaction to low blood glucose concentrations. The impact of β blockade on hypoglycemia has been addressed in several experimental investigations. Some of these studies described a diminished occurrence of tremor and heart pounding under β blockade, but in most of them sweating was increased, as did the total occurrence of symptoms. Until now, no study reported clinically relevant hypoglycemia unawareness associated with BBs treatment. Four recent epidemiological studies have independently confirmed previous findings that cardioselective BBs are not associated with an increased risk of severe hypoglycemia. However, most interestingly, these studies have shown that treatment with ACEI is associated with an increased risk of severe hypoglycemia amongst type 2 diabetes mellitus patients using insulin or sulphonylureas. Hence, BBs do not mask hypoglycemia but may change the pattern of symptoms by increasing the occurrence of sweating. No study has ever reported an increased risk of severe hypoglycemia associated with BB treatment of diabetics [94, 96].

β-blockers and the duration of hypoglycemia

Glycogenolysis and gluconeogenesis in the liver are stimulated through β2-receptors. Blockade of these receptors could prolong recovery time from hypoglycemia. Under unselective BB treatment, such prolongation of hypoglycemia has been described. However, under β1-selective blocker treatment, the recovery from hypoglycemia was not impaired amongst patients with insulin or oral hypoglycemic agents [94, 95, 96].

Renoprotective effects of β-blockers

The initial interventional studies that demonstrated reductions in the rate of deterioration of the glomerular filtration rate in type 1 diabetic patients with nephropathy used β1-blockers and diuretics as antihypertensive medications, frequently with other drugs. In three randomized studies in diabetic hypertensive patients, in which proteinuria was examined, atenolol (a β1 selective blocker) produced similar reductions in proteinuria compared with an ACE inhibitor. In a long-term study (43 patients followed for 3.5 years), atenolol and lisinopril produced similar reductions in the decline of the glomerular filtration rate in patients with type 2 diabetes and nephropathy [12].

Conclusions

Inappropriate attention to surrogate endpoints, at the expense of hard clinical facts, can lead to faulty prescribing [95]. β blockade is at least as effective as "favored" ACE inhibition in the prevention of both macrovascular and microvascular events in young/middle aged hypertensive diabetics [14]. The BB atenolol was less effective than the angiotensin II receptor antagonist losartan in reducing cardiovascular morbidity and mortality and all-cause mortality in mainly elderly hypertensives with or without diabetes [93]. β1 selective blockade should be considered for the first line therapy in younger/middle aged (up to 60–65 years) hypertensives with or without type 2 diabetes. For the elderly hypertensive with or without diabetes, a BB not be first-line therapy but, as in the classic SHEP study [97], should low dose diuretic therapy (which does improve vascular compliance and reduce the risk of cardiovascular events, including myocardial infarction) should be prescribed.

However, very elderly hypertensives with prior myocardial infarction appear to suffer significantly fewer new coronary events when prescribed a BB alone or combined with a diuretic compared to a calcium antagonist or alpha-blocker prescribed alone or combined with a diuretic. Selection of the right type of BB is important; high β1 selectivity will ensure optimal lowering of blood pressure and reduce the risk of potentially dangerous adverse events such as bronchospasm and peripheral vasoconstriction arising from blockade of the β2 receptor [95].

In Table 25.8 the main characteristics of the heterogenous class of BBs are presented.

Table 25.8

β-blockers

β-blockers	Daily dose (mg)	Observations
selective β-blockers		
Propranolol	10–640	Adverse effects on glucose and lipid metabolism, decreased counterregulatory responses to hypoglycemia More frequent peripheral vasoconstriction, bronchospasm
Timolol	20–40	
Carteolol	2.5–10	
β1 selective -blockers without intrinsic sympathetic activity (ISA) (a) and with ISA (b)		
(a) Atenolol	25–100	No clinical significant adverse effects on glucose and lipids metabolism, counterregulatory responses to hypoglycemia, lower risk for peripheral vasoconstriction, bronchospasm With increasing dosage they became less selective
Betaxolol	10–20	
Metoprolol	100–200	
Bisoprolol	5–20	
(b) Acebutolol	200–1200	
Non selective α-β-blockers		
Labetalol	200–1200	peripheral vasodilatation
Carvedilol	6.25–25	
β1 selective blockers with NO dependent vasodilatation action		
Nebivolol	5–10	peripheral vasodilatation

DIURETICS

The principal modality of action of diuretics in hypertension is represented by reduction of cardiac output, of intracellular volume (during the first day of use), decrease of peripheral vascular resistance by reducing vascular reactivity (through decreasing sodium content in the smooth muscle cell), decrease of renal self-regulation, reduction of noradrenergic neuronal activity, and increase of prostaglandin synthesis.

The main diuretics utilized in the treatment of hypertension are: thiazides, that act on the cortical segment of the ascending of Henle loop; loop diuretics, that act on the medullar segment of the Henle loop; indapamide, that besides its diuretic action has also vasodilating activity by modulating NO action and does not interfere with carbohydrate and lipid metabolism; and potassium-sparing diuretics.

Side effects occur especially with the use of thiazides and are represented by: hyperglycemia, hyperuricemia, dyslipidemia, metabolic alkalosis, hypovolemia, hypokalemia, hyponatremia, etc.

In a series of randomized trials, the use of thiazides was associated with a reduction in the risk of stroke and heart failure. In elderly subjects with isolated systolic hypertension diuretics lead to a decrease in cardiovascular morbidity. The SHEP study [97] has demonstrated that low doses of thiazides used for the treatment of high blood pressure in elderly diabetics have produced a significant reduction of cardiovascular events. Diuretics are not efficient in subjects with impaired renal function. The effect of thiazides on the progression of diabetic nephropathy has not been studied in large, randomized clinical trials.

STOP-2 study [47] has shown a reduction of major cardiovascular events of similar magnitude both in hypertensive patients treated with hydrochlorothiazide in association with amiloride and beta blockers and in those treated with enalapril and felodipine. The major determinant of cardiovascular risk reduction was the decrease in blood pressure values.

Low dose thiazides can be used as first line therapy in elderly hypertensive diabetic patients, especially in those with isolated systolic hypertension. They can be also used in association with other blood pressure lowering drugs. The reduction of cardiovascular events in patients treated with chlorthalidone has also been demonstrated by the ALLHAT Study [49].

Indapamide can be used as first line therapy in elderly diabetics, which present the following advantages: does not interfere with carbohydrate and lipid metabolism, is administered in a single daily dose and also exerts a vasodilating effect. Its efficacy as antihypertensive therapy is currently under study, in the HYVET branch, expected to end in 2004.

Table 25.9 presents the types of diuretics used in the treatment of hypertension in diabetes mellitus.

Table 25.9
Diuretics

Drug	Daily dose (mg)	Observations
Thiazides(a) and Related Sulphonamide Compounds(b)		
(a) Hydrochlorothiazide	6.25–50	Low doses (indapamide 1.5 mg, chlorthalidone or hydrochlorothiazide 12.5 mg) do not have adverse metabolic effects. Ineffective when serum creatinine >2.5 mg/dL.
Hydroflumethiazide	12.5–50	
Chlorothiazide	125–500	
(b) Chlorthalidone	12.5–50	
Indapamide	1.5–5	
Loop Diuretics		
Bumetanide	0.5–10	Used when serum creatinine >2.5 mg/dL, usually in combinations
Ethacrynic acid	25–100	
Torsemide	5–10	
Furosemide	20–320	Adverse effects include hypokalemia, hyponatremia, volume depletion
Potassium-sparing agents		
Triamterene	100–300	Used in combinations with other diuretics to counteract hypokalemia; contraindications: hyperkalemia, serum creatinine ≥ 2.5 mg/dL; should not be used with other K^+ conserving agents in renal impairment

CALCIUM CHANNEL BLOCKERS

CCBs have been initially used in the treatment of angina pectoris and of supraventricular arrhythmias but subsequently have also proved effective in the treatment of hypertension.

Although chemically different, CCBs have a common antihypertensive mechanism: they block the sarcolemmal voltage-dependent calcium channels from the vascular smooth muscle cells. The main hemodynamic and cardiovascular effects of CCBs are: peripheral vasodilatation with the consequent decrease of peripheral vascular resistance and reduction of blood pressure, inhibition of the automatism of the sinoatrial and atrio-ventricular nodes, decreased atrioventricular conduction, inotropism inhibition (more pronounced effect for verapamil than for diltiazem), moderate natriuretic effect for dihydropyridines that decrease intrarenal vascular resistance acting predominantly on efferent arteriole. Cardiovascular actions are class-specific: dihydropyridines are mainly peripheral vasodilators, phenylalkylamines act predominantly on the heart, while benzothiazepines have intermediate hemodynamic effects.

Several multicentric studies using CCBs as therapy, such as ALLHAT [49] (amlodipine), Syst-Eur [98] (nitrendipine), HOT [28] (felodipine), NORDIL [99] (diltiazem) have demonstrated that CCBs are well tolerated and decrease the cardiovascular risk in a manner similar to other antihypertensive drugs.

Studies comparing the efficacy of CCBs therapy with that of diuretic or BB therapy have shown that CCBs reduce the risk for stroke but not the one for coronary events. This finding is true both for DCCBs and for non-DCCBs.

In the middle of the 90's, a metanalysis of CCBs studies (Psaty *et al.*, Furberg *et al.*, Pahor *et al.*) reached the conclusion that short-acting CCBs from the first generation would increase the cardiovascular morbidity and mortality as well as the risk for cancer and for hemorrhagic strokes [100].

Further on, numerous subsequent analyses, such as Ad Hoc Subcommittee of the Liaison Committee of the WHO and the International Society of Hypertension [101], have confirmed these observations and have recommended the use of slow release forms (sustained release SR) or of prolonged release forms (extended release ER). Based on these data, rapid-acting nifedipine is not recommended for use in hypertension therapy.

Renoprotective action of CCBs in hypertensive diabetic patients is less clear. It seems that DCCBs act more intensely on the afferent arteriole than on the efferent one, resulting in an increase in filtering pressure and may worsen the evolution of diabetic nephropathy. This observation does not apply however to non-DCCBs that can be thus prescribed in hypertensive diabetic patients with nephropathy.

The effect of CCBs on the renal function and on microalbuminuria in type 1 DM patients has been the subject of multiple studies. The Melbourne Diabetic Nephropathy Study Group [75] has shown an increase in urinary albumin excretion in patients treated with nifedipine, similar to the placebo-treated group, while in perindopril-treated group urinary albumin excretion decreased.

Comparative studies on type 2 diabetes patients have revealed that DCCBs have no effect on proteinuria or the decline of renal function, while non-DCCBs stabilize or even decrease urinary protein excretion. One possible explanation is the different action on glomerular permeability and intraglomerular hemodynamics, and the different effects on proteic matrix as well as the different distribution of calcium channels in glomerular capillary wall. IDNT Study [87] has confirmed the superior renoprotective effect of irbesartan comparative to amlodipine, while in the ABCD Study [51] no significant differences have been found between nitrendipine and enalapril regarding the progression of diabetic nephropathy. FACET Study [52] has demonstrated a significant decrease of cardiovascular events in ACEIs-treated group compared to CCBs-treated group; best protection has been noted in patients treated with amlodipine and fosinopril in association.

CCBs use may be restricted by several side effects: limited vascular selectivity, negative inotropic effect, tachycardia, edema, facial congestion etc. Table 25.10 lists some CCBs used in clinical practice.

Table 25.10

Calcium channels blockers

Drug	Daily dose (mg)	Observations
Dihydropyridine		
Nifedipine	30–90	Second-line drugs used in case of intolerance to ACEIs, diuretics, BBs, ARBs or in combinations Not recommended as monotherapy in the presence of microangiopathy, favorable effect in combination with ARBs/ACEIs Controversial effects on cardiovascular outcomes Neutral metabolic effect Adverse effects: dizziness, flushing, edemas, tachycardia
Nisoldipine	10–60	
Amlodipine	2.5–10	
Felodipine	5–20	
Isradipine	2.5–10	
Nicardipine	60–120	
Non-Dihydropyridine		
Phenylalkylamine Verapamil	80–480	Recommended in diabetic nephropathy in case of intolerance to ACEIs /ARBs
Benzothiasepine Diltiazem	90–360	

α₁-ADRENERGIC BLOCKERS

These drugs selectively block postsynaptic α_1-adrenergic receptors, while the feed-back norepinephrinic loop remains functional, thus producing vasodilatation but without concomitant tachycardia and increase in plasmatic renin activity. Selective α_1-blockers maintain the cardiac output and renal flow within normal limits, and these effects make them useful in patients with heart failure and end-stage renal disease. They do not influence carbohydrate and lipid metabolism. The most frequently utilized drugs of this class are prazosin, doxazosin and terazosin.

One of the most serious side-effects of these drugs is first-dose orthostatic hypotension that may progress even to syncope. That is why the first dose will be very low, 0.5–1 mg, and will be administered at bedtime.

When given in monotherapy, they are efficient in about 50% of the cases.

α_1-blockers are not first-line therapy in hypertensive diabetic patients; however, they may be useful in those with benign prostate hypertrophy.

The ALLHAT study [49], started in 1994, compared the effects of therapy with doxazosin, chlorthalidone or amlodipin in hypertensive patients. In January 2000, the results of an interim analysis showed that in doxazosin-treated patients, there were 25% more cases of congestive heart failure, and the administration of doxazosin was discontinued.

MUSCULOTROPIC VASODILATORS

This class of medication acts directly on resistance vessels, producing the relaxation of arteriolar smooth muscle and consecutively lowers peripheral vascular resistance and blood pressure.

Dihydralazine and endralazine induce peripheral vasodilatation, including the coronary and renal territories. Minoxidil is reserved for severe cases of hypertension that do not respond to other blood-pressure-lowering therapies.

Most common side effects of this class are: tachycardia, increased myocardial oxygen consumption, headache, facial erythema, hydrosaline retention.

They should not be used as first line therapy in the treatment of hypertension in diabetic patients and should be prescribed only in association with β-blockers and diuretics.

CENTRAL ADRENERGIC INHIBITORS

Classic hypotensor agents, with central action, clonidine, guanfacine, guanabenz, α-methyldopa act on central α_2-adrenergic receptors and produce an increase in central inhibitory tonus, followed by the reduction of sympathetic activity with consecutive decrease of arterial constriction and peripheral vascular resistance. They do not interfere with carbohydrate and lipid metabolism. They efficiently decrease blood pressure when given in monotherapy only in 35–50% of the cases. Their use in hypertensive diabetic patients is much limited by their common side effects (occurring in 30% of the cases): sedation, dryness of the mouth, asthenia, fatigability, headache, orthostatic hypotension, etc.

Alpha-methyldopa may be used in the treatment of hypertension in pregnant diabetic women. The use of central adrenergic inhibitors may be considered in diabetic patients who do not respond to other antihypertensive agents, in the third step of therapy, in association.

Moxonidine and rilmenidine act specifically on I1 receptors (imidazolic) from the bulbar centers, resulting in a decrease of central sympathetic tonus and consequently producing arterial vasodilatation. Moxonidine is administered in a single daily dose of 0.2–0.4 mg, has a trough-to-peak ratio of 70% that insures a 24-hour action. It represents an alternative blood-pressure-lowering drug that can be prescribed especially in patients with sympathetic hyperactivity, ventricular dysfunction or marked alteration of renal function.

MONOTHERAPY

Antihypertensive agents most frequently used as monotherapy in the treatment of hypertension in diabetic patients are: ACEIs, BBs, CCBs, and diuretics. Regardless of the class of medication used, only about 50% of the patients respond completely to monotherapy, and many of them present grade 1 hypertension.

In patients with grade 1 or 2 hypertension who have not reached blood pressure target with the first choice medication and who cannot be kept waiting until a more efficient medication is identified, combined therapy is indicated.

Combined therapy is required in most patients since more often it is impossible to identify a single ideal drug that can meet the individual needs of the patients [5, 6, 12].

COMBINED THERAPY

Response rate to blood-pressure-lowering therapy is higher, usually over 70%, if two or more hypotensor drugs are used simultaneously. The physiologic bases of combined therapy are represented by two aspects: each drug may annihilate the counterregulation mechanisms activated by the other drug and more pathogenic pathways of hypertension can be interrupted. Thus, the result of this pharmacological association is a more important reduction of blood pressure than that obtained by the administration of each drug in monotherapy [102].

Clinical trials that have demonstrated the benefits of a tight blood pressure control have used 2 to 4 hypotensor agents, usually in high doses. Thus, in the HOT Study [28], in the group randomized for a diastolic blood pressure less than 80 mmHg, a mean of 3.3 drugs were needed to reach the target. UKPDS [13] has also shown that for a tight blood pressure control (blood pressure under 150/85 mm Hg) more drugs are needed than for a less strict target (less than 180/105 mmHg). After 9 years of follow-up, 29% of those in the tight control group needed three or more drugs to maintain the blood pressure target.

In patients with renal failure, the need for associated therapy is even greater. In the AASK Study [102] a mean of 3.7 hypotensor agents were used, in ABCD trial [51] 2.8 drugs were needed to achieve the target in the group titrated for a diastolic blood pressure of less than 75 mmHg. In RENAAL [86] and IDNT [87] studies, four antihypertensive drugs were needed for an effective blood pressure control.

Most commonly used associations effective for blood pressure control and with renal and cardiovascular protective effects are:

– ACEI + diuretic: useful especially in diabetic patients with heart failure;
– ACEI + CCB: very well tolerated, without metabolic effects;
– ACEI + ARB: protective renal and cardiovascular effects, superior to each drug taken separately;
– ACEI + BB: useful especially in patients with coronary heart disease;
– ARB + diuretic: the diuretic potentates the action of ARB;
– ARB + CCB;
– Diuretic + BB: if given in high doses, may present adverse metabolic effects.

Triple association of antihypertensive drugs is based on utilization of different classes of medications, the use of diuretic in the majority of regimens, and the third medication introduced depending on comorbidity:
– ACEI/ARB + BB + diuretic;
– ACEI/ARB + CCB + diuretic;
– ACEI/ARB + BB + CCB;
– BB + diuretic + CCB.

CONCLUSIONS

Hypertension is extremely common diabetes comorbidity, affecting 20–60% of people with diabetes. Hypertension is also a major risk factor for cardiovascular events, such as myocardial infarction and stroke, as well as for microvascular complications, such as retinopathy and nephropathy. Cardiovascular disease is the most costly complication of diabetes and is the cause of 80% of deaths in persons with diabetes. There is extensive evidence that the treatment of hypertension in diabetes is important for reducing both cardiovascular and microvascular complications; however, the ideal strategy for treating hypertension in persons with diabetes is less clear.

According to our experience, derived from treating thousands of hypertensive diabetic patients, treatment decisions should be individualized based on the clinical characteristics of the patient, including comorbidities as well as tolerability, personal preference, and treatment costs.

Some authors have advanced the idea that, in diabetes, lowering blood pressure is even more important than controlling hyperglycemia. In our opinion both are very important in the management of diabetes.

REFERENCES

1. Stamler J, Vaccaro O, Neaton JD, *et al.* Diabetes, other risk factors and 12-year cardiovascular mortality for men screened in the Multiple Risk Factor Intervention Trial. *Dia Care*, **263**: 2335–2340, 1993.

2. Joint National Committee on Prevention, Detection, Evaluation and Treatment of High Blood Pressure: The Sixth Report of the Joint National Committee on Prevention, Detection, Evaluation and Treatment of High Blood Pressure (JNC VI). *Arch Int Med*, **157**: 2413–2446, 1997.

3. Joint National Committee on Prevention, Detection, Evaluation and Treatment of High Blood Pressure: The Seventh Report of the Joint National Committee on Prevention, Detection, Evaluation and Treatment of High Blood Pressure (JNC VII). *JAMA*, **289**: 2560–2572, 2003.

4. Adler AI, Stratton IM, Neil HA, *et al.* Association of systolic blood pressure with macrovascular and microvascular complications of type 2 diabetes (UKPDS 36): prospective observational study. *BMJ*, **321**: 412–419, 2000.

5. American Diabetes Association: Standards of medical care for patients with diabetes. *Dia Care*, **25** (Suppl. 1): S33–S49, 2002.

6. Hâncu N. Particularitățile managementului clinic în diabetul zaharat. In: Hâncu N (ed.) *Farmacoterapia diabetului zaharat*, Editura Echinox, Cluj-Napoca, 2002, 20–37.

7. Hâncu N, Cerghizan A. Global approach to cardiovascular risk in type 2 diabetic persons. In: Hâncu N (ed) *Cardiovascular Risk in Type 2 Diabetes Mellitus: Assessement and Control*, Springer, Berlin Heidelberg, 2003, 240–276.

8. Ionescu Tîrgoviște C. *Diabetologie Modernă*, Editura Tehnică, București, 1997.

9. Gherasim L, Apetrei E, Carp C *et al.* Hipertensiunea arterială. In: Colegiul Medicilor din România (ed). *Ghiduri de practică medicală*, Vol. I, Editura INFO Medica, 1999, București, 20–35.

10. Wingard DL, Barrett-Connor E. Heart disease and diabetes. In: *Diabetes in America*, Govt. Printing Office, Washington, DC, 1995, 429–448.

11. Hypertension in Diabetic Study (HDS): prevalence of hypertension in newly presenting type 2 diabetic patients and the association with risk factors for cardiovascular and diabetic complications. *J Hyperten*, **11**: 309–317, 1993.

12. Cheța DM. *Preventing Diabetes: Theory, Practice and New Approaches*, Wiley, Chichester, 1999.

13. Tight blood pressure control and risk of macrovascular and microvascular complications in type 2 diabetes: UKPDS 38. UK Prospective Diabetes Study Group. *BMJ*, **317**: 703–713, 1998.

14. Efficacy of atenolol and captopril in reducing risk of macrovascular and microvascular complications in type 2 diabetes: UKPDS 39. UK Prospective Diabetes Study Group. *BMJ*, **317**: 713–720, 1998.

15. Sowers JR, Epstein M. Diabetes mellitus and associated hypertension, vascular disease, and nephropathy: an update. *Hypertension*, **26** (pt 1): 869–879, 1995.

16. Bianchi S, Bigazzi R, Quinones Galvan A, *et al.* Insulin resistance in microalbuminuric hypertension: sites and mechanisms. *Hypertension*, **26**: 189–195, 1995.

17. Reaven GM, Lithell H, Landsberg L. Hypertension and associated metabolic abnormalities – the role of insulin resistance and the sympathoadrenal system. *New Engl J Med*, **334**: 374–381, 1996.

18. DeChaatel R, Weidmann P, Flammer J, *et al.* Sodium, renin, aldosterone, catecholamines and blood pressure in diabetes mellitus. *Kidney Int*, **12**: 412–421, 1977.

19. Băcanu GS, Șerban V, Timar R. Hipertensiunea arterială și diabetul zaharat. Medicina modernă, **9**: 10-14, 1996.

20. Kaplan NM. Treatment of Hypertension: Drug therapy. In: *Clinical Hypertension*. 7th ed., Williams and Wilkens, Baltimore, MD, 1998, 181–265.

21. Resnick LM: Cellular ions in hypertension, insulin resistance, obesity and diabetes: a unifying theme. *J Am Soc Nephrol*, **3**: S78–S85, 1992.

22. Băcanu GS, Babeș K. Hipertensiunea arterială. In: Șerban V (ed). *Diabetul zaharat al vârstnicului*, Editura Brumar, Timișoara, 2003, 83–100.

23. Ginghina C, Băcanu GS, Marinescu M *et al.* *Cordul Diabetic*, InfoMedica, București, 2001.

24. Gherasim L, Dorobanțu M. Actualități in hipertensiunea arterială. In: Gherasim L, Apetrei E (ed). *Actualități în cardiologie*, Editura Medicală Amaltea, București, 1998.

25. Șerban V. *Clinica medicală – Teorie și practică*, Editura de Vest, Timișoara, 1999.

26. Timar R. Șerban V. Hipertensiunea arterială – clasificare, risc cardiovascular și principii de terapie in *Medicina familiei*, **37**: 11–14, 2001.

27. Șerban V. *Medicină internă*, volumul III, Editura Excelsior,Timișoara, 1997.

28. Hansson L, Zanchetti A, Carruthers SG, *et al.* for the HOT Study Group. Effects of intensive blood pressure lowering and low-dose aspirin in patients with hypertension: principal results of the Hypertension Optimal Treatment (HOT) randomized trial. *Lancet*, **351**: 1755-1762, 1998.

29. Feldman RD. The Canadian recommendations for the management of hypertension: on behalf of the Task Force for the Development of the 1999 Canadian Recommendations for the Management

of Hypertension. *Can J Cardiol*, **15:** S57G–S64G, 1999.

30. Sowers JR, Reed J. Clinical advisory treatment of hypertension in diabetes. *J Clin Hypertens,* **2:** 132–133, 2000.

31. Cutler JA, Fohnann D, Allender PS. Randomized trials of sodium reduction: an overview. *Am J Clin Nutr*, **65** (Suppl. 2): 643S–651S, 1997.

32. Trials of Hypertension Prevention Collaborative Research Group. Effects of weight loss and sodium reduction intervention on blood pressure and hypertension incidence in overweight people with high-normal blood pressure: the Trials of Hypertension Prevention, phase II. *Arch Int Med,* **157:** 657-667, 1997.

33. Midgley JP, Matthew AG, Greenwood CM, et al. Effect of reduced dietary sodium on blood pressure: a meta-analysis of randomized controlled trials. *JAMA,* **275:** 1590–1597, 1996.

34. Velussi M, Brocco E, Frigato F, et al. Effects of diet and sodium intake on blood pressure: Subgroup analysis of the DASH-sodium trial. *Ann Intern Med*, **135:** 1019–28, 2001.

35. He J, Whelton PK, Appel LJ, et al. Long-term effects of weight loss and dietary sodium reduction on incidence of hypertension. *Hypertension,* **35:** 544–9, 2000.

36. The Trials of Hypertension Prevention Collaborative Research Group. Effects of weight loss and sodium reduction intervention on blood pressure and hypertension incidence in overweight people with high-normal blood pressure. The Trials of Hypertension Prevention, phase II. *Arch Intern Med.*, **157:** 657-67, 1997.

37. Krezesinki JM, Janssens M, Vanderspeeten F, et al. Importance of weight loss and sodium restriction in the treatment of mild and moderate essential hypertension. *Acta Clin Belg,* **48:** 234–245, 1993.

38. Whelton SP, Chin A, Xin X, et al. Effect of aerobic exercise on blood pressure: A meta-analysis of randomized, controlled trials. *Ann Intern Med*, **136:** 493–503, 2002.

39. Whelton PK, He J, Cutler JA, et al. Effects of oral potassium on blood pressure: meta-analysis of randomized controlled clinical trials. *JAMA*, **277:** 1624–1632, 1997.

40. Houston C, Meador PB, Schipani LM, *Handbook of Antihypertensive Therapy*, 10th Edition, Hanley& Belfus Inc, Philadelphia, 2000.

41. Kalantarinia KM, Siragy HM. The Choice of Antihypertensive Drugs in Patients with Diabetes: Angiotensin II and Beyond. *Curr Diab Rep,* **2:** 423–430, 2002.

42. Michael AM. Drugs That Interrupt the Renin-Angiotensin System Should be Among the Preferred Initial Drugs to Treat Hypertension. *J Invasive Cardiol,* **5:** 137–144, 2003.

43. Biollaz HR, Brunner I, Gavras B, *et al.* Antihypertensive therapy with MK 421: angiotensin II-renin relationships to evaluate efficacy of converting enzyme blockade. *J Cardio Pharmacol*, **4:** 966–972, 1982.

44. Henriksen EJ, Jacob S, Kinnick TR, ACE inhibition and glucose transport in insulin-resistant muscle: roles of bradykinin and nitric oxide. *Am J Physiol*, **277:** R332–R336, 1999.

45. The Heart Outcome Prevention Evaluation Study Investigators. Effects of ramipril on cardiovascular and microvascular outcomes in people with diabetes; results of the HOPE study and the MICRO-HOPE substudy. *Lancet,* **355:** 253–259, 2000.

46. Vijan S, Hayward RA. Treatment of Hypertension in Type 2 Diabetes Mellitus: Blood Pressure Goals, Choice of Agents, and Setting Priorities in Diabetes Care. *Ann Intern Med*, **138:** 593–602, 2003.

47. Hansson L, Lindholm L, Ekborn T, *et al.* Randomized trial of old and new antihypertensive drugs in elderly patients: cardiovascular mortality and morbidity: the Swedish Trial in Old Patients with 2 study. *Lancet*, **354:** 1751–1756, 1999.

48. Hansson L, Lindhol LH, Niskanen L, *et al.* Effect of angiotensin- converting-enzyme inhibition compared with conventional therapy on cardiovascular morbidity and mortality in hypertension: the Captopril Prevention Project (CAPPP) randomized trial. *Lancet,* **353:** 611–616, 1999.

49. Barzilay JI, Jones CL, Davis BR, *et al.* Baseline characteristics of the diabetic participants in the antihypertensive and lipid-lowering treatment to prevent heart attacks trial (ALLHAT) *Dia Care*, **24:** 654–658, 2001.

50. Burnier M. Le point sur le traitement de l'hypertension artérielle: que tirer des grandes études cliniques récentes ? *Med Hyg,* **61:** 1145–52, 2003.

51. Estacio RO, Jeffers BW, Hiatt WR, *et al.* The effect nisoldipine as compared with enalapril on cardiovascular outcomes in patients with non-insulin dependent diabetes and hypertension. *N Engl J Med*, **338:** 645–652, 1998.

52. Tatti P, Pahor M, Byington RP, *et al.* Outcomes results of the Fosinopril versus Amlodipine Cardiovascular Events Randomized Trial (FACET) in patients with hypertension and NIDDM. *Dia Care*, **21:** 597–611, 1998.

53. Pahor M, Psaty BM, Alderman MH, *et al.* Therapeutic Benefits of ACE Inhibitors and Other

Antihypertensive Drugs in Patients with Type 2 Diabetes. *Dia Care,* **23:** 888–892. 2000.

54. Fogari R, Zoppi A, Lazzari P. ACE inhibition but not angiotensin II antagonism reduces plasma fibrinogen and insulin resistance in overweight hypertensive patients. *J Cardiovasc Pharmacol,* **32:** 616–620, 1998.

55. Fukuda N, Satoh C, Hu WY. Endogenous angiotensin II suppresses insulin signaling in vascular smooth muscle cells from spontaneously hypertensive rats. *J Hypertens,* **19:** 1651–1658, 2001.

56. Duka I, Shenouda S, Johns C. Role of the B(2) receptor of bradykinin in insulin sensitivity. *Hypertension,* **38:** 1355–1360, 2001.

57. Rachmani R, Lindar M, Brosh D. Oxidation of low-density lipoprotein normotensive type 2 diabetic patients. Comparative effects of enalapril versus nifedipine: a randomized cross-over study. *Diabetes Res Clin Pract,* **48:** 139–145, 2000.

58. Fogari R, Zoppi A, Lazzari P. ACE inhibition but not angiotensin II antagonism reduces plasma fibrinogen and insulin resistance in overweight hypertensive patients. *Cardiovascular Pharmacol,* **32:** 616–620, 1998.

59. Sowers JR, Lester MA. Diabetes and cardiovascular disease. *Dia Care,* **22:** C14–C20, 1999.

60. O'Driscoll G, Green D, Raskin J. Improvement in endothelial function by angiotensin converting enzyme inhibition in insulin-dependent diabetes mellitus. *J Clin Invest,* **100:** 678–684, 1997.

61. Gasic S, Wagner OF, Fasching P. Fosinopril decreases levels of soluble vascular adhesion molecule-1 in borderline hypertensive type II diabetics with microalbuminuria. *Am J Hypertens,* **12:** 217–222, 1999.

62. Kirpichnikov DR, Sowers JR. Role of ACE Inhibitors in Treating Hypertensive Diabetic Patients. *Curr Diab Rep,* **2:** 251–257, 2002.

63. Lewis EJ, Hunsicker LG, Bain RP, Rohde RD. The effect of angiotensin-converting-enzyme inhibition on diabetic nephropathy. The Collaborative Study Group. *N Engl J Med,* **329:** 1456–1462, 1993.

64. Hermans MP, Birchard SM, Colin I, *et al.* Long-term reduction of microalbuminuria after 3 years of angiotensin-converting enzyme inhibition by perindopril in hypertensive insulin treated diabetic patients. *Am J Med,* **92** (Suppl. 4B): 102S–107S, 1992.

65. Melbourne Diabetic Nephropathy Study Group. Comparison between perindopril and nifedipine in hypertensive and normotensive diabetic patients with microalbuminuria. *BMJ,* **302:** 210–216, 1991.

66. Marre M, Chatellier G, LeBlanc II, *et al.* Prevention of diabetic nephropathy with enalapril in normotensive diabetics with microalbuminuria. *BMJ,* **297:** 1092–1095, 1998.

67. Mathiesen ER, Hommel E, Giese J, Parving HH. Efficacy of captopril in postponing nephropathy in normotensive insulin-dependent diabetic patients with microalbuminuria. *BMJ,* **303:** 81–87, 1991.

68. The ACE Inhibitors in Diabetic Nephropathy Trialist Group. Should all patients with type 1 diabetes mellitus and microalbuminuria receive angiotensin-converting enzyme inhibitors? A meta-analysis of individual patient data. *Ann Intern Med,* **134:** 370–379, 2001.

69. Ravid M, Brosch D, Levi Z. Use of enalapril to attenuate decline in renal function in normotensive normoalbuminuric patients with type 2 diabetes mellitus: a randomized controlled trial. *Ann Intern Med,* **128:** 982–988, 1998.

70. Ruilope LM. Lessons from Trials in Hypertensive Type 2 Diabetic Patients. *Curr Hyperten Rep,* **5:** 322–328, 2003.

71. Lebovitz HE, Wiegmann TB, Cnaan A. Renal protective effects of enalapril in hypertensive NIDDM: role of baseline microalbuminuria. *Kidney Int,* **45**(Suppl): S150–S155, 1994.

72. Bakris GL, Copley JB, Vicknair N. Calcium channel blockers versus other antihypertensive therapies on progression of NIDDM associated nephropathy. *Kidney Int* **50:** 1641–1650, 1996.

73. Agardh CD, Garcia Puig J, Charbonnel B. Greater reduction of urinary albumin excretion in hypertensive type II diabetic patients with incipient nephropathy by lisinopril than by nifedipine. *J Hum Hypertens* **10:** 185–192, 1996.

74. Ravid M, Lang R, Rachmani R, Lischner M. Long-term renoprotective effect of angiotensin-converting enzyme inhibition in non-insulin dependent diabetes mellitus: a 7-year follow-up study. *Arch Int Med,* **156:** 286–289, 1996.

75. Melbourne Diabetic Nephropathy Study Group. Comparison between perindopril and nifedipine in normotensive patients with incipient diabetic nephropathy. *BMJ,* **302:** 210–216, 1991.

76. Velussi M, Brocco E, Frigato F. Effects of cilazapril and amlodipine on kidney function in hypertensive NIDDM patients. *Diabetes,* **45:** 216–222, 1996.

77. Ruggenenti P, Mosconi L, Bianchi L. Long-term treatment with either enalapril or nitrendipine stabilizes albuminuria and increases glomerular filtration rate in non-insulin-dependent diabetic patients. *Am J Kidney Dis,* **24:** 753–761, 1994.

78. Estacio RO, Jeffers BW, Hiatt WR. The effect of nisoldipine as compared with enalapril on cardiovascular outcomes in patients with non-insulin-dependent diabetes and hypertension. *N Engl J Med,* **338:** 645–652, 1998.

79. Lacourciere Y, Belanger A, Godin C, *et al.* Long-term comparison of losartan and enalapril on kidney function in hypertensive type 2 diabetics with early nephropathy. *Kidney Int*, **58**: 762–769, 2000.

80. Hogeboom van Buggenum IM, Polak BC, Reichert-Thoen JW, *et al.* Angiotensin converting enzyme inhibiting therapy is associated with lower vitreous vascular endothelial growth factor concentrations in patients with proliferative diabetic retinopathy. *Diabetologia*, **45**: 203–209, 2002.

81. Moravski C J, Skinner SL, Stubbs A J, *et al.* The renin-angiotensin system influences ocular endothelial cell proliferation in diabetes: transgenic and interventional studies. *Am J Pathol*, **162**: 151–160, 2003.

82. Aiello LM. Perspectives on diabetic retinopathy. *Am J Ophthalmol*, **136**: 122–135, 2003.

83. American Diabetes Association. Treatment of Hypertension in Adults with Diabetes. *Dia Care*, **26**: S80-S82, 2003.

84. Andersen S, Tarnow L, Rossing P, *et al.* Renoprotective effects of angiotensin II receptor blockade in type 1 diabetic patients with diabetic nephropathy. *Kidney Int*, **57**: 601–606, 2000.

85. Lacourcière Y, Bélanger A, Godin C, *et al.* Long-term comparison of losartan and enalapril on kidney function in hypertensive type 2 diabetics with early nephropathy. *Kidney Int*, **58**: 762–76, 2000.

86. Brenner BM, Cooper ME, de Zeeuw D, *et al.* Effects of losartan on renal and cardiovascular outcomes in patients with type 2 diabetes and nephropathy. *N Engl J Med*, **345**: 861–869, 2001.

87. Rodby RA, Rohde RD, Clarke WR, *et al.* The irbesartan type II diabetic nephropathy trial: study design and baseline patient characteristics. *Nephrol Dial Transplant*, **15**: 487–497, 2000.

88. Parving HH, Lehnert H, Brochner-Mortensen J, *et al.* The effect of irbesartan on the development of diabetic nephropathy in patients with type 2 diabetes. *N Engl J Med*, **345**: 870–878, 2001.

89. Brenner BM, Cooper ME, de Zeeuw D. Effects of losartan on renal and cardiovascular outcomes in patients with type 2 diabetes and nephropathy *N Engl J Med*, **345**: 861–869. 2001.

90. Toto RD. Appropriate Drug Therapy for Improving Outcomes in Diabetic Nephropathy. *Curr Diab Rep*, **2**: 545–552, 2002.

91. Mogensen CE, Neldam S, Tikkanen I, *et al*, for the CALM Study Group. Randomised controlled trial of dual blockade of renin-angiotensin system in patients with hypertension, microalbuminuria, and non-insulin dependent diabetes: The Candesartan and Lisinopril Micro-albuminuria (CALM) study. *BMJ*, **321**: 1440–1444, 2000.

92. Cohn JN, Tognoni G. A randomized trial of the angiotensin-receptor blocker valsartan in chronic heart failure. *N Engl J Med*, **345**: 1667–1675, 2001.

93. Lindholm LH, Ibsen H, Dahlof B, *et al.* Cardiovascular morbidity and mortality in patients with diabetes in the Losartan Intervention For Endpoint reduction in hypertension study (LIFE): a randomized trial against atenolol. *Lancet*, **359**: 1004–1010, 2002.

94. Sawicki PT, Siebenhofer A. Beta blocker treatment in diabetes mellitus. *J Intern Med*, **250**: 11–17, 2001.

95. Cruickshank JM. Beta-Blockers and Diabetes: The Bad Guys Come Good. *Cardiovascular Drugs and Therapy*, **16**: 457–470, 2002.

96. Dunne F, Kendall MJ, Martin U. Blockers in the Management of Hypertension in Patients with Type 2 Diabetes Mellitus. Is There a Role? *Drugs*, **61** (4): 429–435, 2001.

97. Perry HM Jr, Davis BR, Price TR, *et al.* Effect of treating isolated systolic hypertension on the risk of developing various types and subtypes of stroke: the Systolic Hypertension in the Elderly Program (SHEP). *JAMA*, **284**: 465–471, 2000.

98. Tuomilehto J, Rastenyte D, Birkenhager WH, *et al.* Effect of calcium channel blockade in older patients with diabetes and systolic hypertension. Systolic Hypertension in Europe Trial Investigators. *N Engl J Med*, **340**: 677–684, 1999.

99. Hansson L, Hedner T, Lund-Johansen P, Kjeldsen SE, *et al.* Randomized trial of effects of calcium antagonists compared with diuretics and beta-blockers on cardiovascular mortality in hypertension: the Nordic Diltiazem Study. *Lancet*, **356**: 359–364, 2000.

100. Pahor M, Psaty BM. Health outcomes associated with calcium antagonists compared with other first–line antihypertensive therapies: a meta analysis of randomized controlled trials. *Lancet*, **356**: 1940–1954, 2000.

101. Ad Hoc Subcommittee of the Liaison Committee of the World Health Organization and the International Society of Hypertension. Effects of calcium antagonists on the risks of coronary heart disease, cancer and bleeding. *J Hypertens*, **15**: 105–115, 1997.

102. Cristodorescu R. Progrese in tratamentul hipertensiunii arteriale. Monoterapie sau terapie combinată, In: Gherasim L (ed). *Progrese în cardiologie*, Editura InfoMedica, Bucureşti, 2002, 35–76.

26

AMBULATORY BLOOD PRESSURE MONITORING IN DIABETES – FOCUS ON DIABETIC NEPHROPATHY

Adrian COVIC, Paul GUSBETH-TATOMIR, David J.A. GOLDSMITH

The prevalence of diabetes mellitus (DM) is growing constantly throughout the world. Along with increased life expectancy, the incidence of type 2 DM is particularly increasing and with this, the incidence of micro- and macrovascular complications. Diabetic nephropathy is a major complication both of type 1 and type 2 diabetes mellitus and it is progressing to end-stage renal disease (ESRD) in most of the cases. Conversely, the prevalence of ESRD due to diabetic nephropathy became impressive, generating a considerable pressure on the renal replacement therapy programs. Moreover, the main cardiovascular morbidity and mortality of the diabetic patient on dialysis is definitely exceeding that of the non-diabetic dialyzed population.

A major determinant of cardiovascular morbidity and mortality (and also of the accelerated progression of diabetic nephropathy) is the arterial hypertension. Casual measurements of blood pressure – as highlighted by recent studies – are less predictive for end-organ damage due to hypertension when compared with ambulatory blood pressure (BP) monitoring.

Ambulatory BP monitoring (ABPM) has emerged in the last decades as a very useful tool in BP evaluation for diagnostic and therapeutic reasons. An abnormal day-night BP profile, resulting from ABPM measurements, is predictive for further development of diabetic nephropathy, and is associated with rapid progression to the proteinuric stage and ESRD. The cardiovascular risk of diabetic patients with abnormal circadian rhythm is also very increased. According to recent studies discussed extensively by the authors, diabetic and nondiabetic patients with impaired lowering of BP during night (mainly due to autonomous neuropathy) have increased the risk of cardiovascular death. An individualized antihypertensive treatment, including measures to correct the abnormal circadian rhythm, may improve significantly the general and cardiovascular prognosis in diabetic patients.

DIABETIC NEPHROPATHY – THE SIZE OF THE PROBLEM

Diabetic nephropathy (DNP) is a serious and frequent complication of both type 1 and type 2 diabetes mellitus (DM). Up to 40% of patients with DM will develop diabetic renal disease with overt proteinuria after 10 to 20 years. With the development of clinically overt DNP, there is a relentless progression to chronic renal failure and eventually to end-stage renal disease (ESRD). Once ESRD reached, survival is not possible in the absence of renal replacement therapy.

The last decade was marked by a progressive and unmistakable shift of the major etiology of ESRD from chronic primary glomerulopathies to diabetic nephropathy in most developed countries. DNP accounts, according to major dialysis registries, for 43 % of all cases of ESRD in the United States [1] and 20–50% in various European countries [2]. This is easily explainable by improvement of medical care in this special population with high morbidity and mortality. Survival of diabetic patients has improved markedly due to a better glycemic control and better management of cardiovascular disease, the major cause of death in this category of patients. As a consequence, most diabetic subjects survivie enough time to develop microvascular complications as retinopathy and nephropathy, two conditions, which develop after several years of chronic hyperglycemia.

On the other hand, the incidence of type 2 DM is growing with older ages. A growing diabetic population parallels longer life expectancy in most parts of the world. A third explanation for the growing diabetic dialyzed population, applicable especially for less developed countries, like the Eastern European countries, is that acceptance of diabetic patients for chronic dialysis has improved markedly. Just a decade ago, due to huge costs of renal replacement therapy (RRT) and the notoriously reduced survival of diabetics on dialysis, nephrologists were reluctant in starting RRT in those patients. This is not so anymore: Eastern European countries have started large national programs for RRT, giving the possibility of initiating dialysis in most uremic diabetic patients. Renal transplantation is a feasible alternative to dialysis in a growing number of diabetics with ESRD.

In recent years, renal replacement therapy programs and the nephrological community has been put under considerable pressure by the constantly increasing incidence of ESRD, especially due to diabetic nephropathy. For example, in 2010, according to recent estimations, there will be about 520,000 patients on RRT in the United States, compared with 300,000 presently [1]. This will enhance costs and medical/logistical efforts, hard to sustain by any national medical system.

As a consequence, the attention of the nephrological community is seriously focused on prevention/slowing progression of chronic kidney disease (CKD). As diabetic nephropathy will account for more than half of CKD cases in most countries, logically a considerable effort has to be attributed to prevention of overt diabetic nephropathy and retarding progression of chronic renal failure to ESRD.

DIABETIC MELLITUS AND HYPERTENSION

Diabetes mellitus and hypertension (HT) are commonly associated, both conditions carrying an increased risk for cardiovascular and renal disease [3–5]. Forty percent of the type 2 DM patients are hypertensives, with the prevalence of hypertension growing with age in this population (60% at 70 years) [6, 7]. In patients with type 1 DM, the presence of hypertension is a hallmark of incipient or already existing diabetic nephropathy, whereas in type 2 DM, HT usually precedes the onset of diabetes by many years. In fact, hypertension in these patients is one aspect of the so-called metabolic syndrome, a condition predisposing to type 2 DM. Studies in special populations, like the diabetes-prone Pima Indians, have shown that hypertension preceding diabetes is a strong determinant of risk for developing later renal disease [8].

Moreover, HT potentates the already high CV risk associated with diabetes [4–6]. Data from the large UKPDS 38 trial [4] in hypertensive type 2 diabetics showed a very impressive difference in several end-points after 9 years of follow-up. The "tight" blood pressure (BP) control group (144/82 mmHg) had a considerable risk reduction when compared with subjects less tight BP control

(154/87 mmHg): 24% in diabetes-related end points, 32% in death related to diabetes, 44% in strokes and 37% in microvascular end points. However, the reduction in all cause of mortality did not reach statistical significance. Noteworthy, "tight" BP control in this study was far from accepted ranges for diabetics in recent years. It should also be emphasised that the "tight" control of BP has been obtained with 3 or more antihypertensives in 29% of patients, pointing out the very difficult task of controlling BP in diabetes mellitus [4].

The presence of HT, in diabetics, is also a risk factor for diabetic nephropathy, as well as retinopathy [8, 9]. Once diabetic nephropathy present, aggressive control of BP reduces albuminuria and deterioration in renal function, both in type 1 and type 2 diabetes [10–12].

There are several modifiable cardiovascular (CV) risk factors in diabetic patients: hypertension, microalbuminuria, smoking, obesity, lipid profile and glycemic control. Very recent data of the Steno-2 Study [13] highlight the effect of targeted, intensified, multifactorial intervention compared with conventional therapy derived from national guidelines in type 2 diabetic patients. This open, parallel trial had as primary end point a composite of death from CV causes, nonfatal myocardial infarction, nonfatal stroke, need for re-vascularisation procedures and amputation. The group randomly allocated to intensive therapy benefited from a stepwise implementation of behaviour modification, secondary prevention of CV disease with aspirin and pharmacological treatment targeting hypertension, hyperglycemia, dyslipidemia and microalbuminuria. The decline in glycosylated Hb values, systolic and diastolic BP, serum cholesterol and triglyceride levels and urinary albumin excretion rate were all significantly greater in the intensive-therapy group than in the conventional-therapy group. Patients receiving intensive therapy also had a significantly lower risk of cardiovascular disease (hazard ratio (HR) = 0.47), nephropathy (HR = 0.39), retinopathy (HR = 0.42) and autonomic neuropathy (HR = 0.37) [13].

According to present evidence, target blood pressure (BP) in patients with diabetic nephropathy should be 120/80 mmHg or less. This is not new: Parving and Mogensen (1984) have obtained a stabilisation of renal function with tight BP control in three of their five patients.

AMBULATORY BLOOD PRESSURE MONITORING – A USEFUL TOOL IN HYPERTENSIVE DISEASES

Ambulatory blood pressure monitoring (ABPM) has slowly become, in the last three decades, a useful adjunct to the management of patients suspected to have or having raised blood pressure. This was facilitated by the development of smaller, cheaper portable and more accurate equipment, provided with more powerful software analysis packages in the late '80s.

For a correct use of ABPM in the daily nephrological practice we need to report to normal standards, derived from the large populational studies. There have been published several large analyses of normo- and hypertensive populations, which, when meta-analysed, have provided a useful normal range for ABPM values. According to the excellent analysis of Staessen et al. [14], the upper limit of normal BP assessed by ABPM is:

– 135/85 mmHg for the mean of daytime BP values;
– 120/75 mmHg for the mean of nighttime BP values;
– 130/80 mmHg for the mean of 24-hours BP values.

Predictably, there is often a good correlation between office-derived and ABPM-derived BP levels. For the same patients, it is difficult to substitute one measure with the other [15]. Many studies have tried to find and to use a single office BP reading that most closely approximates the ABPM data. This has been done mainly in the context of hemodialysis (HD) treatment in end-stage renal disease patients. Pre-, post-, or averaged pre- and post- HD values have been proposed. One of the main problems in assessing BP in these patients is the fact that one relies on single BP measurements taken around the time of dialysis session in an outpatient. There is a very poor correlation between these peri-dialysis BP values and those taken far from the hospital in the dialysis-free interval.

In a recent review, Agarwal [16] showed that, although in some cases, the differences between pre-dialysis BP and ambulatory BP were modest, there were also many patients in which pre-dialysis BP overestimate ABPM by 50 mmHg, or underestimate it by 20 mmHg. Using as a cut-off criterion for hypertension a 2-week average predialysis BP level of > 150/85 mmHg (or postdialysis BP of > 130/75 mmHg) had only 80% sensitivity. Nevertheless, two studies demonstrated that the average of pre-dialysis systolic BP may be equivalent to ABPM as a predictor of target end organ damage [17, 18]. Zoccali and co-workers calculated the average of 12 different pre-dialysis BP values taken carefully by trained nurses, has the same predictive power for left ventricular mass (but not LV internal diameter) as one single APBM session [17].

The classical clinical indications of ABPM are summarized in Table 26.1. We consider that in addition to these classical indications, the assessment of nighttime BP profile in very-high risk cardiovascular patients (*e.g.* diabetics and/or renal failure patients) – see below – is mandatory. The very recently released 2003 European Society of Hypertension – European Society of Cardiology guidelines for the management of arterial hypertension [19], though reviewing briefly rather favourably the advantages of ABPM, was unable to establish firm indications for ABPM. The only exception is "white coat" hypertension [19]. The almost concomitantly released Seventh Report of the Joint National Committee on Prevention, detection, evaluation, and treatment of high blood pressure [20] stated that "Ambulatory BP monitoring is warranted for evaluation of (white-coat) hypertension in the absence of target-organ injury. It is also helpful to assess patients with apparent drug resistance, hypotensive symptoms with antihypertensive medications, episodic hypertension, and autonomic dysfunction. The ambulatory BP values are usually lower than clinical readings. Awaken hypertensive individuals have a mean BP of more than 135/85 mmHg and during the sleep, more than 120/75 mmHg. The level of BP using ambulatory BP monitoring correlates better than office measurements with target-organ injury. Ambulatory

BP monitoring also provides a measure of the percentage of BP readings that are elevated, the overall BP load, and the extent of BP reduction during sleep. In most individuals, BP decreases by 10–20% during the night; those in whom such decreases are not present are at increased risk for cardiovascular events" [20].

Table 26.1

The main indications of ambulatory blood pressure monitoring

Severe hypertension refractory to treatment
Suspected office ("white-coat") hypertension
Patients with intermittent symptoms suggestive for hyper- / hypotension and with normal office BP values
Evaluation of nocturnal symptoms (*e.g.* headache, breathlessness, angina)

THE ABNORMAL BP PROFILE IN DIABETIC PATIENTS

There is a high prevalence of abnormal blood pressure profile in diabetic patients [21]. At the time of diagnosis of type 2 DM, a nocturnal fall of BP of less than 15 % has been recorded in 61% of patients. If the non-dipping status is defined as a nocturnal drop of BP less than 10 % compared with the day-time values, an abnormal day-night rhythm was present in 29% of diabetic patients. Most importantly, this abnormality was progressive with time and with microalbuminuria: after five years, non-dipping status was present in 75 % of patients [22].

Non-dipping is an early phenomenon in diabetes mellitus, long before onset of diabetic nephropathy. In type 1 DM, Lurbe *et al* [23] and subsequently Voros and co-workers [24] have shown that abnormal circadian BP profile is significantly more prevalent in patients without microalbuminuria when compared to healthy controls. Moreover, in both type 1 and type 2 DM with microalbuminuria, there is a very tight correlation between non-dipping and urinary albumin excretion [25]. In a prospective study of young normoalbuminuric diabetics followed-up for two years, the mean systolic BP increased significantly during sleep in patients who later developed microalbuminuria, but not in subjects who maintained a normal urinary albumin excretion. The risk of microalbuminuria was 70% lower in patients with normal circadian BP profile as compared to the non-dippers. In DM type 1 with microalbuminuria, higher night-time BP correlates also with development of retinopathy [26]. Recent data by Lurbe and colleagues [27] showed a clear-cut worsening of the circadian BP profile as diabetic nephropathy worsens; the prevalence of non-dipping status was 10% in healthy controls, 18% in normoalbuminuric diabetics, 58% in diabetics with microalbuminuria and 80% in those with proteinuria.

What is the explanation for the impressive prevalence of this BP profile abnormality in diabetics? First, non-dippers diabetic patients have higher extracellular volume (*i.e.* latent overhydration), a condition known as associated with non-dipping status [28,29]. Second, in DM there is an impaired function of the autonomous nerve system, particularly the parasympathetic. The relationship between abnormal circadian BP and various maneuvers designed to reveal autonomic neuropathy has been well-defined [30]. Higher nocturnal systolic BP is related to a blunted decline of heart rate, which prevents adequate lowering of cardiac output during sleep (van Ittersum *et al.*, study in normoalbuminuric patients with type 1 DM [31]).

At least two small studies have related an abnormal BP profile to poor glycemic control. In Ferreira and co-workers' investigation [32], following metabolic improvement obtained in normotensive diabetic adolescents, the awake-sleep variation of BP became close to the normal pattern. In another study [33], glycosylated hemoglobin inversely correlated with the decline of systolic and diastolic nocturnal BP. A significant association has also been found between a smaller BP nocturnal decrease and ventricular dysfunction and the albumin excretion rate, respectively. It seems reasonable to conclude with the authors that poor glycemic control adversely affects blood pressure and latter may play an important role in cardiac and renal dysfunction in early type 1 DM. The same relationship between poor glycemic control (assessed by glycosylated hemoglobin concentrations) and abnormal BP rhythm has been shown in diabetic pregnant women (see below).

In a very recent trial in diabetic and nondiabetic patients with end-stage renal disease on hemodialysis, Liu and co-workers [34] established also a clear-cut relationship between autonomic neuropathy and non-dipping status. Autonomic nerve function has been evaluated through 24-hour ECG monitoring, with analysis of heart rate variability. This study showed that both sympathetic and parasympathetic functions are depressed in hemodialysis patients when compared to normal controls. However, the normal circadian rhythm of the high frequency and of the ratio high frequency to low frequency components of the HR variability is only preserved in dippers and not in non-dippers [34].

ABNORMAL BP RHYTHM AND OUTCOME

In essential hypertension patients, there is a clear relationship between abnormal circadian BP rhythm and cardiovascular (CDV) morbidity and mortality. As far as 1994, Zweiker *et al.* [35] found that in 116 treated hypertensives, followed for 31 months, there was a significantly higher rate of CDV complications in non-dippers: 4 major events in 29 subjects, as compared with just 1 event in 87 dippers. This was confirmed in the much larger PIUMA study by Verdecchia and co-workers [36]. In the 1187 patients with essential hypertension, followed-up for 3.5 years, the CDV event rate was three times higher in non-dippers. Another interesting finding of this Italian study was that the event rate in the group of patients classified as hypertensives by office BP measurement was similar to the normotensive group. As high blood pressure is a well-known major CDV risk factor, this suggests once again that ABPM is superior to office BP measurement in predicting CDV outcome [36].

These data were confirmed by subsequent studies: Staessen *et al.* [37] found in 808 patients of a substudy, nested in the Syst-Eur trial, that a lack in decline in systolic BP was associated with a greater incidence of myocardial infarction and stroke. In 105 neurological patients with symptomatic lacunar infarcts followed up for 3 years, BP profile has been associated with further neurological events. In the group with subsequent neurological complications, day-to-night ambulatory BP reduction was much less (systolic BP 1.3%, diastolic BP 3.3%) when compared with those without further neurological complications at follow-up (7.2% and 10.4%, respectively) [38]. Extremely interesting are the data of a recent prospective study by Kario and co-workers, in 576 older Japanese patients with sustained hypertension [39]. They classified their patients according to their systolic BP profile in 4 categories: "extreme-dippers", with a >20% SBP nocturnal fall; "dippers", with a >10% but less than 20% SBP; "non-dippers', with >0% but <10 % fall; and "reverse-dippers", who had a higher night than day SBP. The prevalence of cerebral infarcts at baseline as assessed by magnetic resonance was the lowest in the dipper group (29%), significantly higher in the non-dippers (41%) and reverse-dippers (49%), and very high in the extreme-dippers (53%). There was a J-shaped relationship between dipping status and stroke incidence (extreme-dippers 12%, dippers 6.1%, non-dippers 7.6%, and reverse-dippers 22%). The highest stroke incidence for reverse dippers may be explained by the fact that these patients were older, more likely to be male and had a higher 24-hour systolic BP than did the other 3 groups. These 3 factors were all independently associated with stroke prognosis. The worse prognosis of extreme-dippers suggests that cerebral hypoperfusion due to nocturnal fall of BP might trigger ischemic strokes during the night in these patients. On the other hand, in Kario's study, 55% of strokes in extreme-dippers occurred during the morning. These data suggest that exagerated morning rise of BP might also contribute to stroke events [39].

Our group (Covic *et al.*, *Am J Kidney Dis*, **35**: 617–623, 2000, [40]) was able to show that there is a significant correlation between abnormal BP rhythm and ecocardiographically determined left ventricular dilatation, a well-known adverse prognostic element of uremic cardiomyopathy in end-stage renal disease patients. Indeed, those patients with persistently reduced diurnal BP rhythm tended to develop a dilated left ventricle and left atrium in the absence of other known and/or relevant risk factors: persistently elevated sleep BP group – LV end-diastolic diameter 38.2 mm/m^2 *versus* 30.6 mm/m^2 in patients with persistently normal sleep BP group (p < 0.05) [40].

Are these findings relevant for diabetic patients too? This issue has been addressed by Nakano and colleagues [41] in patients with type 2 diabetes. 201 subjects had normal BP profile, whereas the remaining 87 had a reversed one (*i.e.* nocturnal BP higher than day-time BP). Fatal and non-fatal vascular events occurred in 20 subjects with normal BP profile and in 56 out of 87 patients with reversed circadian rhythm. Statistical analysis demonstrated that only circadian BP pattern and age a exhibited significant relative risk for fatal events, while diabetic nephropathy, postural hypotension, and hypertension as well as circadian BP pattern were significantly associated with a relative risk for various nonfatal vascular events [41].

ABNORMAL BP RHYTHM AND RENAL FUNCTION

A very interesting issue is whether an abnormal BP profile increases the renal function decline. This was addressed by Farmer and co-workers [42] in a retrospective investigation in 26 type 1 and type 2 diabetics. There was a more rapid decline in creatinine clearance in non-dippers (–7.9 ml/min/year) when compared with dippers (–2.9 ml/min/year). If this will be confirmed by larger prospective studies, diabetics with nephropathy could be stratified in renal risk groups according to their dipping status. A more aggressive and more adequate – for the particular BP profile of non-dippers – antihypertensive therapy could be of benefit in retarding progression of diabetic nephropathy to end-stage renal disease.

This data confirms more solid evidence obtained from a 3-year longitudinal case-control study performed by Timio *et al.* [43] who have examined 48 hypertensive nondiabetic subjects with renal insufficiency, divided into dippers and non-dippers. There was no difference with respect of demographic data, office BP, mean daytime ABPM values, creatinine clearance and proteinuria at baseline. The nondippers had a significantly faster rate of decline of creatinine clearance when compared with the dippers (0.37 *vs.* 0.27 ml/min/month, p = 0.002). The amount of urinary protein excretion, a recognized factor for accelerated decline of renal function, was also significantly more pronounced in nondippers (993 mg/24 hours versus 691 mg/24 hours in dippers). As stated by the authors, "... a proper nocturnal BP control is an additional aim of anti-hypertensive therapy" [43].

Recently, Knudsen *et al.* [44] performed ABPM and also fundal photography in 80 type 2 diabetic subjects, trying to establish a relationship between retinopathy, nephropathy, macrovascular disease, pulse pressure and diurnal BP variation. They found that increased pulse pressure and blunted diurnal BP variation were hemodynamic abnormalities associated with microvascular and macrovascular complications.

Once both diabetic and non-diabetic patients reaching end-stage renal disease and starting dialysis, abnormal BP profile seems to be a major determinant of survival. Indeed, this was first confirmed by a well-conducted prospective study performed by Amar and colleagues [45] showing that, in non-diabetic ESRD patients, an elevated nocturnal BP increases the cardiovascular mortality by 41%, independently of other confounding factors. Elevated 24-h pulse pressure (as a surrogate marker of arterial stiffness) was also significantly associated with increased risk for cardiovascular death. More recently, Liu *et al.* [23] studied 80 hemodialysis patients (27 with diabetic nephropathy) who underwent ABPM and were categorized as dippers (N = 24) and non-dippers (N = 56). Coronary angiography, 24-hour ambulatory ECG and clinical events over around 3 years were used to compare these two groups. Non-dippers had more coronary artery disease, poorer left ventricular function, impaired circadian heart rhythm, and 3.5 and 9 times the number of cardiovascular events and deaths, respectively compared to dippers. On Cox analysis the non-dipping status had a hazard ratio of 2.5 (p = 0.038) for CV events, and of 9.6 (p = 0.031) for CV deaths.

ABNORMAL CIRCADIAN VARIABILITY OF BP – CAN WE TREAT?

Since the abnormal diurnal rhythm is so frequent in diabetic renal patients and, as discussed, carries an important negative prognostic significance, a central legitimate question for any diabetologist or nephrologist is if we have effective therapeutic strategies today. There are some answers, but clearly the only existing evidence comes from small trials. Czupryniak and co-workers have shown that an angiotensin-converting enzyme inhibitor (ACEI) restores abnormal circadian variability in normotensive, normoalbuminuric type 1 diabetics [46]. The same seems to be true for patients with incipient diabetic nephropathy. Diabetic patients with early microalbuminuria (20–70 μg/min) treated for 2 years with lisinopril had significant reduction of ambulatory BP (primarily of the nocturnal BP) and reversal of microalbuminuria, when compared to the placebo-treated group. There was no difference in office BP between the two groups [47]. In a study of the effect of ACE inhibitor therapy on urinary albumin excretion rate (UAER) and blood pressure assessed by ABPM, Bauduceau and colleagues [48] found that on-drug nighttime diastolic BP was independently predictive for abnormally urinary excretion rate (odds ratio 3.5), whereas office BP was not. The only predictor for UAER decrease was 24-h systolic BP decrease, confirming the superiority of ABPM over clinical BP measurements to predict target organ damage.

ABPM IN DIABETIC PREGNANT WOMEN

Pregnancy in type 1 diabetes is associated with an increased risk of developing pregnancy-induced hypertension (PIH). Ambulatory blood pressure monitoring (ABPM) has been used to screen for preeclampsia in nondiabetic pregnancy.

Flores *et al.* [49] conducted a study regarding ABPM profile during pregnancy in normotensive type 1 diabetic women. ABPM measurements were performed in each trimester in diabetic pregnant women and pregnant nondiabetic controls. The incidence of pregnancy-induced hypertension was fourfold greater in diabetic women than in controls. Diabetic women who developed PIH in the third semester showed significantly higher BP profiles throughout the pregnancy than those who remained normotensive. Nighttime systolic BP showed the best predictive capacity for PIH, with a cut off value of 105 mmHg. The nighttime BP values recorded by ABPM had an excellent sensitivity and specificity (85 and 92%, respectively). This study confirms an early increase in BP of patients who will develop pregnancy-related hypertension. Therefore, the findings that nighttime systolic BP during the second trimester of pregnancy is predictive for PIH in the third trimester suggests that ABPM may be a reliable screening tool for PIH risk assessment in diabetic pregnant women [49].

Indeed, in a recent investigation by Lauszus and co-workers [50], the incidence of preeclampsia was significantly associated with ambulatory BP in 1151 in women with insulin-dependent DM. ABPM values were higher from the first trimester in patients who subsequently developed preeclampsia when compared with patients who do not develop this complication. The best sensitivity and specificity for predicting preeclampsia in primiparous women were cut-off values of daytime BP of 122 and 74 mmHg for systolic and diastolic BP, respectively. The relative risk for preeclampsia increased constantly not only with BP values above the cut-off values, but also with higher urinary albumin excretion rates (UAER). Interestingly, after adjusting for UAER, there was a significant relationship between ambulatory BP values and glycemic control (see previous discussion).

A WORD OF CAUTION – ABPM REPRODUCIBILITY

It is to simplistic to assume that, having arbitrarily categorized subjects into "dippers" and "non-dippers", these labels will always be valid. Peixoto and colleagues have raised recently [51] the issue of reproducibility, performing 48-hour interdialytic ABPM in 21 hemodialysis (HD) patients on two different occasions at about 68 days apart. Reproducibility was determined by analysis of the standard deviation of the differences between the two monitoring periods and the coefficient of variation of each method of BP determination (isolated pre-HD and post-HD values, average pre-HD and post-HD values for the five HD sessions surrounding each monitoring period, and 48-hour interdialytic ABPM values).

This study showed better reproducibility of ABPM compared with isolated pre-HD and post-HD BP and with averaged pre- and post-HD blood pressure values. However, the reproducibility of the decrease in BP during sleep was poor, with up to 43% of the subjects changing dipping category within or between interdialytic periods [51].

Indeed, these concerns about ABPM reproducibility have been confirmed very recently by our group (Covic *et al.*, J Nephrol 2002, [52]) in polycystic kidney disease patients with treated hypertension and mild chronic renal impairment. When comparing a first with a second ABPM measurement (after 3 months), only 43.3% of the patients maintained the initial dipping category. The same proportion of subjects had a similar dipping category when the first ABPM was compared with the third one (after 9 months), but a large (24%) subset of patients had dramatic shifts in their amplitude of nocturnal BP fall, significantly greater than those recorded after shorter inter-measurement intervals. When several ABPM measurements are repeated for the same patients, the repeatability is even worse, since only 36.6% of our study population maintained the initial dipping category across all three ABPM determinations. Equally important, our study revealed that, with time, there isn't a tendency to decreased circadian variation: a similar proportion of patients increased or decreased their amplitude in nocturnal BP fall, at 3 and 9 month. Thus, it would be unwise to extrapolate the impact of a single baseline circadian BP profile on target organ damage [52].

CONCLUSIONS

Given the high prevalence of diabetes mellitus throughout the world, with increasing incidence of type 2 diabetes as life expectancy improves, there is an increasing incidence of micro- and macrovascular complications in the diabetic population. Diabetic nephropathy is a prominent microvascular complication of both type 1 and type 2 diabetes, progressing in most cases to end-stage renal disease. There is an impressive increase of prevalence of end-stage renal disease due to diabetic nephropathy, causing a huge logistical and financial burden on renal replacement therapy systems in most countries.

Moreover, morbidity and mortality on dialysis is clearly more severe in diabetic end-stage renal disease patients when compared with nondiabetic dialysis patients.

One major determinant of cardiovascular and renal outcome in diabetic patients is hypertension. However, office blood pressure seems to be less accurate in predicting target-organ damage in diabetic and non-diabetic patients when compared with ambulatory blood pressure monitoring (ABPM).

ABPM has emerged in the last decades as a very useful tool in assessing blood pressure for diagnostic and therapeutic reasons. Moreover, an abnormal day-night BP profile determined through ABPM is predictive for future development of diabetic nephropathy and is associated with a faster progression to the proteinuric stage and later to chronic renal failure. Concomitantly, cardiovascular risk is determined independently by an abnormal circadian profile. All these translate into a (now) well-defined relationship between non-dippers and less survival. Antihypertensive therapy targeting and correcting the abnormal 24-hours BP profile may improve significantly renal, cardiovascular and overall outcomes in diabetes mellitus patients.

REFERENCES

1. Agodoa LY, Jones CA, Held PJ. End-stage renal disease in the USA: data from the United States Renal Data System. *Am J Nephrol*, **16**: 7–16, 1996.
2. Rychlik I, Miltenberger-Miltenyi G, Ritz E. The drama of the continuous increase in end-stage renal failure in patients with type II diabetes mellitus. *Nephrol Dial Transplant*, **13** (Suppl 8): 6–10, 1998.
3. Perneger TV, Brancati FL, Whelton PK, Klag MJ. End-stage renal disease attributable to diabetes mellitus. *Ann Intern Med*, **121**: 912–918, 1994.
4. ⁎⁎ Tight blood pressure control and risk of macrovascular and microvascular complications in type 2 diabetes: UKPDS 38. UK Prospective Diabetes Study Group. *BMJ*, **317**: 703–713, 1998.
5. Stamler J, Vaccaro O, Neaton JD, Wentworth D. Diabetes, other risk factors, and 12-yr cardiovascular mortality for men screened in the Multiple Risk Factor Intervention Trial. *Diabetes Care*, **16**: 434–444, 1993.

6. ⁎⁎ Hypertension in Diabetes Study (HDS): I. Prevalence of hypertension in newly presenting type 2 diabetic patients and the association with risk factors for cardiovascular and diabetic complications. *J Hypertens*, **11**: 309–317, 1993.
7. ⁎⁎ Hypertension in Diabetes Study (HDS): II. Increased risk of cardiovascular complications in hypertensive type 2 diabetic patients. *J Hypertens*, **11**: 319–325, 1993.
8. Nelson RG, Bennett PH, Beck GJ, Tan M, *et al*. Development and progression of renal disease in Pima Indians with non-insulin-dependent diabetes mellitus. Diabetic Renal Disease Study Group. *N Engl J Med*, **335**: 1636–1642, 1996.
9. Stratton IM, Kohner EM, Aldington SJ, Turner RC, *et al*. UKPDS 50: risk factors for incidence and progression of retinopathy in Type II diabetes over 6 years from diagnosis. *Diabetologia*, **44**: 156–163, 2001.
10. Mogensen CE, Keane WF, Bennett PH, Jerums G, *et al*. Prevention of diabetic renal disease with special reference to microalbuminuria. *Lancet*, **346**: 1080–1084, 1995.
11. Mogensen CE. Systemic blood pressure and glomerular leakage with particular reference to diabetes and hypertension. *J Intern Med*, **235**: 297–316, 1994.
12. Parving HH, Andersen AR, Smidt UM, Hommel E, *et al*. Effect of antihypertensive treatment on kidney function in diabetic nephropathy. *Br Med J* (Clin Res Ed), **294**: 1443–1447, 1987.
13. Gaede P, Vedel P, Larsen N, Jensen GV, *et al*. Multifactorial intervention and cardiovascular disease in patients with type 2 diabetes. *N Engl J Med*, **348**: 383–393, 2003.
14. Staessen JA, Bieniaszewski L, O'Brien ET, Fagard R. Special feature: what is a normal blood pressure in ambulatory monitoring? *Nephrol Dial Transplant*, **11**: 241–245, 1996.
15. Lebel M, Kingma I, Grose JH, Langlois S. Effect of recombinant human erythropoietin therapy on ambulatory blood pressure in normotensive and in untreated borderline hypertensive hemodialysis patients. *Am J Hypertens*, **8**: 545–851, 1995.
16. Agarwal R. Assessment of blood pressure in hemodialysis patients. *Semin Dial*, **15**: 299–304, 2002.
17. Zoccali C, Mallamaci F, Tripepi G, Benedetto FA, *et al*. Prediction of left ventricular geometry by clinic, pre-dialysis and 24-h ambulatory BP monitoring in hemodialysis patients: CREED investigators. *J Hypertens*, **17**: 1751–1758, 1999.
18. Conion PJ, Walshe JJ, Heinle SK, Minda S, *et al*. Predialysis systolic blood pressure correlates

strongly with mean 24- hour systolic blood pressure and left ventricular mass in stable hemodialysis patients. *J Am Soc Nephrol*, 7: 2658–2663, 1996.

19. •*• 2003 European Society of Hypertension – European Society of Cardiology guidelines for the management of arterial hypertension. *J Hypertens*, 21: 1011–1053, 2003.

20. •*•Seventh Report of the Joint National Committee on prevention, detection, evaluation, and treatment of high blood pressure. *JAMA*, 289: 2560–2572, 2003.

21. Keller CK, Bergis KH, Fliser D, Ritz E. Renal findings in patients with short-term type 2 diabetes. *J Am Soc Nephrol*, 7: 2627–2635, 1996.

22. Willenbuecher B, M.D. thesis 2000, University of Heidelberg, Germany, unpublished data.

23. Lurbe A, Redon J, Pascual JM, Tacons J, *et al.* Altered blood pressure during sleep in normotensive subjects with type I diabetes. *Hypertension*, 21: 227–235, 1993.

24. Voros P, Lengyel Z, Nagy V, Nemeth C, *et al.* Diurnal blood pressure variation and albuminuria in normotensive patients with insulin-dependent diabetes mellitus. *Nephrol Dial Transplant*, 13: 2257–2260, 1998.

25. Poulsen PL, Ebbehoj E, Hansen KW, Mogensen CE. 24-h blood pressure and autonomic function is related to albumin excretion within the normoalbuminuric range in IDDM patients. *Diabetologia*, 40: 718–725, 1997.

26. Poulsen PL, Bek T, Ebbehoj E, Hansen KW, *et al.* 24-h ambulatory blood pressure and retinopathy in normoalbuminuric IDDM patients. *Diabetologia*, 41: 105–110, 1998.

27. Lurbe E, Redon J, Pascual JM, Tacons J, *et al.* The spectrum of circadian blood pressure changes in type I diabetic patients. *J Hypertens*, 19: 1421–1428, 2001.

28. Mulec H, Blohme G, Kullenberg K, Nyberg G, *et al.* Latent overhydration and nocturnal hypertension in diabetic nephropathy. *Diabetologia*, 38: 216–220, 1995.

29. Nielsen S, Schmitz A, Poulsen PL, Hansen KW, *et al.* Albuminuria and 24-h ambulatory blood pressure in normoalbuminuric and microalbuminuric NIDDM patients. A longitudinal study. *Diabetes Care*, 18: 1434–1441, 1995.

30. Duvnjak L, Vuckovic S, Car N, Metelko Z. Relationship between autonomic function, 24-h blood pressure, and albuminuria in normotensive, normoalbuminuric patients with Type 1 diabetes. *J Diabetes Complications*, 15: 314–319, 2001.

31. van Ittersum FJ, Spek JJ, Praet IJ, Lambert J, *et al.* Ambulatory blood pressures and autonomic nervous function in normoalbuminuric type I diabetic patients. *Nephrol Dial Transplant*, 13: 326–332, 1998.

32. Ferreira SR, Cesarini PR, Vivolo MA, Zanella MT. Abnormal nocturnal blood pressure fall in normotensive adolescents with insulin-dependent diabetes is ameliorated following glycemic improvement. *Braz J Med Biol Res*, 31: 523–528, 1998.

33. Young LA, Kimball TR, Daniels SR, Standiford DA, *et al.* Nocturnal blood pressure in young patients with insulin-dependent diabetes mellitus: correlation with cardiac function. *J Pediatr*, 133: 46–50, 1998.

34. Liu M, Takahashi H, Morita Y *et al.* Non-dipping is a potent predictor of cardiovascular mortality and is associated with autonomic dysfunction in hemodialysis patients. *Nephrol Dial Transplant*, 18: 563–569, 2003.

35. Zweiker R, Eber B, Schumacher M, Toplak H, *et al.* "Non-dipping" related to cardiovascular events in essential hypertensive patients. *Acta Med Austriaca*, 21: 86–89, 1994.

36. Verdecchia P, Porcellati C, Schillaci G, Borgioni C, *et al.* Ambulatory blood pressure. An independent predictor of prognosis in essential hypertension. *Hypertension*, 24: 793–801, 1994.

37. Staessen JA, Thijs L, Fagard R, O'Brien ET, *et al.* Predicting cardiovascular risk using conventional vs ambulatory blood pressure in older patients with systolic hypertension. Systolic Hypertension in Europe Trial Investigators. *JAMA*, 282: 539–546, 1999.

38. Yamamoto Y, Akiguchi I, Oiwa K, Hayashi M, *et al.* Twenty-four-hour blood pressure and MRI as predictive factors for different outcomes in patients with lacunar infarct. *Stroke*, 33: 297–305, 2002.

39. Kario K, Pickering TG, Matsuo T, Hoshide S, *et al.* Stroke prognosis and abnormal nocturnal blood pressure falls in older hypertensives. *Hypertension*, 38: 852–857, 2001.

40. Covic A, Goldsmith DJ, Covic M. Reduced blood pressure diurnal variability as a risk factor for progressive left ventricular dilatation in hemodialysis patients. *Am J Kidney Dis*, 35: 617–623, 2000.

41. Nakano S, Fukuda M, Hotta F, Ito T, *et al.* Reversed circadian blood pressure rhythm is associated with occurrences of both fatal and nonfatal vascular events in NIDDM subjects. *Diabetes*, 47: 1501–1506, 1998.

42. Farmer CK, Goldsmith DJ, Quin JD, Dallyn P, *et al.* Progression of diabetic nephropathy – is diurnal blood pressure rhythm as important as absolute blood pressure level? *Nephrol Dial Transplant*, 13: 635–639, 1998.

43. Timio M, Venanzi S, Lolli S, Lippi G, *et al*. "Non-dipper" hypertensive patients and progressive renal insufficiency: a 3-year longitudinal study. *Clin Nephrol*, **43**: 382–387, 1995.

44. Knudsen ST, Poulsen PL, Hansen KW, Ebbehoj E, *et al*. Pulse pressure and diurnal blood pressure variation: association with micro- and macrovascular complications in type 2 diabetes. Am *J Hypertens*, **15**: 244–250, 2002.

45. Amar J, Vernier I, Rossignol E, Bongard V, *et al*. Nocturnal blood pressure and 24-hour pulse pressure are potent indicators of mortality in hemodialysis patients. *Kidney Int*, **57**: 2485–2491, 2000.

46. Czupryniak L, Wisniewska-Jaronsinska M, Drzewoski J. Trandolapril restores circadian blood pressure variation in normoalbuminuric normotensive type 1 diabetic patients. *J Diabetes Complications*, **15**: 75–79, 2001.

47. Poulsen PL, Ebbehoj E, Nosadini R, Fioretto P, *et al*. Early ACE-i intervention in microalbuminuric patients with type 1 diabetes: effects on albumin excretion, 24 h ambulatory blood pressure, and renal function. *Diabetes Metab*, **27**: 123–128, 2001.

48. Bauduceau B, Genes N, Chamontin B, Vaur L, *et al*. Ambulatory blood pressure and urinary albumin excretion in diabetic (non-insulin-dependent and insulin-dependent) hypertensive patients: relationships at baseline and after treatment by the angiotensin converting enzyme inhibitor trandolapril. *Am J Hypertens*, **11**: 1065–1073, 1998.

49. Flores L, Levy I, Aguilera E, Martinez S, *et al*. Usefulness of ambulatory blood pressure monitoring in pregnant women with type 1 diabetes. *Diabetes Care*, **22**: 1507–1511, 1999.

50. Lauszus FF, Rasmussen OW, Lousen T, Klebe TM, *et al*. Ambulatory blood pressure as predictor of preeclampsia in diabetic pregnancies with respect to urinary albumin excretion rate and glycemic regulation. *Acta Obstet Gynecol Scand*, **80**: 1096–1103, 2001.

51. Peixoto AJ, Santos SF, Mendes RB, Crowley ST, *et al*. Reproducibility of ambulatory blood pressure monitoring in hemodialysis patients. *Am J Kidney Dis*, **36**: 983–990, 2000.

52. Covic A, Mititiuc I, Gusbeth-Tatomir P, Goldsmith DJ. The reproducibility of the circadian BP rhythm in treated hypertensive patients with polycystic kidney disease and mild chronic renal impairment – a prospective ABPM study. *J Nephrol*, **15**: 497–506, 2002.

27

MYOCARDIAL INFARCTION IN PATIENTS WITH DIABETES MELLITUS

Carmen GINGHINĂ, Dinu DRAGOMIR, Mirela MARINESCU

It is considered that the coronary risk of a diabetic patient is similar to a non-diabetic of the same age who had a previous myocardial infarction. As for the rest of the population, in the diabetic patients the myocardial infarction remains the "privilege" of the over 40 years old persons. In the group of the young age group, the incidence of AMI is higher than in non-diabetic patients. The incidence of the myocardial infarction in diabetics does not depend on the type of antidiabetic treatment but rather on the lack of metabolic control and the duration of diabetes mellitus. Appearance of the myocardial infarction in diabetics has important metabolic implications: excessive sympathetic stimulation, decreased insulin secretion, hyperproduction of cortisol and glucagon, growth of free fatty acids production, emphasis of the glycogenolysis and frequently the diabetic ketoacidosis. The acute metabolic complications of diabetes mellitus have important adverse effects on the evolution and the treatment of the myocardial infarction in this group of patients.

"Diabetic status" of a patient with myocardial infarction is characterized by abnormalities of coagulation, spontaneous thrombolysis and platelet function.

AMI in diabetic patients is more frequently silent and can manifest by acute pump insufficiency, metabolic decompensation or both. The association of early AMI with ketoacidosis (or ketoacidotic coma) is a more rare but very serious, combination. In the diabetic patients, AMI evolves frequently in the acute period with multiple complications, which makes the intra hospital mortality rate to be almost double *versus* the non-diabetics with AMI.

A special attention must be paid to diagnosis of AMI without ST-segment elevation, especially in those situations when the pain is missing and the enzymatic criterion has a great diagnostic importance.

AMI treatment in diabetic patients requires the same general lines as for non-diabetic patients: large-scale use of thrombolytic agents, platelet antiaggregants and ACE inhibitors. Beta-blockers can be used, respecting the specific contraindications. In addition, the therapeutic strategy demands a rigorous metabolic balance. The improvement of the metabolic control with insulin is associated with a better evolution of the diabetic patients after PTCA.

The diabetic patients benefit especially from the therapy with GP IIb/IIIa receptors with results in reducing the postprocedural complications.

It has been noticed that the diabetic patients with myocardial infarction present more frequently a multicoronary affection with diffuse atherosclerotic lesions especially at the level of distal bed. Studies show that it is preferred to use surgical revascularization because the usage of the interventional procedures is associated with a higher rate of restenosis and postprocedural complications. Lately, the use of coronary stents associated to angioplasty in diabetic patients has reduced the restenosis rate.

Frequently the normalization of the lipid profile in the diabetic patient with myocardial infarction cannot be realized with only one class of drugs, therefore it is recommended the statins-fibrates association therapy.

The evolution of the diabetic with myocardial infarction must be considered in relation with the co-existence of other complications of diabetes mellitus, and in the first place of the diabetic microangiopathy and autonomic cardiac neuropathy. The factors of unfavorable prognosis on long-term that should be considered in diabetic patients with myocardial infarction are: the age of the patient, the feminine gender, the association of hypertension, the atherogenic lipoproteic profile (small and dense particles of LDL-cholesterol), ventricular rhythm disorders, diffuse and distal multivascular coronary affection, reduction of the coronary flux reserve, congestive heart insufficiency.

ETIOPATHOGENIC ASPECTS OF THE ACUTE MYOCARDIAL INFARCTION IN DIABETIC PATIENTS

DOES MYOCARDIAL INFARCTION NEED A SPECIAL ATTENTION IN DIABETIC PATIENTS?

At the beginning of this century, the studies regarding the myocardial metabolism showed that the heart of diabetic patients is affected by the disorder of the glucose metabolism. In the latest decades, researchers oriented their effort towards describing as detailed as possible the biochemical mechanisms responsible for metabolic and vascular dysfunction involved in the coronary disease of the patient with diabetes. More than that, in the last ten years the cardiologists, diabetologists, and epidemiologists showed that the diabetic patients present an accelerated process of atherosclerosis, have a higher mortality rate after an acute myocardial infarction, evolve more often towards a cardiac insufficiency after the myocardial injury compared with the non-diabetic patients. During this decade, the prognosis of the non-diabetic patients with coronary heart disease improved considerably, whilst the diabetic coronarian presents, for the same level of coronary status, more frequent major cardiovascular events. These findings support the concept that the diabetic patient with myocardial infarction needs a special approach and a specific treatment according to his diabetes status [1].

Thus, a conclusion has been reached that, in order to improve the prognosis of the diabetic patient with myocardial infarction the reunited efforts of both cardiologist and diabetologists are needed. A unitary approach of those patients is a must, considering that the high number of diabetes mellitus cases (about 150 million world-wide, of which over 90% have diabetes mellitus type 2), will grow significantly in the near future

– it is estimated that in the next 15 years the number will double. About 20% of the patients hospitalized in the coronary intensive care unit are diabetics and in the large clinical trials of cardiovascular diseases a similar share of diabetics can be found.

The recent trials with diabetic patients and the analysis of the subgroups of diabetics from the large clinical trials studying the myocardial infarction and the interventional coronary procedures provided new data regarding the controversial issue "*how do we approach the diabetic patient with myocardial infarction?*" [2].

In this chapter, we tried to summarize and present the currently available data regarding the clinical and therapeutic approach of the diabetic patient with myocardial infarction.

CORONARY RISK FACTORS IN DIABETIC PATIENTS

Diabetes mellitus is considered to be an important risk factor, independent of coronary disease, increasing its relative risk twice for men and over three times for women [3, 4]. As a result, the incidence of the coronary disease is significantly higher for diabetic patients. Additionally, the extensive damages of epicardial coronary vessels is higher for diabetics, for which the coronary graphic data reveal more frequently tri-coronary lesions in the acute myocardial infarction and a more diffuse distribution of the atherosclerotic plaques compared to the non-diabetic patients. Diabetes mellitus has a significant impact on other risk factors. It has been noticed that diabetic patients have multiple coronary risk factors. For example, diabetes mellitus is frequently associated with obesity, arterial hypertension, hypertriglyceridemia and decrease of the HDL-cholesterol level, all of them considered important coronary risk factors; their association in the same patient is common [5, 6].

Diabetes mellitus is frequently associated with increasing VLDL, triglycerides, as well as with reduction of HDL-cholesterol, whilst the total cholesterol and LDL-cholesterol aim to have close values for both diabetic and non-diabetic patients. More than that, HDL-cholesterol and LDL-cholesterol can be the glycosylated, leading to accumulation of LDL in circulation and cholesterol esters in macrophages. The oxidation process of LDL is accentuated in diabetics, contributing to accelerate atherosclerosis [7].

Diabetes mellitus is associated with the alteration of the lipid metabolism and the levels of lipoproteins. The diabetics have more extended, more diffuse and more severe coronary damage than the non-diabetics, fact that can also be explained by the growth of the small, dense particles of LDL-cholesterol. Lipoprotein a – Lp(a) – and the increased oxidation of LDL can also be important factors in accelerating the atherosclerosis in diabetics. Additionally, the glycosylation of apoprotein B, LDL and HDL that can appear in diabetes mellitus, might diminish LDL clearance and increase HDL clearance. The advanced glycosylation products may be involved in the accelerated atherosclerosis in diabetic patients [8].

Changing the risk factors after an acute coronary event of a diabetic patient leads to a reduction of other cardiovascular events at least equal if not higher compared with non-diabetic patients [9].

It is known that smoking aggravates glycemic control and accelerates the micro vascular complications of diabetes mellitus. Unfortunately, diabetics are more addicted smokers than non-diabetics [10].

CORONARY FLUX ADJUSTMENT IN DIABETIC PATIENTS WITH MYOCARDIAL INFARCTION

Though it is well known that the diabetic patients have more severe damage of the coronary arteries, they can show more severe signs and symptoms of myocardial ischemia than non-diabetics having the same level of epicardial coronary damage. This fact is, probably, due to abnormalities at the level of coronary microcirculation (the small vessels' disease). The myocardial distribution of oxygen depends on the coronary flow and it is known that the coronary

vessels with a smaller diameter than 150μm regulate the coronary flow [11]. Therefore, in the patients with similar levels of damage of epicardial coronary vessels, the dysfunction of the coronary microcirculation can explain the big differences between the myocardial distributions of oxygen.

Coronary microcirculation suffers both functional and anatomical changes, similar to anatomical abnormalities met in the microcirculation of other target organs affected by diabetes mellitus [12]. The thickening of the basal membrane of the small coronary vessels is specific, which affects the release of oxygen and nutritional substances at the myocardial level. The histological changes are directly proportional to the duration and severity of diabetes mellitus.

Vascular tonus at the level of the vessels with a diameter smaller than 150μm plays an important role in regulating the coronary blood flow. The micro vascular coronary tonus can be influenced by a series of factors such as the vasodilating prostaglandin, the hyper polarizing factor derived from endothelium, nitric oxide (the relaxing factor derived from endothelium–EDRF). The study of the various vascular beds, including coronary circulation in animals or *in vitro*, proved that the diabetic patients have an insufficient release of nitric oxide derived from endothelium – which contributes to the so-called *endothelial dysfunction.*

Whilst there is enough evidence showing that the release of nitric oxide is less efficient in diabetics than in non-diabetics, the hypothesis of a relative reduction of sensitivity at nitric oxide is less well supported. It seems that the proper nitric oxide production is not significantly affected by diabetes mellitus, a fact that is supported by the observation that administrating arginine – the precursor of nitric oxide – does not influence the endothelial function in diabetics. On the other hand, there is clear evidence that the simultaneous production of a vasoconstrictor factor derived from endothelium is involved in the endothelial dysfunction in diabetics. Moreover, it has been demonstrated that the diabetes status is characterized by the increased production of free radicals of oxygen; it is also well known that superoxide anion interacts with the nitric oxide to form peroxy-nitrite, a substance with relatively poorer vasodilative properties. In the experimental methods in animals, the inhibition of the receptors for vasodilating prostanoids determines the restoration of the normal endothelial function, a fact that is proved as well for the diabetic patients for whom the therapy of reduction of free radicals of oxygen improves the endothelial function in various vascular territories [12, 13, 14].

Researchers paid special attention to the possible mechanism through which vasoconstrictors and free radicals of oxygen production are increasing when it comes for the diabetics with myocardial infarction. The increase of the oxidative stress in diabetes mellitus is realized, on one hand through an increased generation of free radicals of oxygen *via* an increased production of prostaglandin and prostanoid through cyclooxygenase, and on the other hand, through reduction of the free radicals of oxygen clearance. It has been proved that one mechanism involved is represented by the glycosylation of the super-oxide dismutase – which eliminates the free radicals from the circulation, having a role of scavenger – with a result in reduction of the activity of this enzyme. Other mechanisms that might be involved in regulating the coronary flow in the diabetics with myocardial infarction – the implication of proteinkinase C, the final products of advanced glycosylation – are only studied on experimental models in animals and are in progress for research in diabetic patients.

The difficulty in elucidating the mechanisms that occur in flow regulation at the level of the coronary circulation in diabetics is due to the association of diabetes mellitus with several conditions also characterized by endothelial dysfunction: dyslipidemia, arteriosclerosis or hypertension, which in turn associates variable degrees of oxidative stress [12, 15, 16].

COAGULATION DISORDERS AND THROMBUS FORMATION IN DIABETIC PATIENTS WITH MYOCARDIAL INFARCTION

The diabetic status of the patient presenting myocardial infarction is characterized by a pro-coagulating status to which contribute not only the abnormalities from the cascade of the coagulation. The diabetics also present a

hyperaggregability of the platelets mediated by the increase in ADP, arachidonic acid, platelet activating factor and thrombin formation, the growth of thrombocytic factor 4 release and the growth of thromboxane synthesis. In addition, there is a growth of the attachment of fibrinogen with the platelet receptor glycoprotein IIb/IIIa – which is assumed to be due either to the increase of the receptors type IIb/IIIa on the platelet surface, or to the glycosylation process of the receptor. It is interesting to notice that the results of the recent clinical studies show that the diabetics benefit from the administration of blockers for the receptors of glycoprotein IIb/IIIa more than the non-diabetics, possibly because of those mechanisms [12, 17].

It is well known that diabetic patients present with an increase of the fibrinogen concentration and a reduction of fibrinolysis activity. The tissular plasminogen activator (tPA) has normal or increased values in diabetics. However, there is a reduction of the tPA activity, secondary to the concentration of PAI-1 (the inhibitor of the tissular plasminogen activator). It has been also noticed that the level of PAI-1 in atherosclerotic plaques is higher in diabetics. Besides, the plasminogen can be glycosylated, with a result in diminishing the capacity of this enzyme to be activated [21]. Those differences between diabetics and non-diabetics regarding the cascade of coagulation and the platelet functions can contribute to the growth of the ischemia and myocardial infarction incidence in the diabetics.

STATISTICAL DATA

Epidemiological studies show that the middle-aged diabetic patients have a higher risk of coronary disease/events than the non-diabetic patients of the same age: in diabetic men, the coronary mortality risk is 2–3 times higher than non-diabetics of the same age and in diabetic women it is 3–5 times higher. In other words, diabetes mellitus cancels the differences between genders when it comes for the coronary risk [22]. It has been noticed that the coronary risk of a diabetic patient is similar to the one of a non-diabetic of the same age who had myocardial infarction in his history. In the diabetics, the annual absolute risk of fatal and non-fatal coronary events is 2–5%; few epidemiological studies showed that 15–20% of the patients with acute coronary symptoms have documented history of diabetes mellitus when they suffer a coronary accident. As for the rest of the population, in diabetics the myocardial infarction remains the "privilege" of the over 40 years old people. In the group of the young age diabetics, the incidence of AMI is higher than in the non-diabetics, proving the importance of diabetes mellitus as a coronary risk factor [23].

The incidence of the myocardial infarction in diabetics does not depend on the type of diabetes trbeatment but rather on the lack of metabolic control and the duration of diabetes mellitus.

METABOLIC ASPECTS

The appearance of myocardial infarction in diabetics has important metabolic implications: excessive sympathetic stimulation leading to a higher production of catecholamine, decrease of the insulin secretion, hyperproduction of cortisol and glucagon, increased production of the free fatty acids production, excess glycogenolysis and diabetic more frequent ketoacidosis [24]. The acute metabolic complications of diabetes mellitus have important adverse effects on the evolution and the treatment of myocardial infarction in this subgroup of patients.

The glycoregulation disorders occur in a significantly higher percentage in the diabetics with myocardial infarction than in the non-diabetics [25]. The presence of hyperglycemia during the acute phase of myocardial infarction may have the following significance:

– lack of metabolic balance of a known diabetes mellitus under the circumstances of AMI appearance;

– the revealing moment for the diagnosis of a latent diabetes mellitus;

– transitory hyperglycemia.

It has been noticed that a degree of insulin resistance is responsible for the increase in glycemia after a myocardial infarction rather than an insufficiency of insulin secretion. The distinction between an oligosymptomatic diabetes mellitus and a hyperglycemic reaction induced at the moment of AMI can be made based on the identification of glycosylated hemoglobin, which

in first case is high, and in the second situation is normal. In the current clinical practice, we can consider that the hyperglycemia in the acute phase of the myocardial infarction that persists one month after the coronary accident can be interpreted as the expression of diabetes mellitus revealed by the "stress" generated by the acute coronary accident [26].

DIAGNOSTIC CRITERIA OF ACUTE MYOCARDIAL INFARCTION IN DIABETIC PATIENTS

As it is known, the term *myocardial infarction* requires myocardial necrosis secondary to prolonged *ischemia*, as a result of the lack of balance between the demand and the supply of oxygen. The criteria for diagnosing the myocardial infarction in diabetics are similar to the criteria of myocardial infarction in non-diabetics, with the mention that the patient may be known with history of diabetes mellitus or may be detected for the first time with diabetes mellitus at the same time an acute myocardial infarction occurs.

It is possible to diagnose an evolving or recent MI in a patient with diabetes mellitus when at least one of the following criteria is present:

1. Typical increase of serum levels of the biochemical markers of myocardial necrosis (troponin with gradual increase and decline, or CK-MB with faster rise and decline) associated with *at least one* of the following characteristics:

a) Ischemia symptoms;

b) The appearance of the pathological Q waves on ECG;

c) Changes of ECG indicating ischemia (elevation or depression of ST segment), or

d) Intervention on coronary vessels (for example coronary angioplasty).

2. Morphopathological characteristics of acute infarction.

To diagnose the established MI at least one of the following criteria should be present:

1. Appearance of new pathologic Q waves on serial ECG recordings:

– With or without history suggesting AMI;

– Biochemical markers of myocardial necrosis may be normalized depending on the time passed since the beginning of the infarction.

2. Morphologic characteristics of old or new AMI.

CLINICAL CRITERIA

It is not possible to speak about a clinical symptom or sign specific for AMI in patients with diabetes mellitus. Considering the high frequency of the non-painful clinical forms of AMI, some authors consider the loss of balance apparently unmotivated of a diabetic (with the increase of insulin demand) as being "the alarming sign" useful in diagnosing AMI, insisting in those cases to record an ECG and to dose the bio-markers of myocardial necrosis as routine investigation [15, 24]

The association of early AMI with ketoacidosis (or ketoacidosic coma) is a more rare combination but very serious. It is often difficult to establish the succession of the events because, in diabetics, AMI can lead to ketoacidosis, and acidosis through dehydration, hemoconcentration and hypotension can speed up the appearance of a myocardial infarction [21, 24].

The painless form explained through the presence of the autonomic cardiac neuropathy could become manifested by an acute pump insufficiency (even acute pulmonary edema, cardiogenic shock) or through metabolic decompensation or both.

In diabetic patients, AMI evolves frequently in the acute period with multiple complications, which makes the intra hospital mortality rate to be double versus the non-diabetic persons with AMI. There are cases when AMI in diabetics is manifested by digestive symptoms (epigastric pain, nausea, vomiting). In such cases the diagnosis is to be made based on the enzymatic and ECG criteria.

Special attention must be paid to diagnose AMI forms without ST-segment elevation, especially in those situations when the pain is missing and the enzymatic criterion has a great diagnostic importance.

The suggestive forms of myocardial ischemia include pain localized in the chest, epigastrium, arms or jaw, appearing during effort but also at rest, similar to the classical forms of myocardial infarction. Under the circumstances of MI, those symptoms last at least 20 minutes. The pain (discomfort) may appear retrosternal, precordial and radiate to the left upper arm or to the back. Usually, the pain is not localized in a specific point. The pain may appear initially in a non-typical way in the epigastrium, shoulder, arms or back and does not radiate to the chest. The pain is not influenced by mobilization of the chest, or by changing the patient's position. The clinical picture may include dyspnea (secondary to the left ventricle insufficiency), apparently unexplained fatigue, nausea, fainting, syncope or combinations of those symptoms that appear either with chest discomfort or without it.

In the diabetic patient with suggestive chest pain of AMI there are the following issues related to the **differential diagnosis:**
  – Aortic dissection;
  – Pericarditis;
  – Chest pain through relative myocardial ischemia: aortic stenosis, hypertrophic cardiomyopathy, severe HT;
  – GI related pain: esophagus, stomach, duodenum, gallbladder;
    – Lung diseases;
    – Pleural effusion;
    – Pulmonary thromboembolism;
    – Pneumothorax;
    – Hyperventilation syndrome;
    – Musculo-skeletal pain, intercostal neuralgia;
    – Psychogenic pain.

Though there are several studies showing that the diabetic patients more often present silent myocardial infarction than the non-diabetic patients do, this remark does not represent a general rule. If the "silent ischemia" occurs or not more frequently in the diabetic patients compared to with the non-diabetics is still a controversial issue and probably with no clinical relevance because this situation can be met in both categories of patients [21, 24]. However, there is data showing that the silent myocardial infarction is associated with higher mortality rate compared to the "painful" infarction and the silent ischemia has less favorable prognosis.

PARACLINICAL CRITERIA

The presence or absence of the myocardial destruction produced through prolonged ischemia in diabetes mellitus, as well as its level, can be appreciated through several methods that include:
  – Measuring the level of the bio markers of myocardial necrosis in the blood;

– ECG registration (ST segment abnormalities, Q waves);

– Imagistic techniques: myocardial perfusion scintigraphy, echocardiography and radionuclide ventriculography;

– Morpho-pathologic examination.

Each of these techniques aims to make distinction between the minimum necrosis, the small necrosis and the extended necrosis (see Table 27.1). The different sensitivity and specificity of each necrosis detection technique contributes to its quantitative appreciation and the recognition of the evolutionary moment (Table 27.1).

We mention that the myocardial necrosis can occur without symptoms and under these circumstances it can only be highlighted through paraclinical exploration: ECG, biochemical markers, imagistic techniques.

Biochemical Criteria

The myocardial necrosis in diabetics can be recognized the same way as in the non-diabetics through the increase of the serum levels of the *markers of myocardial destruction*: myoglobin, troponins T and I, Creatine phosphokinase (total CK and CK-MB fraction), lactate dehydrogenase and others.

The increase of the serum level of the sensitive and specific bio-markers of the myocardial necrosis, as cardiac troponin and MB fraction of the Creatine kinase are, is *diagnostic* for myocardial infarction *only in the clinical context of myocardial ischemia*, because these bio-markers reflect myocardial lesions, but do not indicate the mechanisms. Thus, an increased value of those, in the absence of the clinical evidence of myocardial ischemia must lead to the search of other causes of myocardial destruction (*e.g.* myocarditis, trauma, electric shock etc.) [24].

The biochemical markers used to detect the myocardial necrosis, in the order of their specificity, are:

– **Cardiac troponins T and I** – recently described, with almost absolute myocardial tissular specificity and high sensitivity (reflecting the microscopic myocardial necrosis as well); because the values of the cardiac troponins may remain high for 7–10 days or even long after the myocardial necrosis, they must be interpreted within the clinical context.

– **CK-MB fraction** – determined within the first hours, represents the best alternative when there is no troponin determination available; it is less tissular-specific than the cardiac troponin, but there are proofs that it has a better specificity when it comes for irreversible lesion.

In order to be significant for an MI diagnosis, the maximum value of CK-MB must exceed two times the superior normal value in the first hours after the clinical event. CK-MB values must grow and decline according to the specific dynamics of the enzyme; the values that are staying permanently high are not due, as a rule, to the myocardial infarction.

– **Total CK** – is not recommended by routine for AMI diagnosis because of the large tissular distribution of this enzyme; it can only be used if troponin and/or CK-MB cannot be determined; a value is considered significant if it is *at least double versus* the reference value.

– **Myoglobin** – marker of "acute phase", with precocious release (1–4 hours), the value of myoglobin for the AMI diagnosis is limited by the short period of its growth (< 24 hours) and the lack of specificity;

– **GOT** (glutamic oxalacetic transaminase, also named aspartate aminotransferase ASAT) and **LDH** (lactate dehydrogenase) with its isoenzymes are not currently recommended for diagnosing the acute myocardial necrosis.

Table 27.1
Methods for highlighting the myocardial necrosis

Methods for highlighting the myocardial necrosis	
Biochemical	Presence of the myocardial cells necrosis markers in the blood
ECG	Evidence of myocardial ischemia (changes ST-T)
	Evidence of losing the electrical function of myocardium (Q wave)
Imaging	Reduction or loss of the tissular perfusion
	Abnormalities of the kinetics of the cardiac wall
Morphopathologic	Myocardial cells necrosis

For most of the patients, the blood sample taken for tests should be obtained immediately after they admission into hospital and repeated at 6–9 hours and 12–24 hours if the precocious determinations are negative and the clinical suspicion is high. For those patients who require a precocious diagnosis, it is recommended to determine a biomarker with fast appearance (*e.g.,* CK-MB or myoglobin), with more reduced specificity, adding – for diagnosis confirmation – a biomarker with higher specificity but that grows later (*e.g.,* cardiac troponin) [24].

Biochemical markers hold an important place in the evaluation of the patients with acute myocardial ischemia, especially in diabetic patients who often present silent myocardial infarction, because they:

– differentiate the entities within the acute coronary syndromes that have a different therapeutic approach (for example, differentiate the unstable angina pectoris from non-Q myocardial infarction);

– have diagnostic value for MI, being useful especially in situations of non-diagnostic ECG;

– differentiate acute MI from recent MI;

– differentiate the *re-infarction of expansion;* under the circumstances of persistent ST segment depression, the re-infarction diagnosis may be difficult if in the first 7–10 days the troponin persists at high levels, in which case the determination of the biomarkers of "acute phase" of MI would orientate the diagnosis. The detection of the re-infarction has clinical importance because it could mean an extra risk for the patient with diabetes mellitus;

– allow the evaluation of the MI extension; the increased level of biomarkers can be used for an orientating evaluation of the myocardial necrosis extent;

– have prognostic value; the level of increased biomarkers is useful for the *risk ranking* in diabetic patients post-MI.

ECG Criteria

Electrocardiogram presents the same characteristics as for non-diabetic patients and can highlight:

– signs of myocardial *ischemia*: evolutionary changes of ST-T;

– signs of myocardial *necrosis*: changes of QRS.

A work definition for recent or acute MI, as it appears on the 12 lead ECG recording, in the presence of the suggestive clinical picture, has been settled based on the studies that correlated the clinical chart with the morphological one.

ECG criteria of myocardial ischemia that can develop towards MI
1) ECG with ST-segment elevation:

An elevation of segment ST newly appeared (or presumably new) from point J, present in 2 contiguous derivations, with values of ≥ 0.2 mV in V1, V2 or V3 or ≥ 0.1 mV in the other derivations, (contiguity in foreground plan is defined through the sequence of derivations I, aVL; II, aVF, III and reversed in aVR)

2) ECG without ST elevation:
• ST-segment depression;
• only changes of T wave.

The new appeared ST depressions (or assumed to be new), changes of T wave or both, must be present in at least one of the contiguous derivations. In addition, negative T waves, symmetric, with amplitude of ≥ 1mm must be present in at least two contiguous derivations on two consecutive ECG, conducted at few hours distance.

The stated ECG criteria reflect the myocardial ischemia and are not sufficient by themselves to define MI. The final diagnosis of myocardial necrosis depends on the identification of the increased serum levels of the biomarkers of the myocardial necrosis.

ST-segment elevation identifies the patients who will benefit of reperfusion therapy. Current data do not support the administration of thrombolytic therapy to the patients without ST elevation or without new LBBB; the benefit of primary coronary angioplasty remains unclear for this category of patients [24].

In the patients with ischemic chest pain, the ST-segment elevation has 91% specificity and 46% sensitivity for diagnosis of the acute MI.

The mortality grows with the number of ECG derivations that present ST elevation.

ST-segment elevation in the diabetic patients with MI probability may regress rapidly, spontaneously or under treatment. The reperfusion therapy effect on the changes of ST segment must be taken into consideration when using ECG for diagnosing MI. Some patients to whom the ST elevation is rapidly reversible will not develop myocardial necrosis.

Table 27.2

Topol classification of myocardial infarction

Topol classification of myocardial infarction				
Category occlusion	**Anatomy**	**ECG**	**30 days Mt(%)**	**1 year Mt (%)**
1. Proximal LAD	Proximal to first perforating branch to interventricular septum	↑ ST V1-6, I, aVL and fascicular block or branch block	19.6	25.62
2. Medium LAD	Distal to first perforating branch to interventricular septum but proximal to the big diagonal branch	↑ ST V1-6, I, aVL	9.2	12.43
3. Distal LAD – distal to the first diagonal or the affection of the first diagonal	Distal to the big diagonal branch or affection of the first diagonal branch	↑ ST V1-4 or ↑ ST I, aVL, V5-V6	6.8	10.24
4. Inferior MI moderate-extended (posterior, lateral, of VD)	RCA proximal or circumflex artery	↑ ST II, III, aVF and any of: a) V1, V3R, V4 R or b) V5-6 or c) R>S V1, V2	6.4	8.45
5. Inferior MI small	RCA distal or CxCA or branches of CxCA	↑ ST only II, III, aVF	4.5	6.7

E. Topol Textbook of Cardiovascular Medicine, 1998.
From the study GUSTO IIa thrombolysed patients.

The topographic classification of AMI with ST-segment elevation in diabetics is similar to the one of non-diabetic patients with AMI and can be realized based on some correlations between the changes of ECG at admission and the angiography as follows (Table 27.2):

MI without ST elevation includes three ECG patterns that are more frequent:

1) Gigantic T waves, reversed in the precordial derivations (frequently characteristic for proximal LAD lesion);

2) Persistent ST depression is much more threatening than reversed T waves for 30 days mortality and the non-fatal reinfarction. The more extended the ischemia, the worst its significance is;

3) The most severe is the "global" ischemia for which ST depression is present in all derivations, with the exception of aVR where there is ST elevation; this often reflects a thrombus in the left coronary or an equivalent ("left main" syndrome).

ST depression maximal in derivations V1-V3 in the absence of elevation in other derivations must be considered as indicative for posterior myocardial ischemia or posterior MI or both, but usually, for confirmation, image and biochemical methods must be used.

In the presence of a new left bundle branch block (or assumed to be new), the ST-segment elevation may accompany left bundle branch block, making difficult or impossible the recognition of an acute MI and, in such situations, in order to confirm the diagnosis of AMI, other diagnostic methods must be used (biological, image) (Table 27.3).

The appearance of sharp T waves, symmetric, with high amplitude (Hyperacute T wave) may be pointed out in the early stages of the AMI.

Table 27.3

Criteria for acute MI diagnosis in the presence of left bundle branch block, after Sgarbossa

Criteria for acute MI diagnosis in the presence of left bundle branch block, after Sgarbossa
ECG criteria
Score↑ ST ≥ 1 mm in accordance with QRS polarity
↓ ST ≥ 1 mm in V1-V2 or V3 ↑ ST ≥ 5 mm in discordance with QRS polarity

The surface electrocardiogram acceptably locates the topography of the infarctions but it is an imperfect method to use for the correct identification of the coronary artery occlusion; the location is more precise for the small, medium or non-transmural infarctions.

LAD occlusion produces infarction at the level of the LV anterior wall, the apex and in two thirds of the anterior inter-ventricular septum.

Circumflex coronary artery occlusion produces infarctions of the lateral and postero-lateral of the LV [24].

Proximal RCA occlusion can be identified when there are direct signs of RV infarction; the obstruction in its medium area frequently catches the inferior wall and/or posterior of the LV, whilst the distal occlusion is associated with the infarction of the inferior wall or the posterior third of the inter-ventricular septum. Though it is generally considered that the inferior infarctions of the LV are generated by the RCA distal occlusion, this is only real for about half of the cases. In most of the cases, if the direct signs of inferior infarction are associated with the lateral ones, the infarction is generated by the CxA obstruction. When the infarction is placed on the inferior and posterior wall, without lateral catch, the RCA obstruction is more frequent than the Cx obstruction [24].

ECG criteria of constituted myocardial infarction:

– Any wave Q R ≥ 30ms, in derivations V1–V3.

– Abnormal Q wave in DI, aVL, DII, aVF, or V4-V6, in two contiguous derivations with at least 1mm depth.

Established myocardial infarction may be defined on ECG criteria – 12 derivations in the absence of other conditions that could change the QRS complex (for example left branch block, left ventricular hypertrophy, WPW syndrome) or immediately after myocardial revascularization surgery (CABG). In these conditions, it is necessary to confirm AMI, suspected through clinical criteria and through other enzymatic or image methods. If only one ECG route meets the criteria described for pathologic Q wave, this is an indication that the patient has myocardial infarction in his history. Q waves with duration below 30 ms associated with the ST-segment depression could represent an infarction but this needs follow up and confirmation. When three or more ECG recordings are accomplished, *at least two* consecutive ECG must prove this change.

Usually LBBB does not allow the expression of Q wave; however, *new* Q waves in the presence of LBBB must be considered pathologic.

Not all the patients who develop myocardial necrosis show ECG changes. *A normal ECG does not exclude the diagnosis of AMI,* a fact that was proved through the appearance of new markers capable to identify that myocardial necrosis that is too small to be associated with abnormal ECG (micro-infarctions).

Imaging Criteria

The imaging exploratory methods are used for:
– Confirmation or exclusion of the AMI or myocardial ischemia in the Hospital department;
– Identification of the non-ischemic conditions that lead to chest pain;
– Evaluation of the prognosis on short and long term;
– Identification of the mechanical complications of AMI.

The usage of imagistic techniques such as echocardiography or radionuclide explorations in "acute" status of the patients with diabetes mellitus and suspicious of acute myocardial infarction is based on the fact that ischemia resulted from regional myocardial hypoperfusion implies a cascade of events. "Ischemic cascade" includes myocardial dysfunction (first diastolic dysfunction and then systolic dysfunction), changes that appear before the ECG changes. In clinical practice, currently used conventional image methods are echocardiography, radionuclide angiography and the perfusion imaging type computerized tomography with emission of unique photon (SPECT).

Imaging "in acute"
Advantages:
– Eco 2D can detect regional abnormalities of parietal kinetic after few moments from the ischemic injury, and can be useful in diagnosing acute MI;
– Identify the place and extent of the MI;

– Ecographic or radionuclide imaging is very helpful in patients with clinical suspicion of acute MI, but with non-diagnostic and un-interpretable ECG;

– Normal Eco and myocardial scintigram of normal perfusion (at rest) in "acute" are useful for the exclusion of the AMI (the negative predictive value of Echocardiography (ECHO) is 95%, and SMP 98%), when CK-MB is used as "golden standard" for diagnosing MI. It remains to elucidate if those have the same negative predictive value in patients with normal CK-MB and increased levels of troponin [12, 15].

Limits:

– The positive predictive value of Eco for diagnosing acute MI is only of 50%, because the regional abnormalities of parietal kinetic highlighted through Eco and radionuclide angiography can appear both in "acute" MI and in other ischemic conditions (old IM, acute myocardial ischemia, hibernating or siderated myocardium or a combination of those) or even in non-ischemic conditions (dilative cardiomyopathy);

– The positive predictive value of the myocardial scintigram type "gated SPECT" is also limited because abnormalities of regional perfusion are also present in old MI, acute ischemia, hibernating or siderated myocardium;

– The frequent artifacts and the difficulties of interpretation can lead to false-positive results [21, 24].

Imaging in established MI

Echocardiography is used for:

– Evaluation of the *residual function* of the LV after the acute moment; the determination of the number of segments with kinetic disorder allowes the calculation of the parietal kinetic score as element of measurement of residual cardiac function; the evaluation of the residual function of LV has an immediate and long term *prognostic* value;

– The evaluation of the myocardial *viability* by stress Echocardiography (exercise or dobutamine);

– The election method for detecting mechanical complications of MI: mitral regurgitation, MI expansion, mural thrombosis, and ruptures of the myocardial structures.

Radionuclide exploration also offers prognostic information in the phase of recent or old MI:

– Evaluation of the size of the infarction through the identification of the size of the perfusion deficiency;

– Evaluation of the LV function through the detection of the increased capture of **radioactive** isotopes by the lungs (expression of the systolic dysfunction of LV) and the ischemic dilatation of the LV;

– May *identify the multi-vascular disease* through detection of the hypoperfusion in more than one coronary artery area;

– Can evaluate the reversibility of the perfusion dysfunction and can estimate the *MI extension* and *myocardial viability* by the nuclear stress imaging (pharmacology or effort) [24]. (Plate 27.1)

Morphopathologic Criteria

IM is defined as the death of the myocardial cells secondary to prolonged ischemia.

The cellular death does not appear immediately after the beginning of the myocardial ischemia (in some animal models after 15 minutes). In order to be possible to identify the myocardial necrosis at standard post-mortem macro- and microscopic examination, a period of about 6 hours is necessary from the beginning of ischemia. It is admitted that the full necrosis of all myocardial cells at risk requires at least 4–6 hours, or more, depending on the presence of collateral circulation in the ischemic area, persistent or intermittent coronary occlusion and the sensitivity of the myocytes.

The morphopathologic identification of the myocardial necrosis is done based on the standard micro and macroscopic standard *examination without reference to the lesions of the epicardial coronary versus the clinical history* [24].

The diagnosis of myocardial infarction in diabetic patients covers in general similar steps as for the non-diabetics; however, the sensitivity and specificity of the diagnostic tests could be different considering the high probability that the coronary disease is present. As it results from the data presented, the unfavorable prognosis of the diabetic with myocardial infarction is given by the multiple abnormalities of the energetic metabolism of the myocardium, best evaluated through positron emission tomography (PET). PET is the only imagistic method that allows the non-invasive evaluation of the myocardial metabolism, coronary flow and receptors density, offering information about the progress *in vivo* of the biochemical and physiological processes. The

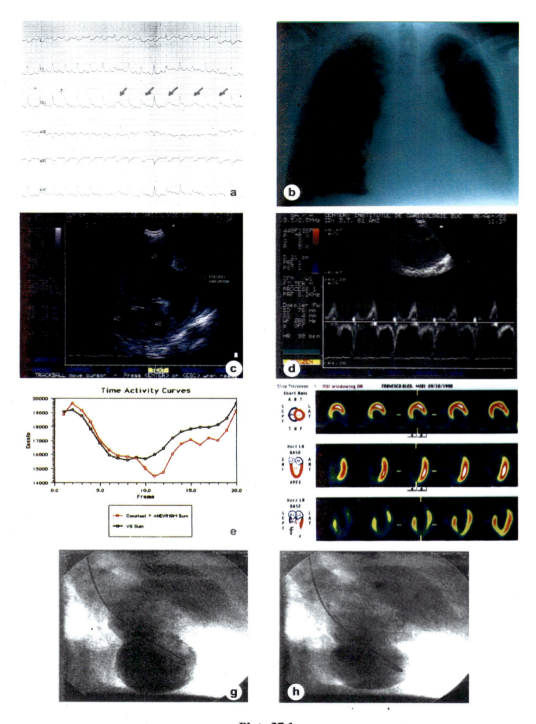

Plate 27.1

D.T., 51 years old. Inferior-lateral acute myocardial infarction complicated with left ventricle pseudoaneurysm (LVPA).
Type 2 diabetes mellitus with metabolic decompensation:

a – 12 lead ECG, electrical alternation of QRS complex and of ST-segment elevation; b – chest radiography: increased cardio-pericardial opacity with prolongation and prominence of the left inferior arch; c – two-dimensional echocardiographic apical four-chamber view: infero-lateral LVPA of large dimensions; d – two-dimensional echocardiographic apical four-chamber view with pulse Doppler flow imaging: the flow passes from the LV into the PAVS during the end-systole and the end-diastole; e – radionuclide angiography of the inferior wall of LVPA: the time-activity curve at the level of LVPA and LV; f – myocardial Tc-MIBI scintigram: the lack of contrast agent at the level of the inferior wall; g and h – ventriculography with contrast agent: gigantic LVPA in systole (g) and diastole (h).

Table 27.4

Morphopathologic classification of MI depending on size, localization and stage of evolution

Morphopathologic classification of MI	
Size	• microscopic MI – focal necrosis • small MI – less than 10% of LV • medium MI – 10–30% of LV • large MI – >30% of LV
Localization	• anterior MI • lateral MI • inferior MI • posterior MI • septal MI • combinations of those localizations
Evolution stage	• Acute MI – 6h–7days – necrosis plus predominant cellular infiltrate with polymorphonuclear leukocytes
	• progress MI (recent) – 7–28 days – necrosis plus predominant cellular infiltrate with mononuclear phagocytes and fibroblasts
	• In old MI > 29 days – fibrous scar without cellular infiltrate

evaluation through PET of the metabolic dysfunction requires the administration of a substance marked with an isotope that emits positrons, intravenous or inhaling, and the PET scanner registers the distribution image of this substance. PET proved to be extremely useful for the study of the myocardial insulin-resistance, the evaluation of the myocardial sanguine flow and the diagnosis of the myocardial viability in the diabetic patients with myocardial infarction [27].

Along with the development of the techniques of pharmacological, interventional and surgical revascularization, it has been proved that the restoration of the blood flow in the myocardial akinetic segments may improve the regional and global left ventricle function, which represents the most important factor in evaluating the prognosis of the coronary patients. The revascularization provides the greatest benefit to the patients with severe left ventricle dysfunction. It is necessary to detect the viable myocardium at the level of dysfunctional ventricular segments; this will allow the selection of the patients who can benefit from revascularization.

Recent studies showed that it is possible to differentiate the ischemia from myocardial necrosis by using PET with nitrogen-13, ammonium (N13H3) and FDG (fluor-deoxy-glucose) after loading with

glucose *per os*. The reduction of both myocardial perfusion and FDG caption ratio (flux-metabolism concordance) showes an infarction area, with irreversible lesion, whilst the ratio of FDG caption is preserved or grown despite a deficit of myocardial perfusion (flux-metabolism discordance) have been considered ischemic and viable. The rate of taking over of FDG by the myocardium depends on several factors such as: diet, cardiac contractility, insulin-resistance, and sympathetic tonus and myocardial ischemia. This method allows comparison of the absolute values of the glucose absorption (μmol/g/min) being useful especially to study the patients with myocardial infarction who associate DM and/or different levels of insulin-resistance. PET is the only non-invasive method of quantitative evaluation of myocardial perfusion; its applicability is limited as it is only available in few specialized centers, is expensive and is used mostly for the stable patients [28].

An alternative method of semi-quantitative evaluation of myocardial perfusion is the echocardiography with contrast substance, administered intra-venously, which allows the evaluation of a high number of patients both stable and unstable (in acute phases), with lower costs and larger availability [29].

THE TREATMENT OF MYOCARDIAL INFARCTION IN DIABETIC PATIENTS

THE IMPORTANCE OF THE ISSUE

Despite the considerable improvement in the treatment of myocardial infarction, it is obvious that the individuals with DM do not have the same benefits as the non-diabetic persons. In addition, the impact of diabetes on the cardiovascular mortality registers a continuous increase. The diabetic patient is frequently met in the coronary care unit, in the services of interventional or surgical myocardial revascularization, an important share of the patients with cardiac insufficiency are diabetic patients and the big clinical trials that take for study cardiovascular patients notice that 15–25% are diabetic patients [24].

Recent epidemiological data show that in the Western-European countries the prevalence of the DM represents about 30% of the acute coronary syndromes and about 40% of the patients with cardiac insufficiency.

The factors of unfavorable prognosis that should be considered in the diabetic patients with myocardial infarction:
– The affection of the diffuse and distal multivascular coronary disease;
  – Coronary microangiopathy;
  – Reduction of the coronary flux reserve;
  – Reduction of the fibrinolytic activity;
  – The increase of the platelet aggregation;
  – The atherogenic lipoproteic profile;
  – Cardiac autonomic dysfunction;
  – The association of the diabetic cardiomyopathy.

The metabolic factors that contribute to the aggravation of the prognosis: decrease of the insulin-secretion associated with the increase of the insulin-resistance and the disorder of the free fat acids metabolism.

The metabolic disorders are emphasized by the aggravation of the cardiac insufficiency and the appearance of the recurrent myocardial ischemia [30].

The stages of treatment for the myocardial infarction in diabetic patients are overlapping with the treatment of myocardial infarction in non-diabetic patients and can be grouped in four stages:

I. Emergency assistance:
  • Pre-hospital assistance
  • Hospital assistance.
  Requires:
    – Initial diagnosis;
    – Treating the pain, dyspnea and anxiety;
    – Prevention and treatment of the cardiac arrest.

II. Early assistance in the hospital – coronary care unit:
  • Continue calming the pain and anxiety.
  • Cardioprotection through restoring the coronary flux: early opening of the artery responsible for the AMI:
    – Fibrinolysis + adjuvants: antithrombotics and antiplatelet;
    – PTCA;
    – CABG.
  • Cardioprotection through decreasing the myocardial consumption of oxygen:
    – Reduction of the size of the infarction;
    – Prevention and treatment of early mechanical, electrical and ischemic complications.
  • Early evaluation of intra-hospital mortality risk.

III. Late assistance in the hospital – post-coronary care unit:
  • Continue with the cardioprotective measures;
  • Late opening of the artery responsible for the infarction;
  • Late complications treatment;
  • Evaluation of the risk before the patient leaves the hospital;
  • Secondary prevention.

IV. Post-hospital assistance
  • Convalescence, rehabilitation;
  • Secondary prevention.

EMERGENCY ASSISTANCE

This period covers the lapse of time since the beginning of the symptoms until the moment of admission in the coronary care unit (CCU). This lapse varies depending on how the care unit is organized and the quality of the medical assistance [24].

Pre-hospital assistance

The activities achieved in this interval are:

- patient or family call, the travel of the ambulance with a doctor to the patient;
- the doctor assigns the diagnostic of certitude, suspicion or exclusion of AMI;
- emergency therapy measures;
- patient surveillance during the transport to the hospital;
- make a choice for the hospital depending on the patient status.

Hospital therapy

The doctor must apply in a short period of time effective therapeutic measures:

- analgesics (Algocalmin, Mialgin, morphine);
- nitroglycerin sublingual or in perfusion;
- aspirin 160–325 mg;
- O$_2$ therapy;
- atropine for severe sinusal bradycardia or/and hypotension;
- for patients under cardiorespiratory arrest, initiation of the cardio-respiratory resuscitation procedures (basic life support);
- it is no longer recommended to administrate xiline and atropine for prophylactic purpose.

Pre-hospital thrombolysis

Thrombolytic treatment became an important therapeutic objective in the pre-hospital period, under the circumstances of existing mobile coronary units. The criteria used for thrombolytic treatment are prolonged precordial pain and ST elevation/LBBB, in the absence of contraindications. The thrombolytic agents commonly used are the streptokinase, tissular activator of plasminogen, APSAC, and urokinase.

The patients treated in the first hour since the beginning of AMI have the highest absolute and relative coefficient of survival. This observation made the first 60 minutes to be called "the golden hour" of reperfusion [31].

Hospital assistance

The protocol in the Hospital for a patient with chest pain suggesting AMI will include:

- clinical examination, ECG and interpretation in the first 10 minutes and then set a venous access line within less than 30 minutes since the patient came.

The first step in treating the patient, while the final therapy is prepared:

- administration of oxygen (usually through nasal tubes at 2 l/min) and morphine (2–4 mg i.v. repeated when necessary);
- aspirin 325mg, if it has not been administered in the pre-hospital phase;
- before using morphine, it is useful to try nitroglycerin sublingual in order to evaluate the potential reversibility of the symptomatology and ST elevation;
- if the patient is from class Killip I or II and does not present bradycardia or hypotension (BPs<110 mm Hg), then using intravenous beta-blockers can be considered as a way to reduce the extent of ischemia;
- if it is necessary, initiate or continue applying the cardiorespiratory resuscitation procedure for the patients that present with cardiorespiratory arrest – advanced measures of supporting the vital functions (advanced life support).

When coming in the Hospital, the patient with prolonged ischemic chest pain can be classified in the following major categories, with different therapeutic approach:

- depending on ECG: with ↑ST and without ↑ST;
- depending on Killip class: with or without hemodynamic deterioration.

EARLY ASSISTANCE IN THE HOSPITAL CORONARY CARE UNIT

– Continue to calm the pain and anxiety: analgesics, nitrates, beta-blockers

– Cardioprotection through restoration of the coronary flow: early opening of the artery responsible for AMI:

    – reperfusion pharmacological + adjuvants: antithrombotics and antiplatelet

    – interventional reperfusion (PTCA)

    – surgical reperfusion (CABG)

– Cardioprotection through decreasing the myocardial consumption of oxygen:

- Reducing the size of the infarction:
  – beta-blockers
  – nitrates
  – ACE inhibitors
  – metabolic support
  – mechanical support

– Prevention and treatment of early mechanical, electrical and ischemic complications

– Hygiene-diet measures

– Early evaluation of the intra-hospital mortality risk [24]

Aspirin, if it has not been administered until this moment!

Using aspirin is the "head stone" of the therapy for the patients with acute myocardial infarction. It has to start as soon as possible. The objective of treatment with aspirin is the fast blockage of the thromboxane A2 formation at the level of the platelets through inhibiting the cyclooxygenase pathway. As the reduced doses (80 mg) require many days for a total antiaggregant effect, it is necessary to administered at least 160–325 mg even in the pre-hospital phase or in the hospital [32].

Analgesia. Supporting measures

The pain – a major symptom in AMI – induces suffering, sympathetic hyperactivity, increased consumption of myocardial oxygen, anxiety and fear of death.

Chest pain control is typically obtained through a combination of analgesics, nitrates, oxygen and beta-blockers.

For pain control, there are used:

A. *regular* analgesics: noraminophenazone (Algocalmin), baralgin (Piafen) or pentazocine (Fortral); in case they are not efficient:

B. *opioid* analgesics: pethidine (Mialgin) or morphine that have the advantage of an intense analgesia, but the disadvantage of some severe adverse effects.

Oxygen

In patients with AMI may develop hypoxemia, which is usually secondary to the ventilation-perfusion abnormalities, secondary to LV dysfunction. It became a regular practice to administrate oxygen to all hospitalized patients with AMI, for at least 24–48 hours, based on the empirical assumption of hypoxemia and the probability that through the increase of the oxygen level in the inspired air the ischemic myocardium will be protected. In general, it is recommended to administrate 2–4 l/minute of oxygen 100% on the mask or nasal probe, for 6–12 hours for the majority of the patients with moderate hypoxemia.

Early cardioprotection in AMI refers to the total of pharmacological or non-pharmacological measures aiming to save the myocardium

The dimension of the infarction is an important factor for prognosis in diabetic patients with AMI. The efforts to limit the size of the infarction (cardioprotection) were oriented towards the following approaches, targeting the improvement of the oxygen balance at the myocardial level:

A. cardioprotection through early opening of the artery responsible for infarction (early reperfusion);

B. cardioprotection through:

– reduction of the energetic needs of the myocardium;

– manipulation of the sources of energy production in the myocardium;

– rhythm disorder, recurrent ischemia, pump dysfunction prophylaxis.

Early opening of the artery responsible for the infarction

Myocardial reperfusion, the most important measure for limiting the size of the infarction, can be initiated in the Hospital and continues in the coronary units.

Although in some patients the reperfusion takes place spontaneously, in most of the patients with AMI the thrombotic occlusion persists with myocardial necrosis. To make the reperfusion in due time for the myocardium at risk represents the most efficient way of restoration of the balance between the supply and the necessary myocardial oxygen demand.

The early opening IRA (arteries responsible for infarction) can be realized through:

1. pharmacological reperfusion;

2. interventional reperfusion:

   – primary PTCA

   – adjuvant PTCA (of consolidation)

   – "rescue" PTCA

3. surgical reperfusion, of exception.

Pharmacological Reperfusion

Angiographic data showed a similar rate of the patency of the vessel responsible for the infarction after thrombolysis in both diabetic and non-diabetic patients. Due to the higher risk, the ratio cost-benefit of the thrombolytic therapy is higher in the diabetic patients *vs.* non-diabetic patients. The revision of the literature data shows that there is no increase of the hemorrhagic complications after the thrombolysis in the diabetic patients and the mortality at 5 weeks after the myocardial infarction is significantly reduced after the thrombolysis in the diabetic group.

For the diabetic patients, a relative contraindication against both thrombolytic treatment and anticoagulant treatment is the diabetic retinopathy (unstable) or a treatment with laser recently applied on the retina, due to the high hemorrhagic risk. The presence of a stable proliferative retinopathy does not represent a contraindication for the thrombolytic treatment [33].

Intra-coronary thrombolysis. It was the first efficient mode of removing the coronary obstruction in AMI. Today, its application is an exception.

Intravenous thrombolysis. Nowadays it is the election treatment for AMI with ST elevation in the first 12 hours.

The selection of the patients for pharmacological thrombolysis. The indications of the thrombolytic treatment are based on the pain and ECG.

1) *Chest pain* suggestive of myocardial ischemia with duration more than 30 minutes, without response at nitroglycerine;

2) *ECG:*

   • ST-segment elevation ≥ 0.1 mV in two peripheral contiguous derivations or

   • New left bundle branch block

3) *Timing*

   • < 12 hours since the beginning – clear indication

   • 12–24 hours since the beginning – when the pain continues or repeats or if new ischemic events appear

4) *Absence of contraindications*

In general, the contraindications must be evaluated individually for each patient; the prolonged resuscitation may or may not be a contraindication in a precise context when the benefit of the thrombolysis is higher than the risk.

Currently there is no age limit; for old patients the reduction of absolute mortality was similar with the reduction obtained for younger patients.

LBBB represent an indication if it is newly appeared or unknown in the past and it is associated with pain suggesting AMI [24, 31].

Thrombolytic agents

In the last few years, several generations of thrombolytics were experimented. (Table 27.5)

The thrombolytic regimes in acute myocardial infarction in diabetic patients are the same as in non-diabetic patients. (Figure 27.1)

Complications of the thrombolytic treatment:

a. Hemorrhagic risk

The most frequent complications and potentially more severe than the hemorrhagic ones:

• Intracranial hemorrhage is the most serious complication of the thrombolytic treatment in diabetic patients – incidence 0.3–1%, its frequency varies depending on the clinical characteristics of the patient and the prescribed thrombolytic agent (higher for rt-PA–0,7% than for SK–0.4%).

• Hemorrhages at the vascular punch biopsy, usually self-limited.

• Digestive hemorrhages in patients with ulcer history (frequency < 5%).

The association of heparin increases the risk of hemorrhage in association with SK, but not in association with rt-PA. The association of aspirin has higher benefits than risks.

b. Arterial hypotension – appears in over 10% of the patients; there is a higher risk of hypotension appearance in case of accelerated administration; they are treated by Trendelenburg position, administration of fluids, occasionally atropine.

Table 27.5

Thrombolytic agent

Generation I	Generation II	Generation III
Streptokinase	rt-PA	Reteplase
Urokinase	Prourokinase	Lanoteplase
APSAC	Staphylokinase	Tenecteplase

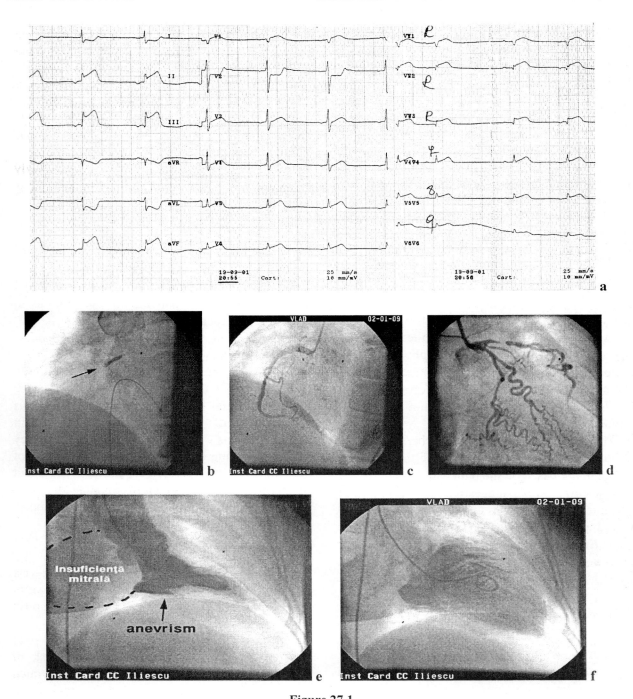

Figure 27.1

V.L., 47 years old.

Inferior, posterior and lateral left ventricular infarction with right ventricular infarction within 3 hours from the onset of AMI, Topol class IV, Killip class III, thrombolysed with Streptokinase, without criteria of reperfusion. The patient is hospitalized after 30 days since the onset of AMI, presenting left ventricular insufficiency NYHA class IV and type 2 diabetes mellitus with metabolic decompensation. a – 18 lead ECG: inferior atrial rate, ST-segment elevation with included T-wave (Pardee wave) in lead II, III and aVF, ST elevation in V4 to V6 and V7 to V9, ST elevation in V1, V2R, V3R, ST depression in V2, ST depression in lead I, aVL; b – Coronary angiography: occlusion of vessel segment I of RCA (arrow); c – Coronary angiography after PTCA with stenting, final result with TIMI grade 3 flow; d – Coronary angiography: stenosis by 80 percent of LAD – segment I/II, stenosis by 70 percent of the intermediary branch at its origin; e and f – Ventriculography: infero-basal (30 percent) left ventricular aneurysm, hypokinesis of the anterior wall; 3rd degree mitral regurgitation.

c. Allergic reactions – in 17% of the patients who receive SK or anistreplase; it is not recommended to administrate hydrocortisol as a routine.

d. Resistance at SK and APSAC, due to antibodies so that a re-administration of those is not possible after 2–5 days and before two years [33].

Adjuvant therapy for pharmacological thrombolysis:

Anti-thrombotic treatment

Heparin does not improve the immediate lysis of the thrombus, but the patent of the coronary artery evaluated after a few hours or days since the thrombolytic therapy with rt-PA seems to be better with intravenous heparin. After administering SK there was no sign of differences between the patients treated with heparin subcutaneous (s.c.) or i.v.

Effects on mortality. The available data suggest that heparin i.v. has probably no effect on the patients who received SK, but can be useful for the patients who received rt-PA.

The effect on the patency of the artery responsible for infarction (ARI). Studies showed a higher rate of patent of the IRA in the patients with AMI treated with rt-PA plus heparin *vs.* the ones treated with rt-PA plus Placebo.

The effects on the LV thrombosis. The anticoagulant treatment reduces significantly the incidence of thrombus in LV; this has been proved by echocardiography, especially in the patients with anterior MI and in the ones with wide areas with abnormal kinetics. In hospital thrombolysis, the incidence of thrombus in LV declined.

It is not to forget that heparin has no effect on the patients with antithrombin III deficit.

The *complications* of the antithrombotic treatment are:

• Major hemorrhagic complications: – intracranial hemorrhage – the most severe complication of the treatment. The risk is higher for the patients with low weight, old age and important prolongation of APTT (over 90–100 seconds). In order to reduce the risk of major hemorrhagic complications it is recommended to monitor frequently the APTT and to adjust the heparin dose. However, we mention that in the first 12 hours after the thrombolysis the APTT growth can only be reduced by the thrombolytic agent (especially SK), which makes difficult to interpret the heparin effects on coagulation.

• Minor hemorrhagic complications: – traumatic hematoma, also at the s.c. injection sites, local or general bleeding.

• Light thrombocytopenia, relatively rare, 2–3%.

Recommendations for anti-thrombotic treatment

Considering the central role played by the thrombin in AMI pathogenesis, the antithrombotic treatment remains an important therapeutic intervention.

A) Unfractionated heparin in the patients who do not receive thrombolytic treatment:

The available data indicate that heparin reduces the cardiovascular mortality and morbidity like re-infarction thromboembolism. Therefore, in the absence of anticoagulation contraindications we recommend to administer heparin as a routine to:

• All the patients with AMI, presenting ST segment elevation and who are not candidates for thrombolysis and primary PTCA.

• To the patients with AMI without ST segment elevation.

B) Heparin in the patients who receive thrombolytic treatment:

• Non-selective thrombolytics of type SK, APSAC or Urokinase.

There is no apparent benefit of heparin administered i.v. on mortality, therefore using it in these circumstances is not recommended.

Patients who have another indication of anticoagulation, as it is an extended previous infarction with significant kinetic abnormalities, atrial fibrillation, recent emboli, etc, represent the only exception. In this case, it is recommended to administer heparin i.v. with target APTT of 60–70 seconds [34].

The routine usage of unfractioned heparin s.c. in doses of 12500 U twice a day remains a disputed issue in the patients who receive SK.

• Fibrinospecific thrombolytics: rt-PA, reteplase, tenecteplase.

It is recommended to associate heparin i.v. at rt-PA based on the principle that rt-PA is a lytic agent more specific for fibrin but with short period of action and important re-occlusion risk and the proof of higher rates of patent of IRA at these patients. It is recommended to administered a bolus of 60 U/kg (maximum 4000 U bolus) followed by continuous perfusion of 12 U/kg/h or 1000 u/h, aiming to obtain a target APTT of 50–70 seconds. The patients must be monitored for any sign of bleeding and there must be conducted frequent determination of APTT (preferably at 6 hours or at least at 12 hours). The administration is done in parallel with the fibrinolytic agent and must be maintained at least 48 hours after the administration of the rt-PA. It may be continued beyond 48 hours only for the patients with high risk of systemic thromboembolism.

C) Low molecular weight heparin has been studied as adjuvant therapy of thrombolysis, starting from the favorable effect proved in the myocardial infarction without ST segment elevation and having in mind their advantages (easy to administer, does not require surveillance, does not depend on the antithrombin III, the stability of the anticoagulant effect, it acts as anti-factor X). It proves to have more and more efficiency in the infarction with ST elevation as adjutant therapy for thrombolysis [31].

Antiplatelet treatment

• Antiaggregation. It has been suggested that the diabetic patients require larger doses of aspirin for TxA2 suppression, considering the pro-aggregate status specific to those patients. However, there is no proof that the aspirin in usual dosage would be less efficient in the diabetic patients. Currently it is recommended that aspirin must be administered with the same indications and with the same dosage for diabetic patients with AMI as well as for non-diabetic patients: 160–325mg.

In practice, it is recommended to administrate aspirin "At the door" for a diabetic patient suspected or diagnosed with myocardial infarction with or without ST segment elevation. It is important to highlight that aspirin has an effect depending on time: the sooner the treatment was given, the higher the reduction of mortality.

The presence of peptic ulcer is a relative contraindication for the antiplatelet treatment. It can be administered in association with a therapy of gastric protection (preferably gastric anti-secretory drugs given i.v.). Aspirin must be continued indefinitely for the patients with AMI [32].

New antiplatelet regimes

Other agents of inhibition of the platelet function have been investigated (inhibitors for Tx synthesis, antagonists of Tx or serotonin receptors and agents with combined action over the Tx and Tx receptor synthesis).

• The most promising class of antiplatelet agents is the antagonists of the GP IIb/IIIa receptor that interfere with the final route common to platelet aggregation.

The atherosclerotic plaques have a very important role in the appearance of the re-occlusion; the platelet activation maintained by various agonists, inclusively on the Tx-A2 route, lead to the exposure of the functional receptors for fibrinogen-receptors GP IIb/IIIa, which is the key element in maintaining the platelet aggregation process. The usage of GPIIb/IIIa receptor blockers (abciximab–Reopro, eptiphybatide-Integrilin, tirophyban–Agrastat) allowed new therapeutic regimes to be tested. These regimes associate a thrombolytic with a GPIIb/IIIa receptor blocker, together with aspirin and heparin. The very good results are not only for the angiographic aspect, but also through evident benefits at the level of microcirculation, benefits that supported through a complete resolution of the ST segment elevation. This last aspect is due to the fact that the maximum inhibition of platelet action through the blockage of the GP IIb/IIIa thrombocyte receptors counteracts the reperfusion injury and the microvascular obstruction secondary to the microembolism generated by the thrombolytic treatment.

The benefits of this standard combination dosed fibrinolytic – GP IIb/IIIa receptor blocker – are shadowed by the unacceptable increase of the major hemorrhagic risk (10% if the dose of thrombolytic is regular and even over 20% if SK is used in usual dose). Therefore, only in well selected cases of patients with AMI following to go through early angioplasty it will be recommended the association of thrombolytic (half does) with GP IIb/IIIa receptor blocker (usual dose), aspirin, heparin (reduced dose 400 U/hour). A combination like that had proved to be efficient and at the same time the only one for the patients with AMI who are going to go through an early angioplasty, without a grown risk of major bleeding.

Ticlopidine acts on the plaques through irreversible blockage of fibrinogen in the plaques, the final pathway of thrombus formation; the inhibition of the platelet aggregation is achieved in proportion of 85%.

It is indicated for the patients with AMI who have contraindication to use aspirin.

• It has been proved that a new blocker for the ADP receptors, clopidogrel, in dose of 75mg/day orally has a thrombolytic effect at least equal if not superior. The clopidogrel (Plavix) has clearly more reduced side effects and a similar efficiency to aspirin [24,32].

The evaluation of the pharmacological reperfusion

The efficiency of the thrombolysis can be appreciated through clinical methods, biological and electrocardiographic and in special cases through invasive or non-invasive imaging methods (coronarography).

The reperfusion syndrome represents the assembly of clinical, electrocardiographic, biological, imaging and angiographic manifestations that accompany the re-permeability of the coronary artery in the acute phase of the infarction. It is accepted that in 20% of the cases there is spontaneous reperfusion. The clinical – electrocardiographic syndrome of reperfusion may appear during the thrombolysis and a few tenths of minutes after the thrombolysis, due to a delayed effect of thrombolytics.

Interventional Reperfusion

Percutaneous transluminal coronary angioplasty in early AMI (PTCA)

It is already well proved that reperfusion can be obtained through emergency PTCA. By using a guide or a balloon catheter, it is easier technically to get through total occlusion produced by a recent thrombus than by an old coronary occlusion.

Angioplasty with balloon is useful in the acute phase of AMI in the following circumstances:

• **Early:**

a) Primary or direct PTCA – without previous thrombolytic: early opening of IRA in order to limit the AMI size;

b) PTCA adjuvant to thrombolysis (of consolidation);

c) "rescue" PTCA in case of thrombolysis failure;

d) PTCA "facilitated" after fibrinolytic in reduced dose ± GP IIb/IIIa receptor blocker.

• **Delayed** PTCA in sub-acute phase of AMI (2–7 days) the delayed opening of the artery in

patients who received or not thrombolytic – aiming to preserve or improve the ventricular function and remodeling (it will be discussed later).

Primary PTCA is defined as the angioplasty without previous or concomitant thrombolytic therapy and it is a therapeutic option only under the circumstances of a fast access in a catheterization laboratory with specialized personnel.

Primary PTCA is efficient in obtaining with success an IRA patency without the bleeding risks of thrombolysis.

The mechanical repermeability of the vessel involved in the infarction does not produce interstitial edema, necrosis with contraction bands and microvascular hemorrhages noticed in the treatment with thrombolytics.

The primary implantation of coronary stent may be seen as an alternative for thrombolysis for the patients with AMI.

Indications. Primary PTCA is recommended in the clinical practice :

• When the thrombolysis is not indicated

• Patients in cardiogenic shock (GUSTO trial, SHOCK trial)

Adjuvant PTCA

PTCA following a thrombolytic treatment with clinical signs of reperfusion has the theoretical advantage of an extra opening of a stenosed coronary artery with the increase of the flow, which can improve the recuperation of the myocardium and can diminish the re-occlusion risk. It may be done immediately or late (2–7 days). However, the existing trials showed that using empirical PTCA as a routine immediately or late after the thrombolysis led to a higher mortality [36].

"Rescue" PTCA

The patients to whom the thrombolytic treatment does not produce reperfusion are candidates for rescue PTCA. It is considered that the patients who benefit from this treatment are those who have continuous chest pain and ST segment elevation persisting more than 90 minutes after the initiation of thrombolytic treatment. The available data show that the patients can successfully benefit from rescue PTCA if this is realized in the first 8 hours since the beginning of the symptoms.

Adjutant therapy for interventional reperfusion:

Antithrombotic treatment

Using antithrombotic agents during and after PTCA is a certain indication for the prevention of early restenosis.

It is recommended to administrate heparin i.v. 24–48 hours after PTCA with or without implantation of stent. The administration depends on the APTT, as it has been described previously. It is possible to continue with low molecular weight heparin.

Antiplatelet treatment

• Aspirin remains a firm indication in preventing a re-occlusion post PTCA.

• Ticlopidine, a blocker for the ADP receptors, has a proved efficiency in preventing the restenosis after the PTCA +/- stent. It is recommended in a therapeutic dose of 250 mg twice a day for a month after the procedure of implanting a stent, associated with aspirin.

• It has been recently demonstrated that the administration of Clopidogrel increases the success in obtaining and maintaining an IRA patent. The dose is 75 mg/day, but in the acute phases, it is possible to administrate a loading dose of 300mg at once, before the procedure.

• In AMI with elevation of ST segment treated interventionally, the administration of GP IIb/IIIa blockers proves to the most promising therapy because they increase the patency and myocardial reperfusion through PTCA – with or without stent implant – they decrease the rate of periprocedural complications and reduce the restenosis rate after PTCA, with a reduction of necessary later revascularizations (Plate 27.2).

Coronary stents

The implant of the coronary stents increases the success rate of reperfusion for the patients with AMI in over 90% of the cases; concomitantly they reduce the restenosis and reinfarction rate. They are indicated in the following cases: primary treatment, when possible; in reperfusion of the coronary occlusion following angioplasty (dissection during PTCA), prevention of restenosis after PTCA [37].

Surgical Reperfusion

The coronary artery bypass grafting (CABG) has a less important place in treating the acute phase of AMI. However, this may be indicated in the following cases:

• Persistent or recurrent chest pain in case of PTCA or thrombolysis failure

• Coronary anatomy with high risk, for example the stenosis of the left common trunk revealed angiographically

• Coronary occlusion during angiography

• When PTCA is not possible

• In mechanical complications of AMI, as interventricular septum rupture or severe mitral regurgitation through rupture or dysfunction of papillary muscle.

For the patients in whom the thrombolysis is efficient, but with persistence of important residual stenosis and whose coronary anatomy better reacts to surgical revascularization than to PTCA the aorto-coronary bypass surgical intervention can be done with low mortality rate (~4%) and low morbidity, with the condition that the surgical intervention should be done after 24 hours since the beginning of AMI. For the patients who require a fast or emergency CABG in the first 24–48 hours after AMI, the mortality rate is much higher – 15–20% and significantly increased when emergency CABG is done under the conditions of persistent ischemia or cardiogenic shock.

The patients who receive emergency CABG in the first 6–12 hours after receiving thrombolytics must get protamine and fresh or frozen plasma to correct the coagulation disorders [38].

It has been noticed that the diabetic patients with myocardial infarction present more frequently a multicoronary affection with diffuse atherosclerotic lesions especially at the level of distal circulation.

It has been proved that the diabetic patients have a lower survival rate after the interventional or surgical myocardial revascularization compared to the non-diabetic patients. However, for the diabetic patients it is preferred to use surgical revascularization because the usage of the interventional procedures is associated with a high rate of restenosis and postprocedural complications (BARI study) [39].

It is well known that the diabetic patients have a lower survival rate after interventional myocardial revascularization (PTCA – Percutaneous Transluminal Coronary Angioplasty) and surgical (CABG) compared to the non-diabetic patients. Data regarding the evolution of the diabetics after the myocardial revascularization is provided by the observational studies because there are no randomized trials to follow the evolution and the long-term prognosis after the PTCA and CABG in the diabetic patients. In the BARI study (Bypass Angioplasty Revascularization Investigation), the 5 years mortality for diabetic patients with bi- and tri-coronary disease was 35% after PTCA, and significantly lower, 19%, after CABG, suggesting that for the diabetic patients with coronary affection it is preferable to use surgical myocardial revascularization.

The results of BARI study provided important arguments for the myocardial revascularization in the patients with diabetes mellitus type 2. Another important issue regarding PTCA in diabetic patients is the high rate of restenosis and periprocedural complications. In this sense, the treatment with derivatives of sulphonylurea may present an interesting issue. The derivatives of sulphonylurea (as well as glibenclamide, currently used) act by inhibiting the opening of the potassium channels ATP-dependent, this way stimulating insulin secretion. However, glibenclamide is not specific for the beta-pancreatic cells, acting at the level of the potassium channels ATP-dependent found at the level of the myocytes and the cells of the vascular endothelium. It is known that the potassium channels ATP-dependent are involved in the process of ischemic pre-conditioning responsible for the cardio-protection after the reperfusion. Besides the inactivation of the ischemic pre-conditioning, through inhibition of the ATP-dependent potassium channels, abnormalities of the coronary vasodilatation and the decrease of the myocardial contraction force appear. These might explain the negative effects of the derivations of sulphonylurea [40].

It has been shown that the improvement of the metabolic control with insulin leads to a more favorable evolution in diabetic patients after PTCA. Several factors, linked with the insulin-resistance and hyperglycemia, are involved in the stenosis process. It seems that insulin therapy decreases the platelet aggregation and activates the fibrinolytic system, two important mechanisms in the restenosis process and probably in unleashing the acute ischemic complications of PTCA. It has been recently proved that diabetic patients benefit especially of the GP IIb/IIIa receptor blockers in reducing the postprocedural complications [41].

It has been proved that using coronary stents during the revascularization procedures leads to a reduction of the restenosis rate both in diabetic and non-diabetic patients. Nonetheless, most of the studies show that the diabetic patients continue to present a higher restenosis and postprocedural complications rate vs. the non-diabetic patients. These findings obtained from the analysis of the subgroups of diabetic patients from the large trials that compare the data after PTCA and CABG are limited and might be changed by prospective studies of some trials that include only diabetic patients [42].

Cardioprotection through decreasing the consumption of myocardial oxygen

In parallel with the myocardium rescue measures, other measures are taken to reduce the consumption of myocardial oxygen, trying to obtain an optimum balance between the demand and the supply with myocardial oxygen in order to save an as large as possible area from the myocardium at risk. This is obtained through specific and non-specific measures.

Non-specific measures:
– Physical and emotional rest, use of light sedatives if necessary.
– Severe anemia must be corrected by careful administration of blood.
– The variation of the systolic blood pressure should not be higher than 25–30 mmHg vs. the usual values of the patient, except for the presence of severe HTA before AMI.
– Marked sinus bradycardia (below 50 b/minute) needs atropine and/or pacing. On the other hand, the administration of atropine as a routine, that leads to an increase of the cardiac frequency in the patients without important bradicardy, is not indicated;
– All forms of tachyarrhythmia require prompt treatment.
– In the absence of complications, the patients with AMI must not remain at rest for more than 12 hours; the progression of physical activity must be individualized based on age, physical capacity and patient status.

Specific measures: beta-blockers, nitrates

Beta-blockers (BB) The aggressive treatment with cardioselective beta-blockers improves significantly the prognosis of diabetic patients with myocardial infarction.

Beta-blockers are used in treating AMI in diabetic patients despite their reputation of masking the symptoms of hypoglycemia and aggravation of metabolic disorders. Avoiding usage of beta-blockers or/and thrombolytics are examples of "myths" that can cost the life of the diabetic with AMI.

If the patient received a beta-blocking agent at the moment when the clinical manifestation of the infarction appeared, this must be continued unless there is a contraindication.

The fast intravenous administration of beta-blockers reduced the cardiac index, cardiac frequency, and blood pressure. The net effect is a reduction of the myocardial oxygen consumption per minute and per beat.

The early beta blockade reduces the size of AMI, fact proved through the reduction of the release of cardiac enzymes, maintaining the R waves and reducing the development of Q waves.

The administration of the beta-blockers is with held in patient with hypotension (BP < 90 mmHg), bradycardia (below 50 b/minute), cardiac blocks (PR > 24), LVI (Killip class > II).

A specific indication of the beta-blockers is atrial fibrillation with fast ventricular response. There are no significant differences between the various types of beta-blockers used.

The current recommendations are to use beta-blockers orally in the diabetic patients with preserved left ventricular function (EFLV estimated at 40%), and initiate this first or second day after admission [43].

The favorable effect of the beta-blocking therapy during and after myocardial infarction in the diabetic patients has several possible explanations; the beta-blocker changes the myocardial metabolism increasing the usage of glucose and reducing the beta-oxidation of fatty acids leading to the reduction of the consumption of myocardial oxygen. The beta-blockers improve the cardiac autonomic dysfunction through the reduction of the sympathetic tonus, improving the sympathetic-vagal balance. Also, they reduce the tachycardia, more frequently met in the post infarction period, more in the diabetic patients than in the non-diabetic patients [44].

Nitrates

The nitroglycerin treatment is applied to the diabetic patients with large anterior AMI, with LV failure, the ones with recurrent or persistent angina and those with HT.

In patients with AMI, the nitrates means a useful pharmacological medication because: they reduce the pressure of ventricular filling, the parietal tension and the wall stress improve the coronary blood flow especially in the ischemia areas, have antiplatelet effects, reduce the size of the infarction, reduce the incidence of mechanical complications.

Nitroglycerin is indicated for two effects:

1) anti-ischemic effect: improves the persistent pain, and

2) hemodynamic effect: vasodilator effect in left ventricle insufficiency from AMI.

Nitroglycerin is contraindicated in: marked arterial hypotension (BPs ≤ 90 mm Hg), especially if it is associated with bradycardia (<50b/min); inferior AMI with suspicion of RV infarction.

The nitrates are not administered orally in the initial phase of AMI.

The duration of nitroglycerin administration is 24–48 hours with prolongation in case of chest pain recurrence and persistence of LV failure. After 48- hours slow release oral Nitroglycerin preparation can be administered (30–60 mg/day) or as ointment (2.5–8 cm at every 6–8 hours for the patients with systolic blood pressure over 120 mmHg).

Many patients show tolerance to NTG when it is administered i.v. (manifested by the increase of the nitroglycerin demand), sometimes at only 12 hours after the first administration. In case of prolonged administration, it is recommended to have minimum 12 hours between administrations [30].

Angiotensin converting enzyme inhibitors (ACE inhibitors)

The studies of the last years showed that ACE inhibitors represent a first class indication of mortality at 6 months for diabetic patients with myocardial infarction.

The reason for using the ACE inhibitors in AMI in diabetic patients:

1. Prevent the ventricular and vascular remodeling, reduce significantly the appearance of cardiac insufficiency, and diminish LV function;

2. Reduce reinfarction;

3. Reduce the mortality due to AMI.

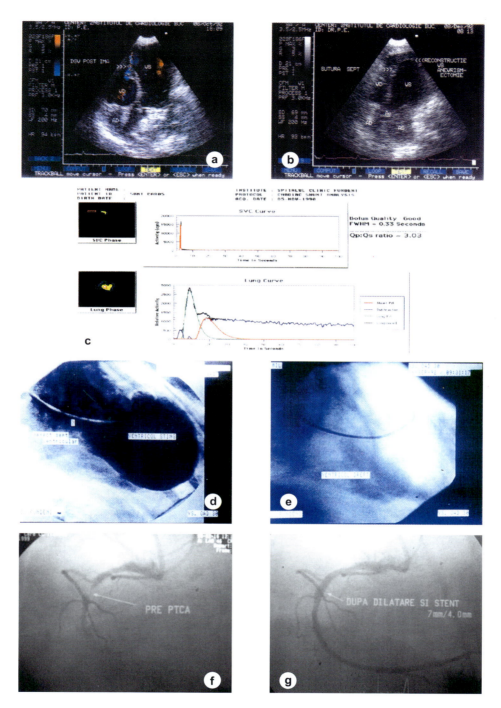

Plate 27.2

P.E., 49 years old. Inferior acute myocardial infarction complicated with ventricular septal rupture. Rescue PTCA on the RCA within the 5th day since the onset of AMI. Type 2 diabetes mellitus with decompensation (ketoacidosis at admission): a – two-dimensional echocardiographic apical four-chamber view shows solution of continuity within the apical third of interventricular septum, at this level reflecting left-to-right shunt using color Doppler flow imaging; b – postsurgical two-dimensional echocardiographic apical four-chamber view; c – radionuclide ventriculography: at the first passage of the contrast agent, confirms the presence of the cardiac shunt and calculates the ratio of the pulmonary blood flow to the systemic blood flow: 3.03/1; d, e – ventriculography with contrast agent proves the presence of the ventricular septal defect out of the opacification of the right ventricle after the injection of the contrast agent into the left ventricle; f – coronary angiography: occlusion of RCA at the level of vessel segment II (univessel coronary artery lesion); g – coronary angiography after PTCA with favorable final result, with TIMI grade 3 flow.

The benefit of ACE inhibitors appears as a class effect because several agents reduced the morbidity and mortality [45].

Significant adverse reaction of ACE inhibitors is represented by hypotension, especially after the first dose and the intolerable coughing in the chronic administration.

Major contraindications of ACE inhibitors include arterial hypotension, in the context of an adequate pre-load, known hypersensitivity, pregnancy, renal insufficiency with creatinine >3 mg%.

Early initiation of the treatment with ACE inhibitors *per os* is recommended within the first 24 hours of AMI. In initial therapy short action, ACE inhibitors (captopril) are recommended. They can be interrupted if hypotension occurs [46].

Although there are not available definite data, yet it seems rational to use blocker for the receptors of the angiotensin II in the patients who do not tolerate ACE inhibitors.

Precautions

Hypotension must be avoided, especially during the reperfusion; therefore we recommend initiating oral therapy with ACE inhibitors after the thrombolysis or primary PTCA. Early administration of the ACE inhibitors plays a very important role especially if the reperfusion therapy was not successful or was not administered.

Recommendations for ACE inhibitors administration

It has to be discussed the ACE inhibitors treatment after administer aspirin, the beginning of the reperfusion strategy and beta blocking in specific cases, for each diabetic patient with AMI [47].

Calcium blockers

Despite some experimental and clinical proofs regarding the anti-ischemic effect, it has not been proved that the calcium antagonists could be useful in the acute phase of AMI, and few studies showed an increase of the mortality risk if prescribed as a routine in AMI.

It is not recommended to use Nifedipine as treatment in early AMI.

Verapamil and diltiazem administered in the acute phase of AMI; it has not been proved a favorable effect of those drugs on the size of the infarction or other important targets for the patients with AMI, with the exception of control of the overt ventricular rhythm disorders [24, 30].

Magnesium

Magnesium deficit must be corrected so that to maintain the serum level on magnesium over 2.0 mEq/l. In the presence of hypokalemia (<4.0 mEq/l) during the treatment of AMI, the serum level of magnesium must be checked and corrected if it is necessary because if there is magnesium deficit, the potassium deficit is difficult to correct.

The episodes of torsade de pointes must be treated with 1–2 g of magnesium in bolus in 5 minutes.

Cardioprotection through metabolic support can be realized through solution glucose-insulin-potassium. The administration of a solution of glucose-insulin-potassium (300 g glucose, 50 units insulin and 80 mEq K^+) in 1000 ml water supplied with a rate of 1.5 ml/kg/hour reduces the plasmatic concentration of free fatty acids and improves the ventricular performance [48].

The rigorous metabolic balance is a beneficial therapeutic strategy in AMI in diabetic patients, because the beginning of AMI in diabetic patients increases the beta-oxidation of the fatty acids simultaneously with the reduction of the glycosylation, with the affection of both the ischemic and non-ischemic myocardial territories. Insulin therapy in the acute phase of the AMI contributes to the decline of the PAI-1 activity, with improvement of the spontaneous fibrinolysis, modulates the platelet activity, corrects the abnormalities of the lipid profile and reduces the beta-oxidation of the free fat acids at the myocardial level [49,50].

The results of the DIGAMI study meant a starting point for the initiation of the treatment with insulin for the diabetic with AMI, under the form of GIK solution (glucose-insulin-potassium), proving the reduction of post-infarction mortality by 28% or 49 lives saved in patients treated with GIK. There is sufficient evidence that support the insulin therapy in diabetic patients with AMI.

The treatment of the myocardial infarction in diabetic patients includes, besides a rigorous metabolic balance, a good control of the risk factors within the measures of secondary prevention.

Normolipemiants

In the diabetic patient with myocardial infarction, the normolipemiant therapy aims to reduce the LDL-C, the studies showing that the diabetic patients benefit to the same extent with the non-diabetic patients from the therapy with statins. The dyslipidemic profile characteristic of the diabetic patients with myocardial infarction responds better to therapy with fibrates; in this sense there are highlighting data provided by the analysis of the subgroup of diabetic patients in the study Helsinki-Heart and the study regarding the fibrates intervention in the diabetes mellitus type 2. The first choice of therapy is based on the level of plasmatic TG. Because most of the available information regarding the normolipemiant therapy in coronary diabetic patients refers to statins, those represent in general the first medicine chosen, with the exception of the cases when the level of TG is high (over 400 mg/dl) when the fibrates are recommended to be the first choice. Frequently the normalization of the lipid profile at the diabetic patient with myocardial infarction cannot be realized with only one class of drugs, therefore statins-fibrates therapy is recommended [7, 51].

The normolipemiant therapy with **HMG-CoA reductase inhibitors (statins)** must be used for all diabetic patients with acute myocardial infarction and high values of LDL-C. This therapy has an important role in stabilizing the atheromatous plaque through the non-lipid effects: anti-swelling dependent on dose, antithrombotic, anticoagulant, increase of the production of NO, increase of the sensitivity of AT1 receptors, decrease of the platelet aggregability, decrease of the apoptosis. The duration of administration for the patients with AMI without ST segment elevation:

– 1–2 weeks for the effect of stabilization of the atheromatous plaque, non lipidic effect;

– 1–2 months for lipid effect: reduces LDL-C and total cholesterol;

– 1–2 years in order to have an effect of reduction of cardiovascular mortality.

Dosage: starts with 20mg/day. Doubling the dose has an extra beneficial effect – 6% higher than the initial one ("the rule of 6"). The doses can grow progressively up to the maximum dose of 80 mg/day, which is the maximum dose accepted for all statins [52, 53].

LATE HOSPITAL ASSISTANCE (POST-CORONARY CARE UNIT PERIOD)

The delayed assistance in the hospital includes the ensemble of pharmacological and non-pharmacological therapeutic measures addressed to the diabetic patient with AMI after moving him from the coronary care unit (CCU) until he is released at home, and assumes:

– To continue the hygiene-diet measures initiated in CCU: early mobilization started in CCU, progressive return to physical activities, adequate diet.

– To continue the cardioprotective measures:

• beta-blockers: continue the administration of BB; if not used until this moment, using them will be considered;

• nitrates: administration 24–48 hours with extension in case of pain recurrence or persistent LV failure;

• ACE inhibitors: to continue the administration started in CCU; if not used until now, the opportunity to introduce them has to be analyzed.

– Delayed opening of the artery responsible for the infarction.

– The treatment of the late complications.

– Evaluation and ranking of the risk.

– Measures of secondary prevention.

Cardioprotection through late opening of the artery responsible for infarction

Both the experimental and clinical proofs indicate that the opening, even late, of the artery responsible for the infarction has a favorable effect on:

– Ventricular remodeling (better healing of the infarcted tissue and prevention of the infarction expansion);

– It also increases the collateral flow;

– Improves the diastolic and systolic function;

– Increases the electrical stability;

– Reduces the long-term mortality.

Early reperfusion (thrombolysis, primary PTCA) shortens the duration of the coronary occlusion and thus limits the size of the infarction, prevents the dysfunction and LV expansion.

Late reperfusion (after 12 hours since the beginning of the coronary occlusion) seems to influence favorably the "healing" process of the infarction and reduces the remodeling of the left ventricle and in the end the appearance of the pump dysfunction and the electrical instability.

The elective PTCA can be taken into consideration for the patients who present ischemia of rest during the hospitalization or during the effort test conducted before leaving home.

It cannot be considered necessary to run a routine coronary angiography for the asymptomatic patients with negative exercise test before release for identification of the patients with severe obstruction, to whom PTCA can be done [36].

Anatomically, the coronary lesions of the diabetic patients with myocardial infarction present distinctive characteristics *vs.* the non-diabetic patients: the coronarographies post-myocardial infarction show that the affection is multivascular, more severe and in several coronary segments than in the non-diabetic patients, and the coronary calcifications have an increased prevalence. The restenosis rate after transluminal coronary angioplasty is also higher in diabetic patients; however, the intrastent restenosis rate is similar in both diabetic and non-diabetic patients. These remarks suggest that the remodeling and the neointimal proliferation after the angioplasty are more emphasized in the diabetic patients *vs.* the non-diabetic patients. The evolution of the diabetic patients after the angioplasty is more serious *vs.* that of non-diabetic patients.

POST-DISCHARGE ASSISTANCE

Convalescence

The *early* recuperation of the diabetic patients with uncomplicated AMI begins in the hospital. The average hospitalization period for these patients is 5 to 7 days since the admission.

On the other hand, the patients with complications, especially those with pump dysfunction, are mobilized with great care after 3–4 days from hemodynamic stabilization.

Recovery in the myocardial infarction

The average period in hospital

The period spent in the hospital by the patients with myocardial infarction is variable from patient to patient. Thus, in patients to whom

the reperfusion was successful, in the absence of the early ventricular tachyarrhythmia, of hypotension or cardiac insufficiency and in the conditions of a good ejection fraction, the risk for late complications is small. These patients can be released from the hospital in 5 days after the beginning of the symptoms.

Most frequently, the discharge is after 7–10 days since the arrival for the patients without complications.

The recovery of the patients with AMI includes the following components:
- Physical exercise;
- Changes of the risk factors;
- Counseling, psychosocial and vocational evaluation.

Discharge Criteria

Before the release, the patients must be evaluated in order to establish the risk class. The evaluation of the diabetic patients with myocardial infarction before release will include clinical and paraclinical evaluation, assessing the pump function of the heart, the risk for myocardial ischemia, the metabolic and arrhythmic risk.

The evaluation of the left ventricle function is based on:
- Clinical data: symptoms, (dyspnea, functional status) and
- Objective data (*e.g.* crepitations, cardiomegaly, protodiastolic gallop);
- Exercise capacity;
- Ejection fraction (measured through: echocardiography, radionuclear ventriculography, possible ventriculography with contrast substance). The evaluation of the telediastolic volume brings prognostic information superior to the ejection fraction in patients with AMI.

The extent of the infarction area; because the affection of the left ventricle function depends on the size of the infarction area, its dimension can be estimated through various paraclinical explorations: serum cardiac enzymatic markers, echocardiography, and techniques with radionuclides (as radionuclear ventriculography, perfusion scintigram).

Secondary prevention

The objectives of secondary prevention post-AMI in diabetic patients are to:
- stabilize the atheromatous plaque at the level of the artery responsible for the infarction (ARI),

and delay the progression (possibly regression) of the atherosclerosis in the non-ARI territory.

– limit the tendency towards complications of the atherosclerotic plaques.

– control of ventricular remodeling.

– provide cardioprotection of the myocardium spared by current MI and of the viable myocardium.

– prevent or at least limit the MI complications.

– diminish the risk of thrombosis and thromboembolism and arrhythmic complications.

– rigorous metabolic control [54].

In the diabetic patients, the complications post-AMI can be systematized after the interval since the appearance of the infarction (see Table 27.6).

The recurrent ischemic events post-AMI can be systematized depending on the coronary territory involved and after the period since the beginning of the AMI (see Table 27.7).

Early myocardial ischemia occurred in the first 2 weeks post-AMI is considered unstable angina (no matter the territory, ARI/non-ARI), therefore it belongs to the category of unstable angina with high risk [55, 56].

PROGNOSTIC PARTICULARITIES

The factors of unfavorable prognostic that should be taken into consideration in diabetic patients with myocardial infarction are:

– Coronary diffuse and distal multivascular affection;

– Coronary microangiopathy;

– Reduction of the coronary flux reserve;

– Reduction of the fibrinolytic activity;

– Increase of the platelet aggregation;

– Lipoproteic atherogenic profile;

– Autonomic cardiac dysfunction;

– Association of the diabetic cardiomyopathy.

The metabolic factors contribute to the aggravation of the prognosis: the decline of the insulin-secretion associated with the increase of the insulin-resistance and disorders of the free fatty acids metabolism.

The aggravation of the cardiac insufficiency and/or the appearance of the recurrent myocardial ischemia accentuate the metabolic disorders.

The size of the infarction is an important element for prognosis in both diabetic patients and non-diabetic patients. However, in diabetic patients, for an equal extension of the infarction area it is noticed a higher mortality rate vs. the non-diabetic patients because diabetic neuropathy and cardiomyopathy, rhythm disorders and congestive cardiac insufficiency are more frequent [57].

The prognosis on medium or long term of the diabetic patients with myocardial infarction is cautious due to the recurrence of the infarction, more frequent ventricular dysfunction and higher mortality rate.

Ketoacidosis is considered a factor of aggravation; its presence at the beginning of the AMI makes the mortality to grow to 35–40%.

The unfavorable prognostic factors on long term for diabetic patients are: patient's age, female gender, hypertension, atherogenic profile of lipoproteins (small, dense particles of LDL-C), ventricular rhythm disorders, diffuse and distal multivascular coronary involvement, reduction of the coronary flow reserve, congestive coronary insufficiency [58, 59].

Table 27.6

Complications after AMI

EARLY COMPLICATIONS (first 2 weeks)	LATE COMPLICATIONS (>2 weeks)
Acute pump dysfunction	Cardiac Insufficiency
Sudden death	Dressler syndrome
Thromboembolic accidents	Rhythm and conduction disorders
Periinfarction pericarditis	Late postinfarction angina
Early postinfarction angina	
Rhythm and conduction disturbances	
Cardiac mechanical complications	

Table 27.7

Recurrent ischemic events post-AMI

RECURRENT ISCHEMIC EVENTS POST-AMI	
After the coronary territory involved	
Artery responsible for infarction (ARI)	Non-ARI
Peri-infarct ischemia Infarction extension = reinfarction	Ischemia at distance Infarction at distance
After the time interval since the beginning of the AMI	
EARLY first 2 weeks	LATE: >2 weeks

The evolution of the diabetic with myocardial infarction must be considered in relation with the co-existence of the other complications of diabetes mellitus, and in the first place of the diabetic microangiopathy and autonomic cardiac neuropathy. The autonomic neuropathy associated to the coronary artery disease in diabetic patients may be an "infirmity" more or less invalidating, especially in the case of association of the orthostatic arterial hypotension [57]. The other forms of manifestation of the autonomic cardiac neuropathy, such as tachycardia at rest, prolonged QT interval and the low variability of the cardiac frequency, give to the diabetic with AMI a strong predisposition for ventricular rhythm disorders and cardiac sudden death [60, 61].

Several recent studies showed that the presence of the autonomic cardiac neuropathy in the patients with MI is correlated with an unfavorable prognosis [62].

CONCLUSIONS

• In diabetic patients, the myocardial infarction has important metabolic implications.

• "Diabetic status" of a patient with myocardial infarction is characterized by important abnormalities of coagulation, spontaneous thrombolysis and platelet dysfunction.

• AMI in the diabetic patients is more frequently silent and can manifest by acute pump insufficiency, metabolic decompensation or both.

• Mortality rate in the hospital is almost double in diabetic patients *vs.* non-diabetics with AMI.

• AMI treatment in diabetic patients requires the same general lines as for the non-diabetic patients: large-scale use of thrombolytic agents, platelet antiaggregants and ACE inhibitors. It is not to avoid beta-blockers, respecting the specific contraindications.

• The "aggressive" treatment with cardioselective beta-blockers improves the prognosis of the diabetic patients with myocardial infarction.

• In addition, the therapeutic strategy demands a rigorous metabolic balance. The improvement of the metabolic control with insulin is associated with a better evolution of the diabetic patients after PTCA.

• The diabetic patients benefit especially from the therapy with GP IIb/IIIa receptors blockers which results in reducing the postprocedural complications.

• Using the coronary stents during the revascularization procedures in diabetic patients reduces the restenosis rate.

• In diabetic patients with coronary affection it is preferred to revascularize through CABG.

• The predictive factors for long term evolution of the diabetic patients with myocardial infarction are: age, cardiac insufficiency and glycemic metabolic status.

REFERENCES

1. Barrett-Connor E, Cohn BA, Wingard DL, Edelstein SL. Why is diabetes mellitus a stronger risk factor for fatal ischemic heart disease in women than in men? The Rancho Bernardo Study. *JAMA*, **265**: 627–631, 1991.
2. Melchior T, Kober L, Madsen CR, *et al.* Accelerating impact of diabetes mellitus on mortality in the years

following an acute myocardial infarction. *Eur Heart J,* **20**: 973–978, 1999.

3. Manson JE, Colditz GA, Stampfer MJ, *et al.* A prospective study of maturity-onset diabetes mellitus and risk of coronary heart disease and stroke in women. *Arch Int Med,* **151**: 1141–1147, 1991.

4. Milan Study on Atherosclerosis and Diabetes (MiSAD) Group. Prevalence of unrecognized silent myocardial ischemia and its association with atherosclerotic risk factors in non-insulin-dependent diabetes mellitus. *Am J Cardiol,* **79**: 134–139, 1997.

5. Long-Term Intervention with Pravastatin in Ischaemic Disease (LIPID) Study Group. Prevention of cardiovascular events and death with pravastatin in patients with coronary heart disease and a broad range of initial cholesterol levels. *N Engl J Med,* **339(19)**: 1349–1357, 1998.

6. Hanefeld M, Fischer S, Julius U, Schulze J, Schwanebeck U, Schmechel H, Ziegelasch HJ, Linder J. Risk factors for myocardial infarction and death in newly detected NIDDM: the Diabetes Intervention Study, 11-year follow-up. *Diabetologia,* **39(12)**: 1577–1583, 1996.

7. Pyörälä K, Pedersen TR, Kjekhus L, *et al.* Cholesterol lowering with simvastatin improves prognosis of diabetic patients with coronary heart disease. A subgroup analysis of the Scandinavian Simvastatin Survival Study (4S). *Diabetes Care,* **20(4)**: 614–620, 1997.

8. Vavuranakis M, Stefanadis C, Toutouzas K, *et al.* Impaired compensatory coronary artery enlargement in atherosclerosis contributes to the development of coronary artery stenosis in diabetic patients. *Eur Heart J,* **18**: 1080–1094, 1997.

9. Abraira C, Colwell J, Nuttall F, *et al.* Cardiovascular events and correlates in the Veterans Affairs Cooperative Study on glycemic control and complications in type II diabetes group. *Arch Intern Med,* **157**: 181–188, 1997.

10. Turner RC, Millns H, Neil HAW, *et al.* Risk factors for coronary artery disease in non-insulin dependent diabetes mellitus: United Kingdom Prospective Diabetes Study (UKPDS: 23). *BMJ,* **317**: 930–942, 1998.

11. Camici PG, Wijns W, Borgers M, *et al.* Pathophysiological mechanisms of chronic reversible left ventricular dysfunction due to coronary artery disease (hibernating myocardium). *Circulation,* **96**: 3205–3214, 1997.

12. Ginghina C, Bacanu GS, Marinescu M, Dragomir D. *Diabetic Heart.* Ed. Infomedica, Bucharest, 2001.

13. Gherasim L, Ionescu-Tîrgoviste C. *Internal Medicine, Cardiovascular and metabolic disease,* volumul II. Ed. Medicală, Bucharest, 1167–1200, 1996.

14. Forrat R, Sebbag L, Wiernsperger N, *et al.* Acute myocardial infarction in dogs with experimental diabetes. *Cardiac Res,* **27**: 1908–1912, 1993.

15. Stanley W, Ryden L (Ed). *The Diabetic Coronary Patient.* Science Press Ltd, London, 29–66, 1999.

16. Smith SC Jr. Blair SN, Criqui MH, Fletcher GF, Fuster V, Gersh BJ, Gotto AM, Gould KL, Greenland P, Grundy SM, *et al.* Preventing heart attack and death in patients with coronary disease. *Circulation,* **92**: 2–4, 1995.

17. C.Paillole *et al.* Detection of coronary artery disease in diabetic patient. *Diabetologia,* **38**: 726–731, 1995.

18. Gray RP, Patterson DLH, Yudkin JS. Plasminogen activator inhibitor activity in diabetic and nondiabetic survivors of myocardial infarction. *Anterioscler Thromb,* **13**: 415–420, 1993.

19. Koskinen P, Mänttäri M, Manninen V, Huttunen J and Hinonon O. Coronary heart disease incidence in NIDDM patients in the Helsinki Heart Study. *Diabetes Care,* **15**: 825–829, 1992.

20. Haffner SM, Lehto S, Ronnemaa T, *et al.* Mortality from coronary heart disease in subjects with type 2 diabetes and in nondiabetic subjects with and without prior myocardial infarction. *N Engl J Med,* **339**: 229–234, 1998.

21. Wilson PW. Diabetes mellitus and coronary heart disease. *Am J Kidney Dis,* **32**: S89–S100, 1998.

22. Diaz R, Paolasso EA, Piegas LS, *et al.* Metabolic modulation of acute myocardial infarction. The ECLA (Estudios Cardiologicos Latinoamerica) Collaborative Group. *Circulation,* **98**: 2227–2234, 1998.

23. Desideri A, Celegon L. Metabolic management of ischemic heart disease: clinical data with trimetazidine. *Am J Cardiol,* **82**: 50K–53K, 1998.

24. Ginghina Carmen, Marinescu M., Dragomir D. *Guide for Diagnosis and Treatment in Acute Myocardial Infarction.* Ed. Infomedica, Bucharest, 2001.

25. Carmen G, Petrescu R., Arsenescu I, Balanica M, Popa A, Rogozea D, Carp C. Acute Myocardial Infarction in diabetic patients. National Meeting of Cardiology, 2–5 Oct., Bucharest, 1991.

26. Macarie C, Ionescu DD. *Urgente Cardiace-Diagnostic si Tratament,* Ed. Militara, 166–242, 1980.

27. De-Silva R, Camici PG. Role of positron emission tomography in the investigation of human coronary circulatory function. *Cardiovasc Res,* **28**: 1595–1612, 1994.

28. Camici PG, Rosen SD. Does positron emission tomography contribute to the management of clinical cardiac problems? *Eur Heart*, **17**: 174–181, 1996.

29. Senior R, Kenny A, Nihoyannopoulos P. Stress echocardiography for assessing myocardial ischaemia and viable myocardium. *Heart*, **78 (suppl 1)**: 12–18, 1997.

30. Scheneider DJ, Sobel BE. Determinants of coronary vascular disease in patients with type II diabetes mellitus and their therapeutic implications. *Clin Cardiol*, **20**: 433–440, 1997.

31. Fibrinolytic Therapy Trialist (FTT) Collaborative Study Group. Indications for fibrinolytic therapy in suspected acute myocardial infarction: collaborative overview of early mortality and major morbidity results from all randomized trials of more than 1000 patients. *Lancet*, **343**: 311–322, 1994.

32. Gregnini L, Marco J, Fajadat *et al.* Ticlopidine and aspirin pretreatment reduces coagulation and platelet activation during coronary dilatation procedures. *JACC*, **29**: 113–120, 1997.

33. Granger CB, Califf RM, Young S, *et al.* Outcome of patients with diabetes mellitus and acute myocardial infarction treated with thrombolytic agens. The Thrombolysis and Angioplasty in Myocardial Infarction (TAMI) study group. *J Am Coll Cardiol*, **21**: 920–925, 1993.

34. Every NR, Persons LS, Hlatky M *et al.* A comparison of thrombolytic therapy with primary coronary angioplasty for acute myocardial infarction. *N Engl J Med*, **335**: 1263–60, 1996

35. Kip KE, Faxon DP, Detre KM, Yeh W, Kelsey SF, Currier JW. Coronary angioplasty in diabetic patients. The National Heart, Lung, and Blood Institute Percutaneous Transluminal Coronary Angioplasty Registry. *Circulation*, **94**: 1818–1825, 1996.

36. Van Belle E, Bauters C, Hubert E, *et al.* Restenosis rates in diabetic patients: A comparison of coronary stenting and balloon angioplasty in native coronary vessels. *Circulation*, **96**: 1454–1460, 1997.

37. Aroson D, Bloomgarden Z, Rayfield EJ. Potential mechanisms promoting restenosis in diabetic patients. *J Am Coll Cardiol*, **27**: 528–535, 1996.

38. Gum PA, O'Keefe LH Jr. Borkon AM, Spertus JA, Bateman TM, McGraw JP, Sherwani K, Vacek J, McCallister BD. Bypass surgery versus coronary angioplasty for revascularization of treated diabetic patients. *Circulation*, **96(suppl II)**: II7–II10, 1997.

39. Influence of diabetes on 5-year mortality and morbidity in a randomized trial comparing CABG and PTCA in patients with multivessel disease: the Bypass Angioplasty Revascularization Investigation (BARI). *Circulation*, **96**: 1761–1769, 1997.

40. Garrat KN, Brady Pa, Hassinger NL, *et al.* Sulfonylurea drugs increase early mortality in patients with diabetes mellitus after direct angioplasty for acute myocardial infarction. *J Am Coll Cardiol*, **33**: 119–124, 1999.

41. O'Keefe JH, Blackstone EH, Sergeant P, McCallister BD. The optimal mode of coronary revascularization for diabetics: a risk-adjusted long-term study comparing coronary angioplasty and coronary bypass surgery. *Eur Heart J*, **19**: 1696–1703, 1998.

42. Thourani VH, Weintraub WS, Stein B, *et al.* Influence of diabetes mellitus on early and late outcome after coronary artery bypass grafting. *Ann Thorac Surg,* **67**: 1045–1052, 1999.

43. Malmberg K, Herlitz J, Hjalmarsson Å, *et al.* Effects of metoprolol on mortality and late infarction in diabetics with suspected acute myocardial infarction: Retrospective data from two large scale studies. *Eur Heart J*, **10**: 4–428, 1989.

44. Gottlieb SS, McCarter RJ, Vogel RA. Effect of beta-blockade on mortality among high-risk and low-risk patients after myocardial infarction. *N Engl J Med*, **339**: 489–497, 1998.

45. ACE Inhibitor Myocardial Infarction collaborative Group. Indications for ACE inhibitors in the early treatment of acute myocardial infarction. Systematic over- view of individual data form 100,000 patients in randomized trials: *Circulation*, **97**: 2202, 1998.

46. Chinese Cardiac Study Collaborative Group. Oral captopril versus placebo among 13,634 patients with suspected acute myocardial infarction. Interim report from the Chinese Cardiac Study (CCS–1); *Lancet*, **345**: 686, 1995.

47. Zuanetti G, Latini R, Maggioni A, *et al.* Effect of the ACE-inhibitor lisinopril on mortality in diabetic patients with acute myocardial infarction: Data from the GISSI-3 study. *Circulation*, **96**: 4239–4245, 1997.

48. Malmberg K, Ryden L, Efendic S, *et al.* A randomized trial of insulin-glucose infusion followed by subcutaneous insulin treatment in diabetic patients with acute myocardial infarction: effects on one year mortality. *J Am Coll Cardiol*, **26**: 57–65, 1995.

49. Malmberg K. Prospective randomized study on intensive insulin treatment on long survival after acute myocardial infarction in patients with diabetes mellitus. DIGAMI (Diabetes Mellitus, Insulin Glucose Infusion in Acute Myocardial Infarction) Study Group [see comments]. *BMJ,* **314**: 1512–1515, 1997.

50. Malmberg K. Prospective randomized study of intensive insulin treatment on long-term survival after acute myocardial infarction in patients with diabetes mellitus. *BMJ*, **315**: 1632–1642, 1997.

51. The Long-Term Intervention with Pravastatin in Ischaemic Disease (LIPID) Study Group: Prevention of cardiovascular events and death with pravastatin in patients with coronary heart disease and a broad range of initial cholesterol levels. *N Engl J Med*, **339**: 1349–1357, 1998.

52. Goldberg RB, Mellies MJ, Sacks FM, Moye LA, Howard BV, Howard WJ, Davis BR, Cole TG, Pfeffer MA, Braunwald E, for the CARE investigators. Cardiovascular events and their reduction with pravastatin in diabetic and glucose-intolerant myocardial infarction survivors with average cholesterol levels: subgroup analyses in the Cholesterol and Recurrent Events (CARE) trial. *Circulation*, **98**: 2513–2519, 1998.

53. Sacks FM, Pfeffer MA, Moye LA, Rouleau JL, Rutherford JD, Cole TG, Brown L, Warnica JW, Arnold JM, Wun CC, Davis BR, Braunwald E, Cholesterol and Recurrent Events Trial investigators. The effect of pravastatin on coronary events after myocardial infarction in patients with average cholesterol levels. *N Engl J Med*, **335**: 1001–1009, 1996.

54. Hulley S, Grady D, Bush T, Furberg C, Herrington D, Riggs B, Vittinghof E, Heart and Estrogen/Progestin Replacement Study (HERS) research group. Randomized trial of estrogen plus progestin for secondary prevention of coronary heart disease in postmenopausal women. *JAMA*, **280**: 605–613, 1998.

55. Turner RC, Millns H, Neil HA, *et al.* Risk factors for coronary artery disease in non-insulin dependent diabetes mellitus: United Kingdom Prospective Diabetes Study (UKDPS: 23). *BMJ*, **316**: 823–828, 1998.

56. Stamler J, Vaccaro O, Neaton JD, *et al.* Diabetes, other risk factors, and 12-yr cardiovascular mortality for men screened in the Multiple Risk Factor Intervention Trial. *Diabetes Care*, **16**: 434–444, 1993.

57. Dragomir D, Ginghina C, Marinescu M, Fotiade B, Bacanu Gh, Apetrei E. Autonomic cardiac neuropathy – marker of prognosis in diabetic patients with AMI. National Symposium "Prof. Dr. Dimitrie Gerota", Bucharest, 5–6 November 2000.

58. Fuller JH, Shipley MJ, Rose G, *et al.* Mortality from coronary heart disease and stroke in relation to degree of glycemia: the Whitehall study. *Br Med J Clin Research Ed*, **287**: 867–870, 1983.

59. Herlitz J, Wognsen GB, Emanuelsson H, Haglid M, Karlson BW, Karlsson T, Albertsson P, Westberg S. Mortality and morbidity in diabetic and nondiabetic patients during a 2-year period after coronary artery bypass grafting. *Diabetes Care*, **19**: 698–703, 1996.

60. Miettinen H, Lehto S, Salomaa V, *et al.* Impact of diabetes on mortality after the first myocardial infarction. *Diabetes Care*, **21**: (1) 69–75, 1998.

61. Morrish NJ, Stevens LK, Fuller JH, *et al.* Incidence of macrovascular disease in diabetes mellitus: the London follow-up to the WHO multinational study of vascular disease in diabetics. *Diabetologia*, **34**: 584–589, 1991.

62. Stone PH, Muller J.E., Hartwell T. *et al.* The effect of diabetes mellitus on prognosis and serial left ventricular function after acute myocardial infarction: Contribution of both coronary disease and diastolic left ventricular dysfunction to the adverse prognosis. *J. Am. Coll. Cardiol,* **14**: 49, 1989.

28

CORONARY ARTERY CALCIFICATION IN DIABETES

Dana DABELEA

Coronary artery calcification represents one of the new subclinical markers of the coronary artery disease which is currently under intense study. The presence of calcium in the coronary arteries intima, in the atherosclerotic plaque, can be radiologically assessed by high-resolution and velocity computed tomography (Electron-Beam Computed Tomography). The coronary calcification correlates significantly with the clinical manifestations of the ischemic heart disease, with the severity of the coronary stenosis and with acute coronary events. Moreover, it can be detected long time before the clinical onset of the coronary disease which makes it useful in predicting the cardiovascular risk and possibly in the ischemic heart disease prevention in patients or populations at high risk. Such a group is that of diabetic patients in which coronary morbidity and mortality are significantly higher than those observed in non-diabetic populations. The following chapter summarizes the current data concerning the role and importance of coronary calcification in diabetes mellitus.

INTRODUCTION

Current epidemiological data indicate that, although widely accepted by the medical community as good indicators or risk, conventional or traditional cardiovascular risk factors, such as cholesterol, smoking, blood pressure, are in fact suboptimal predictors of cardiovascular disease (CVD) and acute coronary events [1]. Recent data have shown that relying excessively on the severity of luminal stenosis as the main determinant of acute events may be wrong since, in fact, the majority of acute events occur in individuals with non-critical arterial stenoses [2, 3].

These observations suggest that new markers of subclinical atherosclerosis, currently under investigation [4], may substantially add in terms of risk stratification of asymptomatic individuals and in terms of defining groups to which prevention efforts should be targeted [5–7].

CORONARY CALCIUM AS A SURROGATE MARKER OF CORONARY ARTERY DISEASE (CAD)

Coronary artery calcification is a useful surrogate marker of CAD that can be measured non-invasively with the electron-beam computed tomography (EBCT) imaging. Electron-beam computed tomography is a cross-sectional imaging technique with high spatial and temporal resolution, currently acknowledged as the gold standard for calcium detection in the coronary arteries [1]. Using a fourth generation ultra-fast computed tomography scanner, imaging is timed to the point in diastole when the motion of the heart is the least (approximately 40–60% of the R-R cycle on the EKG), and each image requires only 50–100 msec for completion [1]. Coronary calcification is quantitated using a score calculated according to the Agatston method [8]. A calcium score for each region is calculated by multiplying the area by the peak density of the calcified lesion. For a density of 130–200 Hounsfield units (HU), the density coefficient is 1, for 201–300 HU it is 2, for 301–400 HU it is 3, and for ≥ 401 HU it is 4. A total calcium score in Agatston units can then be computed by adding up the scores for all slices, separately for left main, left anterior descending, circumflex, and right coronary arteries. The main limitation of this score is its limited reproducibility. For this reason, another scoring method was recently introduced, the calcium volume score, which demonstrates low interscan variability [9].

Coronary calcium accumulates from very early stages of plaque formation, as early as the fatty streak stage [10]. As the atheroma grows and develops into a larger and more mature plaque, with collection of more cholesterol, inflammatory and fibrous cells, calcium accumulates at the base of the intima. At this stage, it becomes easily detectable by means of EBCT surface imaging [1] (Figure 28.1).

Coronary artery calcium was shown to be a good predictor of CAD events. Arad et al. [11] followed 1,173 asymptomatic adults for an average of 19 months. Patients with new CAD events had a significantly higher calcium score at screening than patients without events (764 ± 935 vs. 135 ± 432, p < 0.0001). Detrano et al. [12] studied 491 symptomatic patients referred to sequential cardiac catheterization and EBCT imaging for an average of 30 months. Patients with a score above the median (≥ 75.3) had a 6-fold greater number of events than those with a score below the median. In logistic regression analyses, calcium score was the only significant predictor of events, independent of age, gender and number of diseased vessels. Similarly, following 632 asymptomatic patients screened with EBCT, Raggi et al. [13] noted that the hazard ratio for having an event was significantly higher for patients with a high calcium score than for patients with a high CVD risk profile, suggesting that the presence of high calcium scores carries a severe prognostic implication that appears to be incremental to that provided by the presence of conventional CVD risk factors. Al these are solid evidence that calcium score is a good marker of coronary atherosclerotic disease, especially in asymptomatic individuals at intermediate risks of CAD.

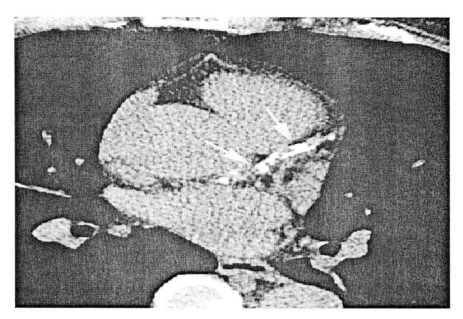

Figure 28.1
Positive coronary calcification.

CORONARY ARTERY CALCIFICATION IN DIABETES

Diabetic patients experience higher CVD incidence, including myocardial infarction, stroke, intermittent claudication [14, 15, 16], as well as shorter survival and increased mortality [17], when compared with the general population. In patients with both type 1 and type 2 diabetes, CVD occurs earlier in life [14, 18] and affects women almost as often as men [19]. However, the basis for the excess CVD risk in patients with diabetes remains unclear. A greater prevalence of classical CVD risk factors (hypertension, high LDL-cholesterol, high triglyceride, low HDL-cholesterol, smoking) as well as of novel CVD risk factors (insulin-resistance, central obesity, impaired fibrinolysis and subclinical inflammation) has been noted among patients with both type 1 and type 2 diabetes than among non-diabetic subjects [16, 20, 21]. Although all contribute to the increased risk, they account for less than half of the excess CVD mortality associated with diabetes [22]. Elevated CVD risk factors may be present years before the diagnosis of diabetes, and clinical CVD is often present at the time of diagnosis of type 2 diabetes [23, 24]. However, little is known about the prevalence of subclinical CVD and the risk factors for its

progression among individuals with diabetes. The information presented below summarizes the current knowledge about the extent and importance of coronary artery calcification in diabetes.

TYPE 2 DIABETES

Hoff *et al.* [25] recently examined the relationship between conventional CVD risk factors and coronary calcification among 30,908 healthy adults aged 30 to 90 years. After age, the strongest predictor of coronary calcification in both men and women was diabetes. History of diabetes was associated with a two-fold higher prevalence of coronary calcification in both genders [odds ratio, 95% confidence intervals 1.83 (1.42–2.34) in men and 2.17 (1.66–2.82) in women], independent of age, smoking, family history of CVD, hypercholesterolemia and hypertension. Among a group of patients referred to Wong *et al.* [26] for EBCT, the patients with self-reported diabetes (6.4%) had a 2.32 (1.06–5.08) higher odds for having any detectable calcification, compared with non-diabetic subjects in the referral sample. Among 103 patients with type 2 diabetes examined by Yoshida *et al.* [27], the mean coronary calcification score was 245 *vs.* 149 (p < 0.05) among matched controls. Similarly,

517

Schurgin and colleagues [28] reported that patients with type 2 diabetes had a significant increase in the prevalence of CAC scores ≥ 400 (25.9%) compared with randomly selected (7.2%) and matched (14.4) non-diabetic individuals. Using clinic-based family data, Wagenknecht et al. [29] reported a high prevalence (27%) of extensive coronary calcification (≥ 400) in subjects with type 2 diabetes compared with non-diabetic siblings (8%, p = 0.003). The extent of coronary calcification was associated with duration of diabetes and was a heritable trait in these families ($h^2 \geq 40\%$). Recent findings from a community-based cohort participating in the Framingham Offspring Study [30] extended these observations, providing further evidence of excessive coronary calcification among participants with diagnosed type 2 diabetes [OR=6.0 (1.4–25.2)], diabetes recently diagnosed during an oral glucose tolerance test [OR=2.1 (0.8–5.5)], and impaired glucose tolerance [OR=1.5 (0.7–3.4)]. Furthermore, Meigs and colleagues [30] found that this excess risk for subclinical coronary atherosclerosis in diagnosed type 2 diabetic patients was independent of elevations in CVD risk factors. These data also point out that there may be excess coronary artery calcification in subjects with pre-diabetes or clinically undetected glucose intolerance, as suggested by the substantially, although not significantly, higher OR in patients with impaired glucose tolerance. This supports the recommendation that it is appropriate to initiate aggressive CVD prevention at the time of diagnosis in all patients with type 2 diabetes.

TYPE 1 DIABETES

Several studies in patients with type 1 diabetes have demonstrated age-specific rates of coronary calcification and associations with a number of classical and emerging CVD risk factors. Among 101 subjects aged 17–28 years with type 1 diabetes of over 5 years' duration and no history of heart disease, Starkman et al. [31] found eleven subjects (10.9%) with calcium scores higher than 0. Smokers were nearly five times more likely than nonsmokers to have calcification (p = 0.03). In addition, each 0.36-mm/l increment of Lp (a) was associated with a 10% increased risk for coronary

artery calcification (p = 0.05), after controlling for potentially confounding factors. Two large studies that included both patients with type 1 diabetes and non-diabetic controls [32, 33] recently reported similar results. In the United Kingdom, Colhoun and colleagues [32] compared coronary artery calcification and CVD risk factors among 199 type 1 diabetic subjects and 201 non-diabetic controls age 30 to 55 years, asymptomatic for CAD. In non-diabetic participants there was a large gender difference in the prevalence of calcification (men 54%, women 21%, OR=4.5 (2.4–6.5), p < 0.001). Type 1 diabetes was associated with increased calcification prevalence in women (47%), but not in men (52%), so that the gender difference in calcification was lost. The odds ratio for diabetes-associated calcification was 3.9 times higher in women than in men, adjusted for age (p=0.002). On adjustment for conventional CVD risk factors (lipids, smoking, blood pressure, body mass index), diabetes remained associated with a threefold higher odds ratio of calcification in women than in men (p=0.02). Dabelea et al. [33] studied 656 patients with type 1 diabetes and 764 non-diabetic controls age 20–55 years, without known CAD, participants in the Coronary Artery Calcification in type 1 diabetes (CACTI) study, in Denver, Colorado. There were more diabetic than non-diabetic people with scores > 0, especially among women. In each age-group examined, diabetes was associated with a higher prevalence of any calcification (Figure 28.2). In men, type 1 diabetes was associated with a 2.1-fold higher age-adjusted prevalence of calcification (48% vs. 39%) while in women, the age-adjusted effect of diabetes on calcification was 3.6 times higher (27% vs. 12%, Figure 28.3). In this study type 1 diabetes was associated with a 1.9 times higher odds for calcification in women than in men. Different from the British study, on adjustment for waist-to-hip ratio, visceral fat (measured with computed tomography), and HDL and LDL-cholesterol, the diabetes-by-gender interaction lost significance. The U.S. CACTI data concluded, therefore, that gender differences in insulin-resistance-associated fat deposition, and HDL and LDL cholesterol distribution may explain why diabetes increases coronary calcification, and likely coronary artery disease, in women more than in men. Another interesting finding of the CACTI study was a significant association between

Prevalence

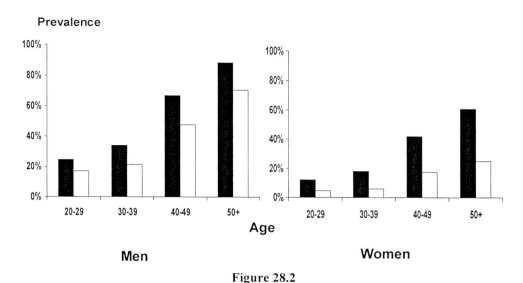

Figure 28.2

Prevalence of coronary calcification (CAC scores > 0) by age group and diabetes status (black bars = type 1 diabetes; white bars = controls) in CACTI men and women [33].

Prevalence

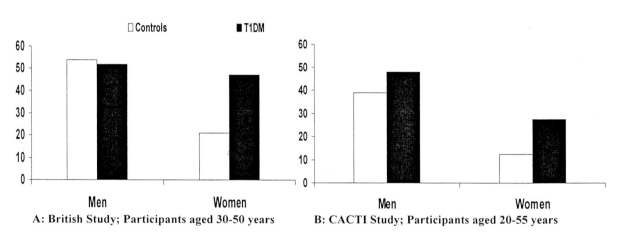

Figure 28.3

Prevalence of coronary calcification (CAC scores > 0) by diabetes status and gender
(black bars = type 1 diabetes; white bars = controls).

Panel A: British Study [32]; Panel B: CACTI Study [33].

insulin resistance, computed with linear regression based on an equation previously validated in type 1 diabetic adults [34], and calcification in both type 1 diabetic subjects (OR=1.6) and controls (OR=1.4), independent of conventional CVD risk factors (lipids, hypertension and smoking).

The ability to track progression of coronary calcification to assess effectiveness of therapy or the need for future cardiac testing are promising

for patients with diabetes [35]. The CACTI study measured calcification twice during an interval of 2.7 years in 109 participants with type 1 diabetes age 20–55 years. Progression of calcification was found in 21 patients, based on change in the square root-transformed volume score [36]. In multiple logistic regression, calcification progression was associated with baseline hyperglycemia (OR=7.11; 1.4–37), after adjustment for presence of calcification at baseline, diabetes duration, sex and age, suggesting that suboptimal glycemic control may be associated with progression of coronary artery disease.

All these recent data are conclusive evidence that coronary calcification is increased in diabetes and is associated with CVD risk factors. However, there is still controversy about whether coronary calcification in patients with diabetes is associated with clinical and angiographic coronary artery disease. At the 10-year follow-up examination of the Pittsburgh Epidemiology of Diabetes Complications (EDC) Study Cohort, 302 adults with type 1 diabetes received EBCT [37]. Coronary calcification correlated with most CVD risk factors and had 84% and 71% sensitivity for clinical CVD in men and women. A coronary artery calcification score of 400 was the most efficient calcium correlate of coronary artery disease. Hosoi *et al.* [38] recently examined the relationship between coronary calcification and angiographic stenosis in 282 symptomatic patients with and without diabetes. The authors were able to show that the sensitivity and specificity of EBCT to detect significant coronary stenosis was not significantly different between diabetic and non-diabetic patients. In patients with diabetes, a calcium score ≥ 90 was associated with 75% sensitivity and 75% specificity, whereas a score ≥ 200 had 64% sensitivity and 83% specificity for significant coronary stenosis.

There is concern that some of the signals detected by EBCT in diabetes represents medial (Mönkeberg's sclerosis) rather than intimal calcification. Although pathology studies suggest that calcification in coronary arteries primarily involves the intimal layer [39], more research is needed to address the EBCT potential to discriminate between medial and intimal calcification in diabetes.

The identification of asymptomatic high-risk individuals can provide the opportunity to initiate preventive actions. Because EBCT is a non-invasive technique and can be performed without the need for exercise testing it may become a useful tool to predict coronary artery disease in patients with diabetes, a population with very high CVD morbidity and mortality.

REFERENCES

1. Raggi P. Coronary calcium on electron beam tomography imaging as a surrogate marker of coronary artery disease. *Am J Cardiol,* **87:** 27A–34A, 2001.
2. Falk E, Shah PK, Fuster V. Coronary plaque disruption. *Circulation,* 92: 657–671, 1995.
3. Davies MJ. Pathophysiology of acute coronary syndromes. *Indian Heart Journal,* **52:** 473–479, 2000.
4. Raggi P, Cooil B, Callister TQ. Use of electron beam tomography data to develop models for prediction of hard coronary events. *American Heart Journal,* **141:** 375–382, 2001.
5. Callister T, Raggi P. Electron-beam computed tomography: a Bayesian approach to risk assessment. *Am J Cardiol,* **88:** 39E–41E, 2001.
6. Raggi P. Coronary-calcium screening to improve risk stratification in primary prevention. *Journal of the Louisiana State Medical Society,* **154:** 314–318, 2002.
7. Raggi P. Electron beam tomography as an endpoint for clinical trials of antiatherosclerotic therapy. *Current Atherosclerosis Reports,* **2:** 284–289, 2000.
8. Agatston AS, Janowitz WR, Hildner FJ, Zusmer NR, Viamonte M Jr., Detrano R. Quantification of coronary artery calcium using ultrafast computed tomography. *Journal of the American College of Cardiology,* 15: 827–832, 1990.
9. Newman AB, Naydeck B, Sutton-Tyrrell K, Edmundowicz D, Gottdiener J, Kuller LH. Coronary artery calcification in older adults with minimal clinical or subclinical cardiovascular disease. *Journal of the American Geriatrics Society,* **48:** 256–263, 2000.
10. Kronmal RA, Smith VE, O'Leary DH, Polak JF, Gardin JM, Manolio TA. Carotid artery measures are strongly associated with left ventricular mass in older adults (a report from the Cardiovascular Health Study). *Am J Cardiol,* **77:** 628–633, 1996.
11. Arad Y, Spadaro LA, Goodman K, Lledo-Perez A, Sherman S, Lerner G, Guerci AD. Predictive value of electron beam computed tomography of the coronary arteries. 19-month follow-up of 1173 asymptomatic subjects. *Circulation,* 93: 1951–1953, 1996.
12. Detrano R, Hsiai T, Wang S, Puentes G, Fallavollita J, Shields P, Stanford W, Wolfkiel C, Georgiou D, Budoff M, Reed J. Prognostic value of coronary calcification and angiographic stenoses in patients undergoing coronary angiography. *Journal of the American College of Cardiology,* **27:** 285–290, 1996.

13. Raggi P, Callister TQ, Cooil B, He ZX, Lippolis NJ, Russo DJ, Zelinger A, Mahmarian JJ. Identification of patients at increased risk of first unheralded acute myocardial infarction by electron-beam computed tomography. *Circulation,* **101:** 850–855, 2000.

14. Krolewski AS, Kosinski EI, Warram JH, Leland OS, Busick EJ, Asmal AC, Rand LI, Christlieb AR, Bradley RF, Kahn CR. Magnitude and determinants of coronary artery disease in juvenile-onset, insulin-dependent diabetes mellitus. *Am J Cardiol,* **59:** 750–755, 1987.

15. Chun BY, Dobson AJ, Heller RF. The impact of diabetes on survival among patients with first myocardial infarction.[comment]. *Diab Care,* **20:** 704–708, 1997.

16. Savage MP, Krolewski AS, Kenien GG, Lebeis MP, Christlieb AR, Lewis SM. Acute myocardial infarction in diabetes mellitus and significance of congestive heart failure as a prognostic factor. *Am J Cardiol,* **62:** 665–669, 1988.

17. Miettinen H, Lehto S, Salomaa V, Mahonen M, Niemela M, Haffner SM, Pyorala K, Tuomilehto J. Impact of diabetes on mortality after the first myocardial infarction. The FINMONICA Myocardial Infarction Register Study Group. *Diab Care,* **21:** 69–75, 1998.

18. Haffner SM, Stern MP, Hazuda HP, Mitchell BD, Patterson JK. Cardiovascular risk factors in confirmed prediabetic individuals. *JAMA,* **263:** 2893–2898, 1990.

19. Lloyd CE, Kuller LH, Ellis D, Becker DJ, Wing RR, Orchard TJ. Coronary artery disease in IDDM. Gender differences in risk factors but not risk. *Arterioscler Thromb Vasc Biol,* **16:** 720–726, 1996.

20. Pyorala K, Laakso M, Uusitupa M. Diabetes and atherosclerosis: an epidemiologic view. *Diabetes-Metabolism Reviews,* **3:** 463–524, 1987.

21. Meigs JB, Mittleman MA, Nathan DM, Tofler GH, Singer DE, Murphy-Sheehy PM, Lipinska I, D'Agostino RB, Wilson PW. Hyperinsulinemia, hyperglycemia, and impaired hemostasis: the Framingham Offspring Study. *JAMA,* **283:** 221–228, 2000.

22. Meigs JB, Stafford RS. Cardiovascular disease prevention practices by U.S. Physicians for patients with diabetes. *Journal of General Internal Medicine,* **15:** 220–228, 2000.

23. Haffner SM, Stern MP, Hazuda HP, Mitchell BD, Patterson JK. Cardiovascular risk factors in confirmed prediabetic individuals. Does the clock for coronary heart disease start ticking before the onset of clinical diabetes? *JAMA,* **263:** 2893–2898, 1990.

24. Kuller LH, Velentgas P, Barzilay J, Beauchamp NJ, O'Leary DH, Savage PJ. Diabetes mellitus: subclinical cardiovascular disease and risk of incident cardiovascular disease and all-cause mortality. *Arteriosclerosis, Thrombosis & Vascular Biology,* **20:** 823–829, 2000.

25. Hoff JA, Daviglus ML, Chomka EV, Krainik AJ, Sevrukov A, Kondos GT. Conventional coronary artery disease risk factors and coronary artery calcium detected by electron beam tomography in 30,908 healthy individuals. *Ann Epidemiol,* **13:** 163–169, 2003.

26. Wong ND, Kouwabunpat D, Vo AN, Detrano RC, Eisenberg H, Goel M, Tobis JM. Coronary calcium and atherosclerosis by ultrafast computed tomography in asymptomatic men and women: relation to age and risk factors. *American Heart Journal,* **127:** 422–430, 1994.

27. Yoshida M, Takamatsu J, Yoshida S, Tanaka K, Takeda K, Higashi H, Kitaoka H, Ohsawa N. Scores of coronary calcification determined by electron beam computed tomography are closely related to the extent of diabetes-specific complications. *Hormone & Metabolic Research,* **31:** 558–563, 1999.

28. Schurgin S, Rich S, Mazzone T. Increased prevalence of significant coronary artery calcification in patients with diabetes. *Diab Care,* **24:** 335–338, 2001.

29. Wagenknecht LE, Bowden DW, Carr JJ, Langefeld CD, Freedman BI, Rich SS. Familial aggregation of coronary artery calcium in families with type 2 diabetes. *Diabetes,* **50:** 861–866, 2001.

30. Meigs JB, Larson MG, D'Agostino RB, Levy D, Clouse ME, Nathan DM, Wilson PW, O'Donnell CJ. Coronary artery calcification in type 2 diabetes and insulin resistance: the Framingham offspring study. *Diab Care,* **25:** 1313–1319, 2002.

31. Starkman HS, Cable G, Hala V, Hecht H, Donnelly CM. Delineation of prevalence and risk factors for early coronary artery disease by electron beam computed tomography in young adults with type 1 diabetes. *Diab Care,* **26:** 433–436, 2003.

32. Colhoun HM, Rubens MB, Underwood SR, Fuller JH. The effect of type 1 diabetes mellitus on the gender difference in coronary artery calcification. *Journal of the American College of Cardiology,* **36:** 2160–2167, 2000.

33. Dabelea D, Kinney G, Snell-Bergeon JK, Hokanson JE, Eckel RH, Ehrlich J, Garg S, Hamman RF, Rewers M. Effect of Type 1 Diabetes on the Gender Difference in Coronary Artery Calcification: A Role for Insulin Resistance? The Coronary Artery Calcification in Type 1 Diabetes (CACTI) Study. *Diabetes,* **52:** 2833–2839, 2003.

34. Williams KV, Erbey JR, Becker D, Arslanian S, Orchard TJ. Can clinical factors estimate insulin resistance in type 1 diabetes? *Diabetes* **49:** 626–632, 2000.

35. Budoff MJ, Lane KL, Bakhsheshi H, Mao S, Grassmann BO, Friedman BC, Brundage BH. Rates of progression of coronary calcium by electron beam tomography. *Am J Cardiol,* **86:** 8–11, 2000.

36. Snell-Bergeon JK, Hokanson JE, Jensen L, Mackenzie T, Kinney G, Dabelea D, Eckel RH, Ehrlich J, Garg S, Rewers M. Progression of Coronary Artery Calcification in Type 1 Diabetes. *Diab Care,* **26:** 2923–2928, 2003.

37. Olson JC, Edmundowicz D, Becker DJ, Kuller LH, Orchard TJ. Coronary calcium in adults with type 1 diabetes: a stronger correlate of clinical coronary artery disease in men than in women. *Diabetes,* **49:** 1571–1578, 2000.

38. Hosoi M, Sato T, Yamagami K, Hasegawa T, Yamakita T, Miyamoto M, Yoshioka K, Yamamoto T, Ishii T, Tanaka S, Itoh A, Haze K, Fujii S. Impact of diabetes on coronary stenosis and coronary artery calcification detected by electron-beam computed tomography in symptomatic patients. *Diab Care,* **25:** 696–701, 2002.

39. Burke AP, Weber DK, Kolodgie FD, Farb A, Taylor AJ, Virmani R. Pathophysiology of calcium deposition in coronary arteries. *Herz,* **26:** 239–244, 2001.

29

HEART FAILURE IN DIABETES MELLITUS

Katalin BABEŞ, Amorin-Remus POPA, Petru Aurel BABEŞ

The increasing comorbidity of diabetes and congestive heart failure becomes a new challenge for cardiological care. Although diabetic cardiomyopathy shows no unique morphological features, profound alterations are found at the biochemical level. Hyperglycaemia induces maladaptative mechanisms that can interfere with efficacy of cardiac energy metabolism, contractile myofibril function, and excitation-contraction coupling, resulting in cytoskeletal changes and increased neurohormonal activity. Metabolic conditions can induce cardiac remodelling and mechanisms, acting in a vicious circle in which both heart failure and insulin resistance contribute.

Diabetic patients have a particularly high risk for developing heart failure, and their prognosis is worse than the already unfavourable outlook for non-diabetic heart failure patients. Identified reasons for this dismal prognosis include the poor outcome of myocardial infarction, the possible existence of a specific diabetic cardiomyopathy, the severity and distribution of coronary artery disease and disturbed autonomic function.

Treatment of symptomatic heart failure in the diabetic patient follows principles outlined in the European Society of Cardiology guidelines on the treatment of congestive heart failure. Few, if any, studies have addressed in detail the therapeutic efficacy of conventional treatment in a diabetic population. In the absence of clinical trials that directly address the subject, it is not known whether there are any strategies that may prevent or at least postpone the development of heart failure among diabetic patients. The implication is that more aggressive metabolic care at an early stage of the disease may delay restructuring of the myocardium and atheromatosis.

Presently, therapeutic efforts are frequently initiated at a late stage of the disease, during which only a modest symptomatic improvement and prolongation of longevity may be obtained. Combined efforts of cardiologists and diabetologists are needed in screening at-risk patients and institution of preventive measures.

INTRODUCTION

Diabetes mellitus (DM), and in particular the type 2 DM, has become an increasingly prevalent disease worldwide. The combination of an ageing population, decreasing levels of physical activity and poor dietary habits (over-consumption) are strong promoting factors. The number of diabetic individuals is predicted to reach 300 million in the 2025, accounting for 5.4% of the global population [1, 2]. Only recently the close interrelation between diabetes and cardiovascular disease was elucidated. Thus, 28% of patients with known coronary artery disease have diabetes, and as many as 70% of patients with acute coronary syndromes have abnormal glucose metabolism, either in the form of diabetes or impaired glucose tolerance [3].

Diabetes and heart failure is also a surprisingly common combination. In some cohorts, antidiabetic drugs were prescribed to approximately 35% of the patients hospitalized because of heart failure.

EPIDEMIOLOGY

Between 0.4 and 2% of the total European population has congestive heart failure; the prevalence increases with age, affecting 6–10% of those older than 65 years of age [4]. The leading causes of chronic heart failure are hypertension and ischaemic heart disease, which comprise 80% of all cases [5]. Another factor that influences this pattern is the increasing prevalence of type 2 diabetes.

The FRAMINGHAM study was the first epidemiological study to demonstrate an increased risk of congestive heart failure in patients with diabetes mellitus. Compared with non-diabetic males and females, the estimated increase in the incidences of heart failure for young diabetic males was fourfold, for females was eightfold [6]. The proportion of diabetic patients with heart failure enrolled in the large randomized controlled clinical trials ranged from 10% in NETWORK [7]-(a trial planned to be representative of a complete heart failure population), through 23% in CONSENSUS [8] (Cooperative North Scandinavian Enalapril Survival Study), and to 35% in RESOLVD [9] (Randomised Evaluation of Strategies for Left Ventricular Dysfunction). The prevalence

of diabetes among patients with more severe heart failure (*i.e.* New York Heart Association [NYHA] functional class III and IV) was even higher, ranging from 47% to 86% [10].

In 1979, Kannel and McGee [6] first reported on the interrelation between diabetes mellitus and congestive heart failure. Another landmark was Campania [11], an Italian cross-sectional study of an elderly population that demonstrated that congestive heart failure was an independent predictor of subsequent type 2 diabetes. In that study a 1% increase in glycosylated haemoglobin A1c (HbA1c), which represents the mean blood glucose concentration over the past 6–12 weeks, increased the risk for developing heart failure by 15%. The association with diabetes was independent of age, sex, blood pressure, body mass index and also of a family history of diabetes. The incidence of diabetes was 29% during 3 years of follow-up among heart failure patients initially free from this disease compared with 18% in a group of matched controls. A possible explanation is that an increased adrenergic drive, caused by heart failure, increases free fatty acid oxidation and insulin resistance, thereby decreasing glucose oxidation and precipitating type 2 diabetes [11].

Diabetes mellitus and congestive heart failure share multiple common subcellular mechanisms that may be tracked at different stages of impaired glucose tolerance and insulin resistance. The presence of hyperglycaemia has in fact been proposed as a causative factor that induces some maladaptive mechanisms, which are common to both heart failure and diabetic cardiomyopathy [12].

HEART FAILURE IN GENERAL

Heart failure is a syndrome that is recognized by a constellation of symptoms and signs that are produced by complex circulatory and neurohormonal responses to cardiac dysfunction. It is a heterogeneous diagnosis, that comprises a various clinical presentation. Heart failure usually comprises a combination of diastolic impairment and systolic dysfunction. These appear to represent different manifestations of the patho-physiological process that underlies left ventricular functional impairment, leading to the clinical manifestations of the heart failure [13]. A recent echo-cardiographical study combining classical recordings with tissue Doppler imaging supported this concept. It revealed a continuous progression of left ventricular dysfunction from asymptomatic diastolic dysfunction through symptomatic diastolic heart failure, and to symptoms mainly related to a significantly impaired systolic function. Approximately half of all patients seen in clinical practice for symptoms of heart failure were reported to have normal left ventricular systolic function in recent surveys such as IMPROVEMENT and the Euro Heart Failure Survey [14].

PROGNOSIS

The overall prognosis of the heart failure is poor, with half of newly diagnosed patients dying within 4 years. In the FRAMINGHAM cohort (1948–1988), the median survival after onset of heart failure was 1.7 years in men and 3.2 years in women [6]. Recent studies reported mortality rates ranging from 14% to 22% within 6 months after hospitalization for heart failure and 35% within 1 year. Patients with the combination of diabetes and heart failure secondary to ischaemic heart disease have substantially greater rates of short-term and long-term mortality. In the DIGAMI (Diabetes mellitus Insulin-Glucose infusion in Acute Myocardial Infarction) study [16], heart failure was the most common cause of death, accounting for 66% of total mortality during the first year of follow-up.

HEART FAILURE MECHANISMS IN DIABETICS

The high prevalence of heart failure in diabetic people cannot be accounted for by the known clustering of traditional risk factors, such as hypertension and hyperlipidaemia, alone. Recent reports indicate that diastolic heart failure is a primary presentation of heart disease, which is often already present in young, apparently 'healthy' diabetic people without additional cardiovascular risk factors [17]. The presentation of diabetic cardiomyopathy may therefore vary from clinically asymptomatic dysfunction to symptomatic impairment in myocardial performance, including increased wall stiffness and restricting ventricular filling, and causing a generalized hypokinesia.

MORPHOLOGY

Numerous investigations have been devoted to morphological alterations in the diabetic heart, as recently discussed by Hardin in an extensive review (mostly derived from autopsy studies) [18]. The most consistent findings were myocyte hypertrophy, deposition of glycoproteins positive for periodic acid-Schiff (PAS) staining, interstitial oedema, extracellular matrix accumulation, and myocyte loss with subsequent replacement by interstitial connective tissue. Vascular abnormalities such as thickening of the arterial intima, formation of microaneurysms and increased thickness of capillary basement have also been observed. However, none of those lesions are characteristic for diabetes as such. This indicates that the reason for diabetic cardiomyopathy may be found at a functional or biochemical level. Interestingly, it appears to be a synergism with structural changes that are usually seen in hypertensive hearts. This may have important therapeutic implications as the effects of antihypertensive therapy are especially favourable in diabetic patients.

DIASTOLIC DYSFUNCTION

The common response in a non-infarcted myocardial area subjected to acut ischemia is a compensatory hyperkinaesia that may almost normalize the ejection fraction. In GUSTO 1 (Global Utilization of Streptokinase and t-PA for Occluded coronary arteries-1), with more than 300 diabetic subjects, coronary angiograms performed 90 min after thrombolysis did not reveal any difference in the global ejection fraction between diabetic and non-diabetic patients. The normal compensatory hyperkinetic response in the non-infarcted area was, however, blunted among diabetic patients [19]. A decreased regional ejection fraction in non-infarcted myocardial areas of diabetic patients has been reported. During follow-up in the GUSTO trial, congestive heart failure was almost twice as common in diabetics compared to the non-diabetic cohort, despite smaller infarct sizes and ejection fraction which were similar to those in subjects without diabetes. These findings probably reflect impaired diastolic function, a finding that seems to be the most characteristic feature of diabetes-associated myocardial disease.

MYOCARDIAL BLOOD FLOW

Another reason for a compromised myocardial blood flow, or an inability to increase this flow when demanded, relates to impaired endothelial dependent vasodilatation. The underlying mechanism that produces endothelial dysfunction in the diabetic patient is not fully understood. Diabetic patients have a reduced myocardial flow reserve compared with matched controls even in the absence of obvious heart disease. Acute hyperglycaemia may impair endothelial-derived vasodilatation in healthy humans [20]. The inability to increase myocardial blood flow is independently related to long-term control of blood glucose, and not to age, blood pressure or blood lipids. Accordingly, it may be assumed that elevated blood glucose by itself is of considerable importance for the impaired vascular response.

GLUCOSE AND MYOCARDIAL FUNCTION

The UK Prospective Diabetes Study (UKPDS) [21] raised concerns that the incidence of heart failure is increased among persons with poor glycaemic control. In a 2-year follow-up of 49 000 adults with type 2 diabetes, an 8% increase in risk for developing heart failure was observed for a 1% increase in HbA1c. Recently acquired evidence goes beyond that finding, indicating that glycaemia represents a risk factor for heart failure even in individuals who, according to established criteria, are not considered diabetic.

Iribarren *et al.* [22] identified abnormal glucose metabolism (diabetes or impaired glucose tolerance) in 43% of patients with stable heart failure. In contrast to left ventricular volume, ejection fraction and neurohormonal activation, abnormal glucose metabolism was the only factor that correlated with increasingly severe symptoms and shorter 6-min walk test [23]. When the association was studied by applying hyperinsulinaemic clamp in patients with chronic heart failure and in healthy individuals, there was a relation between cardiac output and insulin sensitivity, but not with activation of the sympathetic nervous system. It was concluded that insulin resistance probably results from abnormalities at the cellular and molecular level of the skeletal myocyte, rather than from neurohormonal activation. In a recent cross-sectional, population-based study of individuals with no history of diabetes or heart disease [24], fasting and 2-h post-load glucose values were related to left ventricular diastolic dysfunction. However, in that study, increasing glucose levels, still in the upper normal range, had a negative impact on cardiac function.

MYOCARDIAL ENERGY METABOLISM

A number of myocardial structural and biochemical aberrations have been identified in heart failure, independent of the actual aetiology of the disease. Among them there are changes in cardiac energy metabolism, altered expression and function of contractile myofibrils, asynchronized excitation-contraction coupling, dysfunctional cytoskeleton proteins and beta-adrenergic receptor signalling, cardiac myocyte depletion, pathological volume and composition of the extracellular matrix, and increased activity of neurohormonal cytokines [25]. Many of these alterations are found in the diabetic heart.

The heart has a high rate of energy turnover, with adenosine triphosphate (ATP) as a basic source of energy. Stores of ATP are maintained at the required levels by high turnover, fueled by the reduction in $NADH^+$ and $FADH^{2+}$ predominantly generated by oxidation of acetyl coenzyme A. The two coexisting pathways (Figure 29.1) for energy supply are beta-oxidation of free fatty acids (FFA) and breakdown of carbohydrate.

a) The lipolytic pathway includes beta-oxidation of FFA to acetyl coenzyme A (acetyl-CoA), which is transferred to carbon dioxide within the Krebs cycle.

b) The carbohydrate pathway, compound of glycolysis, glycogeno-lysis and lactate oxidation, produces pyruvate, which is decarboxylated by pyruvate dehydrogenase (PDH) to acetyl-CoA and enters the final common pathway of the Krebs cycle.

In the aerobic condition, myocardium generates energy predominantly by oxidation of FFA (70–80%) and only a small part of energy results from glycolysis and pyruvate oxidation (20–30%) from glucose and lactate. In stressed conditions, such as myocardial ischaemia, pressure overload, and hypoxia, glucose and lactate become an important energy source, and there may be a 30-fold increase in glucose uptake [26].

The balance between available energy substrates is preserved by a system originally described by Randle *et al.* [27] in 1963 as a glucose-fatty acid cycle. This system influences energy utilisation in muscular and adipose tissues, controlling the relative blood concentration of the main energy substrates. Glucose utilization is controlled by the availability of insulin and by competition with FFA pathway metabolites. There are several 'checkpoints' in this process. Some of these reactions are controlled by the availability of energy within the cell through the level of ATP or its split products, whereas some are influenced by metabolites that are produced in the FFA pathway, or by citrate concentration, or a combination of several of these factors. Extracellular FFA elevation and intracellular lipid or lipid metabolite accumulation attenuates insulin signalling and impairs intracellular glucose uptake; it also efficiently inhibits PDH activity and limits the availability of glucophosphokinase.

An increase in blood glucose will, on the other hand, induce lipolysis via activation of lipoprotein lipase, with subsequent insulin desensitization. Hyperglycaemia, *via* generation of diacylglycerol, activates also the protein kinase C (PKC) family

(Figure 29. 2). This is a very potent agent that can change the activity of multiple enzymes. One irreversible consequence of increased PKC activity is deactivation of PDH, which causes disturbances in the oxidation chain. Thus, the PDH complex and the PKC family are the most crucial enzymes determining energy utilization in the working heart. The complex interplay between the two main energy substrates, and the activation and deactivation of enzymatic systems heavily impacts on the submolecular processes that are of crucial importance for the function of ion pumps and the permeability of cellular membranes. These effects go beyond the state of cellular metabolism because they involve additional pathways that can interfere with gene expression and change the activity of skeletal and functional proteins and enzymes [25, 27].

Young *et al.* [28] suggested that metabolic conditions play a significant role in cardiac adaptation and remodelling processes. A metabolic milieu characterized by hyperglycaemia and metabolites of FFA may induce foetal gene expression to an extent similar to that induced by increased shear stress and neurohormonal activation.

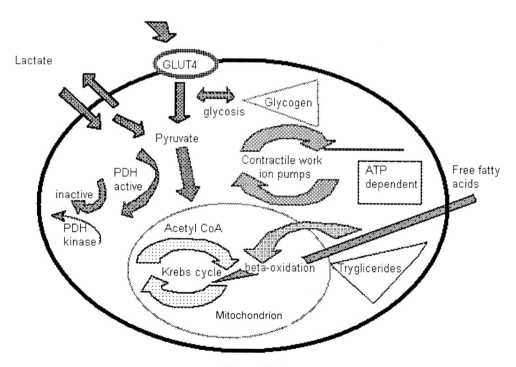

Figure 29.1

Schematic presentation of the myocardial metabolic pathways.

This remodelling leads to increased levels of beta myosin heavy chain, altered troponin T molecules, diminished creatinine phosphatase concentration (energy storage) and decreased sarcoplasmic ATP-ase activity, which results in myocyte hypertrophy associated with impaired myofibril contractile function, diminished energy storage and reduced energy supply [29]. By means of PKC-mediated pathway, hyperglycaemia paradoxically alters the function of endothelial nitric oxide synthase (eNOS) such that it acts as a superoxide generator, which then becomes systematically activated in the whole vascular bed, regardless of the absence of atherosclerotic lesions. Moreover, free radicals are potent stimulators of programmed cell death, which is substantially enhanced in diabetic hearts [28].

It has been suggested that the altered metabolism and impaired insulin action seen in the heart itself and in the skeletal muscles represent both a cause and a consequence of diabetic cardiomyopathy. It has recently been recognized that heart failure can induce insulin resistance of a magnitude that causes similar impairment of myocardial function. An intriguing hypothesis has been proposed, according to which primary heart failure can induce insulin resistance by initiating sympathetic overactivity, endothelial dysfunction, increased activity of cytokines such as tumour necrosis factor-alpha, and decreased skeletal muscle blood flow, which in turn leads to deterioration of skeletal muscle function. This may in turn result in a more sedentary life style, which further worsens the metabolic alterations typical for diabetes. These mechanisms may thus act in a vicious cycle, in which heart failure and insulin resistance worsen one another [28, 29].

TREATMENT OF HEART FAILURE IN DIABETICS

Treatment of symptomatic heart failure in the diabetic patient follows the principles extensively outlined in the European Society of Cardiology guidelines on the treatment of congestive heart failure. Few studies, if any, have addressed in detail the therapeutic efficacy of conventional treatment in a diabetic population.

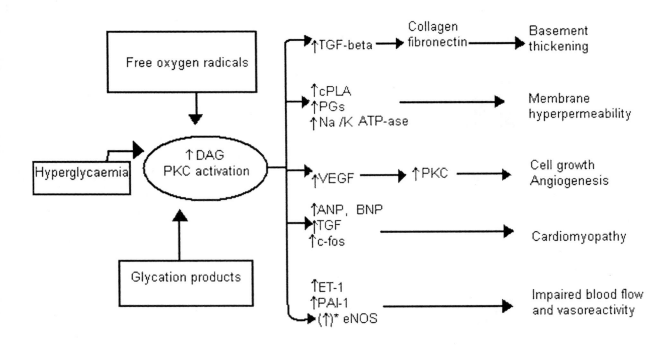

Figure 29.2

Multiple metabolic consequences of hyperglycaemia mediated by altered protein kinase C activity (PKC) and diacylglycerol (DAG).

DIURETICS

Diuretics are mandatory for the symptomatic treatment of heart failure. Whether the use of diuretics will improve or worsen the prognosis of diabetic patients is not known. In the absence of studies in diabetic subjects with heart failure the only available information is derived from antihypertensive trials. Warram *et al.* [30] claimed that diuretic-based antihypertensive treatment of diabetic patients was associated with excess mortality; this observation only related to years of treatment, however, not to the severity of concomitant nephropathy. The type of diuretic was not specified. In contrast, the SHEP (Systolic Hypertension in the Elderly Program) study reported that antihypertensive therapy based on low-dose diuretic (saluretics) effectively prevented major cardiovascular events, including mortality, in patients with type 2 diabetes [31]. Although no studies have specifically looked into the outcome of the use of diuretics in a heart failure population, loop diuretics are recommended rather than diuretics that may further impair the gluco-metabolic state.

ANGIOTENSIN-CONVERTING ENZYME INHIBITORS

The use of ACE inhibitors is a cornerstone in the treatment of congestive heart failure since the landmark CONSENSUS study [8]. Diabetic patients represent a fairly large subgroup of patient cohorts in long-term trials using several angiotensin-converting enzyme (ACE) inhibitors. Analysis of these subgroups reveals that mortality, as may be expected, is higher within the diabetic cohort than among non-diabetic patients. The Studies of Left Ventricular Dysfunction (SOLVD) prevention trial [32] investigated the effects of enalapril in patients with compromised left ventricular function, defined as a left ventricular ejection fraction of 35% or less but without clinical signs of heart failure. The SOLVD treatment study recruited similar patients with signs of heart failure. The ACE inhibitor had similar efficacy in diabetic and non-diabetic subgroups.

The Assesment of Treatment with Lisinopril And Survival (ATLAS) trial [33] compared high and low doses of lisinopril in patients with heart failure of NYHA class II–IV. The cohort included 3164 patients, of whom 611 were diabetic. This trial therefore contains one of the largest diabetic subgroups reported. Mortality and morbidity were considerably greater in diabetic than in non-diabetic patients. The reduction in mortality was 6% for non-diabetic patients versus 14% for the diabetic subgroup and emphasizes the need for appropriate doses of ACE inhibitors when treating diabetic as well as non-diabetic patients.

Hypoglycaemic events have been reported to increase following the administration of ACE inhibitors in diabetic patients. Because some ACE inhibitors have been shown to decrease insulin resistance, it is recommended that blood glucose be monitored in the early phase following the administration of an ACE inhibitor in patients already taking antidiabetic drugs [34].

In conclusion, ACE inhibitors are of value in the treatment of diabetic patients with congestive heart failure. Perhaps the relative efficacy is more apparent in this subgroup than among non-diabetic patients, fitting into the general knowledge that patients at high risk benefit the most. There are data supporting the use of a high-dose ACE inhibitor strategy. Precise knowledge is still lacking on the effect of ACE inhibitors in diabetic patients. Data presented are derived from subgroup analyses of clinical trials in which the diabetic population and their anti-diabetic therapy were poorly defined. The latter may very well influence the effect of other therapeutic measures.

BETA-BLOCKERS

In a subgroup analysis of two studies in which beta-blockers were administered to patients with acute myocardial infarction, starting early with intravenous injections and followed by oral treatment, almost all of the beneficial effects on mortality and non-fatal reinfarction were seen in the diabetic subgroup. Particularly beneficial effects in the diabetic subgroup were also seen in a study that employed the beta-blocker carvedilol, which also has vasodilating and antioxidant properties [35]. It may be speculated that beta-blockade is of particular value in the diabetic group, and that this benefit depends on a reduction in the accumulation of FFA and an increasing myocardial glucose utilization, as shown in clinical studies. The treatment with the most efficacious agent, namely carvedilol, was associated with a substantial (57%) decrease in myocardial use of FFA [36]. A reduction in heart rate, which is increased in diabetic patients, may also contribute to this.

Diabetic patients are often characterized by disturbed cardiac autonomic tone with decreased vagal function, causing sympathetic dominance. Both of these mechanisms would offer relief not only in the post-myocardial infarction phase but also in subjects with heart failure. Evidence to support this hypothesis is provided by subgroup analysis of patients from the recent Metoprolol CR/XL Randomized Intervention Trial in Congestive Heart Failure (MERIT-HF) trial [37]. In this study, 3991 heart failure patients, of whom 24% were diabetic, were randomly assigned to slow release metoprolol or placebo. The patients, who were in NYHA class II-IV and had a left ventricular ejection fraction below 40%, were already being treated with diuretics and ACE inhibitors. The addition of beta-blocker lowered the primary end-point, comprising mortality, and all-cause hospitalization to a similar extent in patients with (-27%) and without diabetes mellitus (-31%). On examining the actual proportion of this end-point reached in the subgroups, there were 21.6% in diabetic cohort and 13.6% in nondiabetic patients. On the currently best possible conventional heart failure treatment, these patients had a considerable less favourable prognosis than did their non-diabetic counterparts.

METABOLIC CONTROL

There are several reasons to assume the prognosis of patients with the combination of heart failure and diabetes mellitus should improve with meticulous metabolic control. For example, the proposed harmful effects of increased FFA oxidation and decreased glucose utilization should both be attenuated by intensive insulin treatment. Bersin *et al.* [38] applied a metabolic concept in the management of non-diabetic patients with severe heart failure by using the drug dichloroacetate. This compound stimulates pyruvate dehydrogenase activity thereby facilitating glucose oxidation and, in parallel, inhibiting free fatty acid metabolism. Myocardial extraction of lactate increased during dichloroacetate infusion. At the same time, there was an improved forward stroke volume, and increased left ventricular minute work, although myocardial oxygen consumption decreased. Another experimental attempt in treating patients with stable heart failure metabolically involved administration of carnitin palmitoyltransferase,

which is believed to counteract foetal reprogramming by increasing expression of sarcoplasmic ATP-ase 2a (SERCA2a) and alpha-myosin heavy chains [39]. After 3 months, a significant increase in maximum stroke volume during exercise and left ventricular ejection fraction was observed. This novel therapeutic approach, aiming at modulating intracellular metabolism, stimulated the interest in agents that can interfere with FFA, such as trimetazidine. Trimetazidine inhibits carnitine palmitoyltransferase 1, which is a key enzyme in a regulation of mitochondrial uptake of fatty acids. This compound therefore facilitates glucose uptake, inducing glycophosphorylation. The open-label Trimetazidine in Poland-1 (TRIMPOL-1) study demonstrated a significant improvement in exercise capacity and decreased frequency of anginal episodes in 50 diabetic patients with confirmed coronary artery disease and stable effort angina [40]. These promising results were supported by a pilot double-blind study conducted in 16 type 2 diabetic patients with advanced ischaemic dilated cardiomyopathy. In addition, a significant decrease in endothelin-1 concentrations was noted, suggesting that the drug can operate both on the heart and vascular endothelium. Futhermore, an activity resembling pharmacologically induced ischaemic pre-conditioning (mediated by adenosin) was recently hypothesized.

Discovering new pharmacological agents that would allow treatment of metabolic perturbations and thus alleviate myocardial dysfunction appears to be an attractive concept. At the same time, a well-known and relatively cheap metabolic modulator – insulin – still awaits to be rediscovered and used more adequately, according to the patients metabolic demands. In the DIGAMI study [16], an insulin-glucose infusion followed by multidose subcutaneous insulin considerably improved the long-term prognosis of diabetic patients with myocardial infarction. Moreover, Von Bibra *et al.* [41] recently found that improved insulin-based metabolic control improved the left ventricular diastolic function and myocardial microvascular perfusion reserve in type 2 diabetic patients studied over a period of 3 months. These findings add to the concept that it would be worthwhile, in a large clinical trial, testing the hypothesis that the outcome of diabetic heart failure patients would improve following meticulous metabolic control by means of insulin.

As early as 1924, Joslin [42] claimed that appropriate treatment of diabetes mellitus may be achieved only by keeping glucose metabolism as close to normal as possible, and similar to levels observed in non-diabetic people. However, insulin still appears to be underused.

CONCLUSION

Diabetic patients have a particularly high risk for developing heart failure, and their prognosis is worse than the already unfavourable outlook for non-diabetic heart failure patients. Reasons for this bad prognosis include the poor outcome of myocardial infarction, the possible existence of a specific diabetic cardiomyopathy, the severity and distribution of coronary artery disease and disturbed autonomic function.

In the absence of clinical trials that directly address the subject, it is not known whether there are any strategies that may prevent or at least postpone the development of heart failure among diabetic patients. It is clear that compromised left ventricular function may precede the clinical presentation of congestive heart failure by a considerable period of time. The implication is that more aggressive metabolic care at an early stage of the disease may delay restructuring of the myocardium and atheromatosis. It appears that such strategy must incorporate a multitude of activities, not in the least including aggressive normalization of the disturbed glucose metabolism, probably with early use of insulin. Such studies are presently being initiated.

Presently, therapeutic efforts are frequently initiated at a late stage of the disease, during which only a modest symptomatic improvement and prolongation of longevity may be obtained. Combined efforts of cardiologists and diabetologists are needed in screening at-risk patients and in institutioning preventive measures. Improved knowledge among diabetologists regarding treatment and prevention of cardiovascular complications, and among cardiologists regarding diabetology is a prerequisite for progress. Considering the large and rapidly increasing number of patients who are at risk, it is certainly urgent that this combined effort be started. The high costs associated with the management of diabetic patients with heart failure suggest that improved therapy is likely to be cost-effective, as for instance has been demonstrated in application of aggressive metabolic care in diabetic patients with myocardial infarction [43].

REFERENCES

1. Bartnik M, Malmberg K, Ryden L. Managing heart disease. Diabetes and the heart: compromised myocardial function-a common challenge; *Eur Heart J,* **5(Suppl B)**: B33–B41, 2003.
2. King H, Aubert RE, Herman WH. Global burden of diabetes 1995–2025. Prevalence, numerical estimates and projections. *Diabetes Care,* **21**: 1414–31, 1998.
3. EUROASPIRE II Group. Lifestyle & risk factors management and use of drug therapies in coronary patients from 15 countries. *Eur Heart J,* **22**: 554–72, 2001.
4. Ho KK, Pinsky JL, Kannel WB, Levy D. The epidemiology of heart failure: the Framingham Study. *J Am Coll Cardiol,* **22**: 6A–13A, 1993.
5. Remme WJ, Swedberg K for the ESC Task Force. Guidelines for the diagnosis and treatment of chronic heart failure. *Eur Heart J,* **22**: 1527–60, 2001.
6. Kannel WB, McGee DL. Diabetes and cardiovascular disease. The Framingham study. *JAMA,* **214**: 2035–8, 1979.
7. The NETWORK investigators. Clinical outcome with enalapril in symptomatic chronic heart failure; a dose comparison. *Eur Heart J,* **19**: 481–9, 1998.
8. The CONSENSUS trial study group. Effect of Enalapril on mortality in severe congestive heart failure. *N Engl J Med,* **316**:1429–35, 1987.
9. McKelvie RS, Yusuf S, Pericak D, *et al.* Comparison of candesartan, enalapril, and their combination in congestive heart failure: randomized evaluation of strategies for left ventricular dysfunction (RESOLVD) pilot study. The RESOLVD Pilot Study Investigators. *Circulation,* **100**:1056, 1999.
10. Reis SE, Holubkov R, Edmundowicz D, *et al.* Treatment of patients admitted to the hospital with congestive heart failure: speciality-related disparities in practice patterns and outcomes. *J Am Coll Cardiol,* **30**: 733, 1997.
11. Amato L, Paolisso G, Cacciatore F, *et al,* on behalf of the Observatorio Geriatrico Regione Campania Group. Congestive heart failure predicts the development of non-insulin dependent diabetes mellitus in the elderly. *Diabetes Metab,* **23**: 213–8, 1997.
12. Suskin N, McKelvie RS, Rolueau J, Sigouin C, Wiecek E, Yusuf S. Increased insulin and glucose levels in heart failure. *J Am Coll Cardiol,* **31** (suppl A): 249A, 1998.
13. Cohen-Solal A. Diastolic heart failure: myth or reality? *Eur J Heart Failure,* **4**: 395–400, 2002.

14. Euro Heart Failure. Report at the Annual Congress of the European Society Of Cardiology, Stockholm, 2001.
15. McGuire DK, Emanuelsson H, Granger CB, *et al,* for the GUSTO-II investigators. Influence of diabetes mellitus on clinical outcomes across the spectrum of acute coronary syndromes. *Eur Heart J,* **21**: 1750–8, 2000.
16. Malmberg K, Ryden L, Efendic S. A randomized study of insulin-glucose infusion followed by subcutaneous insulin treatment in diabetic patients with acute myocardial infarction: effects on 1-year mortality. *J Am Coll Cardiol,* **26**: 57–65, 1995.
17. Zoneraich S, Mollura JL. Diabetes and the heart state of the art in the 1990s. *Can J Cardiol,* **9**: 293–9, 1993.
18. Hardin N. The myocardial and vascular pathology of diabetic cardiomyo- pathy. *Coron Artery Dis,* **7**: 99–108, 1996.
19. Woodfield SL, Lundergran CF, Reiner JS, *et al.* Angiographic findings and outcome in diabetic patients treated with thrombolytic therapy for acute myocardial infarction: the GUSTO-I experience. *J Am Coll Cardiol,* **28**: 1661–9, 1996.
20. Williams SB, Goldfine AB, Timini FK, Ting HH, Roddy MA, Creafer MA. Acute hyperglycemia attentuates endothelium-dependent vasodilatation in humans in vivo. *Circulation,* **97**: 1695–701, 1998.
21. UKPDS-35. Association of glycaemia with macrovascular and microvascular complication of type 2 diabetes: a prospective observational study. *BMJ,* **321**: 405–12, 2000.
22. Iribarren C, Karter AJ, Go AS, *et al.* Glycemic control and heart failure among adult patients with diabetes. *Circulation,* **103**: 2668–73, 2001.
23. Suskin N, McKelvie RS, Burns RJ, *et al.* Glucose and insulin abnormalities relate to functional capacity in patients with congestive heart failure, *Eur Heart J,* **21**: 1368–75, 2000.
24. Holzmann M, Olsson A, Johansson J, Jensen-Urstad M. Left ventricular diastolic function is related to glucose in a middle-aged population. *J Intern Med,* **251**: 415–20, 2002.
25. Braunwald E, Bristow R. Congestive heart failure: fifty years of progress. *Circulation,* **102 (suppl 4)**: 14–23, 2000.
26. Stanley WC. Metabolic dysfunction in the diabetic heart. In: Stanley WC, Ryden L, eds. *The diabetic coronary patient.* Science Press Ltd, London, 1999.
27. Randle PJ, Garland PB, Hales CN, Newsholme EA. The glucose-fatty acid cycle. Its role in insulin sensitivity and the metabolic disturbances of diabetes mellitus. *Lancet,* **13**: 785–9, 1963.
28. Young M, McNulty P, Taegmeyer H. Adaptation and mal-adaptation of the heart in diabetes. Part II. *Circulation,* **105**: 1861–70, 2002.
29. Alpert N, Mulieri L, Warshaw D. The failing human heart. *Cardiovasc Res,* **54**: 1–10, 2002.
30. Warram JH, Laffel LMB, Valsania P, Christlieb AR, Krolewski AS. Excess mortality associated with diuretic therapy in diabetes mellitus. *Arch Intern Med,* **151**: 1350–6, 1991.
31. Curb JD, Pressel SL, Cutler JA, *et al.* for the Systolic in the Ederly Program Cooperative Research Group. Effect of diuretic-based antihyper- tensive treatment on cardiovascular disease risk in older diabetic patients with isolated systolic hypertension. *J Am Med Assoc,* **276**: 1886–92, 1996.
32. The SOLVD investigators. Effect of enalapril on survival in patients with reduced left ventricular ejection fraction and congestive heart failure. *N Engl J Med,* **325**: 293–302, 1991.
33. Ryden L, Armstrong PW, Cleland JGF, *et al,* on behalf of the ATLAS Study Group. Efficacy and safety of high-dose lisinopril in chronic heart failure patients at high cardiovascular risk, including those with diabetes mellitus. *Eur Heart J,* **21**: 1967–78, 2000.
34. Herings RMC, deBoer A, Stricker BHC, Leufkens HGM, Porsius A. Hypoglycemia associated with the use of inhibitors of angiotensin-converting enzyme. *Lancet,* **345**: 1195–8, 1996.
35. Bristow M, Gilbert EM, Abraham WT, *et al.* Effect of carvedilol on LV function and mortality in diabetic versus non-diabetic patients with ischemic or nonischemic dilated cadiomyopathy. *Circulation,* **84 (suppl)**: 664, 1996.
36. Wallhaus TR, Taylor M, DeGrado TR, *et al.* Myocardial free fatty acid and glucose use after carvedilol treatment in patients with congestive heart failure. *Circulation,* **103**: 2441–6, 2001.
37. Hjalmarson A, Goldstein S, Fagerberg B, *et al.* Effects of controlled-release metoprolol on total mortality, hospitalizations, and well-being in patients with heart failure: the Metoprolol CR/XL Randomized Intervention Trial in congestive heart failure (MERIT-HF). MERIT-HF Study Group. *JAMA,* **283**: 1295–302, 2000.
38. Bersin RM, Wolfe C, Kwasman M, *et al.* Improved hemodynamic function and mechanical efficiency in congestive heart failure with sodium dichloroacetate. *J Am Coll Cardiol,* **23**: 1617–24, 1994.
39. Schmidt-Schweda S, Holubarsch C. First clinical trial with etomoxir in patients with chronic congestive heart failure. *Clin Sci,* **99**: 27–35, 2000.
40. Szwed H, Sadowski Z, Pachocki R, *et al.* The anti-ischemic effects and tolerability of trimetazidine in coronary diabetic patients. A substudy from TRIMPOL-1. *Cardiovasc Drugs Ther,* **13**: 217–22, 1999.
41. Von Bibra H, Hansen A, Dounis V, Bystedt, Malmberg K, Ryden L. Diastolic myocardial function and myocardial microvasculature reserve improve with intense insulin treatment in type 2 diabetic patients. *Diabetologia,* **44**: 68, 2001.
42. Joslin EP. *The Treatment of Diabetes Mellitus,* 3rd edition. London, H. Kimpton, 1924.
43. Almbrand B, Johannesson B, Sjostrand B, Malmberg K, Ryden L. Cost-effectiveness of intense insulin treatment after acute myocardial infarction in patiens with diabetes mellitus; results from the DIGAMI study. *Eur Heart J,* **21**: 733–9, 2000.

30

CLINICAL EVOLUTION AND TREATMENT PARTICULARITIES FOR THE DIABETIC PATIENT WITH HEART FAILURE

Dinu DRAGOMIR, Carmen GINGHINĂ, Mirela MARINESCU

A growing trend in the number of diabetic patients with cardiac failure has been noticed lately and increased costs are related to the ambulatory assistance and especially the demand for repeated hospitalization.

Diabetic cardiac failure has well-known cardiac atherosclerotic pathology (coronary macroangiography) frequent association of arterial hypertension (in over 50% of the patients with diabetes mellitus) and last, but not least, a specific myocardial affectation, the so-called diabetic cardiomyopathy. Diabetics with cardiac insufficiency and coronary macroangiopathy frequently present a multi-coronary disease with diffuse atherosclerotic lesions. The presence of myocardial ischemia in diabetic patients can be explained through the insufficiency of the coronary microcirculation, under the conditions of permeable epicardial coronary arteries. Arterial hypertension and diabetes mellitus frequently coexists in the same patient, increasing significantly the cardiac failure risk. The concept of diabetic cardiomyopathy supposes a specific diffuse myocardial affectation, in the absence of epicardial coronary lesions, but most of the authors include in this notion the coronary microangiopathic lesions as well. As it is already known, these coronary microangiopathic lesions are generalized in diabetes mellitus and can be highlighted relatively easy in the early stage, having different other localizations (retinal, renal, etc). The non-invasive exploration (echocardiographic, radio-isotopic) brings valuable diagnostic elements, emphasizing the ventricular dysfunction that is initially diastolic and later systolic dysfunction, first at effort and than at rest.

The severity of the ventricular dysfunction in diabetic patients with cardiac failure is correlated with the level of metabolic control and with the presence of cardiac autonomic dysfunction – diabetic cardiac autonomic neuropathy (CAN) – even when there is no obvious coronary microangiopathy. The pharmacologic treatment of the diabetic patients with cardiac failure is similar to the non-diabetic patients. Diabetics present some particularities about treating heart failure, related to the frequency of renal dysfunction and electrolytic disorders, frequent association with HT and the obscure nature of the coronary atherosclerosis ± diabetic cardiomyopathy. ACE inhibitors and beta-blockers have a therapeutic benefit for the diabetic patients. Diuretic treatment presumes special precautions in the diabetics; thiazide-like diuretics (indapamide) gained an important place.

Metabolic drugs and anti-oxidants associated to the conventional treatment have been proved efficient in improving the prognosis of the diabetic patients with cardiac failure. Using combined alternative treatment strategies (non pharmacological) brings benefits from the cardiovascular mortality and morbidity point of view and can build a bridge for heart transplantation in diabetics with cardiac failure refractory to treatment.

PARTICULAR EPIDEMIOLOGIC ASPECTS OF THE CARDIAC DISEASE IN DIABETUS MELLITUS

IS HEART FAILURE REQUIRING SPECIAL ATTENTION WHEN IT COMES TO DIABETIC PATIENTS?

Diabetes mellitus represents a major risk factor of cardiovascular events in both general population and subjects that already present cardiac affection. About 70% of general mortality of the diabetic population is due to the cardiac affection. Furthermore, though a decrease of the cardiovascular disease has been noticed in general population of industrialized countries, the decrease rate is much lower in type 2 DM; for diabetic women, this rate is actually growing. Diabetes mellitus accelerates and aggravates the evolution of atherosclerosis, and severely affects the life expectancy. In diabetes mellitus type 1, the life expectancy declines by about 50% comparing with general population, and in type 2 diabetes mellitus it is appreciated to about 70% of the non-diabetic population value as a result of the high cardiovascular risk [1].

Epidemiological studies have proved that if no preventive approach and efficient therapeutic method are found, the incidence and prevalence of diabetes mellitus and heart failure will grow in the next decades.

Within the diabetic population, women present a higher risk of cardiac affection than men do, whilst within the general population men are more frequently affected by cardiovascular disease (male sex is considered a risk factor).

As shown previously, diabetes mellitus is a major risk factor for the cardiovascular disease, independent of other risk factors such as hypercholesterolemia, smoking, arterial hypertension, age, gender and body weight indices.

Prospective epidemiological studies showed that for the diabetic men and women the cardiovascular morbidity and mortality risk are 2–3 times, respectively 3–5 times higher than for the non-diabetic individuals of the same age. The frequency of congestive heart failure is 3 times higher in the old patients with diabetes mellitus [2].

The famous Framingham study observed a high morbidity through congestive heart failure in diabetic patients, the risk being about 5.2 times higher for women and 2.4 times higher for men. After excluding the coronary disease or valvular disease risk grew 3.8 times for diabetic men and 6.8 times for diabetic women.

In the last decades of the last century the heart failure became a major public health problem, highly affecting the population with diabetes mellitus or with lower tolerance for glucose. Its prevalence is estimated to continue its growth in the next 2 decades of this century. This growth seems to have no connection with the level of medical assistance because one of the highest rates of heart failure is reported in Western Europe and the United States where there is an excellent level of medical care. It is difficult to explain the explosion registered by the prevalence of this syndrome in the last decades. One of the reasons might be the lack of epidemiological data from the past, but certainly this is not the only explanation [3].

COSTS AND SOCIAL IMPACT

It is appreciated that the cardiac morbidity in diabetes mellitus is mainly due to the heart failure. It has been noticed that there is a trend of increasing number of diabetic patients with heart failure, increased ambulatory assistance and repeated hospitalization costs. As a result of the high prevalence within the diabetic population, of the high morbidity and the high requirement for hospitalization, heart failure in diabetic patients has a very important social impact, overcharging community's care systems in the developed countries [4, 5].

As the diabetic's heart failure is an invalidating disease that affects life quality and has a high mortality (especially sudden death), it remains a matter of public health for the next decades. Even when there is a well-organized medical care system, the high demand for care services, the large number of tests, special programs aiming cardiac transplantation, resynchronization and circulatory assistance are very expensive [6, 7].

To summarize:

– The incidence and prevalence of diabetes mellitus and heart failure in diabetic patients are growing;

– Middle aged diabetic patients have higher cardiovascular morbidity and mortality risk than non-diabetic patients of the same age;

– Diabetes mellitus cancels the gender differences of cardiovascular risk.

THE CONCEPT OF HEART FAILURE IN DIABETIC PATIENTS

THE ETIOLOGIC BASIS OF HEART FAILURE IN DIABETIC PATIENTS

Heart failure in patients with diabetes mellitus is a syndrome that evolves as a result of multiple etiopathological links and it is recognized after a series of signs and symptoms, produced by the complex neuro-hormonal and hemodynamic responses in cardiac dysfunction.

Diabetic's heart failure is found not only associated with known cardiac atherosclerotic pathology (coronary macroangiopathy), but also in the frequent association with arterial hypertension (in over 1/3 of the patients with diabetes mellitus) and in a specific myocardial affection (the so-called diabetic cardiomyopathy). The concept of diabetic cardiomyopathy supposes a specific myocardial affection, diffuse, in the absence of epicardial coronary lesions (coronary macroangiopathy). However, most of the authors also include in this notion the coronary microangiopathic lesions. As it is well known, these are generalized in diabetes mellitus and can be relatively easily highlighted in the early stages, having various localizations (retinal, renal, etc).

The presence of a specific cardiomyopathy in a diabetic person, without a significant coronary disease, HT or other myocardial disease etiologies, seems to contribute to an increased morbidity of the heart failure among the diabetic population. The coexistence of cardiomyopathy with a coronary ischemic disease – especially through macrovascular affection – is frequently met as etiologic substratum of this heart failure [2, 8].

The severity of ventricular dysfunction in diabetic patients with heart failure is correlated with the level of metabolic control and with the presence of an autonomic cardiac dysfunction –

diabetic's cardiac autonomic neuropathy (CAN) – even when there is no obvious coronary macroangiopathy [9].

Therefore, diabetes mellitus is a major risk factor that can contribute through various mechanisms to the heart failure development.

After making reference to the diabetic cardiomyopathy, we will discuss other etiopathogenic links involved in the diabetic's heart failure: coronary macroangiopathy, arterial hypertension, and cardiac autonomic neuropathy [10].

IS DIABETIC CARDIOMYOPATHY A DISTINCTIVE CLINICAL ENTITY?

Besides the known cardiac atherosclerotic pathology (ischemic cardiopathy with classical manifestation – acute myocardial infarction, angina pectoris, silent ischemia, and sudden death) in the last few years appeared the concept of a specific cardiac affection, defined as diabetic cardiomyopathy or, more recently, as the diabetic disease of the cardiac muscle.

Some authors prefer the name of diabetic cardiopathy, but the cardiologists recognize it under the name of diabetic cardiomyopathy (DMCM). This concept defines diffuse myocardial affection, initially subclinical, in the absence of any coronary lesions or arterial hypertension.

The first data regarding a specific cardiomyopathy in diabetic patients dates from 1974 and belongs to Rubler. He described at the necropsy of some young diabetic patients a cardiomegaly with microscopic changes of diffuse fibrosis, with deposits of mucopolysaccharides in the sub-endothelial layer of the intramural arterioles, in the presence of normal coronary arteries. Hamby introduced the term of diabetic cardiomyopathy, describing a myocardial primary idiopathic disease without a coronary implication, in the young diabetic patients. Other data that became reference points in the history of the diabetic cardiomyopathy are: Hamby and Zoneraich – description of diabetic cardiomyopathy; Regan – confirmation of the myocardial interstitial diffuse fibrosis with deposit of positive PAS glycoproteins; Senevirante – description of the pre-clinical phase of the diabetic cardiomyopathy (assigned to microangiopathy) and Fischer – proves a possible mechanism of DMCM as thickening of the basal membrane of the myocardial cell. In 1980, Factor proved the presence of microaneurysms in the arteriolar circulation in the diabetic heart [11, 12].

Recent data confirm the presence of the DMCM and WHO Experts Committee for cardiomyopathies recommends the notion of "diabetic heart muscle disease".

The practical concept of DMCM includes the diffuse myocardial affection in the absence of coronary lesions and microangiopathy. However, several authors (Factor, Fischer) also include in this notion the cardiac microangiopathic lesions that are part of the generalized affection of microangiopathic type in DM (nephropathy, retinopathy, and neuropathy). The existence of a specific diabetic cardiomyopathy in the persons without a significant coronary disease, HT or other etiologies of myocardial disease, seems to be a recognized accepted fact [11, 13].

Arguments supporting the concept of diabetic cardiomyopathy

The epidemiological studies showed that the frequency of the heart failure in the diabetic persons is higher than expected through the atherogenic risk factors. Moreover, the diabetic women have a higher incidence of heart failure than the diabetic men.

The histopathological studies proved that in DM there are typical microangiopathic lesions at the level of the myocardium that can contribute to the myocardial dysfunction. More characteristic to DMCM seems to be extended interstitial fibrosis with preserved myocytes morphology in the early stages. The accumulation of collagen at the level of diabetic myocardium is mainly of insoluble-collagen type, with reduction of the soluble fraction – suggesting that the main mechanism of collagen deposit is the reduction of collagen degradation (due to glycosylation) and not the increase of its synthesis. In the patients with diabetic cardiomyopathy, the changes in the interstitial composition represent the main cause of the ventricular compliance abnormalities. Extracellular matrices changes of myocardium can associate abnormalities of the myocyte membrane and enzymatic system (Ca^{2+}-ATP-ase and Na^+-ATP-ase) as well as accumulation of lipids (free fatty acids) that in advanced stages affects the contractility. Other experimental data have been

brought to support the DMCM concept: in dogs with DM experimentally induced, Regan describes the increase of the LV dimensions with parietal thickening and deposits of positive PAS material. Other authors highlighted the decrease of the cardiac output. Studies of myocardial ultrastructure, performed on rats with induced DM, show changes in the process of myocytes relaxation (change at the level of sarcoplasmic reticulum) and decrease of the contractile proteins that are reversible under insulin treatment. These investigations have created a strong support for the DMCM concept that can explain increased morbidity through congestive heart failure (CHF) in DM [14, 15].

Clinical studies. DMCM develops subclinically for a long time. It can be diagnosed either by mechanic-phonographic evaluation tests (outdated today) or by tracing out the left ventricle diastolic and/or systolic dysfunction by echocardiography evaluation and Doppler exam or by radionuclide ventriculography. Diabetic cardiomyopathy can be more or less symptomatic. In subclinical stage, for the diabetic normotensive persons who do not present other causes of left ventricle (LV) compliance reduction, the diagnosis is suggested by the existence of a diastolic dysfunction – mild or medium – identified with non-invasive methods (echocardiography-Doppler, radionuclide exploration). Advanced diabetic cardiomyopathy will manifest by signs and symptoms of congestive heart failure, but the diagnostic criteria compel to exclude HT, coronary disease or other cardiomyopathies – which is quite difficult to do in clinical practice. From the hemodynamic point of view, diabetic cardiomyopathy points out a predominant diastolic dysfunction, but this may also coexist with abnormal systolic function. Clinically, the diabetic cardiomyopathy presents more frequently with a dilative aspect and very rare with a restrictive one. In current practice, the coexistence with coronary ischemic disease – especially through microvascular affectation – is frequently met [16].

According to several authors, the presence of microvascular lesions is associated in the DMCM pathogenesis. For instance, retinopathy is often an emphasizing factor (marker) for DMCM.

The problem of diabetic microangiopathy (retinal and renal) is complex. Recent data, synthesizing a large experience, says that about 5% of the diabetic patients have a high susceptibility to develop early microvascular lesions, despite the balanced glycemic homeostasis. 20% of the diabetic patients, despite the hyperglycemia that expresses the DM unbalance, have a relative resistance to the appearance of microangiopathy. The rest of 75% of the cases associate those two possibilities, which include a net genetic component [14, 17].

Diabetic cardiomyopathy: clinical - evolutive forms

Four evolutive stages were described for DMCM:

• In the first stage there is an increased cardiac contractility, a true hyperkinetic syndrome with increase of the ejection fraction and of the LV circumferential shortening within a syndrome of tissular hyperperfusion, including renal vascular bed. Robinson (1994) identifies in the patients with DM type 2 with short evolution duration, the alteration of the diastolic function in about 28% of the cases, evaluated with echo-Doppler. This phase seems to be the result of the long-term metabolic unbalance and it is transitory and reversible under a correct treatment with insulin.

• In the second stage, the cardiac functional evaluation shows normal data of the diastolic and systolic function.

• In the third stage, it is noticed a progressive deterioration of the diastolic function, with preservation of the systolic function at rest.

• The fourth stage is characterized by the severe diastolic dysfunction associated with progressive systolic dysfunction [2, 14].

In the DMCM are included, by definition, both the LV functional changes (the diastolic dysfunction occurring early, then the systolic dysfunction, first at effort and later at rest) and morphological changes. For DMCM are considered typical the thickening of the interventricular septum (IVS) and of the posterior wall of LV (PWLV). [Table 30.1]

DMCM develops subclinically for a long time and there are several forms of manifestation:

• *Hypertrophic form of DMCM* (with predominance of IVS and PWLV hypertrophy) can appear relatively early, after several years of disease development, and it is reversible. Several authors (Rio *et al.*, 1992) presented extremely interesting data describing this entity in the newborn babies from diabetic mothers (even in the presence of a compensated DM during the pregnancy), which would be due to excess of maternal growth hormone. This form of unobstructive hypertrophic form of DMCM disappears spontaneously after few months. For both, children and adults, this form is described after several years of disease development (average 5.8 years in type 1 DM). Baandrup and Pierce showed by experimental and clinical studies that there is the possibility of DMCM-generated hypertrophy regression under intensive insulin treatment and some inhibitors of the conversion enzyme. The frequent existence of LV hypertrophy, especially in women with type 2 DM and hyperinsulinism, suggested the existence of other mechanisms as well, that induce left ventricle hypertrophy and the increase of LV mass, due, for instance, to the insulin-like growth factor.

• *Dilative form of DMCM* usually associated with congestive phenomena (initially at effort). This form occurs after a long-term disease development (about 12 years), especially under long-term metabolic unbalance, in parallel with the presence of microangiopathic complications.

• It has also been described a very rare *form of DMCM, restrictive type*, with large atria and normal size ventricles [11, 15].

Table 30.1

Clinical-evolutive stages of diabetic cardiomyopathy

	DMCM early stage Pure diastolic dysfunction	DMCM advanced Systolic + diastolic dysfunction
Pulmonary congestion	Yes	Yes
Cardiac flow	Normal/ ↑	Normal /↓
Ejection fraction	Normal	↓
LV dilatation	No	Yes

Some authors use classifications such as DMCM with manifest heart failure, DMCM with silent myocardial ischemia, DMCM with rhythm disorders.

In reality, these forms are associated and it is extremely difficult to delimitate these forms of DMCM, especially in the advanced forms of the disease, from the coronary ischemia manifestations.

We underline, and it is useful in medical practice, that the cardiac autonomic neuropathy that occurs early in type 1 DM is often associated with the modifications of the ventricular diastolic function, and can be considered an early marker for it. Cardiac autonomic neuropathy frequently manifests by persistent rest tachycardia and/or orthostatic arterial hypotension [2].

Diagnostic particularities in diabetic cardiomyopathy

Besides the clinical exam, in the current practice the pulmonary radiological examination can bring relevant elements regarding the cardiomegaly and pulmonary congestion.

DMCM diagnosis is supported, as we mentioned, by echo-Doppler with evaluation of the systolic and diastolic function. An important condition is the exclusion of the coronary affection, difficult to do in the clinical practice in the absence of coronary angiography. However, the known diagnosis selection elements are ECG at rest, ECG exercise test and especially – when it is possible – myocardial perfusion scintigram with Thallium 201 under effort and at rest.

Positive diagnosis of DMCM is done by evaluation of the left ventricular (LV) systolic and diastolic function parameters with echocardiographic exploration, Doppler examination, and the morphologic data (interventricular septum – IVS – and LV posterior wall thickness).

Loss of working-myocardial mass and alteration of the myocardial contractility in the advanced stages of DMCM produce the alteration of the systolic function. The diastolic disorder occurs as a result of the decreased ventricular compliance. The mechanisms of diastolic affection are not fully clarified. Nowadays a new, more comprehensive concept emerged comprising two forms of heart failure: with preserved systolic function and diastolic dysfunction (early stages of the disease) and with systolic-diastolic dysfunction (advanced stages).

The working group of the European Society of Cardiology has defined echocardiographic criteria of diastolic heart failure as follows:
1. the presence of the symptoms and signs of heart failure;
2. normal or slightly decreased LV systolic function (FE $\geq$ 45%);
3. changes of the ventricular relaxation, filling and/or distensibility.

In the advanced stages of DMCM global ventricular performance can be evaluated by myocardial performance indices described by Tei, that includes the parameters of myocardial systolic and diastolic function and represent the sum of the isovolumetric contraction time and isovolumetric relaxation time reported to the ejection time. In advanced heart failure the aggravation of the ventricular function leads to the increase of the isovolumetric contraction time and the shortening of the isovolumetric relaxation time due to the increase of the filling pressure. The indices of global myocardial performance having normal values of 0.35 ± 0.05, have high diagnosis and prognosis importance in the heart failure of DM. It is recommended to evaluate the global ventricular function of the diabetic with heart failure, considering the fact that all systolic function indices (EF, ventricular volumes, shortening fraction) are dependent on pre and post load. Therefore, in evaluating the global systolic function it has to be taken into consideration the effect of the cardiovascular load and of the medication treatment [2, 18].

Diagnosing the subendocardial dysfunction using tissular Doppler method seems extremely promising for the evaluation of myocardial function in this category of patients, but this method has not been implemented in clinical practice.

Isotopic ventriculography confirmed the decreased ventricular filling. These diastolic abnormalities are the result of diminished LV compliances and are due to a prolonged and uncoordinated LV relaxation.

Radionuclide angiography allows the accurate evaluation of the diastolic function, modified in DMCM by using the following parameters: maximum filling rate and the time until the maximum filling rate is reached, atrial filling, and the isovolumetric relaxation period respectively. Radionuclide exploration using Tc 99-marked red blood cells and the construction of LV's time-radioactivity curves allows the assessment of the systolic function indices at rest and under effort. Non-invasive evaluation through radionuclide exploration of the diabetic with heart failure is limited by the absence of intraventricular pressure data. The combination of radioisotopic activity curves with the pressure curves determined during the hemodynamic study allows the precise evaluation of the LV performance and proves that the non-invasive parameters of the fast diastolic filling are correlated with the invasive parameters: maximum negative rate of dP/dt and the time constant [19] (Plate 30.1).

Regan *et al.,* proved, through cardiac catheterization, the existence of a low LV compliance in diabetic patients with nephropathy and with angiographically normal coronary vessels. For the medical practice, it is important to know that the retinal macroangiography often develops in parallel with DMCM and the clinically manifested nephropathy suggests the presence of a coronary vessel disease [11, 12].

Modern exploration, reserved only for research for the time being, can evaluate DMCM by evaluating the myocardial structural changes with positron emission tomography or nuclear magnetic resonance.

An important role in defining the DMCM diagnosis is due to invasive exploration (determination of the pressures by cardiac catheterization, the evaluation of the ventricular function by contrast ventriculography, exclusion of the epicardial coronary lesions by coronarography) completed with endomyocardial biopsy that can bring valuable information about the specific histological changes of DMCM.

Studies of pathologic anatomy in diabetic patients with heart failure showed a 2.5 times higher frequency of proliferative lesions in the small myocardial intramural vessels, with deposits of positive PAS material.

It seems that the HT accelerates this process both in animals and in humans. In addition, severe interstitial fibrosis with focal scars and myocytes activity is significantly more frequent in the hypertensive diabetic patients with chronic heart failure, examined post-mortem, than in the normotensive diabetic patients. DMCM can also appear in the patients who do not have an obvious large vessel disease or myocardial capillary abnormalities documented by the endomyocardial

biopsy. Common histological abnormalities in DMCM are interstitial myocardial fibrosis and arteriolar hyalinosis [14, 20].

The obvious support of the presence of diabetic cardiomyopathy has been reported even in children with DM. The severity of myocardial dysfunction is linked to the level of metabolic control even when there is an obvious cardiovascular microangiopathy. These studies suggest with strong arguments that in diabetic patients the underlying process in diabetic cardiomyopathy is non-ischemic [18, 21].

To summarize:

• The evolution of diabetic cardiomyopathy is asymptomatic for a long time and signs and symptoms of heart failure are presented in its advanced stages.

• Non-invasive investigations (echocardiographic and isotopic studies) bring valuable elements of diagnosis, highlighting ventricular dysfunction. This dysfunction is initially only diastolic and in evolution, systolic dysfunction appears with effort followed by rest systolic dysfunction.

• The diagnosis of diabetic cardiomyopathy assumes the exclusion of coronary macroangiopathy (through non-invasive and invasive methods), HT and other causes of heart failure.

• The presence of retinal and renal microangiopathy and/or cardiac vegetative neuropathy brings extra arguments for the presence of cardiomyopathy.

ARTERIAL HYPERTENSION IN DIABETIC PATIENTS WITH HEART FAILURE

Arterial hypertension has a high incidence in diabetic patients (over one third of the diabetic patients associate HT). This incidence increases with the patient's age and the diabetes mellitus's (DM) duration. Arterial hypertension (important cardiovascular risk factor) is twice more frequent in diabetic patients than in non-diabetic patients. Arterial hypertension contributes to the increase of morbidity and mortality in diabetic patients with or without heart failure. The reversed relation is also valid, diabetes mellitus leading to an increase of the hypertensive patient's mortality.

Arterial hypertension is a risk factor for diabetic macro- and microvascular complications, the increase of both blood pressure components values (systolic and diastolic) correlating positively with a high mortality rate as well in diabetic patients with heart failure.

Prospective studies continue to prove that the prevalence of diabetes mellitus and arterial hypertension grows along with population age and this association is frequent in the industrialized societies.

It is recognized that the heart failure in diabetic patients is related to arterial hypertension as etiopathologic substratum (hypertensive cardiomyopathy) and to aggravation of the coronary macro and microangiopathic lesions [22].

These observations contributed to a more aggressive therapeutic strategy for the BP values of the patients who associate diabetes mellitus and HT. The purpose of reducing BP values in diabetic patients is the reduction of mortality associated with HT. By consensus, the "target" therapeutic value of BP in diabetic patients is <130/80 mmHg.

The cardiovascular risk for a hypertensive patient is determined not only by the level of BP but also by the level of target organs involvement as well as the sum of other cardiovascular risk factors.

The presence of diabetes mellitus in hypertensive patients classifies them in a high-risk group, regardless of the target organs lesions, presence of other risk factors or other cardiovascular disease [20, 23].

What are the particularities of a hypertensive diabetic with heart failure?

Certain particularities must be taken into consideration when evaluating a diabetic patient with HT.

• For diabetic patients, HT diagnosis must be based on multiple determinations of BP, taken in standard conditions, at least on 3 occasions.

• Considering the variability of the BP, frequently met in diabetic patients, it is recommended to use Holter monitoring of BP in this category of patients.

• Due to the frequency of orthostatic arterial hypotension in diabetic patients, determination of BP must be done both in supine and orthostatism, at each medical exam.

A hypertensive diabetic presents some characteristics that can influence the choice of HT therapy.

• Thus, many patients with type 2 DM do not follow the circadian pattern of BP values and HT remains high during night reflecting the cardiac autonomic dysfunction and the abnormalities of nervous and renal mechanisms.

• Many diabetic patients present hypertension in clinostatism as well as orthostatic hypotension, linked to the cardiac autonomic neuropathy, creating difficulties in the management of those patients.

• Both systolic and diastolic BP has a high variability in the patients with nephropathy, requiring repeated determinations or Holter monitoring.

• Renal dysfunction occurring in about 20% of the patients with type 2 DM and a third of the patients with type 1 DM, is aggravated by hypertension and, in turn, accelerates the progression of the heart failure.

• Additionally, the disproportional increase of the BP values, especially of the systolic BP, is associated with a cardiovascular risk growth and accelerated progression of renal dysfunction in these patients [2, 22, 23].

CORONARY MACROANGIOPATHY IN PATIENTS WITH HEART FAILURE

All types of vascular disease are common in diabetic patients: coronary, cerebral, peripheral. Vascular disease causes death in over 75% of the diabetic patients. In diabetic patients, the involvement of the coronary vascular bed is dominant, over 55% of them having coronary artery disease.

This subchapter refers to particularities of heart failure in diabetic patients with myocardial ischemia produced by:

• Epicardial coronary lesions (coronary macroangiopathy);

• Coronary microvascular disease (coronary microangiopathy).

At the beginning of the last century, studies related to myocardial metabolism showed that the glucose metabolic disorder affects the heart in diabetic patients. In the middle of the century, the term "diabetic cardiac myopathy" was mentioned for the first time. In the last decades, researchers oriented towards a comprehensive description of the biochemical mechanisms responsible for

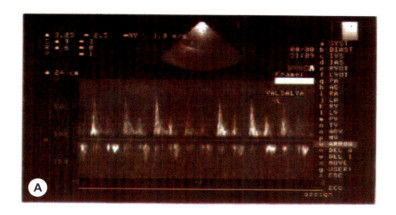

VALSALVA

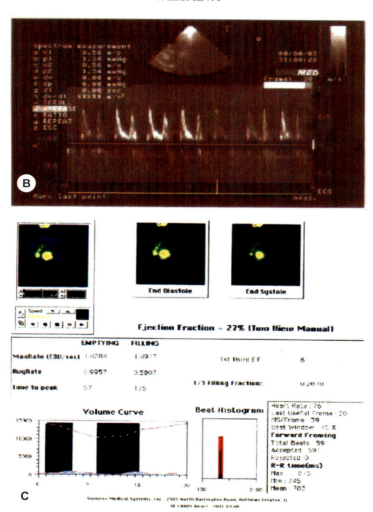

Plate 30.1

N.D., 52 years old. Doppler ultrasonography.

Transmitral diastolic flow with pseudonormal pattern (A) emphasized by Valsalva maneuver (B) in a diabetic patient with NYHA class III heart failure and cardiac macroangiopathy 99mTc pyrophosphate VRI at the same patient shows the following parameters: 1/3 FF=0,2070, T-PFR=175ms, FE=27% (C).

metabolic and vascular disorders in diabetic patients' heart failure. Diabetic patients present an accelerated process of atherosclerosis, have a higher rate of mortality after an acute myocardial infarction, evolve more frequently towards heart failure after myocardial injury, and have a higher rate of restenosis after coronary angioplasty, in comparison with the non-diabetic patient. In these decades, the prognosis for non-diabetic coronary patients improved considerably, whilst the diabetic patients with coronary artery disease present, for the same level of coronary lesions, a higher frequency of major cardiovascular events. These observations support the concept that the diabetic patient with coronary disease who develops heart failure needs a special approach and a specific treatment should be addressed to the diabetic status [24].

About 20% of the patients hospitalized in coronary intensive care units are diabetic patients. A similar proportion of diabetic patients can be found in the large clinical trials for cardiovascular diseases. In the large population studies of heart failure a third of the patients are diabetic. High morbidity and mortality in type 2 diabetes mellitus are correlated with the increased incidence and the severity of the coronary disease.

Recent trials on diabetic patients and the analysis of subgroups of diabetic patients in the large trials that study angina pectoris, myocardial infarction and heart failure post myocardial infarction provided new data regarding the controversial issue "how to approach a diabetic with coronary artery disease?" [2, 25]

The incidence of the coronary disease is significantly higher in diabetic patients with heart failure. Additionally, the expansion of the epicardial coronary disease (coronary macroangiopathy) is much higher in diabetic patients for whom the angiographic data reveal more frequently multiple vessel coronary disease in the acute myocardial infarction and a more diffuse distribution of the atherosclerotic plaques than in non-diabetic patients (Plate 30.2).

Diabetes mellitus is associated with abnormalities of the lipid metabolism and lipoprotein levels. The fact that the diabetic patients have a more extensive, more diffuse and more severe coronary disease than the non-diabetic patients can be explained by the increase of the small, dense particles of LDL-cholesterol. Lipoprotein a (Lp(a))

and increased oxidation of LDL can also be important factors in the acceleration of atherosclerosis in diabetic patients. Furthermore, glycosylation of apoprotein B, LDL and HDL that can occur in diabetes mellitus may reduce the LDL clearance and increase HDL clearance. It is also possible that the advanced glycosylation products are involved in the accelerated atherosclerosis in diabetic patients [26].

From an anatomical point of view, coronary disease in diabetic patients presents distinctive characteristics *vs.* non-diabetic patients. Post myocardial infarction angiography shows that the atherosclerotic disease is multivascular, more severe and involves more coronary segments than in the non-diabetic patients. Also, the coronary calcifications have higher prevalence. Restenosis rate after percutaneous coronary angioplasty is also higher in diabetic patients. However, the intrastent restenosis rate is similar in both diabetic and non-diabetic patients. These observations suggest that the intimal remodeling and proliferation following angioplasty are accentuated in diabetic patients *vs.* nondiabetic patients [27, 28].

CORONARY MICROANGIOPATHY IN DIABETIC PATIENTS WITH HEART FAILURE

It is well known that the diabetic patients with heart failure present more severe symptoms of myocardial ischemia than non-diabetic patients who have the same level of epicardial coronary artery damage. This fact is probably due to the abnormalities at the level of coronary microcirculation (the small vessel disease). In patients with similar levels of affection of the epicardial coronary, the dysfunction of the coronary microcirculation can explain the big differences in myocardial oxygen consumption [29].

In diabetes mellitus the coronary microcirculation suffers both functional and anatomical changes similar to the anatomical abnormalities seen in the microcirculation of other target organs. Thickening of the basal membrane in the small coronary vessel is specific and affects the release of oxygen and nutritional substances at the myocardial level. The histological changes are directly proportional to the duration and severity of diabetes mellitus [20].

The vascular tonus at the level of the vessels with a diameter smaller than 150 μm plays an important role in adjusting the flux of the coronary blood. The coronary microvascular tonus can be influenced by a series of factors, such as the vasodilator prostaglandins, the hyperpolarization factor derived from the endothelium, the nitric oxide (the relaxing factor derived from the EDRF-endothelium). The studies of various vascular beds, including the coronary circulation, in animals or in vivo on patients, proved that in diabetic patients there is not enough release of nitric oxide derived from the endothelium – which leads to the so-called endothelial dysfunction.

Whilst there are enough proofs to show that the release of nitric oxide is less efficient in diabetic patients than in non-diabetic patients, the hypothesis of a relative reduction of the sensitivity to nitric oxide is less well substantiated. Though it is known that in diabetes mellitus the transport of nitric oxide from the production site to the action site is affected, the mechanism is still not clear and is difficult to demonstrate. It seems that the production of nitric oxide is not significantly affected in diabetes mellitus. This fact is substantiated by the observation that administration of arginine – the nitric oxide forerunner – has no influence on the endothelial function in diabetic patients [30].

The role of the endothelial dysfunction in diabetic patients with coronary microangiopathy and heart failure becomes relevant when the consumption of myocardial oxygen increases (for example during physical effort). It is known that the diabetic patients have a lower effort tolerance than the non-diabetic patients. Furthermore, the diabetic patients with no significant lesions of the epicardial coronary present a reduced reserve of the coronary flow and low a coronarodilatator response at pacing, compared to the non-diabetic patients. The mechanisms involved in reducing the vasodilatation response (at the level of coronary microcirculation when the myocardial oxygen demand increases) were studied on experimental models in animals. The increase in myocardial oxygen consumption requires the presence of an anatomically and functionally intact endothelium in order to achieve nitric oxide dependent vasodilatation at the level of coronary microcirculation.

Researchers' attention oriented towards the possible mechanisms that lead to the increased production of vasoconstrictive substances and free radicals of oxygen in diabetic patients.

The increase of the oxidative stress in diabetes mellitus is realized, on the one hand, by the increase of free radicals of oxygen formation generated by increased production of prostaglandins and prostanoids through cyclooxygenase and, on the other hand by reduction of the free oxygen radicals' clearance. It has been proved that one of the mechanisms involved is the glycosylation of superoxide dismutase – that removes the free radicals from circulation, playing the role of scavenger – leading to the reduction of this enzyme activity. Other mechanisms that could be involved in the coronary microcirculation insufficiency in diabetic patients are: the involvement of the proteinkinase C, final products of advanced glycosylation and they are only studied on experimental models in animals and are in progress for research on diabetic patients [31, 32].

The difficulty in elucidating the mechanisms of coronary microcirculation dysfunction in diabetic patients is due to the association of several conditions such as: dyslipidemia, atherosclerosis or arterial hypertension, which in their turn, associate various degrees of oxidative stress.

To summarize, the diabetic status is characterized by:

– The presence of the myocardial ischemia in diabetic patients with permeable epicardial coronary vessels, which can be explained by the coronary microcirculation insufficiency.

– The main mechanisms involved in the coronary microvascular disease are:

• Increased oxidative stress

• Endothelial dysfunction due to the imbalance between vasoconstriction *vs.* vasodilatation processes, having as a result a basal vasoconstrictive tendency and a diminished vasodilatation response due to the increased demand for myocardial oxygen.

It is well known that the silent myocardial ischemia (episodes of myocardial ischemia without angina pectoris, highlighted by rest ECG, exercise ECG or Holter monitoring) is more frequent in diabetic patients with heart failure than in non-diabetic patients. In diabetic patients myocardial ischemia presents more frequently an atypical symptomatology for angina. It has also been noticed that silent myocardial infarction (the

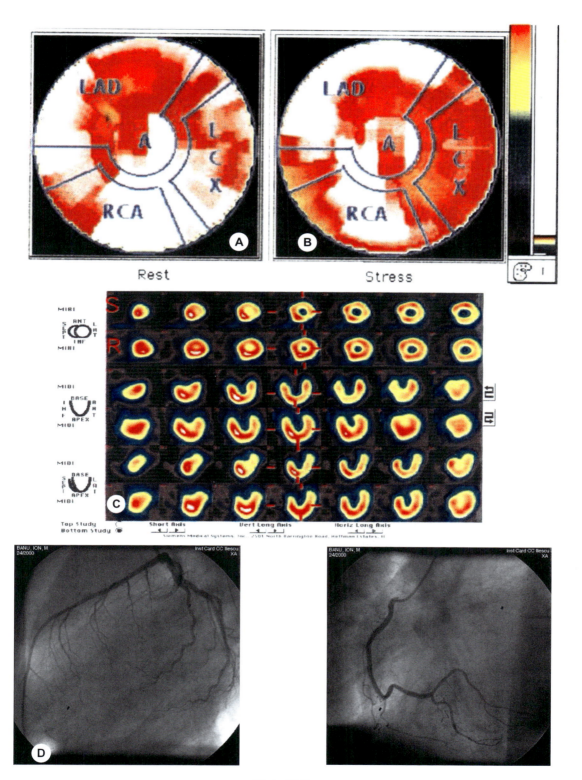

Plate 30.2

Z.E. 46 years old.

99mTc rest myocardial scintigram (A) and stress myocardial scintigram (B,C) with dipiridamol in a diabetic patient with NYHA class II heart failure without cardiac macroangiopathy; coronary angiography shows permeable coronary arteries (D).

presence of evidence and/or increase of enzymes showing infarction in the absence of the characteristic symptomatology) in diabetic patients is met more frequently. The painless infarction in diabetic patients is associated with anatomical and functional evidence of autonomic cardiac neuropathy.

Although there are few studies to show that the diabetic patients with heart failure present more frequent silent myocardial ischemia compared to non-diabetic patients, this observation does not make a general rule.

If "silent ischemia" occurs more frequently in diabetic patients *vs.* non-diabetic patients is still a controversial issue probably without clinical relevance, because this situation is met in both categories of patients. However, there is data showing that the silent myocardial infarction is associated with a higher mortality rate compared with the "painful" infarction, and the silent ischemia has a more unfavorable prognosis in the diabetic patient with heart failure [30, 33].

The diagnosis of coronary disease in diabetic patients, in general, is similar to that in non-diabetic patients. However, the sensitivity and the specificity of the diagnosing tests can be different, considering the high probability for the coronary disease to be present. As previously mentioned, the unfavorable prognostic of the diabetic patients is influenced by multiple abnormalities of the myocardial energetic metabolism, which are best emphasized by the positron emission tomography (PET). PET is the only imagistic method that allows the non-invasive evaluation of the myocardial metabolism, coronary flow and receptors density, offering information regarding the *in vivo* development of the biochemical and physiological processes. In PET a component marker with a positrons-emitting isotope is administered, intravenous or by inhalation to evaluate the metabolic dysfunction by PET scanner which registers the image of this component distribution. PET proves to be extremely useful to study the myocardial insulin-resistance, the evaluation of the myocardial blood flow and the diagnosis of the myocardial viability in both diabetic and non-diabetic patients with coronary disease [19, 24].

The diabetic patients who come with typical symptomatology of myocardial ischemia barely raise diagnosis problems. For a high number of diabetic patients the symptomatology is not typical, therefore the probability of coronary disease is lower than for those who present typical angina pectoris.

ECG exercise testing is the first non-invasive investigation for the diabetic patient with chest pain. There is no available data to compare the accuracy of the diagnosis with ECG exercise test in diabetic *vs.* non-diabetic patients. In the case of the diabetic patient with atypical angina, the probability of coronary disease is much higher than in non-diabetic patients; thus, the ECG exercise test has a higher sensitivity and a higher specificity.

If the ECG exercise test is ambiguous, other non-invasive investigations can be made such as myocardial scintigraphy with thalium-201 or 99mTc sestamibi SPECT (Single-Photon Emission Computed Tomography) at rest and under pharmacological stress and stress echocardiography (physical exercise or pharmacological stress). There is no available data to compare the value of these tests in diabetic *vs.* non-diabetic patients.

The prognostic value of the exercise test and myocardial scintigraphy with thallium SPECT was evaluated in the patients with type 2 diabetes mellitus. The evaluation has shown that in high risk patients, who have limited effort capacity, the 2 years cardiovascular mortality is 8.8% compared to 1.3% in the patients who have a preserved effort capacity. It has been noticed that stress test with dipyridamole had higher mortality in the patients with high perfusion deficiency, whilst the cardiovascular 2 years mortality was 22.3%. The comparison between the sensitivity and specificity of those two methods – myocardial scintigram of perfusion with thallium 201 SPECT and stress echocardiography with dobutamine – proved to have a similar value. Therefore, pharmacological stress test is recommended for the diabetic patients presenting limitation of effort capacity or for whom the electrocardiogram is non-interpretable. The stress echocardiography with dobutamine was assessed to be a valuable technique to diagnose coronary disease, having 90% sensitivity and 94% specificity. A very important issue is the selection of the stress method. The ECG exercise test induces a higher level of ischemia than the administration of dobutamine (with additional administration of atropine if the cardiac frequency does not increase enough) because it has a higher sensitivity [18, 21] (Plate 30.3).

Consequently, the ideal stress test is the ECG exercise test. However, if the patients are incapable of physical effort the dobutamine test can be used, to which, if the theoretical maximum cardiac frequency is reached, the positive predictive value is higher. In diabetic patients the silent myocardial ischemia and the painless myocardial infarctions are frequently met. Considering that the diabetic patients have a higher incidence of the coronary disease it is considered that the asymptomatic patients should also get routine investigation. For the diabetic patients it is necessary to identify the risk factors and then to decide for a more or less aggressive therapy. The interventional or surgical myocardial revascularization in diabetic patients (particularly for women) is associated with an increased mortality and for the asymptomatic patients the risk/benefit ratio must be considered [24, 28].

To summarize:

• Arterial hypertension and diabetes mellitus frequently coexist in the same patient, increasing significantly the risk for heart failure.

• Vascular disease represents a very important issue for the diabetic patient, especially the coronary artery disease that justifies a high percent of the morbidity and mortality of this group.

• The diabetic patients with heart failure and coronary macro-angiopathy frequently present a multicoronary vessel disease with diffuse atherosclerotic lesions.

• Coronary microvascular disease – coronary microangiopathy – can contribute to the appearance of the heart failure in diabetic patients and can explain the myocardial ischemia in the absence of significant lesions at the level of epicardial coronary vessels.

• Diabetic patients with heart failure and coronary disease frequently present atypical symptoms.

• Though the diabetic patients present higher cardiovascular risk, there is no data for screening diabetic patients without symptoms of coronary disease.

PROGNOSTIC ELEMENTS

IS THE PRESENCE OF DIABETIC CARDIOMYOPATHY INFLUENCING THE PROGNOSIS OF THE DIABETIC PATIENTS?

It is considered that the increased prevalence of the heart failure in the patients with diabetes mellitus is due, to a large extent, to this myopathic component. The presence of this entity, frequently associated in the current medical practice with the coronary microangiopathy, HT and cardiac autonomic neuropathy (CAN), contributes to the aggravation of the prognosis in diabetic patients with heart failure. DMCM is associated with coronary artery disease and contributes to the episodes of symptomatic and silent myocardial ischemia in diabetes mellitus. The association with CAN increases the risk of malignant ventricular arrhythmia, aggravating the prognosis of these patients. The severity of the ventricular dysfunction in diabetic patients is correlated with the level of metabolic control even when there is no obvious coronary microangiopathy. This fact supports the idea that the etiopathogenic substratum of diabetic cardiomyopathy is mainly non-ischemic, represented by the metabolic dysfunction [14, 34].

Studies proved an increased prevalence of the post myocardial infarction heart failure compared with the non-diabetic patients that contributes to the aggravation of the prognosis for these patients. The survival in AMI is conditioned by both the extent of the coronary lesion and the myopathic component (difficult to quantify clinically, but suggested by the retinal and/or renal microangiopathy). Furthermore, it has been noticed that the evolution after aorto-coronary by-pass or after renal transplantation depends on the LV performance (a low ejection fraction of the left ventricle leads to unfavorable prognosis).

Sudden death is responsible for about half of the deaths caused by heart failure and this percentage can increase in the case of ischemic etiology (the presence of the coronary macroangiopathy). The increased arrhythmic risk often leads to sudden death produced by malignant ventricular tachyarrhythmia: ventricular fibrillation (VF) and ventricular tachycardia (VT). The asystole can appear, as secondary event, after a prolonged episode of VF or primary as mechanism of the sudden death in the advanced stages of ventricular dysfunction [33, 35, 36].

CARDIAC AUTONOMIC NEUROPATHY IN DIABETIC PATIENTS

The diabetic patients with heart failure, in the absence of the epicardial coronary artery lesions, often present an important ventricular dysfunction. In the absence of the coronary atherosclerosis the

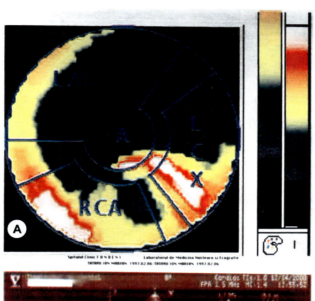

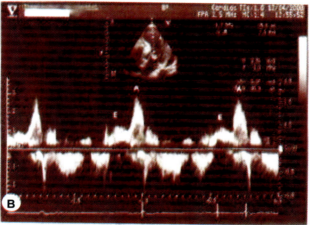

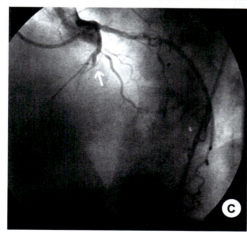

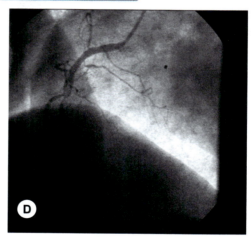

Plate 30.3

T.I., 56 years old.

99mTc myocardial scintigram (polar mapping) in a diabetic patient with NYHA class III heart failure, with acute coronary macroangiopathy shows an important perfusion defect in the anterior territory (A); Doppler ultrasonography – transmitral diastolic flow with "delayed relaxation" pattern type at the same patient (B); Coronary angiography shows occlusion on LAD (left anterior descending coronary artery) – segment II (distal to the origin of the first septal branch) (C) and permeable RCD (right coronary artery) (D).

left ventricular dysfunction appears in one third of the patients with type 2 diabetes mellitus with longer evolution. The diastolic dysfunction usually precedes the systolic dysfunction.

In two studies (Zoneraich, Clarke) the autonomic cardiac neuropathy was present in over one third of the diabetic patients and frequently accompanied by left ventricle dysfunction. The severity of the cardiac dysfunction seems to be linked with the severity of cardiac autonomic neuropathy (CAN). It has been proved that sometimes this can be present before the clinical symptoms of generalized autonomic neuropathy appear. The left ventricle dysfunction, with reduction of the diastolic filling and subsequent reduction of the left ventricular contractility, is the consequence of the diabetic autonomic neuropathy and of the reduction of the catecholamine response, which can lead to sudden death in certain cases [37].

The frequency is appreciated differently in correlation with the criteria used for the diagnosis and varies depending on authors and the selected trial groups, covering a large range of prevalence between 55 and 90%. If the autonomic cardiac dysfunction is appreciated based on modern methods of investigation, the frequency of this localization reaches 30–50% of the cases.

It has been proved that there is a tight link between the appearance of the diabetic neuropathy and age, duration of the diabetes, metabolic status, and presence of retinopathy, smoking and the decrease of the HDL cholesterol [38].

HOW CAN AUTONOMIC CARDIAC NEUROPATHY INFLUENCE THE PROGNOSIS IN DIABETIC PATIENTS WITH HEART FAILURE?

The evolution and the prognostic of the CAN in diabetic patients with heart failure must be considered in relation with the coexistence of the other complications of diabetes mellitus, of which the diabetic micro and macro angiopathy comes first. CAN has a negative influence on the diabetic patients' life duration, leading to higher mortality. Once diabetic autonomic neuropathy manifests clinically, the estimated mortality in 5 years is about 38%. CAN may become extremely severe, leading practically to cardiac de-innervation, that

predisposes to arrhythmias (more frequently ventricular arrhythmias). Hence, the increased risk of sudden death in diabetic patients with highly modified autonomic function test [20, 39].

Other factors that seem to have a direct connection with the severity of CAN in diabetic patients with heart failure are the level of ventricular dysfunction, the low variability of the cardiac frequency, rest tachycardia, orthostatic hypotension, prolonged QT interval, arterial hypertension, the alteration of the physiologic circadian rhythm and even the decline of heat tolerance.

The left ventricular dysfunction with alteration of the diastolic performance (through relaxation disorders) is an important prognostic factor. The severity of the cardiac dysfunction is directly linked with the severity of the cardiac autonomic neuropathy. It has been proved that sometimes it can be present before the clinical symptoms of generalized autonomous neuropathy [38].

Furthermore, CAN may become so severe that it can lead to total cardiac de-innervation. Sometimes, this de-innervation develops arrhythmias (more frequently ventricular arrhythmias). In diabetic patients abnormal tests of autonomic function signal decline of the survival and an increase of the sudden death risk. The syndrome of global cardiac de-innervation is very rare; the cardiac frequency remains unmodified and is not influenced by the physiological or pharmacological stimuli [2, 37].

Therefore, the early detection of the subclinical cardiac autonomic dysfunction is very important for the stratification of the risk and subsequent therapy in the diabetic patient with heart failure.

Are there differences between diabetic patients with cardiac failure in the presence or absence of epicardial coronary lesions?

It is less known whether there are clinical-evolutionary and diagnostic differences between diabetic patients with cardiac failure in the presence or absence of epicardial coronary lesions. However, recent studies show that:

1) There are significant differences between diabetic patients with cardiac failure and coronary macroangiopathy and the ones without coronary epicardial lesions. Characteristic for diabetic patients with cardiac failure and normal epicardial coronary vessels are:

– Young age;
– Predominance of feminine gender;
– More frequent association with type 1DM;

– High frequency of metabolic decompression;

– More frequent association of microangiopathic type lesions;

– More frequent diastolic dysfunction;

– Better systolic function.

2) The prognosis of cardiac failure in diabetic patients in the absence of epicardial coronary lesions is more favorable.

3) The severity of the ventricular dysfunction in diabetic patients with cardiac failure is correlated with the level of metabolic control, even when there is no obvious coronary microangiopathy; this fact supports the idea that the underlying process of diabetic cardiomyopathy is mainly non-ischemic, representing the metabolic dysfunction.

4) A rigorous glycemic control by insulin therapy in diabetic patients during the cardiac decompensation period improves the ventricular systolic and diastolic performance [20, 39, 40].

TREATMENT PARTICULARITIES OF THE HEART FAILURE IN DIABETIC PATIENTS

The therapeutic strategy of the heart failure in diabetic patients contains almost the same general principles as in non-diabetic patients. The complex etiopathologic substratum in diabetic patients will be considered, the heart failure occurring more frequently due to several reasons:

• Diabetes mellitus is a risk factor for the coronary atherosclerosis and its complications

• Diabetes mellitus is frequently associated with the arterial hypertension (over one third of the patients)

• The presence of diabetic cardiomyopathy.

The diabetic patients with heart failure present certain specific features that must be considered in the therapeutic approach:

• Glycemic control and weight loss for the obese diabetic patients

• The diagnosis and the complete evaluation of the co-morbidities

• Renal dysfunction, frequently met in diabetic patients, can raise specific problems for the treatment; the patients with renal insufficiency may not respond to thiazide diuretics, requiring loop diuretics in higher doses than usual; the hypoproteinemia secondary to the diabetic nephropathy contributes to the aggravation of the edematous syndrome.

• Patients with heart failure in general, and especially the diabetic patients, frequently associate abnormalities of the balance between K^+ and Mg^{2+}. K^+ may be higher or lower depending on the renal function; certain medicine as potassium sparing diuretics, angiotensin converting enzyme inhibitors that have positive influences on the balance between K^+ and Mg^{2+} bring a specific benefit to this category of patients [2, 5].

GENERAL TREATMENT MEASURES

General measures of heart failure treatment in diabetic patients

• Correction of the changeable risk factors
  – Stop smoking
  – Weight reduction for obese patients
  – Adequate control of HT
  – Correct dyslipidemia
  – Glycemic control
  – Stop alcohol consumption
• Measures to maintain fluids balance
  – Reduce the salt contribution (3g/day)
  – Daily weight
• Measures to improve the effort capacity
  – Rest in the period of decompensation
  – Daily activity – moderate, progressive, limited by symptoms (except for decompensation)
• The control of ventricular rate for patients with supraventricular tachyarrhythmia
• Anticoagulation for the patients with high thromboembolic risk
• Myocardial revascularization for the patients with active ischemia
• Avoid the antiarrhythmic agents for the control of the asymptomatic ventricular arrhythmia
• Avoid using the non-steroidal anti-inflammatory drugs
• Prophylaxis and treatment of infections

The treatment of the heart failure also includes instructions for patient and his family about diabetes mellitus and heart failure. This is necessary in order to motivate the patient to join permanently and to complete a treatment that is sometimes uncomfortable and expensive. When this is not possible (intelligence level, education, etc.), the presence of a caretaker is necessary to ensure and provide instructions as complete as possible [2, 41].

SPECIFIC TREATMENT MEASURES

The results of the clinical trials showed that four groups of medicine are efficient in treating the heart failure: the angiotensin converting enzyme inhibitors (ACE), diuretics, beta-blockers and digitalis. The algorithm of the treatment for the diabetic patients with heart failure was settled by analyzing the data provided by the study of the subgroups from the large clinical trials (CHF).

Diabetic cardiomyopathy represents a distinctive entity that could be sometimes the physiopathologic substratum in the diabetic patient with heart failure. Therefore, its status evaluation (pure diastolic dysfunction or combined systolic and diastolic dysfunction) involves different prognostic and therapeutic aspects [41, 42].

Angiotensin converting enzyme inhibitors in the treatment of heart failure in diabetic patients

In all the patients with ventricular dysfunction, symptomatic or not, it is recommended to administer ACE in the absence of the contraindications. This recommendation is based on the results obtained in the clinical trials that proved the efficacy of those medicines in reducing the symptoms of heart failure with improvement of life quality and a significant reduction of mortality. As expected, the analysis of the patients in the subgroups of the clinical trials regarding the use of the angiotensin converting enzyme inhibitors in the treatment of the heart failure, showed a favorable influence on the mortality of diabetic patients. The trial HOPE showed a reduction of HF appearance in the patients who received ACE. In the study SOLVD (Studies of Left Ventricular Dysfunction), using enalapril, the efficiency of the angiotensin converting enzyme inhibitors was higher in prevention in diabetic patients compared with the non-diabetic patients and had a similar efficiency in the treatment of the ventricular dysfunction in the diabetic vs. non-diabetic patients.

The study ATLAS (Assessment of Treatment with Lisinopril and Survival) provided data regarding the use of small and large doses of ACE. ATLAS was run on 3164 patients (611 diabetic patients) with heart failure class II-IV NYHA for 45 months. The mortality was considerably increased in the subgroup of diabetic patients vs. non-diabetic patients. Comparing the efficiency of the high doses and respectively the small doses of ACE, a reduction in mortality of 6% for non-diabetic patients and 14% for the group of diabetic patients has been noticed respectively. The study SAVE (Survival and Ventricular Enlargement) that included patients with left ventricular dysfunction post myocardial infarction (EF< 40%) showed a higher total morbidity and mortality in the diabetic patients vs. the non-diabetic patients. It also showed that the treatment with captopril improves the evolution and the prognostic, similar as in non-diabetic patients. It is interesting to highlight that after the introduction of ACE inhibitors, due to the modulation of the insulin-resistance, the diabetic patients with HF show an increase in hypoglycemic events that has been registered with oral anti-diabetic medicine. Although this risk is low, it is not to be ignored. In this sense, during the therapy with ACE inhibitors, it is recommended to monitor the glycemia and adjust the doses of anti-diabetic drugs prescribed per os.

The administration of ACE inhibitors begins with small doses that are titrated up to the maximum tolerated dose because the higher benefit of increased doses of ACE inhibitors has been demonstrated in HF, as shown in the big trials like ATLAS.

When initiating the treatment with ACE inhibitors it has to be taken into consideration that the diabetic patients frequently associate orthostatic hypotension. The doses of ACE inhibitors must be small for the old patients or for those who present low BP values.

In the patients with acute myocardial infarction, the therapy with ACE inhibitors must be started as early as possible, in the absence of contraindications or hemodynamic instability.

The increase in serum creatinine and potassium are the side effects that can appear when administrating ACE inhibitors in diabetic patients with renal dysfunction. However, a slight increase of the serum creatinine is not a reason to stop ACE inhibitor therapy. The changes in the renal function occurring in diabetic patients with HF after administration of ACE inhibitors are the result of the decrease of the renal blood flow and the vasodilatation of the corresponding glomerular arteriole and are not due to the renal "toxic" effect.

In the patients with diabetes mellitus non-steroidal anti-inflammatory medication should be avoided in association with ACE inhibitors.

Sometimes, coughing is described as a side effect of those medicines limiting their use, but its presence can indicate an aggravation of the heart failure as well.

In conclusion, the ACE inhibitors represent a major therapeutic line in diabetic patients with congestive heart failure, having a higher efficiency in the non-diabetic patients. This observation supports the concept that the patients with high risk have the biggest therapeutic benefit [43, 44, 45, 46].

Role of diuretics in diabetic patients with heart failure

It is admitted that the therapy with diuretics improves the symptomatology during the cardiac decompression periods, but it is not yet well established whether it improves or aggravates the prognosis in diabetic patients with heart failure. In the absence of the studies regarding the efficiency of diuretics in diabetic patients with heart failure, the only information available are the ones obtained from the trials regarding hypertension. In SHEP study small doses of diuretics were proved to be efficient in preventing the major cardiovascular events in type 2 DM patients. Loop diuretics are preferable for diabetic patients, because they lead to less metabolic disorders. In the treatment of heart failure in diabetic patients, recent studies have proved the specific efficiency of a thiazide-like diuretic, indapamide.

Diuretics are often used as first line medication in the patients with heart failure and in the presence of a high pulmonary and systemic venous pressure. In the periods of cardiac decompensation, the first option is the loop diuretics administered intravenously. The diabetic patients with renal dysfunction require higher doses of diuretics than the ones used regularly for compensation. As the loop diuretics have short half life (except torsemide) thiazide-like (indapamide) diuretics are preferred for the chronic administration, when renal function is not compromised. In the severe heart failure it is preferred to associate diuretics

with different action mechanism at nephron level, achieving sequential blockage (loop, thiazide, thiazide-like and potassium sparing diuretics). The potassium sparing diuretics are recommended in diabetic patients with heart failure because of their effect of preventing the depletion of potassium and magnesium. Several studies, including RALES (Randomized Aldactone Evaluation Study) showed that the use of spironolactone improves the cardiac remodeling in the patients with advanced heart failure. The association of the spironolactone with ACE inhibitors for the treatment requires monitoring potassium. Diuretics should not be used as monotherapy because they activate the renin-angiotensin-aldosterone system and can lead to electrolyte imbalance that favours arrhythmias. In diabetic patients with heart failure the volume status must be carefully evaluated because both the increase of the capillary permeability and the reduction of the osmotic-colloidal pressure through hypoalbuminemia can reduce the circulating volume [41, 46].

Beta-blockers in diabetic patients with heart failure – legend or reality?

In the previous years there were two big "pharmacological legends" regarding the usage of the beta-blockers: *beta-blockers are contraindicated in heart failure and beta-blockers are contraindicated in patients with diabetes mellitus.* Current data, provided by large clinical trials, recommend beta-blockers use in class II–III NYHA heart failure patients, after titration of the ACE inhibitors up to the maximum efficient dose. The therapy with beta-blockers in heart failure is recommended even for the patients with ACE inhibitors intolerance. However, the beta-blockers should not be used in patients with volume overload or presenting severe hemodynamic deterioration, because in these cases, even small doses of beta-blockers cannot be tolerated by the patients with advanced heart failure. The initiation of the therapy with beta-blockers in heart failure must be done with small doses, with titration in 8 to 26 weeks depending on the chosen beta-blocker.

Similar to ACE inhibitors, in patients with myocardial infarction the beta-blockers must be administered as soon as possible. It has been proved that the diabetic patients with myocardial infarction receiving beta-blockers had a higher benefit compared to the non-diabetic patients. The improvement of the cardiac function after beginning the treatment with beta-blockers is achieved in a long time, weeks or months. It has to be taken into consideration that, in the beginning, the therapy with beta-blockers can be associated with an aggravation of the symptomatology, symptomatic hypotension or severe bradycardia, hypervolemia (highlighted by the increase of the high jugular pressure, edema) requiring an increase of the diuretic dose. The therapy with beta-blockers may require a reduction or the cessation of the treatment with amiodarone or digoxin.

There are no distinctive studies regarding the utility of the beta-blockers for the diabetic patients with heart failure. All the available data are coming from the analysis done on subgroups of patients from trials of heart failure.

For example, the data provided by the American Carvedilol Program showed that using the beta-blockers in the heart failure is more efficient in diabetic patients than in non-diabetic patients.

The pathophysiological reason of using beta-blockers is to prevent the negative effect of very high levels of circulating catecholamines in diabetes mellitus on the heart. Such effects are due to excessive entry of Ca^{2+} in the myocytes in the initial phase of the DM, when the beta-adrenergic receptors are not affected.

In the early stages of diabetic cardiomyopathy small or moderate doses of beta-blockers (atenolol, metoprolol, etc.) are recommended.

The therapy with beta-blockers requires special attention in the type 1 DM because it can increase glycemia. At the same time beta-blockers can hide potential hypoglycemic reactions because many of the symptoms of hypoglycemia recognized by patients are due to the effects generated by adrenaline [2, 41, 47, 48].

The role of digoxin in diabetic patients with heart failure

There are no published data regarding the use of digoxin in diabetic patients with heart failure. If the heart failure symptoms persist after the treatment with diuretics, ACE inhibitors and beta-blockers the therapy with digitalis can be initiated. Digoxin improves the symptomatology in heart failure, but it does not influence the survival. Digoxin is indicated especially for the patients with heart failure and atrial fibrillation [2].

The role of hydralazine/isosorbide-dinitrate in diabetic patients with heart failure

It is proved that associating hydralazine/isosorbide-dinitrate improves the symptomatology and prolongs the survival of the patients with heart failure. There is no proof that this medication is more or less efficient in the patients with diabetes mellitus. Theoretically, diabetes mellitus is characterized by a deficit in nitric oxide; therefore by adding a nitrate the patients with type 2 DM may have a special benefit. For the patients with ACE inhibitor intolerance, this combination can represent a therapeutic alternative. The association hydralazine/isosorbide-dinitrate can also be useful in the patients with heart failure when it is difficult to control BP [2].

Other medication used for heart failure in diabetic patients

Blockers of the angiotensin receptors II. There are studies showing that sartans used in treating patients with heart failure improve the symptomatology and represent an alternative to the inhibitors of the conversion enzyme of angiotensin (ICEA). There are no available data regarding the usage of the angiotensin receptor blockers (ARB) in the diabetic patients with heart failure.

However, the therapeutic future of this class of drugs is to be used together with ICEA and spironolactone, in order to better block the effects of renin-angiotensin-aldosterone system's (RAAS) hyperactivity [49]. One argument would be the fact that there are non-ICEA pathways mediated by the production of angiotensin II, which are important from the clinical point of view and uncontrolled by the administration of the ICEA [50].

Clinical studies where ICEA was used versus ARB II provided contradictory results (Studies ELITE I and II, OPTIMAAL Study) [51]. RESOLVD study, that compared the results of administrating enalapril, candesartan and the combination enalapril+candesartan, showed the considerable favorable effect of the drug association on the ventricular remodeling [52]. The cardioprotective and nephroprotective effect of ARB II was also proved by other important studies such as Val-HeFT (with valsartan) and

549

Table 30.2
Diabetic cardiomyopathy stages – therapeutic possibilities

Medication	Incipient DMCM	Advanced DMCM
Inotropic agents	No	Yes
ACE inhibitors	Yes	Yes
Beta-blockers	Yes	No
Diuretics	Yes	Yes
Metabolic therapy	Yes	Yes
Ca^{2+} channel blockers	Yes	Questionable
Antioxidation therapy	Yes	Yes

effect when administered on long terms for cardiovascular diseases. The majority of the population studies extended on several years do not reveal a reduction of the cardiovascular diseases incidence in the case of diets enriched with beta-carotene.

To summarize, it can be said that the cardiomyopathy in the diabetic is a reality. Knowing this practical concept imposes the diagnostic and evaluation of its stages (pure diastolic dysfunction or combined systolic and diastolic dysfunction) and involves different prognostic and therapeutic aspects (Table 30.2).

Knowing and accepting the clinical entity of diabetic cardiomyopathy, we can act on metabolic balance by early administration of pathogenic treatments. The ACE inhibitors have the main role, along with the calcium channel blockers, beta-blockers, vasodilators, anti-oxidation drugs, etc.

Conventional therapy for the heart failure combined with metabolic therapy also results from the concept of the complex pathogeny of the diabetic cardiomyopathy, centered on lack of insulin. Therefore, the first medicine remains insulin followed in the second therapeutic intention by the association of IEC with beta-blockers. Additionally, the association of calcium channel blockers and use of some drugs aiming to normalize the cholesterol, LDL-cholesterol, etc. is to be taken

for heart transplant is limited and small reported to the number of patients on the waiting list. In this context, the interest for the alternative therapeutic methods is very high.

One of the approached directions is based on the theory that the synchronization of the cardiac contraction can lead to the improvement of the ventricular function and the symptomatology. Along with the demonstration of the efficacy of resynchronization, the trials in progress also address to other aspects such as "multisite" stimulation, the benefit of the defibrillation association with stimulation, new implantation techniques for a higher accessibility [2, 5, 24].

The insufficiency of the pharmacological therapy in diabetic patients with heart failure in advanced stages (refractory congestive heart failure) indicates the necessity of circulation assistance or cardiac transplant. In those cases, the cardiac transplant is the radical solution for treatment, with a survival rate of 70% at 10 years. The major limit of this therapy is the low number of heart donors. Consequently, it is normal that this category of patients to benefit from solutions like the xenotransplant (experimental for the moment) or ventricular assistance (that became reality).

The current use of the circulation assistance

CHARM (with candesartan) in heart failure (HF). Both studies showed that sartans do not decrease the global mortality, but reduce the morbidity and lower the need for re-hospitalization because of HF aggravation, both quality of life and patients' symptomatology being favorably influenced [53].

Aldosterone antagonists. RAAS hyper reactivation generates a secondary hyperaldosteronism in diabetic's HF. Hyperaldosteronism is involved in the evolution of HF because it produces ventricular remodeling, negative electrolytic and hemodynamic effects [54]. The clinical experience showed that administration of ICEA cannot compensate the negative effects of this hormone, because of the "aldosterone-escape" phenomenon and the existence of the non-ICEA ways of producing angiotensin II that make the levels of aldosterone in the blood remain high. Some studies show that aldosterone antagonists would hinder the extension of the myocardial fibrosis and the progression of HF (including in diabetic patients) through the effect on remodeling the extra-cellular matrix at the level of the myocardium. The EPHESUS Study that used eplerenone as anti-aldosterone drug in treating HF post-severe myocardial infarction brought up this kind of arguments. Eplerenone is missing the hormonal effects of spironolactone [53].

As previously mentioned, spironolactone can be useful in the diabetic patients with HF with better benefits than those derived from its diuretic properties. Aldosterone contributes to the cardiac remodeling and the blockage of this effect may explain the benefit on mortality that has also been shown by the RALES trial [55].

To summarize, it is admitted to use blockers of the angiotensin receptors as mono-therapy instead of ICEA only where the intolerance of this was proved (coughing, angioedema). The association between ICEA, ARB II and spironolactone is a therapeutic alternative under investigation especially where there are contraindications for betablockers [56].

Metabolic and antioxidation therapy in diabetic patients with heart failure

It has been proved that prognosis of patients with heart failure is improved by the strict metabolic control, by diminishing the unfavorable effect of increased beta-oxidation of fatty acids

Trimetazidine, a known agent with direct effect in inhibiting the beta-oxidation of the fatty acids and consecutive stimulation of the glucose oxidation, could have a beneficial effect on the severe myocardial metabolic disorders in diabetic patients with heart failure.

Besides, it is interesting to highlight the benefit of the metabolic therapy on the cardiac function by increasing the efficiency of the conventional therapy in diabetic patients with heart failure. There is need for extra studies to bring more arguments to prove that the rigorous metabolic control has a preventive value in heart failure development in diabetic patients with heart failure. Also, some studies have already demonstrated the impact of the rigorous metabolic control on the patients with severe heart failure [20, 57, 58, 59].

The harmful activity of some oxidation products, catecholamines as well as free radicals, is already proved to have toxic effects on the myocardium in diabetic patients. It has been noticed that the activity of the mono-amino-oxidase and catechol-ortho-methyl transferase, that normally inactivates the circulating catecholamines, is low in diabetes mellitus. In the experiments on animals with induced diabetes mellitus, the administration of anti-oxidation agents like ascorbic acid and vitamin E lead to good results. It is suggested that this treatment has to be administered to diabetic patients who associate diabetic cardiomyopathy in order to counteract the negative effects of the free radicals and lipid peroxidation associated to diabetic cardiomyopathy.

Research is oriented towards the completion of the classical treatments with a new dimension, the antioxidation substances. The most powerful inhibition effect on the oxygen free radicals belongs to vitamin E; on the other hand, it has been discovered that the ascorbic acid inhibits specifically the lipid peroxidation initiated by the cytochrome P, NADPH – mediated in the absence of free iron (Fe). The antioxidant treatment improves not only the plasmatic cholesterol level and the progression of atherosclerosis, but also the endothelial response of the vessel to various mediators. Although the antioxidants maintenance of endothelial function, inhibition of platelet aggregation and reduction of the progression of the atheroma plaque had been proved in animals, the effect of the vitamin antioxidant supplement in humans is still under discussion. Beta-carotene

---

ventricular assistance devices have the advantage of a cardiac flow close to normal with the possibility of effort modulation [5, 62, 63].

The surveillance of the patients with ventricular assistance devices is done through clinic examination and ECG exercise tests and simultaneous measurement of the ejection fraction of LV, the opening of the aortic cusps and the ejection velocities, as well as the oxygen consumption by spirometry.

Using a combination of alternative therapies could bring benefits from cardiovascular morbidity and mortality and could be a bridge for cardiac transplantation for the diabetic patient. Future studies remain to establish if the association of a defibrillator and biventricular resynchronization could bring a significant benefit for preventing sudden death and progressive pump failure.

In summary:
- Pharmacological treatment of the diabetic patients with heart failure is, in principal, similar to the one of the non-diabetic patients.
- Diabetic patients present few particularities of the heart failure treatment that are linked with the renal dysfunction, electrolytic disorders, frequent association of HT and the hidden nature of the coronary atherosclerosis ± diabetic cardiomyopathy.
- ACE inhibitors and beta-blockers have particular therapeutic benefits for the diabetic patients with heart failure.
- Diuretic treatment supposes special precautions in diabetic patients; the thiazide-like diuretics hold an important place.
- The efficiency of the metabolic and antioxidation therapy associated with the conventional treatment of the heart failure for the diabetic patients has been shown to improve the prognosis in this category of patients.

Using a combination of some alternative treatment strategies brings benefits for the

3. Report of The Expert Committee on the diagnosis and classification of diabetes. *Diabetes Care*, **20**: 1183–97, 1997.
4. Turner RC, Millns H, Neil HA, *et al.* Risk Factors for Coronary Artery Disease in Non-Insulin Dependent Diabetes Mellitus: United Kingdom Prospective Diabetes Study (UKDPS: 23). *BMJ*, **316**: 823–828, 1998.
5. Macarie C. Carmen Ginghină, E. Apetrei. *Heart Failure from Mechanisms to Treatment*, Ed. Medicală Amaltea, Bucharest, 2002.
6. Ionescu -Tîrgoviște C. *Modern Diabetology*. Ed. Tehnică, Bucuresti, 1997.
7. V. Serban, R. Lichiardopol. *Actualities in Diabetes Mellitus.* Ed Brumar, Timişoara, 2002.
8. Malberg K, Rydén L. Diabetes mellitus and congestive heart failure. Further Knowledge Needed. *Eur Heart J*, **20**: 789–795, 1999.
9. Dhalla Ns, Pierce Gn, Innes Ir, Beamish Re. Pathogenesis of Cardiac Dysfunction in Diabetes Mellitus. *Can J Cardiol* **1**: 263–281, 1995.
10. Mahgoub MA, Abd-Elfattah AS. Diabetes Mellitus and Cardiac Function. *Mol Cell Biochem*, **180**: 59–64, 1998.
11. Regan TJ, Weisse AB. Diabetic Cardiomyopathy. *J Am Coll Cardiol*, **19**: 1165–1166, 1996.
12. Regan TJ, Altszuler N, Eaddy C, *et al.* Relation of Growth Hormone and Myocardial Collagen Accumulation in Experimental Diabetes. *J Lab Clin Med*, **110**: 274, 1997.
13. Regan TJ, Wu GF, Weisse AB, *et al.* Acute Myocardial Infarction in Toxic Cardiomyopathy without Coronary Obstruction. *Circulation*, **51**: 453, 1995.
14. Spector KS. Diabetic Cardiomyopathy. *Clin Cardiol*, **21**: 885–887, 1999.
15. Gotzsche O, Darwish A, Gotzsche L, Hansen LP, Sorensen KE. Incipient Cardiomyopathy in Young Insulin-Dependent Diabetic Patients: A Seven-Year Prospective Doppler Echocardiographic Study. *Diabet Med*, **13**: 834–840, 1999.
16. Raev DC. Evolution of Cardiac Changes in Young Insulin-Dependent (Type I) Diabetic Patients-One More Piece of the Puzzle of Diabetic

20. Dragomir D. Particularities of Heart Failure in Diabetic Patients. Doctorate Thesis, VI, "V. Babeş" University of Medicine and Pharmacy, Timişoara, 2003.

21. Senior R, Kenny A, Nihoyannopoulos P. Stress Echocardiography For Assessing Myocardial Ischaemia And Viable Myocardium. *Heart*, **78 (Suppl 1)**: 12–18, 1999.

22. Gherasim L. *Progresses in Cardiology*. Ed Infomedica, Bucharest, 2002.

23. Garber AJ. Diabetes and vascular disease. *Diabetes, Obesity and Metabolism* **2 (Suppl.2)**: S1–S5, 2000.

24. Stanley W, Ryden L. *The Diabetic Coronary Patient*. Science Press Ltd, London, 1999.

25. Wittels EH, Gotto A. Clinical Features of Ischemic Heart Disease in Diabetes Mellitus. In: *International Textbook Of Diabetes Mellitus*. Ed. J. Willey, Chichester, 1992.

26. Wilson PW. Diabetes Mellitus and Coronary Heart Disease. *Am J Kidney Dis*, **32**: S89–S100, 1998.

27. Chen YT, Vaccario V, Williams CS, *et al.* Risk factors for heart failure in the elderly: a prospective community-based study. *Am J Med*, **106**: 605–612, 1999.

28. Carmen Ginghină, Dragomir D, Mirela Marinescu. *Guide for diagnosis and treatment in Acute Myocardial Infarction*. Ed. Infomedica, Bucharest, 2002.

29. Gerstein HC. Is glucose a continuous risk factor for cardiovascular mortality? *Diabetes Care*, **22**: 659–660, 1999.

30. Lorber D. Complicating matters. *Practical Diabetology*, **19**: 35, 2000.

31. Hammes H-P, Brownlee M. Advanced Glycation End Products and Pathogenesis of Diabetic Complications. In: LeRoith D, Taylor SI, Olefsky JM (eds). *Diabetes Mellitus: A Fundamental and Clinical Text*. Philadelphia, Lippincott-Raven Publishers, 1999, 810–815.

32. Cheţa D. *New insights into experimental diabetes*. Ed. Academiei, Bucureşti, 2002.

33. Gerber P. Diabetes. *Med Et Hyg*, **55**: 25–32, 1997.

34. Savege MP, Krolewski AS, Kenien GG, *et al.* Acute Myocardial Infarction in Diabetes Mellitus and Significance of Congestive Heart Failure as a Prognostic Factor. *Am J Cardiol*, **62**: 665, 1988.

35. Turner R, Stratton I, Horton V, *et al.* For UK Prospective Diabetes Study (UKPDS) Group. UKPDS 25: Autoantibodies to Islet-Cell Cytoplasm and Glutamic Acid Decarboxylase for Prediction of Insulin Requirement in Type II Diabetes. *Lancet*, **350**: 1288–93, 1997.

36. Miettinen H, Lehto S, Salomaa VV, *et al.* Impact of diabetes on mortality after the first myocardial infarction. *Diabetes Care*, **21**: 69–75, 1998.

37. Kempler P. *Neuropathies. Nerve dysfunction of diabetic and other origin*. Springer Verlag, Budapest, Hungary, 1997.

38. Aronson D. Pharmacologic modulation of autonomic tone: implications for the diabetic patient. *Diabetologia*, **40**: 476–481, 2001.

39. Dragomir D, Marinescu M, Ginghină C, Băcanu GS. Could autonomic cardiac dysfunction be a marker of systolic dysfunction in diabetic patients? *Romanian Journal of Diabetes Mellitus, Nutrition and Metabolic Diseases*, **2(3)**: 25–27, 2001.

40. Dragomir D, Marinescu M, Ginghina C, Ilinca R, Apetrei E, Băcanu GS. The role of insulinotherapy on the ventricular performance in cardiac decompensations at diabetic patients. *Romanian Journal of Diabetes, Nutrition and Metabolic Diseases*, **8(5)**: 17–21, 2001.

41. American Diabetes Association. Standards of Medical Care for Patients with Diabetes Mellitus. *Diabetes Care*, **20**: 518–520, 1997.

42. Diabetes Statistics. National Diabetes Information Clearinghouse. Bethesda, National Institute of Diabetes and Digestive and Kidney Disease, NIH Publications, 99–3926. 1999.

43. Solvd Investigators: Effect of Enalapril on Survival in Patients with Reduced Left Ventricular Ejection Fractions and Congestive Heart Failure. *N Engl J Med*, **325**: 293, 1991.

44. Tocchi M, Rosanio S, Anzuini A, *et al.* Angiotensin II Receptor Blockage Combined to ACE Inhibition Improves Left Ventricular Dilatation And Exercise Ejection Fraction in Congestive Heart Failure. *J Am Coll Cardiol*, **31 (Suppl A)**: 188A, 1998.

45. Heart Outcomes Prevention Evaluation (Hope) Study Investigators. Effects of Captopril in Cardiovascular and Microvascular Outcomes in People with Diabetes Mellitus Benefits the Hope Study and Micro-Hope Substudy. *Lancet*, **355**: 253–9, 2000.

46. Scheneider DJ, Sobel BE. Determinants of Coronary Vascular Disease in Patients with Type II Diabetes Mellitus and their Therapeutic Implications. *Clin Cardiol*, **20**: 433–440, 1997.

47. Merit-HF Study Group. Effect of metoprolol CR/XL in chronic heart failure: Metoprolol CR/XL. Randomized Intervention Trail in Congestive Heart Failure (MERIT-HF). *Lancet*, **353**: 2001, 1999.

48. Colucci WS, Packer M, Bristow MR, *et al.*, for the US Carvedilol Heart Failure Study Group. Carvedilol inhibits clinical progression in patients with mild symptoms of heart failure. *Circulation*, **94**: 2800, 1996.

49. Pitt B, Segal R, Martinez FA *et al.* Randomised trial of losartan versus captopril in patients over 65 with heart failure (Evaluation of Losartan in the Elderly Study, ELITE). *Lancet*, **349(9054)**: 747–52, 1997.

50. Davie AP, Dargie HJ, McMurray JJ. Role of bradykinin in the vasodilator effects of losartan and enalapril in patients with heart failure. *Circulation,* **100(3):** 268–73, 1999.51. Pitt B. Evaluation of Losartan in the Elderly (ELITE) Trial: clinical implications. *Eur Heart J,* **18(8):** 1197–9, 1997.

52. McKelvie RS, Yusuf S, Pericak D, Avezum A, Burns RJ, Probstfield J, Tsuyuki RT, White M, Rouleau J, Latini R, Maggioni A, Young J, Pogue J. Comparison of candesartan, enalapril, and their combination in congestive heart failure: randomized evaluation of strategies for left ventricular dysfunction (RESOLVD) pilot study. The RESOLVD Pilot Study Investigators. *Circulation,* **100(10):** 1056–64, 1999.

53. Consensus recommendations for the management of chronic heart failure. On behalf of the membership of the advisory council to improve outcomes nationwide in heart failure. *Am J Cardiol,* **83(A):** 1A–38A, 1999.

54. Heart Failure Society of America (HFSA) practice guidelines. HFSA guidelines for management of patients with heart failure caused by left ventricular systolic dysfunction--pharmacological approaches. *J Card Fail,* **5(4):** 357–82, 1999.

55. Sharma D, Buyse M, Pitt B, Rucinska EJ. Meta-analysis of observed mortality data from all-controlled, double-blind, multiple-dose studies of losartan in heart failure. Losartan Heart Failure Mortality Meta-analysis Study Group. *Am J Cardiol,* **85(2):** 187–92, 2000.

56. Effectiveness of spironolactone added to an angiotensin-converting enzyme inhibitor and a loop diuretic for severe chronic congestive heart failure (the Randomized Aldactone Evaluation Study [RALES]). *Am J Cardiol,* **78(8):** 902–7, 1996.

57. Fleming DR, Jacober SL, Vanderberg MA, *et al.* The Safety Of Injecting Insulin Through Clothing. *J Clin Applied Res Educ,* **20**: 244, 1997.

58. Holleman F, Schmitt H, Rottiers R, Rees A, Symanowski S, Anderson JH. The Benelux UK – Insulin Lispro Study Group. Reduced Frequency Of Severe Hypoglycaemia And Coma In Well-Controlled IDDM Patients Treated With Insulin Lispro. *Diabetes Care,* **20**: 1827–32, 1997.

59. Ikova H, Glaser B, Tunckale A, Bagricik N, Ceraso E. Induction of Long-Term Glycemic Control in Newly Diagnosed Type "Diabetic Patients by Transient Intensive Insulin Treatment". *Diabetes Care,* **20**: 1353–6, 1997.

60. The Diabetes Control and Complications Trial Research Group. The Effect of Intensive Treatment of Diabetes on the Development and Progression of Long-Term Complications in the Insulin-Dependent Diabetes Mellitus. *N Eng J Med,* **329**: 977–86, 1993.

61. Caixas A, Ordonez-Llanos J, Deleiva A, Payes A, Homs R, Perez A. Optimization of Glycemic Control by Insulin Therapy Decreases the Proportions of Small Dense LDL Particles in Diabetic Patients. *Diabetes,* **446**: 1207–13, 1997.

62. Sinclair E. *Diabetes in Old Age.* Wiley, Chichester, 2001.

63. Ebeling P, Jansson PA, Smith U, Lalli C, Bolli GP, Koivisto VA. Strategies Toward Improved Control Insulin Lispro Therapy in IDDM. *Diabetes Care,* **20**: 1287–9, 1997.

31

DIABETIC CARDIOMYOPATHY

Viorel MIHAI

Diabetes mellitus, whether type 1 or type 2, is associated with an excess of cardiovascular morbidity and mortality, factors such as coronary atherosclerosis, hypertension, and microvascular dysfunction being involved. Over the past 30 years, substantial evidence has accumulated (epidemiological, autopsy, experimental animal studies, and non-invasive human studies), supporting the existence of a specific "true" diabetic cardiomyopathy.

In the early stages, diabetic cardiomyopathy is characterized by diastolic dysfunction, often asymptomatic, of the left ventricle. In the pathogenesis of diabetic cardiomyopathy are involved defects in myocardial contractile proteins structure, abnormalities in myocardial calcium handling, lipo- and glucotoxicity, cardiac autonomic neuropathy, and genetic abnormalities. This mild form of cardiomyopathy can become severe in the presence of hypertension and/or ischemic heart disease.

The early diagnostic of the myocardial changes in diabetics is of considerable importance, since the prognosis of patients with diabetes mellitus is generally determined by cardiac complications.

Our echocardiographic study of young asymptomatic insulin dependent diabetes mellitus (IDDM) patients, without evidence of diabetic complications, hypertension, coronary artery disease, and congestive heart failure, found a high incidence (34%) of clinically silent left ventricular diastolic dysfunction. Diastolic dysfunction was related with the degree of metabolic control and was associated with a reduced cardiac reserve.

Left ventricular diastolic dysfunction is considered a marker of evolving heart disease. Therefore, the relatively high prevalence of LV diastolic dysfunction in young asymptomatic IDDM patients revealed by our study (and other ones) supports the necessity of using echocardiography in the early evaluation of subjects with type 1 diabetes.

Diabetes mellitus, whether type 1 or type 2, is associated with an excess of cardio-vascular morbidity and mortality, factors such as coronary atherosclerosis, hypertension and microvascular dysfunction being involved.

The risk of developing congestive heart failure (CHF) is greatly increased in diabetic patients. In the Framingham Heart Study, after adjustment for age, blood pressure, cholesterol level, obesity, and history of coronary artery disease, men (35 to 64 years old) with diabetes had a fourfold risk for CHF, and those over 65 years had a twofold risk for CHF. The risk is even greater in women – eightfold increase in risk for 35 to 64 years of age and fourfold increase in risk for older women [1]. Based on these findings, it appears that the excessive risk of heart failure in diabetic patients is caused by factors other than hypertension, accelerated atherogenesis, and coronary artery disease. Myocardial dysfunction directly attributable to diabetes is one suggested possibility.

After Framingham Heart Study, more recent epidemiological studies have confirmed the association between diabetes and cardiomyopathy [2–4]. In the Studies of Left Ventricular Dysfunction (SOLVD) Trials and Registry, diabetes was found to be an independent risk factor for mortality and morbidity in both symptomatic and asymptomatic heart failure [5]. In men screened for MRFIT Study, for those who had cardiomyopathy, diabetes was an independent risk factor for mortality [6].

A common finding in diabetic patients enrolled in clinical trials of myocardial infarction is a discrepancy between left ventricular systolic function and heart failure symptoms [7, 8]. One putative explanation for this discrepancy is diastolic dysfunction of the left ventricle. The relative impact of diabetes on developing heart failure was found to be greater in women.

In 1928, Root accomplished the first post-mortem study of diabetic heart. The conclusion was that cardiac changes are the result of accelerated atherosclerosis. In 1954, Lundback unified retinopathy, nephropathy, cardiac involvement, and peripheral artery disease of the diabetic patient in a syndrome of diabetic angiopathy.

Based on post-mortem findings in patients with heart failure, free of coronary artery disease or other known cardiac risk factor, Rubler *et al.* first suggested the existence of a specific diabetic cardiomyopathy (1972). They described cardiomegaly with extensive fibrosis, interstitial deposition of periodic acid-Schiff positive material, and normal coronary arteries [9].

Hamby first used the term of "diabetic cardiomyopathy" in 1974.

Over the past 30 years, substantial evidence has accumulated (epidemiological, autopsy, experimental animal studies, and non-invasive human studies) supporting the existence of a specific "true" diabetic cardiomyopathy.

Recently, the WHO Experts Committee in Cardiomyopathy recommended the use of this term: "diabetic heart muscle disease".

PATHOLOGICAL CHANGES

Diabetic cardiomyopathy is characterized, in autopsy studies, by changes in the micro-vasculature and myocardial interstitium, associated with myocellular hypertrophy [10, 11].

Initially, interstitial changes predominate, with deposition of periodic acid-Schiff positive material. Fibrosis and increased collagen content of the myocardium in type 1 diabetic individuals were confirmed by noninvasive studies, such as ultrasound tissue characterization with backscatter analysis [12, 13]. Multiple bioptic samples of left ventricular septum revealed abnormally deposits of cholesterol and triglycerides, in addition to increased collagen content [14]. These interstitial changes with preserved myocardial cells and microvasculature contribute to reduced ventricular compliance.

In patients with advanced stages of congestive heart failure, myocyte hypertrophy and replacement fibrosis, arteriolar or capillary involvement with micro aneurysms and capillary basement membrane thickening, are typically seen.

Studies that are more recent raise doubts about small vessel disease being the cause of cardiac myopathy, because similar changes have been reported to be present in NIDDM subjects. While evidence suggests that occlusive disease of the small vessels is not the cause of diabetic cardiomyopathy [14, 15], the possibility that an imbalance in endothelial factors leading to arterial spasm and subsequent reperfusion injury to the myocardium that may eventually lead to diabetic cardiomyopathy cannot be excluded [16]. In addition, in diabetic patients there may be inadequate reactive angiogenesis in the presence of ischemia [17, 18]. It is also possible that the abnormal permeability seen in diabetic small vessel disease could lead to interstitial edema, fibrosis, and diabetic cardiomyopathy [19].

Coexistence of hypertension and/or myocardial ischemia is considered a major factor in the expression of abnormalities in the myocardium of diabetic patients, with more severe interstitial fibrosis, focal scars and myocytolytic activity [20].

PATHOPHYSIOLOGY

The pathophysiology of diabetic cardiomyopathy remains largely unknown. Results of experimental studies suggest several mechanisms: accumulation of AGEs, abnormal handling of myocardial calcium, defects in myocardial glucose utilization and fatty acid metabolism.

A great deal of attention has been focused on the ability of cardiac cells to handle calcium and several abnormalities have been reported.

The sarcoplasmic reticulum and sarcolemma are important organelles involved in the maintenance of calcium homeostasis within the cardiac cell. In addition, the exchange of calcium for other ions such as sodium and hydrogen is a major factor in regulating the intracellular calcium concentrations. Generally, mechanisms controlling calcium are depressed in the diabetic heart. The ability of the sarcoplasmic reticulum (SR) to take up and release calcium is decreased and the activity of the SR calcium ATPase is depressed [21, 22]. Decreases in Na^+/K^+-ATPase and adenylate cyclase occur, accompanied by decreases in Na^+/Ca^{++} calcium exchange-pump activity and changes in the sarcolemmal membrane [23–25].

Defects in mitochondrial respiratory function accompany the development of diabetic cardiomyopathy [21]. The decrease in Ca^{++} uptake into mitochondria prevents the stimulation of Ca^{++}-sensitive matrix dehydrogenases, decreasing the capacity of mitochondria to up regulate ATP synthesis. The impairment in the augmentation of

ATP synthesis rate accompanies a decreased rate of relaxation.

Decrease in cardiac contractility was shown to result, at least in part, from a dysfunction of the type 2 ryanodine receptor calcium-release channel (RyR2). One of the mechanisms underlying RyR2 dysfunction is non cross-linking of advanced glycation end-products (AGEs) formation on RyR2 [26].

Further support for these hypotheses comes from the beneficial effect of verapamil that prevented diabetes-induced myocardial changes in experimental diabetes [27].

Diabetes is as much a disorder of fatty acid metabolism as it is a disorder of glucose metabolism. In diabetes, the heart is exposed to hyperglycemic and hyperlipidic environment. The heart initially adapts to this environment by increasing the expression of fatty acid metabolizing proteins, thereby increasing the reliance on fatty acids as a fuel [28, 29]. As diabetes progresses, the excessive availability of lipids and fatty acids exceeds the rate of their use by the heart, resulting in lipid accumulation within the cardiomyocyte. Hyperglycemia is associated with a dramatic decrease in the expression of peroxisome proliferator-activated receptor α (PPARα) and PPARα regulating gene, resulting in accelerated lipid accumulation [30].

Lipid accumulation within cells is associated with a phenomenon called "lipotoxicity" [31]. Increased cytosolic levels of long chain fatty acyl-CoAs are utilized in the synthesis of both diacylglycerol and ceramide.

Diacylglycerol is a potent activator of various protein kinase C (PKC) isoforms. Experimental studies showed that chronic activation of PKC in the myocardium causes cardiomyopathy [32].

Increased intracellular ceramide levels can induce accumulation of reactive oxygen species (ROS), inducible NO synthase (iNOS), and apoptosis. Evidence supporting this hypothesis comes from insulin resistant ZDF rat. Hearts isolated from these animals have increased ceramide levels within the cardiomyocytes, DNA laddering indicative of apoptosis, and contractile dysfunction [31].

Carnitine is required for the transport of lipids into mitochondria for subsequent metabolism and low levels of carnitine in diabetic cardiomyocyte will impair lipid utilization, with the consequences described above [33–35].

Diabetic heart has decreased insulin sensitivity. Increased flux through the hexosamine biosynthetic pathway, resulting in increased O-linked glycosylation of specific proteins, such as the insulin receptor substrates, is one current hypothesis for the glucose-induced insulin resistance [36, 37].

Acute hyperglycemia increases inducible NO synthase (iNOS) gene expression and nitric oxide (NO) release in working rat hearts [38]. Up regulation of iNOS and raised NO generation are accompanied by a marked increase of superoxide production, a condition favoring the production of peroxynitrite, a powerful pro-oxidant. The peroxynitrite anion is cytotoxic because it inhibits mitochondrial electron transport, oxidizes sulfhydryl groups in proteins, initiates lipid peroxidation even in the absence of transition metals, and nitrates amino acids such as tyrosine, which affects many signal transduction pathways. The presence of nitrotyrosine residues is a marker of peroxynitrite production. Recent studies demonstrate that the increased apoptosis of myocytes, endothelial cells, and fibroblasts in heart biopsies from diabetic patients and in hearts from streptozotocin-induced diabetic rats is selectively associated with a high level of nitrotyrosine, supporting the hypothesis that high glucose can acutely produce myocardial damage and cardiac cell apoptosis through the formation of nitrotyrosine [38–42].

Oxidative and nitrosative stress in diabetic hearts is accompanied by the increased formation of hydrogen peroxide and peroxynitrite, which are endogenous inducers of DNA single-strand breakage [44]. DNA single-strand breakage is the trigger of poly (ADPribose) polymerase (PARP) activation. Hyperactivation of PARP results in rapid depletion of the intracellular NAD^+ and ATP pools, thus slowing the rate of glycolysis and mitochondrial respiration, eventually leading to cellular dysfunction and death. Based on the results of their studies, Parcher *et al.* conclude that the "reactive oxygen/nitrogen species – DNA injury – PARP activation" pathway also plays a pathogenic role in the development of diabetic cardiomyopathy [45–47].

Accumulation of advanced glycation-end-products (AGE) associated with chronic hyperglycemia induces ROS generation. Excessive free radical generation affects ion channels, Ca^{++} homeostasis, mitochondrial function, transcription factor DNA binding activity, growth, and even initiates apoptosis [48–51].

In vitro and *in vivo* observations support the idea that hyperglycemia is responsible for apoptotic myocyte death associated with diabetes *via* activation of the local renin angiotensin system (RAS). A strong association between the up regulation of cellular RAS and the apoptosis of myocytes, endothelial cells, and fibroblasts has been identified in the diabetic human heart [40].

A biochemical event associated with diabetes is the formation of glycosylated products. Proteins constitute the principal substrate of this reaction, which generates glycoproteins in the extracellular compartment, plasma membrane, cytoplasm, and, ultimately, in the nucleus. The most frequent type of intracellular glycosylation is O-linked N-acetyl-glucosamine. Glycosylation and phosphorylation activate several transcription factors, including p53 [52, 53]. Because p53 binding sites are present in the promoter of angiotensinogen and AT_1 receptor genes, p53 enhances the myocyte renin-angiotensin system (RAS) and the formation of angiotensin II. Moreover, p53 reduces the expression of genes opposing cell death, and up regulates genes promoting apoptosis [54].

AGEs can directly alter the physical and structural properties of extracellular matrix by inducing collagen cross-linking that confers enhanced stiffness [55–58].

The alterations in failing human hearts have been suggested to be, at least in part, a consequence of the increased stimulation of β1-adrenoreceptors by noradrenaline released from the sympathetic nerves in an attempt to restore cardiac function. Similarly, it has been demonstrated that cardiac noradrenaline content is increased in diabetic rats [59]. In addition, it was reported that noradrenaline turnover, uptake, synthesis, and release are all enhanced in diabetic cardiomyopathy [60–62].

Diabetic hearts exhibit decreased responsiveness to stimulation by ß-adrenoreceptor agonists.

Studies performed by Dincer *et al.* showed that the expression of β1-adrenoreceptors decreases, whereas that of β2-ARs increases, in hearts of long-term diabetic rats, thus implicating dysautonomia in the pathogenesis of diabetic cardiac dysfunction [63].

Diabetes mellitus is a heterogeneous disease, caused by both genetic and environmental factors. Diabetes mellitus with the mitochondrial DNA (A–G) mutation is reported to represent 0.5–2.8 % of the general diabetic population. These patients have advanced microvascular complications and mitochondria-related complications, such as cardiomyopathy and cardiac conductance disorders [64].

Diabetes mellitus might be associated with another form of cardiomyopathy. As much as half of the infants of diabetic mothers have signs of congestive heart failure [65]. The cardiomyopathy in these infants is usually transient, and appears to be secondary to hematological, respiratory, and metabolic problems, or to maternal hormonal influences.

Summarizing, in the pathogenesis of diabetic cardiomyopathy are involved: defects in myocardial contractile protein, an increase in collagen formation and accumulation of AGE-modified extracellular matrix proteins, abnormalities in myocardial calcium handling, lipo- and glucotoxicity, cardiac autonomic neuropathy, and genetic abnormalities.

CLINICAL FEATURES

In the first stage of diabetic cardiomyopathy, the pathological and cellular abnormalities in the myocardium discussed above generate diastolic dysfunction of the left ventricle, with the preservation of the systolic performance. On clinical grounds, it is almost unrecognizable, shortness of breath with unusual effort being the only symptom. At this stage, tight glycemic control seems to be the most effective method for treating myocardial dysfunction.

A second stage of diabetic cardiomyopathy is characterized by diastolic dysfunction and progressive deterioration of the systolic performance.

In a third stage, a typical "congestive" cardiomyopathy occurs.

The natural history of diabetic cardiomyopathy is poorly understood. Many diabetic patients have diastolic dysfunction, but only a part will develop systolic dysfunction, producing a typical congestive cardiomyopathy.

It is likely that in diabetics, cardiomyopathy is, per se, usually mild, but when hypertension and/or ischemic heart disease overlap, the cardiomyopathy can become severe.

TREATMENT OF DIABETIC CARDIOMYOPATHY

In preventing and treating diabetic cardiomyopathy glycemic control seems to be essential. Putative ways of improving diastolic dysfunction are exercise, or, pharmacologically, the use of β-blockers and calcium antagonists. At least in part, defects in myocardial glucose utilization and fatty acid metabolism are responsible for the myocardial dysfunction in diabetes. Trimetazidine, which improves myocardial glucose and fatty acids utilization, could be beneficial in this setting.

Aggressive therapy of hypertension with the appropriate antihypertensive agents is essential in preventing, delaying the onset of, and ameliorating the development of myocardial disease.

In addition, tight control of dyslipidemia is mandatory.

Once overt heart failure has occurred, classical therapy, with emphasis on β-blockers and aggressive treatment with ACE inhibitors is highly warranted.

Even with actual aggressive therapy, patients with advanced stages of diabetic cardiomyopathy have a poor prognostic. If asymptomatic left ventricular diastolic dysfunction represents the initial stage of diabetic cardiomyopathy, it is of great importance to detect cardiac involvement from the beginning. In this early stage, cardiac changes may be reversible. Fortunately, diastolic dysfunction of left ventricle is easily diagnosed with Doppler echocardiography.

Numerous studies attempted to determine the prevalence of LV diastolic dysfunction in asymptomatic patients with either type 1 or type 2 diabetes mellitus [66–71]. The results were controversial, one of the possible explanations being that the prevalence of LV diastolic dysfunction assessed by transmitral flow was underestimated, many investigators neglecting to account for pseudonormal patterns of ventricular filling [72, 73]. Valsalva maneuver can be easily used to unmask pseudonormal patterns of filling. Investigators tried to find correlations between glycemic control, microvascular disease and LV diastolic dysfunction. However, a clear relationship has not been clearly established [74–78].

The objectives of this study were to estimate the prevalence of LV diastolic dysfunction in young type 1 diabetic patients using Doppler echocardiography associated with Valsalva maneuver to unmask a pseudonormal pattern, and to evaluate the association between LV diastolic dysfunction and metabolic control.

METHODS

Study population. A total of 29 young patients, aged 21–27 years, mean age 24 ± 2 years, with type 1 diabetes mellitus, were consecutively recruited. The exclusion criteria were clinical evidence of cardiovascular or respiratory disease and presence of diabetic retinopathy, neuropathy or microalbuminuria.

15 age-matched healthy, nondiabetic subjects were recruited.

All subjects were ascertained to be otherwise healthy by medical history and physical examination.

Maximum treadmill exercise testing (Bruce protocol) was used to exclude significant coronary artery disease and to evaluate cardiac performance.

When silent ischemia, arrhythmias or hypertension were suspected, 24-h ambulatory blood pressure and ECG monitoring were performed to rule out these conditions.

Echocardiography. M-mode, two-dimensional and cardiac Doppler studies were performed using a commercially available echo-Doppler unit, equipped with a 3.5 MHz transducer. Subjects were studied in left lateral decubitus, utilizing standard parasternal and apical views.

All recordings were performed at midday to avoid the influence of circadian rhythm on LV diastolic function.

Measurements of interventricular septal thickness (IVST, mm), posterior wall thickness (PWT, mm), LV end-diastolic dimension

(LVEDD, mm), LV end-systolic dimension (LVESD, mm), and left atrial size (LA, mm) were made according to the recommendations of the American Society of Echocardiography [79]. Left ventricular mass (LVM) was calculated using the following formula [80]:

$$LVM = 0.8 \times \{1.04(IVST+LVEDD+PWT)^3 - LVESD^3\} + 0.6g$$

LV mass index was calculated, and LV hypertrophy was considered to be present when it exceeded 104 g/m^2 for women, and 116 g/m^2 for men.

Doppler ultrasound examinations were performed with the transducer at the apex (apical four-chamber view), in pulsed mode, placing the sample volume at the mitral leaflets tips, at the end of the expiration. All the cardiac valves were examined by both spectral and color Doppler to rule out valvular disease.

From the transmitral recordings (100 mm/s), the following measurements were made on three to five consecutive cardiac cycles: peak E velocity in m/s (peak early transmitral filling velocity), peak A velocity in m/s (peak transmitral atrial filling velocity), deceleration time in msec (time elapsed between peak E velocity and the point where the extrapolation of the deceleration slope of the E velocity crosses the zero baseline), and isovolumic relaxation time of LV in msec (measured as the interval from the aortic closure and the onset of the diastolic mitral flow).

Same data were obtained during phase II of the Valsalva maneuver. Patients were instructed to hold a regular breath and to bear down on against closed glottis for at least 10 seconds.

Diastolic physiology was characterized as normal, impaired relaxation, pseudonormal, and restrictive pattern according to widely used criteria. The pseudonormal pattern resembles the normal filling physiology, with E/A ratio > 1, and a deceleration time between 160 and 240 msec. To distinguish these subjects from the normal physiology, the E/A ratio must be < 1 after the Valsalva maneuver. In normal subjects, acute preload reduction induced by the Valsalva strain results in a proportional decrease in both E and A wave velocities; consequently, the E/A ratio is maintained at >1.

No subject had echocardiographically detectable regional wall motion abnormalities, and all subjects had normal ejection fractions and fractional shortening.

STATISTICAL ANALYSIS

Data are presented as mean ± SD and frequency expressed as a percentage. Differences between groups were assessed by Student's paired t test. Subjects with impaired relaxation and pseudonormal patterns were analyzed together when appropriate.

A 2-tailed p value < 0.05 was considered significant.

RESULTS

Table 31.1 lists the clinical characteristics of the control and study group.

Table 31.1

Clinical characteristics of the control and study groups

	Normal (n = 15)	IDDM (n = 29)
Age (years)	25.4 ± 2.2	24.17 ± 2.08
Body mass index (kg/m^2)	24.5 ± 1.79	23.15 ± 1.86
Systolic blood pressure (mmHg)	126 ± 7	128 ± 6
Diastolic blood pressure (mmHg)	72 ± 5	76 ± 6
Exercise (METs)	12.06 ± 2.01	9.89 ± 1.87*
Maximal predicted heart rate (%)	90.6 ± 4	89.37 ± 3.47

* P < 0.05

There were no differences between diabetic patients and control group in body mass index, systolic and diastolic blood pressure. Normal subjects performed 12.06 ± 2.01 METs, whereas as a group, subjects with diabetes attained 9.98 ± 1.87 METs (p < 0.05). There was no difference between groups in predictive heart rate attained during the maximal treadmill test (90.06 ± 4 *vs.* 89.37 ± 3.47 %).

Table 31.2 shows clinical characteristics of diabetic subjects separated into three groups based on left ventricular diastolic function: normal, impaired relaxation or pseudonormal pattern. Normal filling pattern was present in 19 patients (65.51%), impaired relaxation in seven (24.13%), and pseudonormal pattern in three patients (10.34%). There were no differences among groups in diabetes duration, body mass index, systolic and diastolic blood pressure.

There were significant differences in maximal treadmill performance measured in metabolic equivalents (METs), depending on LV diastolic function. Patients with normal diastolic function attained 10.6 ± 1.6 METs, those with impaired relaxation 9.14 ± 1.4, and those with pseudonormal pattern of LV filling, 7 METs. Moreover, subjects in pseudonormal pattern group achieved only 82 ± 2% of predictive heart rate, significantly (P < 0,05) lower than subjects with normal diastolic function (90.5 ± 2.4%) and with impaired relaxation (89.3 ± 2.4%).

Patients with normal LV diastolic function had a better metabolic control of diabetes (HbA1c = 7.4 ± 0.5) compared with patients in impaired relaxation group (HbA1c = 8.6 ± 0.34) and pseudonormal group (HbA1c = 9.5 ± 0.1).

Table 31.3 summarizes the echocardiographic data of the control and IDDM groups. All dimensions were within normal limits. There were no differences between groups in interventricular septum, posterior wall, left atrium, ventricular systolic and diastolic dimensions, left ventricular mass index or left ventricular ejection fraction.

All subjects in control group had normal diastolic function. Patients with diabetes, pooled together, had a longer isovolumic relaxation time of LV and deceleration time of E wave, without reaching statistical significance.

Table 31.4 summarizes the echocardiographic data of the diabetic patients based on LV diastolic function. Left ventricular dimensions, mass index, and ejection fraction were normal, with no differences among the three groups.

Left atrial size in pseudonormal pattern group was larger compared with normal and impaired relaxation groups (P < 0.05). However, LA size was within normal limits in all three groups.

Table 31.2

Clinical characteristics of diabetic patients based on LV diastolic function

	Normal (n=19)	Impaired relaxation (n=7)	Pseudonormal pattern (n=3)
Age (years)	24 ± 1.85	24.8 ± 2.8	23 ± 2
Diabetes duration (years)	4.5 ± 1.42	4.6 ± 1.7	5.3 ± 1.5
Body mass index (kg/m^2)	23.12 ± 1.6	23.04 ± 2.38	23.7 ± 2.8
Systolic blood pressure (mmHg)	128 ± 5	127 ± 6	125
Diastolic blood pressure (mmHg)	75 ± 4	73 ± 5	77 ± 3
Hemoglobin A1c	7.4 ± 0.5	8.6 ± 0.34*	9.5 ± 0.1*
Exercise (METs)	10.6 ± 1.6	9.14 ± 1.4*	7*
Maximal predicted heart rate (%)	90.5 ± 2.4	89.3 ± 2.4	82 ± 2**

* $P < 0.05$ impaired relaxation *vs.* normal, pseudonormal pattern *vs.* normal and impaired relaxation.
** $P < 0.05$ pseudonormal pattern *vs.* normal and impaired relaxation.

Table 31.3

Echocardiographic data of the control and IDDM groups

	Control	IDDM
LV diastolic dimension (mm)	52.8 ± 3.65	51.86 ± 2.43
LV systolic dimension (mm)	32.9 ± 2.18	32.37 ± 2.61
Left atrium (mm)	34.66 ± 3.53	33.24 ± 3.09
Interventricular septum (mm)	10.3 ± 1.06	9.82 ± 1.1
Posterior wall (mm)	9.63 ± 0.99	9.22 ± 0.95
LV mass index (g/m^2)	109.17 ± 16.45	105.70 ± 16.7
Ejection fraction (%)	65.5 ± 2.65	64.9 ± 3.74
Isovolumic relaxation time (ms)	74.66 ± 10.25	87.58 ± 19.34
E velocity (m/s)	1.07 ± 0.22	0.93 ± 0.22
A velocity (m/s)	0.71 ± 0.16	0.78 ± 0.17
Deceleration time E (ms)	175 ± 11.49	183.10 ± 25.3

Table 31.4

Echocardiographic data of the diabetic patients based on LV diastolic function

	Normal (n = 19)	Impaired relaxation (n = 7)	Pseudo-normal pattern (n = 3)
LV diastolic dimension (mm)	52 ± 2.53	51.54 ± 2.63	52 ± 1.73
LV systolic dimension (mm)	32.31 ± 2.56	32 ± 3.21	33.66 ± 1.52
Left atrium (mm)	32.84 ± 2.28	32.85 ± 3.23	36.6 ± 1.5 *
Interventricular septum (mm)	9.94 ± 1.18	9.42 ± 1.01	10 ± 1
Posterior wall (mm)	9.31 ± 1.01	8.85 ± 0.89	9.5 ± 0.5
LV mass index (g/m^2)	107.5 ± 17.8	101.2 ± 15.83	109.06 ± 10.4
Ejection fraction (%)	64.7 ± 2.3	65.8 ± 3.7	64 ± 1
Isovolumic relaxation time (ms)	76.05 ± 10.87	108.57 ± 12.8	110.66 ± 2.88
E velocity (m/s)	1.04 ± 0.19	0.71 ± 0.14	0.8 ± 0.1
A velocity (m/s)	0.75 ± 0.15	0.91 ± 0.19	0.7 ± 0.1
Deceleration time E (ms)	168.94 ± 13.7	216.42 ± 19.3	195 ± 5
E/A ratio	1.41 ± 0.37	0.78 ± 0.08	1.14 ± 0.02
E velocity (m/s) – Valsalva	1.06 ± 0.17	0.71 ±0.13	0.66 ± 0.05
A velocity (m/s) – Valsalva	0.75 ± 0.15	0.95 ± 0.18	0.9 ± 0.1
E/A ratio – Valsalva	1.44 ± 0.38	0.75 ± 0.13	0.74 ± 0.03

* $P < 0.05$ pseudonormal pattern *vs.* normal and impaired relaxation.

The acute preload-reducing maneuver (Valsalva) led to a significant E wave decrease and an A wave increase in subjects with pseudonormal pattern. Consequently, an E/A ratio inversion was noted. In normal and impaired relaxation groups, no changes of E/A ratio were noted.

DISCUSSION

This study demonstrates that as many as 24% of clinically asymptomatic subjects with IDDM, without evidence of hypertension, ischemic heart disease, congestive heart failure, and free of diabetic complications, have impaired relaxation of left ventricle. Using Valsalva maneuver, pseudonormal pattern of LV filling is unmasked in other 10.4% of patients, so the prevalence of diastolic dysfunction of LV is as much as 34.4% in asymptomatic young type 1 diabetics.

Diastolic dysfunction of left ventricle is correlated with diabetes control (HbA1c) and is associated with a lower maximal treadmill performance. Unlike patients with normal and impaired relaxation, those with pseudonormal pattern of LV filling fail to achieve 85% of maximal predicted heart rate, demonstrating a reduced cardiac reserve.

There is no prospective data supporting the benefit or even the need for a specific regimen in diabetics with diastolic dysfunction. If diastolic dysfunction of left ventricle, even asymptomatic, is considered the first step in the evolution of diabetic cardiomyopathy, then better glycemic control is appropriate.

Mild diabetic cardiomyopathy can become severe in the presence of hypertension and/or coronary artery disease. Assessment of diastolic dysfunction is advisable for early detection of left ventricle dysfunction, before clinical symptoms appear. Glycemic control, energetic detection and treatment of hypertension with appropriate antihypertensive agents, detection and aggressive treatment of dyslipidemia, and early detection and treatment of ischemic heart disease are essential in preventing and treating diabetic cardiomyopathy.

STUDY LIMITATION

This study was limited to a small group of young type 1 diabetic patients, without diabetic complications and hypertension, ischemic heart disease or congestive heart failure, to avoid too many confounding variables. Another study including a significantly larger group of patients is needed. This study shows that diabetics with diastolic dysfunction, especially those with pseudonormal pattern of left ventricular filling, have a worse metabolic control. Prospective studies are needed to find out if improving glycemic control will improve myocardial dysfunction.

Left ventricular diastolic dysfunction is considered to be a marker of evolving heart disease. Therefore, the relatively high prevalence of LV diastolic dysfunction in young asymptomatic IDDM patients revealed by this study supports the idea of using echocardiography in the early evaluation of subjects with type 1 diabetes.

REFERENCES

1. Kannel WB, Hjortland M, Castelli WP. Role of diabetes in congestive heart failure: The Framingham study. *Am J Cardiol,* **32:** 29–34, 1974.
2. Coughlin SS, Pearle DL, Baughman KL, *et al.* Diabetes mellitus risk of idiopathic dilated cardiomyopathy. The Washington, DC Dilated Cardiomyopathy Study. *Ann Epidemiol,* **4:** 67–74, 1994.
3. Coughlin SS, Teft MC. The epidemiology of idiopathic dilated cardiomyopathy in women: The Washington, DC Dilated Cardiomyopathy Study. *Epidemiology,* **5:** 449–455, 1994.
4. Galderisi M, Anderson KM, Wilson PW, *et al.* Echocardiographic evidence for the existence of a distinct diabetic cardiomyopathy (The Framingham Heart Study). *Am J Cardiol,* **68:** 85–89, 1991.
5. Shindler DM, Kostis JB, Yusuf S, *et al.* Diabetes mellitus, a predictor of morbidity and mortality in the Studies of Left Ventricular Dysfunction (SOLVD) Trials and Registry. *Am J Cardiol,* **77:** 1017–1020, 1996.
6. Coughlin SS, Neaton JD, Sengupta A, *et al.* Predictors of mortality from idiopathic dilated

cardiomyopathy in 356,222 men screened for The Multiple Risk Factor Intervention Trial. *Am J Epidemiol*, **139**: 166–172, 1994.

7. Stone PH, Muller JE, Turi ZG, Strauss HW, Wilkerson JT, Robertson T. The effect of diabetes mellitus on prognosis and serial left ventricular function after acute myocardial infarction: contribution of both coronary disease and diastolic left ventricular dysfunction to the adverse prognosis: the MILIS Study Group. *J AM Coll Cardiol*, **14**: 49–57, 1989.

8. Gustafson I, Hildebrandt P, Seibæk M, Melchior T, Torp-Pedersen C, Køber L, Kaiser-Nielsen P. Long term prognosis of diabetic patients with myocardial infarction: relation to antidiabetic treatment regimen. *Eur Heart J*, **21**: 1937–1943, 2000.

9. Rubler S, Dluglash J, Uuceoglu YZ, Kumral T, Branwood AW, Grishman A. New type of cardiomyopathy associated with diabetic glomerulosclerosis. *Am J Cardiol* **30**: 595–602, 1972.

10. Fischer VW, Barner HB, and Leskino ML. Capillary basal laminar thickness in diabetic human myocardium. *Diabetes,* **28**: 713–719, 1979.

11. Factor SM, Okun EM, MINASE T. Capillary microaneurysms in the human diabetic heart. *N Engl J Med*, **302**: 384–388, 1980.

12. Perez JE, McGill JB, Santiago JV, *et al*. Abnormal myocardial acoustic properties in diabetic patients and their correlations with the severity of disease. *J Am Coll Cardiol*, **19**: 1154–1162, 1992.

13. Di Bello V, Talarico L, Picano E, *et al*. Increased echodensity of myocardial wall in the diabetic heart: An ultrasound tissue characterization study. *J Am Coll Cardiol*, **25**: 1408–1415, 1995.

14. Sunni S, Bishop SP, Kent SP, and Geer, JC. Diabetic cardiomyopathy. *Arch Pathol Lab Med,* **110**: 375–381, 1988.

15. Shirey EK, Proudfit WL, Hawk WA. Primary myocardial disease: correlations with clinical findings, angiography and biopsy diagnosis: follow-up of 139 patients. *Am Heart J,* **62**: 251–254, 1980.

16. Ahmed SS, Jaferi GA, Narang RM, and Regan TJ. Preclinical abnormality of left ventricular function in diabetes mellitus. *Am Heart J,* **89**: 153–158, 1975.

17. Yarom R, Zirkin H, Stammler G, Rose AG. Human coronary microvessels in diabetes and ischemia: morphometric study of autopsy material. *J Pathol,* **166**: 265–270, 1992.

18. Warly A, Powell JM, and Skepper JN. Capillary surface area is reduced and tissue thickness from capillaries to myocytes is increased in the left ventricle of streptozotocin-diabetic rats. *Diabetologia,* **38**: 413–421, 1995.

19. Bell SH. Diabetic Cardiomyopathy: A Unique Entity or a Complication of Coronary Artery Disease? *Diabetes Care,* **18**: 708–714, 1995.

20. Factor SR, Minase T, Sonnenblick EH. Clinical and morphological features of human hypertensive diabetic cardiomyopathy. *Am Heart J,* **99**: 446–458, 1980.

21. Flarsheim CE, Grupp IL, and Matlib MA. Mitochondrial dysfunction accompanies diastolic dysfunction in diabetic rat heart. *Am J Physiol Heart Circ Physiol,* **221**: H192–H201, 1996.

22. Choi KM, Zhong Y, Hoit BD, Grupp IL, Hahn H, Dilly KW, Guatimosim S, Lederer WJ, Matlib MA. Defective intracellular Ca^{2+} signaling contributes to cardiomyopathy in Type I diabetic rats. *Am J Physiol Heart Circ Physiol,* **283**: H1398–H1408, 2002.

23. Netticadan T, Temsah RM, Elimban V, Dhalla NS. Depressed Levels of Ca^{2+}-Cycling Proteins May Underlie Sarcoplasmic Reticulum Dysfunction in the Diabetic Heart. *Diabetes,* **50**: 2133–2138, 2001.

24. Lagadic-Grossmann D, Buckler KJ, Le Prigent K, Feuvray D. Altered Ca^{2+} handling in ventricular myocytes isolated from diabetic rats. *Am J Physiol Heart Circ Physiol,* **270**: H1529–H1537, 1996.

25. Trost SV, Belke DD, Bluhm WF, Meyer M, Swanson E, Dilman WH. Overexpression of the Sarcoplasmic Reticulum Ca^{2+}-ATPase Improves Myocardial Contractility in Diabetic Cardiomyopathy. *Diabetes,* **51**: 1166–1171, 2002.

26. Bidasee KR, Nallani K, Yu Y, Cocklin RR, Zhang Y, Wang M, Dincer ÜD, Besh HR, Jr. Chronic diabetes increases advanced glycation end-products on cardiac ryanodine receptors/calcium release channels. *Diabetes,* **52**: 1825–1836, 2003.

27. Afzal N, Ganguly PK, Dhalla KS, Pierce GN, Singal PK, Dhalla NS. Beneficial effects of verapamil in diabetic cardiomyopathy. *Diabetes,* **37**: 936–942, 1988.

28. Kersten S, Seydoux J, Peters J, *et al*. Peroxisome proliferator-activated receptor alpha mediates the adaptive response to fasting. *J Clin Invest,* **103**: 1489–1498, 1999.

29. Leone T, Weinheimer C, Kelly D. A critical role for the peroxisome proliferator-activated receptor alpha (PPARα) in the cellular fasting response: the PPARα-null mouse as a model of fatty acid oxidation disorders. *Proc Natl Acad Sci USA,* **96**: 7473–7478, 1999.

30. Young ME, McNulty P, Taegtmeyer, H. Adaptation and Maladaptation of the Heart in Diabetes: Part II. Potential Mechanisms. *Circulation,* **105**: 1861–1883, 2002.

31. Zhou Y, Grayburn P, Karim A, *et al*. Lipotoxic heart disease in obese rats: implications for human obesity. *Proc Natl Acad Sci USA*, **97**: 1784–1789, 2000.

32. Wakasaki H, Koya D, Schoen F, *et al*. Targeted Overexpression of protein kinase C β2 isoform in myocardium causes cardiomyopathy. *Proc Natl Acad Sci USA*, **94**: 9320–9325, 1997.

33. McNeill, JH. Role of elevated lipids in diabetic cardiomyopathy. *Diab Res Clin Pract*, **31**: S67–S71, 1996.

34. Rodrigues B, Ross FR, Farahbakshian S, McNeill JH. Effects of *in vivo* and *in vitro* treatment with L-carnitine on isolated hearts from chronically diabetic rats. *Can J Physiol Pharmacol*, **68**: 1085–1092, 1990.

35. Rodrigues B, Xiang H, McNeill JH. Effect of L-carnitine treatment on lipid metabolism and cardiac performance in chronically diabetic rats. *Diabetes*, **37**: 1358–1364, 1988.

36. Doenst T, Goodwin GW, Cedars AM, *et al*. Load-induced changes *in vivo* alter substrate fluxes and insulin responsiveness of rat heart *in vitro*. *Metabolism*, **50**: 1083–1090, 2001.

37. Sakamoto J, Barr R, Kavanagh K, *et al*. Contribution of malonyl-CoA decarboxylase to the high fatty acid oxidation rates seen in the diabetic heart. *Am J Physiol Heart Circ Physiol*, **278**: H1196–H1204, 2000.

38. Ceriello A, Quagliaro L, D'Amico M, *et al*. Acute hyperglycemia induces nitrotyrosine formation and apoptosis in perfused heart from rat. *Diabetes*, **51**: 1076–1082, 2002.

39. Cai L, Li W, Wang G, *et al*. Hyperglycemia-induced apoptosis in mouse myocardium: mitochondrial cytochrome c-mediated caspase-3 activation pathway. *Diabetes*, **51**: 1938–1948, 2002.

40. Frustaci A, Kajstura J, Cimenti C, *et al*. Myocardial cell death in human diabetes. *Circ Res*, **87**: 1123–1132, 2000.

41. Marfella R, Terrazzo G, Acampora R, *et al*. Glutathione reverses systemic hemodynamic changes by acute hyperglycemia in healthy subjects. *Am J Physiol*, **268**: E1167–E1173, 1995.

42. Mihm MJ, Jing L, Bauer JA. Nitrotyrosine causes selective vascular endothelial dysfunction and DNA damage. *J Cardiovasc Pharmacol*, **86**: 182–187, 2000.

43. Kajstura J, Fiordaliso F, Andreoli AM, *et al*. IGF-1 overexpression inhibits the development of diabetic cardiomyopathy and angiotensin II-mediated oxidative stress. *Diabetes*, **50**: 1414–1424, 2001.

44. Pieper AA, Verma A, Zhang J, Snyder SH. Poly (ADP-ribose) polymerase nitric oxide and cell death. *Trends Pharmacol Sci*, **20**: 171–181, 1999.

45. Zingarelli B, Salzmann AL, Szabo C. Genetic disruption of poly (ADP-ribose) synthetase inhibits the expression of P-selectin and intercellular adhesion molecule-1 in myocardial ischemia / reperfusion injury. *Circ Res*, **83**: 87–91, 1998.

46. Szabo C, Cuzzocrea S, Zingarelli B, *et al*. Endothelial dysfunction in a rat model of endotoxic shock: importance of the activation of poly (ADP-ribose) synthetase by peroxynitrite. *J Clin Invest*, **100**: 723–735, 1997.

47. Parcher P, Liaudet L, Soriano FG, *et al*. The role of poly (ADP-ribose) polymerase activation in the development of myocardial and endothelial dysfunction in diabetes. *Diabetes*, **51**: 514–521, 2002.

48. Morad M, Suzuki YJ. Redox regulation of cardiac muscle calcium signaling. *Antioxid Redox Signal*, **2**: 65–71, 2000.

49. Ide T, Tsutsui H, Hayashidani S, *et al*. Mitochondrial DNA damage and dysfunction associated with oxidative stress in failing hearts after myocardial infarction. *Circ Res*, **88**: 529–535, 2001.

50. Simon HU, Haj-Yehia A, Levi-Schaffer F. Role of reactive oxygen species (ROS) in apoptosis induction. *Apoptosis*, **5**: 415–418, 2000.

51. Dyntar D, Eppenberger-Eberhardt M, Maedler K, *et al*. Glucose and palmitic acid induce degeneration of myofibrils and modulate apoptosis in rat adult cardiomyocytes. *Diabetes*, **50**: 2105–2113, 2001.

52. Shaw P, Freeman J, Bovey R, Iggo R. Regulation of specific DNA binding by p53: evidence for a role for O-glycosylation and charged residues at the carboxy-terminus. *Oncogene*, **12**: 921–930, 1996.

53. Ashcroft M, Kubbutat MHG, Vousden KH. Regulation of p53 function and stability by phosphorylation. *Mol Cell Biol*, **19**: 1751–1758, 1999.

54. Miyashita T, Reed JC. Tumor suppressor p53 is a direct transcriptional activator of the human bax gene. *Cell*, **80**: 293–299, 1995.

55. Avendano GF, Agarwal K, Bashey RI, *et al*. Effects of glucose intolerance on myocardial function and collagen-linked glycation. *Diabetes*, **48**: 1443–1447, 1999.

56. Avendano GF, Agarwal K, Bashey RI, *et al*. Role of TGF-β1 in the collagen accumulation of diabetic myocardium. *J Invest Med*, **44**: 292A, 1996.

57. Vlasara H, Bucala R. Recent progress in advanced glycation end-product receptors. *Diabetes*, **45**: S65–S66, 1996.

58. Mizushige K, Yao L, Noma T, *et al*. Alteration in left ventricular diastolic filling and accumulation of myocardial collagen at insulin-resistant prediabetic

stage of a type II diabetic rat model. *Circulation,* **101**: 899–907, 2000.

59. Paulson DJ, Shetlar D, and Light KE. Catecholamine levels in the heart, serum and adrenals of experimental diabetic rats. *Fed Proc,* **39**: 637, 1980.

60. Ganguly PK, Dhalla KS, Innes IR, *et al.* Altered norepinephrine turnover and metabolism in diabetic cardiomyopathy. *Circ Res,* **59**: 684–693, 1986.

61. Ganguly PK, Dhalla KS, Innes IR, *et al.* Norepinephrine storage, distribution and release in diabetic cardiomyopathy. *Am J Physiol,* **252**: E734–E739, 1987.

62. Akiyama N, Okumura K, Watanabe Y, *et al.* Altered acetylcholine and norepinephrine concentrations in diabetic rat hearts. Role of parasympathetic nervous system in diabetic cardiomyopathy. *Diabetes,* **38**: 231–236, 1989.

63. Dincer ÜD, Keshore RB, Güner Ş, *et al.* The effect of diabetes on expression of β1-, β2-, and β3-adrenoreceptors in rat hearts. *Diabetes,* **50**: 455–461, 2001.

64. Suzuki S, Oka Y, Kadowaki T, *et al.* Clinical features of diabetes mellitus with the mitochondrial DNA 3243 (A–G) mutation in Japanese: Maternal inheritance and mitochondria-related complications. *Diabetes Res Clin Pract,* **59**: 207–217, 2003.

65. Deorari AK, Saxena A, Singh M, *et al.* Echocardiographic assessment of infants born to diabetic mothers. *Arch Dis Child,* **64**: 721, 1989.

66. Tarumi N, Iwasaka T, Takahashi N, *et al.* Left diastolic filling properties in diabetic patients during isometric exercise. *Cardiology,* **83**: 316–323, 1993.

67. Nicolino A, Longobardi G, Furgi R, *et al.* Left diastolic filling properties in diabetes mellitus with and without hypertension. *Am J Hypertens,* **8**: 382–389, 1995.

68. Takenaka K, Sakamoto T, Amano K, *et al.* Left ventricular filling determined by Doppler echocardiography in diabetes mellitus. *Am J Cardiol,* **61**: 1140–1143, 1988.

69. Robillon JF, Sadoul JL, Jullien D, Morand P, Freycet P. Abnormalities suggestive of cardiomyopathy in patients with type 2 diabetes of relatively short duration. *Diabetes Metab,* **20**: 473–480, 1994.

70. Di Bonito P, Cuomo S, Moio N, *et al.* Diastolic dysfunction in patients with non-insulin-dependent diabetes mellitus of short duration. *Diab Med,* **13**: 321–324, 1996.

71. Raev DC. Which left ventricular function is impaired earlier in the evolution of diabetic cardiomyopathy? An ecocardiographic study of young type I diabetic patients. *Diabetes Care,* **17**: 633–639,1994.

72. Rakowski H, Appleton C, Chan KL, *et al.* Canadian consensus recommendations for the measurement and reporting of diastolic dysfunction by echocardiography: from the Investigators of Consensus on Diastolic Dysfunction by Echocardiography. *J Am Soc Echocardiogr,* **9**: 736–760, 1996.

73. Dumesnil JG, Gaudreault G, Honos GN, Kingma JG Jr. Use of Valsalva maneuver to unmask left ventricular diastolic function abnormalities by Doppler echocardiography in patients with coronary artery disease or systemic hypertension. *Am J Cardiol,* **68**: 515–519, 1991.

74. Gough SC, Smyllie J, Barker M, Berkin KE, Rice PJ, Grant PJ. Diastolic dysfunction is not related to changes in glycaemic control over 6 months in type 2 diabetes mellitus: a cross sectional study. *Acta Diabetol,* **32**: 110–115, 1995.

75. Hiramatsu K, Ohara N, Shigematsu S, *et al.* Left ventricular filling abnormalities in non-insulin-dependent diabetes mellitus and improvement by a short term glycaemic control. *Am J Cardiol,* **70**: 1185–1189,1992.

76. Beljic T, Miric M. Improved metabolic control does not reverse left ventricular filling abnormalities in newly diagnosed non-insulin-dependent diabetes patients. *Acta Diabetol,* **31**: 147–150, 1994.

77. Hirai J, Ueda K, Takegoshi T, Mabuchi H. Effects of metabolic control on ventricular function in type 2 diabetic patients. *Intern Med,* **31**: 725–730, 1992.

78. Uusitupa M, Siitonen O, Aro A, *et al.* Effect of correction of hyperglycemia on left ventricular function in non-insulin-dependent (type 2) diabetics. *Acta Med Scand,* **213**: 363–368,1983.

79. Sahn DJ, DeMaria A, Kislo J, Weyman A. Recommendations regarding quantitation in M-mode echocardiography: results of a survey of echocardiographic measurements. *Circulation,* **58**: 1072–1083, 1978.

80. Guidelines from the Canadian Cardiovascular Society and the Canadian Hypertension Society on the echocardiographic determination of left ventricular mass (Consensus Statement). Task Force of the Echocardiography Section. *Can J Cardiol,* **11**: 391–395, 1995.

32

INFLAMMATION AND HEART FAILURE IN DIABETIC PATIENTS

Ioana Maria BRUCKNER, Ilinca SĂVULESCU-FIEDLER, Ion Victor BRUCKNER

The prevalence of diabetes mellitus in patients with heart failure is high, as proved by many clinical trials (SOLVD, NETWORK, V-HeFT, etc.). On the other hand, the Framingham cohort reports an increased incidence of heart failure in diabetic patients, irrespective of associated comorbidities, such as hypertension or coronary artery disease. In fact, the most frequent cause of death in diabetic patients is represented by cardiac disease. Accordingly, the UKPDS study demonstrated that for each 1% increase in glycated hemoglobin levels there is a 16% increase in risk of hospitalization for HF and/or death.

The relation between the two conditions can be partly explained by the occurrence in diabetes of myocardial ischemia due as well to microangiopathy and endothelial dysfunction as to more severe and precocious macroangiopathy, through coassociation with high blood pressure, obesity, dyslipidemia, hyperinsulinemia and a procoagulant state.

But, even in the absence of coronary lesions in persons with diabetes, a diffuse myocardial affection named diabetic cardiomyopathy, is described. The cellular alterations met in this entity, necrosis and apoptosis, are related to an increased oxidative stress resulted from metabolic modifications, increased production of angiotensin, also locally, action of advanced glycation products. Functional alterations in diabetic cardiomyopathy include a decrease in coronary reserve due to endothelial dysfunction and microangiopathy, accumulation of advanced glycation products, oxidative stress and not lastly, metabolic alterations that directly affect the energy supply necessary for myocardial function.

The relation between insulin resistance and heart failure is bi-directional. On the one hand, insulin resistance leads to ventricular dysfunction and, on the other hand, heart failure determines, by different mechanisms, a decrease in insulin sensitivity with an increase in the incidence of type 2 diabetes. These mechanisms are sympathetic overactivity, decrease in muscle mass and muscle blood flow, production of inflammatory cytokines (especially TNFα and IL-6) and last, but not least, an important decrease in exercise. Thus a vicious circle is formed as demonstrated by many clinical studies which underline the relation between insulin resistance, diabetes and inflammation.

The initial cardiac lesion, as well as the increase in ventricular telediastolic stress, induces the formation of cytokines of cardiac origin, which once arrived in the circulation increase the immune reaction. Through macrophage and endothelial activation, amplification of oxidative stress, etc. are created loops of aggravation of heart failure and conditions of an increase in insulin resistance.

The adipose tissue, especially visceral, frequently overdeveloped in diabetes, is also a cytokine source which aggravates the systemic inflammatory reaction.

By this means, inflammation appears as an important mechanism in the relation between heart failure and diabetes mellitus, a relation which is clinically proved, but not yet completely understood.

Abbreviations List

AGEs – advanced glycation end-products
Ang II – angiotensin II
AP-1 – activator protein-1 complex
ApoI-1 – apoptosis inducer 1
ASP – acylation stimulating protein
AT1 – angiotensin receptor 1
AT2 – angiotensin receptor 2
bFGF – basic fibroblast growth factor
BK – bradikinine
CAD – coronary artery disease
CHK – chemokine
Cit. C – cytochrome C
CyK – cytokine
CPK – creatinphosphokinase
CRP – C reactive protein
DAG – diacylglycerol
DCM – diabetic cardiomyopathy
DM – diabetes mellitus
DNA – deoxyribonucleic acid
EF – ejection fraction
EGFR – epidermal growth factor receptor
ERKs – extracellular signal-regulated kinases
FFA – free fatty acids
GLUT4 – glucose transporter protein
GM-CSF – granulocyte-macrophage colony-
    stimulating factor
HETE – hydroxyeicosatetraenoic acid
HF – heart failure
HPETE – hydroperoxyeicosatetraenoic acid
HSL – adipose tissue hormone-sensitive lipase
ICAM-1 – intercellular adhesion molecule-1
ICAP-1 – cellular inhibitor of apoptosis protein-1
IGF-1 – insulin-like growth factor
I-kB – inhibitory-kB
IL – interleukin
IL-1R – IL-1 receptor
IL-1ra – IL-1 receptor antagonist
IP2 – inositol 4,5-biphosphate
IP3 – inositol triphosphate
IRS-1 – insulin receptor substrate
Ly – lymphocyte
Lpt – leptine
LPL – lipoprotein lipase
MAPK – mitogen-activated protein-kinase

MCP-1 – monocyte chemoattractant protein-1
MIP-1α – macrophage inflammatory protein 1α
NADH – nicotinamide adenine dinucleotide
NADPH – nicotinamide adenine dinucleotide
    phosphate
NEFA – nonesterified fatty acids
NF-kB – nuclear factor kB
NIK – NF-kB inducing kinase
NO – nitric oxide
NOs – nitric oxide synthase
iNOs – inducible NOS
NonRTK – nonreceptor tyrosine kinase
OB-Rb – the long isoform of the Leptin receptor
PAI-1 – plasminogen activator inhibitor 1
PDH – pyruvate dehydrogenase
PDK – pyruvate dehydrogenaste kinase
Pg – prostaglandins
PI3K – phosphoinositol 3-kinase
PKB – proteinkinase B (Akt)
PKC – proteinkinase C
PLA2 – phospholipase A2
PLC – phospholipase C
PLD – phospholipase D
PPAR – peroxisome proliferator-activated receptor
PTP – tyrosine phosphatase
RAGE – advanced glycation end-products receptors
RANTES – regulation upon activation normal
    T-cell expressed and secreted
mRNA – messenger ribonucleic acid
RTK – receptor tyrosine kinase
RXR – retinoid X receptors
SAPK – stress-activated protein kinase
SMC – smooth muscle cell
STAT-1 – signal transducer and activation
    of transcription 1
TAG – triacylglycerol
TNFα – tumour necrosis factor α
TNFR – TNFα receptor
sTNFR – soluble TNFR
TGFβ – transforming growth factor β
VCAM-1 – vascular cell adhesion molecule-1
VLDL – very low density lipoproteins

BACKGROUND

The incidence of diabetes mellitus (DM) in the general population is about 4–6%. Nevertheless, many epidemiological trials have demonstrated the increased prevalence of DM in patients with heart failure (HF) which is close to 20% [1], ranging between 10% (in the NETWORK study) and 35% (in the RESOLVD trial). In the Prevention arm of the SOLVD clinical trials, a registry of a large cohort of patients with an ejection fraction (EF) under 45%, 26% of patients had a history of type 1 or 2 DM. In the V-HeFT II trial, the proportion of patients with DM was 20%.

On the other side, an increased risk of heart failure in patients with diabetes was first demonstrated by data obtained from a long follow-up period of the Framingham cohort. This risk was high irrespective of associated comorbidities, such as hypertension or coronary artery disease (CAD). The Framingham cohort results sustain the high mortality in diabetics with heart failure in which the risk level is as high as 5.2 in women and 2.4 in men.

The high prevalence (47–86%) of DM in advanced HF (III-IV NYHA class) stresses the fact that, *per se*, DM is an important risk factor for the occurrence of HF and has also a deleterious impact on its outcome [2]. As a matter of fact, the most frequent cause of death in diabetic patients is represented by cardiac disease. According to this, in the UKPDS study was primarily shown that the incidence of HF significantly correlates with glycated hemoglobin (HbA1c) levels. For each 1% increase in HbA1c levels there is a 16% increased risk of hospitalization for HF and/or death [3].

Despite a clear statistic link between DM and HF, until now, the causative connection is not evident.

WHICH COULD BE THE CONNECTIONS BETWEEN THESE TWO COMORBIDITIES?

Multiple mechanisms of heart involvement in diabetes (irrespective of its types) have been described. The severe heart function impairment in DM is precocious, multicausal, and not necessarily associated with other cardiac insults, such as coronary heart disease (CAD) and hypertension.

Firstly, independent of hypertension and CAD, experimental and clinical studies support the existence in diabetic patients of a diffuse myocardial involvement, leading to myocardial dysfunction [1]. If this specific diabetic cardiomyopathy (DCM) alone may cause HF is unknown and the mechanisms by which it predisposes to heart failure are also not exactly known. The most frequent macroscopic modification found in DCM is concentric left ventricular hypertrophy, but an eccentric hypertrophy can also be found. The most frequent echocardiographic finding is the diastolic dysfunction (symptomatic or not). Many patients without overt HF have diastolic dysfunction, reflected by echo-Doppler patterns suggestive of slowed relaxation and/or decreased compliance. Another echocardiographic aspect is that of dilated cardiomyopathy with systolic dysfunction reflected by low ejection fraction (EF).

Myocardial ischemia represents over 2/3 of the etiology of heart failure [3]. In the Framingham cohort there is an elevated incidence of CAD in diabetic patients. The endothelial dysfunction, the platelet dysfunction, the increasing of fibrinogen, von Willebrand and plasminogen activator inhibitor (PAI-1) levels, all of them found in DM, connect the metabolic disorders to the increased risk for acute coronary events and their worse outcome. All mentioned factors represent atherosclerosis determinants and are related to the atheroma plaques instability. The incidence of plaque rupture and thrombosis in atheroma plaques is amplified in diabetics with HF.

The molecular basis of endothelial dysfunction in the insulin resistance syndrome and in DM are represented by multiple mechanisms such as: increased oxidative stress, ubiquitous nonenzymatic protein glycation, generation and deposition of advanced glycation end-products (AGEs), direct cytokines (CyK) intervention - especially of interleukin-6 (IL-6) and tumour necrosis factor α (TNFα).

Often type 2 DM is associated with other pathologic states such as hypertension, obesity, hypercoagulability and dyslipidemia. Their common basis is insulin resistance, and each of them augments (moreover the association) the risk of HF development. For instance, in patients with DM, the occurrence of hypertension can be expected to initiate the transition from compensated to decompensated cardiomyopathy. This hypothesis is supported by clinical trials which demonstrate that tight blood pressure control dramatically reduces the incidence of HF and mortality in patients with established diabetes [4].

Going back to DCM, the histopathologic picture includes a decrease in number of left ventricular myocytes (with about 28%), associated with an increased volume (with about 13%) for the remaining myocytes. Apart form decreasing of cardiomyocytes mass, other findings include increased PAS+ connective tissue (mainly perivascular), basement membrane thickening also by PAS+ material accumulation, thickening of small arteries and arterioles walls, microaneurysms [5]. The level of interstitial collagen is also high, and is represented mainly by its insoluble component. But this histological aspect is not specific for DCM, many models of HF showing such findings. "Specific" for DCM there are free fatty acids (FFA) settled in left ventricular walls and also a change in location and quantity of serine-protease inhibitors. These serine-protease inhibitors are alpha-1-antitrypsin and antithrombin III. In normal hearts, alpha-1-antitrypsin is distributed mainly in the extracellular matrix, myocytes and smooth muscle cells (SMC) of large arteries and antithrombin III is located especially in the veins and arteries endothelium as in the SMC of large arteries. In contrast, in diabetic hearts, the distribution of these proteases was not uniform and their levels are significantly lower, which might be involved in connective tissues remodeling [6].

In DM, the modifications at cellular level, the myocyte necrosis and the apoptosis, are related to oxidative stress, which is the result of both: angiotensin II (Ang II), which is produced also locally, in cardiac tissue, and products of proteic glycation [4]. Aldosereductase glycation determines decrease in nicotinamide adenine dinucleotide phosphate (NADPH) levels, a process associated to those of reducing in glutathione peroxidase and superoxide dismutase

activities. All these modifications are followed by an increase in oxygen reactive species level. Abnormalities of contractile activity have been detected, including decrease in ionic pumps activity, depressed sarcoplasmic reticulum calcium ATPase-2 (SERCA-2) activation, troponin T alterations, switch from V1 to V3 isomyosin (which has a smaller contractile capacity), decrease in creatinphosphokinase (CPK) level. As functional consequences, result several alterations in excitation-contraction coupling mechanism, prolongation of the action potential, decrease in stocking and energy release. Finally, these develop myocytic hypertrophy and decreases of myofibrils contractile capacity [7]. But, the molecular and cellular abnormalities are not specifically related to DCM; they are generally found in heart failure irrespective of its etiology.

Diabetes is characterized by a major metabolic abnormality which interests all tissues including the heart and vessels.

In a normal aerobic metabolic state, 70–80% of the energy required for myocytes function is supplied by FFA oxidation. On the other hand, the energy required for Na/K pump and calcium ATPase activities are provided by glucose oxidation. In increased mechanical stress, hypoxia or ischemia, glucose and lactate oxidation (the most economic from the point of view of oxygen consumption for one mole of ATP produced) are stimulated. In anaerobiosis, in contracting muscle, pyruvate, resulted from glycolytic Embden-Meyerhof pathway, is reduced to lactate. The last one is reoxidated back to pyruvate, which becomes substrate for gluconeogenesis. The glucose generated from muscular lactate may be delivered to muscle cells, after glucose utilization, resulting lactate again (Cori cycle) [8]. This process is mediated by stimulation of glucose transporter protein (GLUT4) translocation. The translocation of GLUT4 from cytoplasm to sarcolemma takes place under proteinkinase B (PKB), phosphoinositol 3-kinase (PI3K) and proteinkinase C (PKC) control [4]. GLUT4 is expressed by insulin-sensitive tissues, especially by muscle (cardiac and skeletal) and fat. Its action is regulated by insulin.

The relation between the major energy suppliers, glucose and FFA, is "hostile". In other words, glucose inhibits FFA oxidation, by inhibiting carnitine palmitoyl transpherase and, on the other side, FFA inhibit glucose oxidation, followed by rising in lactate level, local acidosis with impaired left ventricular function due to changes in calcium homeostasis [4,7]. This process is as high as the energetic stress, when the energy is supplied by FFA oxidation [4].

Oversimplified, the myocytic metabolic sources are related as follows (Plate 32.1).

The myocytes are taking over the glucose, depending on the local insulin level (because insulin stimulates GLUT4 translocation) and on the intensity of force-contraction relationship. The increase in FFA oxidation (*via* Peroxide Peroxisome Activated Receptors – PPAR) determines rising in AcCoA/CoA ratio in mitochondria and higher pyruvate dehydrogenase kinase (PDK4) levels, both acting together to inhibit pyruvatedehydrogenase (PDH) activity [4]. Insulin inhibits the liberation of FFA from adipose tissue, inhibiting in this way pyruvate oxidation. PDH is the leading enzyme in pyruvate oxidation (through Krebs cycle). The decrease in pyruvate oxidation is followed by a reduction in lactate and glucose oxidation rates [9]. PDH activity is lowered by PKC, so that PDH and PKC are crucial enzymes in cardiac metabolism.

Characteristic for DM are metabolic abnormalities, which affect all these Krebs cycle chain loops. Briefly, they are: increase in FFA level, deficit in GLUT4 translocation, insulin resistance finally.

Concerning the myocyte metabolism, the difference between the heart of a diabetic and nondiabetic person consists in the preferential utilization of FFA and/or ketones as energetic provider instead of glucose by the diabetic heart because of:

– decrease in insulin action in the heart, liver and adipose tissue, with consecutive rising in glucose, FFA and ketone bodies plasmatic level;

– decrease in myocardial glucose uptake, even in the presence of high plasmatic levels, due to diminishing of glucose transmembranar transport insulin depending system;

– decrease in the pyruvatdehydrogenase mitochondrial system with abnormal glucose and lactate oxidation consequences [9]. All these modifications are independent of myocardial ischemia, and the link between them and

endothelial dysfunction has not been clearly understood until now [10].

Another metabolic disturbance, secondary to chronic hyperglycemia, is the polyol pathway activation, expressed by sorbitol and fructose accumulation, decrease in NADPH level and increase in nicotinamide adenine dinucleotide (NADH) titer (see Plate 32.2). Beside their osmotic effects, sorbitol determines also decrease in intracellular myoinositol level, which alters polyphosphoinositides turnover. In consequence, diacylglycerol (DAG) and inositol triphosphate (IP3) levels go down. DAG is involved in intracellular Na content control (*via* proteinkinase C which activates Na/K ATPase).

Decreases in NADPH levels and increases in NADH concentration stimulate *de novo* DAG synthesis (by the pentosophosphate pathway), and on the other hand, activate cyclooxygenases, enzyme involved in prostaglandins (Pg) metabolism. DAG also determines increases in deoxyribonucleotide acid (DNA) synthesis, in SMC number and contraction [11]. More than this, myoinositol depletion is followed by decrease in nitric oxide synthase (NOs), lipooxygenase and cyclooxygenases activities, reflected by a perturbations in nitric oxide (NO) and prostaglandins metabolism.

AGEs bound to smooth muscle cells (SMC) receptors determine cellular proliferation, effect probably mediated by cytokines (CyK) or growth factors.

Myoglobin glycosylation and the glycoprotein depositions in myocardial interstitial space conduce to decrease in myocardial compliance.

Additionally, there are dysfunctionalities in the cardiac nervous system, represented by an increase in cholinergic activity and a decrease in membranar receptors for adrenaline.

The link between insulin resistance and HF is bi-directional; not only that the first leads to left ventricular dysfunction, but also HF determines, by several mechanisms, a decrease in insulin sensitivity, followed by increasing the risk of developing type 2 DM [4]. The means by which this happens are: sympathetic overactivity, decrease in skeletal muscular mass and muscular blood flow, delivering of proinflammatory CyK (especially TNFα and IL-6), and, not the least, impaired physical activity. Here is a pathophysiological self-supported chain. Inflammation is one of this chain's components.

Inflammation can be roughly defined as an answer to injury. Albeit, the initial intention of an inflammatory response is a repairing one, each inflammatory process, by its neuroendocrine, hematopoietic, metabolic and immune responses, leads to functional and after that, to structural modifications, for the first time locally and afterwards, generally. In fact inflammation is not a unitary process, there are different forms of inflammation. The common element is activation through complex cytokine mediation of different "inflammation" cells including monocytes, lymphocytes, leukocytes, but also endothelial and smooth muscle cells.

The innate immune response to inflammation implies leukocyte activation, liberation of CyK under chemokines (CHK) influence. CHK are released by monocytes and endothelial cells. Once arrived into circulation, the CyK intervene in hepatic synthesis of acute phase reactants: fibrinogen, plasminogen, PAI-1, von Willebrand factor, VII and VIII coagulation factors, C-reactive protein (CRP), sialic acid, complement. The inquired immune response implies an antigenic recognition, after the acute response, and specifically involves T (T Ly) and B lymphocytes (B Ly) and immunoglobulins.

The relationship between diabetes mellitus, heart failure and the inflammatory responses is substantiated by multiple paraclinic data, which show an increase in proinflammatory cytokines levels in both conditions. The existence of a chronic "inflammatory" state may contribute to the poor evolution of both diseases.

THE LINK BETWEEN THE INSULIN RESISTANCE SYNDROME/DM AND INFLAMMATION

A lot of clinical trials, few of them will be mentioned, emphasize the relation between the insulin resistance syndrome (IRS), diabetes mellitus (DM) and inflammation mediators. The inflammation in type 2 DM triggers the insulin resistance and does not alter pancreatic cell secretory function [12].

The ARIC study, which analyzed nondiabetic patients aged between 45 and 65 for a period of 7 years, found a positive correlation between leukocytes level and the risk of DM development [12].

The most potent cytokines in the insulin resistance syndrome and type 2 DM are IL-6, TNFα and leptin (Lpt). Their origin is in the adipose tissue, especially in the visceral one. The adipose tissue may release IL-6, TNFα and its receptors (TNFR) [9]. The relationship between obesity (especially the central type) and proinflammatory CyK is proved by the high levels of TNFα, IL-6 and CRP in obesity, and, also, by decreasing the CyK levels as a consequence of weight losing [12, 13].

The visceral adipocytes release double/triple amounts of IL-6 as compared to peripheral adipocytes. Once got into the portal blood, IL-6 stimulates CRP gene expression [13]. Differential adipose tissue distribution appears to have significant effects upon the endocrine function of adipose tissue. Regional variations in adipose tissue signaling functions include increased expression of leptin and binding of acylation stimulating protein (ASP) in subcutaneous adipose tissue, and increased expression of 11-β hydroxysteroids and glucocorticoids receptors in the visceral adipose tissue. Differences in glucocorticoid sensitivity may underline the differences in growth characteristics of visceral and subcutaneous adipose tissue. A large visceral adipose tissue depot is thought to increase hepatic exposure to non esterified fatty acids (NEFA), with secondary impairment of hepatic insulin clearance, increased hepatic synthesis of very low density lipoproteins (VLDL), triglycerides, and impaired peripheral glucose disposal. Furthermore, the increased β_2-adrenoreceptor sensitivity of visceral adipose tissue may account for its increased lipolytic activity and release of NEFA. Obesity is associated also with reduced adipocyte β_2-adrenergic receptor sensitivity and an impaired lipolytic response to adrenergic stimulation. These defects may be caused by adipocytes adrenoreceptor down-regulation in face of an increased sympathetic activation in obesity. Finally, it is possible to speculate that visceral adipose tissue is less effective than subcutaneous adipose tissue in regulating energy balance through its production of leptin [14].

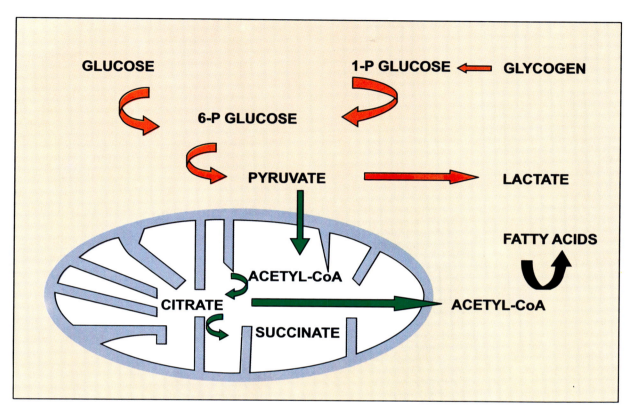

Plate 32.1

The myocytic metabolic sources.

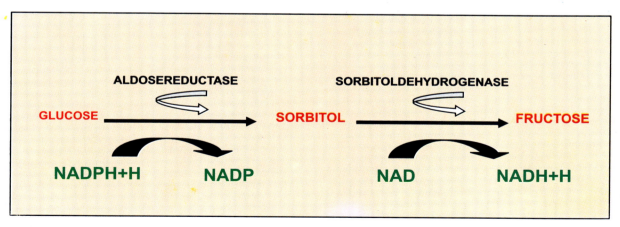

Plate 32.2

The polyol pathway.

TNFα is also involved in insulin signaling. It determines a decrease in insulin receptors and insulin receptor substrate (IRS-1) [15]. TNFα gets down IRS-1 and GLUT4 expressions [15]; so, it is involved in insulin resistance syndrome development. The ways by which TNFα induces insulin resistance, in hepatic and skeletal muscles, are different. Thus, at muscle level, TNFα triggers the decrease in insulin-mediated autophosphorylation of insulin receptors and in tyrosinphosphatase (PTP) activity. PTP has a positive role in insulin signaling regulation. The decrease in glucose utilization at muscular level is followed by an increase in FFA level. The insulin resistance at hepatic level is explained by post receptor mechanism [13]. Also, TNFα stimulates basal glucose uptake into cultured adipocytes (its insulin mimetic effect may be *via* stimulation of PI3K thereby increasing the synthesis of GLUT1), inhibits lipoprotein lipase (LPL) activity and stimulates lipolysis, stimulates glucose and fatty acids oxidation and induces the release of glucagon and cortisol. Alternatively, there is evidence that TNFα may produce insulin resistance by decreasing IRS-1 and GLUT4 expressions [14].

IL-6 and CRP levels correlate with the risk of DM development, according to the Women's Health Study results. This trial registered for 4 years women over 45 years, without DM or evidence of CAD at the time of including [16]. Also, CRP level is inversely proportional to insulin sensitivity and is directly proportional to DM occurrence risk, according to the Cardiovascular Health Study [17].

Leptin is a CyK-like molecule released by the adipose tissue. It is free or bound by seric proteins. It also has growth properties. Insulin and TNFα stimulate Lpt release [14]. Leptin production is influenced by nutritional status, stress and immune activation. The presence of receptors for leptin, not only in the hypothalamus, but also in the peripheral tissues, including the adipose tissue, the liver, skeletal muscle and islet cells, suggests that leptin has peripheral as well as central actions. Leptin can impair insulin signaling, both in the skeletal muscle and adipocytes. Furthermore, leptin was found to inhibit phosphorylation of IRS-1, insulin-mediated glucose uptake, as well as lipogenesis, and to stimulate lipolysis and protein kinase A (PKA)

activation in the skeletal muscle. Leptin stimulates lipogenesis in adipocyte cell lines. Perhaps consistent with an *in vivo* relationship between impaired insulin signaling and increased plasma leptin levels are the results of retrospective studies in Pima Indians, in which insulin resistance was found to be associated with reduced subsequent weight gain, and lower plasma leptin levels to precede weight gain. Thus, insulin resistance may be, in part, a maladaptive consequence of high leptin levels, in response to overfeeding [14]. Glucocorticoid hormones, whose levels are elevated in inflammation, have the same effect on Lpt delivery. Catecholamines inhibit Lpt synthesis [14]. As TNFα and IL-6, Lpt impairs insulin action at hepatic and muscular levels.

The adipose tissue expresses also components of the complement alternative pathway, *e.g.* ASP, which derives from C3. Although ASP exists in preadipocytes and fibroblasts, it is considered as a mature adipocyte marker. Its role is in postprandial fatty acids storage. Although a receptor for ASP has not yet been identified, differences between adipose tissue depots have been observed, with greater degrees of ASP binding in subcutaneous compared to omental fat, in females compared with males, and in morbidity obese compared to non-obese individuals [14, 18].

The local proinflammatory CyK release determines systemic inflammatory responses as shown by the Third National Health and Nutrition Examination Survey 1988–1994 (NHANES III) in which, a positive relation between HbA1c and CRP levels was found, as well as between ferritine (an inflammatory marker) and the prevalence of impaired fasting glucose and DM [19]. As a proof of the same fact in the diabetic population, the level of sialic acid is higher than in nondiabetics [18]. Moreover, the plasmatic sialic acid level correlates with the insulin resistance degree as well as with the magnitude of coronary lesions (higher levels in diabetics with CAD than in those without CAD) [12, 18]. This was the very first observation that linked diabetes and the insulin resistance syndrome to inflammation.

The levels of PAI-1, von Willebrand factor, fibronectine and adhesion molecules are higher in IRS or DM [12]. In fact, actually, in diabetic relatives there have been noted higher PAI-1, fibrinogen and coagulation VII factor levels and also, more frequently, insulin resistance syndrome, unlike in the relatives of nondiabetic patients [20].

In conclusion, all these and other trials stressed that in the insulin resistance syndrome and diabetes mellitus, the level of inflammatory factors is elevated, and also the fact that inflammation predicts DM development. By their action, inflammatory cytokines induce insulin resistance. From these the paradigm is that the insulin resistance syndrome and diabetes are inflammatory conditions.

THE RELATION BETWEEN HEART FAILURE AND INFLAMMATION

Inflammation plays a major role in the pathogenesis of heart failure. The number of proofs regarding the link between proinflammatory CyK, endothelial injury, structural and functional heart modifications, cardiomyocytes and endothelial apoptosis is constantly increasing [21].

The triggers for cardiac CyK release are the initial cardiac injury and the increase of left ventricular telediastolic stress; on the other hand, tissue hypoxia, determined by the low tissue perfusion regimen in HF, determines CyK release. Once arrived into circulation, CyK amplify the immune response. So that, a vicious circle which amplifies the inflammatory response is born.

The mechanical overburden of ventricle is followed by an increase in TNFα, Ang II, as well as other neurohormones (such as endothelin-1, atrial natriuretic peptide, argininevasopressine, catecholamines, etc.) production and oxidative stress. All of them determine the activation of transcription factors, the next step being the genes transcription of inflammatory mediators, leading to hyperproduction of CyK, adhesion molecules, CHK, apoptosis inducers. The final result is the increase in cardiovascular injury and the progression of HF syndrome.

The transcription factors involved are Elk-1, activator protein-1 complex (AP-1), nuclear factor-kB (NF-kB). The last one is regarded as the main factor involved in inflammatory synthesis of mediators, which play a role in HF patho-physiology.

CyKs, whose involvement in HF pathogenesis is proved, are: TNFα, IL-6, IL-1, IL-2 [21].

TNFα is released mainly by activated macrophages, but also by other cells: lymphocytes, neutrophils, mast cells, SMC and fibroblasts. It has been found in two forms: bound to cell membrane and secreted. Hypoxia and mechanical stress are inducers of myocytic TNFα synthesis. At cardiac level, TNFα binds to its receptors: TNFR1 and TNFR2. The expression of these two receptors seems to be regulated by separate mechanisms, as they differ in their cellular and tissue distribution. The circulating levels of both soluble receptors correlate with measures of adiposity. By detaching of the extracellular TNFRs domain result soluble TNFα receptors (sTNFR1 and sTNFR2). Their role is to bind TNFα, diminishing in this way its negative cellular effects. So, sTNFR act like cell protectors. The level of sTNFR, as expression of local CyK activation, is increased in patients with HF. TNFα stimulates the production of various CyK (IL-1, IL-6). TNFα stimulates myocytic necrosis, extracellular matrix production and apoptosis; so it has been involved in the appearance of left ventricular dysfunction. TNFα promotes free oxygen radicals generation and nitric oxide (NO) production, by stimulation of inducible nitric oxide synthase (iNOs). NO is a depressor of contractile function.

IL-6 is synthesized by activated macrophages, T lymphocytes and endothelial cells, and also, by monocytes and fibroblasts. IL-6 binds to a receptor complex (which has two glycoproteic subunits) and is involved in the occurrence of myocytic hypertrophy and apoptosis. The high IL-6 plasmatic level is considered to be the best predictor of poor HF evolution (superior in evaluation to the TNFα level, neurohormones or EF of left ventricle).

IL-1 is synthesized mainly by myocytes, but all cells have the ability to synthesize IL-1. The effects of IL-1 are achieved by binding to its receptors, IL-1RI and IL-1RII. IL-1RI is the only receptor able to transduce the signal. This CyK plays a prominent part in inflammatory response, intervening in prostaglandins (Pg) generation. IL-1 stimulates the activity of interstitial metalloproteinases, playing a role in the process of cardiac remodeling. Additionally, IL-1 impairs β-adrenoreceptors-adenylatecyclase coupling, decreasing the myocytic contractility sympathetic-mediated. The myocytes synthesize also the IL-1 receptor antagonist (IL-1ra). This has a protector effect, inhibiting IL-1 binding to its receptors.

IL-2, whose synthesis is stimulated by IL-1, is an endogenic mitogen of T Ly. IL-2 self stimulates the expression of its own receptors on T Ly, amplifying in this way its effects. Its important role is in the direction of raising the immune response [21]. IL-2 also stimulates the synthesis of TNFα and granulocyte-macrophage colony stimulating factor (GMCSF) by the activated macrophages. By its actions it is implied in the pathogenesis of dilated cardiomyopathy and viral myocarditis.

Beside CyK, in HF pathophysiology CHK, adhesion molecules, hematopoietic factors and apoptosis mediators are involved.

CHK respond for the directional migration of leukocytes. Local increased release of CyK and amplification of inflammatory response follow this. CHK involved in HF pathogenesis are: monocyte chemoattractant protein-1 (MCP-1), macrophage inflammatory protein-1α (MIP-1α), regulation upon activation normally T-cell expressed and secreted factor (RANTES) and IL-8.

MCP-1, whose expression is provoked by mechanical requirements, plays a role in directional migration of monocytes and macrophages. The MCP-1 level correlates with the extent of monocyte activation and the level of oxidative stress.

MIP-1α is released by various inflammatory cells and is an important chemoattractant for monocytes and Ly. The level of MIP-1α is high in HF, and correlates with left ventricle EF.

RANTES, whose release depends on thr interaction between platelets and inflammatory cells, are involved in free radicals and CyK releasing. Its level is overnormal in advanced HF.

IL-8, chemoattractant for neutrophils, is produced by monocytes, platelets, T Ly, neutrophils, endothelial cells, fibroblasts and SMC. IL-8 is generated by monocyte-platelet interaction. There is a positive association between IL-8 level and HF severity, evaluated by NYHA class.

The endothelial layer and the activated macrophages express soluble adhesion molecules, which mediate inflammatory cell adhesion on the endothelial surface. Two of them, whose level is high in HF, intracellular adhesion molecule-1 (ICAM-1) and vascular cell adhesion molecule-1 (VCAM-1), by their soluble forms, mediate the interaction between vessel and inflammatory cells.

The inflammatory hematopoietic factors operate the interaction between monocytes and endothelial cells. GMCSF has the main contribution in this process. GMCSF also stimulates cells growing. It intervenes, also, in free radicals generation and amplifies CyK production. There is a good correlation between GMCSF high level in HF and the magnitude of neurohumoral activation.

Fas (ApoI-1) belongs to TNFα receptors superfamily. Fas is a membrane protein whose function consists in apoptosis signaling. By binding of ligand, it generates FasL, which is a CyK TNFα-related. By extracellular Fas domain cleavage it generates soluble Fas (sFas), which acts by blocking the interaction between Fas and its ligand. Fas level is high in severe HF. sFas intervenes in left ventricular remodeling. The soluble form of FasL, sFasL, is delivered into circulation, and plays a role in intracellular calcium homeostasis regulation and in caspase activation, an enzyme which intervenes directly in apoptosis [21].

All of the presented mediators of inflammation (CyK, CHK, etc.) lead to transcription factors activation, which promotes cardiac remodeling, by interventions in myocytic viability, in modifications of interstitial matrix structure and so lead on to heart failure. Thus, the progressive evolution and poor prognosis of heart failure is linked to a chronic "inflammatory" state. Modern therapy of heart failure tries to diminish this state.

SIGNAL TRANSDUCTION

Ang II mediates its effects by acting directly through Ang II receptors (mainly on AT1 and AT2 receptors), indirectly through the release of various factors and also *via* cross talk with intracellular signaling cascades of growth factors and CyK. The binding of Ang II to AT1 receptors promotes the activation of many receptor and nonreceptor tyrosine kinases (RTK and non-

RTK). As follows, we will refer only to that which activates directly the transcription factors.

The transcription factors are responsible for the vascular and cellular trophic responses in HF, for the increased interstitial collagen synthesis (followed by interstitial fibrosis), as well as the myocytic damage through necrosis and apoptosis in this syndrome. The transcription factors are represented especially by NF-kB and, in addition, by Elk-1 and AP-1. NF-kB is localized intracytoplasmically, as an inactive form, coupled with inhibitory-kB (IKB). By detaching of IKB from NF-kB–IKB complex, under transactivated transforming growth factor β (TGFβ) and free radical actions, NF-kB becomes activated. Once

activated, NF-kB enters the nucleus, where it promotes gene transcription. The activation of NF-kB is stimulated by the binding of TNFα to TNFR1, which are localized in the myocardium [21]. This binding is followed by NF-kB activation (*via* NF-kB inducing kinase-NIK) and by stress-activated protein-kinase (SAPK) activation. The activation of NF-kB determines rising in NO production (*via* iNOs) [22]. NO has a negative inotrop effect and decreases the positive inotrop effect of β-adrenergic stimulation [10]. By the interaction between NO and free radicals result peroxynitrites, which activate further NF-kB, generating free radicals.

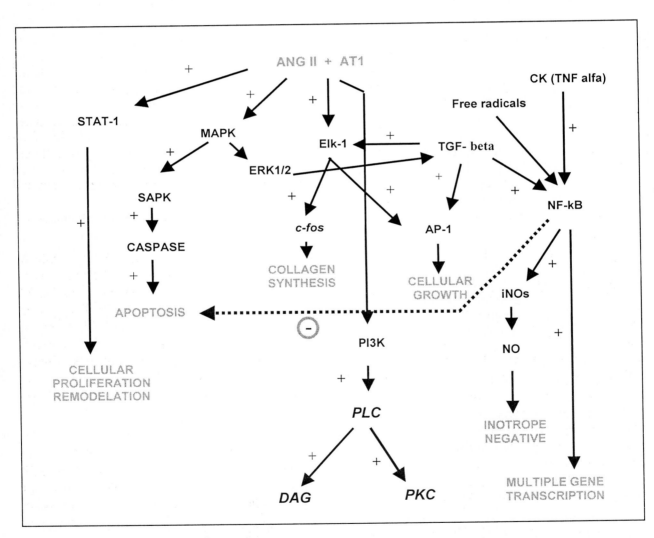

Figure 32.1

The signal transduction.

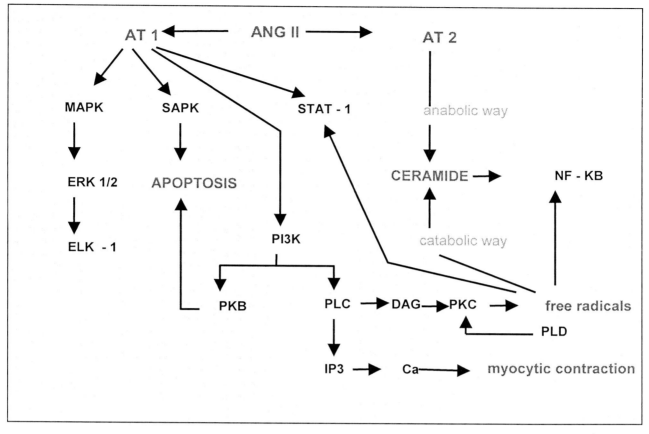

Figure 32.2

The contributions of Ang II and proinflammatory factors to heart damage.

Via AT1, Ang II stimulates phosphorylation of nuclear mitogen-activated protein-kinase (MAPK) system, which intervenes in intracellular protein phosphorylation, mediating in this way the nuclear transduction of extracellular signals [22]. This kinase family includes many subfamilies, *e.g.*, extracellular signal-regulated kinases (ERK1/2), SAPK. ERK1/2, activated in response to growth and differentiation factors intervenes in extracellular signaling and in phosphorylation, and so, in activation of transcription factor Elk-1 which in turn determines *c-fos* proto-oncogene expression and AP-1 generation. *C-fos* also increases Iα2 collagen gene expression. AP-1 is a transcription factor which mediates cell growing [22]. Moreover, ERK1/2 determines TGFβ transactivation, this factor contributing to the increase in collagen synthesis and in activation of NF-kB. On the other hand, the cellular stress and the proinflammatory cells activate SAPK, which stimulates AP-1 activation. NF-kB and SAPK have opposite effects regarding apoptosis initiation. NF-kB stimulates cellular inhibitor of apoptosis protein-1 (ICAP-1). ICAP-1 inhibits procaspase-8, so inhibiting apoptosis. SAPK activation determines caspase activation, promoting the apoptotic process [22] (see Figure 32.1).

NF-kB activation determines rising in mRNA for TNFα level, amplifying in this way its synthesis [21]. SAPK hyperactivation is realized also by the ceramide pathway (see below).

By phosphorylation of kinases that belong to Src family, the system STAT1 (signal transducer and activation of transcription 1), that intervenes in cellular growth, proliferation and repairing, will become activated [22].

By binding to AT1, Ang II triggers PI3K activation, enzyme involved in cytoskeleton growth and organization and in cellular metabolism. PI3K activation determines protein-kinase B (PKB/Akt) activation, which, by caspase inhibition and by stimulation of Bcl-2 and c-Myc expressions, has antiapoptotic function. The activated form of PI3K stimulates phospholipase C (PLC), which intervenes in inositol 4,5 biphosphate (IP2) metabolism. Under PLC action will generate inositol triphosphate (IP3) and diacylglycerol (DAG). IP3, rising intracellular calcium, triggers phosphorylation, calcium-dependent, calmodulin-activated of the light myosin chain, thus promoting myocytic contraction. DAG activation stimulates PKC activation, which regulates intracellular pH, acting on Na/K exchanger [22]. Actually, DAG synthesis may be obtained by phospholipase D (PLD) pathway. PLD becomes activated by Ang II-AT1 coupling (see Figure 32.1).

PKC is an enzyme with intracellular localization, which plays the role of intracellular transducer for CyK synthesis. The consequences of PKC activation are increasing in CyK production, augmentation in extracellular matrix production and Na/K ATPase activity inhibition. The decrease in Na/K ATPase activity has implications in cellular growth and differentiation. It intervenes in altering of muscular contractility, in myocytic necrosis and interstitial fibrosis. Activated PKC stimulates the expression of type IV collagen, as much as the accumulation of fibronectine and laminine [10]. PKC also stimulates the production of free radicals, by activation of NAD(P)H oxidase.

The free radicals, generated under activated PKC, determine further NF-kB, STAT1 and epidermal growth factor receptor (EGFR)s activation. The last one activates further ERK1/2, so the process goes on and on.

The binding of Ang II to AT1 does not represent the only way of transcription factors (particularly NF-kB) activation. By AT2 receptors fixing, Ang II opens another signaling way, that of ceramide, which seems to be the common signaling way for CyK, free oxygen species and Ang II by which the molecular ways of heart failure development come together.

Ceramide belongs to the sphingomyelin family and acts as an intracellular second messenger. It is generated by sphingomyelin hydrolysis, under sphingomyelinase action (the catabolic pathway), or by cellular uptake of serine and its condensation with palmitoyl-CoA (the anabolic pathway). The catabolic generation of ceramide is done under CyK (TNFα, IL-1β) and oxygen free radicals action [23]. The coupling of Ang II with AT2 receptors promotes ceramide synthesis – the anabolic pathway. Ceramide has proapoptotic effects, realized by SAPK activation [23]. So that, NF-kB and SAPK activation have molecular effects, represented by myocytic loss through necrosis and apoptosis (Figure 32.2).

THE LINKS BETWEEN DIABETES MELLITUS AND THE UNFAVORABLE EVOLUTION AND HIGHER INCIDENCE OF HEART FAILURE IN DIABETIC PATIENTS

Which are the mechanisms responsible for the higher incidence of HF in diabetics and why in diabetic patients the evolution of HF is more severe? We are trying to answer these challenging questions by the inflammatory process point of view, knowing that also other explanations (such as neurohumoral contributions) are possibly involved and linked to inflammation.

In diabetes mellitus there are many disturbances in carbohydrates, lipid and protidic metabolisms. The modifications in quantitative responses to insulin have an additional role in the occurrence of complications in DM.

HYPERGLYCEMIA

Hyperglycemia determines changes in intracellular calcium and glycosylation of intracellular and extracellular proteins, as well as increase in oxidative stress. All these result in intracellular signal transcription, on PKC pathway [5]. PKC level is elevated using IP3 as source, or by tyrosine kinase receptors phosphorylation's way, under Ang II influence. Both glucose and FFA have destructive effects on cytoskeleton and on myofibrils. FFA induces apoptosis in adult myocytes, proved in rats, on the ceramide way. The chronic hyperglycemia determines apoptosis in many ways. Firstly, by rising in intracellular calcium, it activates the intracellular proteases (caspases). Caspase determines mitochondrion membrane depolarization, allowing thus the entrance of cytochrome C (Cyt C) into the cell and its binding to an apoptosis inducer (Apol-1). Secondly, by activation of a protein-phosphatase which acts on the mitochondrion membrane and stimulates Cyt C delivery in cytosol. Thirdly, by calpaines activation, calcium-dependent proteases, which have apoptotic virtues [18]. On the other hand, hyperglycemia, *per se*, may have antiapoptotic action, by modifications in Bcl-2 expression/phosphorylation (proved on new-born myocytes cultures) [5].

Hyperglycemia alters cellular function in many ways, which are:

The generation of intracellular and extracellular AGEs

The intracellular AGEs formation is more rapid than that of the extracellular AGEs. All intracellular proteins undergo functional changes by glycation, but the most ample effect is on basic fibroblast growth factor (bFGF), with consequences on decreasing in cytoplasmic mitogen activity. Intracellular AGEs trigger DNA lesions. Extracellular AGEs determine modifications in extracellular matrix and in its intercellular interactions, as much as in the interactions between matrix cells and other cellular types. The subendothelial glycosylated proteins accumulation is followed by decreasing in vascular cross section area. Type I and IV collagen and laminine glycosylation have important unfavorable effects. Type IV collagen glycosylation determines decrease in endothelial cells adhesion. Laminine glycation is followed by a decrease in its autopolymerisation, as well as decrease in its binding by IV type collagen. The vitronectin glycation determines diminishing in cells interactions [14].

AGEs receptors also exist on the surface of monocytes and macrophages. By AGEs binding on macrophages receptors, the CyK (IL-1, TNF α), CHK (MCSF, TGFβ) and insulin-like growth factor-1 (IGF-1) production are stimulated. The scavenger macrophage receptors play a role in AGEs scavenge.

On the endothelial surface there are specific AGEs receptors (RAGE), which intervene in signal transduction mediation, *via* free radicals, followed by transcription factors activation. The glucose autooxidation triggers NAD(P)H/NAD systems oxidation in this way, increasing the free radicals production on myeloperoxidase system and mitochondrion metabolism [14].

Hyperglycemia and the oxidative stress

The insulin resistance in type 2 DM is associated with an increment in oxidative stress, due to rise in free radicals production and decrease in antioxidant mechanisms functionality. The last event is linked to the glycation phenomenon of the involved enzymes: aldosereductase, glutathion-ereductase, glutathioneperoxidase, superoxide-dismutase. The free oxygen radicals represent highly reactive species, which alter proteins, lipids and DNA. The most sensible surface at their action is the endothelium, as blood-tissue interface. The free oxygen species (the most aggressive are O_2^-, H_2O_2, OH^-) oxidize the fatty acids (process named lipoperoxidation), the resulted lipohydroperoxides having a cytotoxic effect. By free radicals-NO coupling generates peroxynitrites, aggressive species, which generate OH^-. The free radicals are protooncogenes inducers and amplify non RTK Ang II action on AP-1, and that of TNFα on NF-kB activation.

Free radicals are generated in many ways: the polyols pathway, nonenzymatic glycation and glucose autooxidation. The glucose autooxidation determines NAD(P)H/NAD oxidation, with free radicals delivery and cellular NAD(P)H depletion. Hyperglycemia stimulates, by increasing in lipooxygenase-12 activity in SMC, the synthesis from arachidonic acid of hydroperoxyeicosatetraenoic acid (HPETE) and hydroxyeicosatetraenoic acid (HETE). Both metabolites activate PKC, raise the proto-oncogene expression, induce SMC hypertrophy and migration, and stimulate the extracellular matrix production [11]. The endothelium itself is a source of free radicals in diabetic patients, due to endothelial NOs dysfunction, which is related to tetrahydrobiopterin depletion [24]. The free radicals inhibit endothelial NOs activity, so enduring production of free radicals.

There are theories which sustain that oxidative stress precedes DM installation [25]. The relatives of type 1 DM have a higher free radicals level compared to those without DM family records. The association between type 1 DM and the higher CAD risk (in the absence of dyslipidemia) suggests the negative pathophysiologic role of free radicals in DM. The free radicals synthesis is initiated and amplified by AGEs [11, 18].

Hyperglycemia raises DAG concentration in blood vessels, heart, liver, skeletal muscle

The DAG synthesis is realized from phosphatidylcholine under PLD action, or by synthesis from phosphatidilinositol under PLC action, or under free radicals intervention. More than this, DAG is generated *de novo*, from glycolytic intermediary metabolism. Binding of DAG to PKC determines activation of PKC. The PKC isoforms involved in cardiac complications of DM belong to conventional, calcium-dependent, DAG-sensible isoforms. They are βI and βII PKC isoforms.

By β PKC activation, TGFβ factor, which increases fibronectine and IV type collagen synthesis, becomes transactivated. Additionally, there is an activation in *c-fos* and TGFβ expressions. The changes in Na/K ATPase and the high NO synthesis, both with the above-mentioned modifications determine the histological changes recorded in DM [10].

DYSLIPIDEMIA

Hypertriglyceridemia

In the insulin resistance syndrome there are noted *à jeun* and postprandial hypertriglyceridemia. The insulin resistance triggers adipose tissue hormone-sensitive lipase (HSL) inhibition, hormone responsible by FFA from adipose tissue releasing. FFA determine rising in hepatic VLDL production and their content in triglycerides, which explains *à jeun* hypertriglyceridemia. Postprandial hypertriglyceridemia is due to chilomicrons production and reduction in lipoprotein lipase activity. The high hepatic FFA flow inhibits pancreatic insulin secretion and stimulates hepatic glucose production. FFA metabolisation in skeletal muscle is followed by a decrease in muscular glucose uptake. Dyslipidemia

is associated with an increase in NF-kB disponibility and endothelial expression of leukocytes adhesion molecules. Additionally, hypertriglyceridemia raises the oxidative stress level, which activates PKC pathway and transcription factors.

Lipotoxicity

Lipotoxicity refers to functional impairment of nonadipocytes. The impairment is variable in amplitude, until cellular destruction-apoptosis. Lipotoxicity is due to triacylglycerol (TAG) excess. TAG results from FFA esterification in nonadipocytic cells. Nonadipocytes do not have the ability to eliminate the fatty acids, which come from circulation, TAG remaining intracytoplasmic until fatty acids are hydrolyzed and oxidized. Overloading of nonfat cells with TAG precedes alterations in cellular functionality. A protector mechanism against steatosis in nonadipose tissues is FFA oxidation, in this process Lpt having a stressed role. Lpt determines nonadipocytes TAG accumulation, having a role against steatosis. The modifications in Lpt receptors determine heart, liver, muscle TAG overaccumulation [22]. By binding Lpt to the long isoform of the leptin receptor (OB-Rb), STAT-3 becomes activated. STAT-3, in its activated form, stimulates the catabolic factor-PPARα. PPARα determines the excess of FFA oxidation, with heat production [22]. PPARs are located intranuclearly and are represented by three isoforms: α (in the liver, muscles, endothelial cells, macrophages), γ (in the adipose tissue, endothelial cells, macrophages) and β (in many tissues). PPARs exist as heterodimers coupled with retinoid X receptors (RXR). The complex PPAR/RXR has inhibitory activity on transcription. By PPAR/RXR dissociation, the genes transcription is promoted. PPARα actions, especially on those genes which mediate fatty acids uptake (by carnitine palmitoyl transferase) and fatty acids oxidation (by AcCoA synthase) and also on genes that intervene in lipoproteins metabolism. PPARα stimulates Apo I and Apo II synthesis (rising in HDL and cholesterol levels), the Apo V synthesis (followed by decrease in triglycerides level), stimulates lipoprotein lipase gene (triggering lipolysis) and inhibits Apo-C III synthesis (decreasing VLDL triglycerides content). A very important PPARα property is that of transcription of NF-kB and

Ap-1 genes, by IKB stimulation and direct inhibition of nuclear translocated NF-kB. PPARα decreases metalloproteinases and CyK production by NF-kB, AP-1 and STAT inhibition [18]. PPARγ determines adipose tissue free fatty acids deposits. These receptors have widespread distribution (in the skeletal muscle, heart, kidney, bowel, endothelium, macrophages), but the highest level is recorded in the adipose tissue. It seems that PPARγ is involved in insulin resistance development. More than this, PPARγ mediates Lpt gene suppression. Modifications in Lpt receptors are followed by PPARα activity blockage and by PPARγ overexpression, event that is followed by oversynthesis of TAG, initiating the lipoproteic cascade. The excess of TAG is followed by ceramide synthesis (from serine and palmitoyl-CoA), the common Ang II and CyK signaling pathway. Ceramide is also the common signaling way for both type 1 and 2 DM. In type 1 DM, the ceramide production is increased due to sphingomyeline catabolism and in type 2 DM, the ceramide production is increased in the anabolic manner [22].

HYPERINSULINEMIA IN TYPE 2 DM

In this type of DM the insulinemia level is high. But, a prothrombotic and hypofibrinolytic status must be noted with associated platelet dysfunction, high fibrinogen and PAI-1 levels and low thrombomodulin values. In these patients, the acute reactants phase protein level is high [22]. But how does this happen, when insulin, a hormone with vasodilatatory, antithrombogenetic, fibrinolytic and acute inflammation mediators' inhibitory properties, is high? The answer consists in tissular insulin resistance.

The common fact to all metabolisms signaling pathway is PKC. PKC is involved in insulin resistance by decreasing the tyrosinekinase activity of the insulin receptor, which is due to IRS-1 and glucose transporter activity impairments as well as insulin mediated glucose metabolism. The activation of PKC precedes AGEs and free radicals synthesis, as long as it is involved in insulin resistance pathogenesis [22]. The PKC effects are realized by stimulation of angiotensin converting enzyme activity (via MAPK activation and by inferences with NOs),

resulting an increase in Ang II production and high bradikinin destruction. Besides its vasodilatatory virtue, bradikinin, binding to B2 receptors, directly increases glucose transport and cellular utilization, actions that are realized through insulin receptors phosphorylation and rising in insulin stimulated GLUT4 translocation from cytosol to membrane [22]. Those are demonstrated by that the treatment with converting enzyme inhibitors augments not only the glucose insulin mediated transport, but also the cellular glucose utilization. PKC overexpression, resulted from Ang II hyperproduction, is traduced in terms of myocytic losing, associated to remained myocytic hypertrophy and interstitial fibrosis. But PKC also determines an increase in CK production, with an overproduction of interstitial matrix, by connective tissue growth factor expression stimulation [22]. By PLA2 activation, PKC determines a decrease in Na/K ATPase activity, fact that is involved in cellular growth and differentiation, myocardic contractility and viability, and interstitial fibrous tissue production. By TGFβ stimulation, PKC increases type IV collagen, laminine and fibronectine expressions. TGFβ transactivation is done by the link between Ang II and AT1 [10]. PKC inhibits IP3K activity, enzyme involved in endothelial NOs production.

Ang II and proinflammatory factors interact in contributing to structural with functional heart damage leading to the appearance and progression of heart failure.

CONCLUSIONS

The heart failure syndrome occurs more frequently and is more severe in diabetic patients. The precise mechanisms are unknown, until now, but it seems, based on presented data, that the inflammatory reaction plays a peculiar high role. There is a proved link between heart failure and inflammatory mediators. The involvement of inflammation in diabetes is also known. As was presented in the preceding pages, diabetes as well as heart failure are involved in inflammatory factors activation. The same factors that lead to insulin resistance are also involved in the progression of heart failure (TNFα and IL-6 being the most studied). May be, the association of these inflammatory conditions explains the worse evolution of heart failure in diabetic patients, as well as the greater incidence of diabetes in heart failure patients.

Inflammation modifies the equilibrium between the protein phosphorylation level and that of phosphatase activation. It is a condition which highly activates the transcription factors, leading to increases in cellular growth and proliferation. This phenomenon is strernghened in DM, mainly due to the high level of free radicals, which activates receptor and nonreceptor tyrosine kinases, receptor and nonreceptor serine/threonine kinases.

On the other hand, removal of incorporated phosphates by phosphatases turns off the proliferative signals. Or, in DM, the activity of protein tyrosine phosphatases is lower; the result will be the loss of control over growth genes.

A peculiar role as transcription factor may be atributed, in DM, to NF-kB, because its activation is closely related to the level of free radicals. NF-kB activation is blocked by AT1 receptor antagonists or antioxidants.

The multiple ways of PKC activation in DM and the fact that PKC determines a decrease in PDH activity, put into a causal relationship the level of PKC and the switch of energetic myocardium substrate from lactate and glucose to FFA.

In this way, diabetes may aggravate the energetic deficiency of heart failure on the one hand and, on the other, strenghtens the inflammatory reaction, which contributes to the unfavorable evolution of heart failure.

REFERENCES

1. Bauters C, Lamblin N, McFadden EP, van Belle E, Millaire A, de Groote P. Influence of diabetes mellitus on heart failure risk and outcome. *Cardiovasc Diabetol,* **2**(1): 1, 2003.
2. Gheorghiade M, Bonow RO. Chronic heart failure in the United States: a manifestation of coronary artery disease. *Circulation,* **97**: 282–289, 1998.
3. Stratton IM, Adler AI, Neil HA, Matthews DR, Manley SE, Cull CA, Hadden D, Turner RC, Holman RR. Association of glycaemia with macrovascular and microvascular complications of type 2 diabetes (UKPDS 35): prospective observational study. *BMJ,* **321**: 405–412, 2000.
4. Taegtmeyer H, McNulty P, Young ME. Adaptation and maladaptation of the heart in diabetes: Part I: general concepts. *Circulation,* **105**: 1727–1733, 2002.
5. NHLBI working group on cellular and molecular mechanisms of diabetic cardiomyopathy. http://www.nhlbi.nih.gov/meetings/workshops/diab min.htm.
6. Schiaffini R, Pantaleo A, Battocletti T, Vaccari V, Brufani C, Martuscelli E, Gargiulo P. Serine-protease inhibitors in diabetic cardiomyopathy. Abstract 1064, 2003, http://www.diabetolognytt.com/abstracts 2000/1062.pdf.
7. Bartnik M, Malmberg K, Ryden L. Managing heart disease. Diabetes and the heart: compromised myocardial function a common challenge. *Eur Heart J* Supplement 5(Supp B): B33–B41, 2003
8. Cristea-Popa E, Popescu A, Trutia E, Dinu V. *Tratat de biochimie medicală,* Ed Medicală, Bucureşti, 1991.
9. Ionescu-Tîrgovişte C. *Diabetologia modernă,* Ed. Tehnică, Bucureşti, 1997.
10. Pickup JC, Mattock MB, Chusney GD, *et al.* NIDDM as a disease of the innate immune system: association of acute-phase reactants and interleukin-6 with metabolic syndrome X. *Diabetologia,* **40**: 1286–1292, 1997.
11. Kelly RA, Smith TW. Cytokines and cardiac contractile function. *Circulation,* **95**: 778–781, 1997.
12. Barzilay J, Freedland E. Inflammation and its association with glucose disorders and cardiovascular disease. *Treatments in Endocrinology,* **2** (2): 85–94, 2003.
13. Cheng AT, Ree D, Kolls J, Fuselier J, Coy DH, Bryar-Asch M. An *in vivo* model for elucidation of the mechanism of tumor necrosis factor α (TNF-α)–induced insulin resistance: evidence for a differential regulation of insulin signaling by TNF-α. *Endocrinology,* **139**: 4928–4935, 1998.
14. Mohamed-Ali V, Pinkney JH, Coppack SW. Adipose tissue as an endocrine and paracrine organ. *Int J Obes Relat Metab Disord,* **22**: 1145–1158, 1998.
15. Dronca Maria. *Glicozilarea nonenzimatică a proteinelor.* Casa cărţii de ştiinţă, Cluj, 2000.
16. Pradhan AD, Manson JE, Rifai N. C-reactive protein, interleukin 6, and risk of developing type 2 diabetes mellitus. *JAMA,* **286**: 327–334, 2001.
17. Barzilay JI, Abraham L, Heckbert SR *et al.* The relation of markers of inflammation to the development of glucose disorders in the elderly: the Cardiovascular Health Study. *Diabetes,* **50**: 2384–2389, 2001.

18. Kahn CR, Weis G. *Joslin's Diabetes Mellitus*. Lea & Febiger, Philadelphia, 13th Ed, 1994.
19. Ford ES. Leukocyte count, erythrocyte sedimentation rate, and diabetes incidence in a national sample of US adults. *Am J Epidemiol*, **155:** 57–64, 2002.
20. Herlihy OM, Barrow BA, Grant PJ. Hyperglycaemic siblings of type II (non-insulin-dependent) diabetic patients have increased PAI-1, central obesity and insulin resistance compared with their paired normoglycaemic siblings. *Diabetologia*, **45:** 635–641, 2002.
21. Parissis JT, Adamapoulos S, Karas SM, Kremastinos DT. An overview of inflammatory cytokine cascade in chronic heart failure. *Hellenic J Cardiol*, **43:** 18–28, 2002.
22. Lehtonen JY, Horiuchi M, Daviet L, Akishita M, Dzau VJ. Activation of the *de novo* biosynthesis of sphingolipids mediates angiotensin II type 2 receptor-induced apoptosis. *J Biol Chem,* **274:** 16901–16906, 1999.
23. Berry C, Touyz R, Dominiczak AF, Webb RC, Johns DG. Angiotensin receptors: signaling, vascular pathophysiology, and interactions with ceramide. *Am J Heart Physiol Circ Physiol*, **281,** H2337–H2365, 2001.
24. Makimattila S, Liu ML, Vakkilainen J, Schlenzka Anna, Lahdenpera S, Syvanne M, Mantysaari M, Summanen P, Bergholm R, Taskinen MR, Yki-Jarvinen H. Impaired endothelium-dependent vasodilatation in type 2 diabetes. Relation to LDL size, oxidized LDL, and antioxidants. *Diabetes Care*, **22:** 973–981, 1999.
25. Matteucci E, Giampietro O. Oxidative stress in families of type 1 diabetic patients. *Diabetes Care,* **23:** 1182–1186, 2000.

33

CARDIAC FUNCTION IN DIABETES – ECHOGRAPHIC EVALUATION

Ion Victor BRUCKNER, Adriana Luminiţa GURGHEAN, Ioana Maria BRUCKNER

Diabetes mellitus is the most important independent risk factor for cardiovascular disease, with a continuously increasing incidence and prevalence. It represents the leading cause for poor outcome of cardiovascular diseases. Many epidemiological studies showed that diabetic patients have a worse short and long-term prognosis compared to non-diabetic patients with known cardiac disease.

In type 2 diabetes, macrovascular complications are frequent early findings, mainly coronary artery disease, stroke and peripheral vascular disease, through its strong association with atherosclerosis. On the other hand, in type 1 diabetes, at least in its early stages, microvascular complications dominate. The presence of myocardial fibrosis without evident cardiac disease represents the substrate for diabetic cardiomyopathy, frequently seen in this setting.

Regardless of the type of diabetes, cardiovascular lesions become rapidly irreversible, leading to heart failure – the end-stage of all cardiovascular diseases. Therefore, it is mandatory to evaluate diabetic patients with or without evidence of cardiac disease in order to prevent the occurrence or to delay the progression to heart failure. A thorough evaluation is, in fact, necessary for early detection of myocardial and vascular damage.

Echocardiography, among other non-invasive investigations, has an important place in the evaluation of these patients due to its high accuracy and availability.

The value of echocardiography resides in its ability to detect early morphological anomalies (myocardial hypertrophy, left ventricular geometry and dimensions), and also functional changes (diastolic dysfunction, regional motion abnormalities, global systolic dysfunction).

New echocardiographic techniques, such as contrast echocardiography, tissue Doppler echocardiography, improved the accuracy of this method, allowing for better diagnosis.

DIABETES AND CARDIOVASCULAR DISEASES

INTRODUCTION

Diabetes is by far the most powerful risk factor for heart disease, even when not associated with other well-known cardiovascular risk factors. Beside these elements, some other emerging risk factors in diabetes such as albuminuria, high serum free fatty acids, hypercoagulability, and the insulin resistance syndrome seem to be involved in the developing or the outcome of heart diseases. Despite the fact that the incidence of heart disease tends to decrease in the general population, this is not the case in the presence of diabetes.

In diabetic patients, cardiovascular diseases are associated with a poorer short- and long-term outcome as compared to nondiabetic subjects. In addition, coronary lesions in diabetic patients are more extensive and complex, leading to more severe forms of coronary heart disease (unstable angina, myocardial infarction) and, by consequence, to a higher rate of heart failure.

Although overt hyperglycemia is recognized as the most important independent risk factor for heart disease, recent studies suggest that dysglycemic states (impaired fasting glucose or impaired glucose tolerance) preceding diabetes, may be associated with a higher incidence of cardiovascular damage. Out of the two entities mentioned above, post-prandial glucose level seems to be more strongly related to cardiovascular outcomes than is the fasting level. It seems that the degree of dysglycemia, measured by the plasma glucose level or by HbA1c is related to the risk for a new or recurrent cardiovascular event. Even so, the efficiency of lowering the glucose or HbA1c level in order to reduce cardiovascular events remains under debate.

In terms of cardiovascular mortality, data show a two to three fold increase in men with diabetes and even more in diabetic women. In addition, the rate of heart failure is significantly higher, independent of other risk factors such as age, gender, hypercholesterolemia, smoking or hypertension.

The relationship between diabetes and heart disease is not unidirectional, but rather a reciprocal one, since it was observed that heart failure may be an independent predictor of subsequent type 2 diabetes.

The deleterious effects of diabetes on the heart and vessels are based upon the important metabolic changes (due to hyperglycemia, hyperinsulinemia, oxidative stress, dyslipidemia) that occur at this level, associated to the procoagulant state and genetic factors.

Both effects (on heart and vessels) may be responsible for the poor outcome of ischemic heart disease in these patients.

THE DIABETIC HEART STRUCTURE AND FUNCTION – A BRIEF REVIEW

The heart is a continuously working pump, which necessitates a large amount of energy to assure contraction and associated ionic changes, including those involved in relaxation and impulse conduction. The main source of energy for these processes is adenosine triphosphate (ATP). ATP concentration in the cardiomyocyte is relatively constant due to the matching of its use and resynthesis. The main sources of energy for resynthesis in the normal heart are the oxidative breakdown of fatty acids (60–80%), glucose (10–30%), and lactate (10–30%). Ketone bodies may also contribute, but insignificantly, in the normal heart [1].

In contrast, the major energy sources in the diabetic heart are represented by free fatty acids and ketone bodies due to impaired insulin stimulation of cardiac glucose uptake associated with elevation of circulating fatty acids, ketone bodies and glucose levels.

The abnormalities in myocardial carbohydrate and lipid metabolism due to insulin deficiency may result in decreased ATP activity, changes in calcium homeostasis and increased myocardial oxygen consumption (Figure 33.1).

The consequences are myocyte hypertrophy, progressive loss of myofibrils and replacement by fibrosis leading to impaired myocardial contractility. These histopathological findings are present in diabetes even in the absence of hypertension or coronary artery disease and their combination is particularly damaging to the heart.

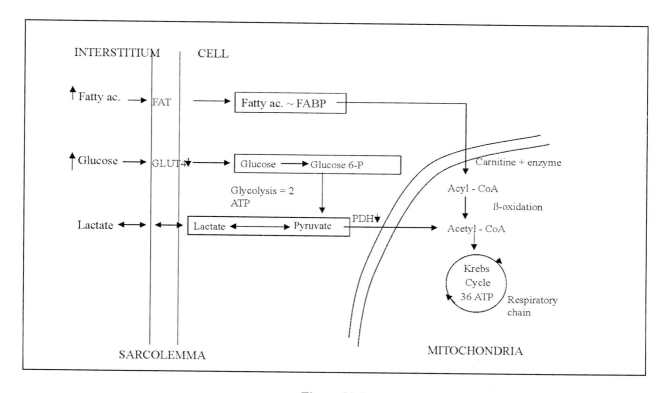

Figure 33.1
Cardiac metabolic changes in diabetes.
FABP = fatty acid binding protein.

In the diabetic heart, there is also an increase in extracellular collagen probably related to the degree of hyperglycemia and to the impaired collagen degradation. This condition accounts for an increase of myocardial stiffness and subsequent diastolic and systolic dysfunction.

In addition, the presence of diabetes is predisposing to early atherosclerosis, a process that is more severe, extensive and has some peculiarities in this situation.

The effect of diabetes on enhancing athero-sclerosis has multiple explanations. Alteration in lipoprotein composition, especially an increase in small dense LDL, glycation and oxidation accelerate the atherosclerotic process. A very special role in this process is occupied by the endothelial dysfunction. If diabetes *per se* is an important risk factor for coronary disease, it is also frequently associated with other coronary risk factors such as hyperinsulinism, obesity, hypertension, hypertriglyceridemia and decreased high-density lipoprotein (HDL) levels, the so-called metabolic syndrome.

Among all vascular territories, the coronary territory is by far the most affected one, leading to different types of myocardial ischemia, which overlap with the myocardial changes previously described.

The inadequate oxygen supply in myocardial ischemia also leads to metabolic changes mainly by increasing the anaerobic glycolysis and impaired pyruvate oxidation. Depending upon the degree of the coronary stenoses, the myocardial metabolic substrate may be different. In complete obstruction leading to necrosis, the coronary flow ceases and there is no delivery of glucose to the myocardium. Therefore, the only source of glycolysis in this situation is glycogen. In mild or moderate stenoses, the reduction of coronary flow leads to a decrease in myocardial oxygen consumption and the tissue damage is reversible. Even if there is contractile dysfunction, the main source of energy to synthesize ATP is represented by fatty acids.

In diabetic patients, coronary artery disease has some peculiar functional and anatomic characteristics, as compared to the non-diabetic population, at multiple levels: macrovascular and microvascular. The imbalance of coagulation factors, increased platelet aggregation and decreased thrombolysis that are present in patients with diabetes, contributes to the increased incidence of ischemia.

The macrovascular level is characterized by a greater extent of coronary lesions, which involves in a diffuse pattern more than one vessel (evidenced by coronary angiography and morphopathological observations). In addition, calcification within atherosclerotic plaques is more common in this situation. One aspect must be emphasized: the remodeling process appears decreased in diabetic patients in contrast to the increased neo-intimal proliferation post-angioplasty responsible for higher rates of re-stenosis.

Coronary microcirculation presents anatomical and functional abnormalities in diabetes and the consequence is the decreased vasodilator reserve. Anatomically, the basal lamina is thickened in coronary microvessels correlating, among other factors, with the duration of diabetes. A number of factors influence the microvascular tonus through nitric oxide derived from the vascular endothelium. The hallmark is endothelial dysfunction through several mechanisms involved in diabetes, such as impaired production and transport of nitric oxide, relative insensibility to nitric oxide or production of constricting factors. Coronary microangiopathy in combination with subendocardial fibrosis and glycoprotein deposits is involved in diabetic cardiomyopathy. The autonomic dysfunction present in diabetes also seems to play an important role in this entity.

Myocardial ischemia, due to macro- as well as micro-angiopathy, has an important impact on the cardiac function; depending on its extension and severity, it may alter the diastolic function (delayed relaxation) or, in its severe forms, may depress the systolic function (expressed by a low ejection fraction).

ECHOCARDIOGRAPHIC EVALUATION OF CARDIAC FUNCTION

When we analyze cardiac function, we refer to both the contractile and lusitropic status of the heart. Both are active processes that require energy. The complex abnormalities described above lead to a large energy shortage, resulting in both diastolic and systolic myocardial dysfunction.

Cardiac function can be assessed invasively or by using noninvasive methods, the former remaining the golden standard, but due to their possible side effects, are reserved for unclear or complex situations. Among the multitude of noninvasive methods, echocardiography has many advantages in terms of availability, accuracy, reproducibility and cost-effectiveness. Even more, modern echocardiographic techniques like stress echocardiography, myocardial contrast echocardiography, strain-Doppler echocardiography improved significantly the accuracy of this method when evaluating the cardiac function. If the acoustic window is good, the accuracy of cardiac echography in the evaluation of the systolic function – either global or regional – is comparable to that of other methods like magnetic resonance imaging or radionuclide angiography.

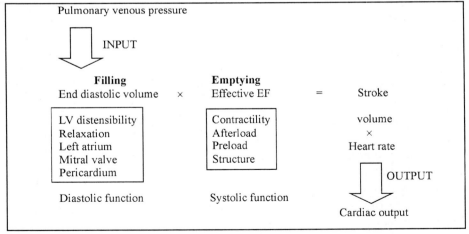

Figure 33.2
Diagram of left ventricular pump performance.

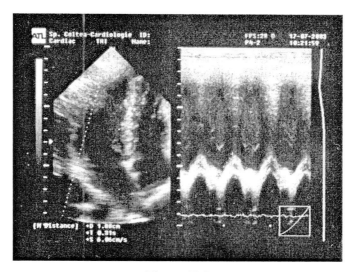

Figure 33.3
"MAPSE" – at the level of the lateral wall. Apical four-chamber view.

In addition, it is a very good method for diastolic dysfunction detection, even if there is quite high investigator dependence.

The pump performance of the left ventricle depends on both its ability to fill (diastolic function) and to empty (systolic function) [2] (Figure 33.2).

Global systolic performance is influenced not only by myocardial contractility, but also by load and ventricular geometry. It can be quantified by using many algorithms with M mode and two-dimensional echocardiography. The most commonly used is the determination of the left ventricular ejection fraction (LVEF) which represents the percent of left ventricular diastolic volume that is ejected in systole. The commonly used methods in quantifying LVEF are the area-length and Simpson's methods. The area-length method requires manual tracing of the endocardial border in diastole and systole and the measurement of the left ventricular long axis from the plane of the mitral annulus to the apex in apical 4 or 2-chamber view sections. The Simpson's method principle is the evaluation of the volume of an irregular, ovoid object (the left ventricle) by summing multiple regularly distributed circular sections. This operation is done automatically on most echographic machines. Ejection fraction (EF) is the ratio between stroke volume (SV) and end-diastolic volume (EDV). Stroke volume is the difference between end-diastolic and end-systolic volumes (EDV-ESV). The resulting formula is EF = SV/EDV × 100. Normal values are considered 63–69%. An ejection fraction of 40–50% is considered abnormal, but with a limited clinical significance. Generally, by convention, depressed systolic function is represented by an ejection fraction below 40%. To simplify, one can use linear dimensions using M mode or 2D echo to calculate fractional shortening, which is the difference between the telediastolic (LVTDtd) and telesystolic (LVIDts) dimension divided by the telediastolic dimension (LVIDtd – LVIDts / LVIDd × 100). Normal fractional shortening is between 18 and 42% [3].

If the endocardium is well delineated, systolic function can also be assessed by using a very easy method, *i.e.* M-mode echocardiography in apical 4-chamber or 2-chamber views. With this method one can evaluate the mitral annulus plane systolic excursion (MAPSE) at the level of the LV anterior, lateral, inferior or septal wall as the difference of end-diastolic and end-systolic lines (in mm) (Figure 33.3). In general, an average value greater than 10 mm correlates with a normal ejection fraction.

Regional systolic function must be evaluated in the presence of myocardial ischemia or infarction, situations in which wall thickening abnormalities may be suspected. For quantitative assessment, it requires the division of the left ventricle into segments. The American Society of Echocardiography recommends the 16 segments model. The location of these segments follows the distribution of the major epicardial arteries to facilitate the diagnosis of myocardial ischemia. For each segment, a wall motion score is assigned. Normal wall motion consists of simultaneous myocardial thickening and inward motion of the endocardium towards the left ventricular cavity; the score for normal motion is 1. Abnormal wall motion extends from hypokinesis (decreased contractility) – score 2, akinesis (absence of contractility) – score 3 to dyskinesis (wall motion is opposite to the other segments) – score 4, for aneurismal segments – score 5. The average score is then calculated and the number resulted is directly proportional to the extent and severity of wall motion abnormalities [4].

Contrast echocardiography is based on the principle of introducing a very echogenic material (microbubbles) in the blood stream. It was developed as a method to detect congenital or acquired intracardiac shunts and in the diagnosis of complex congenital heart diseases. This was due to the size of the microbubbles used to provoke contrast, which was larger than the capillaries diameter.

infarct size, myocardial viability, hibernating myocardium, coronary flow reserve and, by improving two-dimensional echocardiography images, allows for a more accurate evaluation of the left ventricular function.

Doppler echocardiography can also be used for determining global systolic function. The peak velocity (V_{max}) on the aortic flow in systole or the velocity time integral (VTI) can be determined by tracing the entire aortic flow envelope (Figure 33.4). Another method is to examine Doppler flow in patients who have mitral regurgitation. The rate with which the left ventricular pressure rises (dp/dt) is a measure of the left ventricular contractility. To calculate dp/dt, two points on the slope of the mitral regurgitant flow (conventionally, the two points are at 1m/sec and respectively at 3m/sec) must be taken and the pressure gradient between the left ventricle and the left atrium at each point calculated using the modified Bernoulli equation (4 mmHg, respectively 36 mmHg), and divide by the time between those two points (dt).

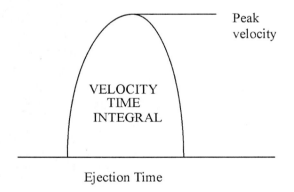

Figure 33.4

Left ventricular systolic function
by aortic Doppler flow.

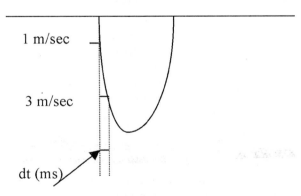

Figure 33.5

Doppler-derived rate of left ventricular pressure rise
using mitral regurgitation jet (dp/dt).

Pressure at 1m/sec is 4 mmHg and at 3m/sec 36 mm Hg (by the simplified Bernoulli equation), so dp between this points is 32 mm Hg.

In time, this technique has spectacularly evolved since microbubble ultrasound contrast agents improved (microbubbles small enough to pass through the capillaries) in order to provide opacification of the left ventricle cavity, better delineation of the endocardial border, detection and quantification of the myocardial perfusion. Myocardial contrast echocardiography with microbubbles is a very useful tool in assessing the

Thus, one can calculate dp/dt (mmHg/sec) by dividing the difference between pressure gradients (32 mmHg) by dt (ms) (Figure 33.5). Poor contractility is reflected by a dp/dt under 1800 mmHg/sec [5].

Cardiac function can also be assessed with Doppler techniques by calculating the Doppler index of myocardial performance (IMP) (Tei-index) based on measurement of Doppler derived time intervals. It is calculated by measuring three time-intervals: the isovolumic contraction time between cessation of mitral inflow and onset of the aortic flow (ICT); the isovolumic relaxation time (IRT) and the ejection time (ET) between onset and cessation of the aortic flow. The formula is IMP = (ICT+IRT)/ET. Tei-index offers data about systolic contraction, ejection and diastolic relaxation (Figure 33.6). The value of the index increases as global myocardial dysfunction progresses.

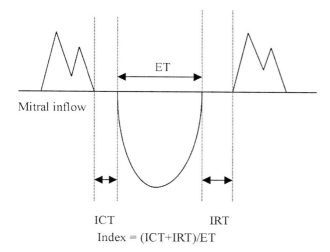

Index = (ICT+IRT)/ET

Figure 33.6

Schematic representation of Doppler intervals for calculation of Tei-index.

ET= ejection time; ICT= isovolumetric contraction time; IRT= isovolumetric relaxation time.

A very new echo technique in evaluating cardiac function, which is much less load-dependent, is tissue Doppler echocardiography (TDE). This imaging modality allows quantification of myocardial velocities by using pulsed and color Doppler.

Systolic wall motion velocities (S_m), obtained with pulsed Doppler, can provide information about both segmental and global ventricular contractility, but they are influenced by heart translation. Myocardial strain and strain rate – estimated as the spatial derivative of velocities (dV/ds) with TDE – seem to be better noninvasive indexes of cardiac contraction. Myocardial strain reflects the ability of the fiber to shorten, while the strain rate is the velocity change in myocardial fiber length (in other words, it represents an index of the speed of contraction) [6].

Concerning diastolic dysfunction, its prevalence in the general population is not very clear, even though new methods and parameters were developed for its evaluation. However, data exist to sustain that approximately half of all patients with symptoms of heart failure have normal left ventricular systolic function (IMPROVEMENT study – 51% and Euro Heart Failure Survey – 47%) [7, 8].

The diastolic dysfunction diagnosis (impaired filling of the left ventricle in order to provide an adequate cardiac output) requires special attention because it seems to be present in a higher proportion than systolic dysfunction, especially in the elderly. Accurate evaluation of the diastolic function is not very easy. It becomes at least as important as the evaluation of the systolic function since it was observed that diastolic dysfunction *per se* has also an important impact on cardiac morbidity and mortality.

Echocardiographic advances in the assessment of the diastolic function can now replace invasive methods in most of the cases.

The left ventricular filling pattern is commonly assessed by Doppler echocardiographic measurement of the mitral inflow velocities. The normal pattern is characterized by rapid filling early in diastole (E wave) and an additional filling during atrial contraction (A wave). The normal filling pattern can be quantified by measuring the peak early velocity and the peak velocity during atrial contraction. E/A ratio expresses the contribution of early and atrial filling and is normally greater than 1.0. Other parameters currently measured are the time required for deceleration of the early diastolic flow (DT_E), the rate of this deceleration (E/DT_E), the isovolumetric relaxation time (IVRT) – the time from aortic valve closure to mitral valve opening (Figure 33.7).

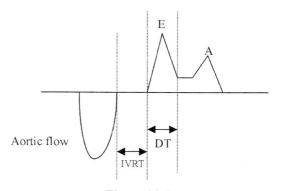

Figure 33.7

Normal diastolic filling pattern.

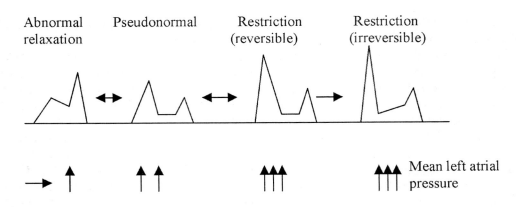

| Abnormal relaxation | Pseudonormal | Restriction (reversible) | Restriction (irreversible) |

Figure 33.8

Abnormal diastolic filling patterns. Progression of diastolic dysfunction.

There are three abnormal diastolic patterns of mitral filling (Figure 33.8) representing progressively worsening of LV diastolic performance. With "impaired relaxation", E/A ratio is less than 1.0. (E < A); DT_E and IVRT are prolonged; deceleration rate of the early filling is slower.

In the "pseudonormalized" pattern, E wave is larger than A wave, but DT_E is shortened, and in the "restricted" pattern, E is much larger than A (E>>A) with a very short DT_E. The presence of the restrictive pattern correlates with the poorest prognosis.

Pulmonary venous flow pattern can be used to complement the mitral valve inflow. With pulsed Doppler in apical 4-chamber view, one can measure the peak pulmonary venous systolic (S) and diastolic (D) wave velocities and the peak pulmonary venous atrial reverse (AR) wave velocity. They provide additional information about diastolic filling. Normally, S wave is greater than D wave and the AR wave velocity is under 35 cm/sec (Figure 33.9).

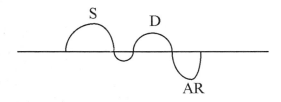

Figure 33.9

Normal pattern of pulmonary venous flow.

S > D; AR <35 cm/sec.

When left ventricular stiffness is increased, the AR wave velocity and duration are augmented,

systolic velocity decreases and becomes smaller than the diastolic velocity. Thus, pseudonormalized and mostly restrictive patterns are associated with large and prolonged AR waves, with peak flow velocity greater than 35 cm/sec, unless atrial systolic failure is present (small AR waves).

It must be emphasized that the parameters described above can be used only when there is no atrial fibrillation and are load dependent.

Noninvasive assessment of myocardial relaxation, independent of loading conditions, became an important goal in order to measure the diastolic function more accurately. The propagation of flow into the LV cavity in early diastole, assessed by color M-mode echocardiography, correlates better with the time constant of relaxation (tau) measured invasively, unless important mitral or aortic regurgitation are present. Normal relaxation has quick flow propagation into the left ventricle.

Based on recent publications [9], the propagation velocity (Vp) seems to be relatively load independent and does not vary with maneuvers known to influence the filling pressure (*e.g.* Valsalva, nitroglycerine); also, the degree of systolic performance has no influence on this parameter.

Using the combination of the mitral deceleration (DT) and Vp, Moller and coauthors [10] characterized diastolic function as normal when DT = 140–240 ms and Vp is greater than 45 cm/sec. Pseudonormal and restrictive patterns, both with worse prognosis, have Vp under 45 cm/sec (delayed flow propagation). A ratio of mitral E velocity over Vp (E/Vp) greater than 1.5

in combination with DT under 130 msec were demonstrated to be the strongest predictors of in-hospital heart failure post myocardial infarction [11].

A more recent noninvasive load independent method that estimates myocardial relaxation is tissue Doppler echocardiography (TDE) which assesses mitral annular velocities in diastole with the Doppler sample volume at different portions of the mitral annulus (septal, lateral, or average of several sites) in apical views. TDE pattern in diastole is characterized by two negative waves – early (Em) and atrial (Am). Diastolic indexes include Em and Am peak velocities (m/s), Em/Am ratio (normally greater than 1), deceleration time (DTm) and relaxation time (Rm) – the time interval between the end of peak systolic velocity (Sm) and the onset of Em. The combination between Em and E velocity of the transmitral flow, *i.e.* E/Em was demonstrated to be the single best predictor of LV filling pressure and independent of systolic function. Patients with E/Em greater than 15 have elevated filling pressure, while E/Em less than 8 denotes low or normal filling pressure [12]. Another important utility of TDE is in the differentiation between normal and pseudonormal diastolic filling patterns. In pseudonormal pattern, Em/Am remains below 1, while on diastolic transmitral flow, E/A is above 1 (and thus may be interpreted as normal diastolic pattern) [13].

In order to evaluate the diastolic function, the measurement of an isolated, single parameter is insufficient. As patients with depressed systolic function always associate diastolic dysfunction, to distinguish between normal and pseudonormal does not represent a problem. In contrast, in patients with preserved systolic function, the distinction can be made only by measuring multiple parameters and using both Doppler and two-dimensional echocardiography.

THE IMPORTANCE OF ECHO EVALUATION OF CARDIAC FUNCTION IN DIABETES

The main role of echocardiography in diabetes is supposed to be the detection of early myocardial anatomic or functional changes, before the onset of clinical heart failure. Once overt heart disease is present, echography allows its precise diagnosis and follow-up.

In diabetes, an important risk factor aggregation increases the risk for cardiac heart disease (UKPDS study has provided important data in this direction). The frequent association of diabetes with hypertension and coronary artery disease leads to heart failure more rapidly than in nondiabetic subjects. However, it was observed that myocardial structural alteration (interstitial fibrosis, myocyte hypertrophy) and/or dysfunction (systolic and diastolic) exist even in the absence of a known cardiac disease [14]. Therefore, diabetic myocardial disease became a distinct entity and a disputed subject of debate.

ECHO EVALUATION OF MYOCARDIAL HYPERTROPHY

Left ventricular hypertrophy is present in diabetes in the absence of hypertension and it can be assessed by two-dimensional (apical, parasternal long and short axis views) and M-mode echocardiography (parasternal long/short axis view) as thickening of the interventricular septum (IVS), posterior wall (PW), anterior wall; abnormal values are greater than 11 mm. The consequence is the elevation of the left ventricular mass or mass-index (g/m^2) – over 131 g/m^2 in men, or over 100 g/m^2 in women – determined by Devereux's formula (LVEDd is the left ventricular end-diastolic dimension): LV mass = 1.04 $[(LVEDd + IVS + PW)^3 - LVEDd^3] - 13.6$.

Left ventricular hypertrophy is one of the most frequent conditions that lead to diastolic dysfunction because it decreases myocardium elasticity, increases stiffness and, by consequence, impairs relaxation. Left ventricular hypertrophy may be found early in diabetes even in the absence of systemic hypertension, although left ventricular hypertrophy and hypertension are common comorbidities of diabetes mellitus. Echocardiography may reveal its presence, being a very sensitive method as compared to electrocardiography in this respect. However, when electrocardiography meets the criteria of left ventricular hypertrophy (voltage score plus secondary changes of ventricular repolarization), there is good correlation with myocardial hypertrophy found on echocardiography.

Diastolic dysfunction, the consequence of myocardial hypertrophy, may be therefore present in diabetes in the absence of an overt cardiac disease. Impaired relaxation, the early stage of diastolic dysfunction, is characterized by:

– E/A ratio less than 1 (<50 years), or less than 0.5 (>50 years);

– prolonged isovolumic relaxation time (IVRT): over 100ms (<50 years), or >105ms (>50 years);

– prolonged DT: over 220ms;

– AR under 35cm/sec (echo Doppler in pulmonary veins);

– Vp under 45cm/sec; elevation of E/Vp ratio (M-mode color Doppler) [15].

In time, diastolic dysfunction may progress on its own, but mainly when coronary artery disease or hypertension coexist, at echo, one may find patterns of pseudonormal (E/A = 1–2; IVRT < 100ms; DT = 150–200ms; AR > 35cm/sec; Vp < 45cm/sec) or even restrictive filling (E/A >2; IVRT < 60ms; DT < 150ms; AR > 35cm/sec; Vp < 45cm/sec; E/Vp > 1.5).

It is very important to emphasize that evidence of preserved or only mildly impaired systolic function (ejection fraction of the left ventricle > 40%) is mandatory in order to assert isolated or "pure" diastolic dysfunction.

In the stage of impaired relaxation and maybe in pseudonormal filling, systolic function can be normal or nearly normal. This is not the case when a restrictive pattern is present (left ventricle compliance significantly impaired), in which case systolic dysfunction is always present (ejection fraction < 40%) [16].

EVALUATION OF CORONARY HEART DISEASE IN DIABETES

The diagnosis of coronary heart disease (CHD) in patients with diabetes is very important because its presence in this subset of patients is at least twice as common as in nondiabetic individuals. The overall prevalence of CHD, in all of its forms (myocardial infarction, acute coronary syndrome, angina pectoris, and sudden death) is as high as 55% among adults with diabetes. The prognosis of CHD in diabetic patients is much worse than in nondiabetic subjects. CHD mortality in patients with type 2 diabetes is two to four times higher than that in nondiabetic people (over 50% of diabetic patients die from CHD) [17].

When typical symptoms of CHD (such as angina) are present, the diagnosis is not difficult. However, many diabetic patients present with either atypical symptoms or no symptoms at all – the so-called silent ischemia, its major form being silent myocardial infarction. In this situation, echocardiography, among other investigations (standard ECG, 24 hours ambulatory ECG monitoring) may be a very useful tool in order to diagnose the presence of CHD, or to evaluate its severity.

Transthoracic echocardiography can find regional anomalies of myocardial motion by using the standard dividing of the left ventricle. These anomalies can vary from hypokinesis to more severe changes such as myocardial akinesis or dyskinesis when myocardial infarction is present. At the same time, global systolic myocardial function can be evaluated by measuring the left ventricular ejection fraction or fractional shortening, which are the most used parameters in daily practice.

When systemic hypertension is present in diabetic patients, the association of CHD can first aggravate a preexisting diastolic dysfunction. With the progression of ischemia, the systolic function may become impaired as well.

Systolic dysfunction is proportional to the extent and the severity of the ischemic burden. This feature is expressed in terms of echocardiography by a low ejection fraction. In this stage, the prognosis of these patients worsens because the progression to heart failure is more rapid in this population than in nondiabetic subjects.

EVALUATION OF HEART FAILURE IN DIABETES

Diabetes mellitus, mainly type 2, is associated with heart failure, mostly through its association with hypertension and coronary artery disease [18]. As it is now recognized, the prevalence of heart failure in diabetic patients is significantly greater than in nondiabetic subjects (the proportion varies from 10% in NETWORK to 35% in RESOLVD study) [19, 20]. On the other hand, the prevalence of diabetes among patients with severe heart failure (NYHA III, IV class) was even higher (47–86%) [21].

In this respect, data obtained from a study performed in the Cardiology Department of "Colţea" Hospital showed similar results – from 442 patients with heart failure, 54.23% associated diabetes mellitus (unpublished data).

Concerning the pathophysiological type of heart failure (systolic or diastolic), when we compared this data with those from another study performed in a Department of Diabetes ("N. Malaxa" Hospital), the results showed significant differences. In the first group we found a predominance of systolic dysfunction (59.7%) *vs.* diastolic dysfunction (40.3%), whereas in the other study group diastolic dysfunction was predominant (64%) *vs.* systolic dysfunction (36%). We considered that these differences might be at least partly explained by the predominance of type 2 diabetes among patients in the study group of a cardiology department. These patients also associated important cardiovascular risk factors like hypertension and coronary artery disease (including myocardial infarction). On the other hand, the higher prevalence of type 1 diabetes and younger patients in the other study group, with probable diabetic cardiomyopathy, may explain the predominance of diastolic dysfunction [22, 23].

Heart failure in the presence of diabetes has a multifactorial etiology and can appear due to epicardial atherosclerotic coronary artery disease, small vessel disease, or diabetes itself [24]. As compared to nondiabetic subjects, patients with diabetes have a significantly greater risk for developing heart failure (risk ratio 7.2 *vs.* 3.8). Heart failure seems to be the most common cause of death in diabetic patients; the data from DIGAMI study showed that heart failure accounted for 66% of total mortality during the first year of follow-up [25].

Cardiac dysfunction in diabetes, beyond the atherosclerotic process, may also be due to specific myocardial damage described, in fact for a very long time. It is known as *diabetic cardiomyopathy*. The diagnosis of diabetic cardiomyopathy is not very easy because it implies exclusion of hypertension, coronary artery disease or other cardiomyopathies, which may be difficult in practice. It is often already present in young diabetic people (especially type 1), without additional cardiovascular risk factors [26, 27]. There are various forms of diabetic cardiomyopathy, from clinically asymptomatic dysfunction to symptomatic impairment of myocardial performance.

The value of echocardiography consists in the fact that it may reveal non-invasively the presence of structural and/or functional myocardial changes that appear in this setting in early, asymptomatic stages.

Based on echocardiographic findings, several forms of diabetic cardiomyopathy were described, the most frequent one being the *dilated cardiomyopathy*, which occurs after a long period of evolving diabetes with frequent metabolic decompensation. The other two forms described are *hypertrophic cardiomyopathy, which* occurs early and may be reversible and *restrictive cardiomyopathy*, which is much less frequently observed [28].

Several morphological echocardiographic features characteristic for diabetic cardiomyopathy are the thickening of ventricular walls, (especially interventricular septum and posterior wall) and the increase of the end diastolic left ventricular dimensions and of the left ventricular mass (it was noted that these changes were more important in women than in men with diabetes) [29]. The consequences of these morphological changes are delayed and uncoordinated ventricular relaxation, which lead to diastolic dysfunction. In early stages, the common pattern seen is delayed relaxation (E<A, prolonged DT and IVRT). Once wall stiffness increases, ventricular compliance decreases and the pattern becomes pseudonormal and even restrictive (E>>A, short DT and IVRT). At the same time, impaired diffuse myocardial contractility occurs, with developing of systolic dysfunction (low ejection fraction, depressed Doppler indexes of systolic performance). In early stages, systolic dysfunction may be asymptomatic or symptoms may occur only at effort, but it rapidly evolves towards heart failure.

INDICATIONS OF ECHO EVALUATION IN DIABETIC PATIENTS

The present guidelines of the European Society of Cardiology do not have clear recommendations about the moment of the initial echographic evaluation and the necessity of subsequent echographic follow-up in heart failure, hypertension or ischemic heart disease.

Our point of view is that an echographic heart evaluation in diabetes is indicated in the following situations:

– any diabetic patient (type 1 or 2) with symptoms of heart failure should be evaluated by echocardiography in order to point out the presence and quantify the severity of the morphological (cavity dimensions, wall thickness, ventricular mass) and functional (parameters of diastolic function, systolic performance – ejection fraction) myocardial changes;

– asymptomatic diabetic patient with evidence of cardiovascular disease (hypertension and/or coronary artery disease); echo evaluation in these patients is mandatory because of the very rapid progression towards severe heart failure. Early stages of diastolic dysfunction or asymptomatic systolic dysfunction, detected by echocardiography may benefit from specific medical treatment (angiotensin converting enzyme inhibitors, diuretics, beta-blockers) proved to delay the occurrence of heart failure;

– diabetic patients without evidence of cardiovascular disease, but with familial history of myocardial infarction, sudden death, stroke, systemic hypertension. Many of these patients may have silent ischemia or even silent myocardial infarction, which can be detected by echocardiography as anomalies of myocardial motion (severe hypokinesis, akinesis);

– the presence of micro- and/or macro-angiopathic complications which represent an increased risk for cardiovascular events and/or death;

– asymptomatic type 1 diabetes – in order to early diagnose structural and/or functional changes suggestive for diabetic cardiomyopathy (probable indication);

– any change in clinical status generally requires a new echographic evaluation.

REFERENCES

1. Stanley WC. Metabolic dysfunction in the diabetic heart. In: Stanley WC (ed). *The Diabetic Coronary Patient*, Science Press, London, 1999, 13–28.

2. Little WC. Assessment of normal and abnormal cardiac function. In: Braunwald E (ed). *Heart Disease*, 6th edition, WB Saunders, 2001, 479–500.

3. Feigenbaum H. Echocardiographic evaluation of cardiac chambers. In: *Echocardiography*, 5th edition, Lea & Febiger, 1994, 134–180.

4. Sheehan FH. Quantitative evaluation of regional left ventricular systolic function. In: Otto CM (ed). *The Practice of Clinical Echocardiography*, 2nd edition, WB Saunders, 2002, 88–113.

5. Chung N, Nishimura RA, Holmes Jr. DR and Tajik AJ. Measurement of left ventricular dp/dt simultaneous Doppler echocardiography and cardiac catheterization. *J Am Soc Echocardiogr*, **5**: 147, 1992.

6. Greenberg NL, *et al*. Doppler–derived myocardial systolic strain rate is a strong index of left ventricular contractility. *Circulation*, **105**: 99–105, 2002.

7. Cleland J. Improvement of heart failure. Presented at the Annual Meeting of the European Society of Cardiology, Amsterdam, 2000.

8. Euro Heart Failure. Report at the Annual Congress of the European Society of Cardiology, Stockholm, 2001.

9. Moller J, Poulsen S, Sondergaard E, *et al*. Preload dependence of color M-mode Doppler flow propagation velocity in controls and in patients with left ventricular dysfunction. *J Am Soc Echocardiogr*, **13**: 902–909, 2000.

10. Moller J, Sondergaard E, Seward J, Appleton C, Egstrup K. Ratio of left ventricular peak E wave velocity to flow propagation velocity assessed by color M-mode Doppler echocardiography in first myocardial infarction: prognostic and clinical implications. *J Am Coll Cardiol*, **35**: 363–370, 2000.

11. Moller J, Sondergaard E, Poulsen S, *et al*. Pseudonormal and restrictive filling patterns predict left ventricular dilation and cardiac death after a first myocardial infarction: a serial color M-mode Doppler echocardiographic study. *J Am Coll Cardiol*, **36**: 1841–1846, 2000.

12. Ommen SR, Nishimura RA, Appleton CP, *et al*. Clinical utility of Doppler echocardiography and tissue Doppler imaging in the estimation of left ventricular filling pressures: A comparative simultaneous Doppler-catheterization study. *Circulation*, **102**: 1788–1794, 2000.

13. Nishimura RA, Tajik A. Evaluation of diastolic filling of left ventricle in health and disease: Doppler echocardiography is the clinician's Rosetta Stone. *J Am Coll Cardiol*, **30**: 8–18, 1997.

14. Mehta S, Nuamah I, Kalhan S. Altered diastolic function in asymptomatic infants of mothers with

gestational diabetes. *Diabetes*, 40 Suppl., **2:** 56–60, 1991.

15. Fischer M. *et al*. Prevalence of left ventricular diastolic dysfunction in the community. *Eur Heart J*, **24:** 320–328, 2003.

16. Pinamonti B, Zecchin M, Di Lenarda A, *et al*. Persistence of restrictive left ventricular filling pattern in dilated cardiomyopathy: An ominous prognostic sign. *J Am Coll Cardiol*, **29:** 604, 1997.

17. Laakso M., Kuusisto J. Understanding patient needs. Diabetology for cardiologists. *Eur Heart J*, **5** Suppl. B: B5–B13, 2003.

18. Grundy SM, Benjamin IJ, Burke GL, *et al*. Diabetes and cardiovascular disease: a statement for healthcare professional from the American Heart Association. *Circulation*, **100:** 1134–46, 1999.

19. The NETWORK investigators. Clinical outcome with enalapril in symptomatic chronic heart failure; a dose comparison. *Eur Heart J*, **19:** 481–9, 1998.

20. McKelvie RS, Yusuf S, Pericak D, *et al*. Comparison of candesartan, enalapril and their combination in congestive heart failure: randomized evaluation of strategies for left ventricular dysfunction (RESOLVD) pilot study. The RESOLVD Pilot Study Investigators. *Circulation*, **100:** 1056–64, 1999.

21. Reis SE, Holubkov R, Edmundowicz D, *et al*. Treatment of patients admitted to the hospital with congestive heart failure: speciality-related disparities in practice patterns and outcomes. *J Am Coll Cardiol*, **30:** 733–8, 1997.

22. Bruckner IV, Gurghean A, Negrila A, Manolache D. *et al*. Observations concerning the diagnosis and treatment of heart failure: epidemiological study. Report at Romanian National Congress of Cardiology, Sinaia, 2002.

23. Bruckner IM, Vlaiculescu M, Dodan R, Grozavu P. Epidemiological aspects of heart failure in diabetic patients. Report at Romanian National Congress of Diabetes, Nutrition and Metabolism, Craiova, 2003.

24. Lutton SR, Ratliff, NB, Yung JB. Cardiomyopathy and myocardial failure. In: Topol EJ (ed). *Textbook of Cardiovascular Medicine*, 2nd edition, Lippincott Williams & Wilkins, 2002, 1819–37.

25. Malmberg K, Ryden L, Efendic S. A randomized study of insulin-glucose infusion followed by subcutaneous insulin treatment in diabetic patients with acute myocardial infarction: Effects on 1- year mortality. *J Am Coll Cardiol*, **26:** 57–65, 1995.

26. Dubrey SW, Raeveley DR, Seed M, *et al*. Risk factors for cardiovascular disease in IDDM. A study of identical twins. *Diabetes*, **43:** 831–5, 1994.

27. Zoneraich S, Mollura JL. Diabetes and the heart: state-of-the-art in the 1990s. *Can J Cardiol*, **9:** 293–9, 1993.

28. Gotzsche O, Darwish A, Gotzsche L, Hansen LP, Sorensen KE. Incipient cardiomyopathy in young insulin dependent diabetic patients: a seven-year prospective Doppler echocardiographic study. *Diabetes Med*, **13:** 834–40, 1996.

29. Nesto RW, Libby P. Diabetes Mellitus and the Cardiovascular System. In: Braunwald E (ed). *Heart Disease*, 6th edition, WB Saunders, 2001, 2133–46.

34

SILENT MYOCARDIAL ISCHEMIA IN DIABETIC PATIENTS

Igor TAUVERON, Françoise DESBIEZ, Laurence MARTEL-COUDERC, Philippe THIEBLOT

Coronaropathy represents the major cause of death in diabetic patients. Silent myocardial ischemia occurs frequently in diabetics. Yet, the implication of autonomous neuropathy in the pathophysiology remains debated. Its prognosis is as worse as the prognosis of painful angina.

Risk factors associated with silent myocardial ischemia in diabetics are close to those previously described for non diabetic coronary disease: age, male gender, dyslipidemia, hypertension, smoking, familial history of cardiovascular disease. Beyond, peripheral arterial disease and proteinuria (to a smaller extent – microalbuminuria) appear as major factors in diabetics. Insulin therapy (in type 2 diabetics) and retinopathy are also evoked. The selection of diabetic patients who need screening for silent myocardial ischemia remains debated. A tendency would be to screen diabetics with at least two risk factors. The validation of a scale of risk (based on a score according to the relative influence of each individual risk factor) seems essential.

The screening tools are many. In the absence of base line ECG change, we suggest the exercise treadmill test, as the first diagnosis step. A negative test under maximal effort conditions provides reassuring information on the lack of ischemic heart disease. When sub-maximal or impossible, a second test is required. Holter ECG recording is not reliable enough. The diagnosis value of myocardial scintigraphy is not as good as in the general population, but its prognosis value remains satisfactory. Stress echocardiography has a sensitivity and specificity similar to those of scintigraphy, but must be performed by experienced groups. Electron beam computed tomography and cardiovascular magnetic resonance imaging need to be validated. A significant abnormality will lead to coronary angiography, with a diagnosis, prognosis and therapeutic aim.

INTRODUCTION

For years, diabetes mellitus has been recognized as a major risk factor for ischemic heart disease. Cardiovascular disease represents the leading cause of death in patients with diabetes [1, 2].

These dramatic reports of high links between diabetes and cardiovascular disease are valid for both type 1 and type 2 diabetes [3, 4], also for men and women. This excess mortality for age is induced by an increased prevalence of myocardial infarction, but also because of the higher severity and poorer prognosis of myocardial infarction in diabetics.

Major intervention studies, among which DCCT, UKPDS, HOT, HOPE, HPS, and many more, have demonstrated that a better control of diabetes and other risk factors would lead to a reduction in cardiovascular disease.

A stage between prevention of all vascular risk factors (ideal, but practically hard to succeed) and care of patent cardiovascular disease (efficient, but obviously too late) should not be missed: early diagnosis of coronary disease, when it is limited to silent myocardial ischemia (SMI).

SMI is a term usually used to describe myocardial ischemia in the absence of pain, but in the presence of other evidence of ischemia.

The aim of this paper, after a review of the prevalence, mechanism and prognosis of SMI in diabetics is to approach factors related to SMI in order to decide who to screen. The second part of the paper is a discussion of the suggested screening tests.

IS SILENT ISCHEMIA MORE FREQUENT IN DIABETICS?

Several studies have suggested that silent ischemia is more common in diabetics than in the general population. Yet, all studies must be taken with care, since they consider heterogeneous diabetics (type 1 or 2, complicated or not, presenting with no or numerous risk factors...), and are based on various tests. A prevalence of 13.5% to 58% occurred. Note that only one study is population based [5] and reveals the lowest prevalence. The risk ratio of diabetics compared to controls reached 1.78, but remained not significant. Only two studies performed a coronary angiography in all subjects [6,7]. Both report a significantly increased prevalence of SMI in diabetics, respectively 9 and 12.1%, when compared to non-diabetics, respectively 1.3 and 5.3% (the latter being recruited for hypertension).

In type 2 diabetes, the prevalence of SMI ranges from 12 to 52%. Interestingly, a greater prevalence is noted in diabetics with abnormal angiograms [7] – up to 2.2 times – with microalbuminuria [8] or on insulin [7] – 2.6 times greater prevalence (this can probably be explained by the fact that type 2 diabetics are often switched to insulin when complicated). In contrast, the Milano study [9] concerning young (mean age 54 years) type 2 diabetics without complications reveals a prevalence of SMI of 12.5%. This figure is even reduced to 6.4% if patients presenting basal abnormalities of ST segment are withdrawn.

In type 1 diabetics, results are also variable, with a prevalence of SMI ranging from 10.9 to 30% [see 10]. Most studies concerned elderly type 1 diabetics or patients with long duration (above 20 years) of diabetes. Note that microalbuminuria was linked with SMI in one paper [11].

PATHOPHYSIOLOGY OF SILENT ISCHEMIA

Autonomic neuropathy has for a long time been implicated in the pathophysiology of silent ischemia. Pathologists demonstrated in 1977 that diabetics who had died from painless myocardial infarction presented neuropathic lesions of the myocardial nervous fibers, in contrast with diabetics with painful infarction, who had no lesion [12]. Clinical studies are not fully concordant. Langer [13] demonstrated that silent myocardial ischemia in diabetic men occurred frequently in association with autonomic dysfunction. He further developed an evaluation of the sympathetic innervation in diabetics, using metaiodobenzyl-guanidine (MIBG) imaging, demonstrating a diffuse reduction in MIBG uptake, on the basis of autonomic dysfunction [14]. Another approach was the measurement of anginal perceptual threshold (defined as the time interval from onset of 1 mm ST depression to the onset of pain) in patients with typical effort angina during an ETT. The threshold was prolonged in diabetics with autonomic and sensorial neuropathy [15], leading to the conclusion that altered perception of myocardial ischemia might result from damage to the sensorial innervation of the heart. In contrast, Valensi [16] and MISAD [9] showed an equivalent prevalence of autonomic neuropathy in diabetics with or without silent ischemia. Others failed to demonstrate any link with peripheral neuropathy [17].

Central pain perception disorder was also involved in the mechanism of SMI. PET (Positron Emission Tomography) scanning of the brain can be used to assess regional blood flow. The induction of myocardial ischemia by dobutamine infusion increases blood flow in the thalamus of all subjects. But only patients with painful ischemia increase frontal cortical flow [18], in contrast with patients with silent ischemia. In another study [19], beta endorphin levels and pain thresholds during exercise were higher in non diabetic patients with silent ischemia than in diabetics.

Therefore, several explanations could be given for the different clinical presentations of myocardial ischemia in diabetics, associating changes in thresholds of pain sensitivity, beta endorphin levels and peripheral mechanisms, among which is autonomic neuropathy.

In contrast, some papers, among which the Asymptomatic Cardiac Ischemia Pilot (ACIP) [20], demonstrated a similar prevalence of silent ischemia in diabetics and non diabetics (yet note that a previous cardiac event was required to enter ACIP, so the disease was not consistently silent). Airaskinen [21] considers SMI mainly as a reflection of accelerated coronary atherosclerosis.

PROGNOSIS OF SMI

In the general population, the Coronary Artery Surgery Study (CASS) followed patients for 7 years. The survival rates were similar in patients with angina or SMI [22], leading to the idea that unrecognized disease had a similar poor prognosis as recognized disease.

In diabetes, limited data is available. In general, the mortality rate is increased by a two-fold factor in diabetic men and four-fold in diabetic women [1]. More recently, it was demonstrated that when myocardial ischemia

(silent or painful) was present during exercise testing, the long-term survival among diabetics was worse than for non-diabetics [23]. In contrast, in the absence of ischemia, mortality was similar between diabetics and non-diabetics. Importantly, the survival rates of patients with silent ischemia were similar to those of symptomatic patients. Therefore, since asymptomatic diabetics have an as poor prognosis as symptomatic diabetics, early screening and care of SMI seems commendable [24].

WHICH FACTORS ARE LINKED TO SMI?

In most studies concerning coronary disease in diabetics, age and male gender are regularly related to SMI. In the MISAD study [9], the only multivariate study including 925 patients, SMI is independently related both to male sex (odd ratio 3.64) and aging (odd ratio increased by 1.5 every 5 years of age). These data are confirmed by smaller studies [5, 8, 11], although inconstantly for age [10, 16, 25, 26].

Insulin treatment [7] and long term glucose control [27] are associated with SMI (odd ratio 3.2) in only one study. Surprisingly, duration of diabetes and body mass index do not seem to be correlated to SMI.

Among complications of diabetes, nephropathy has been associated to coronary atherosclerosis; therefore, the presence of macroproteinuria occurs as an independent risk factor of SMI (odd ratio 8.25 in MISAD) [9]. The position concerning microalbuminuria [28] should be more debated. If an odd ratio of 1.65 and 6.5 is reported by Rutter [8] and Earle [11], three studies do not establish any increase in the risk [9, 10, 16]. Retinopathy is also associated with SMI (odd ratio 3.17) in the Marseilles study [10]. Statistical significance is not obtained in other four studies [7, 9, 26, 29]. When analyzing, all 5 studies, 25% of patients with SMI have retinopathy while only 10% without SMI have retinopathy.

Since atherosclerosis is a general disease, it is not surprising to observe a strong correlation between peripheral arterial disease and SMI. 57% of patients with lower limb arterial disease present SMI [26], reflecting an approximately 5 fold risk increase [10].

RECOMMENDATIONS FROM SCIENTIFIC SOCIETIES

Various medical societies have made an attempt to classify the individual role of each risk factor, and presented various recommendations. In North America, the American Diabetes Association (ADA) and the American College of Cardiology (ACC) presented in 1998 their common consensus statement [30], which can be summarized as follows: screening for SMI should be performed in diabetics (type 1 or 2) with lower limb arteritis, a carotid stenosis or presenting with two or more of the following risk factors: hypertension above 149/90 mm Hg, smoking, LDL-cholesterol above 1.60 g/l, HDL-cholesterol below 0.35 g/l, total cholesterol above 2.4 g/l, microalbuminuria (or proteinuria), familial history of coronary disease, autonomic neuropathy.

In France, the Association de Langue Française pour l'Etude du Diabete et des Maladies Metaboliques (ALFEDIAM) presented a series of recommendations in the late 90's. The statement [31] established in 1995 was very close to the later suggested American propositions and recommended to explore diabetics complicated by or associated with peripheral vascular disease, proteinuria or microalbuminuria, hypertension, dyslipidemia, heavy smoking, familial history of premature cardiovascular death, without forgetting diabetics aged over 65 years and women. The French health care ministry evaluated that this recommendation would lead to systematic SMI screening in about 90% of diabetics. A few years later, the French Agence National d'Accreditation et d'Evaluation en Santé (ANAES), among which members belong to ALFEDIAM experts and public health specialists, presented its recommendations for the care of type 2 diabetics [32]. It was suggested not to screen for SMI asymptomatic type 2 diabetics with normal rest ECG. This position is supported by a recent editorial by Airaksinen [21], who wrote: "In my view large-scale hunting for silent coronary artery disease in diabetic or non diabetic population with normal exercise tolerance, a sign of good prognosis, is not justified. At the present time, we do not know if we do more harm than good with the goal of making asymptomatic people (= « healthy » in their own perception) feel they are sick and start to treat them with methods not proven to be useful". In a more neutral but optimistic view, the next step is probably to try and establish scores (which are not yet validated) for coronary risk, extrapolated from the Framingham study and improved, in order to optimize the cost/efficacy ratio to detect SMI in diabetics.

WHICH SCREENING TEST SHOULD BE USED?

Various tools have been used in order to diagnose cardiovascular disease. The exercise treadmill test (ETT) still represents a central exploration. Yet, ST depression is unable to localize the territory of the implicated coronary. By contrast, imaging tests may localize ischemia and diagnose coronary disease, especially in patients unable to perform an effort or with resting ST depression (>1 mm), left bundle branch block or Wolf-Parkinson-White syndrome. Stress echography has also recently been developed, and is now rather widely available. However, coronary angiography is still referred as the gold standard, and it is used to evaluate the sensitivity and specificity of all other tests. Yet, its conclusion only relates to macroangiopathy and the relationship between the intensity of narrowing and risk is not absolute [33].

EXERCISE TREADMILL TEST

Simple to perform but time consuming, ETT was frequently evaluated both in symptomatic and asymptomatic patients. Few data are available in the asymptomatic diabetics. Sensibility and specificity of the test seem comparable in diabetic (respectively 47 and 81%) and non-diabetic patients (52 and 80%), presenting with pain as a clinical symptom [34]. The positive predictive value of the test to detect coronary disease (when compared to coronary angiography) remains weak, and occurrence of ST depression during exercise is only synonymous of coronary disease in 50%. If other data, such as blood pressure profile during exercise, chronotropic failure, occurrence of ventricular extrasystoles, precocity and intensity of ST depression are taken into account, the positive predictive value increased.

Note that since diabetics are often hypertensive with left ventricular hypertrophy, the specificity of the test might be reduced. In a paper by Gerson [35], an ETT result that was either abnormal or inconclusive because of failure to achieve 90% of predicted maximal heart rate, pointed out patients who developed coronary heart disease within 4 years. Further predictability was limited to 4 years, suggesting the need for repeated testing. In another paper [36], it was demonstrated, both in the general population and in diabetics, that inability to perform a more than 6 mets effort was associated with increased mortality (4.6% *versus* 1% in patients with negative maximal ETT) within 2 years. In contrast, the negative predictive value of the ETT is robust. A negative maximal ETT can be reassuring.

However, conventional ETT cannot be performed in many diabetics with multiple risk factors, especially in elderly and inadapted persons to muscular efforts [37].

In summary, ETT remains the most widely accessible test in the detection of SMI. In diabetics, as in the general population, a negative maximal ETT is strongly reassuring. In contrast, when ETT is impossible or physically limited or if severe ST depression occurs, a second screening test should be performed.

CONTINUOUS ECG MONITORING (HOLTER ECG)

Among all methods used to detect SMI, continuous monitoring has the lowest sensibility and specificity. In diabetics, it can be used to detect autonomic neuropathy. In patients with known coronaropathy, it can also be used to evaluate the 24 hours ischemic load or detect transient arrhithmias. In contrast, it is not further used for the detection of SMI in diabetics [38].

NUCLEAR TECHNIQUES

Thallium-201 or technetium-99 m are available to obtain information about cardiac diseases. The aim of perfusion imaging is to quantify regional blood flow, using a comparison of the relative distribution of isotopes at rest and under stress. Stress can either be induced by exercise (the limitations described above (see ETT) then apply)

or by pharmacological drugs, using either inotropes (mostly dobutamine) [39] or vasodilators, such as adenosine or dipyridamole. The isotope is injected during stress. Images are immediately performed using a gamma-camera, followed by resting images a few hours later. The comparison of images can lead to "fixed" perfusion defects (reflecting the scan of a previous myocardial infarction) or to "reversible" defects (reflecting ischemic coronary disease). Although, thallium-201 has been used for many years, the recent trend is to prefer technetium-99m labelled molecules, especially sestamibi, which provide higher resolution for a lower radiation dose. Recently, three-dimensional images were available using a head of gamma-camera rotating around the patient (so-called single photon emission computed tomography SPECT).

The diagnosis and prognosis values of nuclear techniques have been evaluated in a limited number of studies. It occurs that its specificity is lower in diabetics than in non-diabetics. For example, a normal coronary angiography was discovered in almost 50% of diabetics presenting abnormal scintigraphy [6]. A limited predictive value was also reported for significant coronary artery disease and perioperative cardiac events in diabetics with end-stage renal failure [40]. This can be explained by an abnormal capacity of coronary dilatation or a highly prevalent left ventricular hypertrophy. In contrast, recent data suggest that when adjusted for clinical variables and SPECT, the difference of predictive value of abnormal images between diabetics and non-diabetics disappeared [41]. However, in subjects with normal SPECT, the 2 year-event rate was higher in diabetics [42]. Beyond positive or negative SPECT, interesting data are available on the extension of the infusion defect. For example, in high risk type 2 diabetics, a perfusion defect below 15% of the myocardium is associated with good prognosis, in contrast to wider hypoperfusion (>20 to 30%) [36]. In the latter condition, the simultaneous existence of microalbuminuria was associated with a 60% probability of cardiovascular event within 2 years.

STRESS ECHOCARDIOGRAPHY (SE)

SE has been developed as an alternative to ETT. It is based on the fact that ischemic myocardium moves less than non-ischemic myocardium. It therefore allows the detection of ischemic disease reflected by segmental defects. Stress is generally induced by infusion of dobutamine. In the general population and when compared to ETT, a general trend to lower sensibility, but higher specificity to detect coronary stenosis is reported. In terms of prognosis, it results in lower negative predictive value contrasting with higher positive value. These results are consistent with pathophysiology of ischemia, since infusion abnormalities occur before contraction abnormalities. Note that this technique is highly dependent on the experience of the practitioner, and this point clearly is the discriminant factor. Data in diabetic patients are scarce [43, 44]. They tend to demonstrate similar or even better performance, when tampered to the general population. Yet, its prognosis value remains unclear, although Elhendy [44] demonstrated by a multivariate model that a prior history of myocardial infarction, treadmill exercise capacity, ejection fraction and the percentage of ischemic segments were most predictive of cardiac events.

ELECTRON BEAM COMPUTED TOMOGRAPHY (EBCT)

EBCT is a radiographic technique, which can quantitatively measure coronary artery calcification [45]. Its interpretation in terms of diagnosis and prognosis remains controversial. Although coronary artery calcium scores are higher in diabetic patients [46], no clear association between score and risk was demonstrated. Yet, an absolute calcium score above 400 seems to be highly predictive for coronary events. Before this technique can be regularly applied, the existence of a relationship between coronary calcium and plaque stability must be confirmed. Further, considerations of cost and irradiation must be evoked.

CARDIOVASCULAR MAGNETIC RESONANCE IMAGING (MRI)

Considered as the future of non-invasive cardiology imaging [see 47 for a review], MRI is not yet widely available. In the heart, anatomy and

morphology can be analyzed with high spatial resolution using the so-called "black blood" imaging. A greater resolution than bidimensional echo can be obtained in kinetic mode in less than 1 minute. An analysis of the left ventricular function in basal condition, but also under exercise or pharmacological stress, can be obtained during one breath stop, by calculating circumferential shortening. So-called "tagging" techniques allow the detection of localized wall motion abnormalities, and can be combined with perfusion imaging. Eventually, although MR angiography of the large vessels has been possible recently, MR angiography of the coronary arteries seems to be far away from routine application.

CORONARY ANGIOGRAPHY (CA)

CA remains the gold standard to analyze coronary disease. Yet, it cannot be considered as a first line-screening test for SMI. It is generally performed once a screening test is positive, in order to quantify the lesions and to offer the best available treatment.

CONCLUSION

SMI is common in diabetic patients. It could be related to autonomic dysfunction, and probably occurs more commonly than in the general population. SMI seems to be associated with poorer prognosis than the non-silent disease. Therefore, the interest of detecting SMI in diabetics is worthwhile. The first question remains the choice of the diabetic patients to screen, with respect to cost / efficacy ratio. Recommendations remain debated. In our practice, although not validated by a clinical study, we expect to screen all patient with "clinical or ECG suspicion". This includes patients mentioning effort dyspnea or non-typical pain, but also basal ST segment changes. In fully asymptomatic patients, we consider risk factors, possibly distinguishing major risk factors, such as peripheral vascular disease or proteinuria and regular risk factors (age, gender, hypertension, lipid profile, smoking, familial history, duration according to type of diabetes...). We feel the need for a validated score of risk (*i.e.* based on the Framingham score for the risk of cardiovascular event, but adapted to diabetic populations), rather than selecting patients with more than two risk factors (almost 100% diabetic patients referred to our Regional University Diabetes Department). When accepted, we suggest an ETT as the first choice. It is cheap, safe and has a predictive value similar to that in the non-diabetic population. In many patients ETT remains inappropriate or insufficient, and we then turn either to nuclear perfusion imaging or stress echocardiography (which can also inform about left ventricular dysfunction). If the first selected test is normal, we suggest to continue the optimization of blood glucose control, eradicate or take care of other risk factors and perform a new test after a 3 to 5 years period. By contrast, should any screening test for SMI be abnormal, we perform coronary angiography, to which we have easy access, in order to provide the best medical, vascular or surgical therapy available.

Acknowledgements: Authors thank Mrs Regine Reignat for her expert secretarial assistance.

REFERENCES

1. Kannel WB, Mc Gee DL. Diabetes and cardiovascular disease: the Framingham study. *Jama*, **241**: 2035–2038, 1979.

2. Stamler J, Vaccaro L, Neaton JD, *et al*. Diabetes, other risk factors, and 12 year cardiac mortality for men screened in the multiple risk factor intervention trial. *Diabetes Care*, **16**: 434–444, 1993.

3. Wilson PW, D'Agustino RB, Levy D, Belanger AM, Silbershatz H, Kannel WB. Prediction of coronary heart disease using risk factor categories. *Circulation*, **97**: 1837–1847, 1998.

4. Alexander MC, Landsman PB, Teutsch SM, Haffner SM. NCEP-defined metabolic syndrome, diabetes, and prevalence of coronary heart disease among NHANES III participants age 50 years and older. *Diabetes*, **52**: 1210–1214, 2003.

5. May O, Arildsen H, Damsgbaard EM, Mickley H. Prevalence and prediction of silent ischemia in diabetes mellitus: a population based study. *Cardiovasc Res*, **34**: 241–247, 1997.

6. Koistinen MJ. Prevalence of asymptomatic myocardial ischaemia in diabetic subjects. *Br Med J*, **301**: 92–95, 1990.

7. Naka M, Hiramatsu K, Aizawa T, *et al*. Silent myocardial ischemia in patients with non insulin-dependent diabetes mellitus as judged by treadmill exercise testing and coronary angiography. *Am Heart J*, **123**: 46–53, 1992.

8. Rutter MK, McComb JM, Brady S, Marshall SM. Silent myocardial ischemia and microalbuminuria in asymptomatic subjects with non insulin-dependent diabetes mellitus. *Am J Cardiol*, **83**: 27–31, 1999.

9. Milan Study on Atherosclerosis and Diabetes (MISAD) Group. Prevalence of unrecognized silent myocardial ischemia and its association with atherosclerosis risk factor in non insulin-dependent diabetes mellitus. *Am J Cardiol*, **79**: 134–139, 1997.

10. Janand-Delenne B, Savin B, Habib G, Bory M, Vague P, Lassman-Vague V. Silent myocardial ischemia in patients with diabetes. *Diabetes Care*, **22**: 1396–1400, 1999.

11. Earle KA, Mishra M, Morocutti A, *et al*. Microalbuminuria as a marker of silent myocardial ischemia in IDDM patients. *Diabetologia*, **39**: 854–856, 1996.

12. Faerman, Faccio E, Milei J, *et al*. Autonomic neuropathy and painless myocardial infarction in diabetic patients. *Diabetes*, **26**: 1147–1158, 1977.

13. Langer A, Freeman R, Josse RG, *et al*. Detection of silent myocardial ischaemia in diabetes mellitus. *Am J Cardiol*, **67**: 1037–1038, 1991.

14. Langer A, Freeman MR, Josse RG, *et al*. Metaiodobenzyl-guanidine imaging in diabetes mellitus: assessment of cardiac sympathetic denervation and its relation to autonomic dysfunction and silent myocardial ischaemia. *J Am Coll Cardiol*, **25**: 610–618, 1995.

15. Ambepityia G, Kopelman PG, Ingram D, *et al*. Exertional myocardial ischaemia in diabetes: a quantitative analysis of anginal perceptual threshold and the influence of autonomic function. *J Am Coll Cardiol*, **15**: 72–77, 1990.

16. Valensi P, Sachs RN, Lormeau B, *et al*. Silent myocardial ischaemia and left ventricle hypertrophy in diabetic patients. *Diabete Metab (Paris)*, **23**: 409–416, 1997.

17. Hume L, Oakley GD, Boulton AJM, Hardisty C, Ward JD. Asymptomatic myocardial ischaemia in diabetes and its relationship to diabetic neuropathy: an exercise electrography study in middle-aged diabetic men. *Diabetes Care*, **9**: 384–388, 1986.

18. Rosen SD, Paulesu E, Nihoyannopoulos P, *et al*. Silent ischaemia is a central problem: regional brain activation compared in silent and painful myocardial ischaemia (comment). *Ann Intern Med*, **124**: 939–949, 1996.

19. Hikita H, Kurita A, Takase B, *et al*. Usefulness of plasma beta-endorphin level, pain threshold and autonomic function is assessing silent myocardial

ischaemia in patients with and without diabetes mellitus. *Am J Cardiol*, **72:** 140–143, 1993.

20. Caracciolo EA, Chaitman BR, Forman SA, *et al.* Diabetics with coronary disease have a prevalence of asymptomatic ischaemia during exercise treadmill testing and ambulatory ischaemia monitoring similar to that of non diabetic patients. An ACIP database study. Asymptomatic Cardiac Ischaemia Pilot (ACIP). Investigators. *Circulation*, 93: 2097–2105, 1996.

21. Airaskinen KEJ. Silent coronary disease in diabetes. A feature of autonomic neuropathy or accelerated atherosclerosis. *Diabetologia*, **44:** 244–266, 2001.

22. Weiner DA, Ryan TJ, McCabe CH, *et al.* Risk of developing an acute myocardial infarction or sudden coronary death in patients with exercise-induced silent myocardial ischemia (CASS Registry). *Am J Cardiol*, 62: 1155–1158, 1988.

23. Weiner DA, Ryan TJ, Parsons L, *et al.* Significance of silent myocardial ischaemia during exercise testing in patients with diabetes mellitus: a report from the Coronary Artery Surgery Study (CASS). Registry. *Am J Cardiol*, **68:** 729–734, 1991.

24. Cosson E, Guimfack M, Paries J, Paycha F, Attali JR, Valensi P. Prognosis for coronary stenoses in patients with diabetes and silent myocardial ischemia. *Diabetes Care*, **26:** 1313–1314, 2003.

25. Koistinen MJ, Huikiri HV, Pirttiaho H, *et al.* Evaluation of exercise electrocardiography and thallium tomographic imaging in detecting asymptomatic coronary artery disease in diabetic patients. *Br Heart J*, **63:** 7–11, 1990.

26. Nesto RW, Watson FS, Kowalchuk GJ, *et al.* Silent myocardial ischemia and infarction in diabetics with peripheral vascular disease: assessment by dipyridamole Thallium-201 scintigraphy. *Am Heart J*, **120:** 1073–1077, 1990.

27. Larsen J, Brekke M, Sandvik L, Arnesen H, Hanssen KF, Dahl-Jorgensen K. Silent coronary atheromatosis in type 1 diabetic patients and its relation to long-term glycemic control. *Diabetes*, **51**: 2637–2641, 2002.

28. Rutter WK, Wahid ST, McComb JM, Marshall SM. Significance of silent ischemia and microalbuminuria in predicting coronary events in asymptomatic patients with type 2 diabetes. *J Am Coll Cardiol*, **40:** 56–61, 2002.

29. Inoguchi T, Yamashita T, Umeda F, *et al.* High incidence of silent myocardial ischemia in elderly patients with non insulin-dependent diabetes mellitus. *Diabetes Res Clin Pract*, **47:** 37–44, 2000.

30. Barrett E, Ginsberg H, Parker S, *et al.* Consensus development conference on the diagnosis of coronary heart disease in people with diabetes. *Diabetes Care*, **21:** 1551–1559, 1998.

31. Passa Ph, Drouin P, Issa-Sayegh M, *et al.* Recommendations de l'ALFEDIAM. Coronaires et Diabète. *Diabete Metab (Paris)*, **21:** 446–451, 1995.

32. Recommendations de l'ANAES. Suivi du patient diabétique de type 2 à l'exclusion du suivi des complications. *Diabete Metab (Paris)*, **25** (suppl 2): 1–64, 1999 or www.anaes.fr

33. Topol EJ, Nissen SE. Our preoccupation with coronary luminology. The dissociation between clinical and angiographic findings in ischemic heart disease. *Circulation*, **92:** 2333–2342, 1995.

34. Lee DP, Fearon WF, Froelicher VF. Clinical utility of the exercise ECG in patients with diabetes and chest pain. *Chest*, **119:** 1576–1581, 2001.

35. Gerson MC, Khoury JC, Hertzberg VS, Fischer EE, Scott RC. Prediction of coronary artery disease in a population of insulin-requiring diabetic patients: results of an 8-year follow-up study. *Am Heart J*, **116:** 820–826, 1988.

36. Vanzetto G, Halimi S, Hammoud T, *et al.* Prediction of cardiovascular events in clinically selected high-risk NIDDM patients. Prognostic value of exercise stress test and thallium 201 single-photon emission computed tomography. *Diabetes Care*, **22:** 19–25, 1999.

37. Bacci S, Villella M, Villella A, Langialonga T, Grilli M, Rauseo A, Mastriaonno S, De Cosmo S, Fanelli R, Trischitta V. Screening for silent myocardial ischaemia in type 2 diabetic patients with additional atherogenic risk factors: applicability and accuracy of the exercise stress test. *Eur J Endocrinol*, **147:** 649–654, 2002.

38. Henry P, Le Heuzey JY. Holter et cardiopathie ischémique chez le diabétique. In Valensi P (ed). *Cœur et diabète*. Frison-Roche, Paris, 1999, 193–204.

39. Elhendy A, Schinkel AF, Van Domburg RT, Bax JJ, Poldermans D. Comparison of late outcome in patients with *versus* without angina pectoris having reversible perfusion abnormalities during dobutamine stress technetium-99m sestamibi single-photon emission computed tomography. *Am J Cardiol*, 91: 264–268, 2003.

40. Holley HL, Fenton RA, Arthur RS. Thallium stress testing does not predict cardiovascular risk in diabetic patients with end-stage renal disease undergoing cadaveric renal transplantation. *Am J Med*, 90: 563–570, 1991.

41. Giri S, Shaw L, Murthy D, Travin M, *et al.* Impact of diabetes on the risk stratification using stress single-photon emission computed tomography

myocardial perfusion imaging in patients with symptoms suggestive of coronary artery disease. *Circulation*, **105**: 32–40, 2001.

42. Wackers F, Zaret B. Detection of myocardial ischemia in patients with diabetes mellitus. *Circulation*, **105**: 5–7, 2002.

43. Bates JR, Sawada SG, Ryan T, *et al*. Evaluation using dobutamine stress echocardiography in patients with insulin-dependent diabetes mellitus before kidney and/or pancreas transplantation. *Am J Cardiol*, **77**: 175–179, 1996.

44. Elhendy A, Arruda A, Mahoney D, Pellikka P. Prognostic stratification of diabetic patients by exercise echocardiography. *J Am Coll Cardiol*, **37**: 1551–1557, 2001.

45. O'Rourke RA, Brundage BH, Froelicher VF, *et al*. American College of Cardiology/American Heart Association Expert Consensus document on electron-beam computed tomography for the diagnosis and prognosis of coronary artery disease. *Circulation*, **102**: 126–140, 2000.

46. Shurgin S, Rich S, Mazzone T. Increased prevalence of significant coronary artery calcification in patients with diabetes. *Diabetes Care*, **24**: 335–338, 2001.

47. Task Force of the European Society of Cardiology in collaboration with the Association of European Paediatric Cardiologists. The clinical role of magnetic resonance in cardiovasculair disease. *Eur Heart J*, **19**: 19–39, 1998.

35

STATINS AND DYSLIPIDEMIA IN DIABETES

Ioan Mircea COMAN, Anca Ileana COMAN

The starting point of cardiovascular morbidity in diabetics is early atherosclerosis (ATS) and arguments for diabetes mellitus (DM) association with ATS come from epidemiological studies. The pre-existing insulin-resistance (IR) and hyperinsulinemia may be the primary events in a cascade of secondary changes that converge finally to define diabetes mellitus (DM) as an independent major risk factor (RF).

Premature coronary heart disease (CHD) in diabetics is mainly multifactorial. Beside DM, other factors (especially those defining the metabolic syndrome) remain relevant; dyslipidemia seems to be the most important modifiable risk factor in (especially type 2) diabetes.

Moderately elevated total and low-density lipoprotein (LDL) cholesterol plasma levels, elevated triglycerides and low high-density lipoprotein (HDL) cholesterol characterize the typical diabetic dyslipidemia.

Statins are competitive inhibitors of HMG-CoA reductase, key enzyme in cholesterol's metabolic pathway. By decreasing its synthesis, statins lower initially the concentration of intracellular cholesterol; secondarily, by feedback mechanisms, an overexpression of LDL-cholesterol receptors appears and increases plasma lipoproteins transfer. Studies also show a non–lipidic protective effect (pleiotropic action) partially linked to the inhibition of the mevalonate pathway; whether the pleiotropic component of the statin's action could be greater in diabetics than in the general population remains to be speculated.

Interventional studies bring arguments for statin therapy. In spite of low percent of diabetics, the SSS Study strongly suggests that cholesterol lowering with simvastatin improves prognosis in this subgroup. A recent metaanalysis of the pravastatin studies (including CARE and LIPID) has shown that, where LDL cholesterol is < 3 mmol/L, most of the benefit of statin therapy appears in patients with diabetes and not in normoglycemics. HPS provides impressive evidence that statin therapy produces substantial reductions in the risk of heart attacks, strokes and revascularization of people with diabetes, even if they do not already have diagnosed coronary or other occlusive arterial disease. According to these data, therapy could be considered routinely for all diabetic patients at sufficiently high risk of major vascular events, irrespective of their initial cholesterol concentrations. The Anglo-Scandinavian Cardiac Outcomes Trial (ASCOT) using atorvastatin was stopped early, due to a better outcome of patients under atorvastatin. Using the same drug, GREACE Study showed the risk decrease of diabetics being the greatest among different subgroups analyzed.

The Position Statement of the American Diabetes Association (ADA) and The Third Report of the National Cholesterol Education Program (NCEP) Expert Panel (NCEP/ATPIII) recommended statins as the main option in diabetics with LDL >130 mg/dl (or non-HDL >160 mg/dl) (representing the vast majority of the general diabetic population) and as one of the possible therapies for almost all others (100–130 mg/dl LDL or 130–160 mg/dl non HDL-cholesterol). The use of statins as "plaque stabilizers" in acute coronary syndromes has to be mentioned in order to clarify their full clinical impact on diabetics.

DIABETES AND THE CARDIOVASCULAR BURDEN. RISK FACTORS AND THEIR RELATIVE IMPACT

It has been estimated that incidence and number of diabetic patients are growing in both developed and developing countries [1], with an estimate of more than 235 million cases worldwide in 2010 (3 % of world's population).

Almost 80 years ago, (the 3rd decade of XXth century), cardiovascular events exceeded coma and ketoacidosis as main cause of death in diabetes patients. In the Framingham cohorts, a more than double incidence (39.1% *versus* 19.1% for men, 27.7% *versus* 10.2 % for women) and even a more significant mortality difference (17.4 % → 8.5 %, 17.0 % → 3.6%) between diabetics and non-diabetics were reported [2]. The difference is even greater in women (5 to 6 fold) and recent USA data confirm this trend [3].

The starting point of cardiovascular morbidity is early atherosclerosis (ATS), and a comprehensive debate of causes can be found elsewhere [4]. Just for a summary of the currently accepted data, we should notice – without doubt – that diabetes mellitus (DM) *per se* is an independent major risk factor (RF).

Specific diabetic metabolic peculiarities (such as hyperglycemia, glycation of proteins, coagulation abnormalities and subsequent endo-thelial dysfunction) [5], may play a role, but, most of all, the preceding insulin-resistance (IR) and hyperinsulinemia may be the primary event in a cascade of secondary changes which converge to typical atherosclerotic profile [6].

Confirmation of diabetes mellitus effect on ATS comes from epidemiological studies. In the OASIS population [7], incidence of CHD events in NIDDM patients without CHD (average age 65) has been reported to be comparable with that of non-diabetic subjects with established CHD. In the HOPE trial [8], patients with type 2 diabetes with no previous cardiovascular disease, but with one or more cardiovascular risk factors, had a high annual event rate for CHD (2.5 %).

That the increased risk for premature CHD in diabetics is not due only to a higher level/number of other associated risk factors was confirmed by Stamler *et al.* [9]; they evaluated mortality in diabetics *versus* non-diabetics – all subjects with similar levels of other well-known factors (smoking, dyslipidemia, and diet) – and demonstrated a major difference exists. Similarly, in a Finish (high risk) population study [10] (which included 1059 subjects with type 2 diabetes mellitus), the authors found a similar risk ratio (RR) for CHD death for diabetic subjects with no previous myocardial infarction and non-diabetic subjects with previous myocardial infarction; the adjustment for age, sex, total cholesterol, arterial hypertension and smoking preserved a RR not significantly different from 1.0, therefore attesting the impact of NIDDM.

The results of these and other trials further support the idea that patients with type 2 diabetes, even without clinical CHD, fit in the group of CHD risk equivalent and this concept is one of the major changes of the NCEP-ATP III recommendations [11] in comparison to ATP II.

There are still some doubts whether in older persons diabetes justifies the designation of CHD risk equivalent. Prospective studies [12] illustrated that the relative risk for CHD of patients with diabetes decreases with age. Nonetheless, the combined risk factors of age plus diabetes appear to raise absolute risk for CHD to above 20 percent per decade.

In some ethnic groups (*e.g.* people with East Asian origin), where the baseline risk of coronary heart disease is very low, the presence of adult hyperglycemia is a weak predictor of CHD [13].

Improved blood glucose levels delay the onset and slow the progression of microvascular complications (retinopathy, nephropathy, and neuropathy) in patients with type 1 and type 2 diabetes [14], but tight glycemic control does not seem to be sufficient to significantly control macrovascular ATS disease [15, 16]. Intensive treatment with sulphonylureas or insulin reduced the risk of myocardial infarction by 16% in 3 867 patients with newly diagnosed type 2 diabetes, but this reduction was of borderline statistical significance [15].

Consequently, there is some intriguing mismatch between the initial observed importance of diabetes mellitus as a risk factor and less relevant changes of cardiovascular burden achieved by decreasing glycemic levels. This – by itself – does not seem to solve problems. Several explanations could be discussed according to existing data.

First of all, diabetes means much more than hyperglycemia: atypical complex metabolic pathways (insulin resistance, excessive glycation of cellular proteins, increased amounts of advanced glycation end-products), increased proinflammatory and prothrombotic factors are not (not immediately/not entirely) influenced by glycemic control. More than that, there is the clear established link between prediabetic metabolic conditions – especially insulin resistance and dyslipidemia – "classic" RF to be discussed below. Hyperinsulinemia (irrespective of glycemic levels) is preceding hypertriglyceridemia (HTG) and low plasma HDL levels, suggesting IR as the trigger for secondary changes that converge to the typical diabetic lipid profile. As suggested several years ago [6], hyperinsulinemia and not diabetes mellitus should be considered as an independent risk factor for ischemic heart disease.

Secondly, macrovascular disease antedates the overt decompensation of glucidic metabolism. Stratton et al [17] – in a prospective observational analysis of UKPDS patients – showed a very high percent of them having clinically relevant ATS at time of first abnormal glucidic control; so, at first DM diagnosis, the ATS disease is quite advanced and needs more aggressive and more complex therapeutic measures.

Third – and the most important probably – in spite of significant influence of diabetes mellitus *per se*, the high risk for premature CHD of diabetes patients is mainly multifactorial. Other factors (especially those that define the metabolic syndrome) have a higher incidence in diabetic populations and remain equally relevant for ATS development in diabetics. There is clear evidence that controlling them is important. The UKPDS [18] showed that treatment of hypertension improved cardiovascular outcome in persons with type 2 diabetes. Which is the impact of the main modifiable factor in the general population – dyslipidemia? Evidence that it maintains a fundamental role comes out from both observational and interventional studies. The Framingham Heart Study [2], the CCAIT [19], the Multiple Risk Factor Intervention Trial (MRFIT) [20], and the Lipid Research Clinics (LRC) trial

[21], all established a direct relationship between levels of LDL cholesterol (or total cholesterol) and the rate of new-onset CHD in both diabetic and non-diabetic patients. Data supporting the predictive value of TG and HDL levels came from other sources. Interventional studies – in both primary [22, 23] and secondary prevention [24, 25, 26] – showed diminishing of ATS when lipids were reduced with fibrates and / or nicotinic acid; even more convincing data came from the studies that used statins, as discussed later. Concluding, dyslipidemia seems to be the most important modifiable risk factor of atherosclerosis in (especially type 2) diabetics. Therefore, understanding and treating it remains essential in controlling the cardiovascular complications of the disease.

Besides early onset in diabetes, ATS gives some secondary reasons for concern and aggressive treatment. Confirming prior reports [27], UK Prospective Diabetes Study (UKPDS) (with absolute 10-year risk for "hard" CHD events of 15–20 % depending on the subgroup) showed one year case fatality rate for the first myocardial infarction (from the onset of symptoms, including pre-hospitalization mortality) of 45 % in men and 39 % in women with diabetes, compared to 38 % and 25 % for men and women without diabetes, respectively. Of the diabetics who died, 50 % of men and 25 % of women did so before hospitalization. In such conditions, secondary prevention strategies are inadequate and primary prevention is essential.

DIABETIC DYSLIPIDEMIA

Dyslipidemia in diabetes has both quantitative and qualitative peculiarities. Diabetics have lipid metabolism disturbances in higher percentages than non-diabetics (matched for age and sex).

The typical diabetic dyslipidemia is characterized by moderately elevated total and low-density lipoprotein (LDL) cholesterol plasma levels, elevated triglycerides and low high-density lipoprotein (HDL) cholesterol.

Moderately elevated total and low density lipoprotein (LDL) cholesterol plasma levels in NIDDM patients with good glycemic control do not generally exceed the mean values for matched non-diabetic groups but, due to their high incidence in the general population, are very common [28].

Small LDL particles have higher incidence in NIDDM patients. It has been postulated that high plasma triglyceride levels influence LDL size and density through a cycle of lipid exchange [29].

A number of recent prospective studies showed the small dense LDL is a risk factor for coronary artery disease [30, 31]. LDL size may contribute to an increased risk of atherosclerosis in a number of ways. Small dense LDL bind to the arterial wall with greater affinity than bigger ones [32] and are more prone to glycation and oxidation [33]; along with intermediate density lipoprotein (IDL), these oxidized LDL can easier be taken up by arterial wall macrophages that become foam cells.

NCEP /ATPIII "continue to identify elevated LDL cholesterol as the primary target of cholesterol-lowering therapy".

Increased triglycerides (>150mg %) and reduced HDL-cholesterol levels (< 40%) are – from the epidemiological point of view – more characteristic for dyslipidemia in NIDDM.

Hypertriglyceridemia in type 2 diabetes is due to both hepatic VLDL overproduction and impaired catabolism of triglyceride-rich particles.

Mechanisms involved include:

1. Genetic apoprotein peculiarities: apoprotein E A4 isoform dominance shows protecting effects (lower TG levels at same hyperinsulinemia) [34].

2. Low level of LPL activity, favoring elevated and prolonged postprandial (but also fasting) HTG. LPL, key enzyme in removal and degradation of triglycerides from the circulation, is low in both insulin deprived (type 1 diabetes) and insulin resistant (type 2 diabetes) patients [35].

3. Increased peripheral lipolysis, with growing FFA efflux to the liver (and high circulating FFA).

In spite of some suggestive data [36], it is still questionable to consider HTG as an independent risk factor. Nevertheless, as mentioned, triglycerides are proved predictors of cardiovascular disease in diabetes [9, 37].

The ATP III statements accept that "Elevated serum triglycerides are associated with increased risk for CHD and are commonly associated with other lipid and non-lipid risk factors". Some species of triglyceride–rich lipoproteins, notably cholesterol-enriched remnant lipoproteins, promote athero-

sclerosis and predispose to CHD (level of evidence C1).

Elevated triglycerides are relevant in ATS management in two ways: (a) as markers for atherogenic remnant lipoproteins and (b) as markers for other lipid and non-lipid risk factors in the metabolic syndrome. The former leads to non-HDL cholesterol as a secondary target of therapy when triglycerides are high, whereas the latter calls for more intensive lifestyle therapies.

Third component of diabetic dyslipidemia is low HDL.

HDL levels are influenced by the rate of production, lipolysis and catabolism of the VLDL-IDL-LDL system and are known for a long while as reversely correlated with TG [38].

Low HDL concentrations may imply defects in the reverse cholesterol transport (RCT) system, with cholesterol ester transfer protein (CETP) and lecithin-cholesterol acyl transferase (LCAT) as main components [39], loss of protection against atherogenicity of LDL and reduction in HDL-carried anti-atherogenic factors [40, 41].

Epidemiological studies show low HDL cholesterol to be an independent risk factor for CHD. In some prospective studies [42], HDL proved to be the lipid factor most highly correlated with CHD risk, with an estimated 1 percent decrease in HDL cholesterol associated with a 2–3 percent increase in CHD. In fact, its independence is partially underscored because of the association of low HDL with other atherogenic factors.

The benefit of intervention on isolated HTG or low HDL patients (without high LDL) is actually unknown, due to lack of evidence from randomized study of such (quite rare) condition.

A2 evidence level supports the NCEP statement that "clinical trials provide suggestive evidence that raising HDL-cholesterol levels will reduce the risk for CHD". However, it remains uncertain whether raising HDL-cholesterol levels per se, independent of other changes in lipid and/non-lipid profile, would bring a real benefit.

Besides diabetics, the three lipid disorders mentioned above are also typical in patients with metabolic syndrome; due to its pathogenic impact, their association was called "atherogenic dyslipidemia" [43]. This atherogenicity is linked simultaneously to low HDL, small LDL, and remnant lipoproteins. In epidemiological studies of high-risk populations, the contributions of individual components of atherogenic dyslipidemia to CHD risk cannot reliably be dissected from the sum of lipid risk factors. For this reason, "it is reasonable to view the lipid triad as a whole as a risk factor" [11].

In type 1 diabetes, there is a modest overall difference between the plasma lipid levels of patients who are under adequate glycemic control and those of nondiabetic subjects. Abnormalities in lipoprotein composition are observed in these patients [44–46]. In very poorly controlled type 1 diabetic subjects marked hypertriglyceridemia or even chylomicronemia may result.

STATINS AND CARDIOVASCULAR PROTECTION: LIPID AND PLEIOTROPIC EFFECTS

Discovery of statins is linked to the works of Endo *et al.* [47] published in the late 70s; shortly after, the experimental impact of the drugs was reported [48]. Since than, a huge amount of research and impressive data from clinical trials have established them a preeminent place in the treatment of dyslipidemia and atherosclerosis.

These pharmacologic agents are competitive inhibitors of HMG-CoA reductase, key enzyme in the cholesterol synthesis pathway. Molecular cloning and full understanding of HMG-CoA reductase role [49] were accomplished parallel to – and amplified by – statin studies.

Hepatic cells have two modalities to enrich in cholesterol: first, the endogenic cholesterol synthesis pathway, starting with acetyl-CoA (where HMG-CoA reductase interferes with conversion of HMG-CoA to mevalonate), and subsequently, the exogenous pathway, using the extracellular cholesterol supplied by LDL and IDL particles-which are captured, internalized and metabolized.

By decreasing HMG-CoA reductase synthesis, statins lower initially the concentration of intracellular cholesterol; secondarily, by feedback mechanisms, an overexpression of LDL-cholesterol receptors appears and increases plasma lipoproteins transfer.

In fact, statins trigger the increase in expression of genes that contain the information for certain enzymes responsible for cholesterol synthesis (HMG-CoA synthase, HMG-CoA reductase), and of LDL receptor genes.

Regulating expression of genes that control the extracellular cholesterol supply depends on transcriptional factors bound to the sarcoplasmic membrane: sterol regulatory element-binding proteins: SREBP1 and SREBP2 [50].

Decreased intracellular cholesterol supply [51] (as the one determined by statins) favors the link between cytoplasm–COOH end of SREBPs and the COOH end of another membrane protein, SREBP cleavage activity protein (SCAP); this initiates SREBP splitting. Resulting molecular segments migrate into the nucleus and bind to sterol regulatory elements (SRE 1 a.s.o.) located on promoter's gene, mainly the regulatory genes of HMG-CoA reductase and the genes for LDL receptors [52].

Increased expression of membrane receptors improves plasma clearance of atherogenic molecules, not only LDL; intermediate density lipoprotein (IDL) and VLDL remnants are also removed via the LDL receptor. The latter effect contributes to lowering of triglyceride-rich lipoproteins by statins.

Statins also appear to reduce hepatic release of lipoproteins into the circulation; this effect may be due in part to enhanced removal of lipoproteins by LDL receptors within hepatocytes or in the space of Disse [53].

Six members of the statin family are currently on the market: lovastatin, pravastatin, simvastatin, fluvastatin, atorvastatin, rosuvastatin; an increasing number of related chemical compounds will probably be available in the future [54].

Most statins have a high first-pass clearance by the liver and a short half-life (except atorvastatin and rosuvastatin, with very long half-lives). Metabolic peculiarities of each product, drug interactions [55] and rare statin-produced myopathy and rhabdomyolysis have to be taken into consideration when initiating, monitoring and evaluating results of statin treatment.

Lipid/lipoprotein effects of available statins include [11] LDL cholesterol lowering of 18–55% (dose-dependent) and HDL-cholesterol increase by 5–15 % (0.06 mmol/l to 0.08 mmol/l) on average, with no detectable dose-effect. Triglycerides are influenced by 7–30 %; when triglyceride levels are >200 mg/dl, triglycerides fall in direct proportion to LDL-cholesterol lowering.

It was initially assumed that any beneficial effect of statins on coronary events is linked only to their hypocholesterolemic properties. However, experimental in vivo studies showed a protective effect of this group of drugs despite no significant lipid lowering [56, 57]. Clinical trials also suggest that – despite comparable reduction in serum cholesterol levels – the risk of cardiovascular events in statin-treated patients is lower compared with other agents or modalities used to decrease serum cholesterol [58]. This data support the presence of non-lipidic mechanisms. In the WOSCOPS study, it was anticipated that reduction in LDL would give a 24 % reduction of events, whereas a 35 % reduction occurred. Furthermore, the Myocardial Ischemia Reduction with Aggressive Cholesterol Lowering (MIRACL) trial showed that statin therapy reduces the recurrence rate of cardiac events following acute coronary syndrome from within 4 weeks and new ischemic events by 16 weeks following initiation. Although at this time point a considerable reduction in serum cholesterol was observed, it is unlikely that any significant vascular remodeling could have occurred. Theoretically, because mevalonic acid (MVA) – an intracellular product of HMG-CoA reductase – is the precursor of numerous metabolites, inhibition of the enzyme potentially results in pleiotropic effects and thus explains some of the anti-atherosclerotic properties of statins.

Recent evidence from in vitro or in vivo experiments confirms that a number of statin actions is correlated to the inhibition of the mevalonate pathway, as well as modified endothelial nitric oxide synthetase [59], and endothelin-1 synthesis and expression [60]. Acting on the cellular components of ATS, statins decrease leuco-endothelial cell adhesion [61], modify natural killer T-cell function in transplanted hearts [62], and alter tissue factor activity and expression in human macrophages [63]. The macrophage growth induced by oxidized LDL is blocked by statins [64], and some proteins involved in growth factor signal transduction have been shown to be lipid-modified by the covalent attachment of mevalonate-derived isoprenoid groups [65].

Involvement in migration and proliferation of arterial myocytes has been reported. Experimental complete inhibition of cholesterol biosynthesis correlates with 50% inhibition of myocyte cell growth, while adding mevalonate or its isoprenoid derivatives, F-OH and GG-OH, could restore smooth muscle cell (SMC) proliferation [66], confirming that inhibition of MVA and other intermediates of cholesterol synthesis (isoprenoids) are essential for blocking processes such as cell migration, proliferation and deposition of lipids.

Hence, it is conceivable that statins can directly affect major events occurring in the arterial wall during atherogenesis. Lesser superoxide generation [67], higher scavenger receptor expression [68], and increased fibrinolytic activity [69] are other noticed actions, but unhappily, their relevance in clinical settings was not clarified. Some secondary lipid effects as influencing lipoprotein secretion through modified apoprotein B levels [70] and reduced susceptibility of LDL to peroxidation [71] are to be noticed.

The non-lipid-related properties of statins may explain to a certain extent the early significant cardiovascular event reduction reported in several clinical trials [4S] and angiographic and clinical benefit in normocholesterolic patients, as in the Lipoprotein and Coronary Atherosclerosis Study [72]. Overall, theoretical, experimental and clinical evidence clearly confirm that statins, beyond their lipid-lowering properties, have a direct anti-atherosclerotic effect on the arterial wall and this could explain some (not yet clearly defined) part of their protection.

Whether the pleiotropic component of the statins action might be greater in diabetics than in the general population could be speculated. Some peculiar non-lipid vascular alteration mechanisms in NIDDM (such as glycation of proteins and coagulation abnormalities) could be clearly influenced by the above-mentioned statin properties.

What has to be noticed is that pleiotropic actions (although common to statins as a group) are not equal for all chemical compounds.

The LCAS mentioned results – as well as laboratory data – argue for active pleiotropic action of fluvastatin. Experimentally, there are striking differences – for example in SMC proliferation inhibition – between cerivastatin and pravastatin (> 100/1).

There are also sometimes significant differences between animal/human *ex vivo* tissue actions, suggesting caution in extrapolating experimental data to clinical practice.

DIABETES AND STATINS: CLINICAL STUDIES

A huge amount of clinical work has been done during the 80s to get necessary evidence for the theoretically positive effects of statins in the "real" world. Unhappily, the number of diabetic patients in the first relevant studies was too low and post hoc analysis of diabetic subgroups had minor statistical significance. Deceiving few data come from the primary prevention trials. To exemplify, the extremely small number of diabetics enrolled in WOSCOPs [73] (only 76 patients) makes the study unuseful for our discussion. In the AFCAPS/TexCAPS [74], a primary prevention study of lovastatin, only 155 subjects had a clinical diagnosis of diabetes. From this small number, a 42 percent reduction in CHD was observed *versus* 37 percent reduction in CHD in the overall study population, but the difference was not statistically significant.

In spite of low percent of diabetics in its 4 444 patients (four times lower than DM prevalence in the total population of involved countries!), the Scandinavian Simvastatin Survival Study (4S) [75] post hoc subgroup analysis carried out by Pyorala [76] on data from 202 diabetes patients with previous myocardial infarction or angina pectoris, showed encouraging scores. Over the 5.4-year mean follow-up period (with initial serum total cholesterol of 5.5–8.0 mmol/l and triglycerides < 2.5 mmol/l) simvastatin produced mean changes in diabetic patients' lipids similar to those observed in non-diabetics. The relative risks (RR) in main endpoints in simvastatin-treated diabetic patients *versus* non-diabetics were as follows:

1. total mortality **0.57** (95% CI, 0.30–1.08; p = 0.087) *versus* **0.71** (95% CI, 0.58–0.87; p = 0.001);

2. major CHD events **0.45** (95% CI, 0.27–0.74; p = 0.002) / **0.68** (95% CI, 0.60–0.77; p < 0.0001);

3. any atherosclerotic event **0.63** (95% CI, 0.43–0.92; P = 0.018) / **0.74** (95% CI, 0.68–0.82; p < 0.0001).

There is a poorer statistical significance of scores in the DM group (due to less patients), but still the figures strongly suggest that cholesterol lowering with simvastatin improves the prognosis.

In the extension of 4S published in 1999, Haffner [77] (including 483 diabetes or impaired fasting glucose patients) finds an even more significant RR (42 *versus* 32%, p < 0,001).

The absolute clinical benefit obtained by lowering cholesterol may be greater in diabetic than in non-diabetic patients with CHD because diabetic patients have a higher absolute risk of recurrent CHD events and other atherosclerotic events.

The CARE study results were published in 1996 [78]. Pravastatin or placebo was given to 4 159 patients (3583 men and 576 women) with myocardial infarction, with plasma total cholesterol levels below 240 mg% and LDL cholesterol levels of 115 to 174 mg%. The primary end point was a fatal coronary event or a nonfatal myocardial infarction.

A 14 % of diabetic patients (586) was present, in spite of exclusion of patients with glucose levels of >220 mg. The frequency of the primary end point was 10.2 percent in the pravastatin group and 13.2 percent in the placebo group, an absolute difference of 3 percentage points and a 24 percent reduction in risk (95 percent confidence interval, 9 to 36 percent; p < 0.003). Pravastatin lowered the rate of coronary events more among women than among men. The reduction in coronary events was also greater in patients with higher pretreatment levels of LDL cholesterol.

These results clarified that the benefit of cholesterol-lowering therapy extends to patients with coronary disease who have average cholesterol levels.

Analysis of the diabetic subgroup (Goldberg 1998) [79] showed that the mean baseline LDL of 136 mg% was reduced by 28% with a resulting 25% overall CHD risk reduction (p < 0.05). The decrease was 23% for the others, a result clearly not worse, but also not significantly better than for non-diabetics.

Equally using pravastatin (40 mg daily) or placebo, but this time including unstable angina patients, LIPID [80] was a double-blind, randomized trial, comparing over a mean follow-up period of 6.1 years 9014 patients who had initial plasma total cholesterol levels of 155 to 271 mg %. A number of 784 diabetics were included and subgroup analysis defined a 19 % risk reduction of cardiovascular death (95% CI – 10 to 41) compared with 25% in non-diabetics.

A quite big rate of crossover from the allocated treatment at the midpoint of the trial (20 percent) determined a surprisingly low difference in LDL levels (13% at 6 years).

Apparently, there is no additional benefit in NIDDM over non-diabetics in the CARE and LIPID trials. It has been suggested this could be due to the lower baseline total cholesterol level compared to the 4S trial or the hydrophilicity of pravastatin (with lower diffusion into the arterial wall and blunted direct anti-atherosclerotic properties). However, a recent metaanalysis of the pravastatin studies (the Pravastatin Pooling Project) [81] has shown that, where LDL cholesterol < 3 mmol/L, most of the benefit of statin therapy accrues to patients with diabetes and not to those with normoglycemia.

Pooling the data of the main publications till 2002 [82], only about 1 500 diabetic patients with symptomatic coronary disease and 200 without coronary disease had been included in randomized outcome trials of statin therapy. Luckily, a much more impressive population was randomized in recently published papers.

The most important data – in order of statistic significance and significant conclusions – came from the HPS [83].

As mentioned, the main study's advantage is the involvement of 5963 patients with known diabetes – by far the greatest number ever included in a randomized study. They were allocated to receive 40 mg simvastatin daily or placebo. First major coronary event (non-fatal myocardial infarction or coronary death), first major vascular event and subsequent vascular events during the treatment period were analyzed.

Comparison was made between all simvastatin-allocated (40 mg/d) *versus* all placebo-allocated participants (*i.e.*, intention to treat), average difference in LDL cholesterol of 1.0 mmol/L (39 mg/dL) during 5-year treatment period.

Results for the diabetic population of the trial could give some good answers to major questions: "do we use statins in DM?", "when do we use them?", "which diabetics have the greatest benefit?", and "which mechanism is mainly involved?"

A 22% (95% CI 13–30) reduction in the global event rate (20.2% simvastatin-allocated *vs* 25.1% placebo allocated, p < 0.0001) was noted, similar to that among the other high-risk individuals studied). For the HPS diabetics, this represented a 20% reduction in coronary mortality [6.5% simvastatin *vs* 8.0% placebo, p = 0.02], a 37% reduction in first non-fatal myocardial infarction [3.5% *vs* 5.5%, p = 0.0002] and a 28% reduction in strokes attributed to ischemia [3.4% simvastatin *vs* 4.7% placebo, p = 0.01], this is once again supporting the benefit of statins in DM.

The highly significant reductions of events – 33% (p = 0.0003) – among the 2 912 diabetic participants who did not have any diagnosed occlusive arterial disease at entry is a major point for the early introduction of the drug in order to prevent further vascular ATS involvement.

The proportional reduction in risk (about a quarter) was similar in various subcategories of diabetic patients studied, including: those with different duration, type or control of diabetes; those aged over 65 years at entry, with hypertension and those with total cholesterol below 5.0 mmol/L. This suggests that almost all categories of diabetics could benefit of statin therapy. The 27% (p = 0.0007) reduction of events among the 2426 diabetic participants whose pretreatment LDL cholesterol concentration was below 3.0 mmol/L (116 mg/dL) underlines the nonlipidic (pleiotropic) effects of simvastatin. In addition, among participants who had a first major vascular event following randomization, allocation to simvastatin reduced the rate of subsequent events during the scheduled treatment period.

Summarizing, HPS provides impressive evidence that cholesterol lowering statin therapy can produce substantial reductions in the risk of heart attacks, strokes, and revascularizations in people with diabetes, even if they have not already been diagnosed coronary or other occlusive arterial disease. Therapy should now be considered routinely for all diabetic patients at sufficiently high risk of major vascular events, irrespective of their initial cholesterol concentrations.

In the Antihypertensive and Lipid-Lowering Treatment to Prevent Heart Attack Trial (ALLHAT) [84], 40 mg pravastatin daily was compared with usual care among 10,355 hypertensive patients. 3,638 of the participants had type 2 diabetes, with/without additionally known occlusive arterial disease.

The average difference in LDL cholesterol concentrations measured between the two treatment groups was only about 0.6 mmol/L (4.8 years follow-up) due to widespread use of non-study statin therapy in the usual care group. This probably explains only a small and non-significant 9% reduction in the coronary event rate, with similar proportional reductions in the presence or absence of diabetes.

It might be speculated that this lack of significant effect (when LDL differences are low) also reflects a non-significant pleiotropic action of pravastatin in this population.

In the Anglo-Scandinavian Cardiac Outcomes Trial (ASCOT), [85] 10 mg atorvastatin daily was compared with placebo among 10,305 hypertensive patients, of whom 2532 had type 2 diabetes and cholesterol levels less than 6.5 mmol/l; the LDL reduction at the end of the study was 29% (1 mmol/L).

Due to better outcome of patients receiving statin, the study stopped early; after 3.3 years of follow-up, atorvastatin was associated with a highly significant 36% (95% CI 17–50, p = 0.0005) reduction in major coronary events. Surprisingly, the relative reduction on primary endpoint (nonfatal infarction and cardiovascular death) was less significant among the diabetic than non-diabetic participants in that trial. The explanation may be the low absolute number of events in this subgroup (underpowered) and the quite short time of follow-up; a longer time may be needed to influence people with early-established vascular lesions.

The DALI Study [86] offered some new data on the effect of aggressive *versus* standard lipid lowering by atorvastatin on diabetic dyslipidemia. In 217 patients with type 2 diabetes and fasting triglyceride levels between 1.5 and 6.0 mmol/l, administration of atorvastatin 10 and 80 mg resulted in significant reductions (25 and 35%, respectively) of plasma triglyceride levels (both

p < 0.001). The effects seem not to be dose-related for HDL and triglycerides. Suggestive for the pleiotropic effect would be the reported strong decrease in C-reactive protein.

In order to reach the NCEP goal of LDL-cholesterol < 100 mg, 152 diabetics with established heart disease (19% of total population) were included in the atorvastatin arm of the GREACE Study [87]. With a mean dose of 24 mg of statin over 3 years of follow-up, a risk ratio of 0.42 (p < 0.0001) of atorvastatin-treated patients *versus* the "usual care" arm (which included hypolipidemic treatment in only 14%) was found for all CV events (death, MI, unstable angina, CHF, revascularization and stroke); the risk decrease of diabetics was the greatest among different subgroups analyzed.

Including some diabetic patients (but with glycaemia not higher than 180 mg%) a recent small study using rosuvastatin [88] seems to show a greater impact on LDL at baseline doses *versus* pravastatin and simvastatin. Higher increase in HDL *versus* pravastatin and atorvastatin was also reported [89].

In a meta-analysis [11] prepared for ATP III by panel members and statistical consultants (including AFCAPS, POSCH, VAHIT, CARE, LIPID, 4S) on 2,443 diabetics and 25,147 non-diabetics, a 31% CHD risk reduction (95% CI 17–42 %) *versus* 27% (CI 21–32 %) was found.

In terms of P-interaction (where the higher the number, the more homogeneous the effect between the two subgroups) the 0.596 value shows a clear better trend of improvement for diabetics.

None of the trials reported higher incidents or secondary effects of drug in diabetic subgroups and the increased tendency to cancer diagnosis in the pravastatin arm of the PROSPER trial [90] was not confirmed by others.

Classically, fibrates were first-line therapy in diabetes dyslipidemia but – as mentioned – recent years brought us a huge amount of clinical data about the use of statins in diabetics. There is nowadays a significant statistical support to use the new results for supporting evidence–based recommendation in this domain.

In the light of the above resumed trials, we favor the use of statins before fibrates in most persons. Still, the combination of statin + fibrate is attractive in persons with diabetes who have atherogenic dyslipidemia.

Recent evidence supports the presence of a specific transporter that facilitates the movement of cholesterol from bile acid micelles into the brush border membrane of enterocyte. This mechanism of cholesterol transport has been exploited as a therapeutic target in the development of new drugs such as ezetimibe. The mechanism of action of ezetimibe is complementary to that of statins. Using both agents could therefore produce additive effects on LDL-cholesterol reduction [91]. Moreover, the addition of ezetimibe to a lower dose of a statin can avoid the risk of potentially serious adverse effects associated with the use of higher doses of statins.

Simvastatin, pravastatin, atorvastatin and, to a lesser extent, fluvastatin [72] lovastatin [74], and rosuvastatin [88, 89] were safely used in diabetic patients.

Every statin keeps the common features of the group; it has also, however, a peculiar metabolic behavior. Extrapolating valid, positive data of a certain compound to others can favor misinterpretations or even negative clinical events, as proved by the cerivastatin "story".

The statin impact on clinical events could be even greater than it was shown by the main trials. Some statins achieve larger reductions (for example, 2.6 mmol/l with atorvastatin 80 mg/day and 2.8 mmol/l with rosuvastatin 80 mg/day) and could lead to greater reductions in cardiovascular events; this was not directly proved by randomized trials, as no trial achieved such a large reduction. Some of the extended statin trials used pravastatin, which is relatively less effective.

Secondly, non-adherence to the protocol (placebo patients taking statins and treated patients not taking them) makes the intention to treat analysis to underscore the true preventive pharmacological effect: both a smaller than expected difference in LDL cholesterol concentration and a smaller than expected difference in the number of cardiovascular events will be registered.

Last but not least, the risk decreases relatively little within the first two years, and inclusion of these early events in the results underestimates the full preventive effect of the drugs.

CURRENT RECOMMENDATIONS FOR USE OF STATINS IN DIABETIC PATIENTS

The most up-to-date recommendations at this moment are:

The Position Statement: "Standards of Medical Care for Patients With Diabetes Mellitus" of the American Diabetes Association [92] and The Third Report of the National Cholesterol Education Program (NCEP) Expert Panel on Detection, Evaluation and Treatment of High Blood Cholesterol in Adults (Adult Treatment Panel III) (NCEP/ATPIII) [11].

Evidence-based analysis of cardiovascular risk in diabetics pointed that type 2 diabetes should be managed as a CHD risk equivalent. Diabetics are very high-risk patients, and we should protect them as early and as aggressive as possible, interfering as many risk factors as possible; controlling their dyslipidemia has to be one of the main goals.

Using the P-interaction to study differences between high/low LDL, respectively HDL and triglyceride group results, the NCEP/ATPIII found a striking lower value for LDL, showing once again that this molecule remains the main target of therapy.

We have A-level evidence that lowering LDL cholesterol is associated with a reduction in cardiovascular events; we have only B-level evidence that lowering triglycerides and increasing HDL cholesterol favor the same trend. This is why ADA states, that "the first priority of pharmacological therapy is to lower LDL cholesterol".

As a result, the goals of therapy and the cut points for initiating treatment are stated in terms of LDL.

"Treatment for LDL cholesterol in NIDDM should follow ATP III recommendations for persons with established CHD". If the patient also has high triglycerides (> 200 mg/dL), non-HDL cholesterol will be considered as a secondary target.

The level of evidence for the target-goal of LDL<100 mg/dl (2.6 mmol/l) for adults is B, while triglycerides to <150 mg/dl (1.7 mmol/l) and HDL cholesterol to > 45 mg/dl (1.15 mmol/l) in men and > 55 mg/dl (1.40 mmol/l) in women are scored as C-level of evidence.

The treatment recommendations (A-level of evidence) state that patients who do not achieve lipid goals with lifestyle modifications require pharmacological therapy. Statins should be used as first-line pharmacologic therapy for LDL lowering; moreover, lowering VLDL remnants as well as LDL often can achieve the secondary goal for non-HDL cholesterol in hypertriglyceridemic persons with diabetes.

As a rule in type 2 diabetes, management of atherogenic dyslipidemia is delayed until LDL goal has been achieved.

For type 1 diabetes, NCEP/ATPIII accepts that intensity of LDL-lowering therapy should depend on clinical judgment.

Recent onset type 1 diabetes need not be designated a CHD risk equivalent; hence reduction of LDL cholesterol to <130 mg/dL is sufficient.

With increasing duration of disease, a lower goal (<100 mg/dL) should be considered. Regardless of duration, LDL-lowering drugs should be considered in combination with lifestyle therapies when LDL-cholesterol levels are >130 mg/dL.

To summarize, statins are recommended as the main option for diabetics with LDL >130 mg (or non-HDL >160) (representing the vast majority of the general diabetic population) and as one of the possible therapies for almost all others (100–130 mg LDL or 130–160 non HDL-cholesterol).

Therefore, a very high percent of diabetics, mainly NIDDM patients, fall into the indication of statin therapy of the NCEP. To have in mind the full clinical impact of this class of drugs, we should also add the use of statins as "plaque stabilizers" in acute coronary syndromes of diabetic patients. However, just a couple years ago, the diabetic patients of the Losartan Intervention For Endpoint Reduction In Hypertension Study (LIFE), for instance, reported the use of statins at baseline below 10%, increasing to only 30% during the trial. Therefore, many steps are still missing in the process of implementing the guidelines.

The gap would be even greater if one accepted the suggestions of the investigators of HPS that statin therapy should be considered routinely for all diabetic patients at sufficiently high risk of major vascular events, irrespective of their initial cholesterol values. With more evidence on such a protective effect, standard use of statins in diabetics could be accepted as a rule.

As a general rule, the intensity of risk-reduction therapy should be adjusted to a person's absolute risk, but using or not using statins in a certain category of patients is not only a medical challenge, but also a cost-efficiency problem to be solved according to the limit of the community's or individual's health budget. A recently published paper [93] on long-term benefits and cost-effectiveness of lipid level modification with atorvastatin 10 mg (including 28% and 38% reductions in total cholesterol and LDL cholesterol levels, respectively, and a 5.5% increase in HDL cholesterol level) analysis showed (when only direct medical care costs were considered) the incremental cost-effectiveness ratios for lifelong therapy were generally positive, ranging from a few thousand to nearly $ 20,000 per year of life saved. When the societal point of view was adopted and indirect costs were included, the total costs were generally negative, representing substantial cost savings (up to $ 50,000) and increased life expectancy for most groups of individuals.

REFERENCES

1. King H. Diabetes Mellitus: a growing international health care problem. *Intern.Diabet.Monit.* 9: 1–6, 1997.
2. Kannel WB, McGee DL. Diabetes and glucose tolerance as risk factors for cardiovascular disease: the Framingham Study. *Diabetes Care,* 2: 120–6, 1979.
3. Gu K, Cowie CC, Harris MI. Diabetes and heart disease mortality in US adults. *JAMA,* 281: 1291–97, 1999.
4. Fuster V, Ross R, Topol E. *Atherosclerosis and Coronary Artery Disease.* New York, Lippincott-Raven Ed., 1996.
5. Wautier JR, Guillausseau J: Diabetes, advanced glycation end-products and vascular disease. *Vasc. Med.* 3: 131–137, 1998.
6. Despres JP, Lamarche B, Mauriege P, Hyperinsulinemia as an independent risk factor for ischemic heart disease. *N Engl J Med,* 334: 952–957, 1996.

7. Malmberg K, Yusuf S, Gerstein HC, Brown J, Zhao F, Hunt D, Piegas L, Calvin J, Keltai M, Budaj A, for the OASIS Registry Investigators. Impact of diabetes on long-term prognosis in patients with unstable angina and non-Q-wave myocardial infarction: results of the OASIS (Organization to Assess Strategies for Ischemic Syndromes) Registry. *Circulation,* **102:** 1014–9, 2000.

8. Heart Outcomes Prevention Evaluation Study Investigators. Effects of an angiotensin-converting enzyme inhibitor, ramipril, on cardiovascular events in high-risk patients. *N Engl J Med,* **342:** 145–53, 2000.

9. Stamler J, Vaccaro O, Neaton JD, Wentworth D. Diabetes, other risk factors and 12 years cardiovascular mortality for men screened in the Multiple Risk Factor Intervention Trial (MRFIT). *Diabetes Care,* **1:** 434–444, 2001.

10. Haffner SM, Lehto S, Rönnemaa T, Pyörälä K, Laakso M. Mortality from coronary heart disease in subjects with type 2 diabetes and in nondiabetic subjects with and without prior myocardial infarction. *N Engl J Med,* **339:** 229–34, 1998.

11. Third Report of the National Cholesterol Education Program (NCEP) Expert Panel on Detection, Evaluation, and Treatment of High Blood Cholesterol in Adults (Adult Treatment Panel III) Final Report. National Cholesterol Education Program, National Heart, Lung, and Blood Institute, National Institutes of Health NIH Publication No. 02–5215 September 2002.

12. Kannel WB, McGee DL. Diabetes and cardiovascular disease: the Framingham Study. *JAMA,* **241:** 2035–8, 1979.

13. Keys A, Menotti A, Aravanis C, Blackburn H, Djordjevic BS, Buzina R, Dontas AS, Fidanza F, Karvonen MJ, Kimura N, Mohacek I, Nedeljkovic S, Puddu V, Punsar S, Taylor HL, Conti S, Kromhout D, Toshima H. The Seven Countries Study: 2,289 deaths in 15 years. *Prev Med,* **13:** 141–54, 1984.

14. The Diabetes Control and Complications Trial Research Group. The effect of intensive treatment of diabetes on the development and progression of long- term complications in insulin-dependent diabetes mellitus. *New Engl J Med,* **329:** 977–86, 1993.

15. Turner RC, Holman RR, Cull CA, Stratton IM, Matthews DR, Frighi V, *et al.* Intensive blood-glucose control with sulphonylureas or insulin compared with conventional treatment and risk of complications in patients with type 2 diabetes (UKPDS 33). *Lancet,* **352:** 837–53, 1998.

16. UK Prospective Diabetes Study (UKPDS) Group. Effect of intensive blood-glucose control with metformin on complications in overweight patients with type 2 diabetes (UKPDS 34). *Lancet,* **352:** 854–65, 1998.

17. Stratton IM, Adler AI, Neil AW, *et al.* Association of glycaemia with macrovascular and microvascular complications of type 2 diabetes (UKPDS 35): prospective observational study. *BJM* **321:** 405–412, 2000.

18. UK Prospective Diabetes Study Group. Tight blood pressure control and risk of macrovascular and microvascular complications in type 2 diabetes: UKPDS 38. *BMJ,* **317:** 703–13, 1998.

19. Waters D, Higginson L, Gladstone P, Boccuzzi SJ, Cook T, Lespérance J, for the CCAIT Study Group. Effects of cholesterol lowering on the progression of coronary atherosclerosis in women: a Canadian Coronary Atherosclerosis Intervention Trial (CCAIT) Substudy. *Circulation,* **92:** 2404–10, 1995.

20. Stamler J, Wentworth D, Neaton JD, for the MRFIT Research Group. Is relationship between serum cholesterol and risk of premature death from coronary heart disease continuous and graded? Findings in 356,222 primary screening of the Multiple Risk Factor Intervention Trial (MRFIT). *JAMA,* **256:** 2823–8, 1986.

21. Lipid Research Clinics Program. The Lipid Research Clinics Coronary Primary Prevention Trial results I: Reduction in the incidence of coronary heart disease. *JAMA,* **251:** 351–64, 1984.

22. Frick MH, Elo MO, Haapa K, Heinonen OP, Heinsalmi P, Helo P, Huttunen JK, Kaitaniemi P, Koskinen P, Manninen V, Mäenpää H, Mälkönen M, Mänttäri M, Norola S, Pasternack A, Pikkarainen J, Romo M, Sjoblom T, Nikkila EA. Helsinki Heart Study: primary prevention trial with gemfibrozil in middle-aged men with dyslipidemia: safety of treatment, changes in risk factors, and incidence of coronary heart disease. *N Engl J Med,* **317:** 1237–45, 1987.

23. Committee of Principal Investigators. A co-operative trial in the primary prevention of ischemic heart disease using clofibrate: Report from the Committee of Principal Investigators. *Br Heart J,* **40:** 1069–118, 1978.

24. Rubins HB, Robins SJ, Collins D, Fye CL, Anderson JW, Elam MB, Faas FH, Linares E, Schaefer EJ, Schectman G, Wilt TJ, Wittes J, for the Veterans Affairs High-Density Lipoprotein Cholesterol Intervention Trial Study Group. Gemfibrozil for the secondary prevention of coronary heart disease in men with low levels of high-density lipoprotein cholesterol. *N Engl J Med,* **341:** 410–8, 1999.

25. Coronary Drug Project Research Group. Clofibrate and niacin in coronary heart disease. *JAMA,* **231:** 360–81, 1975.

26. Diabetes Atherosclerosis Intervention Study Investigators. Effect of fenofibrate on progression of coronary-artery disease in type 2 diabetes: the Diabetes Atherosclerosis Intervention Study, a randomized study. *Lancet,* **357**: 905–10, 2001.

27. Abbott RD, Donahue RP, Kannel WB, Wilson PW. The impact of diabetes on survival following myocardial infarction in men *vs* women: the Framingham study. *JAMA,* **260**: 3456–60, 1988.

28. Syvänne M, Taskinen MR. Lipids and lipoproteins as coronary risk factors in non-insulin-dependent diabetes mellitus. *Lancet,* **350**: S120–23, 1997.

29. Taskinen MR, Lahdenpera S, Syvanne M. New insights into lipid metabolism in NIDDM. *Ann Med,* **28**: 335–40, 1996.

30. Gardner CD, Fortmann SP, Krauss RM. Association of small low-density lipoprotein particles with the incidence of coronary artery disease in men and women. *JAMA,* **276**: 875–81, 1996.

31. Mykkänen L, Kuusisto J, Haffner SM, Laakso M, Austin MA. LDL size and risk of coronary heart disease in elderly men and women. *Arterioscler Thromb Vasc Biol,* **19**: 2742–8, 1999.

32. Camejo G, Hurt-Camejo E, Bondjers G. Effect of proteoglycans on lipoprotein-cell interaction: possible contribution to atherogenesis. *Curr Opin Lipidol,* **1**: 431–6, 1990.

33. De Graaf J, Hak-Lemmers HLM, Hectors MPC, Demacker PNM, Hendriks JCM, Stalenhoef AFH. Enhanced susceptibility to in vitro oxidation of the dense low-density lipoprotein subfraction in healthy subjects. *Arterioscler Thromb,* **11**: 298–306, 1999.

34. Despres JP, Verdon MF, Moorjani S, Pouliot MC, Nedeau A, Bouchard C, Tremblay A, Lupien PJ. A Apoprotein E polymorphism modifies relation of hyperinsulinemia to hypertriglyceridemia. *Diabetes,* **42**: 1474–1481, 1993.

35. Eckel RH. LPL: A multifunctional enzyme relevant to common metabolic diseases. *N Engl J Med,* **32**: 1060–1068, 1989.

36. Fontbonne A, Eschwege E, Cambien F, Richard JL, Ducimetiere P, Thibult N *et al.* Hypertriglyceridaemia as a risk factor of coronary heart disease mortality in subjects with impaired glucose tolerance or diabetes. Results from the 11-year follow-up of the Paris Prospective Study. *Diabetologia,* **32**: 300–4, 1989.

37. Uusitupa MI, Niskanen LK, Siitonen O, Voutilainen E, Pyorala K. Ten-year cardiovascular mortality in relation to risk factors and abnormalities in lipoprotein composition in type 2 (non-insulin-dependent) diabetic and non-diabetic subjects. *Diabetologia,* **36**: 1175–84, 1993.

38. Davis CE. Gordon D, laRosa J, Woods PDS, Halperin M. Correlations of plasma HDL-cholesterol with other plasma lipid and lipoprotein concentrations: the LRCPP Study. *Circulation,* **62 Suppl IV**: 24–30, 1980.

39. Quintao ECR, Medima WL, Passarelli M. Reverse cholesterol transport in diabetes mellitus. *Diabetes Metab Res Rev,* **16**: 237–45, 2000.

40. van Lenten BJ, Hama SY, de Beer FC, Stafforini DM, McIntyre TM, Prescott SM, La Du BN, Fogelman AM, Navab M. Anti-inflammatory HDL becomes pro-inflammatory during the acute phase response: loss of protective effect of HDL against LDL oxidation in aortic wall cell cultures. *J Clin Invest,* **96**: 2758–67, 1995.

41. Navab M, Hama SY, Anantharamaiah GM, Hassan K, Hough GP, Watson AD, Reddy ST, Sevanian A, Fonarow GC, Fogelman AM. Normal high density lipoprotein inhibits three steps in the formation of mildly oxidized low density lipoprotein: steps 2 and 3. *J Lipid Res,* **41**: 1495–508 2000.

42. Assmann G, Schulte H, von Eckardstein A, Huang Y. High-density lipo-protein cholesterol as a predictor of coronary heart disease risk: the PROCAM experience and pathophysiological implications for reverse cholesterol transport. *Atherosclerosis,* **124 (suppl 6)**: S11–S20, 1996.

43. Verges BL. Dyslipidaemia in diabetes mellitus: review of the main lipoprotein abnormalities and their consequences on the development of atherogenesis. *Diabetes Metab,* **25(suppl 3)**: 32–40, 1999.

44. Sosenko JM, Breslow JL, Miettinen OS, Gabbay KH. Hyperglycemia and plasma lipid levels. *New Engl J Med,* **302**: 650–4, 1980.

45. Patti L, Di Marino L, Maffettone A, Romano G, Annuzzi G, Riccardi G *et al.* Very low-density lipoprotein subfraction abnormalities in IDDM patients: any effects of blood glucose control? *Diabetologia,* **38**: 1419–24, 1995.

46. Winocour PH, Durrington PN, Bhatnagar D, Ishola M, Arrol S, Mackness M. Abnormalities of VLDL, IDL, and LDL characterize insulin-dependent diabetes mellitus. *Arterioscler Thromb,* **12**: 920–8, 1992.

47. Endo A, Kuroda M, Tsujita Y. ML236A, ML236B, and ML236C, new inhibitors of cholesterol genesis is produced by Penicilinium citrinum. *Antibiot (Tokyo),* **29**: 1346–1348, 1976.

48. Alberts AW, Chen J, Kuron G, *et al.* Mevinolin-a highly potent competitive inhibitor of HMG-CoA reductase and a cholesterol–lowering agent. *Proc. Natl. Acad. Sci. USA,* **77**: 3957–61, 1980.

49. Chin DJ, Luskey KL, Faust JR, *et al.* Molecular cloning of HMG-CoA reductase and evidence for

regulation in its mRNA. *Proc. Natl. Acad. Sci. USA,* **79:** 7704–7708, 1982.

50. Vallett SM, Sanchez HB, Rosenfeld JM, Osborne TF. A direct role for sterol regulatory element-binding protein in activation of HMG-CoA reductase gene. *J Biol Chem,* **271:** 12247–53, 1996.

51. Nohturfft A, DeBose-Boyd RA, Scheek S, Goldstein JR, Brown MS. Sterols regulate cycling of sterol regulatory element-binding cleavage-activating protein (SCAP) between endoplasmic reticulum and Golgi. *Proc. Natl. Acad. Sci. USA,* **96:** 11235–40, 1999.

52. Brown MS, Goldstein JR. A proteolytic pathway that controls the cholesterol content of membranes, cells and blood. *Proc. Natl. Acad. Sci. USA,* **96:** 11041–48, 1999.

53. Twisk J, Gillian-Daniel DL, Tebon A, Wang L, Barrett PHR, Attie AD. The role of the LDL receptor in apolipoprotein B secretion. *J Clin Invest,* **105:** 521–32, 2000.

54. Davignon J, Montigny M, Dufour R. HMG-CoA reductase inhibitors: a look back and a look ahead. *Can J Cardiol,* **8:** 843–64, 1992.

55. Hanston PD, Horn JR. Drug interactions with HMG-CoA reductase inhibitors. *Drug Interactions Newsletter,* 103–6, 1998.

56. Bandoh T, Mitani H, Niihashi M, Bandoh T, Mitani H, Niihashi M, Kusumi Y, Ishikawa J, Kimura M, Totsuka T, Sakurai I, Hayashi S. Inhibitory effect of fluvastatin at doses insufficient to lower serum lipids on the catheter-induced thickening of intima in rabbit femoral artery. *Eur J Pharmacol,* **315:** 37–42, 1996.

57. Igarashi M, Takeda Y, Mori S, Ishibashi N, Komatsu E, Takahashi K, Fuse T, Yamamura M, Kubo K, Sugiyama Y, Saito Y: Suppression of neointimal thickening by a newly developed HMG-CoA reductase inhibitor, BAYW6228 and its inhibitory effect on vascular smooth muscle cell growth. *Br J Pharmacol,* **120:** 1172–1178, 1997.

58. Buchwald H, Varco RL, Matts JP, Long JM, Fitch LL, Campbell GS, Pearce MB, Yellin AE, Edmiston WA, Smik RD Jr. Effect of partial ileal bypass surgery on mortality and morbidity from coronary heart disease in patients with hypercholesterolemia: report of the Program on the Surgical Control of the Hyperlipidemias (POSCH). *N Engl J Med,* **323:** 946–955, 1990.

59. Endres M, Laufs U, Huang Z, Nakamura T, Huang P, Moskowitz MA, Liao JK: Stroke protection by 3-hydroxy-3-methylglutaryl (HMG)-CoA reductase inhibitors mediated by endothelial nitric oxide synthase. *Proc Natl Acad Sci USA,* **95:** 8880–8885, 1998.

60. Hernandez-Perera O, Perez-Sala D, Navarro-Antolin J, Sanchez-Pascuala R, Hernandez G, Diaz C, Lamas S: Effects of the 3-hydroxy-3-methylglutaryl-CoA reductase inhibitors, atorvastatin and simvastatin, on the expression of endothelin-1 and endothelial nitric oxide synthase in vascular endothelial cells. *J Clin Invest,* **101:** 2711–2719, 1998.

61. Masaaki K, Kurose I, Russell J, Granger DN. Effect of fluvastatin on leukocyte-endothelial cell adhesion in hypercholesterolemic rats. *Arterioscler Thromb Vasc Biol,* **17:** 1521–1526, 1997.

62. Kobashigawa JA, Katznelson S, Hillel L, Johnson JA, Yeatman L, Wang XM: Effect of pravastatin on outcomes after cardiac transplantation. *N Engl J Med,* **333:** 621–627, 1995.

63. Colli S, Eligini S, Lalli M, Camera M, Paletti R, Tremoli E: Vastatins inhibit tissue factor in cultured human macrophages: a novel mechanism of protection against atherothrombosis. *Arterioscler Thromb Vasc Biol* **17:** 265–272, 1997.

64. Sakai M, Kobori S, Matsumura T, Biwa T, Sato Y, Takemura T, Hakamata H, Horiuchi S, Shichiri M. HMG-CoA reductase inhibitors suppress macrophage growth induced by oxidized low density lipoprotein. *Atherosclerosis,* **133:** 51–59, 1997.

65. Bellosta S, Bernini F, Ferri N, Quarato P, Canavesi M, Arnaboldi L, Fumagalli R, Paoletti R, Corsini A. Direct vascular effects of HMG-CoA reductase inhibitors. *Atherosclerosis,* **137 (Suppl.):** S101–S109, 1998.

66. Bellosta S, Ferri N, Arnaboldi L, Bernini F, Paoletti R, Corsini Al. Pleiotropic Effects of Statins in Atherosclerosis and Diabetes. *Diabetes Care,* **23 (Suppl. 2):** B72–B78, 2000.

67. Giroux LM, Davignon J, Naruzewicz M. Simvastatin inhibits the oxidation of low-density lipoproteins by activated human monocyte-derived macrophages. *Biochim Biophys Acta,* **1165:** 335–338, 1993.

68. Umetani N, Kanayama Y, Okamura M, Negoro N, Takeda T. Lovastatin inhibits gene expression of type-I scavenger receptor in THP-1 human macrophages. *Biochim Biophys Acta,* **1303:** 199–206, 1996.

69. Essig M, Nguyen G, Pri D, Escoubet B, Sraer JD, Friedlander G. 3-Hydroxy-3-methylglutaryl coenzyme A reductase inhibitors increase fibrinolytic activity in rat aortic endothelial cells. *Circ Res,* **83:** 683–690, 1998.

70. La Ville A, Moshy R, Turner PR, Miller NE, Lewis B. Inhibition of cholesterol synthesis reduces low-density-lipoprotein apoprotein B production without decreasing very-low density lipoprotein apoprotein B synthesis in rabbits. *Biochem J,* **219:** 321–323, 1984.

71. Hussein O, Schlezinger S, Rosenblat M, Kheidar S, Aviram M. Reduced susceptibility of low density lipoprotein (LDL) to lipid peroxidation after fluvastatin therapy is associated with the hypocholesterolemic effect of the drug and its binding to the LDL. *Atherosclerosis,* **128:** 11–18, 1997.

72. Herd JA, Ballantyne CM, Farmer JA, Ferguson JJ III, Jones PH, West MS, Gould KL, Gotto AM Jr. Effects of fluvastatin on coronary atherosclerosis in patients with mild to moderate cholesterol elevations. (Lipoproteins and Coronary Atherosclerosis Study [LCAS]). *Am J Cardiol,* **80:** 278–286, 1997.

73. Shepherd J, Cobbe SM, Ford I, Isles CG, Lorimer AR, MacFarlane PW *et al.* Prevention of coronary heart disease with pravastatin in men with hypercholesterolemia. West of Scotland Coronary Prevention Study Group. *N Engl J Med,* **333:** 1301–7, 1995.

74. Downs JR, Clearfield M, Weis S, Whitney E, Shapiro DR, Beere PA, Langendorfer A, Stein EA, Kruyer W, Gotto AM Jr, for the AFCAPS/TexCAPS Research Group. Primary prevention of acute coronary events with lovastatin in men and women with average cholesterol levels: results of AFCAPS/TexCAPS. *JAMA,* **279:** 1615–22, 1998.

75. Scandinavian Simvastatin Survival Study Group. Randomized trial of cholesterol lowering in 4444 patients with coronary heart disease: the Scandinavian Simvastatin Survival Study (4S). *Lancet,* **344:** 1383–9, 1994.

76. Pyorala K, Pedersen TR, Kjekshus J, Faergeman O, Olsson AG, Thorgeirsson G. Cholesterol lowering with simvastatin improves prognosis of diabetic patients with coronary heart disease. A subgroup analysis of the Scandinavian Simvastatin Survival Study (4S). *Diabetes Care,* **20(4):** 614–620, 1997.

77. Haffner SM, Alexander CM, Cook TJ, Boccuzzi SJ, Musliner TA, Pedersen TR, Kjekshus J, Pyörälä K, for the Scandinavian Simvastatin Survival Study Group. Reduced coronary events in simvastatin-treated patients with coronary heart disease and diabetes or impaired fasting glucose levels: subgroup analyses from the Scandinavian Simvastatin Survival Study. *Arch Intern Med,* **159:** 2661–7, 1999.

78. Sacks FM, Pfeffer MA, Moye LA, Rouleau JL, Rutherford JD, Cole TG, Brown L, Warnica JW, Arnold JMO, Wun C-C, Davis BR, Braunwald E, for the Cholesterol and Recurrent Events Trial Investigators. The effect of pravastatin on coronary events after myocardial infarction in patients with average cholesterol levels. *N Engl J Med,* **335:** 1001–9, 1996.

79. Goldberg RB, Mellies MJ, Sacks FM, *et al,* for the CARE Investigators. Cardiovascular events and their reduction with pravastatin in diabetic and glucose-intolerant myocardial infarction survivors with average cholesterol levels: subgroup analyses in the Cholesterol and Recurrent Events (CARE) trial. *Circulation,* **98:** 2513–19, 1998.

80. Long-Term Intervention with Pravastatin in Ischaemic Disease (LIPID) Study Group. Prevention of cardiovascular events and death with pravastatin in patients with coronary heart disease and a broad range of initial cholesterol levels. *N Engl J Med,* **339:** 1349–57, 1998.

81. Sacks FM, Tonkin AM, Craven T, Pfeffer MA, Shepherd J, Keech A, Furberg CD, Braunwald E. Coronary heart disease in patients with low LDL-cholesterol: benefit of pravastatin in diabetics and enhanced role for HDL-cholesterol and triglycerides as risk factors. *Circulation,* **105:** 1424–28, 2002.

82. Armitage J, Collins R. Need for large scale randomized evidence about lowering LDL cholesterol in people with diabetes mellitus: MRC/BHF heart protection study and other major trials. *Heart,* **84:** 357–60, 2000.

83. MRC/BHF Heart Protection Study of cholesterol lowering with simvastatin in 5963 people with diabetes: a randomized placebo controlled trial. *Lancet,* **361:** 2005–16, 2003.

84. The ALLHAT officers and coordinators for the ALLHAT Collaborative Research Group. Major outcomes in moderately hypercholesterolemic, hypertensive patients randomized to pravastatin *vs.* usual care: the Antihypertensive and Lipid-Lowering Treatment to prevent Heart Attack Trial (ALLHAT-LLT). *JAMA,* **288:** 2998–3007, 2002.

85. Sever PS, Dahlöf B, Poulter NR, *et al,* for the ASCOT investigators. Prevention of coronary and stroke events with atorvastatin in hypertensive subjects who have average or lower-than-average cholesterol concentrations, in the Anglo-Scandinavian Cardiac Outcomes Trial-Lipid lowering arm (ASCOT-LLA): a multicenter randomized controlled trial. *Lancet,* **361:** 1149–58. 145–53, 2003.

86. The Effect of Aggressive *Versus* Standard Lipid Lowering by Atorvastatin on Diabetic Dyslipidemia The DALI Study: a double-blind, randomized, placebo-controlled trial in patients with type 2 diabetes and diabetic dyslipidemia. *Diabetes Care,* **24:** 1335–1341, 2001.

87. Athyros VG, Papageorgiou AA, Mercouris BR, *et al.* Treatment with atorvastatin to the NCEP goal *versus* "usual" care in secondary coronary heart disease prevention: the GREACE Study. *Curr Med Research and Opp,* **18(4):** 220–228, 2002.

88. Brown WV, Bays HF, Hassman DR, *et al*. Efficacy and safety of rosuvastatin compared with pravastatin and simvastatin in patients with hypercholesterolemia: A randomized, double blind, 52–weeks study. *Am Heart J,* **144:** 1036–43, 2002.

89. Davidson M, Ma P, Stein EA, *et al*. Comparison of effects on LDL with cholesterol and HDL cholesterol with rosuvastatin *versus* atorvastatin in patients with type II A and II B hypercholesterolemia. *Am J Cardiol,* **89:** 268–275, 2002.

90. Prosper Study Group. Pravastatin in elderly individuals at risk of vascular disease (PROSPER): a randomized controlled trial. *Lancet,* **360:** 1623–30, 2002.

91. Gagne C, Bays HE, Weiss SR, *et al*. Efficacy and safety of ezetimibe added to ongoing statin therapy for treatment of patients with primary hyper-cholesterolemia. *Am J Cardiol,* **90:** 1084–1091, 2002.

92. Position Statement: Standards of Medical Care for Patients with Diabetes Mellitus. American Diabetes Association. *Diabetes Care,* **25:** S33–S49, 2002.

93. Grover SA, Ho V, Lavoie F, Coupal L, Zowall H, Pilote L. The Importance of Indirect Costs in Primary Cardiovascular Disease Prevention. Can We Save Lives and Money With Statins? *Arch Intern Med,* **163:** 333–339, 2003.

36

GLYCOSAMINOGLYCANS IN DIABETIC VASCULOPATHY: HYPOTHESES AND CURRENT EVIDENCE

Gabriela NEGRIŞANU, Laura DIACONU

Increasing evidence has shown abnormalities of glycosaminoglycans (GAGs) content and function in diabetes mellitus. The loss of GAGs, especially of heparan sulfate (HS), from the vessel wall may play an important role in the development of vascular complications in diabetes. HS is a strongly negatively charged molecule that is structurally similar to heparin, but its base polymer has a lower degree of processing (sulphation, epimerization). HS forms anionic sites in the matrix and are thought to restrict the passage of macromolecules through the basement membrane (including albumin, fibrinogen and atherogenous lipoproteins). HS also participates in the antithrombotic endothelial activity and has inhibitory action on the synthesis and activity of growth factors (such as TGF-β) which are enhanced by hyperglycaemia and are responsible for the synthesis of collagen and other fibrotic proteins of the extracellular matrix and the regulation of smooth muscle cells growth. The altered GAGs metabolism in the vessel intima and luminal endothelial membrane may be a consequence of endothelial dysfunction in microalbuminuric diabetic patients and may further contribute to the development of diabetic micro- and macroangiopathy. Numerous experimental and clinical studies have demonstrated that GAGs are able to reduce vascular risk factors induced by hyperglycaemia, improve the clinical status of the patients with vascular disease and counteract the onset of thromboembolic complications. Although only limited studies have been conducted, the favorable effects of GAG treatment on albuminuria in diabetic nephropathy are encouraging. Clearly, dose-finding and long-term studies are needed to demonstrate that these drugs are capable of curing human diabetic nephropathy and not simply albuminuria. Several studies have shown that GAGs effects depend on their non-sulphated molecular backbone or are reached at non-anticoagulant dosages or both. This may provide the opportunity to select new derivatives with specific effects on diabetic nephropathy and macroangiopathy, possibly and most importantly without anticoagulation suitable for long term use to prevent or treat diabetic vascular disease. In this chapter we reviewed the postulated hypotheses and current available evidence regarding the role of abnormal GAGs metabolism in vascular complications of diabetes.

Vascular complications are the main cause of morbidity and mortality in diabetic patients [1]. Diabetic vasculopathy involves both small and large vessels. The most important macrovascular complications are coronary heart disease, cerebrovascular disease and peripheral occlusive artery disease and represent the cause of death for nearly 80% of diabetic population [2]. The most important microvascular complications are nephropathy, which is the main cause of end stage renal disease, retinopathy, the leading cause of acquired blindness and neuropathy accompanied with serious disabilities [3]. Although data from the Diabetes Control and Complications Trial establish that hyperglycemia has a central role in diabetic complications, strict metabolic control can be difficult to achieve. Therefore, new approaches to the pathogenesis and prevention of diabetic complications have been proposed. Evidence has been provided [4,5] that the alterations of the glycosaminoglycan (GAG) metabolism in diabetes may be important for the development of chronic complications and also may have therapeutic significance [6].

PATHOGENESIS OF DIABETIC VASCULOPATHY

Although macroangiopathy is considered the result of accelerated atherosclerosis and microangiopathy is a more specific diabetes complication, their onset and progression are stimulated by common pathogenetic factors [1] present in the abnormal metabolic state that accompanies diabetes. Hyperglycaemia, insulinresistance and the associated metabolic abnormalities such as accumulation of advanced glycation end products, increased diacylglycerol concentrations, overactivity of protein kinase C (PKC), increased oxidative stress, excess of free fatty acid release, increased levels of oxidized and glycoxidized low density lipoprotein (LDL) cholesterol and triglyceride rich lipoproteins impair the function of several cells including the endothelium, vascular smooth muscle cells and platelets [7]. Consecutively, the endothelial synthesis of nitric oxide (NO) is decreased while increased levels of superoxide anion directly quenche NO [8]. In addition, endothelial synthesis of endothelin-1 and angiotensin II is increased [9], thus promoting vasoconstriction, vascular smooth muscle cell growth and migration. Activation of the transcription factors nuclear factor kappa-beta (NF-κβ) and activator protein-1 induces inflammatory gene expression, with release of leukocyte-attracting chemokines, increased production of inflammatory cytokines, and augmented expression of adhesion molecules [10]. Increased endothelial production of von Willebrand factor and tissue factor, a potent procoagulant, in addition to increased levels of plasma coagulation factors such as factor VII and decreased levels of endogenous anticoagulants such as anthithrombin III and protein C [11, 12] creates a procoagulant state. Moreover, the increased endothelial production of plasminogen activator inhibitor 1 (PAI 1) decreases fibrinolysis [7]. Also, platelet adhesion and aggregation is increased. In conclusion, endothelial dysfunction induces a state of augmented vasoconstriction, inflammation and permeability of vascular wall, increased activation of growth factors, increased thrombosis and decreased fibrinolysis may represent the primary alteration in diabetic micro- and macrovasculopathies [7, 13].

Data from epidemiological studies revealed that albuminuria is associated not only with diabetic nephropathy, but also with cardiovascular morbidity and mortality, proliferative retinopathy and diabetic cardiomyopathy [14]. This suggested the existence of a common pathogenetic pathway for both micro- and macroangiopathy, which probably is the endothelial dysfunction [14]. In support of this hypothesis are the findings of increased plasma levels of von Willebrand factor and thrombomodulin, and reduced fibrinolytic capacity in diabetic patients with even slightly increased urinary albumin excretion, suggesting that albuminuria reflects a generalized vascular disease [14].

The altered GAGs metabolism in the vessel intima and luminal endothelial membrane may be a consequence of endothelial dysfunction in microalbuminuric diabetic patients and may further contribute to the development of diabetic micro- and macroangiopathy.

THE ROLE OF GAGs IN THE PATHOGENESIS OF DIABETIC VASCULOPATHY

GAGs STRUCTURE AND FUNCTION

GAGs are highly glycosylated and sulfatated glycoproteins, consisting of dimeric repeated units containing an uronic acid (iduronic or glucuronic acid) and an aminosugar (glucosamine or galactosamine) [15]. Three major classes of GAGs have been described: a predominant large chondroitin sulphate (CS), a small dermatan sulphate (DS) and a polydisperse heparan sulphate (HS). These molecules are widely distributed in the body and are prominent in extracellular matrices. GAGs are vital in maintaining the structural integrity of the tissues.

Basement membranes contain a HS in the form of a proteoglycan (PG) unique to that tissue. HS is a strongly negatively charged molecule that is structurally similar to heparin, but its base polymer has a lower degree of processing (sulphation, epimerization) [15]. HS forms anionic sites in this matrix and are thought to restrict the passage of macromolecules through the basement membrane (including albumin, fibrinogen and atherogenous lipoproteins). HS also participates in the antithrombotic endothelial activity an have inhibitory action on the synthesis and activity of growth factors (such as TGF-β) which are enhanced by hyperglycaemia and are responsible for the synthesis of collagen and other fibrotic proteins of the extracellular matrix and the regulation of smooth muscle cells growth [2].

GAGs METABOLISM IN DIABETES

In diabetic patients, the increased macromolecular permeability within the glomeruli that precedes the onset of established renal lesions and the increased vascular permeability to albumin seem to be related to structural alterations in the macromolecular pathway, i.e. the extracellular matrix, between the endothelial cells [5]. A number of reports indicate that HS metabolism is impaired in diabetes and this is responsible for the extracellular

matrix negative charge loss [5]. The reduction in HS negative charges may depend on either a decreased sulphation of the glycosaminoglycan molecule or an absolute reduction in the heparan sulphate proteoglycan (HSPG) [16]. Studies using biochemical techniques to measure GAG content of kidneys obtained at autopsy demonstrated that glomerular basement membrane of patients with diabetic nephropathy contained less GAG than kidneys of nondiabetic control subjects [17,18]. Similar changes in HS content in the intima of the aortas of patients with diabetes mellitus have been observed [19], suggesting that the abnormalities in HS metabolism are not necessarily restricted to the kidney. Studies on muscle have demonstrated that the HS content of the basement membrane in muscle capillaries is reduced in diabetic patients with nephropathy and, notably, is inversely correlated to the degree of albuminuria [14]. In addition, the concentration of acid GAGs is reduced by 50% in extramural coronary arteries in type 2 diabetic patients [20]. The cause of the reduced vascular and extracellular content of HS in susceptible diabetic patients is unknown. The altered HSPG metabolism in the vessel intima and luminal endothelial membrane may be a consequence of endothelial dysfunction in microalbuminuric diabetic patients [21].

The Steno Hypothesis [22] postulated that diabetic patients susceptible to nephropathy and macroangiopathy have a genetic defect in regulation of HS production by endothelial, myomedial and mesangial cells, leading to a lower activity of the enzymes responsible for GAG sulfation under high glucose conditions. The resulting undersulfated GAG chains would then play a crucial role in the pathogenesis of proteinuria (due to the loss of anionic charges in the glomerular basement membrane [GBM]) and its morphologic substrate, diabetic nephropathy, as well in the pathogenesis of diabetic micro- and macroangiopathy. Although genes have been cloned for N-deacetylase/ N-sulfotransferase, 3-O-sulfotransferase, and 6-O-sulfotransferase enzymes [23], it is still unclear whether different allotypes of these enzymes with a different susceptibility to high glucose concentrations really exist. Although the Steno hypothesis has not been formally proved, it has stimulated in vitro studies and therapeutical trials both in animal models and in humans [24].

627

THE ROLE OF GAGs ABNORMAL METABOLISM IN DIABETIC VASCULOPATHY

The alterations of GAG structure and function may contribute to the development of diabetic micro- and macroangiopathy.

The loss of GAGs from the vessel wall, in particular the endothelium, the basement membrane and the extracellular matrix, is responsible for abnormal increase in vessel permeability. Decreased GAGs, especially HS – a strongly anionic molecule – causes a loss of negative charged ions from the membrane. The qualitative and quantitative changes in the PG composition of the renal extracellular matrix could also deeply affect the growth and protein synthesis of renal endothelial, mesangial, and glomerular and tubular epithelial cells, thus inducing glomerulosclerosis. The cell-extracellular matrix interaction plays an important role in regulating the adhesion, migration and proliferation of these cells [24]. Moreover, extracellular matrix and cell-associated PGs may modulate the activity of growth factors. In particular, it was suggested that the cell surface and extracellular matrix HSPG may act together to regulate the bioavailability of otherwise diffusible effector molecules to their signal transducing receptor [25]. At the same time, this causes a reduction in GAG inhibitory action on the synthesis and activity of growth factors (TGF β). These factors are activated by hyperglycemia and are responsible for the synthesis of collagen and other fibrotic proteins of the extracellular matrix [25, 26].

The loss of GAGs is also responsible for a decrease in endothelial antithrombogenic activity, with consequent platelet adhesion and microthrombus formation, which in turn causes an increase in the concentration of platelet growth factors. HSPG stimulates thrombin-antithrombin complex formation and regulates, together with vascular cell-secreted heparin-like products, fibroblast growth factor activity [27]. The fall in endothelial cell HS contents might also influence local fibrinolysis. Endothelial cells synthesize specific HS and chondroitin sulphate to which tissue plasminogen activator (t-PA) can bind [28]. This t-PA binding capacity might be important in forming a t-PA storage pool, from which t-PA is released and made locally available under certain circumstances [28]. HS-bound t-PA released from endothelial cells would provide an additional mechanism for locally increased fibrinolytic activity and render endothelial cells resistant to fibrin deposition. Thus, the derangement in this fibrinolytic mechanism could lead to increased fibrin deposition on the vascular wall in diabetes.

The multiplicity of effects of HS may also explain the association between generalized vascular dysfunction and nephropathy.

EXOGENOUS GAGs ADMINISTRATION

In view of the important role of GAGs loss in the pathogenesis of diabetic vascular damage, the use of exogenous GAGs would appear justified in the therapy as an attempt to increase and at least partially restore the content and biological effects of GAGs in the vessel walls.

The effects of several GAGs have been studied in diabetic patients: heparin, low molecular weight heparin, dermatan sulfate, danaparoid (a mixture of GAGs consisting mostly of HS), sulodexide.

A major point of concern in the treatment of diabetic patients with GAGs and heparin has been the risk of bleeding, particularly in subjects with retinal neoangiogensis, due to the fragility of new vessels. In a recent study it was demonstrated that therapy with the GAG danaparoid was safe, although the dosages used were relatively low, sufficient only to inhibit factor X [29]. Moreover, in this study, a reduction in retinal hard exudates was observed. Because a spontaneous reduction in such abnormalities is not likely to occur within a few months, the effect of danaparoid on hard exudates might well be related to the modulation of sequestered VEGF in the retina [24].

Anticoagulation may also constitute a critical problem in long-term treatment with heparin-related drugs. The anticoagulant properties of heparin and heparin-derived GAGs depend on both the chemical structure of the molecule and the route of administration. The chemical structure is certainly very important; anticoagulant activity is largely dependent on the degree and pattern of GAG sulfation, so that chemical desulfation of GAG might be essential for safe chronic use. On the other hand, anticoagulant activity also depends on the type of molecular repeat, *i.e.*, heparin is anti-coagulant, whereas chondroitin and dermatan sulfate are not anticoagulant. In long-term experiments, in either desulfated heparin-treated or dermatan sulfate-treated animals no hemorrhagic deaths were observed [30, 31]. To achieve therapeutic anticoagulation, heparin must be administered intravenously; when it is administered through other routes, anticoagulant levels cannot be reached. Thus, to expand the use of these drugs as well as increase patient compliance, it would be relevant to study the pharmacokinetics and pharmacodynamics of heparin and GAG administered through different routes. A few reports have demonstrated that heparin and dermatan sulfate have oral bioavailability. After oral administration of heparin to rats, Larsen *et al.* [32] found fragments as large as octasaccharides with anti-factor Xa activity in the plasma. Furthermore, heparin was shown to be rapidly absorbed at the gastric level in quantities sufficient to prevent venous thrombosis in rats, but with no clinically significant anticoagulant effect due to its rapid sequestration by the endothelium [33, 34]. Dermatan sulfate is also absorbed in active form at the gastrointestinal level with a 3 to 9% oral bioavailability [35]. These investigations addressed the possibility of oral bioavailability of GAG in terms of the anticoagulant and antithrombotic activity, but two clinical studies in microalbuminuric diabetic patients treated with sulodexide [36, 37] showed that after oral administration GAG maintain their effects not only on fibrinolytic parameters, but, interestingly, also on albuminuria.

Osteopenia is frequently reported as a possible adverse effect of long-term heparin administration, but few studies have evaluated this issue. Interestingly, contrary to the basic assumption, it was reported that a 12 weeks course of heparin therapy in rats with chronic renal failure did not influence bone metabolism [38].

The risk of antibody induction is very low with GAG therapy because low molecular weight GAG are poor antigens. Therefore, the use of GAG structure-based anti-TGF-β agents certainly carries a lower risk of inducing antibody formation, compared with protein-based anti-TGF-β agents (*e.g.*, antibodies or decorin). Heparin-induced thrombocytopenia is a well-recognized complication of heparin therapy that is frequently associated with severe thrombotic events due to the formation of immune complexes between IgG, heparin, and platelet factor 4 (PF4). Although about 5% of patients receiving standard unfractionated heparin may develop this complication, its prevalence is

significantly lower in patients treated with low molecular weight heparin and heparin-related GAG [39] probably because of the lower affinity for PF4. Therefore, these agents have been used to replace standard heparin to avoid thrombocytopenia and thrombosis [40, 41]. The use of other GAG, such as chondroitin or dermatan sulfate, remains an interesting possibility because thrombocytopenia is much less likely to occur; however, there is no experience with these compounds in patients [24].

Sulodexide is a heparin-like GAG that can be administered both parenterally and orally, characterisitic that makes it particularly suitable for chronic treatment. It is composed of a fast-moving heparin fraction (iduronil – glucosaminoglycan sulfate) (80%) and a dermatan sulfate fraction (20%). Sulodexide has complex vasculoprotective effects: it counteracts thrombus formation and growth, improves blood flow, maintains the selective vascular permeability, has antilipaemic and antiproliferative effects. In contrast to heparin and low molecular weight heparins (LMWHs), sulodexide can activate both AT III, which acts mainly on circulating thrombin, and heparin II cofactor (HC II), which inhibits mostly thrombin bound to the fibrin present in the thrombus and in the vessel wall, resulting therefore an increase of the antithrombotic effect. This characteristic of sulodexide is very important, because thrombin formation, within the trombus can persist well beyond the acute phase in ischemic syndromes. In addition to the antithrombinic activity, sulodexide enhances fibrinolytic activity through activation of local tPA and inhibition of PAI 1 release [1, 42, 43, 44]. A study [45] carried out in healthy subjects and type 1 diabetic patients evaluated the effects of sulodexide on fibrinopeptide A (FPA) a marker of thrombin activity, PAI and tPA plasma levels, during glucose infusion. Administration of sulodexide during hyperglycaemia decreased FPA levels and improved the fibrinolytic response both in healthy and in diabetic patients, decreasing PAI and increasing tPA levels. Thus, sulodexide was able to counteract the prothrombotic state induced by hyperglycaemia by inhibiting thrombin activation and enhancing the impaired fibrinolytic response [5]. Sulodexide also has platelet antiaggregant effect. It prevented platelet activation induced by catepsin G and inhibited thrombin-induced platelet aggregation with equivalent potency as heparin. The favorable haemorrheologic effect of sulodexide consists in lowering blood viscosity by reducing fibrinogen and very low density lipoprotein (VLDL) levels. Sulodexide restores the normal negative charge of the vessel wall and inhibits basement membrane and extracellular matrix expansion, thus maintaining the selective vascular permeability. Oral and parenteral administration of sulodexide induces the release of lipoprotein lipase and reduced total cholesterol plasma levels, low density lipoproteins (LDL) and VLDL. *In vitro* experiments have shown effective antiproliferative effects of sulodexide in cultured smooth muscle, fibroblast-like cells and epithelial cells [1, 42, 44].

The main pharmacokinetic characteristics of sulodexide, which favours its complex pharmacological activity, is its high vessel wall tropism, manifested by a large uptake of fluorescent marker by the vessel wall after injection of marker in laboratory animals [46].

THE ROLE OF GAGs IN MACROVASCULAR COMPLICATIONS

THE ROLE OF SUBENDOTHELIAL HSPG IN ATHEROGENESIS

The role of proteoglycans in atherosclerosis has been the subject of intense investigations largely owing to the observation that CS/DS proteoglycans associate with apoB-containing lipoproteins *in vitro* [47]. Since the content of CS/DS proteoglycans is increased in atherosclerosis, it was postulated that CS/DS PG in vessels contribute to this latter part of lipoprotein retention. Heparan sulfate proteoglycans (HSPG), in contrast, negatively correlate with human atherosclerosis, aging and diabetes [48, 49]. In addition, the amount of cholesterol accumulated in the lesion is inversely proportional to the concentration of HS in the aorta. Research that spans more than two decades has clearly shown that HSPG can modulate events related to atherogenesis such as lipoprotein metabolism, monocyte recruitment, smooth muscle cell proliferation and thrombosis.

Subendothelial matrix, which is the center stage of essential events in the development of atherosclerosis, is composed of adhesion proteins and proteoglycans [50]. Matrix HSPG not only provide a physical barrier to the movement of cells and other large molecules such as lipoproteins into tissues, but the HS chains of the

HSPG bind and sequester a variety of bioactive proteins, including growth factors, chemokines, cytokines, and enzymes [51]. The major HSPG in the subendothelial matrix is perlecan [52]. Perlecan consists of a core protein to which three HS chains are attached to one end of the molecule. Perlecan core protein has a complex functional organization that can potentially influence events related to atherosclerosis. The core protein consists of five consecutive domains with homologies to molecules involved in the control of cell proliferation, lipoprotein uptake and cell adhesion. The N-terminal domain I contains attachment sites for HS chains. Although HS chains are not required for correct folding and secretion of the protein, lack of HS or decreased sulfation can decrease perlecan's ability to interact with matrix proteins. Thus, removal of HS chains may affect matrix organization and endothelial barrier function [53, 54]. Domain II comprises four repeats homologous to the ligand-binding portion of the LDL receptor, with six conserved cysteine residues and a pentapeptide, which mediates ligand binding by the LDL receptor. Surprisingly, whether this domain indeed mediates lipoprotein binding has never been tested. Domain III has homology to the domain IVa and IVb of laminin. This domain contains a tripeptide RGD that can promote integrin-mediated cell attachment. Although this sequence is not conserved in humans, both mouse and human perlecan protein core can mediate cell attachment. Domain V, which has homology to the G domain of the long arm of laminin, is responsible for self-assembly and may be important for basement membrane formation *in vivo*. Thus, perlecan core protein and HS chains could modulate matrix assembly, cell proliferation, lipoprotein binding and cell adhesion [53].

Subendothelial HSPG potentially inhibits several events related to atherogenesis, such as:

Lipoprotein transport

Perlecan core proteins and HS interact with surrounding matrix proteins and stabilize matrix organization and barrier function and thus limit lipoprotein transport in subendothelial matrix [53].

Lipoprotein retention

Perlecan HS can inhibit Lp(a) binding to the fibronectin from the subendothelial extracellular matrix and inhibit minimally oxidized LDL binding to other matrix proteins. Removal of subendothelial HS but not CS and DS by enzymatic treatment increased the binding of three different atherogenic lipoproteins: LDL, minimally oxidized LDL and lipoprotein(a) by 1.5 to 3 fold [54]. A careful analysis of this increase showed that removal of HS chains exposed lipoprotein-binding sites within the matrix. Fibronectin is an adhesion protein in the subendothelial matrix that can bind Lp(a) via its heparin binding domain and the lysine binding sites of Apo(a) [55]. Fibronectin is an early marker of atherogenesis and co-localizes with Lp(a) in early atherosclerotic lesions and plaques. Consistent with this, the increased Lp(a) binding after HS removal was significantly inhibited by anti-fibronectin antibodies. Because HSPG are in a network with fibronectin and other matrix adhesion proteins that have HS binding domains, it is possible that removal of HS leads to those sites being exposed. Alternatively, since apo(a) is a negatively charged protein, removal of negatively charged HS in the matrix may decrease charge repulsion, leading to increased binding. The mechanism behind the increase in the binding of LDL and minimally oxidized LDL is less clear. Matrix collagen [56] or perlecan core protein (domain II) could interact with LDL and oxidized LDL, and it is conceivable that in normal matrix HS masks these domains. Removal of HS exposes such domains leading to accumulation of lipoproteins.

Monocyte recruitment

Perlecan HS inhibits monocyte binding to subendothelial matrix either by inhibiting integrin-matrix interactions or by inhibiting monocyte cell surface HSPG interactions with matrix. Removal of HS also increased the association of monocytes with the subendothelial matrix [57]. Monocyte recruitment, retention and differentiation play a central role in the development of atherosclerosis [58]. Transendothelial migration (diapedesis) and passage through extracellular matrix (interstitial migration) are distinct and separable phases of monocyte migration [59]. Studies have shown that HS affected monocyte interaction only with matrix but not with endothelial monolayer. It is conceivable that in the absence of specific interactions with matrix proteins, monocytes may fail to enter the subendothelial space. The ability of HS to inhibit monocyte binding to matrix could

be due to inhibition of binding either to a matrix protein (e.g., fibronectin) or to perlecan core protein. HS may inhibit monocyte cell surface integrin binding to RGD domains of matrix proteins [60]. In addition to integrin binding domains, matrix proteins contain sequences that bind HS. Thus, monocyte surface HSPG could play a role in cell binding to these proteins and HS in matrix could potentially inhibit monocyte HSPG-mediated cell binding [61].

Macrophage differentiation

Perlecan HS can sequester several cytokines and regulate their bioavailability, thus modulating macrophages differentiation.

Smooth muscle cell proliferation

Perlecan can directly inhibit smooth muscle cells proliferation or bind and regulate the bioavailability of smooth muscle cells mitogens. Proliferation and migration of smooth muscle cells is a key event in the development of vascular lesions. *In vitro*, HSPGs maintain smooth muscle cells in a quiescent state by inhibiting phenotypic changes and DNA synthesis [62]. Arterial HSPG were shown to be more effective than heparin in inhibiting neointima in a rabbit model of restenosis [63]. Although *in vitro* all isolated HSPG are effective inhibitors of mesangial cells proliferation, the identity of the antiproliferative HSPG *in vivo* is not known. Cell surface HSPG are required for the mitogenic activity of several growth factors. Extracellular HSPG, on the other hand, can inhibit cell proliferation by regulating growth factor availability or by directly inhibiting signaling molecules associated with cell proliferation without interfering with early events in growth factor signaling [64]. Perlecan negatively correlates with smooth muscle cells proliferation [65]. Also, it is required to mediate the effects of antiproliferative agents. The antiproliferative effect of perlecan is likely due to the HS chains. However, a monoclonal perlecan antibody that reacts with domain III of perlecan completely blocked the antiproliferative effect of perlecan [65]. Domain III is thought to mediate cell adhesion; and attachment to the matrix and spreading is a key part of cell growth [66]. Vascular cells produce a variety of growth promoters and inhibitors. Atherosclerosis-relevant agents that stimulate smooth muscle cells proliferation include platelet-derived growth factor (PDGF), thrombin, oxidized LDL, and lysolecithin. Vascular cell derived growth inhibitors include: TGF-β, NO/cyclic guanosine monophosphate (cGMP) and ApoE. A review of literature on perlecan regulation identified an interesting possibility that perlecan may be the key for modulation of smooth muscle cell growth. PGDF [67], thrombin [68], serum oxidized LDL [69], and lysolecithin [60], which stimulate smooth muscle cells growth, decrease perlecan. In contrast, antiproliferative agents, TGF-β [62], ApoE and even heparin stimulate perlecan expression.

Thrombosis

Subendothelial HS are enriched in antithrombin binding sequences, thus potentiate antithrombin inhibition of thrombin activity. Reduced HS synthesis by endothelial cells might cause thrombophilia in diabetes mellitus because, due to its negative charge, HS regulates the development of pericellular thrombotic phenomena at the level of the endothelial membrane, by interacting with antithrombin III [70]. This hypothesis is supported by studies which found an increased ratio between fibrinogen and antithrombin III, due to a decrease in antithrombin III in the aorta of diabetic rats [71] and the observation of increased levels of markers of thrombin activation in diabetic patients [72]. As recently suggested, this last condition may produce an increase in fibrinogen [73], a well recognized cardiovascular risk factor also in diabetes [74]. The fall in endothelial cell HS content might also influence local fibrinolysis. Endothelial cells synthesize specific HS and chondroitin sulphate to which tissue plasminogen activator (t-PA) can bind [75]. This t-PA binding capacity might be important in forming a t-PA storage pool, from which t-PA is released and made locally available under certain circumstances [76]. HS-bound t-PA released from endothelial cells would provide an additional mechanism for locally increased fibrinolytic activity and render endothelial cells resistant to fibrin deposition. Thus, the derangement in this fibrinolytic mechanism could lead to increased fibrin deposition on the vascular wall in diabetes [14].

Regulation of HSPG by HDL and oxidized LDL cholesterol

Recent studies showed that HSPGs are negatively regulated by atherogenic molecules and positively regulated by antiatherogenic agents.

Extracellular matrix HSPG, perlecan, appears to be an important target of regulation by these agents. At least two levels of regulation appear to control perlecan HSPG in matrix: a change in core protein expression or a change in heparan sulfate metabolism. Atherogenic levels of LDL, oxidized LDL and lysolecithin decrease not only perlecan core protein synthesis but also enhance heparan sulfate degradation by stimulating endothelial secretion of heparanase. In contrast, apoE and apoE-HDL increase perlecan core protein as well as sulfation of heparan sulfate [53] (Figure 36.1).

CLINICAL EFFICACY OF GAGs TREATMENT IN MACROVASCULAR COMPLICATIONS

Acute myocardial infarction

A large multicentre, prospective randomised trial evaluated the efficacy of sulodexide in the prevention of cardiovascular events (death and thromboembolism) during the 12 months following an acute myocardial infarction [76]. Standard therapy did not include anticoagulants or anti-aggregants. Patients treated with sulodexide showed a statistically significant reduction, compared to the control group, of the following parameters: mortality (from 7.1% to 4.8%, risk reduction = 32%), reinfarction (from 4.6% to 3.35%; risk reduction = 28%) intraventricular thrombosis (from 1.3% to 0.6%; risk reduction = 53%). These results are similar to those obtained with antiaggregannts and oral anticoagulants. Sulodexide was well tolerated, with no relevant side effects [1].

Peripheral occlusive arterial disease

To assess the effect of sulodexide on peripheral occlusive arterial disease of the lower limbs in diabetic patients, we performed a randomized, placebo controlled study on eighty two patients with type 2 DM and Leriche-Fontaine stage II peripheral arterial disease. Subjects were randomized to receive sulodexide (60 mg, intramuscularly, once a day, for 10 days, followed by 25 mg, orally, twice a day for another 80 days) or placebo for 90 days. At the beginning and the end of the study, we assessed the pain-free walking distance with a standardized treadmill test, plasma levels of fibrinogen, total cholesterol, HDL cholesterol and triglycerides. The average pain-free walking distance

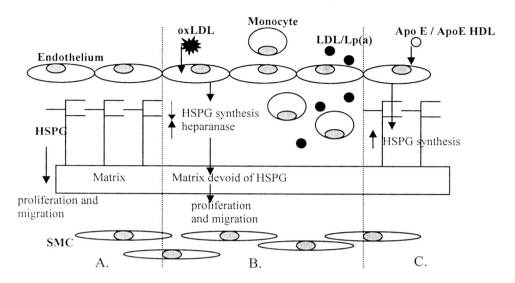

Figure 36.1.

Atheroprotective effects of subendothelial HSPG (modified after Pillarisetti, 2000 [53]).

A. Normal situation: subendothelial matrix contains HSPG and adhesion proteins. HSPG are atheroprotective: 1) stabilize matrix organization and barrier function; 2) inhibit atherogenic lipoproteins and monocytes interactions with adhesion proteins within the matrix; 3) inhibit smooth muscle cells (SMC) and migration; 4) bind antithrombin III providing locally antithrombotic effects. B. 1) ox LDL decreases core protein synthesis and stimulates endothelial secretion of heparanase, which degrades HSPG, generating a matrix devoid of HSPG. 2) Reduced HSPG within subendothelial matrix leads to increased retention of LDL, Lp(a) and circulating monocytes, promotes smooth muscle cells proliferation and migration in the subendothelial intima. C. Apo E and Apo E HDL may counter these events by increasing HSPG expression.

(±SD) increased with the sulodexide from 171.5 ± 30.41 m to 295.24 ± 34.14 m, while with placebo it increased from 167.48 ± 29.52 m to 208.54 ± 26.73 m. The increase of average pain-free walking distance in the sulodexide treated group was 123.74 ± 11.6 m (72.15%) *vs.* 41.06 ± 9.3 m (24.52%) in the placebo treated group (p < 0.001). Moreover, sulodexide significantly reduced the main vascular disease risk factors: plasma levels of fibrinogen (reduced by 14.25% compared to baseline, p < 0.001), total cholesterol (reduced by 20.22%, p < 0.001), triglycerides (reduced by 31.5 %, p < 0.001) and increased plasma levels of protecting HDL -cholesterol (by 23.6 %, p < 0.001). Our results were similar to other studies that evaluated the effects of sulodexide on peripheral artery disease and included both nondiabetic and diabetic patients.

In a randomized, multicenter, double-blind, placebo-controlled study performed in 286 patients with Leriche-Fontaine stage II peripheral arterial obstructive disease, the doubling of the pain-free walking distance was achieved in 23.8% of patients treated with sulodexide for 27 weeks *vs.* in 9.1% of those treated with placebo (p = 0.001). The pain-free walking distance increased by 64.7% from baseline with sulodexide and by 29.9% with placebo (p = 0.001). The maximum walking distance increased by 76.0% from baseline with sulodexide and by 27.9% with placebo (p < 0.001). Plasma fibrinogen decreased with sulodexide, but increased with placebo. Results for patients with type 2 diabetes (25%) were similar to those for non-diabetic patients [77].

A meta-analysis [78] of 19 double blind and placebo controlled trials on the effects of sulodexide in patients with chronic occlusive arterial diseases of the lower limbs confirmed the efficacy of sulodexide in significantly reducing claudication (the pain-free walking distance increased by 36% compared to controls, p = 0.009), improving blood flow and pressure values, and significantly reducing important vascular disease risk factors such as plasma fibrinogen (reduced by 15% compared to baseline, p < 0.0001), hypertriglyceridemia (reduced by 28% , p < 0.0015) and blood viscosity, while simultaneously increasing plasma levels of protecting factors such as HDL -cholesterol (by 24%, p = 0.0007). All the above parameters were unchanged in the placebo treated group. In most of these studies, sulodexide was administered intramuscularly for the first 10–20 days and, subsequently, orally for 60–180 days. In other studies it was administered either orally or intramuscularly.

On the basis of these results it seems that sulodexide could be particularly indicated in diabetic patients, who have numerous concomitant vascular risk factors [79].

THE ROLE OF GAGs IN DIABETIC NEPHROPATHY

THE ROLE OF ABNORMAL GAGs IN PATHOGENESIS OF DIABETIC NEPHROPATHY

Possible GAG metabolism abnormalities in diabetic nephropathy were originally investigated for the following reasons: 1) albuminuria and proteinuria appear in diabetic nephropathy; 2) this phenomenon suggests abnormal glomerular basement membrane (GBM) permeability; and 3) GAG, in particular HS, were thought to be important determinants of GBM permeability. Biochemical techniques as well as immunohistology and histochemical staining procedures, combined with electron microscopy morphometric studies, have been used to examine glomerular HSPG and GAG content in diabetic nephropathy. Studies using biochemical techniques to measure GAG content of kidneys obtained at autopsy demonstrated that GBM of patients with diabetic nephropathy contained less GAG than kidneys of nondiabetic control subjects [80, 81]. Using electron microscopy, Vernier et al. [82] described a reverse correlation between GBM HSPG expression and mesangial expansion in diabetic nephropathy. JM-403, a very interesting monoclonal antibody which reacts with HS-GAG chains, mainly stains the GBM in normal kidneys, but largely fails to stain tubular basement membranes. Using this antibody, one could show that a decreased GBM staining intensity correlated with proteinuria, expressed as a function of creatinine clearance in patients with diabetic nephropathy [83]. Also, it was shown that staining of skin basement membrane was significantly reduced in patients with diabetic nephropathy compared to patients with long-standing diabetes without nephropathy [84]. It should be noted that the exact meaning of a decreased staining by this antibody under pathologic conditions in relation to total GAG content or sulfation is not yet known.

Several groups reported a decreased ^{35}S sulfate incorporation in the glomerular basement membrane of diabetic glomeruli [85, 86]. In mice and rats with diabetes, reduced synthesis of glomerular proteoglycans and basement membrane HSPG was found [87]. However, the findings of the numerous sulfate incorporation experiments are not without controversy, and a marked increase in radiolabeled sulfate incorporation in proteoglycans in diabetic tissues has also been reported [88].

The effects of the diabetic milieu on glomerular HSPG synthesis have been studied in vitro, using glomerular cell cultures [89]. When human glomerular visceral epithelial and mesangial cells were cultured under normal (5 mM) and high (25 mM) glucose conditions, and then stained with the same monoclonal antibody (JM-403) that had been used on the tissue sections of diabetic kidneys, a decreased extracellular matrix staining after culture in 25 mM glucose was observed [90]. The rise of metabolic labeling also disclosed an altered proteoglycan production under high glucose conditions, predominantly with a decrease in HS, compared with dermatan or chondroitin sulfate proteoglycan. N-sulfation analysis of HSPG produced under high-glucose conditions revealed less di- and tetra-saccharides, compared with larger oligosaccharides, indicating an altered sulfation pattern.

Renal function deterioration and proteinuria in diabetic patients are correlated with mesangial expansion as the main morphologic parameter [24].

Metabolic labeling studies revealed that angiotensin II induced a decrease in HSPG synthesis, with a decrease in N-sulfation of the GAG side chains. Enzyme linked immunosorbent assay measurements using JM-403 confirmed that angiotensin II decreased HS production. Angiotensin II increased TGF-β production in a dose-dependent manner. Specific mRNA for perlecan HSPG decreased, while mRNA for TGF-β increased after incubation with angiotensin II. Blockade of the subtype 1 angiotensin II receptor (ATR1) reversed the effects of angiotensin II on both HSPG and TGF-β production. Coincubation of the mesangial cells with neutralizing antibodies against TGF-β did not prevent the angiotensin II - induced reduction of HS. These results indicate that the decrease in HS synthesis induced by angiotensin II is not mediated by an increase in TGF-β, but, on the contrary, the increase in TGF-β partially counteracts the inhibition of HS production by angiotensin II .

Because defects in HS-GAG synthesis are so striking in *in vitro* models of diabetic nephropathy (induced either by high glucose concentrations or angiotensin II), and because decreased renal and extrarenal JM-403 staining seems to be a rather specific marker for nephropathy in patients with diabetes, treatment of diabetic nephropathy with HS-GAG-like substances can be viewed as an experiment to test the Steno hypothesis [24].

GAGs RENOPROTECTIVE EFFECTS IN EXPERIMENTAL DIABETIC NEPHROPATHY

The treatment of diabetic nephropathy with GAGs was originally proposed on the basis of the somewhat simple idea that restoring the lacking anionic charges and GAGs to the diabetic kidney could cure the albuminuria and putatively return the above described cell functional anomalies to normal [91]. The observation of pathophysiological similarities between diabetic nephropathy and the so-called remnant kidney, *i.e.* reduced functioning tissue after a renal lesion, was also considered. In the classical model reproducing this kind of lesion, the 5/6 subtotal nephrectomized rat, heparin and derived drugs were shown effective in slowing the progression to uremia. In view of these considerations, the effect of heparin and GAGs on diabetic nephropathy was studied in the streptozotocin diabetic model. Despite differences in drug formulation and dosage, some effects were constant, especially the effects on the ultrastructure of the glomerulus, whereas others, such as those on albuminuria, were contradictory. GAGs reduced glomerular basement membrane thickening and anionic charge loss, as well as mesangial area expansion, and prevented the onset of albuminuria and the disorder in charge permselectivity [92]. However, Marshall *et al.* were not able to confirm a reduction of albumin excretion in female streptozotocin diabetic Wistar rats on a twice daily

dose of 200 units heparin over a period of 6 months. They did, though, report that basement membrane thickness, mesangial volume fraction and absolute mesangial volume were lower in heparin-treated diabetic animals compared with untreated diabetic animals [15]. The difference in the results may be mainly due to different qualities and quantities of drugs in the different protocols [93]. At high dosages, heparin appears in the glomerular ultrafiltrate; it then may interfere with the charge-dependent proximal tubule reabsorption of albumin due to its high degree of sulfation, thereby increasing albuminuria [24]. Furthermore, it should be emphasized that when referring to heparin, it is generally overlooked that heparin is a heterogeneous group of polysaccharides, with varying degrees of sulfation, molecular weights, and biologic activities. Commercial heparins are similar regarding their anticoagulant activity, but not with respect to many other activities. For example, although heparins from different suppliers have the same anticoagulant activity, they show a broad range of anti-mitogenicity, and some are even mitogenic. Furthermore, depending on its dosage, the same heparin preparation may be both antiproliferative and proliferative [3].

THE MECHANISMS OF GAGs RENOPROTECTIVE EFFECT

Numerous reports showed that heparin and more generally GAGs prevent and cure experimental diabetic nephropathy [91, 92, 94, 95]. However, it soon became clear that the activity of these drugs could not be explained, according to the Steno hypothesis [22], only in terms of recovery of the diabetes-induced abnormalities in HSPG metabolism, and restoration of anionic-HS charges in glomerular and other basement membranes [3]. There are several hypotheses on the mechanisms responsible for the protective effect of GAGs. Other than restoring the GBM anionic charge, effects on the coagulation cascade, on various proteases, on cellular proliferation or synthesis of extracellular matrix components may be involved [96] (Figure 36.2).

Heparin and GAG improve glomerular permselectivity to proteins, as deduced by evaluating the fractional clearances of neutral and anionic dextrans [97]. This has been indirectly confirmed by a number of investigators reporting a reduction in the albumin excretion rate after

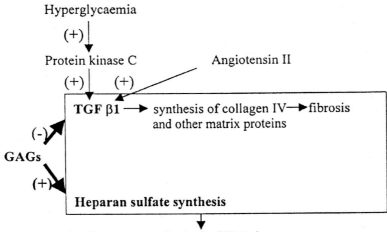

Figure 36.2
Renoprotective effects of GAGs therapy in diabetes mellitus.

heparin treatment in diabetic animals. This effect is probably related to the activity of heparin on extracellular matrix and GBM protein synthesis, rather than adhering to the GBM and thereby correcting the charge deficiency [24].

It was demonstrated that exogenous GAGs stimulates the glomerular synthesis of HS and sulphur (S) incorporation. S incorporation in glomeruli is a process strictly related to the synthesis of HS. In the glomeruli of diabetic rats there is a reduction of ^{35}S incorporation, which was reversed after GAGs treatment [96]. GAGs may also play a role in the synthesis of some extracellular matrix compounds which typically accumulate in the glomeruli in diabetic nephropathy. Indeed, diabetic animals show an increase of type IV collagen, in terms of either gene expression (increased mRNA levels) or increased protein synthesis, with consequent accumulation of collagen. GAGs treatment, either preventive or curative, reduced collagen IV glomerular cell synthesis and its accumulation in the extracellular matrix and glomerular basement membrane. Moreover, GAGs normalise type III collagen expresion in glomeruli, another parameter which is increased in diabetic rats [96]. The activity of GAGs on the sulfation and synthesis of HSPG [97] and on the collagen IV/perlecan mRNA ratio might be relevant to maintaining the authentic architecture of the membrane with normal permeability characteristics [97, 24].

Immunohistochemistry analyses have highlighted an increased expression of TGF-β1 in the glomeruli of animals and patients with diabetic nephropathy, both at protein and mRNA levels, while no immunoreactivity was evident in glomeruli of healthy controls [98]. This data suggest that TGF-β might play an important role in the pathogenesis of diabetic nephropathy [97]. In diabetes, hyperglycaemia and the related metabolic abnormalities such as accumulation of advanced glycation end products, production either *de novo* or by hydrolysis of diacylglycerol, and oxidative stress increases or activates PKC. The β I and II isoforms are predominantly increased in the vascular cells of diabetic patients. Activation of PKC is known to induce transcription of c-fos and c-jun which are protooncogenes, regulating gene transcription through the AP-1 binding site. Promoter regions of TGF-β1 contain AP-1 binding consensus sequences, supporting the hypothesis that hyperglycaemia-induced PKC activation is responsible for the increased expression of extracellular matrix proteins, through overexpression of TGF-β1. TGF-β1 is involved in several functions: matrix protein synthesis, matrix degradation (decreased synthesis of plasminogen activator and type IV collagenase, increased synthesis of plasminogen activator inhibitor), effects on integrins (increased synthesis of $\alpha5$ and $\beta1$ subunits), antiproliferative effects and apoptosis induction [96]. Although TGF-$\beta1$ was shown to increase HSPG synthesis, a potentially favorable effect according to the Steno hypothesis, as a whole it has a more prominent and pivotal role in the pathogenesis of glomerulosclerosis [24]. TGF-$\beta1$ stimulates production of extracellular matrix components such as type IV and VI collagen, fibronectin, and laminin in cultured endothelial, mesangial and glomerular epithelial cells, resulting in mesangial expansion and capillary membrane thickening. *In vitro* studies on mesangial cells exposed to high glucose concentrations showed that incubation of these cells with GAGs reversed the increased TGF-$\beta1$ in glomerular and tubular cells of diabetic animals, as assessed by immunohistochemical and in situ hybridisation techniques [96]. Renoprotective GAGs (modified heparins and dermatan sulfate) inhibit the PKC-dependent induction of TGF-$\beta1$ mRNA obtained with phorbol myristate acetate [24]. GAGs therapy in long-term diabetic rats prevents characteristic manifestations of diabetic nephropathy that are possibly related to TGF-β activity, mesangial matrix expansion, and deposition of periodic acid-Schiff-positive material, collagen III and IV [96]. Together, these findings support the view that GAGs are directly involved in the inhibition of TGF-$\beta1$ overexpression, most likely, as ongoing experiments indicate, by inhibiting stimulated TGF-$\beta1$ promoter activity without reducing basal activity. Interestingly, in unstimulated mesangial cells, the addition of renoprotective GAG has no effect on basal TGF-$\beta1$ mRNA levels. This observation mirrors the fact that GAGs treatment has no effect on TGF-$\beta1$ mRNA levels in nondiabetic animals. Together, the data indicate that GAG treatment prevents overexpression of TGF-$\beta1$ mRNA in mesangial cells induced by different stimuli, but does not affect basal levels. In theory, the chronic blockage of all TGF-$\beta1$ activity may be deleterious because of the risk of autoimmune-like diseases and malignant cell transformation [99]. The fact that GAG inhibit TGF-$\beta1$ overexpression leaving its basal expression unaffected seems to argue against such risks. Indeed, *in vivo* long-term (8 to 12 months) studies showed that GAG treatment prevents diabetes-induced overexpression of TGF-$\beta1$ with no occurrence of autoimmune-like disease, excess mortality, or cancer [94, 24].

Recent studies have shown that angiotensin II is a potent inducer of TGF-$\beta1$ synthesis *in vitro*. The most likely hypothesis is that TGF-$\beta1$ synthesis by angiotensin occurs by a different mechanism from that induced by hyperglycaemia. The cascade of events that leads to hyperstimulation of TGF-β synthesis by hyperglycaemia seems to be counteracted by GAGs, including sulodexide. It can be stated that in diabetic nephropathy, there are two targets counteracting TGF-$\beta1$ upregulation; both targets could be reached by associating ACE-inhibitors and GAGs, which should presumably show a synergistic effect [96].

GAGs antiproliferative role was evaluated by means of immunohistochemical techniques using anti PCNA (proliferating cell nuclear antigen) antibodies. Since PCNA is a cyclin, active during mitosis, nuclei of dividing cells will be PCNA-positive. In glomerular cells from diabetic animals treated *vs.* nontreated with GAGs, no differences in PCNA positivity were apparent, thus indicating that GAGs did not modify cell proliferation [96].

GAGs RENOPROTECTIVE EFFECTS IN HUMAN DIABETIC NEPHROPATHY

Previous experimental findings and the observation that increased TGF-ß1 expression exists in humans with diabetic nephropathy [100] suggest that the results obtained in animal studies may also be relevant to human disease. Recent reports have indeed described favorable results of GAG treatment on proteinuria in diabetic nephropathy. Treatment with a low molecular weight heparin reduced albuminuria in both micro- and macroalbuminuric patients with type 1 DM [101]. Danaparoid, a mixture of sulfated GAG consisting mainly of HS, also could lower proteinuria in a small, double-blind cross-over study in patients with type 1 DM and albumin excretion rates exceeding 300 mg/24 h [102]. A minimum of 6 weeks was necessary for the antiproteinuric effect to become manifest with no modifications in blood pressure and creatinine clearance. Sulodexide, a formulation composed of the two GAGs (80% fast-moving heparin and 20% dermatan sulfate) that were active in preventing diabetic nephropathy in the experimental model [95], was reported to reduce albuminuria in patients with type 1 or type 2 DM [103, 104, 105], and this effect lasted several weeks after its withdrawal [103, 105]. Although sulodexide treatment in type 1 DM seems to be consistently effective in reducing microalbuminuria, this hypoalbuminuric effect is observed in only 30 to 50% of patients with type 2 DM. It is known that microalbuminuria in patients with type 2 DM is not always caused by the typical diabetic nephropathy, because different, nondiabetic histologic changes were reported in two-thirds of the patients. Because the antiproteinuric effects of heparin differ among the various nephropathies (e.g., experimental diabetic nephropathy is much more sensitive to heparin than puromycin-induced nephrosis), it was suggested that in some patients with type 2 DM, GAGs did not reduce albuminuria due to a dosage that is low relative to the underlying renal lesion. The relatively low dosages could also be related to differences in the type of administered heparin.

The double blind, crossover and placebo-controlled study by Solini *et al.* is particularly interesting because of the methods used. Sulodexide 1000 LSU/day was administered orally for 4 months to 12 patients with albuminuria, hypertension and type 2 diabetes mellitus. Sulodexide significantly reduced albuminuria and this reduction was maintained stable for 4 months after withdrawal [36].

Diabetic Nephropathy-Albuminuria-Sulodexide trial, a multicentre, multinational, randomised, double-blind, placebo controlled trial have shown that oral treatment with sulodexide for 4 months reduced micro- and macroalbuminuria in a significant dose-dependent manner both in patients with type 1 and type 2 diabetes. Moreover, the dose - dependent eficacy of sulodexide was maintained for up to 4 months after treatment withdrawal, for the daily dose regimens of 100 and 200 mg [106].

Although promising, the studies published thus far were too short-term to clarify whether GAG treatment in diabetic patients is capable of curing diabetic nephropathy, instead of simply influencing one of its surrogate end points, albuminuria.

The Steno hypothesis [22] postulated a crucial role for heparin-like structures in the pathogenesis of diabetic nephropathy. There are some specific structures in the GAG chains of heparin molecules, which are useful for renoprotection and do not necessarily have a relationship with the anticoagulant activity of heparin.

THE ROLE OF GAGs IN DIABETIC RETINOPATHY

PHYSIOPATHOLOGY OF DIABETIC RETINOPATHY

One of the earlier signs of retinal damage induced by high plasma glucose concentrations is the appearance of permeability and selectivity alterations of capillary basal membranes due to GAGs substitution with collagen, fibronectin and hyaline compounds, and consequent microvascular leakage. This pathogenetic event is characteristic not only of diabetic retinopathy but also of nephropathy and any other microvascular complication of diabetes. In the retina, microvascular leakage is responsible for the formation of hard exudates that are widespread and represent a loss of lipids and proteins from the damaged vessels. Moreover, haemorrhagic areas and accumulation of soft exudates (cotton wool spots) appear. Vascular lesions are acccompanied by the proliferation of endothelial cells and the loss of pericytes which, in physiological conditions, surround and support the vessels. From a morphological point of view, microscopic analysis of endothelial cells of retinal capillaries in diabetic patients shows a large thickening of the basal membrane and the presence of ghost pericytes, the latter feature being another typical sign of diabetic retinopathy.

The pathogenetic mechanisms of retinopathy, which are very complex and not well understood, appear to be similar to those of nephropathy.

In fact, the fundamental pathogenetic event is an increase of collagen, accumulation of fibrous and hyaline material in the basement membrane and loss of GAGs, with basement membrane thickening and modification of anionic charge [107].

POSSIBLE ROLE OF GAGs IN DIABETIC RETINOPATHY

HSPG is the most abundant GAG in endothelial basement membrane and the major constituent of TGF-β1 receptor, highly expressed in the endothelial cells. This receptor, apart from being involved in coagulation processes, in antioxidant activity and in glucose uptake, seems to modulate pericytes growth. The proteoglycans, interfering with TGF-β1 and other growth factors, like a FGF (fibroblast growth factor a) and b FGF, could regulate retinal capillary metabolism determining an up- or downregulation of pericytes of endothelial cells and basement membrane. A recent study on animal models [108] has shown that synthesis and mRNA expression of HSPG are reduced in endothelial BM in the retina of diabetic rats, causing a reduction of basement membrane anionic sites and an increase of capillary permeability, which are typical vascular complications of diabetes. Moreover, the existence of a relationship between urinary albumin excretion and development of microangiopathy in type 1 diabetic patients was shown [109]. Such link has been demonstrated in type 2 diabetic patients as well [110], indicating that urinary albumin excretion can be considered a predictor of diabetic retinopathy, neuropathy and cardiovascular diseases associated with diabetes. Furthermore, a significant correlation between microalbuminuria and diabetic retinopathy progression has been demonstrated [107]. Microalbuminuria is associated with two-fold increase of the risk of background retinopathy in type 2 diabetic patients, while in type 1 diabetes albuminuria is associated with three-fold risk increase of proliferative retinopathy.

GAGs have been shown to reduce microalbuminuria in type1 diabetic patients, suggesting that exogenous administration of these compounds may also prove to be more effective in diabetic retinopathy.

A preliminary study on 30 patients with type 1 or type 2 diabetes treated for 16 weeks with sulodexide (600 LSU/day i.m. for the first 3 weeks followed by oral treatment with 1000 LSU/day for 13 weeks) reported a significant reduction of hard exudates, intraretineal microvascular abnormalities and haemorrhages in patients affected by background diabetic retinopathy, and this effect was independent of arterial blood pressure or metabolic status [107].

In a recent study, the reduction in retinal hard exudates was attributed to danaparoid therapy, because a spontaneous reduction in such abnormalities is not likely to occur within a few months. Overexpressed vascular endothelial growth factor (VEGF) plays a pivotal role in the pathogenesis of increased vascular permeability and neovascularization in diabetic retinopathy. Under physiologic conditions, some VEGF isoforms are sequestered and modulated by extracellular matrix-sulfated GAG. Alterations in the sulfation of GAGs in diabetes could thus lead to an altered disposal of VEGF, and exogenous GAGs could reverse this phenomenon [94]. The effect of danaparoid on hard exudates might well be related to the modulation of sequestered VEGF in the retina [24].

More double blind, placebo controlled studies are needed to clarify the effects of sulodexide treatment in diabetic retinopathy.

CONCLUSIONS

Increased vessel permeability to macromolecules such as albumin, fibrinogen and atherogenous lipoproteins may represent a primary alteration in diabetic micro- and macrovasculopathies. The loss of GAGs from the vessel wall may concur to the development of vascular complications in diabetes. Numerous experimental and clinical studies have demonstrated that GAGs are able to reduce vascular risk factors induced by hyperglycaemia, improve the clinical status of the patients with vascular disease, and counteract the onset of thromboembolic complications.

Although only small studies have been conducted, the favorable effects of GAG treatment on albuminuria in diabetic nephropathy are encouraging. Clearly, dose-finding and long-term studies are needed to demonstrate that these drugs are capable of curing human diabetic nephropathy and not simply albuminuria [3].

Also, additional studies will be needed in diabetic retinopathy to confirm interesting positive results of preliminary studies suggesting that GAG may restore metabolic activity and functions of endothelial basement membrane in patients with type 1 and type 2 diabetes mellitus.

Some of the previous studies reported that GAGs effects depend on their non-sulphated molecular backbone or are reached at non-anticoagulant dosages or both. Studies of the structure-function relationship of heparin and GAGs and their optimal dosage may provide the opportunity to select new derivatives with specific effects on diabetic nephropathy and macroangiopathy, possibly and most importantly without anticoagulation effect [1]. Such a compound is sulodexide, a heparin-like GAG (composed of 80% fast moving heparin and 20% dermatan sulfate) with increased antithrombotic efficacy and lower anticoagulant activity than low-molecular weight heparin, which has also oral bioavailability. Therefore sulodexide is particularly useful for long term treatment and has demonstrated its efficacy and safety in all the clinical studies performed.

REFERENCES

1. Harenberg J. Vascular complications of diabetes and treatment with sulodexide. In: *Highlights of Satellite Symposium "Diabetic microangiopathy and sulodexide"*. Adis International, Milan, 2001, 6–11.
2. Colwell JA. Vascular thrombosis in types II diabetes mellitus. *Diabetes*, **42**: 8–11, 1993.
3. Ragucci E, Zonszein J, Frishman H. Pharmacotherapy of Diabetes Mellitus; Implications for the Prevention and Treatment of Cardiovascular Disease. *Heart Dis*, **5**: 18–33, 2003.
4. Deckert T, Kofoed-Enevoldsen A, Norgaard K. Microalbuminuria. Implications for micro- and macrovascular disease. *Diabetes Care*, **15**: 1181–11913, 1992.
5. Gambaro G, Baggio B. Role of glycosaminoglycans in diabetic nephropathy. *Acta Diabetol*, **29**: 149–155, 1992.
6. Gambaro G, Skrha J, Ceriello A. Glycosaminoglycan therapy for long-term diabetic complications? *Diabetologia*, **41**: 975–979, 1998.
7. Beckman JA, Creager MA, Libby P. Diabetes and atherosclerosis: epidemiology, Pathophysiology and management. *JAMA*, **287**: 2570–2581, 2002.
8. Kashihara N, Wanatabe Y, Makino H, *et al.* Selective decreased de novo synthesis of glomerular proteoglycans under the influence of reactive oxygen species. *Proc Natl Acad Sci USA*, **89**: 6309–6313, 1992.
9. Sowers JR, Epstein M. Diabetes mellitus and associated hypertension, vascular disease, and nephropathy: an update. *Hypertension*, **26** (pt 1): 869–879, 1995.
10. Bianchi S, Bigazzi R, Quinones Galvan A, *et al.* Insulin resistance in microalbuminuric hypertension: sites and mechanisms. *Hypertension*, **26**: 189–195, 1995.
11. Fogari R, Zoppi A, Lazzari P. ACE inhibition but not angiotensin II antagonism reduces plasma fibrinogen and insulin resistance in overweight hypertensive patients. *Cardiovascular Pharmacol*, **32**: 616–620, 1998.
12. Sowers JR, Lester MA: Diabetes and cardiovascular disease. *Diabetes Care*, **22**: C14–C20, 1999.
13. Guerci B, Bohme P, Kearney-Schwartz A, *et al.* Endothelial dysfunction and type 2 diabetes. *Diabetes metab*, **27**: 436–447, 2001.
14. Jensen T. Pathogenesis of diabetic vascular disease; Evidence for the role of reduced Heparan Sulfate Proteoglycan. *Diabetes*, **46**: S98–S100, 1997.
15. Muir H, Hardingham TE. Structure of proteoglycans. In: Whelan Butterworths WJ (ed). *MTP Inter Rev Sci Biochemistry of Carbohydrates*, Biochemistry Series One Vol 5, University Park Press, 1976.
16. Born van den J, Berden JHM. Is microalbuminuria in diabetes due to changes in glomerular heparan sulphate? *Nephrol Dial Transplant*, **10**: 1277–1296, 1995.
17. Parthasarathy N, Spiro R. Effect of diabetes on the glycosaminoglycan component of the human glomerular basement membrane. *Diabetes*, **31**: 738–741, 1982.
18. Shimomura H, Spiro R. Studies on macromolecular components of human glomerular basement membrane and alterations in diabetes: Decreased levels of heparan sulfate proteoglycans and laminin. *Diabetes*, **36**: 374–381, 1987.
19. Wasty F, Alavi MZ, Moore S. Distribution of glycosaminoglycans in the intima of human aortas: Changes in atherosclerosis and diabetes mellitus. *Diabetologia*, **36**: 316–322, 1993.
20. Dybahhl H, Ledet T. Diabetic microangiopathy; quantitative histopathological studies of the extramural coronary arteries from type 2 diabetic patients. *Diabetologia*, **30**: 882–886, 1987.
21. Jensen T. Albuminuria: a marker of renal and generalised vascular disease in insulin-dependent diabetes mellitus. *Dan Med Bull*, **38**: 134–144, 1991.
22. Deckert T, Feldt-Rasmussen B, Borch-Johnsen K, *et al.* Albuminuria reflects widespread vascular damage. The Steno hypothesis. *Diabetologia*, **32**: 219–226, 1989.
23. Rosenberg RD, Shworak NW, Liu J. Heparan sulfate proteoglycans of the cardiovascular system: Specific structures emerge but how is synthesis regulated? *J Clin Invest*, **100**: S67–S75, 1997.
24. Gambaro G, van der Woude FJ. Glycosaminoglycans: use in treatement of diabetic nephropathy. *J Am Soc Nephrol*, **11**: 359–368, 2000.
25. Ruoslahti E. Proteoglycans in cell regulation. *J Biol Chem*, **264**: 13369–13372, 1989.
26. Yamamoto T, Nakamura T, Noble NA *et al.* Expression of transforming growth factor beta is

elevated in human and experimental diabetic nephropathy. *Proc Natl acad Sci*, **90**: 1814–1818, 1993.

27. Nungent MA, Karnovsky MJ, Elderman ER. Vascular cell derived heparan sulfate shows coupled inhibition of basic fibroblast growth factors binding and mitogenesis in vascular smooth muscle cells. *Circ Res*, **73**: 1051–1060, 1993.

28. Böhm T, Geiger M, Binder BR. Isolation and caracterisation of tissue-plasminogen activator-binding proteoglzcans from human umbilical vein endothelial cells. *Arterioscler Thromb Vasc Biol*, **16**: 665–672, 1996.

29. van der Pijl JW, van der Woude FJ, Swart W, *et al.* Effect of danaparoid sodium on hard exudates in diabetic retinopathy. *Lancet*, **350**: 1743–1745, 1997.

30. Gambaro G, Cavazzana AO, Luzi P *et al.* Glycosaminoglycans prevent morphological renal alterations and albuminuria in diabetic rats. *Kidney Int*, **42**: 285–29, 1992.

31. Crepaldi G, Fellin R, Calabrò A, *et al.* Double-blind multicenter trial on a new medium molecular weight glycosaminoglycan. Current therapeutic effects and perspectives for clinical use. *Atherosclerosis*, **81**: 233–243, 1990.

32. Larsen AK, Lund DP, Langer R, *et al.* Oral heparin results in the appearance of heparin fragments in the plasma of rats. *Proc Natl Acad Sci*, **83**: 2964–2968, 1986.

33. Jaques LB, Hiebert LM, Wice SM. Evidence from endothelium of gastric absorption of heparin and of dextran sulfates 8000. *J Lab Clin Med*, **117**: 122–130, 1991.

34. Hiebert LM, Wice SM, Jaques LB. Antithrombotic activity of oral unfractionated heparin. *J Cardiovasc Pharmacol*, **28**: 26–29, 1996.

35. Dawes J, Hodson BA, MacGregor IR. Pharmacokinetic and biological activities of dermatan sulfate (Mediolanum MF701) in healthy human volunteers. *Ann NY Acad Sci*, **556**: 292–303, 1989.

36. Solini A, Vergnani L, Ricci F, *et al.* Glycosaminoglycans delay the progression of nephropathy in NIDDM. *Diabetes Care*, **20**: 813–817, 1997.

37. Velussi M, Cernigoi AM, Dapas F, *et al.* Glycosaminoglycans oral therapy reduces microalbuminuria, blood fibrinogen levels and limb arteriopathy clinical signs in patients with non-insulin dependent diabetes mellitus. *Diabetes Nutr Metab*, **9**: 53–58, 1996.

38. Obata H, Inoue Y, Kojiro S, *et al.* Influence of heparin administration on bone metabolism in experimental chronic renal failure rats. *Nephrol Dial Transplant*, **11**: 46a, 1996.

39. Warkentin TE, Levine MN, Hirsh J. Heparin-induced thrombocytopenia in patients treated with low-molecular weight heparin or unfractionated heparin. *N Engl J Med*, **332**: 1330–1335, 1995.

40. Magnani HN. Heparin-induced thrombocytopenia (HIT): An overview of 230 patients treated with organan (Org 10172). *Thromb Haemostasis*, **70**: 554–561, 1993.

41. Hill GR, Hickton C, Henderson S. The use of organan in heparin-induced thrombocytopenia associated with *in vitro* platelet aggregation at higher organan concentrations. *Clin Lab Haematol*, **19**: 155–157, 1997.

42. Harenberg J. Review of pharmacodynamics, pharmacokinetics and therapeutic properties of sulodexide. *Med Res Rev*, **18**(1): 1–20, 1998.

43. Velussi M, Cernigoi AM, Dapas F, *et al.* Glycosaminoglycans oral therapy reduces microalbuminuria, blood fibrinogen levels and limb arteriopathy clinical signs in patients with non-insulin dependent diabetes mellitus. *Diabetes Nutr Metab*, **9**: 53–58, 1996.

44. Karnovsky MJ, Wright TC, Castellot JJ, *et al.* Heparin, heparan sulfate, smooth muscle cells, and atherosclerosis. *Ann NY Acad Sci*, **556**: 268–281, 1989.

45. Cerrielo A. Quatraro A, Marchi E, *et al.* Impaired fibrinolytic response to increased thrombin activation in type 1 diabetic patients; effects of glycosaminoglycan sulodexide. *Diabete Metab*, **19**: 225–229, 1993.

46. Ruggeri A. Guizzardi S, Franchi M, *et al.* Pharmacokinetics and distribution of a fluoresceinated glycosaminoglycan, sulodexide, in rats. *Arzneim-Forch/Drug Res*, **35**: 1517–1519, 1985.

47. Hurt-Camejo E, Olsson U, Wiklund O, *et al.* Cellular consequences of the association of apoB lipoproteins with proteoglycans. *Arterioscler Thromb Vasc Biol*, **17**: 1011–1017, 1997.

48. Schwenke DC, Carew TE. Initiation of atherosclerotic lesion in cholesterol-fed rabbits. II. Selective retention of LDL *vs.* selective increases in LDL permeability in susceptible sites of arteries. *Arteriosclerosis*, **9**: 908–918, 1989.

49. Hollman J, Schmidt A, von Bassewitz D, *et al.* Relationship of sulfated glycosaminoglycan and cholesterol content in normal and atherosclerotic aorta. *Arteriosclerosis*, **9**: 154–158, 1989.

50. Wight TN. The extracellular matrix and atherosclerosis. *Curr Opin Lipid*, **6**: 326–334, 1995.

51. Lindahl U, Lindholt K, Spillman D, *et al.* More to heparin than anticoagulation. *Thrombosis Res*, **75**: 1–32, 1994.

52. Iozzo RV, Cohen IR, Grassel S, *et al.* The biology of perlecan. *Biochem J*, **302**: 625–639, 1994.

53. Pillarisetti S. Lipoprotein Modulation of Subendothelial Heparan Sulfate Proteoglycans (Perlecan) and Atherogenicity. *Trends Cardiovasc Med*, **10**: 60–65, 2000.

54. Pino RM: Perturbation of the blood-retinal barrier after enzyme perfusion. A cytochemical study. *Lab Invest*, **56**: 475–480, 1987.

55. Van der Hoek Y, Sangarar W, Cote GP, *et al*. Binding of recombinant apo(a) to extracellular matrix proteins. *Arterio Thromb*, **14**: 1792–1798, 1994.

56. Hoover GA, McCormick S, Kalant N. Interaction of native and cell-modified low density lipoprotein with collagen gel. *Arteriosclerosis*, **8**: 525–534, 1988.

57. Pillarisetti S, Obunike JC, Goldberg IJ. Lysolecithin induced alterations of subendothelial heparan sulfate proteoglycans increases monocyte binding to matrix. *J Biol Chem*, **270**: 29,760–29, 765, 1995.

58. Ross R. Atherosclerosis: an inflammatory disease. *N Engl J Med*, **340**:115–126, 1999.

59. Liao F, Huynh HK, Eiroa A, *et al*. Migration of monocytes across endothelium and passage through extracellular matrix involve separate molecular domains of PECAM-1. *J Exp Med*, **182**:1337–1343, 1995.

60. Hayashi K, Madri JA, Yurchenco PD. Endothelial cells interact with the core protein of basement membrane perlecan through beta 1 and beta 3 integrins: an adhesion modulated by glycosaminoglycan. *J Cell Biol*, **19**: 945–959, 1992.

61. Woods A, Couchman J, Syndecans R. Synergistic activators of cell adhesion. *Trends Cell Biol*, **8**: 189–192, 1998.

62. Iozzo RV, Pillarisetti J, Sarma B, *et al*. Structural characterization of perlecan gene promoter. *J Biol Chem*, **272**: 5219–5228, 1997.

63. Bingley JA, Hayward IP, Campbell JH, *et al*. Arterial heparan sulfate proteoglycans inhibit vascular smooth muscle cell proliferation and phenotype change *in vitro* and neo intimal formation *in vivo*. *J Vasc Surg*, **28**: 308–318, 1998.

64. Daum G, Hedin U, Wang Y, *et al*. Diverse effects of heparin on mitogen-activated protein kinase-dependent signal transduction in vascular smooth muscle cells. *Circ Res*, **81**: 17–23, 1997.

65. Paka S, Obunike JC, Kako Y, *et al*. Apo E stimulates endothelial production heparan sulfate rich in biologically active heparin-like domains. *J Biol Chem*, **274**: 4816–4823, 1999.

66. Aplin AE, Howe AK, Juliano RL. Cell adhesion molecules, signal transduction and cell growth. *Curr Opin Cell Biol*, **11**: 737–744, 1999.

67. Koyama N, Kinsella MG, Wight TN, *et al*. Heparan sulfate proteoglycans mediate a potent inhibitory signal for migration of vascular smooth muscle cells. *Circ Res*, **83**: 305–313, 1998.

68. Fuji N, Kaji T, Akai T, *et al*. Thrombin reduces large heparan sulfate proteoglycan molecules in cultured vascular endothelial cell layers through inhibition of core protein synthesis. *Thromb Res*, **88**: 299–307, 1997.

69. Brown CT, Nugent MA, Lau FW, *et al*. Characterization of proteoglycans synthesized by cultured corneal fibroblasts in response to transforming growth factor beta and fetal calf serum. *J Biol Chem*, **274**: 7111–7119, 1999.

70. Stern DM, Esposito C, Gerlach H, *et al*. Endothelium and regulation of coagulation. *Diabetes Care*, **14** [Suppl 1]: 160–166, 1991.

71. Witmer MR, Hadcock SJ, Peltier, *et al*. Altered levels of antithrombin III and fibrinogen in the aortic wall of the alloxan-induced diabetic rabbit: evidence of a prothrombotic state. *J Lab Clin Med*, **119**: 221–230, 1992.

72. Ceriello A. Coagulation activation in diabetes mellitus: the role of hyperglycaemia and therapeutic prospects. *Diabetologia*, **36**: 1119–1125, 1993.

73. Ceriello A, Taboga C, Giacomello R, *et al*. Fibrinogen plasma levels as a marker of thrombin activation in diabetes. *Diabetes*, **43**: 430–432, 1994.

74. Ceriello A. Fibrinogen and diabetes mellitus: is it time for intervention trials? *Diabetologia*, **40**: 731–734, 1997.

75. Böhm T, Geiger M, Binder BR. Isolation and characterization of tissue type plasminogen activator-binding proteoglycans from human umbilical vein endothelial cells. *Arterioscler Thromb Vasc Biol*, **16**: 665–672, 1996.

76. Condorelli M, Chiariello M, Dagianti A *et al*. IPO-V2: a prospective, multicenter, randomized, comparative clinical investigation of the effects of sulodexide in preventing cardiovascular accidents in the first year after acute myocardial infarction. *J Am Coll Cardiol*, **23**: 27–34, 1994.

77. Coccheri S, Scondotto G, Agnelli G. Sulodexide in the treatment of intermittent claudication. *European Heart Journal*, **23**: 1057–1065, 2002.

78. Gaddi A, Galetti C, Illuminati B, Nascetti S. Meta-analysis of some results of clinical trials on sulodexide therapy in Peripheral Occlusive Arterial Disease. *J Intl Med Res*, **24**: 389–406, 1996.

79. Cooper Me, Gilbert RE, Jerums G. Diabetic vascular complications. *Clin Exp Pharmacol Physiol*, **24**: 770–775, 1997.

80. Parthasarathy N, Spiro R. Effect of diabetes on the glycosaminoglycan component of the human

glomerular basement membrane. *Diabetes,* **31**: 738–741, 1982.

81. Shimomura H, Spiro R. Studies on macromolecular components of human glomerular basement membrane and alterations in diabetes: Decreased levels of heparan sulfate proteoglycans and laminin. *Diabetes,* **36**: 374–381, 1987.

82. Vernier RL, Steffes MW, Sissons-Ross S, *et al.* Heparan sulfate proteoglycan in the glomerular basement membrane in type I diabetes mellitus. *Kidney Int,* **41**: 1070–1080, 1992.

83. Tamsma JT, van den Born J, Bruijn JA, *et al.* Expression of glomerular extracellular matrix components in human diabetic nephropathy: Decrease of heparan sulphate in the glomerular basement membrane. *Diabetologia,* **37**: 313–320, 1994.

84. Van der Pijl JW, Daha MR, Van den Born J, *et al.* Extracellular matrix in human diabetic nephropathy: Reduced expression of heparan sulphate in skin basement membrane. *Diabetologia,* **41**: 791–798, 1998.

85. Cohen MP, Surma ML. 35S sulfate incorporation into glomerular basement membrane glycosaminoglycans is decreased in experimental diabetes. *J Lab Clin Med,* **98**: 715–722, 1981.

86. Brown DM, Klein DJ, Michael AF, *et al.* 35S-glycosaminoglycan and 35S glycopeptide metabolism by diabetic glomeruli and aorta. *Diabetes,* **31**: 418–425, 1995.

87. Kanwar YS, Rosenzweig LJ, Linker A, *et al.* Decreased de novo synthesis of glomerular proteoglycans in diabetes: Biochemical and autoradiographic evidence. *Proc Natl Acad Sci USA,* **80**: 2272–2275, 1983.

88. Iozzo RV, Cohen IR, Grassel S, Murdoch AD. The biology of perlecan: The multifaceted heparan sulphate proteoglycan of basement membranes and pericellular matrices. *Biochem J,* **302**: 625–639, 1994.

89. Van der Woude FJ, van Det NF. Heparan sulphate proteoglycans and diabetic nephropathy. *Exp Nephrol,* **5**: 180–188, 1997.

90. Van Det NF, van den Born J, Tamsma JT, *et al.* Effects of high glucose on the production of heparan sulfate proteoglycan by human mesangial and glomerular visceral epithelial cells *in vitro. Kidney Int,* **49**: 1079–1089, 1996.

91. Gambaro G, Cavazzana AO, Luzi P, *et al.* Glycosaminoglycans prevent morphological renal alterations and albuminuria in diabetic rats. *Kidney Int,* **42**: 285–29, 1992.

92. Gambaro G, Venturini AP, Noonan, DM, *et al.* Treatment with a glycosaminoglycan formulation ameliorates experimental diabetic nephropathy. *Kidney Int,* **46**: 797–806, 1994.

93. Gambaro G, Baggio B. Heparin and diabetic nephropathy. *Am J Physiol,* **274**: E192, 1998.

94. Oshima Y, Isogai S, Mogama K, *et al.* Protective effect of heparin on renal glomerular anionic sites of streptozocin-injected rats. *Diabetes Res Clin Pract.* **25**: 83–89, 1995.

95. Oturai PS, Rasch R, Hasseleger E, *et al.* Effect of heparin and aminoguanidine on glomerular basement membrane thickening in diabetic rats. *Acta Patol Microbiol Immunol Scand.* **104**: 259–264, 1996.

96. Gambaro G. Glycosaminoglycans in the pathogenesis and treatment of diabetic nephropathy. In: *Highlights of Satellite Symposium "Diabetic microangiopathy and sulodexide".* Adis International, Milan, 2001: 12–19.

97. Ceol M, Nerlich A, Baggio B, *et al.* Increased glomerular a1(IV) collagen expression and deposition in long-term diabetic rats is prevented by chronic glycosaminoglycan treatment. *Lab Invest,* **74**: 484–495, 1996.

98. Yamamoto T, Nakamura T, Noble NA, *et al.* Expression of transforming growth factor beta is elevated in human and experimental diabetic nephropathy. *Proc Natl acad Sci,* **90**: 1814–1818, 1993.

99. Myrup B, Hansen PM, Jensen T, *et al.* Effect of low-dose heparin on urinary albumin excretion in insulin dependent diabetes mellitus. *Lancet,* **345**: 421–422, 1995.

100. Ketteler M, Noble NA, Border WA. Transforming growth factor-b and angiotensin II. The missing link from glomerular hyperfiltration and glomerulo-sclerosis? *Annu Rev Physiol,* **57**: 279–295, 1995.

101. Tamsma JT, van der Voude FJ, Lemkes HHPJ. Effect of sulfated glycosaminoglycans on albuminuria in patients with overt diabetic (type-1) nephropathy. *Nephrol Dial Transplant,* **11**: 182–185, 1996.

102. Van der Pijl JW, van der Woude FJ, Geelhoed-Duijvestijn PHLM, *et al.* Danaparoid sodium lowers proteinuria in diabetic nephropathy. *J Am Soc Nephrol,* **8**: 456–462, 1997.

103. Skrha J, Perusicova J, Pontuch P, *et al.* Glycos-aminoglycan sulodexide decreases albuminuria in diabetic patients. *Diabetes Res Clin Pract,* **38**: 25–31, 1997.

104. Poplawska A, Szelachowska M, Topolska J, *et al.* Effect of glycosaminoglycans on urinary albumin excretion in insulin-dependent diabetic patients with micro- or macroalbuminuria. *Diabetes Res Clin Pract,* **38**: 109–114, 1997.

105. Szelanowska M, Poplawska A, Jopdska J, *et al.* A pilot study of the effect of the glycosaminoglycan sulodexide on microalbuminuria in type I diabetic patients. *Curr Med Res Opin,* **13**: 539–545, 1997.

106. Manitius J, *et al.* Albuminuria reduction by oral sulodexide in micro- and macroalbuminuric DM 1 and DM 2 diabetic patients: The Di. N.A.S. trial. In: *Highlights of Satellite Symposium "Diabetic microangiopathy and sulodexide".* Adis International, Milan, 2001: 20–23.

107. Rubbi F. The effects of sulodexide on diabetic retinopathy. In: *Highlights of Satellite Symposium "Diabetic microangiopathy and sulodexide".* Adis International, Milan, 2001: 24–27.

108. Bollinieni JS, Alluru I, Reddi AS. Heparan sulfate proteoglycan synthesis and its expression are decreased in the retina of diabetic rats. *Curr Eye Res,* **16**:127–130, 1997.

109. Cruickshanks KJ, Ritter LL, Klein R, *et al.* The association of microalbuminuria with diabetic retinopathy. The Wisconsin Epidemiologic Study Of Diabetic Retinopathy. *Ophthalmology,* **100**: 862–867, 1993.

110. Savage S. Estacio RO, Jeffers B, *et al.* Urinary albumin excretion as a predictor of diabetic retinopathy, neuropathy and cardiovascular disease in NIDDM. *Diabetes Care,* **19**(11): 1243–1248, 1996.

37

PROTECTION FROM THE VASCULAR COMPLICATIONS OF DIABETES, INDEPENDENT OF GLYCAEMIC CONTROL: THE ROLE OF GLICLAZIDE

Paul JENNINGS

Diabetic vascular disease or angiopathy is a combination of the microvascular processes that are unique to diabetes and the macrovascular processes that lead to accelerated atherosclerosis and premature death. Both micro- and macro-angiopathy share factors in common such as changes in endothelial cell structure and function, enhanced platelet reactivity and an increase in oxidative stress which may all be properties of free radical reactions. Lipid peroxides, which are products of free radical reactions, also modulate the arachidonic acid cascade demonstrating a relationship between oxidative stress and the thrombotic tendency.

Gliclazide is a second-generation sulphonylurea with a unique structure due to its amino-AZA bicyclo[3.3.0] octane ring which has been grafted onto the molecule. Gliclazide not only lowers blood glucose, but also has been shown *in vitro* to be a general free radical scavenger. Gliclazide is also effective against the formation of oxidised low density lipoprotein cholesterol as elucidated by a series of studies both *in vitro* and *in vivo*. An expanding body of research has examined the effects of gliclazide on vascular function, specifically vascular permeability and endothelium-dependent relaxation. These basic research studies have been supported clinically by demonstrations of beneficial effects on lipid peroxidation and other aspects of free radical activity have been found to be independent of effects on glycaemic control. These studies offer a possible explanation as to observations which have noted clinical end-points such as proliferative retinopathy, to be seen less commonly in patients treated with gliclazide. Therefore, using gliclazide for its haemovascular properties independent of its hypoglycaemic action, have demonstrated improvements in the abnormalities in oxidative stress, hyper-coagulability, endothelial function and platelet function, which have not been demonstrated by other sulphonylureas.

INTRODUCTION

Vascular disease is the major cause of morbidity and mortality in type 2 diabetes. The development of diabetic complications is positively associated with prolonged hyperglycaemia, hence poorly controlled long duration diabetic patients are more likely to suffer vascular disease than well controlled patients. Improving diabetic control is now well established to prevent complications and delay the progression of vascular disease [1,2]. Gliclazide, a second generation sulphonylurea, has been used in similar studies in different populations and has been demonstrated to maintain diabetic control for at least five years of maintenance therapy [3]. Furthermore, the use of gliclazide in a randomised intensive multifactorial management regime demonstrates its role in reducing the progression to nephropathy of a group of microalbuminuric type 2 diabetic patients [4]. During the 3.8 years of the study, significant reductions in the risk of progression of retinopathy, autonomic neuropathy and peripheral vascular disease occurred. These studies refer back to earlier evidence that gliclazide may have vascular protective properties independent of its hypoglycaemic actions.

Diabetic vascular disease or angiopathy is a combination of the microvascular processes that are unique to diabetes and the process that leads to accelerated atherosclerosis and premature death. Many factors have been implicated in the development of complications including functional abnormalities within the microcirculation, the physiological consequences of enhanced glucose metabolism *via* different pathways of non-glycolytic metabolism and genetic susceptibility. Both micro- and macro-angiopathy share common factors such as changes in endothelial cell structure and function, enhanced platelet reactivity and an increase in oxidative stress. However, damage to endothelial cells, modification of platelet reactivity and modulation of the arachidonic acid cascade are all properties of free radicals and their reaction products, the lipid peroxides [5]. Lipid peroxides also modulate the arachidonic acid cascade reducing the synthesis of prostacyclin whilst stimulating cyclooxygenase to promote platelet production of thromboxane A2 [6]. This demonstrates there is a relationship between oxidative stress and the thrombotic tendency.

OXIDATIVE STRESS

Oxidative stress occurs when there is an imbalance between oxygen derived free radical production and scavenging. Free radicals are naturally produced by normal metabolism, but are scavenged effectively. In diabetes, however, several factors lead to an increase in the production of free radicals and a reduction in the ability to scavenge them, leading to oxidative stress. Evidence for the involvement of reactive oxygen species in type 1 and type 2 diabetes has recently been reviewed [7]. There is considerable evidence that diabetic patients are under oxidative stress [8]. Most early evidence came from measurement of lipid peroxidation [9], protein modification [10], evidence of DNA damage and lower anti-oxidant defences. Superoxide dismutase (SOD), for example, is a specific anti-oxidant which is widespread but its activity is impaired by glycosylation [8]. Also, glutathione in its reduced form detoxifies organic peroxides. Following this reaction the then oxidised glutathione is rapidly reduced back to its active form by reactions utilising NADPH. NADPH is a key element formed by a series of oxidation and reduction reactions known as "redox cycling". NADPH may be lacking in hyperglycaemia as it is a co-factor for aldose reductase in the polyol pathway [11]. The polyol pathway is of particular relevance in insulin insensitive tissues (retina, lens, nerve, etc.) where hyperglycaemia drives the over-expression of the enzyme aldose reductase which converts glucose to sorbitol. Consumption of NADPH by increased flux through this pathway leaves insufficient remaining to regenerate antioxidants such as glutathione or vitamin C and leaves the tissues susceptible to free reactive oxygen species attack.

ADVANCED GLYCOSYLATION END-PRODUCTS AND ENDOTHELIAL CELL FUNCTION

While inducing oxidative stress, hyperglycaemia leads to the accumulation of advanced glycosylation end-products (AGE) as well. The process leading to protein glycosylation generates free radicals and further reaction products that react with nitric oxide (NO). The reaction with NO prevents its usual vasodilator and anti-coagulant actions. AGE modification of proteins in the vascular wall also changes its structure and function, leading to, for example, trapping of proteins and immunoglobulins and a loss of elasticity. The AGE modification of low density lipoprotein promotes its up-take by macrophages leading to the formation of foam cells which are important in the development of atherosclerotic plaques [12].

Both oxidative stress and AGE have been linked to endothelial cell dysfunction, particularly to an imbalance that has led to defective endothelium dependant vasodilatation and increased endothelium dependant vasoconstriction. The evidence supporting the abnormalities in vascular function in type 2 diabetes has recently been reviewed [13]. One of the most important factors leading to impaired vasodilatation is a decrease in nitric oxide, which is known to be quenched by free radicals, thereby preventing nitric oxide to diffuse effectively to target smooth muscle cells. This abnormality can be reversed by adding free radical scavengers in studies on isolated blood vessels from diabetic animals [14].

Other factors responsible for abnormalities of vascular endothelium in type 2 diabetes include abnormalities of tumour necrosis factor-alpha, transforming growth factor-beta and vascular endothelial growth factor. Yet, in addition to the abnormalities of the vascular endothelium is the demonstration that diabetic patients are in a hypercoagulable state. There is a shift in the balance between coagulation and fibrinolysis, several different mechanisms contributing to these abnormalities [15]. Type 2 diabetic patients have elevated levels of fibrinogen, coagulation factors and inhibitors of plasminogen activation. Some patients have low levels of plasminogen activator which is important in fibrinolysis [16]. In addition, the fibrin network within clots may be altered in diabetic patients making this network more resistant to fibrinolysis [17]. So, there is evidence that diabetic patients exhibit a shift in the balance between coagulation and fibrinolysis towards increased blood clot formation. Furthermore, the platelets in diabetic patients are hyper-reactive showing a greater than normal tendency to adhere and aggregate [18]. This factor may well be attributed to increased oxidative stress due to the known effects of lipid peroxidation on the

thromboxane to prostacyclin ratio. They modulate the arachidonic acid cascade reducing the synthesis of prostacyclin whilst stimulating cyclooxygenase to promote platelet production of thromboxane A2 [6, 19]. On the other hand, nitric oxide, which normally inhibits platelet activation, is not as available in diabetes because of the reduced output of NO by the endothelial cells.

Hence, in type 2 diabetes, there is a substantial body of evidence showing increased free radical production and reduced anti-oxidant defences, with the promotion of LDL cholesterol oxidation. This, associated with AGE depositing around the blood vessels, is linked to dysfunction of the endothelial cells both structurally and functionally, with reduced production of NO, impaired vasodilatation and increased platelet aggregation. A highly pro-thrombotic situation is thus induced. This pathological process is clearly manifested in the diabetic patient by the widespread microvascular changes, readily appreciated in the retina and kidney. In addition, these changes promote accelerated atherosclerosis which is the main reason for the reduced life expectation in patients with type 2 diabetes. Vascular abnormalities can be changed or even eliminated by maintaining normal blood glucose levels, as has been demonstrated in the landmark clinical studies DCCT [2] and the UK PDS [1].

NON-GLYCAEMIC EFFECTS OF GLICLAZIDE

Gliclazide is a second-generation sulphonylurea with a unique structure due to its amino-AZA bicyclo[3.3.0]-octane ring which has been grafted onto the molecule. Hence, gliclazide not only lowers blood glucose but also has been shown *in vitro* to be a general free radical scavenger. The similarity of this ring structure to hydrazine (H_2N-NH_2) [20] which has been demonstrated recently to scavenge radicals and interfere with lipid peroxidation, gives a molecular basis for the *in vitro* demonstrations of its antioxidant properties at therapeutic concentrations. Gliclazide was initially demonstrated to be a general free-radical scavenger by its ability to inhibit the photo-oxidation of dianisidine with concentrations well below the expected therapeutic level [21].

Glibenclamide and other sulphonylureas however have no free radical scavenging effect even at very high concentrations *in vitro*. This effect against specific reactive oxygen species has been assayed using electron spin resonance spectroscopy [22] showing that not only did gliclazide scavenge the superoxide radical but also it was effective against the more reactive hydroxyl radical. Again this was in a dose dependent manner, whereas glibenclamide was not effective.

One of the major causes of the accelerated atherosclerosis in type 2 diabetes is the enhanced formation of oxidised low-density lipoprotein (LDL). Gliclazide is effective against the formation of oxidised low density lipoprotein cholesterol, as elucidated by a series of studies both *in vitro* and *in vivo*. Gliclazide reduces the chemically induced oxidation of LDL taken from diabetic patients in a manner similar to that seen with vitamin C in contrast to other sulphonylureas which had no effect [23]. In a clinical study type 2 diabetic patients previously poorly controlled on glibenclamide, (with HbA1c levels greater than 9%), were switched to an equipotent dose of gliclazide for 3 months' treatment. All patients were also taking metformin throughout this study before and after the exchange of therapy. Lipid peroxide levels, serum cytokine levels, monocyte cytokine production and monocyte adhesion to endothelial cells were assessed and compared with results from healthy non-smoking control subjects matched for sex and body mass index. Both high lipid peroxide levels and monocyte adhesion to endothelial cells were completely reversed by gliclazide treatment and an associated reduction in production of the pro-atherogenic tumour necrosis factor-α was observed [24]. Subsequently, an *in vitro* study employing human monocytes and cultured human endothelial cells extended these findings [25]. Incubation of these cells in the presence of glycated albumin was associated with a time-dependent increase in monocyte adhesion, which could be significantly reduced by pre-incubation with gliclazide in therapeutic concentration. A probable molecular mechanism for the inhibition of monocyte adhesion by gliclazide was suggested by demonstration of marked reductions in induction of both soluble and cell-associated adhesion molecules: ELAM-1, ICAM-1 and VCAM-1. Inhibition of expression of these adhesion molecules by gliclazide appeared to be exerted at the transcriptional level, as a concurrent suppressive effect on the activation of the transcriptional factor NF-κB was observed.

An expanding body of research has examined the effects of gliclazide on vascular function, specifically vascular permeability and endothelium-dependent relaxation. The effects of gliclazides on the capillary macromolecular permeability and reactivity were studied in a hamster cheek-pouch preparation [26]. Gliclazide, applied topically, dose-dependently inhibited increases in vascular permeability induced both by histamine in non-diabetic hamsters and by ischaemia/re-perfusion in streptozotocin-treated hamsters with no residual pancreatic function. No changes in glycaemia were observed in either model and in the post-ischaemic model the effect of gliclazide was comparable to that of equimolar vitamin C, supporting the hypothesis that reduced vascular permeability is a glycaemia-independent effect mediated *via* reduction in oxidative stress.

Another similar animal model of diabetes [27], the alloxan-treated rabbit, was employed to further study the effects of gliclazide on the vasculature. Again, gliclazide had no effect on glycaemia or insulinaemia in this model, so any effect identified can be considered glycaemia-independent. Relaxation responses of sections of pre-contracted aorta were recorded in a number of experimental conditions, before and after 6 weeks treatment with gliclazide at 10mg/kg/day. Diabetes was associated with significant impairment of acetylcholine-induced endothelium-dependent relaxation of the abdominal aorta, these responses being restored to a level that was not different from non-diabetic controls during gliclazide treatment. Similarly, augmented aortic contractions to acetylcholine in the presence of the NO synthase inhibitor, L-NAME, were significantly reduced by gliclazide to a level that was not different from that of normal rabbits.

This effect of gliclazide appears to be specific to the abnormality arising in diabetes, as 6 weeks' gliclazide treatment of non-diabetic rabbits did not affect vessel responses.

Dose-dependent improvement of diabetic endothelial dysfunction by gliclazide has also been observed in human microvessels [28]. Omental microvessels were obtained from non-diabetic, normotensive, non-smokers undergoing surgical intervention (Plate 37.1).

Glycated oxyhaemoglobin at 10% or more was found to inhibit relaxation responses of pre-contracted vessels to bradykinin, this effect appearing to be NO-mediated, as it mirrored the effects seen with L-NAME, but not with indomethacin, in the same model. The impaired relaxation induced by glycated oxyhaemoglobin could be dose-dependently inhibited by gliclazide in concentrations within the therapeutic range, or by either equimolar vitamin C or superoxide dismutase at 100 U/L.

Neither glibenclamide nor indomethacin alone showed any effect on impaired relaxation responses. Besides showing for the first time a deleterious effect of glycated haemoglobin on endothelial function in human vessels, these data support the view that gliclazide has its protective effect on the endothelium *via* reduction of oxidative stress, thus preserving NO-mediated vessel relaxation responses.

NORMALISING THE PROTHROMBOTIC TENDENCY

Thromboxane A_2 (TXA$_2$) is a potent platelet derived vasoconstrictor that is promoted by the effects of lipid peroxides on the arachidonic acid cascade. This is done by modulating the arachidonic acid cascade, reducing the synthesis of prostacyclin whilst stimulating cyclooxygenase to promote platelet production of thromboxane A_2 [6]. This demonstrates there is a relationship between oxidative stress and the thrombotic tendency, which may be important in the development of vascular complications. Studies in animals have indicated that gliclazide corrects this balance. This was further supported in a Chinese study looking at the effect of gliclazide on the balance between thromboxane and prostacyclin. This used a study design where patients crossed over from glibenclamide to gliclazide. Diabetic control at three months remained constant both fasting plasma glucose and insulin levels had not changed but the TXA$_2$: prostacyclin ratio decreased almost to the normal range in the gliclazide treated patients [29]. Similarly, an open study looking at the effect on not only thromboxane, but also on parameters of free radical activity such as lipid peroxidation, again documented a decline in the

vasoconstrictor TXA$_2$ together with a decline in lipid peroxides, which was independent of glycaemic control [30].

IMPROVING OXIDATIVE STRESS

The hypothesis that the beneficial haemovascular effects were secondary to its free radical scavenging and independent of glycaemic control was further investigated in a blinded glibenclamide controlled study over a six month period [31]. (Plate 37.2). In this study 30 type 2 patients were studied, 20 were male of a mean age 58. All patients had been treated for diabetes for more than 2 years (mean 8 years) and had been established on glibenclamide for at least two years, with or without adjunctive metformin. On entering into the study half the patients were randomly allocated to change to gliclazide at equipotent dose to those remaining on glibenclamide. At 3 months, diabetic control was unaltered, but there were significant improvements in the oxidative status of the gliclazide-treated patients.

Lipid peroxides decreased (8.3 ± 1.1 to 7.0 ± 0.6 µmol, $P < 0.01$) and red blood cell SOD increased (135 ± 21 to 152 ± 36 µg/mL, $P < 0.05$). PSH levels were unaltered at 458 ± 38 µmol/L, while they had decreased significantly in the glibenclamide patients (414 ± 34 µmol/L, $P < 0.05$), resulting in a significant difference between the two treatment groups ($P < 0.004$). Platelet reactivity to collagen also improved in the gliclazide-treated patients, decreasing from $65.1\% \pm 14\%$ to $50.8\% \pm 24\%$ ($P < 0.01$). The reactivity of the platelets remained unaltered in the glibenclamide patients. At 6 months, the significant differences between the two treatment groups remained, although there were no further improvements in the gliclazide patients (Plate 37.3).

Similar clinical effects were seen during a recent study in 45 diabetic patients over 10 months using both the standard and the new sustained release formulation of gliclazide. In this study 8-isoprostanes, a maker of lipid peroxidation, fell significantly together with improvements in the antioxidant properties of the patients [32]. Interestingly, oxidative parameters continued to fall throughout the study, despite a plateau in glycaemic control after 4 months of treatment. (Table 37.1).

Table 37.1

Reduction in oxidative stress demonstrated in a study using modified-release preparation of gliclazide [32]

	n	Baseline	4 months	10 months	P value*
8-Isoprostanes (pg/ml)	19	158±65	81±52	14±4.1	<0.001
TPAC (mmol/Ltrolox)	18	0.69±0.06	0.84±0.07	0.88±0.05	0.03
SOD (U/Hb/L)	16	453±46	569±60	684±37	0.01
Thiols (mmol/L)	12	0.61±0,02	0.64±0.01	0.76±0.03	<0.001

* Statistical analysis performed using Friedman (nonparametric) test

EFFECTS OF GLICLAZIDE ON HAEMOSTATIC VARIABLES

The clinical studies [30, 31] also showed that gliclazide had an effect at reducing the hyper-reactivity of the platelets. This was first shown in a short-term study in 1982 on 18 diabetic patients treated for 30 days [33]. This initial study monitored platelet function in isolation determining the minimum dose of adenosine diphosphate (ADP) required to induce irreversible platelet aggregation *in vitro* both before and after gliclazide treatment. After 30 days of treatment with gliclazide, the dose of ADP required was significantly higher than at baseline, and was close to normal. The other studies either used reaction products released from platelets upon activation [30] or relied on the more physiological effects of collagen on platelet numbers in whole blood [31].

In addition to these effects seen in the clinical studies on platelet activity and free radicals, benefits have also been shown in correcting the imbalance seen between blood coagulation and fibrinolysis. For example patients switched from chlorpropamide to gliclazide normalised their previously low vascular plasminogen activator activity and the inhibitors of plasminogen activator were significantly reduced after 48 months of therapy [34]. A similar study showed significant improvements in TPA activity in patients previously treated with tolbutamide [16].

Tolbutamide-treated type 2 diabetic patients were switched from their previous treatment to gliclazide for 12 months [14]. Sustained increases in tissue-type plasminogen activator (t-PA) activity were seen in those with no detectable t-PA activity at baseline. Interestingly, no changes in this variable were observed in a subgroup of patients with marked t-PA activity at baseline. As plasminogen activator inhibitor (PAI-1) remained constant throughout the study, increased endothelial cell production or release of t-PA was thought likely, this theory being supported by a significant increase in t-PA antigen following venous occlusion. As metabolic control was unchanged during the study, this effect seems to be glycaemia-independent, further evidence for this coming from another study showing increased activity of both t-PA and pre-kallikrein during 6 months of treatment of male type 1 diabetics with gliclazide [35].

Other effects of gliclazide on the thrombotic process include alterations in fibrin structure and fibrinolysis seen during treatment. *Ex vivo* studies were performed in platelet-free plasma from diabetic subjects and age, sex-matched controls [17]. In plasma from uncontrolled diabetics, using turbidity and permeability measures, reduced fibrin fiber thickness and permeability of fibrin networks were found, this being attributed to inhibition of lateral polymerisation, and probably related to glycation of plasma proteins including fibrinogen. This altered fibrin network structure is associated with resistance to lysis [36]. Pre-treatment with a therapeutic concentration of gliclazide was found to significantly increase fibrin fiber thickness, diminish tensile strength and reduce permeability. These effects were attributed to enhanced lateral polymerisation and enhanced cross-linking within the network and were not reproduced by metformin, glibenclamide or insulin pre-treatment. Gliclazide was also

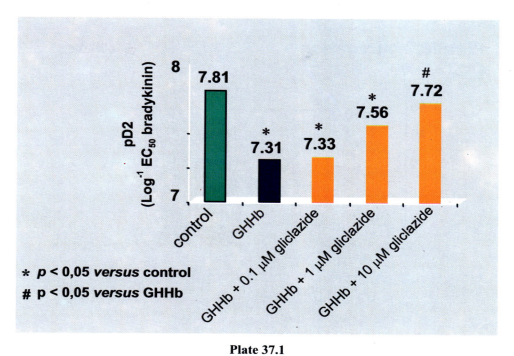

Plate 37.1
Effect of gliclazide on endothelial dysfunction (expressed as pD_2 values for bradykinin [28]).

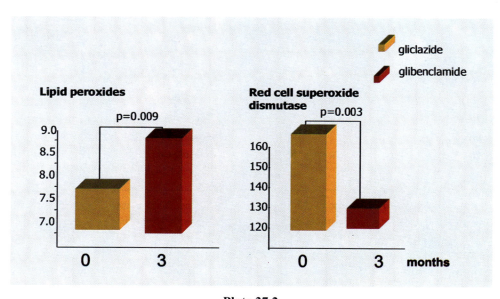

Plate 37.2
Effect of sulphonylurea treatment on lipid peroxide levels and superoxide dismutase activity over the first 3 months of study [31].

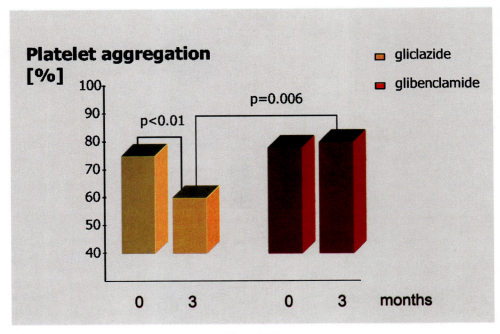

Plate 37.3

Platelet aggregation significantly decreased in the gliclazide group compared to baseline values and to glibenclamide group at 3 months. This was maintained for 6 months [31].

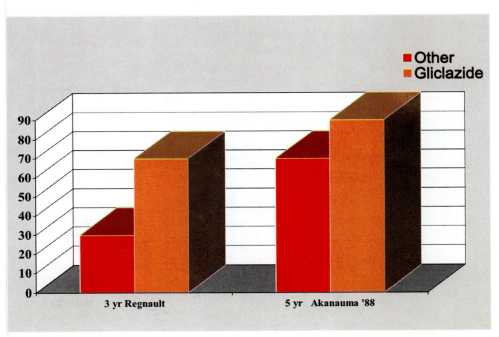

Plate 37.4

The percentage of patients showing improvement or stabilisation in retinal appearances during clinical studies comparing sulphonylurea treatments (all p<0.05) [37, 38].

associated with some enhancement of fibrinolysis in this model, this fitting in with previous results from several studies specifically dedicated to fibrinolytic activity in diabetes and the effect of gliclazide treatment.

CLINICAL EFFECT OF GLICLAZIDE ON VASCULAR COMPLICATIONS

Using gliclazide for its haemovascular properties, independent of its hypoglycaemic action, has demonstrated improvements in the abnormalities in oxidative stress, hyper-coagulability, endothelial function and platelet reactivity which has not been demonstrated by other sulphonylureas. This may have clinical relevance as suggested by the Japanese Retinopathy Programme, which in studying the progression of retinopathy over a five year period, found a lower rate of deterioration of retinopathy with significantly lower incidence of pre-proliferative retinopathy occurring in the group of patients receiving gliclazide, compared to other patients despite equivalent metabolic control [37]. This finding followed on from an interesting early study where, over a mean follow-up period of 39 months, patients randomised to gliclazide had fewer capillary occlusions and microaneurysms than glibenclamide-treated patients. That this was a glycaemia independent finding was further suggested by the small subgroup of type 1 patients that showed similar results [38] (Plate 37.4).

CONCLUSION

Much of the morbidity and mortality of type 2 diabetes is due to the micro- and macro-vascular abnormalities. The changes that are induced by prolonged hyperglycaemia are wide ranging. Fundamental to these, are the changes induced by excess reactive oxygen species. This increase in free radical activity coupled to an impairment of anti-oxidant defences produces changes to the function of the endothelium and the endothelial cells which may be central to the process leading to end stage vascular disease. These vascular complications can be prevented or their progression slowed by achieving good diabetic control. Yet, in type 2 diabetes, clinical benefits have been difficult to demonstrate because of the multi-factorial nature of large vessel complications such as ischaemic

heart disease in particular. Nevertheless, improving the oxidative status of patients by using gliclazide for its haemovascular properties independent of its hypoglycaemic action, has demonstrated improvements in the abnormalities in oxidative stress, hyper-coagulability, endothelial function and platelet reactivity which has not been demonstrated by other sulphonylureas. Therefore, in type 2 diabetes where hyperglycaemia and oxidation are fundamental to the ultimate thrombotic complications of diabetes, agents such as gliclazide with anti-oxidant activities in addition to hypoglycaemic actions may have an enhanced therapeutic role.

REFERENCES

1. UKPDS. UK Prospective Diabetes Study (UKPDS) Group. Intensive blood glucose control with sulphonylureas or insulin compared with conventional treatment and risk of complications in patients with type 2 diabetes (UKPDS 33). *Lancet*, **352**: 837–853, 1998.
2. DCCT. The Diabetes Control and Complications Trial Research Group. The effect of intensive treatment of diabetes on the development and progression of long-term complications in insulin-dependent diabetes mellitus. *N Engl J Med*, **329**: 977–986, 1993.
3. Guillausseau P-J. An evaluation of long-term glycaemic control in non-insulin dependent diabetes mellitus: the relevance of glycated hemoglobin. *Am J Med*, **90**(6A): 46–49, 1991.
4. Gaede P, Vedel P, Parving H-H, Pedersen O. Intensified multifactorial intervention in patients with type 2 diabetes mellitus and microalbuminuria: the Steno type 2 diabetes study. *Lancet*, **353**: 617–622, 1999.
5. Procter PH, Reynolds ES. Free radicals and disease in man. *Physiol Chem Phys*, **16**: 175–195, 1984.
6. Warso MA, Lands WEM. Lipid Peroxidation in relation to Prostacyclin and thromboxane physiology. *Br Med Bull* **39**: 277–280, 1983.
7. West CI. Radicals in oxidative stress in diabetes. *Diabetic Medicine,* **17**: 171–180, 2000.
8. Wolff SP. The potential role of oxidative stress in diabetes and its complications; novel implications for theory and therapy. In: Crabbe MJC (ed). *Diabetic complications; Scientific and clinical aspects,* Churchill Livingstone, Edinburgh, 1987, 167–221.
9. Jennings PE, Jones AF, Florkowski CKM, Lunec J, Barnett AH. Increased diene conjugates in diabetic subjects with microangiopathy. *Diabetic Medicine,* **5**: 111–117, 1988.

10. Jones AF, Jennings PE, Wakefield A, Winkles JW, Lunec J, Barnett AH. The fluorescence of serum proteins in diabetes mellitus. Relationship to microangiopathy. *Diabetic Medicine*, **5**: 547–551, 1988.

11. Cogan DG. Aldose Reductase and complications of diabetes. *Annal Int Med*, **101**: 82–91, 1984.

12. Brownlee M, Vlassara H, Cerami A. The pathogenetic role of non-enzymatic glycosylation in diabetic complications. In: Crabbe MJC (ed). *Diabetic complications; Scientific and clinical aspects*, Churchill Livingstone, Edinburgh, 1987, 94–139.

13. Tooke JE, Goh KL. Vascular function in type 2 diabetes mellitus and pre-diabetes: The case for intrinsic endotheliopathy. *Diabetic Medicine*, **16**: 710–715, 1999.

14. Tesfamariam B, Cohen RA. Free radicals mediate endothelial cell dysfunction caused by elevated glucose. *Am J Physiol*, **262**: H321–H326, 1992.

15. Grant PJ. Risk factors for arterial disease in diabetes: coagulopathy. In: Tooke JE (ed). *Diabetic Angiopathy*, Arnold, London, 1999, 93–111.

16. Gram J, Kold A, Jespersen J. Rise of plasma t-PA fibrinolytic activity in a group of maturity onset diabetic patients shifted from a first generation (tolbutamide) to a second generation sulphonylurea (gliclazide). *J Intern Med*, **225**: 241–247, 1989.

17. Nair CH, Azhar A, Wilson JD, Dhall DP. Studies on fibrin network structure in human plasma. Part II – clinical application: diabetes and antidiabetic drugs. *Thromb Res*, **64**: 477–485, 1991.

18. Wincour PD. Platelet abnormalities in diabetes mellitus. *Diabetes*, **41**: 26–31, 1992.

19. Davi G, Catalano I, Averna M. Thromboxane biosynthesis and platelet function in type II diabetes mellitus. *N Engl J Med*, **322**: 1769–1774, 1990.

20. Zhou S, Dickinson LC, Yang Li, Decker EA. Identification of hydrazine in commercial preparations of carnosine and its influence on carnosine's antioxidative properties. *Analyst Biochem*, **261**: 79–86, 1998.

21. Scott NA, Jennings PE, Brown J, Belch JJF. Gliclazide a free radical scavenger. Eur J *Pharm*, **208**: 175–177, 1991.

22. Noda Y, Mori A, Packer L. Gliclazide scavenges hydroxyl, superoxide and nitric oxide radicals: an ESR study. *Res Comm Mol Pathol Pharmacol*, **96**: 115–124, 1997.

23. O'Brien RC, Luo M. The effects of gliclazide and other sulfonylureas on low-density lipoprotein oxidation *in vitro*. *Metabolism*, **46**: 1–5, 1997.

24. Desfaits A-C, Serri O, Renier G. Normalization of plasma lipid peroxides, monocyte adhesion and tumour necrosis factor-alpha production in NIDDM patients after gliclazide treatment. *Diabetes Care*, **21**: 487–493, 1998.

25. Desfaits A-C, Serri O, Renier G. Gliclazide reduces the induction of human monocyte adhesion to endothelial cells by glycated albumin. *Diabet Obes Metab*, **1**: 113–120, 1999.

26. Bouskela E, Cyrino F, Conde C, Garcia A. Microvascular permeability with sulfonylureas in normal and diabetic hamsters. *Metabolism*, **46**: 26–30, 1997.

27. Pagano PJ, Griswold MC, Ravel D, Cohen RA. Vascular action of gliclazide in diabetic rabbits. *Diabetologia*, **41**: 9–15, 1998.

28. Vallejo S, Angulo J, Peiró C. Highly glycosylated oxyhaemoglobin impairs nitric oxide relaxations in human mesenteric microvessels. *Diabetologia*, **43**: 83–90, 2000.

29. Fu ZZ, Yan T, ChenY-J, Sang JQ. Thromboxane/prostacyclin balance in type11 diabetes: gliclazide effects. *Metabolism*, **41** (Suppl 1): 33–35, 1992.

30. Florkowski CM, Richardson MR, Le Guen C, Jennings PE, O'Donnell MJ, Jones AF, Lunec J, Barnett AH. Effect of gliclazide on thromboxane B₂, parameters of haemostasis, fluorescent 1gG and lipid peroxides in non-insulin dependent mellitus. *Diabetes Research*, **9**: 87–90, 1988.

31. Jennings PE, Scott NA, Saniabadi AR, Belch JJF. Effects of Gliclazide on Platelet Reactivity and Free Radicals in Type II Diabetic Patients Clinical Assessment. *Metabolism*, **41**(5): 36–39, 1992.

32. O'Brien RC, Luo M, Balazs N, Mercuri J. *In vitro* and *in vivo* antioxidant properties of gliclazide. *J Diab Comps*, **14**: 201–206, 2000.

33. Violi F, De Mattia GC, Alessandri A, Vezza E. The effects of gliclazide on platelet function in patients with diabetes mellitus. *Curr Med Res Opin*, **8**: 200–203, 1982.

34. Almer L-O. Effect of chlorpropamide and gliclazide on plasminogen activator activity in vascular walls in patients with maturity onset diabetes. *Thromb Res*, **35**: 19–25, 1984.

35. Gram J, Jespersen J, Kold A. Effects of an oral anti-diabetic drug on the fibrinolytic system of blood in insulin-treated diabetic patients. *Metabolism*, **37**: 937–943, 1988.

36. Nair CH, Sullivan JR, Singh D, Azhar A, Van Gelder J, Dhall DP. Fibrin network structure as a determinant of fibrinolysis. *Thromb Haemos*, **62**: 86, 1989.

37. Akanuma Y, Kosaka K, Kanazawa Y, Kasuga M, Fukuda M, Aoki S. Long Term Comparison on Oral Hypoglycaemic Agents in Diabetic Retinopathy. *Diabetes Research and Clinical Practice*, **5**: 81–90, 1988.

38. Régnault AF. Prognosis of non-proliferative diabetic retinopathy during treatment with gliclazide. *Roy Soc Med Int Congr Symp Ser*, **20**: 249–57, 1980.

38

INSULIN AND CARDIOVASCULAR DISEASE IN TYPE 2 DIABETES

Rodica POP-BUŞUI, Martin STEVENS

The past several years have witnessed a major surge of interest in the cardiovascular actions of insulin. This interest has stemmed, on the one hand from epidemiological studies that demonstrated an association between obesity, insulin resistance and hypertension, leading to the so-called insulin hypothesis of hypertension. On the other hand, this interest has been stimulated by experimental evidence suggesting that the vascular actions of insulin may play a role in its main action, namely the promotion of glucose uptake in the skeletal muscle. However, the vascular actions of insulin extend beyond its ability to increase skeletal muscle blood flow and glucose uptake. Current data suggest that insulin modulates vascular tone, as well as vascular smooth muscle cell proliferation and migration, *via* the release of nitric oxide and other yet unidentified mechanisms.

Thus, the effects of insulin on the vascular system may be important in the prevention or delay of cardiovascular disease progression.

Cardiovascular disease is the major cause of morbidity and mortality in patients with both type 1, insulin-dependent and type 2, non-insulin-dependent diabetes mellitus (DM). While in type 1 DM patients cardiovascular complications are usually secondary to the development of diabetic nephropathy, in type 2 DM atherosclerotic lesions are often already present at the time of diagnosis of diabetes.

The underlying pathophysiological mechanisms leading to cardiovascular complications in both types of diabetes are poorly understood. Numerous epidemiological studies have focused on the description of risk markers independently associated with the development and progression of macrovascular complications in diabetes.

It has been well established that diabetes is an independent risk factor for the development of coronary heart disease (CHD). In the western world, the risk for endpoints of cardiovascular disease is increased two- to seven-fold among diabetic patients when compared to non-diabetic subjects. Some earlier large prospective studies have demonstrated a 1.5 to three-fold increased risk of CHD in subjects with diabetes compared

with those without diabetes even after adjustment for other CHD risk factors [1–3].

The excess risk for CHD associated with diabetes is more marked in women than in men [1]. In the Framingham study, 18-year follow-up results showed that total CHD, MI, angina and sudden death were all increased in diabetic men and women aged 45–74 years compared with non-diabetics [4]. Furthermore, it has been demonstrated that in type 2 diabetes, the large majority of all mortality is as a result of CHD [5].

The greater incidence of atherosclerotic cardiovascular disease in patients with diabetes mellitus is associated with increased mortality and morbidity compared with nondiabetic patients with cardiovascular disease [6–11]. Patients with diabetes mellitus are more likely to die after an acute myocardial infarction than patients without diabetes [10, 12].

Haffner et al. have shown that diabetic patients without a previous myocardial infraction have as high a risk of myocardial infarction as nondiabetic patients with previous myocardial infarction [13] (Figure 38.1). People with diabetes are also at higher risk of re-infarction compared with non-diabetic controls [12].

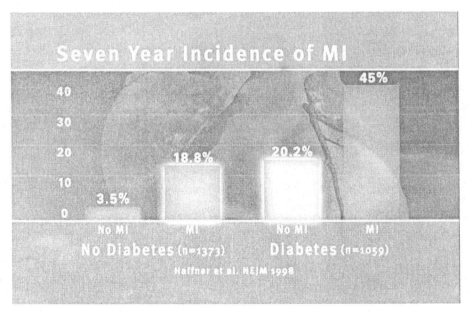

Figure 38.1

Incidence of cardiovascular events during a seven-year follow-up in relation to History of myocardial infarction in subjects with type 2 diabetes and in nondiabetic subjects (adapted from Haffner et al., [13]).

In both diabetic and nondiabetic subjects, a history of myocardial infarction at base line was significantly associated with an increased incidence of myocardial infarction (fatal and nonfatal), stroke (fatal and nonfatal), and death from cardiovascular causes. The incidence of myocardial infarction among nondiabetic subjects was 18.8 percent in those with prior myocardial infarction and 3.5 percent in those without prior myocardial infarction. Among diabetic subjects, the incidence of myocardial infarction was 45.0 percent in those with prior myocardial infarction and 20.2 percent in those without prior myocardial infarction.

The increased mortality is seen both in the acute phase and during one year of follow up after MI [14, 15].

Of particular interest is that it has been also reported that the greatest increase in relative risk of death acutely following an MI was in those patients with diabetes in the lowest preinfarction risk profile [16].

In addition, diabetes is an independent risk factor for lesion progression, graft occlusion, and cardiac mortality after CABG [17–20].

In two recent studies, a history of diabetes was associated with a two-fold increase in mortality over 5 to 8 years after percutaneous transluminal coronary angioplasty (PTCA) compared with patients without diabetes [21–23]. Diabetes mellitus has been also identified as an independent risk factor for the development of restenosis after balloon angioplasty or stent placement [24, 25]. And although recent evidence, from randomized trials that involve subgroups of patients with diabetes, showed a survival advantage associated with bypass surgery as compared with angioplasty [26–29], patients with diabetes have a much poorer adjusted long-term survival than similarly treated patients without diabetes [22, 27, 30, 31].

PROCESS OF ATHEROGENESIS IN TYPE 2 DIABETES

Recent observations have focused attention on additional mechanisms that may be relevant to atherogenesis both in patients with type 2 diabetes and obesity. Patients with type 2 diabetes and/or obesity have an increase in oxidative stress and inflammation. Increased oxidative stress in type 2 diabetes is indicated by an increase in reactive oxygen species (ROS) generation by circulating mononuclear cells [32], increased lipid peroxidation [33], protein carbonylation [34], nitro-tyrosine formation [35], and DNA damage [36]. More recently, increased oxidative stress was also demonstrated in obese patients, as reflected by increased lipid peroxidation, protein carbonylation, and ortho-tyrosine and meta-tyrosine formation. These changes reversed after caloric restriction to 1,000 calories/day for 4 weeks, as did ROS generation by leukocytes [37]. Similarly, glucose and macronutrient intake set up a state of oxidative stress and inflammation [38]. Thus, there is a close link between type 2 diabetes and macronutrient intake, oxidative stress, inflammation, and obesity.

There is also evidence that both diabetes and obesity are associated with inflammation. Plasma interleukin 6 (IL-6), tumor necrosis factor α (TNFα), and tumor necrosis factor receptor (TNF-R) are elevated in the obese and in type 2 diabetes [39–42]. Plasminogen activator inhibitor (PAI-1) is also increased in both [43, 44]. PAI-1 is known to be regulated by the key proinflammatory transcription factors nuclear factor-kB (NF-kB) and Egr-1 [45] and, thus, should be considered an inflammatory product.

Atherosclerosis is now recognized as an inflammation of the arterial wall (Plate 38.1) [46]. It starts with abnormalities in the endothelium, resulting in the adhesion of circulating monocytes and T cells, and in the formation of an inflammatory nidus. The adherent monocytes are then activated and move into the subendothelial space, where they form "foam cells" loaded with oxidized low-density lipoprotein. These foam cells are active and secrete matrix metalloproteinases, which may lyse the fibrous cap of the atherosclerotic plaque to make the plaque unstable and to cause plaque rupture. Such a rupture, characteristic for unstable plaques that are loaded with many foam cells and have thin fibrous caps, leads to initiation of the thrombotic process [47–49]. Tissue factor, expressed on the surface of foam cells now exposed to the bloodstream, activates factor VII, which eventually leads to the formation of thrombin. Thrombin activates platelet aggregation and converts fibrinogen to fibrin, initiating thrombosis [50, 51]. It is noteworthy that the expression of metalloproteinases is regulated by the proinflammatory transcription factor AP-1, and expression of tissue factor is regulated by the transcription factor Egr-1, in addition to other proinflammatory transcription factors [45, 52].

Thus, inflammation triggered by proinflammatory transcription factors can account for evolution of the process of atherosclerosis, plaque rupture, and the thrombotic process. It also accounts for the diminished fibrinolysis caused by elevated PAI-1. This would suggest that anti-inflammatory agents could play an important role in the prevention and treatment of atherosclerosis in general and, in diabetes and obesity, in particular.

Considerable data have accumulated during the past few years to show that thiazolidinediones (TZDs) may have a series of effects on the atherogenic process in the vessel wall, including effects on endothelial function, monocyte/ macrophage function, lipid abnormalities, smooth muscle cell migration, and fibrinolysis (Table 38.1). All of

Table 38.1

Proposed mechanisms linking TZD with inflammation
(Adapted from Dandona *et al.* [172])

Suppression of ROS generation
Reduction of 9-and 13-HODE
Reduction in plasma concentration of CRP, ICAM-1, MCP-1, TNFα, PAI-1
Reduction in intranuclear NF-κB
Enhanced expression of inhibitor κβα
Increase in IL 10 and TH_2

these functions are believed to be abnormal as a part of insulin resistance. Independent of these effects, TZDs also have been shown to possess anti-inflammatory properties [53, 54]. This has profound implication for atherosclerosis, because atherosclerosis is an inflammatory process.

INSULIN AS AN ANTI-INFLAMMATORY AGENT

The available data with TZDs prompted a series of experiments with insulin to test the hypothesis that if insulin sensitizers are anti-inflammatory, insulin is also anti-inflammatory. *In vitro* data obtained from human aortic endothelial cells showed that insulin suppressed intracellular adhesion molecule 1 expression and secretion and that this effect was nitric oxide mediated [55]. Insulin is known to induce nitric oxide release and to enhance nitric oxide synthase expression in endothelial cells [56, 57]. Insulin also was shown to suppress intranuclear NF-κB and monocyte chemotactic protein 1 expression [58]. These data suggest an anti-inflammatory effect of insulin.

The first comprehensive description of an anti-inflammatory effect of insulin in the obese human, *in vivo*, was made recently [58]. A low-dose infusion of insulin (2 IU/hour), resulting in plasma concentrations of 24 to 28 μU/mL, caused suppression of intranuclear NF-κB, increased IκB, decreased ROS generation by polymorphonuclear leukocytes and mononuclear cells, and decreased plasma concentrations of soluble intracellular adhesion molecule 1, monocyte chemotactic protein 1, and CRP. This effect was observed within 2 hours of insulin infusion and reversed within 2 hours after the end of the infusion. This rapid and comprehensive anti-inflammatory effect of insulin at the cellular and molecular levels suggests that it would be important to rethink the

entire issue of inflammation and atherosclerosis with respect to insulin.

In view of the epidemiologic relationship between hyperinsulinemia and CAD, [59–61], a number of *in vitro* studies have been published to justify a role for insulin in the pathogenesis of atherosclerosis. Insulin has been shown at 10 nM/mL to stimulate mitogen-activated protein kinase activity, which leads to mitogenesis and atherogenesis [62–64]. Concentrations of 10 nM/mL (1,600 μU/mL) do not occur in humans, *in vivo*, except in a few extremely rare syndromes of insulin resistance. Clearly, it is important to rethink the mechanisms underlying insulin resistance. They are proinflammatory, and the putative candidates for induction of insulin resistance may well be proinflammatory cytokines, such as TNFα or IL-6. TNFα has been shown to interfere with insulin action by inhibiting phosphorylation of the insulin receptor in the adipocyte [65] and human aortic endothelial cells [66]. Furthermore, TNFα reduces insulin-receptor content in human aortic endothelial cells [66]. Although infusion of soluble TNFα receptor restores the sensitivity to insulin in a rodent model of obesity [67], a neutralizing antibody against TNF-α has not yielded changes in insulin sensitivity in patients with established type 2 diabetes [68].

It is thus possible that insulin resistance is mediated by a series of proinflammatory cytokines and mediators. Recent work has focused on IκB-kinase β (IKK-β), the enzyme that phosphorylates IκB to cause its ubiquitousness. This releases NF-κB, which then translocates into the nucleus, initiating the transcription of proinflammatory genes. Aspirin, a classic anti-inflammatory drug, inhibits this enzyme and causes a reduction in insulin resistance in animal models of obesity and in the obese human [69–71]. In view of recent observations, we suggest a new

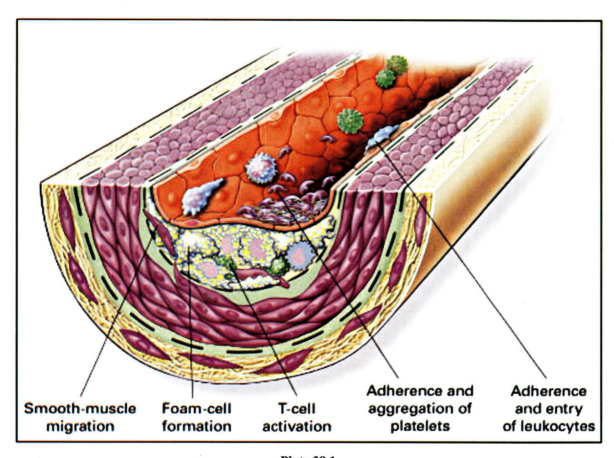

| Smooth-muscle migration | Foam-cell formation | T-cell activation | Adherence and aggregation of platelets | Adherence and entry of leukocytes |

Plate 38.1

Fatty streak formation in atherosclerosis.

Fatty streaks initially consist of lipid-loaded monocytes and macrophages (foam cells) together with T lymphocytes. Later they are joined by various numbers of smooth muscle cells. The steps involved in this process include smooth muscle migration, which is stimulated by platelet-derived growth factor, fibroblast growth factor 2, and transforming growth factor β; T-cell activation, which is mediated by TNF α, interleukin 2, and granulocyte-macrophage colony-stimulating factor; foam cell formation, which is mediated by oxidized low-density lipoprotein, macrophage colony-stimulating factor, TNF α, and interleukin 1; and platelet adherence and aggregation, which are stimulated by integrins, P-selectin, fibrin, thromboxane A_2, and tissue factor. These processes are comprehensively inhibited by insulin and thiazolidine diones. (Reprinted with permission from Ross R. *et al.*) [46].

paradigm that the states of insulin deficiency (type 1 and type 2 diabetes) and insulin resistance (type 2 diabetes and obesity) are proinflammatory and proatherogenic. Although there is evidence that insulin therapy has profound beneficial effects in acute myocardial infarction [72–77], evidence regarding its long-term beneficial effects as an anti-inflammatory agent is still to be obtained.

VASCULAR ACTIONS OF INSULIN

Even though insulin-induced sympathetic activation is thought to be, at least in part, sympathetic vasoconstrictor [78], there is abundant evidence that insulin stimulates the blood flow and decreases vascular resistance in the skeletal muscle. Insulin-induced vasodilation was first reported, shortly after its introduction into clinical practice [79]. These early studies used injection of large doses of insulin, and the vasodilation was thought to be mediated at least in part by hypoglycemia-induced stimulation of epinephrine release [80]. Subsequently, it has been shown that insulin-induced stimulation of muscle blood flow is not dependent on epinephrine release because it occurs in adrenalectomized humans [81] and during euglycemic hyperinsulinemia [82–87] situations in which there is no stimulation of epinephrine release. At the beginning of the present decade, independent findings by Laasko and colleagues [82, 88–90] and Anderson and colleagues, firmly established the concept that in lean subjects, euglycemic hyperinsulinemia [84] at high physiological concentrations stimulates the blood flow in the skeletal muscle tissue. Such stimulation is related primarily to insulin itself rather than to stimulation of carbohydrate metabolism [83]. Insulin-induced increases in the blood flow are comparable in the upper and the lower limbs [87] and have been demonstrated with the use of both invasive measurement techniques such as thermodilution [82, 88–90] and dye dilution [91] and noninvasive techniques such as plethysmography [92–95], positron emission tomography [96, 97], and B-mode ultrasound [87]. Insulin-induced stimulation of limb blood flow occurs selectively in the skeletal muscle tissue but not in the skin [87, 97]. The relative limb muscle content is an important determinant of the interindividual variation in the blood flow response to insulin in normal subjects.

MECHANISM(S) OF INSULIN-INDUCED VASODILATION

In 1994, two independent reports have provided conclusive evidence that in lean subjects, inhibition of nitric oxide (NO) release by the stereospecific inhibitor of nitric oxide synthase N^G-monomethyl-L-arginine (L-NMMA) abolishes insulin-induced vasodilation [93, 98]. In healthy humans, insulin has a stimulating effect on NO-dependent basal blood flow [93, 98] and on agonist-stimulated endothelium-dependent vasodilation [99, 100]. Consistent with these observations *in vivo*, insulin induces vasorelaxation mediated by endothelium-derived nitric oxide (NO) in isolated rat skeletal muscle arterioles [101], and increases cyclic guanosine monophosphate content by a NO-dependent mechanism and activates L-arginine transport and NO-synthase [102] in human vascular smooth muscle cells and stimulates nitric oxide release in cultured vascular endothelial cells *in vitro* [56]. While these studies establish the major role played by NO in the mediation of insulin-induced vasodilation, two important questions remain to be answered. Does insulin stimulate NO release by a local (vascular) or a systemic (*i.e.*, stimulation of neuronal vasodilation) action? Do other mechanisms contribute to insulin-induced vasodilation?

Regarding the former question, comparison of insulin-induced vasodilation during local, intra-arterial, and systemic intravenous insulin infusion should provide some clues. Although this approach appears compelling, the evidence is conflicting. Indeed, while insulin-induced vasodilation has been a consistent finding in the large majority [82–87, 89, 103], but not all [104, 105] of the studies using systemic insulin infusion at both physiological [83–85, 87, 103] and pharmacological [87, 97] concentrations, during local insulin infusion many studies did not find a vasodilation [106–113], but others did [94, 95, 114, 115]. The observations that insulin infusion produces hypotension in patients with autonomic failure [115] and vasodilation in patients having undergone regional sympathectomy for hyperhidrosis [116] argue against sympathetic neural vasodilation as the only mechanism. We find it interesting that vasodilation occurs much more rapidly in the denervated than in the innervated limb, which suggests that in innervated limbs, sympathetic vasoconstrictor tone may mask the local vasodilator action of insulin [116].

Earlier reports had suggested that β-adrenergic mechanisms could contribute to insulin-induced vasodilation [117, 118]. Interpretation of these studies was difficult, however, because of potential confounding effects of hypoglycemia-induced stimulation of epinephrine release. Recent observations in humans indicate that in the absence of hypoglycemia, β-adrenergic mechanisms do not appear to contribute importantly to insulin-induced vasodilation [86]. Similarly, cholinergic vasodilator mechanisms do not appear to play a role because atropine infusion did not alter insulin-induced stimulation of the blood flow [86].

A final unresolved issue relates to the prolonged time course of insulin-induced vasodilation. During insulin infusion at stepwise increasing rates over several hours, muscle blood flow increases progressively throughout the infusion, an observation that has been used to indicate that stimulation of the blood flow is both time dependent and dose dependent [87]. This experimental approach, however, does not allow determination of the respective roles of time and dose on insulin-induced vasodilation. Recent observations are consistent with the hypothesis that within the physiological range, infusion time rather than infusion rate is the main determinant of the vasodilator response to insulin. In lean subjects, when compared at the same time point, vasodilator responses were comparable during low and high physiological hyperinsulinemia [119], and during insulin infusion at a constant rate over a prolonged 3- to 6-hour period, the muscle blood flow continued to increase roughly linearly throughout the entire infusion [86, 92]. It is possible, however, that in subjects who are resistant to the vasodilator action of insulin and/or when insulin is infused at pharmacological concentrations, the dose may be an important determinant of the response, as evidenced by the stimulation of the blood flow by pharmacological, but not by physiological hyperinsulinemia in insulin-resistant obese subjects.

In summary, in healthy subjects, insulin-induced vasodilation is mediated chiefly by stimulation of nitric oxide release. Further studies are needed to determine whether additional mechanisms contribute to insulin-induced vasodilation *in vivo*.

Although earlier studies reported that these effects are blunted in patients with obesity-associated insulin resistance or type 2 diabetes [82, 89, 100], recent evidence demonstrated that insulin therapy can ameliorate [120] or restore [121] endothelial function in patients with type 2 DM and coronary artery disease.

The most important trials on the effect of hypoglycemic drug therapy on clinical cardiovascular end points in type 2 diabetes are the U.K. Prospective Diabetes Study (UKPDS) [122], which included patients with newly diagnosed type 2 diabetes, and the Diabetes Mellitus, Insulin Glucose Infusion in Acute Myocardial Infarction (DIGAMI) trial [75], which included patients with diabetes (> 80% with type 2 diabetes) and myocardial infarction. The UKPDS showed a nonsignificant 16% reduction of relative risk of myocardial infarction in patients managed with an intensive treatment policy of blood glucose control during a mean follow-up time of 8.4 years, whereas the DIGAMI trial showed a significant 28% reduction of relative risk of 1-year total mortality in patients who received an insulin-glucose infusion in the acute phase, followed by subcutaneous insulin injections during at least 3 months after discharge. The DIGAMI trial, as opposed to the UKPDS, may have been able to show a statistically significant benefit because it included high-risk patients. It is possible that the beneficial effect of insulin therapy in the DIGAMI trial was due to an improvement of the vascular endothelial function.

With the results of the DIGAMI trial in mind, Rask-Madsen *et al.* [121] examined the effects of 2 months of insulin therapy on endothelial function and insulin-stimulated endothelial function in patients with type 2 diabetes and stable ischemic heart disease and showed that in patients with type 2 diabetes and ischemic heart disease, long-term insulin therapy improves insulin-stimulated endothelium-dependent vasodilation. These results constitute an argument for the concept that endothelial insulin resistance is an aspect of insulin resistance [100], which has traditionally been thought to be primarily confined to the skeletal muscle, the liver, and fat. Because of the central role of metabolic insulin resistance in the pathogenesis of type 2 diabetes, endothelial insulin resistance may be a mechanism that explains the particular risk for vascular disease in type 2 diabetes. It is also a possible physiological explanation for the fact that insulin resistance is an independent risk factor for atherosclerotic disease and its complications.

However, the survival of endothelial cells critically determines vessel growth and inflammatory processes in the vessel wall. Survival of the cells is counterbalanced by the induction of physiological cell death, apoptosis. Besides the contribution of apoptosis to endothelial injury, apoptotic cell death regulates vessel growth. Thus, recent studies have provided evidence that inhibition of endothelial cell apoptosis in combination with enhanced proliferation is implicated as the basis for angiogenesis. Angiogenesis, the development of new blood vessels, is a highly regulated process that is important for the neovascularization of new tissue and revascularization after ischemic infarction and counteracts the vascular regression after injury of the blood vessel. In this respect, in a recent study, Hermann et al. have demonstrated that insulin prevents TNFα-induced apoptosis of endothelial cells and that apoptosis-suppressive effects of insulin are mediated by PI3K-dependent activation of protein kinase Akt [123].

INSULIN AND MYOCARDIAL INFARCTION IN TYPE 2 DM

The management of patients with acute myocardial infarction has improved dramatically with the restoration of arterial perfusion with thrombolytic and antiplatelet therapy. However, recently attention has turned to adjunctive pharmacological treatments to enhance myocardial tolerance to ischemia/reperfusion injury, in an attempt to further reduce mortality in conjunction with reperfusion therapy [124]. Ideally, as this cytoprotective therapy would usually be administered after the onset of ischemia, candidate agents would need to be effective when administered during reperfusion. Cellular protection or tolerance against ischemia has been postulated as the new challenge for patient management in cardiovascular diseases [124].

The most practical therapeutic approach to achieve this cardioprotection would be if the candidate therapy could be administered during reperfusion therapy after acute myocardial ischemia. In a recent study, Jonassen et al. demonstrated that insulin given at the onset of reperfusion reduces infarct size in the isolated perfused rat heart [125]. Moreover, the administration of this mitogen was only required for a 15 minute period to confer this cardiac-protected phenotype. Conversely, the delay in administration of insulin by 15 minutes after the onset of reperfusion abrogated these cardioprotective effects [125].

The concept that the metabolic cocktail glucose-insulin-potassium (GIK) may protect ischemic cardiomyocytes was initially introduced by Sodi-Pallares et al. in 1962 [126]. The rationale for the use of this metabolic therapy was further delineated by Opie [127] in 1970, where he

described two chief mechanisms: i.e., the promotion of cardiac glycolysis and the inhibition of free fatty acids (FFA) in the serum. Eventually, De Leiris et al. described a direct cardioprotective effect of insulin in the absence of glucose [128], since insulin administration attenuated LDH release in the isolated perfused working rat heart during sustained ischemia in the absence of glucose or glycolytic intermediates in the perfusate [128].

During the mid 1960s and 1970s, several clinical trials of GIK therapy in acute myocardial infarction were performed [72, 129–141].

However, results were inconclusive because of several factors, including a low number of recruits, poor design, and methodological discrepancies between different clinical trials, including varying times to the initiation of GIK therapy and the use of different GIK regimens. Many trials continued recruitment as late as 48 hours after the onset of chest pain, and several trials used oral glucose therapy with subcutaneous insulin injections, whereas others used continuous intravenous infusions (Table 38.2). Many of these studies may have used inadequate GIK regimens. Of the optimally randomized placebo-controlled trials, only 1 study [129] showed a significant benefit from GIK therapy. In the majority, a nonsignificant reduction in mortality with the use of this therapy could be demonstrated. Individually, however, none of these trials was sufficiently large to have power to be able to show a significant difference between the treated and control groups.

Many factors have been proposed to explain the worse prognosis in people with diabetes following MI. Differences in the severity of coronary artery disease do not appear to explain the increased mortality. The infarction size does not offer an explanation either, since diabetic subjects appear to have an increased risk of post-infarct congestive cardiac failure (CCF), despite a smaller infarction size [142].

Some have postulated that diabetic cardiomyopathy may contribute to the adverse outcome but this remains unproved [143]. Diabetes mellitus is an independent marker of mortality after acute myocardial infarction [10, 144, 145].

In the DIGAMI study, the unfavorable long-term prognosis was improved by intensive insulin treatment, which tended to favorably influence all cardiovascular causes of death (Figure 38.2) [75]. Age and previous heart failure were the only conventional risk markers that independently predicted long-term mortality in the complete

Table 38.2
Randomized Placebo-Controlled Trials of GIK Therapy in Acute Myocardial Infarction
(Adapted from Fath-Ordoubadi *et al.* [160])

Study	Year	Design	Delays Between Onset of MI and Treatment (h)	Exclusion criteria	Regimen	Duration of treatment
Heng	1977	Open	<12	CS, RF	High-dose IV	6-12 h
Stanley	1978	Open	<12	1	High-dose IV	48 h
Rogers	1979	Open	<12	Age >75 y, IDDM, RF	High-dose IV	48 h
Satler	1987	DB	<24	Age >75 y, IDDM	High-dose IV	48 h
Mittra	1965	Open	<48	IDDM, RF	Oral GK and SC insulin	14 d
Pilcher	1967	Open	1	DM	Oral GK and SC insulin	14 d
Pentecost	1968	Open	<48	IDDM, severe LVF	IV	48 h
MRC	1968	Open	<48	DM, RF	Oral GK and SC insulin	14 d
Hjermann	1971	DB	<48	Age >75 y, IDDM, RF	Oral GK and SC insulin	10 d

DB indicates double-blind; CS, cardiogenic shock; RF, renal failure; IDDM, insulin-dependent diabetes mellitus; G, glucose; K, potassium; DM, diabetes mellitus; LVF, left ventricular failure; and high-dose IV, regimen of 30% glucose, 50 U insulin, and 80 mmol potassium at a rate of ≥1.5 mL/kg/*per* hour.

[1] No information available.

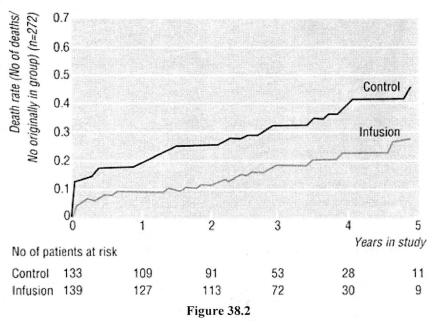

No of patients at risk

Control	133	109	91	53	28	11
Infusion	139	127	113	72	30	9

Figure 38.2
Mortality curves during long term follow-up in patients receiving insulin-glucose infusion and in control group among total DIGAMI cohort.
Absolute reduction in risk was 11%; relative risk 0.72 (0.55 to 0.92); P=0.011 adapted after Malmberg *et al.* [75].

DIGAMI cohort. Previous myocardial infarction and hypertension, known risk factors in nondiabetic patients [146], did not add prognostic power. Admission hyperglycemia is a predictor of poor in-hospital outcome after acute MI according to several studies of diabetic and nondiabetic patients. Hyperglycemia has been linked to extensive myocardial damage causing heart failure and secondary stress [147–150]. In the DIGAMI control subjects, there was an almost linear relationship between blood glucose tertiles and long-term mortality. The most powerful predictor of blood glucose at admission was previous metabolic control (HbA1c). This indicates that blood glucose at admission is not only a marker of acute stress but also reflects the present glucometabolic state. The relationship between a high admission blood glucose and poor long-term outcome did not reach statistical significance in the group on intensive insulin. Thus, the harmful effect of elevated blood glucose was attenuated. In the total DIGAMI cohort, baseline HbA1c level tended to independently predict mortality in the control group, but not in the group on intensive insulin. Thus, strict insulin treatment with improved metabolic control seems to reduce the adverse effect of an initially poor metabolic control.

Many studies suggest that metabolic control is an important determinant of future development of coronary heart disease among NIDDM patients [151–154]. Intensive treatment with insulin caused a 40% reduction in cardiovascular events in the Diabetes Control and Complications Trial. This indicates that regardless of a causal relationship, improved metabolic care reduces the progression of the atherothrombotic process. During the first year of follow-up in the DIGAMI trial, a reduction in HbA1c was most apparent in patients without previous insulin and at low cardiovascular risk. The most pronounced early and long-term mortality improvement was achieved in this group, supporting the assumption that glycemic control is mandatory for secondary prevention of ischemic complications in diabetic patients, including NIDDM patients.

It is debatable whether improved metabolic control with insulin or decreased use of possibly harmful sulfonylureas caused the beneficial effects in DIGAMI. Data from the recently published UK Prospective Diabetes Study (UKPDS) of intensive blood glucose control by either sulfonylureas or insulin are of interest in this regard [122]. In UKPDS, there was a significant decrease in the risk of microvascular but not macrovascular disease

in NIDDM patients regardless of the type of antidiabetic therapy. In any case, the reduction in myocardial infarctions reached borderline significance ($P = 0.052$), indicating that the beneficial effect of intensive glucose control outweighed the theoretical risk of the antidiabetic agent and supporting the idea that improved metabolic control is of crucial importance.

CLINICAL USE OF INSULIN

Insulin can be used in type 2 diabetes for the maintenance of euglycemia at any stage in the evolution of this disease. However, it is usually used when maximal doses of oral agents have failed to restore HbA1c levels to the target of less than 7%. The initial approach to starting insulin therapy is to provide a basal insulin preparation, usually injected at night, to obtain fasting glucose concentrations of 90–110 mg/dl. The previous oral hypoglycemic agents are left on board because they may control postprandial glucose concentrations during the day. Should this not happen, additional insulin therapy with fast-acting preparations may be added during the day as necessary. The previous hesitation about the use of insulin therapy for fear of increasing hyperinsulinemia is unjustified because the underlying insulin resistance, and not hyperinsulinemia, is the probable cause of atherosclerosis. Insulin should also be the treatment of choice in hospitalized patients with uncontrolled hyperglycemia and when subjects are admitted to the critical care unit with or without acute coronary syndromes. Treatment with insulin in the setting of severe symptomatic hyperglycemia or when it is added to oral agents, when the latter are unable to achieve adequate glycemic targets, or in the hospitalized and critically ill patients has a dual benefit from both a reduction in glycemia and the direct antiinflammatory effect of insulin.

It is estimated that 20% of the subjects admitted with acute myocardial infarction (MI) have diabetes, and of those not known to have diabetes, 65% have either undiagnosed diabetes or impaired glucose tolerance [155]. Hyperglycemia at the time of acute MI has been correlated to increased mortality in diabetic patients and nondiabetic subjects [156]. Impaired glucose metabolism, increased free fatty acid concentration, and preferential myocardial fatty acid use have been suggested as mechanisms for aggravating ischemia and inducing arrhythmias in these populations

[157]. Hyperglycemia has also been associated with increased incidence of no-reflow after successful reperfusion [158]. Insulin infusion of 5 U/h has been shown to reduce long-term mortality by 30–50% in diabetic patients and nondiabetic subjects, presumably based on its glucose- and free fatty acid-lowering metabolic effect [159–161]. The ECLA group reports the largest prospective, randomized trial of GIK for the treatment of acute MI ever performed and the only such trial done in the era of thrombolytic therapy [159]. They observed a remarkable 66% reduction (2P = 0.008) in the relative in-hospital mortality risk when GIK was added to reperfusion (95% of those reperfused had thrombolysis, 5% had primary PTCA) relative to reperfusion alone; the absolute mortality risk decreased from 15.2% to 5.2%. Considering the relatively long average time from the onset of acute MI symptoms until the start of treatment (10 to 11 hours), the magnitude of the mortality reduction was even more remarkable. Moreover, a survival benefit persisted during a 1-year follow-up period in the group that received high-dose GIK plus reperfusion as acute MI treatment [159].

However, a prothrombotic milieu promoted by proinflammatory mediators resulting in the persistence of an unstable plaque, and an increase in matrix metalloproteinases (MMPs) affecting left ventricular remodeling could also lead to failure of reperfusion, reocclusion, and congestive heart failure post MI [162–165]. Commensurate with this hypothesis are the observations that CRP and PAI-1 are markers of thrombolytic efficacy in acute MI and that suppression of MMP decreases left ventricular remodeling after MI in animals [166, 167]. Anti-inflammatory properties of insulin as mentioned above as well as its vasodilatory (arterial and venous) and antiplatelet properties could thus improve prognosis after acute MI, independent of its metabolic effect [168]. On the basis of these hypotheses and the observation that insulin is most beneficial when given with thrombolysis and at the onset of reperfusion, an insulin infusion should be started to control hyperglycemia, preferably with the commencement of thrombolysis and reperfusion in type 2 diabetes [125]. We recommend initiating therapy with blood glucose in the impaired fasting or impaired glucose tolerance range and maintaining blood glucose between 100 and 140 mg/dl with the use of a minimum of 2.5 U insulin *per* hour for a period of time that the subjects are in the critical care unit.

The anti-inflammatory action of insulin may have a beneficial role in inflammatory conditions, unrelated to traditional hyperglycemia. Patients with critical illness including sepsis, as well as experimental endotoxemia, often have hyperglycemia and an insulin-resistant state even in the absence of diabetes [169]. Sepsis and endotoxin administration impair insulin-mediated glucose uptake in the skeletal muscle, and it has been suggested that lipopolysaccharides may alter multiple steps in the insulin signal transduction pathway [170]. In fact, a recent prospective, randomized trial of insulin infusion in 1548 mechanically ventilated, critically ill patients (only 13% were diabetic) in an intensive care unit (ICU) setting has shown remarkable benefit [171]. Insulin infusion to maintain normal blood glucose in the range of 80–110 mg/dl reduced ICU mortality by 43%, hospital mortality by 34%, and bacteremia by 46%. The greatest reduction in mortality involved deaths due to multiple-organ failure with a proved septic focus. There was also a significant reduction in the duration of ICU stay, need for dialysis, and need for prolonged ventilator support.

Whether these benefits of insulin infusion in conditions of acute coronary events or critically ill patients of diverse etiologies, including sepsis, are related to both improvement in glucose concentrations and the antioxidative and antiinflammatory actions of insulin needs to be explored further.

REFERENCES

1. Garcia MJ, *et al.* Morbidity and mortality in diabetics in the Framingham population. Sixteen year follow-up study. *Diabetes*, **23**(2): 105–11, 1974.
2. Jarrett RJ, Shipley MJ. Mortality and associated risk factors in diabetics. *Acta Endocrinol Suppl* (Copenh), **272**: 21–6, 1985.
3. Reunanen A, Loikkanen M, Pyorala K. Cardiovascular and coronary heart disease mortality of diabetes and non-diabetics: impact of risk factors. *J Am Coll Cardiol*, **1**(2): 600, 1983.
4. Kannel W. Role of diabetes in cardiac disease: conclusions from population studies. In: Zoneraich S (ed). *Diabetes and Heart*, Springfield, 1978, 97–122.
5. Panzram G. Mortality and survival in type 2 (non-insulin-dependent) diabetes mellitus. *Diabetologia*, **30**(3): 123–31, 1987.
6. Abbott RD, *et al.* The impact of diabetes on survival following myocardial infarction in men vs women. The Framingham Study. *JAMA*, **260**(23): 3456–60, 1988.

7. Butler L. The inheritance of diabetes in the Chinese hamster. *Diabetologia*, **3**: 124–129, 1967.

8. Jarrett RJ. Type 2 (non-insulin-dependent) diabetes mellitus and coronary heart disease-chicken, egg or neither? *Diabetologia*, **26**: 99–102, 1984.

9. Jarrett RJ, Shipley MJ. Type 2 (non-insulin-dependent) diabetes mellitus and cardiovascular disease-putative association via common antecedents; further evidence from the Whitehall Study. *Diabetologia*, **31**: 737–740, 1988.

10. Malmberg K, Ryden L. Myocardial infarction in patients with diabetes mellitus. *Eur Heart J*, **9**(3): 259–64,1988.

11. Stamler J, *et al.* Diabetes, other risk factors, and 12-yr cardiovascular mortality for men screened in the Multiple Risk Factor Intervention Trial. *Diabetes Care*, **16**(2): 434–44, 1993.

12. Herlitz J, *et al.* Mortality and morbidity during a five-year follow-up of diabetics with myocardial infarction. *Acta Med Scand*, **224**(1): 31–8, 1988.

13. Haffner SM, *et al.* Mortality from coronary heart disease in subjects with type 2 diabetes and in nondiabetic subjects with and without prior myocardial infarction. *N Engl J Med*, **339**(4): 229–34, 1998.

14. Malmberg K, Bavenholm P, Hamsten A. Clinical and biochemical factors associated with prognosis after myocardial infarction at a young age. *J Am Coll Cardiol*, **24**(3): 592–9, 1994.

15. Malmberg KA, Efendic S, Ryden LE. Feasibility of insulin-glucose infusion in diabetic patients with acute myocardial infarction. A report from the multicenter trial: DIGAMI. *Diabetes Care*, **17**(9): 1007–14, 1994.

16. Singer DE, Moulton AW, Nathan DM. Diabetic myocardial infarction. Interaction of diabetes with other preinfarction risk factors. *Diabetes*, **38**(3): 350–7, 1989.

17. Verska JJ, Walker WJ. Aortocoronary bypass in the diabetic patient. *Am J Cardiol*, **35**(6): 774–7, 1975.

18. Manske CL. Coronary revascularization may improve short term survival in insulin-dependent diabetics considered for renal transplantation. *Circulation*, **84(suppl II)**(II): 516, 1991.

19. Engelman RM, *et al.* The influence of diabetes and hypertension on the results of coronary revascularization. *Am J Cardiol*, **35**: 135, 1975.

20. Chychota NN, *et al.* Myocardial revascularization. Comparison of operability and surgical results in diabetic and nondiabetic patients. *J Thorac Cardiovasc Surg*, **65**(6): 856–62, 1973.

21. Kip KE, *et al.* Differential influence of diabetes mellitus on increased jeopardized myocardium after initial angioplasty or bypass surgery: bypass angioplasty revascularization investigation. *Circulation*, **105**(16): 1914–20, 2002.

22. Kip KE, *et al.* Coronary angioplasty in diabetic patients. The National Heart, Lung, and Blood Institute Percutaneous Transluminal Coronary Angioplasty Registry. *Circulation*, **94**(8): 1818–25, 1996.

23. Stein B, *et al.* Influence of diabetes mellitus on early and late outcome after percutaneous transluminal coronary angioplasty. *Circulation*, **91**(4): 979–89, 1995.

24. Carrozza JP, *et al.* Restenosis after arterial injury caused by coronary stenting in patients with diabetes mellitus. *Ann Intern Med*, **118**(5): 344–9, 1993.

25. Califf RM, *et al.* Restenosis after coronary angioplasty: an overview. *J Am Coll Cardiol*, **17**(6 Suppl B): 2B–13B, 1991.

26. King SB 3rd, *et al.* Eight-year mortality in the Emory Angioplasty versus Surgery Trial (EAST). *J Am Coll Cardiol*, **35**(5): 1116–21, 2000.

27. Weintraub WS, *et al.* Outcome of coronary bypass surgery versus coronary angioplasty in diabetic patients with multivessel coronary artery disease. *J Am Coll Cardiol*, **31**(1): 10–9, 1998.

28. Weintraub WS, Kosinski A, Culler S. Comparison of outcome after coronary angioplasty and coronary surgery for multivessel coronary artery disease in persons with diabetes. *Am Heart J*, **138**(5 Pt 1): S394–9, 1999.

29. Influence of diabetes on 5-year mortality and morbidity in a randomized trial comparing CABG and PTCA in patients with multivessel disease: the Bypass Angioplasty Revascularization Investigation (BARI). *Circulation*, **96**(6): 1761–9, 1997.

30. Barsness GW, *et al.* Relationship between diabetes mellitus and long-term survival after coronary bypass and angioplasty. *Circulation*, **96**(8): 2551–6, 1997.

31. Halon DA, *et al.* Late-onset heart failure as a mechanism for adverse long-term outcome in diabetic patients undergoing revascularization (a 13-year report from the Lady Davis Carmel Medical Center registry). *Am J Cardiol*, **85**(12): 1420–6, 2000.

32. Orie NN, Zidek W, Tepel M. Increased intracellular generation of reactive oxygen species in mononuclear leukocytes from patients with diabetes mellitus type 2. *Exp Clin Endocrinol Diabetes*, **108**(3): 175–80, 2000.

33. Nishigaki I, *et al.* Lipid peroxide levels of serum lipoprotein fractions of diabetic patients. *Biochem Med*, **25**(3): 373–8, 1981.

34. Aljada A *et al.* Increased carbonylation of proteins in diabetes mellitus. *Diabetes*, **44**(Suppl 1): 113, 1995.

35. Aydin A, *et al.* Oxidative stress and nitric oxide related parameters in type II diabetes mellitus: effects of glycemic control. *Clin Biochem*, **34**(1): 65–70, 2001.

36. Dandona P, *et al.* Oxidative damage to DNA in diabetes mellitus. *Lancet*, **347**(8999): 444–5, 1996.

37. Dandona P, *et al.* The suppressive effect of dietary restriction and weight loss in the obese on the generation of reactive oxygen species by leukocytes, lipid peroxidation, and protein carbonylation. *J Clin Endocrinol Metab*, **86**(1): 355–62, 2001.

38. Mohanty P, *et al.* Glucose challenge stimulates reactive oxygen species (ROS) generation by leucocytes. *J Clin Endocrinol Metab*, **85**(8): 2970–3, 2000.

39. Kern PA, *et al.* Adipose tissue tumor necrosis factor and interleukin-6 expression in human obesity and insulin resistance. *Am J Physiol Endocrinol Metab*, **280**(5): E745–51, 2001.

40. Dandona P, *et al.* Tumor necrosis factor-alpha in sera of obese patients: fall with weight loss. *J Clin Endocrinol Metab*, **83**(8): 2907–10, 1998.

41. Vozarova B, *et al.* Circulating interleukin-6 in relation to adiposity, insulin action, and insulin secretion. *Obes Res,* **9**(7): 414–7, 2001.

42. Nilsson J, *et al.* Relation between plasma tumor necrosis factor-alpha and insulin sensitivity in elderly men with non-insulin-dependent diabetes mellitus. Arterioscler *Thromb Vasc Biol,* **18**(8): 1199–202, 1998.

43. Matsuda T, *et al.* Plasminogen activator inhibitor in plasma and arteriosclerosis. *Ann N Y Acad Sci,* **748**: 394–8, 1995.

44. Panahloo A, Yudkin JS. Diminished fibrinolysis in diabetes mellitus and its implication for diabetic vascular disease. *Coron Artery Dis,* 7(10): 723–31, 1996.

45. Mackman N. Regulation of the tissue factor gene. *Faseb J,* **9**(10): 883–9, 1995.

46. Ross R. Atherosclerosis - an inflammatory disease. *N Engl J Med*, **340**(2): 115–26, 1999.

47. DiCorleto PE. Cellular mechanisms of atherogenesis. *Am J Hypertens,* **6**(11 Pt 2): 314S–318S, 1993.

48. Faruqi RM, DiCorleto PE. Mechanisms of monocyte recruitment and accumulation. *Br Heart J,* **69**(1 Suppl): S19–29, 1993.

49. Raines EW, Ross R. Biology of atherosclerotic plaque formation - possible role of growth factors in lesion development and the potential impact of soy. *J Nutr*, **125**(3 suppl): 624S–630S, 1995.

50. Petersen LC, Freskgard J, Ezban M. Tissue factor-dependent factor VIIa signaling. *Trends Cardiovasc Med,* **10**(2): 47–52, 2000.

51. Rauch U, Nemerson Y. Circulating tissue factor and thrombosis. *Curr Opin Hematol*, **7**(5): 273–7, 2000.

52. Westermarck J, Kahari VM. Regulation of matrix metalloproteinase expression in tumor invasion. *Faseb J,* **13**(8): 781–92, 1999.

53. Ricote M, *et al.* The peroxisome proliferator-activated receptor-gamma is a negative regulator of macrophage activation. *Nature,* **391**(6662): 79–82, 1998.

54. Jiang C, Ting AT, Seed B PPAR-gamma agonists inhibit production of monocyte inflammatory cytokines. *Nature,* **391**(6662): 82–6, 1998.

55. Aljada A, *et al.* Insulin inhibits the expression of intercellular adhesion molecule-1 by human aortic endothelial cells through stimulation of nitric oxide. *J Clin Endocrinol Metab*, **85**(7): 2572–5, 2000.

56. Zeng G, Quon MJ. Insulin-stimulated production of nitric oxide is inhibited by wortmannin. Direct measurement in vascular endothelial cells. *J Clin Invest*, **98**(4): 894–8, 1996.

57. Aljada A, Dandona P. Effect of insulin on human aortic endothelial nitric oxide synthase. *Metabolism*, **49**(2): 147–50, 2000.

58. Aljada A, *et al.* Insulin inhibits NFkappaB and MCP-1 expression in human aortic endothelial cells. *J Clin Endocrinol Metab*, **86**(1): 450–3, 2001.

59. Welborn TA, Wearne K. Coronary heart disease incidence and cardiovascular mortality in Busselton with reference to glucose and insulin concentrations. *Diabetes Care*, **2**: 154–160, 1979.

60. Fontbonne AM, Eschwege EM. Insulin and cardiovascular disease. Paris Prospective Study. *Diabetes Care*, **14**(6): 461–9, 1991.

61. Pyorala M, Miettinen H, Laakso M, Pyorala K. Plasma insulin and all-cause, cardiovascular, and noncardiovascular mortality - the 22–year follow-up results of the Helsinki Policemen Study. *Diabetes Care,* **23**: 1097–1102, 2000.

62. Carel K, *et al.* Insulin stimulates mitogen-activated protein kinase by a Ras-independent pathway in 3T3-L1 adipocytes. *J Biol Chem,* **271**(48): 30625–30, 1996.

63. Indolfi C, *et al.* Effects of balloon injury on neointimal hyperplasia in streptozotocin-induced diabetes and in hyperinsulinemic nondiabetic pancreatic islet-transplanted rats. *Circulation*, **103**(24): 2980–6, 2001.

64. Golovchenko I, *et al.* Hyperinsulinemia enhances transcriptional activity of nuclear factor-kappaB induced by angiotensin II, hyperglycemia, and advanced glycosylation end products in vascular smooth muscle cells. *Circ Res*, **87**(9): 746–52, 2000.

65. Hotamisligil GS, *et al.* IRS-1-mediated inhibition of insulin receptor tyrosine kinase activity in TNF-alpha- and obesity-induced insulin resistance. *Science,* **271**(5249): 665–8, 1996.

66. Aljada A, *et al.* Tumor necrosis factor-alpha inhibits insulin-induced increase in endothelial nitric oxide synthase and reduces insulin receptor content and phosphorylation in human aortic endothelial cells. *Metabolism,* **51**(4): 487–91, 2002.

67. Hotamisligil GS, *et al.* Reduced tyrosine kinase activity of the insulin receptor in obesity-diabetes. Central role of tumor necrosis factor-alpha. *J Clin Invest*, **94**(4): 1543–9, 1994.

68. Ofei F, *et al.* Effects of an engineered human anti-TNF-alpha antibody (CDP571) on insulin sensitivity and glycemic control in patients with NIDDM. *Diabetes*, **45**(7): 881–5, 1996.

69. Yuan M, *et al.* Reversal of obesity- and diet-induced insulin resistance with salicylates or targeted disruption of Ikkbeta. *Science*, **293**(5535): 1673–7, 2001.

70. Kim JK, *et al.* Prevention of fat-induced insulin resistance by salicylate. *J Clin Invest,* **108**(3): 437–46, 2001.

71. Baron SH. Salicylates as hypoglycemic agents. *Diabetes Care*, **5**(1): 64–71, 1982.

72. Rogers WJ, *et al.* Reduction of hospital mortality rate of acute myocardial infarction with glucose-insulin-potassium infusion. *Am Heart J,* **92**(4): 441–54, 1976.

73. Lazar HL. Enhanced preservation of acutely ischemic myocardium and improved clinical outcomes using glucose-insulin-potassium (GIK) solutions. *Am J Cardiol,* **80**(3A): 90A–93A, 1997.

74. Jonassen AK, *et al.* Glucose-insulin-potassium reduces infarction size when administered during reperfusion. *Cardiovasc Drugs Ther,* **14**(6): 615–23, 2000.

75. Malmberg K. Prospective randomised study of intensive insulin treatment on long term survival after acute myocardial infarction in patients with diabetes mellitus. DIGAMI (Diabetes Mellitus, Insulin Glucose Infusion in Acute Myocardial Infarction) Study Group. *Br Med J,* **314**(7093): 1512–5, 1997.

76. Malmberg K, McGuire DK. Diabetes and acute myocardial infarction: the role of insulin therapy. *Am Heart J,* **138**(5 Pt 1): S381–6, 1999.

77. Malmberg K, *et al.* Randomized trial of insulin-glucose infusion followed by subcutaneous insulin treatment in diabetic patients with acute myocardial infarction (DIGAMI study): effects on mortality at 1 year [see comments]. *J Am Coll Cardiol,* **26**: 57–65, 1995.

78. Lembo G, *et al.* Abnormal sympathetic overactivity evoked by insulin in the skeletal muscle of patients with essential hypertension. *J Clin Invest,* **90**(1): 24–9, 1992.

79. Abramson D, *et al.* Influence of massive doses of insulin on peripheral blood flow in man. *Am J Physiol,* **128**: 124–132, 1939.

80. DiSalvo R, *et al.* A comparison of the metabolic and circulatory effects of epinephrine, norepinephrine and insulin hypoglycemia with observations on the influence of autonmic blocking agents. *J Clin Invest,* **35**: 568–577, 1956.

81. Ginsburg J, Paton A. Effects of insulin after adrenalectomy. *Lancet,* **271**: 491–494, 1956.

82. Laakso M, *et al.* Decreased effect of insulin to stimulate skeletal muscle blood flow in obese men. A novel mechanism for insulin resistance. *J Clin Invest,* **85**(6): 1844–52, 1990.

83. Scherrer U, *et al.* Suppression of insulin-induced sympathetic activation and vasodilation by dexamethasone in humans. *Circulation,* **88**(2): 388–94, 1993.

84. Anderson EA, *et al.* Hyperinsulinemia produces both sympathetic neural activation and vasodilation in normal humans. *J Clin Invest,* **87**(6): 2246–52, 1991.

85. Vollenweider P, *et al.* Differential effects of hyperinsulinemia and carbohydrate metabolism on sympathetic nerve activity and muscle blood flow in humans. *J Clin Invest,* **92**(1): 147–54, 1993.

86. Randin D, *et al.* Effects of adrenergic and cholinergic blockade on insulin-induced stimulation of calf blood flow in humans. *Am J Physiol,* **266**(3 Pt 2): R809–16, 1994.

87. Utriainen T, *et al.* Methodological aspects, dose-response characteristics and causes of interindividual variation in insulin stimulation of limb blood flow in normal subjects. *Diabetologia,* **38**(5): 555–64, 1995.

88. Laakso M, *et al.* Kinetics of *in vivo* muscle insulin-mediated glucose uptake in human obesity. *Diabetes,* **39**(8): 965–74, 1990.

89. Laakso M, *et al.* Impaired insulin-mediated skeletal muscle blood flow in patients with NIDDM. *Diabetes,* **41**(9): 1076–83, 1992.

90. Laakso M, *et al.* Effects of epinephrine on insulin-mediated glucose uptake in whole body and leg muscle in humans: role of blood flow. *Am J Physiol,* **263**(2 Pt 1): E199–204, 1992.

91. Capaldo B, *et al.* Epinephrine directly antagonizes insulin-mediated activation of glucose uptake and inhibition of free fatty acid release in forearm tissues. *Metabolism,* **41**(10): 1146–9, 1992.

92. Lundgren F, *et al.* Insulin time-dependent effects on the leg exchange of glucose and amino acids in man. *Eur J Clin Invest,* **21**(4): 421–9, 1991.

93. Scherrer U, *et al.* Nitric oxide release accounts for insulin's vascular effects in humans. *J Clin Invest,* **94**(6): 2511–5, 1994.

94. Neahring JM, *et al.* Insulin does not reduce forearm alpha-vasoreactivity in obese hypertensive or lean normotensive men. *Hypertension,* **22**(4): 584–90, 1993.

95. Jamerson KA, *et al.* Reflex sympathetic activation induces acute insulin resistance in the human forearm. *Hypertension,* **21**: 618–623, 1993.

96. Nuutila P, *et al.* Role of blood flow in regulating insulin-stimulated glucose uptake in humans. Studies using bradykinin, [15O]water, and [18F]fluoro-deoxy-glucose and positron emission tomography. *J Clin Invest,* **97**(7): 1741–7, 1996.

97. Raitakari M, *et al.* Evidence for dissociation of insulin stimulation of blood flow and glucose uptake in human skeletal muscle: studies using [15O]H2O, [18F]fluoro-2-deoxy-D-glucose, and positron emission tomography. *Diabetes,* **45**(11): 1471–7, 1996.

98. Steinberg HO, *et al.* Insulin-mediated skeletal muscle vasodilation is nitric oxide dependent. A novel action of insulin to increase nitric oxide release. *J Clin Invest,* **94**(3): 1172–9, 1994.

99. Taddei S, *et al.* Effect of insulin on acetylcholine-induced vasodilation in normotensive subjects and patients with essential hypertension. *Circulation,* **92**(10): 2911–8, 1995.

100. Steinberg HO, *et al.* Obesity/insulin resistance is associated with endothelial dysfunction. Implications for the syndrome of insulin resistance. *J Clin Invest,* **97**(11): 2601–10, 1996.

101. Chen YL, Messina EJ. Dilation of isolated skeletal muscle arterioles by insulin is endothelium dependent and nitric oxide mediated. *Am J Physiol*, **270**(6 Pt 2): H2120–4, 1996.

102. Sobrevia L, *et al*. Activation of L-arginine transport (system y+) and nitric oxide synthase by elevated glucose and insulin in human endothelial cells. *J Physiol* (Lond). **490**: 775–781, 1996.

103. Tack CJ, *et al*. Effects of insulin on vascular tone and sympathetic nervous system in NIDDM. *Diabetes*, **45**(1): 15–22, 1996.

104. DeFronzo RA, *et al*. Effects of insulin on peripheral and splanchnic glucose metabolism in noninsulin-dependent (type II) diabetes mellitus. *J Clin Invest*, **76**(1): 149–55, 1985.

105. Kelley DE, *et al*. Effects of insulin on skeletal muscle glucose storage, oxidation, and glycolysis in humans. *Am J Physiol*, **258**(6 Pt 1): E923–9, 1990.

106. Chisholm DJ, *et al*. Interaction of secretin and insulin on human forearm metabolism. *Eur J Clin Invest*, **5**(6): 487–94, 1975.

107. Ferrannini E, *et al*. Independent stimulation of glucose metabolism and Na+–K+ exchange by insulin in the human forearm. *Am J Physiol*, **255**(6 Pt 1): E953–8, 1988.

108. Natali A, *et al*. Effects of insulin on hemodynamics and metabolism in human forearm. *Diabetes*, **39**(4): 490–500, 1990.

109. Capaldo B, *et al*. Dual mechanism of insulin action on human skeletal muscle: identification of an indirect component not mediated by FFA. *Am J Physiol*, **260**(3 Pt 1): E389–94, 1991.

110. Sakai K, *et al*. Intra-arterial infusion of insulin attenuates vasoreactivity in human forearm. *Hypertension*, **22**(1): 67–73, 1993.

111. Lembo G, *et al*. Insulin reduces reflex forearm sympathetic vasoconstriction in healthy humans. *Hypertension*, **21**(6 Pt 2): 1015–9, 1993.

112. Lembo G, *et al*. Insulin blunts sympathetic vasoconstriction through the alpha 2-adrenergic pathway in humans. *Hypertension*, **24**(4): 429–38, 1994.

113. Fujishima S, *et al*. Effects of intra-arterial infusion of insulin on forearm vasoreactivity in hypertensive humans. *Hypertens Res*, **18**(3): 227–33, 1995.

114. Gelfand RA, Barrett EJ. Effect of physiologic hyperinsulinemia on skeletal muscle protein synthesis and breakdown in man. *J Clin Invest*, **80**(1): 1–6, 1987.

115. Mathias CJ, *et al*. Hypotensive and sedative effects of insulin in autonomic failure. *Br Med J* (Clin Res Ed), **295**(6591): 161–3, 1987.

116. Sartori C, Trueb L, Scherrer U. Insulin's direct vasodilator action in humans is masked by sympathetic vasoconstrictor tone. *Diabetes*, **45**: 85A, 1996.

117. Liang C, *et al*. Insulin infusion in conscious dogs. Effects on systemic and coronary hemodynamics, regional blood flows, and plasma catecholamines. *J Clin Invest*, **69**(6): 1321–36, 1982.

118. Creager MA, Liang CS, Coffman JD. Beta adrenergic-mediated vasodilator response to insulin in the human forearm. *J Pharmacol Exp Ther*, **235**(3): 709–14, 1985.

119. Vollenweider P, *et al*. Impaired insulin-induced sympathetic neural activation and vasodilation in skeletal muscle in obese humans. *J Clin Invest*, **93**(6): 2365–71, 1994.

120. Gaenzer H, *et al*. Effect of insulin therapy on endothelium-dependent dilation in type 2 diabetes mellitus. *Am J Cardiol*, **89**(4): 431–4, 2002.

121. Rask-Madsen C, *et al*. Insulin therapy improves insulin-stimulated endothelial function in patients with type 2 diabetes and ischemic heart disease. *Diabetes*, **50**(11): 2611–8, 2001.

122. Intensive blood-glucose control with sulphonylureas or insulin compared with conventional treatment and risk of complications in patients with type 2 diabetes (UKPDS 33). UK Prospective Diabetes Study (UKPDS) Group [see comments]. *Lancet*, **352**: 837–853, 1998.

123. Hermann C, *et al*. Insulin-mediated stimulation of protein kinase Akt: A potent survival signaling cascade for endothelial cells. *Arterioscler Thromb Vasc Biol*, **20**(2): 402–9, 2000.

124. Theroux P. Myocardial cell protection: a challenging time for action and a challenging time for clinical research. *Circulation*, **101**(25): 2874–6, 2000.

125. Jonassen AK, *et al*. Myocardial protection by insulin at reperfusion requires early administration and is mediated *via* Akt and p70s6 kinase cell-survival signaling. *Circ Res*, **89**(12): 1191–8, 2001.

126. Sodi-Pallares D, Testelli M, Fishelder F. Effects of an intravenous infusion of a potassium-insulin-glucose solution on the electrocardiographic signs of myocardial infarction. *Am J Cardiol*, **9**: 166–181, 1962.

127. Opie L. The glucose hypothesis: relation to acute myocardial ischemia. *J Mol Cell Cardiol*, **1**: 107–114, 1970.

128. De Leiris J, Opie LH, Lubbe WF. Effects of free fatty acid and enzyme release in experimental glucose on myocardial infarction. *Nature*, **253**(5494): 746–7, 1975.

129. Mittra B. Potassium, glucose, and insulin in treatment of myocardial infarction. *Lancet*, **2**(7413): 607–9, 1965.

130. Potassium, glucose, and insulin treatment for acute myocardial infarction. *Lancet*, **2**(7583): 1355–60, 1968.

131. Lundman T, Orinius E. Insulin-glucose-potassium infusion in acute myocardial infarction. *Acta Med Scand*, **178**(4): 525–8, 1965.

132. Sievers J, *et al*. Acute myocardial infarction treated by glucose-insulin-potassium (GIK) infusion. *Cardiology*, **49**(4): 239–47, 1966.

133. Autio L, *et al.* Anticoagulants and Sodi-Pallares infusion in acute myocardial infarction. *Acta Med Scand*, 179(3): 355–60, 1966.

134. Malach M. Polarizing solution in acute myocardial infarction. *Am J Cardiol*, 20: 363–366, 1967.

135. Pilcher J, *et al.* Potassium, glucose and insulin in myocardial infarction. *Lancet*, 1: 1109, 1967.

136. Pentecost BL, Mayne NM, and Lamb C, Controlled trial of intravenous glucose, potassium, and insulin in acute myocardial infarction. *Lancet* 1(7549): 946–8, 1968.

137. Iisalo E, Kallio V. Potassium, glucose and insulin in the treatment of acute myocardial infarction. *Curr Ther Res Clin Exp*, 11(5): 209–15, 1969.

138. Hjermann I. A controlled study of peroral glucose, insulin and potassium treatment in myocardial infarction. *Acta Med Scand*, 190(3): 213–8, 1971.

139. Heng MK, *et al.* Effects of glucose and glucose-insulin-potassium on haemodynamics and enzyme release after acute myocardial infarction. *Br Heart J*, 39(7): 748–57, 1977.

140. Stanley A, Prather J. Glucose-insulin-potassium, patient mortality and the acute myocardial infarction: results from a prospective randomized study. *Circulation*, 57(suppl II): II–62, 1978.

141. Rogers W, *et al.* Prospective randomized trial of glucose-insulin-potassium in acute myocardial infarction: effects of hemodynamics, short and long-term survival. *J Am Coll Cardiol*, 1: 628, 1983.

142. Jaffe AS, *et al.* Increased congestive heart failure after myocardial infarction of modest extent in patients with diabetes mellitus. *Am Heart J*, 108(1): 31–7, 1984.

143. Celentano A, *et al.* Early abnormalities of cardiac function in non-insulin-dependent diabetes mellitus and impaired glucose tolerance. *Am J Cardiol*, 76(16): 1173–6, 1995.

144. Abbud ZA, *et al.* Effect of diabetes mellitus on short- and long-term mortality rates of patients with acute myocardial infarction: a statewide study. Myocardial Infarction Data Acquisition System Study Group. *Am Heart J*, 130(1): 51–8, 1995.

145. Orlander PR, *et al.* The relation of diabetes to the severity of acute myocardial infarction and post-myocardial infarction survival in Mexican-Americans and non-Hispanic whites. The Corpus Christi Heart Project. *Diabetes*, 43(7): 897–902, 1994.

146. Gustafsson F, *et al.* Long-term prognosis after acute myocardial infarction in patients with a history of arterial hypertension. TRACE study group. *Eur Heart J*, 19(4): 588–94, 1998.

147. Oswald GA, *et al.* Determinants and importance of stress hyperglycaemia in non-diabetic patients with myocardial infarction. *Br Med J* (Clin Res Ed), 293(6552): 917–22, 1986.

148. O'Sullivan JJ, *et al.* In-hospital prognosis of patients with fasting hyperglycemia after first myocardial infarction. *Diabetes Care*, 14(8): 758–60, 1991.

149. Bellodi G, *et al.* Hyperglycemia and prognosis of acute myocardial infarction in patients without diabetes mellitus. *Am J Cardiol*, 64(14): 885–8, 1989.

150. Fava S, *et al.* The prognostic value of blood glucose in diabetic patients with acute myocardial infarction. *Diabet Med*, 13(1): 80–3, 1996.

151. Kuusisto J, *et al.* NIDDM and its metabolic control predict coronary heart disease in elderly subjects. *Diabetes*, 43: 960–967, 1994.

152. Uusitupa MI, *et al.* Ten-year cardiovascular mortality in relation to risk factors and abnormalities in lipoprotein composition in type 2 (non-insulin-dependent) diabetic and non-diabetic subjects. *Diabetologia*, 36: 1175–1184, 1993.

153. Klein R. Hyperglycemia and microvascular and macrovascular disease in diabetes. *Diabetes Care*, 18(2): 258–68, 1995.

154. Andersson DK, Svardsudd K. Long-term glycemic control relates to mortality in type II diabetes. *Diabetes Care*, 18(12): 1534–43, 1995.

155. Norhammar A, *et al.* Glucose metabolism in patients with acute myocardial infarction and no previous diagnosis of diabetes mellitus: a prospective study. *Lancet*, 359(9324): 2140–4, 2002.

156. Wahab NN, *et al.* Is blood glucose an independent predictor of mortality in acute myocardial infarction in the thrombolytic era? *J Am Coll Cardiol*, 40(10): 1748–54, 2002.

157. Aronson D, Rayfield EJ, Chesebro JH. Mechanisms determining course and outcome of diabetic patients who have had acute myocardial infarction. *Ann Intern Med*, 126(4): 296–306, 1997.

158. Iwakura K, *et al.* Association between hyperglycemia and the no-reflow phenomenon in patients with acute myocardial infarction. *J Am Coll Cardiol*, 41(1): 1–7, 2003.

159. Diaz R, *et al.* Metabolic modulation of acute myocardial infarction. The ECLA (Estudios Cardiologicos Latinoamerica) Collaborative Group. *Circulation*, 98(21): 2227–34, 1998.

160. Fath-Ordoubadi F, Beatt KJ. Glucose-insulin-potassium therapy for treatment of acute myocardial infarction: an overview of randomized placebo-controlled trials. *Circulation*, 96(4): 1152–6, 1997.

161. Malmberg K, *et al.* Randomized trial of insulin-glucose infusion followed by subcutaneous insulin treatment in diabetic patients with acute myocardial infarction (DIGAMI study): effects on mortality at 1 year. *J Am Coll Cardiol*, 26(1): 57–65, 1995.

162. Topol EJ. Toward a new frontier in myocardial reperfusion therapy: emerging platelet preeminence. *Circulation*, 97(2): 211–8, 1998.

163. Paganelli F, *et al*. Relationship of plasminogen activator inhibitor-1 levels following thrombolytic therapy with rt-PA as compared to streptokinase and patency of infarct related coronary artery. *Thromb Haemost*, **82**(1): 104–8, 1999.

164. Ott I, *et al*. Proteolysis of tissue factor pathway inhibitor-1 by thrombolysis in acute myocardial infarction. *Circulation*, **105**(3): 279–81, 2002.

165. Libby P, Lee RT. Matrix matters. *Circulation*, **102**(16): 1874–6, 2000.

166. Andreotti F, *et al*. Von Willebrand factor, plasminogen activator inhibitor-1 and C-reactive protein are markers of thrombolytic efficacy in acute myocardial infarction. *Thromb Haemost*, **68**(6): 678–82, 1992.

167. Rohde LE, *et al*. Matrix metalloproteinase inhibition attenuates early left ventricular enlargement after experimental myocardial infarction in mice. *Circulation*, **99**(23): 3063–70, 1999.

168. Tomlinson DR, Fernyhough A, Diemel LT. Role of neurotrophins in diabetic neuropathy and treatment with nerve growth factors. *Diabetes*, **46 Suppl 2**: S43–9, 1997.

169. Agwunobi AO, *et al*. Insulin resistance and substrate utilization in human endotoxemia. *J Clin Endocrinol Metab*, **85**(10): 3770–8, 2000.

170. Fan J, *et al*. Endotoxin-induced alterations in insulin-stimulated phosphorylation of insulin receptor, IRS-1, and MAP kinase in skeletal muscle. *Shock*, **6**(3): 164–70, 1996.

171. Van den Berghe G, *et al*. Intensive insulin therapy in the critically ill patients. *N Engl J Med*, **345**(19): 1359–67, 2001.

172. Dandona P, Aljada A. A rational approach to pathogenesis and treatment of type 2 diabetes mellitus, insulin resistance, inflammation, and atherosclerosis. *Am J Cardiol*, **90**(5A): 27G–33G, 2002.

39

NEW INSIGHTS INTO THE TREATMENT OF ACUTE CORONARY SYNDROMES IN DIABETIC PATIENTS

Maria DOROBANȚU, Şerban BĂLĂNESCU

Patients with diabetes mellitus mainly those with type 2, non-insulin dependent have a high prevalence of coronary artery disease (CAD) and especially acute coronary syndromes (ACS). They have diffuse CAD with long lesions in small vessels, display a hypercoagulability state with increased procoagulant factors and decreased fibrinolytic activity and have dysfunctional platelets. All these are associated with an inflammatory vasculopathic state, partly due to hyperglycemia, with decreased endothelium dependent vasodilative response and increased levels of pro-inflammatory cytokines and adhesion molecules that accelerate the atherosclerotic process and destabilize chronic lesions. On this background there is a higher risk of subsequent cardiovascular events and mortality after the index coronary event in diabetic patients as compared with non-diabetics. Constantly increasing prevalence of type 2 diabetes, the high prevalence of CAD and ACS and poor long term outcome of this group of patients represent a major challenge for cardiovascular medicine. The future of the diabetic patient with an ACS depends dramatically on therapeutic measures undertaken at the time of admission. An aggressive strategy with early angiography and percutaneous coronary intervention (PCI) appears justified despite a higher rate of acute complications, incomplete revascularization and poorer outcome when compared to non-diabetics. The best revascularization treatment that should be used in diabetics is the association between stent implantation and administration of a Gp IIb/IIIa inhibitor, particularly abciximab. There is a large amount of data supporting aggressive metabolic treatment with insulin, glucose and potassium to rapidly reverse glucose metabolic disorders in ACS that confers major long term survival benefits. No evidence-based treatment that showed effective in ACS should be withheld from diabetics because of fear of adverse events, if otherwise indicated. This is the case of thrombolytic therapy and beta blockade. Surgery performs clearly better than PCI as revascularization method in stable diabetics, but new PCI strategies have not been compared with CABG yet. Drug eluting stents that significantly reduce the incidence of restenosis may eventually prove effective even in diabetics and thus cancel the major drawback of PCI in these patients that is high incidence of target vessel revascularization.

INTRODUCTION

The number of patients with diabetes mellitus (DM) particularly of those with type II, non insulin dependent disease (which is responsible for about 90% of cases) is rapidly expanding. Progressive ageing of the population, obesity and lack of physical activity are among the main culprits of this epidemic. The prevalence of DM at the end of 2005 is expected to be 5.5% while doubling of the number of diabetics is anticipated during the first quarter of the 21st century [1].

Although major advances in the glycemic control of patients with DM have been achieved in recent years, cardiovascular complications represent the main cause of death and morbidity in this particular population. The risk of cardiovascular death in diabetics is two- to six times greater than that of non diabetic subjects and the incidence of coronary artery disease (CAD) is twice as frequent the age-adjusted prevalence of the disease in normal individuals [2]. Cardiovascular death is the major cause of mortality in these patients, as 75 to 80% of them will die because of acute myocardial infarction (AMI), stroke or peripheral artery disease [3]. A troubling epidemiological observation showed that in recent years patients with diabetes do not experience a reduced mortality rate with improved medical care in contrast with general population [2].

The increased cardiovascular risk of diabetic patients is emphasized by two epidemiological observations. The first demonstrated that diabetics with no history of CAD have the same risk of death as individuals with prior MI and no diabetes [4]. The second one showed that type 2 diabetics have a two- to three times increase of atherosclerotic arterial complications than non diabetics [5].

Because of their increased cardiovascular risk, including that of ACS, diabetic patients should be aggressively treated with the specific aim to fully achieve glycemic control, normal blood pressure, LDL and HDL cholesterol, and triglycerides. Such an aggressive strategy was associated with a significant decrease in cardiovascular complications (OR = 0.47; 95% CI = 0.24 – 0.73) *versus* conventional treatment according to national guidelines at a mean follow-up of 7.8 years in patients with type 2 DM [6].

One of the most important issues of cardiovascular complications in diabetic patients is treatment of acute coronary syndromes (ACS),

including ST segment elevation AMI (STEMI). Despite progress in drug therapy and increased use of invasive treatment in these clinical settings, diabetic patients continue to have poorer outcome in ACS with a survival rate at 5 years of 50% [7, 8]. Furthermore, percutaneous intervention (PCI) adopted as revascularization strategy in diabetics has significant drawbacks with increased rates of major adverse cardiovascular events (MACE). These include recurrent ischemia or MI, target lesion revascularization (TLR) or target vessel revascularization (TVR) because of an increased risk of restenosis and may culminate in cardiac death [9, 10].

All of the above: increased incidence of systemic atherosclerotic disease, CAD and cardiovascular complications, increased risk of cardiovascular mortality and poorer outcome of revascularization strategies in diabetic patients, represent a major challenge for cardiovascular medicine. No other clinical situation is so relevant by its potential life threatening complications as an ACS in a diabetic patient. The following topic will deal with particular pathophysiological, clinical and therapeutic aspects of ACS in diabetes.

EPIDEMIOLOGICAL ASPECTS OF ACS IN DIABETES

Initial reports found that 10% of patients with AMI had DM, but recent studies found a much higher prevalence of 20 to 25% of the disease in this selected population [11, 12]. The OASIS registry (Organization to Assess Strategies for Ischemic Syndromes) identified a 21% prevalence of DM among patients with unstable angina and non ST segment elevation myocardial infarction (NSTEMI) [7]. There were significant differences between countries, patients with ACS from the USA having the highest incidence of DM (more than 30% of the whole group). When patients with ACS that had impaired oral glucose tolerance test were included in the prevalence analysis, two thirds of these patients had an abnormality of glucose metabolism. Thus only about 30% of subjects with previous MI have normal blood glucose levels at three months after infarction [13]. The conclusion of these epidemiological observations is that insulin resistance and DM are the most frequent risk factors for development of ACS.

In patients with diagnosed DM the prevalence of MI is higher than that found in control population. Irrespective of their previous coronary status, the 2175 diabetics included in the GUSTO IIb study [14] had a twice greater risk of developing an ACS than control population at 6 months, even after adjustment for age and other multivariate predictors of outcome [8].

A study performed on 2432 patients, of whom 1059 had diabetes, has demonstrated at a mean follow-up of 7 years that the incidence of MI in diabetics was virtually the same with that of non diabetics that previously had a major coronary event (20.2% vs. 18.8%) [4]. Such studies clearly demonstrated that isolated DM is associated with the same cardiovascular risk as previous MI in an otherwise healthy population and determined the designation of DM as a CAD equivalent by the National Cholesterol Education Program in Adult Treatment Panel III (ATP III) [15].

MORBIDITY AND MORTALITY IN DIABETICS WITH ACS

Initial studies reported a 50% 1-year mortality rate in consecutive unselected diabetic patients with AMI [11]. Despite reduction in mortality with recent therapeutic advances in ACS, diabetics have an increased relative risk for mortality of 1.5–2.5 times higher than non-diabetics. A study performed on more than 25.000 Swedish diabetic patients enrolled in the RIKS-HIA trial found a 1-year mortality of 30% after 65 years of age [12]. The impact of diabetes on mortality was higher in younger patients: the odds ratio for dying was 1.7 in elderly patients and 3.0 in those under 65 years, despite overall mortality was lower in the latter. There is strong evidence that DM is an independent predictor of mortality in patients with non ST segment elevation ACS. The OASIS registry demonstrated that DM was independently predicting not only cardiovascular death, but also cardiovascular adverse events, like new MI, stroke and heart failure [7].

The most frequent cause of death in diabetics with ACS is heart failure, despite most studies showed consistently that infarction size in diabetics was identical or even smaller than in non-diabetics. This paradox may be explained by diffuse myocardial disease with almost universal diastolic dysfunction in DM and no compensatory reserve of non infarcted myocardium related mostly to metabolic derangements specific to the disease.

A recurrent major coronary event is the second most frequent cause of death in DM. This can be easily understood from the well-known diffuse coronary atherosclerosis found in diabetics and to their propensity to destabilize atherosclerotic lesions and to coronary thrombosis.

The third most frequent cause of death in DM is sudden death. Many mechanisms may interact in leading to sudden death in diabetics. Decreased or abolished ischemic pain perception may be responsible for ignored severe episodes of myocardial ischemia that can result in malignant ventricular tachyarrhythmia. Diabetics with autonomic neuropathy have decreased vagal output to the heart resulting in severely decreased indexes of heart rate variability and constantly increased heart rate. This is a well-known risk factor for ventricular arrhythmias and it has been independently correlated with sudden cardiac death [16, 17].

WHY DO DIABETICS HAVE A PROPENSITY TO DESTABILIZE ATHEROSCLEROTIC LESIONS?

Not only cardiovascular risk factors have a higher impact on development and progression rate of atherosclerotic lesions in diabetics, but they also tend to have unstable complicated plaques responsible for ACS and other acute atherothrombotic manifestations. The mechanisms for this tendency to complicated atherosclerotic lesions resulting in increased cardiovascular risk are apparently related to hypertension, dyslipidemia, smoking or obesity in only 25% of cases [18]. The presence of advanced glycation end-products (AGEs) determined by uncontrolled hyperglycemia promote a vascular inflammatory response by interacting with AGEs receptors (RAGEs) in the vessel walls [19]. This leads to proliferation of inflammatory cells, influence the redox state of the endothelium [20] and adversely influence the generation of subintimal extracellular matrix resulting in accelerated progression of atherosclerotic lesions and acute complications [21].

Inflammation and hypercoagulability are the two faces of unstable atherosclerotic lesions and they influence one another in a continuum that determines the occurrence of an ACS [22].

Inflammation is perhaps the most important link between diabetes and unstable atherosclerosis [23]. An early stage of the atherosclerotic process is characterized by increased expression of genes involved in the redox phenomenon in endothelium and smooth muscle cells [24]. The nuclear factor kappa-beta (NF-κβ) is a monocyte chemotactic protein involved in transcription of many cytokines and stimulates expression of vascular adhesion molecule-1 (VCAM-1) [25]. The transcription factor NF-κβ, the macrophage-colony stimulating factor (M-CSF) and interleukin-6 are highly expressed in the monocytes of diabetics [26], and they are the main culprits involved in the chronic inflammatory vasculopathic state. By increased expression of adhesion molecules, like VCAM-1 and selectins, monocytes accumulate at the site of atherosclerotic lesions [24]. They then transform into macrophages and produce collagen-degrading enzymes (like metalloproteinases – MMPs), contributing to plaque ulceration by transforming atherosclerotic lesions into "thin-cap atheromas". A high percentage of macrophages were seen in the atherosclerotic plaques of persons with DM obtained by atherectomy compared to culprit lesions of non-diabetic patients [3].

High serum levels of M-CSF are strongly correlated with the development of an ACS [27] and cardiac event-free survival is lower in patients M-CSF higher than 1 γ/liter [28]. This growth factor modulates monocyte adherence and proliferation and may directly influence SMC death by apoptosis [29]. This reduces the ratio between macrophages and SMCs in atherosclerotic lesions, which characterizes unstable plaques [30]. Abciximab has been shown to inhibit the killing effect of M-CSF-activated macrophages on SMCs [28]. This effect has been attributed to inhibition of the Mac-1 receptor on the macrophages with abciximab preventing their adhesion to the intercellular adhesion molecule-1 (ICAM-1) on the membrane of SMCs. The macrophages of patients with DM are particularly sensitive to the action of M-CSF and express high activity of peroxisome proliferator activated receptor-gamma (PPARγ), that is responsible for the activity of DM and its complications [31].

The chronic inflammatory state is associated to an increased risk of plaque ulceration, but also determines endothelial dysfunction and altered vasodilator response, both responsible for the increased risk for development of an ACS in DM.

Platelet dysfunction is common in DM and may be responsible for acute complications during PCI and difficulty in efficiently controlling an ACS with conventional drug approach. The platelets of diabetic patients have a greater number of Gp IIb/IIIa receptors with up to 26% [32], are more frequently activated [33] and show greater ability to aggregate [34] and higher thromboxane A2 synthesis [35] than those of non diabetics. *In vitro* studies have previously shown that diabetic platelets excessively react in all phases of activation, adhesion and ability to aggregate [36]. All these anomalies are encountered despite normal platelet counts compared to healthy controls; however, the platelet of a diabetic has a larger volume [32]. All these modifications occur irrespective of glycemic control and depend on the chronic hyperinsulinemia [36].

Hypercoagulability is also encountered in diabetes and has a major role both in progression of atherosclerotic lesions [37] and in acute complications of unstable plaques [38]. Some coagulation factors, like fibrinogen, thrombin, factor VIIa and endothelium related plasminogen activator-inhibitor (PAI-1) are increased in the serum obtained from diabetics. At the same time natural anticoagulants, like tissue plasminogen activator (t-PA), have lower plasma concentrations, while AGEs modify the endothelial receptor sites for tPA [38].

Inflammation, increased thrombin generation, reduced fibrinolytic potential and activated platelets are responsible for a systemic prothrombotic state [36] and explain why 75% of diabetic patients die because of atherothrombotic disease [37].

CHARACTERISTICS OF CAD IN DIABETICS

One of the most important pathologic characteristics of coronary atherosclerosis in DM is that these patients tend to have longer lesions in smaller vessels. This has a particular impact on the acute results of PCI and on the increased rate of restenosis observed at 6 months after the initial procedure.

An intriguing observation about coronary atherosclerosis and plaque formation in diabetes is that negative remodeling is a frequently encountered phenomenon at the site of plaque development.

This has been attributed to insulin treatment, probably as a result of a dysfunctional adaptive phenomenon [39]. This phenomenon occurs not only in native arteries, but also in vessels treated with simple balloon PCI and contributes to the increased incidence of restenosis in DM, when no stent has been implanted during the index procedure. This contrasts with a process of progressive outwards wall expansion as a positive remodeling phenomenon that occurs with accumulation of the lipid core, described by Glagov [40]. This tends to reduce the impact of subintimal plaque accumulation on luminal surface, which is reduced in later stages.

Diabetic patients have a reduced propensity to form collateral vessels with chronic myocardial ischemia [41], that might be life saving in the presence of an acute coronary event. Impaired metabolism of NO and other promoters of angiogenesis may be responsible for this defect.

CONVENTIONAL TREATMENT OF ACS IN DIABETICS

Insulin significantly improves myocardial metabolism by increasing glucose uptake and oxidation and by reducing the use of free fatty acids for energy production. This is essential mainly for the vulnerable not-infarcted myocardium in ACS. Rapid amelioration of glucose metabolism by insulin leads also to improvement in spontaneous fibrinolytic mechanisms and to improved endothelial function.

It is also well recognized that the occurrence of an ACS can suddenly worsen the metabolic state of an otherwise stable diabetic. The most frequent biological finding in a diabetic patient suffering from an ACS is hyperglycemia and this most frequently due to relative insulin deficiency determined by acute stress. Stress hyperglycemia is related to short term mortality in both diabetic and normal controls [42]. In another study (Diabetes Mellitus Insulin-Glucose Infusion in Acute Myocardial Infarction – DIGAMI) a direct relationship between long-term cardiovascular mortality and admission blood glucose was identified in patients with AMI [43]. A similar correlation was observed in non-diabetic patients at long-term follow-up after AMI [44]. In conclusion abnormal blood glucose during an ACS is indicating patients at risk for development of future cardiovascular events and mortality. Interestingly "blood glucose is a continuous risk factor that operates well below the diabetic threshold" [45].

The survival effect of reestablishing metabolic balance with insulin, glucose and potassium infusion during AMI in diabetic patients was tested in the DIGAMI study [43]. Diabetics were randomly assigned to aggressive metabolic treatment with glucose-insulin-potassium (GIK) infusion followed by subcutaneous multiple insulin injections and to "conventional treatment" left to the decision of the treating cardiologist. A high percentage of patients with AMI included in this study received thrombolytic (80%) and beta-blocker (70%) therapy. Almost 90% of patients initially assigned to insulin therapy were left on it at hospital discharge *versus* 44% of those treated conventionally. The patients that received GIK and insulin during the index event had a 1-year mortality rate of 19% *versus* 28% of those that received the so-called standard treatment. This difference persisted at 3.4 years follow-up with a 33% mortality in the insulin group *versus* 44% in the conventional treatment arm (RR = 0.72; 95% CI = 0.92–0.55; p = 0.011). The most important survival advantage in insulin treated patients was observed among those who never received insulin prior the acute coronary event and who were thought at lower cardiovascular risk.

The utility of insulin treatment in AMI in non diabetics has been addressed in some small studies. A meta-analysis performed on few studies that included 1932 non-diabetic patients demonstrated a mortality reduction of 25% in those treated with GIK infusion [46]. Other studies reported a striking decrease of mortality in patients treated with GIK infusion and reperfusion therapy (RR = 0.34; 95% CI = 0.15–0.78; p = 0.008) [47]. Another study performed on 1 548 patients with MI, of whom only 13% were diabetics, were randomized to insulin therapy [48]. The trial was prematurely interrupted because of a major decrease in CCU (Coronary Care Unit) mortality (RR = 0.58; 95% CI = 0.38–0.78; p = 0.05) and reduction of in-hospital mortality.

The mechanisms for the clinical benefit seen with insulin treatment in patients with abnormal glucose metabolism during ACS are very diverse. Acute hyperglycemia is responsible for impaired endothelium dependent vasodilatation even in healthy subjects. Type 2 diabetic patients show no increase in myocardial blood flow reserve which is independently related to blood glucose control [49]. There is a positive relationship between the severity of hyperglycemia and arterial stiffness in type 2 DM which varies between impaired glucose metabolism and decompensated diabetes [50]. In a study on type 2 diabetics intensive treatment with associated insulin and metformin not only resulted in a significant reduction of fasting glucose, free fatty acids and HbA1c, but also led to normal forearm blood flow response to acetylcholine at 6 months follow-up [51].

Insulin treatment can also favorably influence coagulation-lysis equilibrium during ACS. A study performed in type 2 diabetics with AMI randomly assigned to receive GIK infusion followed by subcutaneous insulin injections showed significant reductions of plasma PAI-1 and fibrinogen concentrations as compared to the control group [52].

Another beneficial effect of insulin treatment is related to its newly described anti-inflammatory actions responsible for progression and destabilization of atherosclerotic lesions. Insulin may reduce the vascular inflammatory status as expressed by reduced levels of intranuclear nuclear factor kappa-beta (NF-κβ) with consequent reduction in endothelial adhesion molecules and plasma PAI-1 activity [53].

Thus there is a large amount of data about the paramount importance to rapidly normalize the altered metabolic function in an ACS in diabetics and non-diabetic patients. Consequently, all recently discovered or previously diagnosed diabetics with aggravated metabolic dysfunction should be treated with insulin during an ACS, irrespective of their previous medication. This is extremely beneficial for the vascular status and myocardial function during the ACS and it may avoid future vascular events. Continuation of insulin therapy should be individually decided in the convalescence period after the ACS.

Conventional medical treatment of ACS with aspirin, heparin, thrombolytics, angiotensin-converting enzyme inhibitors, beta-blockers and statins proved equally effective in diabetics as in non-diabetics. For example, statin therapy may increase endothelium-dependent vasodilatation without altering lipid profile as early as three days after an ACS [54]. However, some very efficient medication has been inexplicably not given to some diabetics during ACS because of concern of adverse reactions. This holds particularly true for thrombolytics and beta-blockers. Despite proved increased benefit interventional revascularization procedures are still underused in diabetics, because of otherwise justified fear of poorer outcome, incomplete revascularization, diffuse coronary disease, contrast-induced nephropathy and vascular access complications. There is proof that evidence-based beneficial treatment during ACS is underused in diabetics, which should be a matter of concern.

SPECIFIC PROBLEMS IN THE TREATMENT OF ACS IN DIABETICS

FIBRINOLYTIC THERAPY IN ACUTE MYOCARDIAL INFARCTION

Large scale clinical trials have proved a major survival benefit with thrombolytic therapy in all categories of patients with AMI including diabetics. In the GUSTO study reperfusion therapy with streptokinase or tPA was associated with the same patency rate in diabetics as in non diabetic patients. However, 30-day mortality rate was almost double in diabetics (10.5% vs. 6.2%), and it was surprisingly 1.3 times higher in insulin dependent subjects compared to non insulin dependent patients.

Although there were doubts about the efficiency of fibrinolytics in diabetes because of baseline high platelet ability to aggregate, which can be increased by the thrombolytic drug, high coagulant activity and the increased synthesis of PAI-1 all clinical trials have proved significant benefits in the diabetic subgroups. Fear of hemorrhagic complications was not confirmed by higher incidence of intracranial (0.6%) or intraocular bleeding in diabetic patients in all major studies. Also there is no significant difference in the incidence of TIMI (Thrombolysis in Myocardial Infarction) 3 flow 90 minutes after thrombolytic therapy between diabetic and non diabetic population. Although a higher rate of reocclusion and recurrent infarction after fibrinolysis has been observed in diabetics it has not reached statistical significance in all trials; recurrent ischemia is more frequent in diabetics treated with fibrinolysis.

We have to emphasize the importance of administration of thrombolytic therapy in diabetic patients with AMI, as clinical trials report frequently data about underutilization of this tremendously important therapy in myocardial infarction. There have been reports of thrombolytic therapy being given to only 50% of diabetics with AMI that had clear indication to receive it, mainly because of concern of hemorrhagic complications. At the same time it has to be considered the frequent late presentation of the diabetic patient with AMI and atypical chest pain that makes the immediate diagnosis difficult and delays administration of efficient therapy.

BETA-BLOCKERS AND ANGIOTENSIN CONVERTING ENZYME INHIBITORS IN DIABETIC PATIENTS WITH AMI

Early beta-blocker therapy in AMI is associated with smaller infarct size, lower rates of recurrent ischemia and reinfarction and sudden cardiac death. Some trials have reported a lower rate of free wall rupture in AMI with the use of beta-blocker therapy. Despite all these advantages there is concern that beta-blockers given to diabetic patients with AMI can worsen glycemic control or mask hypoglycemic symptoms. If used with care beta-blockers show the same advantages in diabetics and should not be withheld from this patient subgroup.

When the data on 45 308 patients with AMI older than 65 (26% were diabetics) enrolled in the National Cooperative Cardiovascular Project have been analyzed, beta-blocker therapy was associated with a lower mortality rate both in insulin dependent and in non insulin dependent patients. The survival benefit was equal to that observed in non diabetic patients with no increase in diabetes-related complications.

Angiotensin converting enzyme inhibitors (ACE-I) given to patients with AMI are responsible for smaller infarcts, prevent LV (Left Ventricular) remodeling and reduce mortality. These effects are more prominent in patients with anterior AMI and in those with early systolic dysfunction. In the GISSI-3 trial that included 2 790 diabetic subjects with AMI lisinopril treatment reduced 6-month mortality from 16.1% to 12.9%. The survival benefit was higher in the diabetic subgroup and occurred independently from insulin treatment during the acute phase. Analysis of data obtained from diabetics enrolled in the TRACE trial showed also a survival advantage in this population: the relative risk was 0.64 for all-cause mortality and 0.38 for new onset LV failure in diabetics treated with ACE-I.

USE OF GP IIB/IIIA INHIBITORS IN ACS IN DIABETIC PATIENTS

Platelet membrane expresses glycoprotein receptors from the integrin family, responsible for platelet adhesion and aggregation [55]. Glycoprotein (GP) IIb/IIIa suffers conformational changes in contact with agonists such as thrombin, adenosine diphosphate or epinephrine that allows it to bind fibrinogen together with increased phenotypic expression of its own molecule [56]. All agonists of platelet aggregation interact in activating and increasing expression of Gp IIb/IIIa as a final common pathway for white platelet thrombus formation. Cross linking of platelets by fibrin strands results in formation of thrombus at the site of arterial injury. Fibrinogen is the most important ligand for Gp IIb/IIIa because of its relatively high plasma concentration which is further increased in diabetics [55].

There are three different available drugs that inhibit the Gp IIb/IIIa receptor that have been approved for clinical use: abciximab, eptifibatide and tirofiban. They differ significantly in the way they antagonize the Gp IIb/IIIa receptors due to their different molecular structure. Antithrombotic efficacy translated into marked reduction in adverse ischemic cardiac events is evident when more than 80% of platelet aggregation capacity is inhibited [57]. These drugs are of tremendous importance in treating diabetic patients with an ACS, either managed medically or treated by PCI.

Abciximab is a human murine chimeric monoclonal antibody fragment with high molecular weight of approximately 48,000 Da, short plasma half-life of 15–30 min, but prolonged platelet-bound half-life (6–12 hours) due to high-affinity for the Gp IIb/IIIa receptor and stable binding in a 1.5-2.0 ratio; at steady state it is predominantly receptor bound with little unbound drug present in the plasma [58]. Abciximab binds to a complex ligand site on the Gp IIb/IIIa receptor, and also blocks the vitronectin receptor ($\alpha_v\beta_3$ integrin) from endothelial and smooth muscle cells and the CD11b/18 ($\alpha_m\beta_2$ or MAC 1) receptor found on granulocytes, monocytes and natural killer cells [59]. Thus abciximab is able not only to block platelet aggregation, but also to interfere with the interaction between platelets and endothelial cells and platelets and white cells as demonstrated in few studies [60–62]. More than that abciximab reduces serum levels of C-reactive protein (CRP), demonstrating a potent anti-inflammatory effect [63].

Eptifibatide is a small-molecule cyclic heptapeptide with a molecular weight of 800 Da with extended plasma half-life of 2.5 hours due to reversible binding to the Gp IIb/IIIa platelet receptor and a large unbound, plasma concentration at steady state [64]. It binds directly to the arginine-glycine-aspartic acid (RGD) component of the β_3 subunit of the Gp IIb/IIIa receptor [59]. It is a low-affinity agent with relatively long plasma half-life and short duration of action at the target receptor site.

Tirofiban is a small, non peptide molecule with a short plasma half-life and marked specificity for Gp IIb/IIIa receptor very similar to eptifibatide from the pharmacodynamic point of view [65].

All these drugs have been clinically tested in large scale trials in conjunction with aspirin and i.v. heparin, both in ACS managed medically and in interventional settings in patients treated by PCI.

A meta-analysis of 16 randomized trials that enrolled more than 32,000 patients treated with Gp IIb/IIIa inhibitors showed a marked reduction in clinical endpoints (death, death/MI, and combined endpoints) as early as 48 to 96 hours after inclusion, that were sustained at 6 months follow-up [66]. Another meta-analysis was performed on the 6 randomized trials with Gp IIb/IIIa inhibitors used in patients with ACS that were not scheduled to be treated by an early revascularization procedure (PRISM, PRISM-PLUS, PARAGON A and B, GUSTO IV ACS and PURSUIT) [67]. This study demonstrated that treatment with Gp IIb/IIIa inhibitors is associated with a relative risk reduction of death or MI at 30 days of 9% (n = 31 402; p = 0.015), even in this population of patients that were not treated by early revascularization.

Another meta-analysis was performed on 6 458 diabetic patients with non ST segment elevation ACS included in the same 6 previous studies (PRISM and PRISM-PLUS with tirofiban, PURSUIT with eptifibatide, GUSTO IV ACS with abciximab, and PARAGON A and B with lamifiban). A significant reduction in 30-day mortality was observed in patients treated with Gp IIb/IIIa inhibitors from 6.2% to 4.6% (p = 0.007) [68]. The survival advantage was not observed in the 23.072 non diabetic patients. There was a significant correlation between Gp IIb/IIIa blockage and the presence of diabetes (p = 0.036).

USE OF GP IIB/IIIA INHIBITORS DURING PCI IN DIABETIC PATIENTS

As already mentioned above, PCI in diabetic patients is technically demanding mainly because of the presence of long lesions in small vessels and extensive vessel injury at the site of angioplasty. Diabetics have increased mortality rates after PCI [69].

Two treatment strategies have been shown to dramatically improve outcome after PCI in diabetics. Stent implantation was associated with increased 6-month survival rates than plain balloon angioplasty [70]. When used together, Gp IIb/IIIa inhibitors and stents are particularly useful during PCI in DM [71].

EPISTENT was a study in which three revascularization strategies were tested in 2 399 patients: PCI + abciximab, stent + abciximab and stent + placebo [72]. There was a significant reduction in the 6-month combined clinical endpoint in the abciximab treated patients against those treated with stents alone. A subsequent analysis performed on the 491 diabetic patients enrolled in EPISTENT demonstrated that combination between abciximab and coronary stenting was the best percutaneous revascularization strategy in diabetics, neutralizing their excessive risk relative to non-diabetics with regard to short and long-term complications after PCI [73]. Abciximab and stenting provided a greater absolute risk reduction in the combined endpoint at 30 days in diabetics, 6.5% *versus* 5.3% in non-diabetic subjects [74].

Most benefit of abciximab in diabetic patients enrolled in EPISTENT was obtained mainly in the rate of late target vessel revascularization [74]. Divergence in the TVR event-curves began to occur 90 days after PCI, not depending at all on suppression of acute ischemic complications with abciximab. It can be speculated that interference with endothelial and smooth muscle cells integrins by abciximab is responsible for this benefit in the late need for revascularization, which is not evident at 30 days after PCI. There was a strong trend of a reduced one-year mortality rate in diabetics treated with a stent and abciximab (1.2%; p = 0.11) compared to those receiving a stent and placebo (4.1%).

The meta-analysis by Roffi *et al.*, performed on 1279 diabetic patients with non ST segment elevation ACS included in 6 randomized studies with Gp IIb/IIIa inhibitors, showed a larger benefit in mortality reduction in those treated with PCI and a Gp IIb/IIIa inhibitor. Mortality at 30 days was 4% with PCI *vs.* 1.2% with PCI and Gp IIb/IIIa inhibition (p = 0.002) [68], similar to the results obtained in EPISTENT with abciximab. The data emerging from this meta-analysis confirmed that the best therapeutic strategy in non ST segment elevation ACS in diabetics is early revascularization associated with administration of a Gp IIb/IIIa inhibitor.

OUTCOME OF DIABETIC PATIENTS TREATED WITH PCI

The same poorer outcome observed for diabetic patients with conservatively treated AMI compared with multivariate risk factor-adjusted control population with no diabetes is noted after PCI in diabetics. In-hospital mortality after PCI, irrespective of the urgency of the procedure, either elective or urgent, is increased two times in DM [75]. In a randomized study comparing outcome of patients treated with PCI *vs.* CABG 8-year survival was lower in diabetics treated with PCI *versus* non-diabetics treated with the same revascularization method (60.1% *vs.* 82.6%; p=0.02) (the EAST study) [76]. The incidence of TLR or TVR was also higher in DM patients. Other major trials comparing PCI with CABG showed the same results in diabetic patients treated by angioplasty [77].

REVASCULARIZATION STRATEGIES IN DIABETIC PATIENTS: STENT OR SCALPEL?

Some major trials compared PCI and CABG in the effort to clarify the issue of long term outcome of coronary patients treated by one of these revascularization methods. In the Bypass Angioplasty Revascularization Investigation (BARI)

1829 patients with multivessel CAD have been randomized to either PCI or CABG [78]. In non diabetic patients the 5-year outcome was virtually the same with both methods. Diabetics with multivessel CAD treated by PCI had a 5-year survival rate of 65.5% *versus* 80.6% of those treated by CABG (p = 0.003).

In the EAST study although 3 years after the index revascularization procedure there was no difference between PCI and CABG in DM patients, survival curves started to separate at 5 years and at 8 years a trend showing an advantage of CABG emerged (75.9% *vs.* PTCA 60.1%; p = 0.23) [76].

Also in the Arterial Revascularization Therapy Study (ARTS) diabetics randomized to be stented had worse outcome at one year than CABG patients (event free survival 63.4% *vs.* 84.4%; p < 0.001), mainly because of the increased need of repeated intervention [79]. However, stroke and death rate were the same with both treatment methods.

Although stents have been shown to reduce the incidence of restenosis after PCI both in non-diabetics and in diabetic patients, the latter have increased rates of restenosis because of increased neointimal hyperplasia after the initial vessel wall injury [80] and increased late luminal loss [81]. Rates of restenosis as high as 47–71% have been described [80]. This is associated with increased clinical events, including mortality [82].

A high rate of asymptomatic reocclusion of the treated vessel of 15% has also been described in diabetics treated with PCI [83]. This has been associated with lower ejection fraction and increased mortality [9].

Even if we know that diabetics treated with PCI tend to have worse outcomes than those treated by surgery, the best revascularization strategy in these patients is still to be defined. CABG-treated diabetics also have poorer outcomes than their normal controls and this has been seen in the ARTS study. Just like in their PCI-treated counterparts, diabetics revascularized by CABG had higher 5-year mortality rate than operated non-diabetics. A significant higher rate of stroke accompanied surgery in CABG-treated patients with DM (6.3% *vs.* 2.4% in non-diabetics) [79]. We also have no data randomly comparing the best interventional revascularization strategies, stents and Gp IIb/IIIa inhibitors *versus* CABG in diabetics.

At the same time we have no data concerning the incidence of restenosis in diabetics treated with drug eluting stents that have been shown to markedly reduce restenosis rate, *versus* surgery. In the RAVEL trial in which bare stents have been randomly compared with sirolimus-eluting stents, restenosis occurred in 0% of diabetic patients treated with a coated stent and in 41.7% of those who received standard stents (p = 0.002) [84]. In the SIRIUS study the rate of TVR in diabetic patients was 18% with a drug eluting stent and 50% with bare stents that reduces the gap against the better results of CABG in diabetics compared to coronary stenting.

Thus, current recommendations for coronary revascularization in diabetics should rely on a combination between coronary anatomy (lesion length, vessel diameter), LV function and estimated risk of restenosis as far as recently proved highly efficient PCI therapies (stents + Gp IIb/IIIa inhibitors, drug eluting stents) have not been compared with CABG yet.

REFERENCES

1. King H, Aubert R, Herman W. Global burden of diabetes, 1995–2005. Prevalence, numerical estimates, and projections. *Diabetes Care,* 21: 1414–1431, 1998.
2. Gu K, Cowie C, Harris M. Diabetes and decline in heart disease mortality in US adults. *JAMA,* 281: 1291–1297, 1999.
3. Moreno P, Murcia A, Palacios I, *et al*. Coronary composition and macrophage infiltration in atherectomy specimens from patients with diabetes mellitus. *Circulation,* 102: 2180–2184, 2000.
4. Haffner S, Lehto S, Rönnemaa T, Pyörälä K, Laakso M. Mortality from coronary heart disease in subjects with type 2 diabetes and in nondiabetic subjects with and without prior myocardial infarction. *N Engl J Med,* 339: 229–234, 1998.
5. Turner R, Millns H, Neil H, *et al*. Risk factors for coronary artery disease in non-insulin dependent diabetes mellitus: United Kingdom Prospective Diabetes Study (UKPDS: 23). *BMJ,* 316: 823–828, 1998.
6. Gæde P, Vedel P, Larsen N, Jensen G, Parving H, Pedersen O. Multifactorial intervention and cardiovascular disease in patients with type 2 diabetes. *N Engl J Med,* 348: 383–393, 2003.
7. Malmberg K, Yusuf S, Gerstein H, *et al*. Impact of diabetes and long-term prognosis in patients with unstable angina and non-Q-wave myocardial infarction. Results of the OASIS registry. *Circulation,* 102: 1014–1019, 2000.
8. McGuire D, Emanuelsson H, Granger C, *et al*. Influence of diabetes mellitus on clinical outcomes across the spectrum of acute coronary syndromes. Findings from the GUSTO-IIb study. GUSTO IIb Investigators. *Eur Heart J,* 21: 1750–1758, 2000.
9. Van Belle E, Ketelers R, Bauters C, *et al*. Patency of percutaneous transluminal coronary angioplasty sites at 6-month angiographic follow-up: a key determinant of survival in diabetes after coronary balloon angioplasty. *Circulation,* 103: 1218–1224, 2001.
10. Kip K, Faxon D, Detre K, Yeh W, Kelsey S, Currier J. for the Investigators of the NHLBI PTCA Registry. Coronary angioplasty in diabetic patients: the National Heart, Lung, and Blood Institute Percutaneous Transluminal Coronary Angioplasty Registry. *Circulation,* 94: 1818–1825, 1996.
11. Malmberg K, Ryden L. Myocardial infarction in patients with diabetes mellitus. *Eur Heart J,* 9: 256–264, 1988.
12. Norhammar A, Malmberg K, Tornvall P, Ryden L, Senestrand U, Wallentin L and the RIKS-HIA group. The unfavourable prognosis in diabetic patients with acute myocardial infarction relates to under-utilisation of evidence-based treatment. *Circulation,* 104: 2962, 2001.
13. Norhammar A, Tenerz A, Nilsson G, Hamsten A, S. E, Ryden L, Malmberg K. Abnormal glucose metabolism: unexpectedly common in patients with acute myocardial infarction and no previous diagnosis of diabetes mellitus. *Lancet,* 359: 2140–2144, 2002.
14. The Global Use of Strategies to Open Occluded Coronary Arteries (GUSTO) IIb Investigators. A comparison of recombinant hirudin with heparin for the treatment of acute coronary syndromes. *N Engl J Med,* 335: 775–782, 1996.
15. Expert Panel on Detection, Evaluation, and Treatment of High Blood Cholesterol in Adults: Executive Summary of the Third Report of the National Cholesterol Education Program (NCEP) Expert Panel on Detection, Evaluation, and Treatment of High Blood Cholesterol in Adults (Adult Treatment Panel III). *JAMA,* 285: 2486–2487, 2001.
16. Singh N, Mironow D, Armstrong P, *et al*. for the GUSTO ECG Substudy Investigators. Heart rate variability assessment early after acute myocardial infarction. Pathophysiological and prognostic correlates. *Circulation,* 93: 1388–1395, 1996.
17. Hohnloser S, Klingenheben T, van de Loo A, Hablawetz E, Just E, Schwartz P. Reflex *versus* tonic vagal activity as a prognostic parameter in patients with sustained ventricular tachycardia or ventricular fibrillation. *Circulation,* 89: 1068–1073, 1994.
18. Keaney J, Loscalzo J. Diabetes, oxidative stress, and platelet activation. *Circulation,* 99: 189–191, 1999.
19. Schmidt A, Stern D. RAGE: a new target for the prevention and treatment of the vascular and inflammatory complications of diabetes. *Trends Endocrinol Metab,* 11: 368–375, 2000.

20. Bierman E. George Lyman Duff Memorial Lecture. Atherogenesis in diabetes. *Arterioscler Thromb,* **12**: 647–656, 1992.

21. Park L, Raman K, Lee K, *et al.* Suppression of accelerated diabetic atherosclerosis by the soluble receptor for advanced glycation endproducts. *Nat Med,* **4**: 1025–1031, 1998.

22. Libby P, Simon D. Inflammation and thrombosis. The clot thickens. *Circulation,* **103**: 1718–1720, 2001.

23. Libby P, Ridker P, Maseri A. Inflammation and atherosclerosis. *Circulation,* **105**: 1135–1143, 2002.

24. Ross R. Atherosclerosis - an inflammatory disease. *N Engl J Med,* **340**: 115–126, 1999.

25. Dechend R, Maass M, Gieffers J, *et al.* Chlamydia pneumoniae infection of vascular smooth muscle and endothelial cells activates NF-kB and induces tissue factor and PAI-1 expression: a potential link to accelerated arteriosclerosis. *Circulation,* **100**: 1369–1373, 1999.

26. Pickup J, Chusney G, Thomas S, Burt D. Plasma interleukin-6, tumour necrosis factor a and blood cytokine production in type 2 diabetes. *Life Sci,* **67**: 291–300, 2000.

27. van der Wal A, Becker A, van der Loos C, Das P. Site of intimal rupture or erosion of thrombosed coronary atherosclerotic plaques is characterized by an inflammatory process irrespective of the dominant plaque morphology. *Circulation,* **89**: 36–44, 1994.

28. Saitoh T, Kishida H, Tsukada Y, *et al.* Clinical significance of increased plasma concentration of macrophage colony-stimulating factor in patients with angina pectoris. *J Am Coll Cardiol,* **35**: 655–665, 2000.

29. Clinton S, Underwood R, Hayes L, Sherman M, Kufe D, Libby P. Macrophage colony stimulating factor gene expression in vascular cells and in experimental and human atherosclerosis. *Am J Pathol,* **140**: 301–316, 1992.

30. Seshiah P, Kereiakes D, Vasudevan S, *et al.* Activated monocytes induce smooth muscle cell death: role of macrophage colony–stimulating factor and cell contact. *Circulation,* **105**: 174–180, 2002.

31. Berger J, Moller D. The mechanisms of action of PPARS. *Annu Rev Med,* **53**: 409–435, 2002.

32. Tschoepe D, Roesen P, Kaufmann L, *et al.* Evidence for abnormal platelet glycoprotein expression in diabetes mellitus. *Eur J Clin Invest,* **20**: 166–170, 1990.

33. Tschoepe D, Roesen P, Esser J, *et al.* Large platelets circulate in an activated state in diabetes mellitus. *Semin Thromb Hemost,* **17**: 433–438, 1991.

34. Knobler H, Savion N, Shenkman B, *et al.* Shear-induced platelet adhesion and aggregation on subendothelium are increased in diabetic patients. *Thromb Res,* **90**: 181–190, 1998.

35. Tschoepe D, Rauch U, Schwippert B. Platelet-leukocyte cross-talk in diabetes mellitus. *Horm Metab Res,* **29**: 631–635, 1997.

36. Tschoepe D. The activated megakaryocyte-platelet-system in vascular disease: focus on diabetes. *Semin Thromb Hemost,* **21**: 152–160, 1995.

37. Tschoepe D, Roesen P. Heart disease in diabetes mellitus: a challenge for early diagnosis and intervention. *Exp Clin Endocrinol Diabetes,* **106**: 16–24, 1998.

38. Jokl R, Colwell J. Arterial thrombosis and atherosclerosis in diabetes. *Diabetes Reviews,* **5**: 316–330, 1997.

39. Kornowski R, Mintz G, Lansky A, *et al.* Paradoxic decreases in atherosclerotic plaque mass in insulin-treated diabetic patients. *Am J Cardiol,* **81**: 1298–1304, 1998.

40. Glagov S, Weisenberg E, Zarins C, *et al.* Compensatory enlargement of human atherosclerotic coronary arteries. *N Engl J Med,* **316**: 1371–1375, 1987.

41. Abaci A, Oguzhan A, Kahraman S, *et al.* Effect of diabetes mellitus on formation of coronary collateral vessels. *Circulation,* **99**: 2239–2242, 1999.

42. Capes S, Hunt D, Malmberg K, Gerstein H. Stress hyperglycemia and prognosis of myocardial infarction in non-diabetic and diabetic patients: a systematic overview. *Lancet,* **355**: 773–778, 2000.

43. Malmberg K, Norhammar A, Wedel H, Ryden L. Glycometabolic state at admission: important risk marker of mortality in conventionally treated patients with diabetes mellitus and acute myocardial infarction: long-term results from the Diabetes Mellitus Insulin-Glucose Infusion in Acute Myocardial Infarction (DIGAMI) study. *Circulation,* **99**: 2626–2632, 1999.

44. Norhammar N, Ryden L, Malmberg K. Admission glucose plasma-independent risk factor for long-term prognosis after myocardial infarction even in non-diabetic patients. *Diabetes Care,* **22**: 1827–1831, 1999.

45. Ryden L, Malmberg K. Who are the enemies? Diabetes mellitus - a major risk factor for ischemic myocardial injury: new directions in the management of acute coronary syndromes in the diabetic patient. *Eur Heart J Supplements,* **4**: G21–G25, 2002.

46. Fath-Ordoubadi F, Beatt K. Glucose-insulin-potassium therapy for treatment of acute myocardial infarction: an overview of randomized placebo-controlled trials. *Circulation,* **96**: 1152–1156, 1997.

47. Diaz E, Romero G. on behalf of the ECLA collaborative group. Metabolic modulation of acute myocardial infarction. The ECLA glucose-insulin-potassium Trial. *Circulation,* **98**: 2227–2234, 1998.

48. Van den Berge G, Wouters P, Weekers F, *et al.* Intensive insulin therapy in critically ill patients. *N Engl J Med,* **345**: 1359–1367, 2001.

49. Youkoyama I, Momomura S, Ohtake T, *et al.* Reduced myocardial flow reserve in non-insulin-dependent diabetes mellitus. *J Am Coll Cardiol,* **30**: 1472–1477, 1997.

50. Henry R, Kostense P, Spijkerman A, *et al.* Arterial stiffness increases with deteriorating glucose tolerance status. The Hoorn Study. *Circulation,* **107**: 2089–2095, 2003.

51. Vehkavaara S, Makimattila S, Schlenzka A, *et al.* Insulin therapy improves endothelial function in type 2 diabetes. *Arterioscler Thromb Vasc Biol,* **20**: 545–550, 2000.

52. Melidonis A, Stefanidis A, Tournis S, *et al.* The role of strict metabolic control by insulin infusion on fibrinolytic profile during an acute coronary event in diabetic patients. *Clin Cardiol,* **23**: 160–164, 2000.

53. Dandona P, Aljada A, Mohanty P, *et al.* Insulin inhibits intranuclear nuclear factor kappa B and stimulates I kappa B in mononuclear cells in obese subjects: evidence for an anti inflammatory effect? *J Clin Endocrinol Metabol,* **86**: 3257–3265, 2001.

54. Tsunekawa T, Hayashi T, Kano H, Sumi D, Matsui-Hirai H, Thakur N, *et al.* Cerivastatin, a hydroxymethylglutaryl coenzyme A reductase inhibitor, improves endothelial function in elderly diabetic patients within 3 days. *Circulation,* **104**: 376–379, 2001.

55. Vorchheimer D, Badimon J, Fuster V. Platelet glycoprotein IIb/IIIa receptor antagonists in cardiovascular disease. *JAMA,* **281**: 1407–1414, 1999.

56. Scarborough R, Kleiman N, Phillips D. Platelet glycoprotein IIb/IIIa antagonists. What are the relevant issues concerning their pharmacology and clinical use? *Circulation,* **100**: 437–444, 1999.

57. Steinbuhl S, Kottke-Marchant K, Moliterno D, *et al.* Attainment and maintenance of platelet inhibition through standard dosing of abciximab in diabetic and nondiabetic patients undergoing percutaneous coronary intervention. *Circulation,* **100**: 1977–1982, 1999.

58. Tcheng J, Ellis S, George B, *et al.* Pharmacodynamics of chimeric glycoprotein IIb/IIIa integrin antiplatelet antibody Fab 7E3 in high-risk coronary angioplasty. *Circulation,* **90**: 1757–1764, 1994.

59. Kereiakes D, Runyon J, Broderick T, *et al.* IIb's are not IIb's. *Am J Cardiol,* **85**: 23C–31C, 2000.

60. Thompson R, Wakelin M, Larbi K, *et al.* Divergent effects of platelet-endothelial cell adhesion molecule-1 and B3 integrin blockade on leukocyte transmigration *in vivo. J Immunol,* **165**: 426–434, 2000.

61. Neumann F, Zohlnhöfer D, Fakhoury L, Ott I, Gawaz M, Schömig A. Effect of glycoprotein IIb/IIIa receptor blockade on platelet-leukocyte interaction and surface expression of the leukocyte integrin Mac-1 in acute myocardial infarction. *J Am Coll Cardiol,* **34**: 1420–1426, 1999.

62. Mickelson J, Ali M, Kleiman N, *et al.* Chimeric 7E3 Fab (Reo-Pro) decreases detectable CD11b on neutrophils from patients undergoing coronary angioplasty. *J Am Coll Cardiol,* **33**: 97–106, 1999.

63. Lincoff A, Kereiakes D, Mascelli M, *et al.* Abciximab suppresses the rise in levels of circulating inflammatory markers after percutaneous coronary revascularization. *Circulation,* **104**: 163–167, 2001.

64. Philips D, Scarborough R. Clinical pharmacology of eptifibatide. *Am J Cardiol,* **80**: 11B–20B, 1997.

65. Topol E, Byzova T, Plow E. Platelet GPIIb-IIIa blockers. *Lancet,* **353**: 227–231, 1999.

66. Kong D, Califf R, Miller D, *et al.* Clinical outcomes of therapeutic agents that block the platelet glycoprotein IIb/IIIa integrin in ischemic heart disease. *Circulation,* **98**: 2829–2835, 1998.

67. Boersma E, Harrington R, Moliterno D, *et al.* Platelet glycoprotein IIb/IIIa inhibitors in acute coronary syndromes: a meta-analysis of all major randomised clinical trials. *Lancet,* **359**: 189–198, 2002.

68. Roffi M, Chew D, Mukherjee D, *et al.* Platelet glycoprotein IIb/IIIa inhibitors reduce mortality in diabetic patients with non-ST-segment-elevation acute coronary syndromes. *Circulation,* **104**: 2767–2771, 2001.

69. Bhatt D, Marso S, Lincoff A, *et al.* Abciximab reduces mortality in diabetics following percutaneous coronary intervention. *J Am Coll Cardiol,* **35**: 922–928, 2000.

70. Serruys P, de Jaegere P, Kiemeneij F, *et al.* for the Benestent Study Group: A comparison of balloon-expandable-stent implantation with balloon angioplasty in patients with coronary artery disease. *N Engl J Med,* **331**: 489–495, 1994.

71. Lincoff A. Important triad in cardiovascular medicine: diabetes, coronary intervention, and platelet glycoprotein IIb/IIIa receptor blockade. *Circulation,* **107**: 1556–1559, 2003.

72. The EPISTENT Investigators. Randomised placebo-controlled and balloon-angioplasty-controlled trial to assess safety of coronary stenting with use of platelet glycoprotein IIb/IIIa blockade. *Lancet,* **352**: 87–92, 1998.

73. Marso S, Lincoff A, Ellis S, *et al.* Optimizing the percutaneous interventional outcomes for patients with diabetes mellitus. Results of the EPISTENT (Evaluation of Platelet IIb/IIIa Inhibitor for Stenting Trial) Diabetic Substudy. *Circulation,* **100**: 2477–2484, 1999.

74. Lincoff A. Potent complementary clinical benefit of abciximab and stenting during percutaneous coronary revascularization in patients with diabetes mellitus: results of the EPISTENT trial. *Am Heart J,* **139**: S46–S52, 2000.

75. Marso S, Huber K, Coen M, Giorgi L, Laster S, Rutherford B. Insulin treated diabetes mellitus is associated with a marked increase in in-hospital mortality following urgent PCI: a continuation of the oral *vs.* insulin treatment debate. *Circulation,* **102**: II-391, 2000.

76. King S, Kosinski A, Guyton R, Lembo N, Weintraub W. Eight-year mortality in the Emory Angioplasty *versus* Surgery Trial (EAST). *J Am Coll Cardiol,* **35**: 1116–1121, 2000.

77. Niles N, McGrath P, Malenka D, *et al.* for the Northern New England Cardiovascular Disease Study Group. Survival of patients with diabetes and multivessel coronary artery disease after surgical or percutaneous coronary revascularization: results of a large regional prospective study. *J Am Coll Cardiol,* **37**: 1008–1015, 2001.

78. The Bypass Angioplasty Revascularization Investigation (BARI) Investigators. Influence of diabetes on 5-year mortality and morbidity in a randomized trial comparing CABG and PTCA in patients with multivessel disease: the Bypass Angioplasty Revascularization Investigation (BARI). *Circulation,* **96**: 1761–1769, 1997.

79. Abizaid A, Costa M, Centemero M, *et al.* Clinical and economic impact of diabetes mellitus on percutaneous and surgical treatment of multivessel coronary disease patients. *Circulation,* **104**: 533–538, 2001.

80. Kornowski R, Mintz G, Kent K, *et al.* Increased restenosis in diabetes mellitus after coronary interventions is due to exaggerated intimal hyperplasia: a serial intravascular ultrasound study. *Circulation,* **95**: 1366–1369, 1997.

81. Carrozza J, Kuntz R, Fishman R, Baim D. Restenosis after arterial injury caused by coronary stenting in patients with diabetes mellitus. *Ann Intern Med,* **118**: 344–349, 1993.

82. Stein B, Weintraub W, Gebhart S, *et al.* Influence of diabetes mellitus on early and late outcomes after percutaneous transluminal coronary angioplasty. *Circulation,* **91**: 979–989, 1995.

83. Van Belle E, Abolmaali K, Bauters C, McFadden E, Lablanche J-M, Bertrand M. Restenosis, late vessel occlusion and left ventricular function six months after balloon angioplasty in diabetic patients. *J Am Coll Cardiol,* **34**: 476–485, 1999.

84. Morice M, Serruys P, Serruys J, *et al.* A randomized comparison of a sirolimus-eluting stent with a standard stent for coronary revascularization. *N Engl J Med,* **346**: 1773–1780, 2002.

40

CORONARY REVASCULARIZATION STRATEGIES IN DIABETES

Claude HANET

Diabetes mellitus is a well-established risk factor for atherosclerotic cardiovascular disease which, when present, is associated with increased mortality and morbidity compared to non-diabetic patients with coronary artery disease. The absolute risk of death from cardiovascular disease has indeed been shown to be much higher for diabetic than for non-diabetic patients of every age stratum, ethnic background and risk factor level [1].

Compared with non-diabetics, diabetic patients also have a worse long-term outcome after coronary revascularization by either bypass surgery (CABG) or percutaneous coronary intervention (PCI). Diabetes is an independent risk factor for lesion progression and cardiac mortality after CABG [2, 3]. After PCI, diabetes has been identified as a risk factor for the development of restenosis. Furthermore, the incidence of occlusive restenosis after balloon angioplasty is dramatically higher in diabetic patients than in non-diabetic subjects and is associated with a negative effect on left ventricular function [4].

Several multicenter trials have been designed to determine the optimal revascularization strategy in patients with coronary artery disease. Considering the high rate of adverse events after myocardial revascularization in diabetic patients, this subpopulation has been particularly studied with special attention to the factors susceptible to affect both short- and long-term outcome.

CORONARY ARTERY BYPASS SURGERY

Approximately 20 to 30% of patients undergoing coronary artery bypass surgery have diabetes. Most follow-up studies identified diabetes as an independent risk factor for both short-term and long-term morbidity and mortality after bypass surgery.

SHORT-TERM OUTCOME

In a retrospective large-scale cohort study, Carson et al. [3] reported an increased risk of in-hospital morbidity, defined as infection, myocardial infarction, renal failure, stroke or multisystem failure, in diabetic compared to non diabetic patients (13.0 vs. 9.1%). The 30-day mortality was 3.74% in patients with diabetes and 2.70% in those without diabetes, the majority of patients dying from cardiac causes. Diabetic patients treated with insulin had the highest risk of early post-operative mortality and morbidity compared to patients using oral medications. The adjusted risk for each of these outcomes was 50% to 61% higher for insulin-treated diabetics compared to non-diabetics.

LONG-TERM OUTCOME

Diabetic patients have a mortality rate during the 2-year period after CABG that is about twice that of non-diabetic patients during both the early and late phase after the operation [5]. At 5 years, in the study by Morris et al. [6], the overall survival probability was 0.91 in non-diabetic and 0.80 in diabetic patients (p < 0.0001). Not surprisingly, insulin-requiring patients fare worse than diabetic patients treated with oral agents [3]. More than an independent direct effect of insulin therapy, this observation probably reflects a more advanced state and/or longer duration of diabetes resulting in more advanced atherosclerosis. The worse outcome reported in patients with diabetic retinopathy as compared to diabetic patients without retinopathy also probably reflects the deleterious consequences of a longer period of poor-controlled diabetes and a higher incidence of additional comorbidities [7].

Technical aspects such as the use of internal mammary artery grafts are known to influence the long-term outcome after bypass surgery in the general population. The superior long-term patency rate of the internal mammary artery graft compared to saphenous vein graft is thought to result from specific biological properties protecting this vessel against atherosclerosis [8]. Based on the demonstrated superiority of the internal mammary artery conduit over saphenous vein, bilateral internal mammary artery grafting is recommended in several centers for patients requiring surgical revascularization of both the left anterior descending and left circumflex coronary arteries. This approach appears to give an additional survival benefit over the use of a single mammary artery graft in combination with one or more saphenous vein grafts [9].

In diabetic patients, the relation of the presence of an internal mammary artery graft to cardiac mortality is particularly striking. In the "Bypass Angioplasty Revascularization Investigation" (BARI), the 5-year postoperative cardiac mortality was 2.9% in diabetic patients when at least one internal mammary artery graft was used and 18.2% when only saphenous vein grafts were used [10]. Although the use of internal mammary artery graft was not assigned at random in this study, the difference remained significant after adjustment for selection factors (likelihood of receiving a mammary artery graft). These data directly support the use of the internal mammary artery as conduit graft in diabetic patients, particularly for revascularization of the left anterior descending coronary artery. They also provide indirect arguments for the use of bilateral mammary artery grafts when technically feasible. A controversy however exists about a possible increased incidence of sternal wound problems in diabetic patients in whom both internal mammary arteries are harvested. An adequate surgical technique seems able to prevent this problem in diabetic patients who have the most to gain from bilateral internal mammary artery grafts [9].

PERCUTANEOUS INTERVENTIONS

Since its introduction by Gruentzig in 1977, coronary angioplasty has enjoyed explosive growth and popularity. Initially restricted to patients with single, discrete and concentric stenoses, percutaneous revascularization has progressed to the point that is now considered a safe alternative to coronary artery bypass surgery in some complex anatomical situations previously considered to be solely the realm of the cardiovascular surgeon. Specific problems have been identified in diabetic patients, such as an increased risk of recurrence resulting in a greater need for additional revascularization procedures and a higher rate of myocardial infarction.

SPECIFIC PROBLEMS OF DIABETIC PATIENTS

In a review of 1 133 diabetic and 9 300 non-diabetic patients undergoing elective angioplasty from 1980 to 1990, Stein *et al.* [11] analyzed the influence of diabetes on early and late post-procedural outcome. No significant difference in angiographic success or in-hospital complication rate was observed between diabetic and non-diabetic patients. Within the group of diabetics, only a trend toward increased Q-wave myocardial infarction (1.14% *vs.* 0.38%) and death (0.85% *vs.* 0.26%) was observed in insulin-requiring patients compared to non-insulin-requiring patients, but these differences remained insignificant by multivariate analysis. Despite similar major in-hospital complication rates, the long-term outcome was adversely affected by the presence of diabetes mellitus. Survival at 5 years was 93% for patients without and 88% for those with diabetes (p < 0.0001). Coronary bypass surgery and additional percutaneous procedures were more frequently required in diabetic than in non-diabetic patients (respectively 23% *vs.* 14% and 43% *vs.* 32%; p < 0.0001). Survival free of myocardial infarction, bypass surgery and additional angioplasty was present in 53% of non-diabetic patients and only 36% of diabetics (p < 0.001). Multivariate analysis confirmed the influence of diabetes as a significant independent correlate of reduced 5-year survival even after correction for other comorbid factors.

Angiographic follow-up studies illustrated the role of restenosis and disease progression in the target coronary vessel in this late outcome. In a consecutive series of 377 diabetic patients, Van Belle *et al.* [12] reported a rate of restenosis (defined as a >50% diameter stenosis at the dilated site 6 months after the initial procedure) of 62%, much higher than the rate generally reported for the general population. This study also showed that late vessel occlusion was a frequent mode of restenosis in diabetic patients affecting 13% of dilated segments. Late vessel occlusion was associated with a decrease in ejection fraction at follow-up and could explain the poor long-term clinical outcome reported in such patients after traditional balloon angioplasty. Other studies [13] reported a higher incidence of new narrowings in diabetic patients, particularly in the angioplasty artery both proximal and distal to the site of balloon inflation.

Several factors could contribute to the worse outcome of diabetic patients, among which an increased vascular response to injury. Insulin is known to promote the proliferation of human vascular smooth muscle cells and to increase the synthesis of growth factors. The hyperinsulinemia in treated diabetic patients could accelerate the proliferative response to the vascular injury caused by balloon dilatation, stimulating the development of new narrowings in the treated coronary vessels. The increased procoagulant state in diabetics could also contribute to accelerate disease progression. In addition, endothelial dysfunction, reduced synthesis of prostacyclin, increase in plasminogen activator inhibitor type 1, increased blood viscosity and decreased red cell deformability may impair the vascular mechanisms aimed at reducing the consequences of intravascular clotting [11, 13].

RECENT IMPROVEMENT IN TECHNIQUES AND IN ADJUNCTIVE PHARMACOLOGICAL TREATMENT

During the last decade, technical improvements in percutaneous revascularization, particularly coronary stents, allowed to achieve higher procedural success rates while decreasing the incidence of long-term restenosis. The clinical benefit 6 months after stent implantation appears particularly relevant in diabetic patients with rates of restenosis (27% *vs.* 62%; p < 0.0001) and occlusion (4% *vs.* 13%; p < 0.005) lower than in a matched group of patients treated with balloon angioplasty [14]. Stent implantation could also reduce long-term mortality after percutaneous coronary revascularization as suggested by a trend toward a reduced rate of death and large MI at one year (4.9% *vs.* 10.4%)

reported among diabetics receiving abciximab randomized to stent implantation compared to those treated with balloon angioplasty [15]. However, despite these encouraging results, the presence of diabetes mellitus still remained the key predictor of outcome by multivariate Cox regression analysis in the ARTS trial after coronary stenting [16].

New adjunctive pharmacological treatments have recently shown their ability to improve the outcome after percutaneous coronary interventions in diabetic patients. In the EPISTENT study, the use of the platelet GP IIb/IIIa inhibitor abciximab (ReoPro® Centocor, Malvern, Pa) during stent implantation significantly reduced the 6-month combined death or myocardial infarction rate and the need for repeated percutaneous or surgical revascularization [15, 17]. In a pooled analysis, diabetic patients who were randomized to receive abciximab at the time of intervention demonstrated one-year mortality rates similar to that of non-diabetic patients receiving placebo [18]. The mechanisms involved in these protective effects of GP IIb/IIIa blockade have not been clearly identified, but prevention of distal embolization and microvascular damage, attenuation of the endothelial response to the injury caused by vessel instrumentation and modulation of cell adhesion molecules may be of particular importance in diabetic patients. Based on these findings, the prophylactic use of abciximab should be strongly considered at the time of intervention in diabetic patients, especially those who are treated with insulin.

COMPARISON BETWEEN CORONARY ARTERY BYPASS SURGERY AND PERCUTANEOUS INTERVENTION

Coronary balloon angioplasty was initially introduced as a catheter-based technique for treating simple concentric lesions involving a single coronary artery. Progressively, growing experience of interventional cardiologists, improvements in percutaneous technologies and progress in adjunctive pharmacological treatment allowed considering percutaneous interventions for more complex cases including patients with multivessel coronary artery disease. Consequently, the lines of demarcation for patients suited for

bypass surgery or angioplasty became blurred. Routine stent implantation further increased the dilemma by allowing treating very complex coronary lesions with a low risk of *bailout* emergency bypass surgery and an acceptable incidence of long-term restenosis.

Several randomized trials have been designed to compare bypass surgery and percutaneous interventions in patients with coronary artery disease thought to be suitable for either form of revascularization [2, 16, 19–26]. In the early nineties, six major trials [2, 19–23] compared the efficacy of balloon angioplasty and bypass surgery; more recently, three trials [16, 25, 26], compared bypass surgery with routine stent implantation for the treatment of multivessel coronary artery disease.

In all these trials, the baseline characteristics were similar between patients randomized to surgery and those randomized to percutaneous intervention; patients were enrolled if the consensus view of the surgeon and interventional cardiologist was that revascularization was clinically indicated and appropriate by either strategy. All studies excluded very high-risk patients and most excluded patients with prior revascularization. Consequently, the percentage of screened patients enrolled in these trials ranged from 2% to 12% [27], which limits their clinical implications to this carefully selected population. The vast majority of screened patients were not enrolled because their coronary anatomy or clinical status was considered to be in favor of one or the other approach.

BALLOON ANGIOPLASTY *VERSUS* BYPASS SURGERY

Most of the initial randomized studies failed to show any significant difference in long-term mortality between patients randomized to either approach. An increased need for subsequent percutaneous or surgical target vessel revascularization was however consistently observed for patients initially randomized to percutaneous intervention.

In the EAST trial [22], survival at 8 years was 79.3% in the angioplasty group and 82.7% in the surgical group (NS). The percents of patients with subsequent revascularization were 65.3% and 26.5% respectively (p < 0.001), the first additional procedure occurring primarily within the first three years. Long-term results of the RITA [19],

ERACI [20], GABI [21] and CABRI [23] trials confirmed similar rates of mortality for both approaches and an increased need for subsequent revascularization in patients who were randomized to initially undergone percutaneous intervention.

The BARI trial [24] is of particular interest with regard to the role of diabetes in long-term outcome since the size of the population and the proportion of randomized patients with treated diabetes allowed considering the outcome of diabetic patients after either revascularization strategy. At five years, survival rate was 89.3% in the surgical group compared to 86.3% in the angioplasty group (NS). However, within the subgroup of patients with treated diabetes mellitus – a subgroup not specified a priori – a significant difference in survival was observed in favor of surgery. At seven years, the benefit of surgery over percutaneous intervention was even more pronounced, with overall survival rates of 76.4% and 55.7% respectively (p = 0.0011). Among non-diabetic patients, there was no difference in seven-year survival (86.4% *vs.* 86.8%).

As mentioned earlier, among diabetic patients who were assigned to surgery in the BARI trial, those who received at least one internal mammary artery graft had better seven-year survival compared to those who received only saphenous vein grafts. The survival rate in the group of diabetics who received only saphenous vein grafts was almost identical to that for diabetics treated by percutaneous intervention.

Interestingly, the BARI study also includes a registry of patients who were considered to be eligible for the trial but refused randomization. Among the BARI registry patients with treated diabetes, those with the most extensive disease were preferentially referred to surgery whereas those with a lower angiographic risk profile were selected for percutaneous intervention. The survival rates were similar in these two non-randomized treatment groups, which suggests that physicians correctly identified those patients with diabetes who would do well with percutaneous intervention.

STENTING *VERSUS* SURGERY

Recent improvements in both percutaneous and surgical techniques may limit the validity of the conclusions drawn from earlier studies. The routine use of coronary stents has reduced the risk of early complications and the need for subsequent revascularization. Simultaneously, refinements in surgical techniques, particularly the growing use of the internal mammary artery as conduit graft may enhance freedom from ischemic events and confer greater longevity in selected patients. Three randomized studies were designed to compare the current techniques of surgical and catheter-based myocardial revascularization [16, 25, 26]. Most patients (88.5% to 93%) randomized to bypass surgery received at least on mammary artery graft and stents were implanted in most attempted lesions (78% to 89%) of patients randomized to percutaneous intervention.

The results of these studies confirmed the findings of previous trials, the rate of repeated intervention remaining lower with surgery. However, the rate with stenting was lower than had been seen in previous trials with balloon angioplasty, tending to decrease the gap between both approaches. Differences in mortality were observed at 1 and 2 years in favor of stenting in the ERACI II trial [25] and in favor of surgery in the SOS trial [26]. In the ARTS study [16], no difference in the incidence of death, myocardial infarction or stroke was observed at one-year but the proportion of patients requiring an additional revascularization procedure was higher after stenting than after bypass surgery (21.0% *vs.* 3.8%).

The impact of diabetes on the outcome was specifically addressed in the ARTS trial [28]. At 1 year, diabetic patients treated with stenting had the lowest event-free survival rate (63.4%) compared to both diabetic patients treated with surgery (84.4%, p < 0.001) and non-diabetic patients treated with stents (76.2%, p < 0.04). The incidence of 1-year mortality was twice as high in the diabetic patients assigned to stenting as that in those assigned to surgery (6.3% *vs.* 3.1%, NS). The difference in repeated revascularization rates in favor of surgery was almost twice as great in diabetics as in the non-diabetic group (21.6% *vs.* 12.4%, respectively). It is worth noting that the protective effects of GP IIb/IIIa [17] had not been reported and that only a small proportion (3.5%) of diabetic patients received abciximab at the time of the procedure. Extrapolation of the reported benefit of GP IIb/IIIa blockade [18] to the ARTS diabetic substudy would close the gap in mortality rates between surgery and percutaneous intervention.

RECOMMENDATIONS IN DIABETIC PATIENTS

Considering the greater incidence of adverse events in diabetic than in non-diabetic patients regardless of revascularization strategy, the selection of the optimal treatment in every specific situation is essential.

For diabetics with single vessel disease requiring revascularization, the optimal strategy has not been specifically studied. In these patients, the use of revascularization should be considered for treatment of ischemia, relief of angina and improvement in quality of life. Percutaneous intervention when technically feasible seems reasonable as an initial strategy, just as in non-diabetics.

In multivessel disease, coronary bypass surgery is the preferred approach for those borderline cases that, based on current experience and practice, are considered suitable for both approaches and would actually have similar outcomes in the absence of diabetes. The presence of multivessel disease however does not preclude percutaneous intervention when lesions are discrete and approachable with a high likelihood of success. In the BARI registry, the majority of the patients who were determined to be eligible for the clinical trial but refused randomization were treated with percutaneous intervention. As expected, these patients had fewer complex lesions than the patient selected for bypass surgery. In contrast to the randomized trial, the 7-year mortality rate of treated diabetics in the registry was equally high (26%) with percutaneous intervention or bypass surgery. This demonstrates that physicians could identify those patients with diabetes who would do well with percutaneous intervention. Percutaneous intervention can thus be recommended in those diabetic patients with multivessel disease who, based on coronary anatomy, are though to be good candidates for a low-risk percutaneous intervention.

A particular situation is that of diabetic patients needing revascularization after previous bypass surgery. In these high-risk patients, redo bypass surgery is associated with higher initial mortality and similar long-term results than percutaneous intervention [29]. It seems thus appropriate to have an initial bias toward percutaneous intervention in these cases, the surgical option being based on individual patients characteristics, such as the ability to replace an old dysfunctional venous by new arterial graft conduits or the presence of an unprotected left main.

Finally, whatever the technique selected for myocardial revascularization, the procedure must be performed following the recommendations derived from clinical studies which include the use of at least one internal mammary artery graft conduit for surgical revascularization and the prophylactic use of GP IIb/IIIa inhibitors in all diabetic patients at the time of percutaneous intervention.

CONCLUSION AND PERSPECTIVES

Patients with diabetes mellitus referred for myocardial revascularization represent a major challenge for the cardiac surgeon and for the interventional cardiologist. Diabetes is associated with more diffuse and more complex forms of coronary artery disease and is an independent predictive parameter of bad outcome after any form of treatment. Continuous improvements in techniques and in adjunctive medical treatment have improved the outcome of diabetic patients without closing the gap between them and non-diabetics.

Further major improvements are progressively integrated in our clinical practice and could at short notice influence our approach. Surgical techniques become less invasive; off-pump surgery could reduce the morbidity, particularly the cognitive decline noted after bypass surgery. Drug-eluting stents reduce restenosis to an unprecedented low level and could decrease revascularization rates after percutaneous intervention close to the values reported after bypass surgery. The comparison of coronary bypass surgery and percutaneous coronary intervention will certainly be the object of new clinical trials in the near future. Meanwhile, diabetes will remain an important clinical parameter influencing the choice of the revascularization strategy and the technical aspects of the procedure itself.

REFERENCES

1. Stamler J, Vaccaro O, Neaton JD, Wentworth-D. Diabetes, other risk factors, and 12-yr cardiovascular mortality for men screened in the Multiple Risk Factor Intervention Trial. *Diabetes Care*, **16**(2): 434–44, 1993.

2. The BARI Investigators. Comparison of coronary bypass surgery with angioplasty in patients with multivessel disease. *N Engl J Med*, **335**: 217–225, 1996.

3. Carson JL, Scholz PM, Chen AY, Peterson ED, Gold J, Schneider SH. Diabetes mellitus increases short-term mortality and morbidity in patients undergoing coronary artery bypass graft surgery. *J Am Coll Cardiol*, **40**: 418–23, 2002.

4. Van Belle E, Abolmaali K, Bauters C, McFadden EP, Lablanche J-M, Bertrand ME. Restenosis, late vessel occlusion and left ventricular function six months after balloon angioplasty in diabetic patients. *J Am Coll Cardiol*, **34**: 476–485, 1999.

5. Herlitz J, Wognsen GB, Emanuelsson H, Haglid M, Karlson BW, Karlson T, Albertsson P. Westberg S. Mortality and morbidity in diabetic and nondiabetic patients during a 2-year period after coronary artery bypass grafting. *Diabetes Care*, **19**: 698–703, 1996.

6. Morris JJ, Smith LR, Jones RH, Glower DD, Morris PB, Muhlbaier LH, Reves JG, Rankin JS. Influence of diabetes and mammary artery grafting on survival after coronary bypass. *Circulation*, **84**: III 275–284, 1991.

7. Ono T, Kobayashi J, Sasako Y, Bando K, Tagusari O, Niwaya K, Imanaka H, Nakatani T, Kitamura S. The impact of diabetic retinopathy on long-term outcome following coronary artery bypass graft surgery. *J Am Coll Cardiol*, **40**: 428–36, 2002.

8. Hanet C, Robert A, Wyns W. Vasomotor response to ergometrine and nitrates of saphenous vein grafts, internal mammary artery grafts and grafted coronary arteries late after bypass surgery. *Circulation*, **86**: II–210–216, 1992.

9. Taggart DP, D'Amico R, Altman DG. Effect of arterial revascularization on survival: a systematic review of studies comparing bilateral and single internal mammary arteries. *Lancet*, **358**: 870–75, 2001.

10. The BARI Investigators. Influence of diabetes on 5-year mortality and morbidity in a randomized trial comparing CABG and PTCA in patients with multivessel disease. *Circulation*, **96**: 1761–1769, 1997.

11. Stein B, Weintraub WS, Gebhart SSP, Cohen-Bernstein CL, Grosswald R, Liberman HA, Douglas JS, Morris DC, King III SB. Influence of diabetes mellitus on early and late outcome after percutaneous transluminal coronary angioplasty. *Circulation*, **91**: 979–989, 1995.

12. Van Belle E, Abolmaali K, Bauters C, McFadden EP, Lablanche JM, Bertrand ME. Restenosis, late vessel occlusion and left ventricular function six months after balloon angioplasty in diabetic patients. *J Am Coll Cardiol*, **34**: 476–85,1999.

13. Rozenman Y, Sapoznikov D, Mosseri M, Gilon D, Lotan C, Nassar H, Weiss AT, Hasin Y, Gotsman MS. Long-term angiographic follow-up of coronary balloon angioplasty in patients with diabetes mellitus. *J Am Coll Cardiol*, **30**: 1420–1425, 1997.

14. Van Belle E, Périé M, Braune D, Chmaït A, Meurice T, Abolmaali K, Mc Fadden EP, Bauters C, Lablanche JM, Bertrand ME. Effects of coronary stenting on vessel patency and long-term clinical outcome after percutaneous coronary revascularization in diabetic patients. *J Am Coll Cardiol*, **40**: 410–417, 2002.

15. Topol EJ, Mark DB, Lincoff AM, for the EPISTENT investigators. Outcomes at 1 year and economical implications of platelet glycoprotein IIb/IIIa blockade in patients undergoing coronary stenting: results from a multicenter randomised trial. *Lancet*, **354**: 2019–24, 1999.

16. Serruys PW, Unger F, Sousa E, Jatene A, Bonnier HJ, Schönberger JP, Buller N, Bonser R, Van den Brand MJ, van Herwerden LA, Morel MA, van Hout BE for the ARTS investigators. Comparison of coronary-artery bypass surgery and stenting for the treatment of multivessel disease. *N Engl J Med*, **344**: 1117–24, 2001.

17. Marso SP, Lincoff AM, Ellis SG, Bhatt DL, Tanguay JF, Kleiman NS, Hammoud T, Booth JE, Sapp SK, Topol EJ. Optimizing the percutaneous interventional outcome for patients with diabetes mellitus. Results of the EPISTENT diabetic substudy. *Circulation*, **100**: 2477–2484), 1999.

18. Bhatt DL, Marso SP, Lincoff AM, Wolski KE, Ellis SG, Topol EG. Abciximab reduces mortality in diabetics following percutaneous coronary intervention. *J Am Coll Cardiol,*, **35**: 922–928, 2000.

19. Henderson RA, Pocock SJ, Sharp SJ, Nanchahal K, Sculpher MJ, Buxton MJ, Hampton JR for the RITA-1 trial investigators. Long-term results of RITA-1 trial: clinical and cost comparisons of coronary angioplasty and coronary-artery bypass grafting. *Lancet*, **352**: 1419–1425, 1998.

20. Rodriguez A Mele E, Peyregne E, Bullon F, Perez Balino N, Liprandi MI, Palacios IF. Three-year follow-up of the Argentine randomized trial of percutaneous transluminal coronary angioplasty versus coronary artery bypass surgery in multivessel disease (ERACI). *J Am Coll Cardiol*, **27**: 1178–1184, 1996.

21. Hamm CW, Reimers J, Ischinger T, Rupprecht HJ, Berger J, Bleifeld W for the German angioplasty bypass surgery investigation (GABI). A randomized study of coronary angioplasty compared with

bypass surgery in patients with symptomatic multivessel coronary disease. *N Engl J Med,* **331**: 1037–1043, 1994.

22. King SB III, Kosinski AS, Guyton RA, Lembo NJ, Weintraub WS for the emory angioplasty versus surgery trial (EAST) investigators. Eight years mortality in the Emory angioplasty *versus* surgery trial (EAST). *J Am Coll Cardiol,* **35**: 1116–1121, 2000.

23. CABRI Trial Participants. First-year results of CABRI (Coronary Angioplasty *versus* Bypass Revascularisation Investigation). *Lancet,* **346**: 1179–1184, 1995.

24. The BARI investigators. Seven-years outcome in the bypass angioplasty revascularization investigation by treatment and diabetic status. *J Am Coll Cardiol,* **35**: 1122–9, 2000.

25. Rodriguez A, Bernardi V, Navia J, Baldi J, Grinfeld L, Martinez J, Vogel D, Grinfeld R, Delacasa A, Garrido M, Oliveri R, Mele E, Palacios I, O'Neill W for the ERACI II investigators. Argentine randomized study: coronary angioplasty with stent *versus* coronary bypass surgery in patients with multiple-vessel disease (ERACI II): 30-day and one-year follow-up results. *J Am Coll Cardiol,* **37**: 51–8, 2001.

26. The SoS investigators. Coronary artery bypass surgery versus percutaneous coronary intervention with stent implantation in patients with multivessel coronary artery disease (the Stent or Surgery trial): a randomized controlled trial. *Lancet,* **360**: 965–970, 2002.

27. Hoffman SN, Tenbrook JA, Wolf MP, Pauker SG, Salem DN, Wong JB. Analysis of randomized controlled trials comparing coronary artery bypass graft with percutaneous transluminal coronary angioplasty: One- to eight years outcome. *J Am Coll Cardiol,* **41**: 1293–1304, 2003.

28. Abizaid A, Costa M, Centemero M, Abizaid AS, Legrand VM, Limet RV, Schuler G, Mohr FW, Lindeboom W, Sousa AG, Sousa JE, van Hout B, Hugenholtz PG, Unger F, Serruys PW. Clinical and economic impact of diabetes mellitus on percutaneous and surgical treatment of multivessel coronary disease patients. *Circulation,* **104**: 533–538, 2001.

29. Cole JH, Jones EL, Craver JM, Guyton RA, Morris DC, Douglas JS, Ghazzal Z, Weintraub WS. Outcome of repeat revascularization in diabetic patients with prior coronary surgery. *J Am Coll Cardiol,* **40**: 1968–75, 2002.

41

SMOKING CESSATION PROGRAMS IN DIABETIC PATIENTS

Laurence GALANTI

Smoking is an important public health concern and a major risk factor for many chronic and life threatening illnesses, particularly for diabetes. The great majority of smokers are chronically dependent on tobacco. A variety of stages may be identified in the smoking career. The addictive potential of tobacco smoking is strongly related to the presence of nicotine. This dependence arises from the rituals and sensory associations of smoking reinforced within seconds by a rapid burst of nicotine from the cigarette. Guidelines describe recommendations designed to assist clinicians in delivering and supporting effective treatments for smokers to stop smoking. These strategies involve different actions: to ask each patient about tobacco use and to advice to quit, to assess willingness to make a quit attempt, to assist in quit attempt and to arrange follow up. The interventions should be adapted according to the stage of maturation of the smoker. Several pharmacological strategies have been developed for the treatment of nicotine addiction including nicotine replacement therapy and bupropion to increase smoking cessation rates in the short-and long-terms. The effectiveness of drug treatments is better when associated with effective counseling and behavioral treatments.

INTRODUCTION

Tobacco use has been cited as the chief avoidable cause of illness and death in developed countries [1]. Smoking is known as a cause of cancer, stroke, complications of pregnancy and chronic obstructive pulmonary disease. It is also an independent risk factor for cardiovascular disease [2]. Diabetes mellitus results in accelerated macrovascular and microvascular atherosclerotic disease, doubling the risk of stroke, myocardial infarction and peripheral vascular disease. In the presence of smoking, this risk increases from four to eleven fold [3]. Diabetes has been found to increase the risk of hyperlipidemia [4] and hypertension [5]. The combination of these two risk factors with smoking increases the risk of death from coronary disease eleven fold [6]. Cigarette smoking contributes to the presence of arterial vasoconstriction, increasing the risk of peripheral vascular disease in diabetes [7]. Diabetic patients who stop smoking for at least 2 years have 30% lower prevalence of lower extremity arterial disease than those who continued to smoke. Given the health dangers it presents and the public's awareness of those dangers, tobacco use remains surprisingly prevalent, particularly in diabetic patients for whom smoking prevalence appears similar to the non-diabetic population [8]. Furthermore, giving the high rates of smoking found among diabetic patients and the obvious deleterious effects of smoking and diabetes, it is striking that almost no research has been published on smoking cessation in this group.

Tobacco dependence must be recognized as a chronic disease with an expectation that patients may have periods of relapse and remission. Although a minority of tobacco users achieve permanent abstinence in an initial quit attempt, the majority relapse for weeks, months or years. Clinician must remain motivated to treat tobacco use consistently. Indeed, 70% of smokers want to quit smoking completely, 46% try to quit each year, more than 70% of smokers visit a health care setting each year. The physician's advice to quit is an important motivator for attempting to stop smoking, and effective treatments now exist [9].

Although most primary care clinicians are often bound by time constraints, it is essential to provide at least a brief intervention to all tobacco users at each clinical visit, especially to patients with a chronic disease such as diabetes. Specific strategies are described to guide clinicians in their work.

It is now widely accepted that a large majority of regular tobacco smokers become addicted to the nicotine present in tobacco smoke. This addiction plays an important role in maintaining the tobacco smoking habit and is bounded to pharmacological and behavioral processes similar to those observed in illicit drugs addiction. Physical and behavioral dependences must be treated at the same time to increase the successful rate of tobacco smoking cessation interventions. Cessation is a process in which the smoker progresses through several stages of change, the "smoker's career", including precontemplation, contemplation, action, maintenance and relapse [10]. Knowledge of this process is needed for the health care team, particularly for diabetes care team, to effectively individualize smoking prevention and cessation strategies.

SMOKER'S CAREER

During its lifetime, a smoker's career has been previously described [10, 11]. After a period of some experiences of tobacco use, the non-smokers become occasional smokers. A very few number of these smokers stop smoking although the most progress toward regular smokers. These smokers remain "happy smokers" most often for a long time (precontemplation stage): they do not want to stop smoking. After this period, the smokers perceive more acutely the positive but also the negative effects of tobacco smoke and become "ambivalent smokers": they hesitate between smoking and not smoking. Later on, some prepare to stop (contemplation stage) and start to make a quit attempt (action stage), which is sometimes followed by perseverance (maintenance stage). But in most cases, cessation is followed by a relapse and the smoker progresses further, often several times, into the cessation cycle through the stages of "ambivalent smoker" and "smoker ready to stop" before finally succeeding with cessation. They become persistent "happy ex-smokers". Some of them, unable to quit completely tobacco use, become occasional smokers or reduce their daily cigarette consumption in order finally to quit. However, some remain continuing smokers until their death (Plate 41.1) [11].

CLINICAL PRACTICE GUIDELINES

Several guidelines [9, 12–19] have been published containing strategies and recommendations designed to assist clinicians in delivering and supporting effective treatments for tobacco use dependence to smokers willing to quit. The strategy called the "5 As" (Table 41.1) has been proposed and consists of five steps:

– A1. Ask about tobacco use: Identify and document tobacco use for every patient at every visit. It is important for the clinician to ask the patient if he or she uses tobacco.

– A2. Advise to quit: In a clear, strong and personalized manner urge every tobacco user to quit.

– A3. Assess willingness to make a quit attempt: Is the tobacco user willing to make a quit attempt at this time?

– A4. Assist in quit attempt: For the patient willing to make a quit attempt, use counseling and pharmacotherapy to help him or her quit.

– A5. Arrange follow-up: Schedule a follow-up contact preferably early within the first week after the quit date.

Table 41.1

The 5 As strategy

A1	Ask about tobacco use
A2	Advise to quit
A3	Assess willingness
A4	Assess in quit attempt
A5	Arrange follow-up

The Tobacco Use and Dependence Clinical Practice Guideline Panel, Staff, and Consortium Representatives (5).

These strategies are consistent with those produced by the NCI [12–13] and the American Medical Association [14], as well as others [15–16].

TOBACCO SMOKING

PHYSICAL DEPENDENCE

Nicotine addiction [17]

The World Health Organization described drug dependence as "a behavioral pattern in which the use of a given psychoactive drug is given a sharply higher priority over other behaviors which once had a significantly higher value".

Table 41.2

Summary of Diagnostic and Statistical Manual of Mental Disorders (DSM IV) and International Classification of Diseases (ICD-10) criteria for substance dependence

DSM IV	ICD-10
At least 3 of the following phenomena are necessary:	A cluster of behavioral, cognitive and physiological phenomena that develop after repeated substance use and that typically include:
Substance often taken in larger amounts or over a longer period than intended	A strong desire to take the drug
Persistent desire or unsuccessful efforts to cut down or control use	Difficulty controlling use
A great deal of time spent in activities necessary to obtain the substance, use the substance or recover from its effect	
Important social, occupational or recreational activities given up or reduced because of substance use	A higher priority given to drug use than to other activities and obligations
Continued substance use despite knowledge of having a persistent or recurrent social, psychological or physical problem that is caused or exacerbated by the use of the substance	Persisting in use despite harmful consequences
Tolerance: need for markedly increased amounts of the substance to achieve intoxication or desired effect or markedly diminished effect with continued use of the same amount.	Increased tolerance
Withdrawal: the characteristic withdrawal syndrome or the same (or a closely related) substance is taken to relieve or avoid withdrawal symptoms	Sometimes, a physical withdrawal state

In other words, the drug comes to control behavior to an extent considered detrimental to the individual or to society. In addition to highly controlled or compulsive use of the drug, the Surgeon General's criteria require the drug to produce psychoactive effects, and there must be evidence that drug-taking behavior is reinforced by effects of the drug.

Based on the specific criteria listed in the DSM IV (The American Psychiatric Association Diagnostic and Statistical Manual of Mental Disorders) and the ICD-10 (World Organization International Classification of Diseases) (Table 41.2), nicotine intake through smoking meets standard diagnostic criteria for addiction:

1. A strong desire to take the drug. The desire to smoke, important in the relapse of smokers trying to give up smoking, is a manifestation of nicotine withdrawal and clearly related to underlying dependence on nicotine.

2. Substance taken in larger amounts or longer than intended. Although smokers are 'likely to find that they use up their supply of cigarettes faster than originally intended', this criterion probably does apply so clearly to nicotine.

3. Difficulty in controlling use. The majority of smokers want to stop smoking but a majority also believe that if they were to try to give up they would fail. Only a tiny proportion of quit attempts succeed.

4. A great deal of time is spent in obtaining, using or recovering from effects of substance. Because smoking is legal and can be engaged in while doing other things, this criterion is less clear for smoking than other drugs or alcohol. However, as a result of recent smoking restrictions in public places and working area, smokers are becoming less able to smoke where and when they choose and they must spend more time in activities specifically related to smoking.

5. A higher priority given to drug use than to other activities and obligations. This criterion is in general not applicable to smoking because smoking is socially relatively acceptable. But priority given to smoking appears when smokers expose their children to the passive smoke at home or when smokers forgo the interdiction to smoke in restricted areas.

6. Continued use despite harmful consequences. Most smokers are aware of the health risks,

although the majority of smokers continue to smoke after diagnosis of smoking related disease.

7. Tolerance. Tolerance to nicotine is manifested by absence of nausea, dizziness.

8. Withdrawal.

Nicotine absorption and metabolism [20–21]

Tobacco can be used in several presentation forms, mainly by inhalation route with cigarettes, pipe and cigar smoking, or by dipping and chewing tobacco. Tobacco smoke is inhaled into the lungs from which it is absorbed into the pulmonary circulation. Delivery of nicotine can thus be expected to move quickly from inhaled cigarette smoke to the brain, effectively within as low as 10 seconds. Nicotine concentrations in the arterial blood and the brain rise quickly following exposure, and decline over 20 to 30 minutes as it is redistributed to other body tissues, particularly skeletal muscle. Rapid passage into the brain provides for the possibility of rapid behavioral reinforcement from smoking. By using smokeless tobacco, the total blood nicotine content achieved can be comparable to that achieved by smoking cigarettes, but the blood level concentration obtained after oral route administration increases more slowly and remains longer than by inhalation. The concentration of nicotine in the plasma of regular smokers tends to rise during the day. Approximately 80 to 90% of nicotine is metabolized mainly by the liver. The major metabolites of nicotine are cotinine and cotinine-1-N-oxide formed by oxidation. The nicotine half-life is approximately 2 hours. The kidneys rapidly eliminate nicotine and its metabolites. Smokers regulate levels of nicotine in their body within certain limits; they change the way they puff a cigarette depending on nicotine yield, as determined by a cigarette smoking machine. People smoke to deliver the desired doses of nicotine to their bodies, with certain rates of delivery and intervals between doses; these behaviors tend to be consistent for a person from day to day.

Nicotinic receptors [22–23]

Nicotine binds stereospecifically to the nicotinic acetylcholine receptor, a heterogeneous five subunits ligand-gated ion channel, located in different organs of the body (brain, skeletal muscle, autonomic ganglia, adrenal medulla, neuromuscular junction, lymphocytes, etc.). Specific neuronal nicotinic receptors are observed in various parts of the brain (hypothalamus, hippocampus, thalamus, cerebral cortex, nigrostriatal, ventral tegmentum and nucleus accumbens). Nicotine acts on the synapse sites to enhance the release of neurotransmitters such as acetylcholine, norepinephrine, serotonin, beta-endorphin, gamma-amino-butyric acid and dopamine. Dopamine, acting through the dopaminergic mesolimbic pathway, has been implicated in the behavioral reinforcing effects of nicotine. Chronic exposure to nicotine causes nicotinic receptor desensitization and compensatory receptor up-regulation, which may account for tolerance to the psychopharmacological effects of nicotine observed in regular smokers.

Withdrawal syndrome [24–25]

Nicotine withdrawal occurs abruptly on the cessation of nicotine use and includes all nicotine forms and routes of administration. Changes in mood and performance due to withdrawal can be detected within 2 hours of the last nicotine use. They most often peak within 24 hours, and gradually subside within a few days to several weeks. The signs and symptoms of withdrawal are craving for tobacco, irritability, anxiety, difficulty concentrating, restlessness, bradycardia, increased

appetite, but can be also frustration, anger, depression, impatience, somatic complaints, and insomnia. The number, frequency and intensity of these symptoms varied across the studied lot. Tobacco withdrawal is associated with nicotine tolerance and is suppressed by the resumption of nicotine use, as is the case with other drugs that produce pharmacological dependence. Even though most nicotine is cleared from the body within 1 to 2 days of abstinence, mental dysfunction and other signs of withdrawal can persist for weeks. Powerful cravings can resurge for months and years.

Evaluation

Questionnaire [26–27]

A frequently used marker of dependence is daily cigarette consumption, based on the assumption that the more cigarettes smoked per day the harder people should find it to stop. Questionnaire methods have also been used to measure nicotine dependence. The most widely used is the Fagerström Test for Nicotine Dependence (FTND) or its two-item version, the Heaviness of Smoking Index (HIS), which measures the number of cigarettes per day and the time to the first cigarette of the day. A threshold of 6 on the FTND is generally used to divide smokers into high and low-dependence categories (Table 41.3).

Table 41.3
The Fagerström test for nicotine dependence

Question	Answer	Score
How soon after you wake up do you smoke your first cigarette	Within 5 minutes	3
	6–30 minutes	2
	31–60 minutes	1
	> 60 minutes	0
Do you find it difficult to refrain from smoking in places where it is forbidden?	Yes	1
	No	0
Which cigarette would you hate to give up most?	The first one in the morning	1
	Others	0
How many cigarettes per day do you smoke?	< 10	0
	11–20	1
	21–30	2
	> 30	3
Do you smoke more frequently during the first hours after waking than during the rest of the day?	Yes	1
	No	0
Do you smoke if you are so ill that you are in bed most of the day?	Yes	1
	No	0

Scores are totaled to yield a single value.

Other questionnaires evaluate subjective feelings of dependence and craving during abstinence, predicting the severity of urges to smoke during quit attempts and the failure of these attempts.

Biological measurements

The validity of self-reported smoking can be questioned because of the belief that smokers are sometimes inclined to underestimate the amount smoked or to deny smoking at all [28]. Denial of smoking will vary according to circumstances, for example diabetes is a disease known to be susceptible to misclassification of smoking [29]. Biochemical measurement of smoking by-products in body fluids can be used to validate self-reports of smoking, to evaluate the exposure to tobacco smoke and to adapt the nicotinic replacement therapy. The most commonly used biochemical assessments are carbon monoxide in expired air [30], thiocyanates [31, 32] and cotinine in plasma, saliva or urine. Rapid, inexpensive, expired air carbon monoxide monitoring is a near-patient technique using hand-held instruments. It allows evaluating the smoking inhalation depth. Unfortunately, carbon monoxide has a short half-life (2–4 hours) and is also observed after combustion of other organic substances than tobacco. It remains a good indicator of short-term tobacco use. Thiocyanates are end-products of detoxification of cyanide present especially in cigarette smoke and also in some other exogenous components. Saliva tests are the most stable and sensitive procedure for obtaining thiocyanates measures of smoking exposure [33]. The half-life of salivary thiocyanates is 10 to 14 days, allowing the evaluation of exposure to the toxic components of tobacco smoke during the preceding 3 weeks. Nicotine and cotinine, its main metabolite, are the most specific markers of tobacco smoke. Urinary or salivary cotinine [34] are the most widely used because of their relatively long half-life (1–2 days).

PSYCHOLOGICAL AND BEHAVIORAL DEPENDENCES

From early on their smoking career, smokers perceive that smoking provides certain psychological benefits. Most smokers agree that smoking produces arousal, particularly with the first few cigarettes of the day, and relaxation particularly in stressful situations. They are more inclined to smoke when they feel tense, embarrassed, depressed, angry or bored, smoking reducing these unpleasant emotions. Smokers may also experience the relief from hunger and prevention of weight gain by smoking. Studies have shown improvement in attention, learning, reaction time, and problem solving by smoking nicotine cigarettes [35]. However, the magnitude of this effect of nicotine is comparable to the effects obtained by consuming caffeinated beverages [36]. Although many smokers believe that smoking nicotine cigarettes lifts their mood and performance, it remains unclear if these positive rewards are due to relief of symptoms of abstinence or/and to an intrinsic enhancement effect of nicotine [37]. At the same time, smokers begin to associate specific moods, situations or environmental factors with the rewarding effects of tobacco consumption. People often smoke cigarettes in specific situations, such as after a meal, with a cup of coffee or an alcoholic beverage, or with friends who smoke. The association between smoking and these events, repeated many times, causes the environmental situations to become powerful cues for the urge of smoke. Manipulation of smoking materials, taste, smell, or feel of smoke in the throat, can be also associated with the pleasure of smoking. Even unpleasant moods can become conditioned cues for smoking, like irritability after nicotine abstinence, relieved by tobacco use. After repeating this experience, a smoker may come to regard irritability from any source, such as stress or frustration, as a cue for smoking. This conditioning develops exclusively because of the association between pharmacological actions of tobacco smoke and behaviors. Drug-taking behavior within a family or among friends is a strong motivator and reinforcer of drug use. Conditioning loses its power without the presence of nicotine but there are other factors in nicotine addiction including personality, social setting and also sociologic factors [38].

SMOKING CESSATION GUIDELINES

Cigarette smoking is the most avoidable cause of illness in the general population as well as in

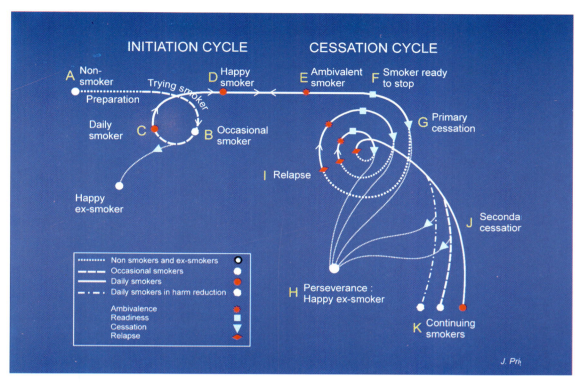

Plate 41.1

Smokers' career reproduced from J. Prignot (A tentative illustration of the smoking initiation and cessation cycles. Tobacco Control, Letter 9: 113, 2000) with permission.

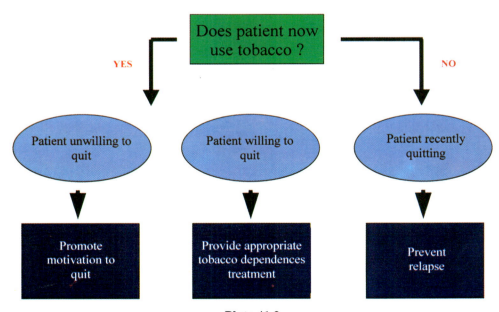

Plate 41.2

Algorithm for treating tobacco use.

patients with diabetes. The danger of developing late complications is much higher for smoking than for non-smoking diabetic patients. Health care professionals must advise all the patients to improve their health by stopping smoking, particularly patients with a chronic disease like diabetes. Such advice may be brief, or part of more intensive interventions. The care approach must include preventive, behavioral and pharmacological strategies as components of routine diabetes education [39]. Changing a behavioral pattern which relates to pharmacological dependence, and which is reinforced many times each day, is difficult. Most people with diabetes, who smoke, do wish to stop and many have made several attempts, only to relapse back to the smoking habit.

BRIEF INTERVENTION

Any clinician can provide brief interventions. Tobacco use status could be queried for every patient at every clinic visit and clearly documented in the medical record. Clinicians should advice all smokers to quit in a clear, strong and personalized manner. They should assess the patient's willingness to make a quit attempt within the next 30 days. Schematically, three maturation stages can be considered: current smokers unwilling at this time to make a quit attempt (precontemplation/contemplation stage), smokers now willing to make a quit attempt (action stage), and former smokers who have recently quit (maintenance stage). Accordingly, three types of intervention could be described (Plate 41.2).

Smokers unwilling to make a quit attempt

For patients unwilling to make a quit attempt, clinicians should use an intervention to promote the motivation to quit. For this purpose, the clinician must be empathic, inform and educate the patient, promote patient autonomy and support its self-efficacy. Information must be given about the harmful effects of tobacco and the dependence process. Motivational information has the greatest impact, if it is relevant to the patient's disease status or risk, family or social situation, age, gender, prior quitting experience, health concerns, etc. The clinician should ask the patient to identify

potential negative consequences of tobacco use and potential benefits of its stopping. It is necessary to identify barriers to quitting like withdrawal symptoms, enjoyment of tobacco, stress control, fear of failure, weight gain, etc. The motivational intervention should be repeated at each visit of an unmotivated patient. Smokers who have failed in previous attempts must know that, frequently, people make repeated quit attempts before they are successful.

Smokers willing to quit

For smokers willing to quit rapidly, within the next 30 days, clinician should aid the patients with a quit plan: to set a quit date, to remove tobacco products from their environment, to request support from their family and friends, to plan pleasant activities to compensate tobacco smoking enjoyment, to change usual behavior patterns, to anticipate triggers or challenges in upcoming attempt. Clinician should clearly notify that total abstinence is important, not even a single puff after the quit date. Smokers in a quitting attempt should identify from previous quit experiences what helped and what hurt, should often limit or abstain drinking alcohol beverages since alcohol can frequently cause relapse and should encourage other smokers in the household to quit smoking or not to smoke in their presence. The clinician should provide a supportive clinical environment and schedule a follow-up contact, either in person or *via* telephone. The first follow-up contact should occur soon after the quit date, preferably during the first week; further contacts should be scheduled according to the needs of each patient. During the follow-up contact, the clinician should congratulate success and if tobacco use has occurred, he should review the circumstances of relapse and remind the patient that a lapse can be used as a learning experience. He should also identify problems encountered and anticipate challenges in the future. Anxiety about weight gain is often an impediment to smoking cessation, particularly for diabetes patients who often feel restricted by treatment regimens. The clinician should neither deny the likelihood of this gain nor minimize its significance to the patient but should prepare the patient for this occurrence and give the relatively moderate weight gain that typically occurs. Although intensive weight control strategies are not recommended during the quit attempt, the patient should be encouraged to maintain or adopt a healthy lifestyle that includes moderate exercise, eating plenty of fruits and vegetables, and limiting alcohol consumption [40]. Tobacco addiction is a complex process. Many smokers are able to quit by themselves or with behavioral therapies but a substantial number of smokers are unable to do so. Because the pharmacological action of nicotine is an important factor in maintaining smoking consumption, every smoker should be encouraged to use pharmacotherapies except in the presence of special circumstances (pregnant women, adolescents). The first-line pharmacotherapy agents include bupropion SR and nicotinic substitution.

Smokers who have recently quit

Because of the chronic relapsing nature of tobacco dependence, clinicians should provide brief effective relapse prevention treatment. Relapses occur mostly within the first 3 months but also several months or even years after the quit date. The clinicians should reinforce the patient's decision to quit, provide cessation-counseling support, assist the patient in resolving any residual problems arising from quitting, anticipate threats to maintain abstinence and review the benefits of quitting. These interventions should be delivered by means of either clinic visits or telephone calls. Recovering nicotine addicts sometimes fantazise about smoking one cigarette now and then. They should be reminded that nicotine addicts do not become 'social smokers', that addiction to nicotine is permanent and that progression to compulsive use is the rule after smoking one cigarette. A recovering nicotine addict always avoids smoking a cigarette, pipe, chewing tobacco, or cigars. Because weight gain after quitting could often be a cause of relapse, clinicians should recommend starting or increasing physical activity, should reassure the patient that this gain is common and self-limiting. Although clinicians emphasize the importance of a healthy diet, it is sometimes necessary to refer the patient to a dietician. It could be useful to maintain the patient on pharmacotherapy known to delay weight gain. A negative mood or depression could induce smoking again. Clinicians should provide counseling, prescribe appropriate medications or refer the patient to a specialist if necessary.

INTENSIVE CLINICAL INTERVENTION

Intensive clinical intervention produces higher success rates than do less intensive intervention, but implies resource availability and time constraints. These interventions are appropriate for any tobacco user willing to participate and not only for specific populations. Intensive interventions should be provided by specialists in the treatment of tobacco dependence who possess the skills, knowledge and training to provide efficacious interventions and who conduct research on tobacco dependence and its treatment. The tobacco dependence interventions offered by specialists represent an important resource for patients who do not receive tobacco dependence treatment from their primary care clinician. Interventions may be made more intense by increasing the length of individual treatment sessions (longer than 10 minutes) and the number of sessions (4 or more). Multiple types of providers like physicians, nurses, psychologists are effective and should be involved. A medical care clinician will deliver messages about health risks and benefits and will prescribe pharmacotherapy. Non-medical clinicians will deliver psychosocial and behavioral interventions. Either individual or group and telephone counseling may be used.

MANAGEMENT OF NICOTINE ADDICTION

NON-PHARMACOLOGICAL APPROACHES

Behavioral interventions

As previously described, the behavioral therapy consists of a multimodal approach to self-management techniques aimed at assisting the smokers to 'unlearn' their habit and to develop alternative forms of behavior. Recording cigarette consumption, systematic control of smoking situations, agreement on a contract and relapse prevention are included in the process.

Hypnosis and acupuncture

Among the existing treatments for smokers, hypnosis and acupuncture hold a special place. Although the Cochrane group reviewing studies of hypnosis [41] and of acupuncture [42] has concluded that evidence of specific efficacy is lacking, some people can be helped by numerous different unproven procedures *via* placebo effect.

PHARMACOLOGICAL APPROACHES [43]

All smokers trying to quit should receive pharmacotherapy for smoking cessation. Specific precautions should be taken for populations with medical contraindications, for light smokers smoking fewer than 10 cigarettes per day, for pregnant or breastfeeding women and for adolescent smokers. Bupropion SR and nicotinic replacement therapy are recommended as first-line pharmacotherapies and are approved by the FDA. The choice of a specific first-line pharmacotherapy must be guided by factors such as the clinician's familiarity with the medications, contraindications for selected patients, patient preference, previous patient experience or patient characteristics. Long-term use of pharmacotherapies may be helpful with smokers with persistent withdrawal symptoms. It may be possible to combine different pharmacotherapies. The pharmacological approach is most effective when used as part of a comprehensive program that includes behavioral therapy.

Nicotine replacement therapy [44–48]

Nicotine replacement therapy (NRT) is widely used for smoking cessation. A variety of delivery vehicles have been introduced, including nicotine chewing gum, transdermal patch, oral inhaler, sublingual tablet, nasal spray and more recently lozenge. In controlled trials, smoking cessation rates obtained with NRT have consistently been approximately twice those obtained with placebo or no therapy. There were no significant differences between the NRT systems although the patch appeared to be slightly more effective than gum. Given the apparent equivalence in efficacy among the available NRT systems, the choice of product depends on the individual smoker's preference. Cigarette smoking rapidly produces high nicotine concentrations in the venous circulation (5–7 min), providing the euphoric effect associated with the development of addiction. In contrast, peak venous nicotine concentrations achieved with NRT systems are lower and considerably delayed, limiting their attraction to smokers. Chewing nicotine gum (4 mg) produces the highest nicotine concentrations. The oral inhaler and nasal spray devices produce intermediate nicotine levels. Nicotine absorption is faster with the nasal spray and the inhaler could replace some of the behavioral and hand-to-mouth activity associated with cigarette smoking. Each of these systems has been shown to aid smoking cessation but also have certain drawbacks: constant chewing of gum may induce local adverse events such as jaw ache; the nasal spray has been associated with sneezing and local irritation usually transient. NRT are safe medications. The most common side effects are local or topical, depending on the specific nicotine delivery device and not caused by the low systemic nicotine levels attained. Smokers often under-dose NRT during treatment, resulting in an insufficient dose of nicotine to prevent withdrawal symptoms and leading to treatment failure. NRT appears to be more effective if multiple delivery methods are combined: a steady-state delivery system (transdermal patch) together with a self-administrated and self-controlled faster-acting system (gum, tablets, a.s.o.) may yet prove to be a superior treatment than either treatment alone. Although smokers often use NRT for a short period, there are instances when a prolonged duration of use is desirable to maintain abstinence from smoking (smokers with depression, etc). NRT used to reduce the cigarette consumption of smokers who will not stop smoking, may increase their motivation to quit, which must remain the ultimate goal of NRT while reducing the incidence of tobacco-related disease.

Hydrochloride Bupropion [49–56]

Bupropion sustained release (SR) is recommended as first-line treatment in both the UK and US guidelines for smoking cessation.

Bupropion is a norepinephrine and dopamine reuptake inhibitor, and is thought to work by enhancing dopaminergic activity in the mesolimbic system and the nucleus accumbens. Treatment with bupropion alleviates craving, withdrawal symptoms and attenuates the weight gain associated with smoking cessation. At the recommended dose of 300 mg/day for 7 to 9 weeks, bupropion SR, in conjunction with motivational support, is significantly more effective than placebo as an aid to smoking cessation in patients with or without a history of prior bupropion SR or NRT use. Bupropion SR alone or together with a nicotine patch seems to be significantly superior to the nicotine patch alone. It is effective in the prevention of relapse to smoking in patients who have successfully quit and also in smokers who have returned to smoking after a previous administration of bupropion SR. Treatment with bupropion SR is generally well tolerated. The adverse reactions reported were gastrointestinal (dry mouth, nausea, vomiting), neurological (dizziness, headache, tremor), psychiatric (anxiety, depression, insomnia) and skin (angioedema, pruritus, rash, urticaria) events. More frequently occurring events were insomnia and dry mouth, but the most clinically significant adverse reactions of bupropion SR were seizures and hypersensitivity reactions. The risk of seizures occurring with the use of bupropion SR appears to be strongly associated with the presence of predisposing risk factors. Therefore, bupropion SR should be contraindicated in patients with one of these predisposing conditions such as history of seizures or head trauma, central nervous system tumor and association with other medications known to lower the seizure threshold. Caution should be used in alcohol abuse, abrupt withdrawal from alcohol or benzodiazepines, use of stimulants or anorectic products and diabetes treated with hypoglycemic drugs or insulin. In diabetic patients 150 mg once a day is the recommended dose.

Others [9]

Other non-nicotine medications have been reported as second-line medications. Although there is evidence that these pharmacotherapies present some efficacy for treating tobacco dependence, they have a more limited role than the first-line medications. The FDA has not approved them for a tobacco dependence treatment indication and there are more concerns about potential side effects than exist with first-line medications. Second-line treatments should be considered for use on a case-by-case basis after first-line treatments have been used or considered.

Primarily used as an antihypertensive medication, clonidine delivered either transdermally or orally is an efficacious smoking cessation treatment but specific dosing regimen for its use has not been established, varying from 0.1 to 0.75 mg/day. It should be noted that abrupt discontinuation can result in symptoms such as nervousness, agitation, headache, and tremor, accompanied or followed by a rapid rise in blood pressure and elevated catecholamines levels. Therefore, clinicians need to be aware of the specific warnings regarding this medication as well as its side-effect profile.

Nortriptyline is used primarily as an anti-depressant. The use of nortriptyline seems to increase abstinence rates when compared to a placebo. Side-effects profile includes the risk of arrhythmia, sedation and dry mouth, limiting its use.

CONCLUSION

Smoking causes a wide range of diseases but many of the adverse health effects for smoking are reversible. Smoking cessation treatments represent some of the most cost effective of all healthcare interventions. Nicotine is physically and psychologically addictive, with multiple factors contributing to the initiation and continuation of the habit. Since smoking duration is the principal risk factor for smoking-related morbidity, the treatment goal should be early cessation and prevention relapse [57]. A common characteristic of diabetes and smoking is that both are chronic disorders with careers determined for an individual by the interaction between family, personal and external factors. There is little research that directly addresses smoking among those with diabetes. Combining what we know about smoking and diabetes raises the following problems:
- exacerbation of general underestimation of risks of smoking prompted by attention to risk of diabetes;

- distraction from smoking cessation by professionals' attention to metabolic control;
- fear of weight gain which may be exacerbated by concern for weight control in diabetes management;
- utility of nicotine's mood elevating effects in reducing depressed moods commonly found in diabetes;
- smoking ameliorating stress associated with poor metabolic control or with efforts to maintain good metabolic control and high levels of family stress or diminished social support, which may be exacerbated in diabetes;
- use of smoking to enhance task performance frequently required to manage a complex diabetic regimen of medication, diet and activity [58].

In order to improve smoking cessation rates, effective behavioral and pharmacological treatments, coupled with professional counseling and advice are required. Although patient's motivation to quit is necessary, physicians can play over time a critical role in increasing patient motivation so that he/she becomes ready to set a target quit date. Once the patient reaches this stage, medical treatment can double to triple short- and long-term treatment outcome. If the physician treats tobacco dependence as a chronic medical disease and manages relapse in the same fashion as other chronic disease recurrence, long-term, outpatient 'cure' rates of 30 to 40% are possible. Although the greatest benefit accrues from ceasing smoking when young, even quitting in middle age avoids much of the excess healthcare risk associated with smoking [59].

REFERENCES

1. Peto R, Lopez AD, Boreham J, Thun M, Health C. *Mortality from smoking in developed countries 1950–2000*, Oxford University Press, 1994.
2. US Department of Health and Human Services. The health benefits of smoking cessation: A report of the Surgeon General. Atlanta (GA): US Department of Health and Human Services. Public Health Service, Centres for Disease Control, Centre for Chronic Disease Prevention and Health Promotion, Office of Smoking and Health. *DHHS Publication* N° (CDC) 90–8416: 1990.
3. Rytter L, Troelsen S, Beck-Nielsen H. Prevalence and mortality of acute myocardial infarction in patients with diabetes. *Diabetes Care*, 8: 230–234, 1985.
4. Gordon T, Castelli WP, Hjortland MC. High density lipoprotein as a protective factor against coronary heart disease: the Framingham study. *Am J Med*, 62: 707–714, 1977.
5. Christlieb AR. Diabetes and hypertension vascular disease. *Am J Cardio*, 32: 592–606, 1973.
6. Kannell WB, Schatzkin A. Factor analysis. *Prog Cardiovasc Dis*, 26: 309–332, 1984.
7. Lithner F. Is tobacco of importance for the development and progression of diabetic vascular complications? *Acta Med Scand (Suppl)*, 687: 33–36, 1983.
8. Jones RB, Hedley AJ. Prevalence of smoking on a diabetic population: the need for action. *Diabetic Med*, 4: 233–236, 1987.
9. The Tobacco Use and Dependence Clinical Practice Guideline Panel, Staff, and Consortium Representatives. A Clinical Practice Guideline for Treating Tobacco Use and Dependence. A US Public Health Service Report. *JAMA*, 283: 3244–3254, 2000.
10. Prochaska JO, Di Clemente CG. Towards a comprehensive model of change. In: Miller WR, Heather N. eds. Treating addictive behaviour: process of change. New York, Plenum Press, 1986.
11. Prignot J. A tentative illustration of the smoking initiation and cessation cycles. *Tobacco Control*, Letter 9: 113, 2000.
12. Glynn TJ, Manley MW. How to help your patients stop smoking: a National Cancer Institute manual for physicians. Bethesda, MD: *NIH Publication*, N° 89–3064, 1989.
13. Glynn TJ, Manley MW, Pechacek TF. Physician-initiated smoking cessation program: the National Cancer Institute trials. *Prog Clin Biol Res*, 339: 11–25, 1990.
14. American Medical Association. American Medical Association guidelines for the diagnosis and treatment of nicotine dependence: how to help patients stop smoking. Washington DC: *American Medical Association*, 1994.
15. Mecklenburg RE, Christen AG, Gerbert B, Gift MC. How to help your patients stop using tobacco: a National Cancer Institute manual for the oral health team 1990. US DHHS Public Health Service, National Institutes of Health, National Cancer Institute. *NIH Publication* N° 91–3191, 1991.
16. American Psychiatric Association. Practice guideline for the treatment of patients with nicotine dependence. *Am J Psychiatry*, 156 (10 suppl): S1–S31, 1996.

17. Royal College of Physicians. Nicotine Addiction in Britain. *A report of the Tobacco Advisory Group of the Royal College of Physicians*, 2000.

18. British Thoracic Society. Smoking cessation guidelines and their cost-effectiveness. *Thorax*, **53 (suppl 5, part 1):** S1–S38, 1998.

19. The Cochrane Collaboration. Cochrane Database of Systematic Reviews. *The Cochrane Library*, 4, 1999.

20. Benowitz NL. Pharmacologic aspects of cigarette smoking and nicotine addiction. *N Engl J Med*, **319:** 1318, 1988.

21. Miller NS, Cocores JA. Nicotine dependence: diagnosis, pharmacology and treatment. *J. Addictive Diseases*, **11(2):** 51–65, 1991.

22. Leonard S, Bertrand D. Neuronal nicotinic receptors: from structure to function. *Nicotine and Tobacco Research*, **3:** 203–223, 2001.

23. Paterson D, Nordberg A. Neuronal nicotinic receptors in the human brain. *Progress in Neurobiology*, **61:** 75–111, 2000.

24. Hughes JR, Hatsukami D. Signs and symptoms of tobacco withdrawal. *Arch Gen Psychiatry*, **43:** 289–294, 1986.

25. Henningfield JE, Fant RV, Shiffman S, Gitchell J. Tobacco dependence: scientific and public health basis of treatment. *TEN*, **2(1):** 42–46, 2000.

26. Heatherton TF, Kozlowski LT, Frecker RC, Fagerström KO. The Fagerström Test for Nicotine Dependence: a revision of the Fagerström Tolerance Questionnaire. *British. Journal of Addiction*, **86:** 1119–1127, 1991.

27. Hughes JR, Higgins ST, Bickel WK. Nicotine withdrawal versus other drug withdrawal syndromes: similarities and dissimilarities. *Addiction*, **89:** 1461–1470, 1994.

28. Patrick DL, Cheadle A, Thompson DC, Diehr P, Koepsell T, Kinne S. The validity of self-reported smoking: a review and meta-analysis. *Am. J. of Public Health*, **84:** 1086–1093, 1994.

29. Holl RW, Grabert M, Heinze E, Debatin KM. Objective assessment of smoking habits by urinary cotinine measurement in adolescents and young adults with type 1 diabetes. Reliability of reported cigarette consumption and relationship to urinary albumin excretion. *Diabetes Care*, **13:** 996–999, 1996.

30. Jarvis MJ, Russell MAH, Saloojee Y. Expired air carbon monoxide: a simple breath test of tobacco smoke intake. *Br Med J*, **281:** 484–485, 1980.

31. Barylko-Pikielna N, Pangborn RM, Calif D. Effect of cigarette smoking on urinary and salivary thiocyanates. *Arch Environ Health*, **17:** 739–745, 1968.

32. Luepker RV, Pechacek TF, Murray DM, Johnson CA, Hund F, Jacobs DR. Saliva thiocyanate: a chemical indicator of cigarette smoking in adolescents. *AJPH*, **71:** 1320–1324, 1981.

33. Galanti LM, Delwiche JP, Dubois P, Somville M, Pouthier F, Prignot J. Effect of storage conditions on saliva thiocyanate concentration. *Clin Chem*, **35:** 496, 1989.

34. Haufroid V, Lison D. Urinary cotinine as a tobacco-smoke exposure index: a minireview. *Int Arch Occup Environ Health*, **71:** 162–168, 1998.

35. Wesnes K, Warburton DM. Smoking, nicotine and human performance. *Pharmacol Ther*, **21:** 189–208, 1983.

36. Cohen C, Pickworth WB, Bunker EB, Hennigfield JE. Caffeine antagonises EEG effects of tobacco withdrawal. *Pharmacol Biochem Behav*, **47:** 919–926, 1994.

37. Pomerleau CS, Pommerleau OF. Cortisol response to a psychological stressor and/or nicotine. *Pharmacol Biochem Behav*, **35:** 211–213, 1990.

38. Benowitz NL. Cigarette smoking and nicotine addiction. *Medical clinics of North America*, **76(2):** 415–437, 1992.

39. Haire-Joshu D. Smoking cessation and the diabetic health care team. *Diabetes Educ*, **17(1):** 54–64, 1991.

40. The smoking cessation clinical practice guideline panel and staff. The Agency for health care policy and research smoking cessation clinical practice guideline. *JAMA*, **275(16) :** 1270–1280, 1996.

41. Abbot NC, Stead LF, White AR, Barnes J, Ernst E. *Hypnotherapy for smoking cessation (Cochrane review)*. The Cochrane Library, Issue 2, Oxford: Update software, 1999.

42. White AR, Rampes H. *Acupuncture for smoking cessation (Cochrane review)*. The Cochrane Library, Issue 2, Oxford: Update software, 1999.

43. National Institute for Clinical Excellence. Guidance on the use of nicotine replacement Therapy (NRT) and bupropion for smoking cessation. *Technology Appraisal Guidance*, **39:** 1–21, 2002.

44. World Health Organization Regional Office for Europe. Regulation of nicotine replacement therapies: an expert consensus, 2001.

45. McNeill A, Foulds J, Bates C. Regulation of nicotine replacement therapies (NRT): a critique of current practice. *Addiction*, **96:** 1757–1768, 2001.

46. Fagerström KO, Schneider NG, Lunell E. Effectiveness of nicotine patch and nicotine gum as individual versus combined treatments for tobacco withdrawal symptoms. *Psychopharmacology*, **111:** 271–277, 1993.

47. Balfour D, Benowitz N, Fagerström KO, Kunze M, Keil U. Diagnosis and treatment of nicotine dependence with emphasis on nicotine replacement therapy. *Eur Heart J*, **21:** 438–445, 2000.

48. Fagerström KO. Nicotine replacement: present and future. *CVD Prevention*, **2**: 145–149, 1999.

49. Hurt RD, Sachs DPL, Glover ED, Offord KP, Johnston JA, Dale LC, Khayrallah MA, Schroeder DR, Glover PN, Rollynn Sullivan C, Croghan IT, Sullivan PM. A comparison of sustained-release bupropion and placebo for smoking cessation. *N Engl J Med*, **337**: 1195–1202, 1997.

50. Jorenby DE, Leischow SJ, Nides MA, Rennard SI, Johnston JA, Hughes AR, Smith SS, Muramoto ML, Daughton DM, Doan K, Fiore M, Baker TB. A controlled trial of sustained-release bupropion, a nicotine patch, or both for smoking cessation. *N Engl J Med*, **340**: 685–691, 1999.

51. Tashkin DP, Kanner R, Bailey W, Buist S, Anderson P, Nides MA, Gonzales D, Dozier G, Patel MK, Jamerson BD. Smoking cessation in patients with chronic obstructive pulmonary disease: a double-blind, placebo-controlled, randomised trial. *Lancet*, **357**: 1571–1575, 2001.

52. Shiffman S, Johnston JA, Khayrallah M, Elash CA, Gwaltney CJ, Paty JA, Gnys M, Evoniuk G, DeVeaugh-Geiss J. The effect of bupropion on nicotine craving and withdrawal. *Psychopharmacology*, **148**: 33–40, 2000.

53. Gonzales DH, Nides MA, Ferry LH, Kustra RP, Jamerson BD, Segall N, Herrero LA, Krishen A, Sweeney A, Buaron K, Metz A. Bupropion SR as an aid to smoking cessation in smokers treated previously with bupropion: a randomised placebo-controlled study. *Clin Pharmacol Ther*, **69**: 438–444, 2001.

54. Hays JT, Hurt RD, Rigotti NA, Niaura R, Gonzales D, Durcan MJ, Sachs DPL, Walter TD, Buist AS, Johnston JA, White JD. Sustained-release bupropion for pharmacologic relapse prevention after smoking cessation. *Ann Intern Med*, **135**: 423–433, 2001.

55. Holm KJ, Spencer CM. Bupropion. A review of its use in the management of smoking cessation. *Drugs*, **59(4)**: 1007–1024, 2000.

56. Jorenby D. Clinical efficacy of bupropion in the management of smoking cessation. *Drugs*, **62(suppl 2)**: 25–35, 2002.

57. Fagerström KO. The epidemiology of smoking. Health consequences and benefits of cessation. *Drugs*, **62(suppl 2)** : 1–9, 2002.

58. Fiore MC, Novotny TE, Pierce JP, Giovino GA, Hatziandreu EJ, Newcomb PA, Surawicz TS, Davis RM. Methods used to quit smoking in the United States. Do cessation programs help? *JAMA*, **263(20)**: 2760–2765, 1990.

59. Sachs DPL, Fagerström KO. Medical management of tobacco dependence: practical office considerations. *Current Pulmonology*, **16 (9)**: 239–249, 1995.

42

THE ROLE OF THE VASCULATURE IN DIABETIC FOOT ULCERS

Lawrence Chukwudi NWABUDIKE

Diabetic foot ulcers are a dreaded complication of diabetes mellitus. Foot ulcers can be neuropathic, ischaemic or neuroischaemic. Associated factors are infection and trauma. Ischaemia is an aetiologic factor in 30.4% of our cases. Parts of the foot without collateral circulation, such as the toes, are more frequently affected and 76.0% of cases were at the level of the toes. The toes were also the site of the majority of cases of multiple ulcers (85.7%). The pathogenesis of ischaemia at the level of the lower limbs is *via* sympathetic nerve damage, which results in increased vessel wall stiffness and medial arterial sclerosis (MAC), as well as *via* arteriovenous shunting that bypasses the capillary circulation thus predisposing to tissue ischaemia. Direct vascular factors, like atherosclerosis, stenosis and microvascular changes, such as decreased blood pressure at the level of the ankle and toes, as well as reduced capillary blood flow and diminished partial pressure of oxygen, all predispose to ischaemia. Trauma, infection and trophic changes all contribute, against a backdrop of ischaemia, to the production of foot ulcers.

INTRODUCTION

The incidence and prevalence of diabetes mellitus continue to grow at an alarming rate especially in the industrially developed countries of the world. The improved standards of health care that are now available as well as the constantly refined treatment possibilities offered by modern technology have ensured a brighter prognosis of this disorder for those who suffer from it. Albeit a source of joy and hope for those afflicted with this disease and their families, this improved life expectancy is not without a serious drawback. This comes in the form of an increase in the potential for the development of long-term complications of diabetes mellitus such as ocular, renal, cardiovascular and neurological disorders.

Another area of diabetes care that is of great concern is the diabetic foot. This is because of the potential for lower extremity amputations that result, in the main part, from foot ulcers. In Bucharest, the prevalence of foot ulcers in a group of outpatients studied for the cutaneous manifestations of diabetic neuropathy was estimated at 3.7%, while 6.8% of another study group of Bucharest inpatients for the skin manifestations of diabetes mellitus had foot ulcers [1, 2]. Other authors, using different recruitment criteria and target points, had an incidence of 12.7% for foot ulcers [3]. This is closer to the 15% figure reported by our surgical colleagues in a Bucharest center [4]. The higher figures reported by both groups are also a reflection of the different clinical profiles and case varieties that differ between a medical and a surgical center.

It is generally accepted that most foot ulcers are neuropathic in aetiology, although ischemia plays an important role. In this paper, some clinical data concerning foot ulcers in patients with diabetes mellitus is analyzed together with the role played by the vasculature in ulcer pathogenesis. The relevant literature in this field is then examined in the light of this clinical data.

RESEARCH DATA

A clinical study was carried out involving 46 patients presenting at our outpatient footcare clinic for diabetic foot ulcers. The clinical characteristics of these patients were observed.

Predisposing factors were determined with a view to defining therapeutic and prophylactic approaches to management.

METHODOLOGY AND CLINICAL MATERIAL

A total of 46 patients with diabetes mellitus presenting consecutively to our outpatient footcare center for foot ulceration were recruited into the study. Their ulcers were assessed for probable cause by using symptomatology related to neuropathy or vasculopathy, clinical examination (location, depth, margins, base, presence of infection, and nature of surrounding skin), as well as simple neurologic and vascular tests, such as pulse palpation, oscillometry, vibration perception thresholds and thermal sensitivity. Each ulcer was also staged according to the Wagner staging method. This study was presented at the IDF 18th Congress, Paris, 2003 [5].

Table 42.1

Characteristics of the patient group studied

Characteristics	Numbers
Male:Female ratio	33:13 (71.7% : 28.3%)
Average age at presentation	59.9 years (range 32–86 years)
Average duration of diabetes	10.8 years (0–28 years)
Type of diabetes (T1:T2)	(1:45)

From Table 42.1 it can be seen that there was a male predominance in this group (33 vs. 13). This may be explained by a number of factors such as occupation, which may predispose male patients to trauma. Other predisposing factors such as arteriopathy and neuropathy, tend to be more frequent in male patients. Female patients are also known to pay much greater attention to the care of their feet than male patients and would therefore have a smaller risk of developing foot ulcers.

The average age at presentation was 59.9 years with an upper limit of 86 years showing that most patients were in the older age bracket. This increased age is correlated with a greater likelihood of inability to attend to the care of their feet in a proper manner as a result of age-

Table 42.2

The results of the study

Cause of ulcers	Location of ulcer	Wagner classification
Neuropathy – 32 (69.6%) Mixed ulcers – 12 (26.1%) Arteriopathy – 2 (4.3%) [1]Infection – 7 (15.2%) [2]Trauma – 5 (10.8%)	Toes 51 (76%) Foot 9 (13.4%) Heels 4 (5.9%) Plantar area 2 (2.8%) Metatarsal area 1 (1.5%) *Single ulcers = 32 (69.6%)* *Multiple ulcers= 14 (30.4%)* Toe = 12 (85.7%) Heel = 1 (7.1%) Plantar area = 1(7.1%)	W1 = 1 (2.1%) W2 = 21 (45.7%) W3= 22 (47.8%) W4 = 2 (4.2%)

[1] Associated factors.
[2] Associated factors.

associated infirmities such as diminished visual acuity, decreased physical ability and impaired manual dexterity. The incidence of vascular disease and neuropathy also increases with age even in populations without diabetes. Experience at the "N. Paulescu" Institute of Diabetes Footcare Clinic shows that most patients of older age present with lesions that are discovered by the physician rather than reported by the patient. This underscores the necessity for regular foot examinations in this subgroup of patients.

The average duration of diabetes was 10.8 years in this study group, which implies a long average duration of diabetes. Increased duration of diabetes mellitus is correlated with the risk of development of complications.

RESULTS OF THE STUDY

Based on the assessment of each ulcer, the probable cause for each ulcer was given as neuropathy, arteriopathy or mixed (neuro-ischaemic). Trauma and infection were noted as associated factors. The Wagner category was assessed for each ulcer.

A total of 67 ulcers were noted for the 46 patients, thus forming an average of 1.45 ulcers *per* patient with a range of 1–6 ulcers *per* patient. A number of patients (14/30.4%) presented with multiple ulcers while the remaining 32 (69.6%)

had only one ulcer each. Most patients (12/85.7%) with multiple ulcers presented with these ulcers in the toe area. Previous amputation was seen in 5 (10.8%) of patients, while 41 (90.2%) of patients had no amputation prior to presentation.

DISCUSSION

In this study group, most ulcers were neuropathic (69.6%). Arteriopathic and mixed (neuroischaemic) ulcers comprised 4.3% and 26.1% respectively. Thus, ischaemia was an aetiologic factor in 30.4% of cases. AJM Boulton, on the other hand, reported that 7% and 45% of patients studied by his team had ischaemic and neuroischaemic foot ulcers respectively [6], *i.e.* ischaemia was a factor in 52% of cases.

Also, 76% and 5.9% of ulcers were located in the toe and heel areas respectively (with a predilection for ischaemic change), and 15.2% of patients had associated infection. Trauma was a factor in 10.8% of cases. The toe and heel areas were also most likely to present with ischaemic and neuroischaemic ulcers with a high risk of trauma and infection (see Table 42.2).

Ischaemia can result directly from macrovascular and microvascular disease as well as from the effect of autonomic denervation on the vasculature.

Ischaemic and neuroischaemic ulceration may therefore result from one of several pathways:

1. Sympathetic nerve failure – This brings about medial arterial calcification as well as arteriovenous shunting at the level of the feet. This may be compounded by trophic changes such as plantar fissures that may, against the background of predisposition to diminished blood flow, lead to ulcers.

2. Arteriopathy – This may result from microvascular or macrovascular disease. The ischaemia may bring about ulceration by itself, depending upon severity, or it may aggravate the ulcer.

3. Infection and trauma – They may compound any of these processes and trigger the onset of necrosis as well as gangrene.

1. Sympathetic nerve failure. The sympathetic nerve fibers travel with the small, unmyelinated C fibers that are known to be responsible for nociception. Diabetic autonomic neuropathy or sympathetic failure is known to be strongly associated with medial arterial calcification (MAC) and many patients that have undergone unilateral sympathectomy develop MAC on the affected side only [7]. There is some debate on the significance of this disorder in the aetiology of ischaemic changes in the lower limb. The work of other authors showed that there is an increase in post-exercise transcutaneous oxygen tension [tcPO$_2$] in the feet of diabetic patients with MAC without peripheral ischaemic vascular disease as opposed to diabetic patients with peripheral ischaemic vascular disease while controls showed no change [8]. On the other hand, some workers have been able to show that increased arterial wall stiffness limits blood flow volume to the affected limb [9]. These authors were able to show an increased pulse wave velocity, in other words, a decreased flow volume in the popliteal arteries of patients with diabetes mellitus. Arterial wall stiffness is a direct consequence of MAC and leads to increased resistance to blood flow and hence to limitation of blood supply. This limitation in blood supply is especially important in critical situations where a constant increase in blood flow is required to prevent or correct ischemic damage.

The limited blood flow noted in [9] may not translate to a decrease in tcPO$_2$ in the foot as might be expected, but this may even be increased, as was shown by Chantelau *et al.* [8]. An explanation of this apparent paradox can be found in the work of Edmonds and Watkins who showed that there is an increase in total blood flow in the neuropathic foot as a result of the opening of arteriovenous shunts to the feet. The opening of these arteriovenous shunts results from decreased sympathetic tonus that is a consequence of neuropathy [10, 11]. Their viewpoint is supported by a more recent work in which capillary blood velocity and skin temperature were measured at the 2nd and 5th finger before and after ulnar blockage [12]. The results showed that following ulnar block (by implication autonomic block) there was a significant increase in blood flow and skin temperature in the 5th finger as compared to the 2nd finger.

This increase in blood flow, through the arteriovenous shunts, results in a venous tcPO$_2$ that is almost equal to that of arterial tcPO$_2$ as well as to increased total blood flow to the skin of the foot [10, 11]. These observations, combined with the fact that arterial wall stiffness and MAC are also strongly associated with sympathetic failure, may help explain the observations of increased tcPO$_2$ observed in the feet of diabetic patients with MAC following exercise [8] with a limitation of total blood flow through the major vessels [9].

Increased arteriovenous shunting is thought to be responsible for a "capillary steal" syndrome that results in the diversion of blood from the capillaries, which are primarily responsible for nutrient and oxygen supply to the foot [10]. This could bring about tissue ischaemia in spite of raised total cutaneous blood flow and increased venous tcPO$_2$, a situation of "starvation in the midst of plenty". The effect of autonomic neuropathy and arteriovenous shunting in foot ulcers is supported by the work of Uccioli *et al.* [13]. These workers showed that arteriovenous shunting was greater in diabetic patients with neuropathy than without neuropathy. Also, they found that arteriovenous shunting was greater in neuropathic patients with ulcers than without ulcers. Thus, both these factors, *i.e.* increased blood vessel stiffness as well as diminished capillary blood flow could contribute to ischaemia and thus increase the risk of foot ulcer production.

Arteriovenous shunts are most frequently found in the circulation of the fingers and toes. The toes are not supplied with collateral vessels and are very prone to trauma especially in patients with neuropathy. Neuropathy found in most patients (44/95.6%) in our study causes sensory loss and this, together with ischaemia from arteriovenous shunting, predisposes patients to trauma, tissue damage and necrosis as well as to gangrene. Most of the patients in our study (76%) had foot ulcers in the toe area. In fact, most patients presenting with multiple ulcers (12/85.7%) also had these ulcers in the toe area.

Further support for the role of neuropathy as a "vasculopathic" factor in foot ulcer aetiology comes from work carried out by some authors who used capillary microscopy to study the capillary blood flow in type 2 diabetic patients with and without polyneuropathy as well as in a control group [14]. Their results showed that capillary blood flow was lower in patients with polyneuropathy than in patients without polyneuropathy. Transient peak circulatory flow as measured by laser-Doppler fluxmetry following dependency was the greatest in patients with type 2 diabetes and polyneuropathy, suggesting a loss of reflex vasoconstriction that is a consequence of sympathetic neuropathy. The groups with type 2 diabetes showed a greater reduction in laser-Doppler fluxmetry measurements compared to the control group and this reduced blood flow was most marked in patients with polyneuropathy. These differences were enhanced in patients with a history of polyneuropathy and foot ulceration. This diminution in the cutaneous blood flow of patients with diabetes is supported by work that demonstrated that patients with diabetes mellitus displayed blunted vasodilatory responses to local heating to 44 °C at the dorsum of the feet [15, 16]. This would appear to contradict the research discussed above [8] that indicates an increased total cutaneous blood flow with exercise. However, it was also shown [16] that this blunting was not evident at the level of the toe pulps, an area of prominent arteriovenous anastomosis. The increased total cutaneous blood flow could be the result of increased blood flow through the arteriovenous anastomoses in the finger and toe pulps, that may more than compensate for the diminished blood flow through the predominantly nutritional vasculature of the dorsum of the hand and foot [14–16] and clearly explain the findings observed by other workers [8].

Therefore, autonomic neuropathy is an indirect cause of ischaemia at the level of the lower limbs *via* large vessel stiffness and MAC as well as *via* by-pass of the nutritional capillaries due to increased arteriovenous shunting. This by-pass may be the cause of the diminished capillary blood velocity observed in patients with diabetes and neuropathy especially in patients with a history of foot ulceration. In spite of this, the neuropathic foot is warm, with increased venous $tcPO_2$, but with lower maximal blood flow through the large (sclerotic) blood vessels and, hence, a greater risk of ischaemic tissue damage.

Sympathetic failure is a cause of dry, fissured skin and, together with ischaemia, could lead to severe local tissue necrosis (see Plate 42.1).

2. Arteriopathy. As stated above, patients with diabetes mellitus suffer from a greater incidence and prevalence of macrovascular pathology than do patients without diabetes. The incidence of peripheral artery disease was estimated in one study to be 15% at 10 years and this increased to 45% at 20 years after diagnosis of diabetes mellitus. In the same study, 8% of patients with diabetes mellitus already had peripheral vascular disease at the time of diagnosis of diabetes mellitus [17]. There is an increased frequency of vascular disease in other organs in diabetic patients with foot ulcers as opposed to diabetic patients without foot ulcers. In a study of 8,905 patients with diabetes mellitus, 514 patients presented with foot ulcers. The incidence of peripheral vascular disease, hypertension, end-stage renal disease and stroke was higher in diabetic patients with ulcers (23.1% *vs.* 13.0%; 56.4% *vs.* 30.1; 2.6% *vs.* 1.4%; 13.0% *vs.* 8.7%) than in the general population of patients with diabetes [18]. There is therefore a significantly greater incidence of morbidity from peripheral vascular disease and therefore risk of ischaemic damage in diabetic patients with foot ulcers than in the general population of patients with diabetes.

Toe blood pressure, an indicator of the severity of foot perfusion and thus of large vessel disease, was found to be diminished in a study of patients with impaired ulcer healing (57 ± 31 mmHg) as compared to patients that healed (75 ± 31 mmHg] [19]. In the same study, transcutaneous partial pressure of oxygen [$tcPO_2$] measured in patients with impaired ulcer healing at the level of the dorsum of the foot was 13 ± 14 mmHg and, for patients that healed, it was 50 ± 20 mmHg. In the same study, it was found that tcPO$_2$ was a more specific indicator of healing than toe blood pressure. In addition, even in patients with chronic non-healing foot ulcers in which ischaemia did not appear to play a major causative role, increased tcPO$_2$ following hyperbaric oxygen therapy was found to be associated with improved ulcer healing. In fact, during this treatment, patients were found to have increased tcPO$_2$ levels (21.9 ± 12.1 to 454.2 ± 128.1 mmHg) at the margins of the ulcers [20]. Ankle blood pressure readings are another indicator of macrovascular function and other workers [21] found that there was no healing in patients with ankle blood pressure below 40 mm Hg and that 85% of patients with ankle blood pressure greater than 45 mm Hg experienced ulcer healing. The severity of arterial occlusive disease is also related to the risk for major amputation. In patients with only one total occlusion, there was a 3.6% (1 of 28 patients) amputation rate. This rose to 54.5% (6 of 11 patients) when there were two occlusions and 100% (10 of 10 patients) as well as 83.7% (5 of 6 patients) with 3 and 4 total occlusions respectively [22].

Foot ulcers are a defect in cutaneous coverage that affects the basement membrane.

Some authors studied the vascular density of the skin of the dorsum of the foot and found no significant difference between vascular (capillary, venule and arteriole) density in patients with diabetes compared to those without diabetes [23]. In a more recent study, capillary microscopy was used to measure capillary density in subjects with and without diabetes in the supine position and after 50 minutes with the legs suspended [14]. This study found that the patients all had similar capillary densities in the supine position but patients with peripheral neuropathy had the lowest capillary densities after 50 minutes in the sitting position with their legs suspended. This, together with the changes discussed earlier with regard to arteriovenous shunting, would imply that patients with diabetes mellitus do not suffer a "quantitative channel deficit" but, under certain circumstances, may suffer a "qualitative channel deficit" with regard to the microvasculature.

Other factors affecting microvascular flow include endothelial reactivity, basement membrane thickness and capillary permeability. It is well established, for instance, that diabetes mellitus is associated with basement membrane thickening as well as increased capillary permeability [24]. These have been thought to affect nutrient and oxygen transfer at the tissue level thus enhancing the ischemic changes.

As has been stated earlier, sympathetic nerve abnormalities may also adversely affect microvascular function. Sympathetic nerves are carried by the C-fibers, which are also responsible for pain transmission. Earlier, Boulton et al. had shown that patients with painful diabetic neuropathy, a sign of intact C-fiber function, had a greater capacity to constrict blood vessels than patients with painless neuropathy [25]. More recent work using sodium nitroprusside and acetylcholine that directly and indirectly influence endothelial reactivity, has demonstrated that there is a deficit in C-fiber-mediated axon-related vasodilation in patients with diabetic neuropathy as compared to subjects without neuropathy [26, 27].

Endothelial reactivity is a measure of microvascular function and may be indicative of the degree of blood flow in the affected member. Some authors, using laser Doppler fluximetry to measure capillary blood flow, have been able to show that endothelial reactivity is diminished in patients with diabetes compared to controls [28]. This diminution is also related to increased levels of endothelin-1, a potent vasoconstrictor as well as to increased levels of von Willebrand's factor. Other workers were also able to show that endothelial reactivity was diminished in the lower limbs of diabetic patients after exercise and that this decrease was directly related to hyperglycaemia [29]. Using video capillaroscopy, some workers were able to show that peak capillary blood velocity was lower in insulin-dependent diabetic patients with poor glycaemic control compared to insulin-dependent patients with good glycaemic control [30]. It has also been shown that there is a decrease in capillary reactivity in the foot as compared to the forearm [31]. This latter observation may also help explain why there is a greater morbidity from vascular pathology at the level of the lower limbs than at the level of the upper limbs. The conclusion that can be drawn here is that although there is probably no microvascular "occlusive" pathology, there are functional disorders such as decreased reactivity as well as diminished flow and these are aggravated by hyperglycaemia and attenuated by good glycaemic control. This decreased functionality of the microcirculation is associated with increased levels of vasoconstrictor substances such as endothelin-1 and coagulative principles such as von Willebrand's factor. The combined effect of these is to predispose to, or bring about, a degree of tissue ischaemia that could increase risk of ulceration, cause foot ulceration or diminish the capacity of already existing wounds to heal.

Unilateral ischaemia may causing ulceration at the base of the toe (see Plate 42.2).

3. Trauma and infection are significant associated factors in the pathogenesis of ischaemic foot ulcers. Infection brings about the release of vasotoxic and tissue necrotic factors that cause intravascular thrombosis thus resulting in compromise of blood supply. Trauma causes tissue destruction and the release of substances that would promote intravascular coagulation. Both factors would therefore aggravate the ischaemic process. Trauma is more frequent at the toes as shown in our study [5] and the toes themselves are at the greatest risk of ischaemic damage.

Trauma may precipitate acute ischaemia and gangrene (Plate 42.3).

Thus, in summary, the role of ischaemia in the pathogenesis of ulceration is two-fold:

– Indirectly, *via* sympathetic dysfunction leading to arterial wall stiffness and medial calcification. This could bring about impaired blood flow through the affected limb especially in conditions of increased demand. Sympathetic dysfunction also causes arteriovenous shunting and a diversion of flow from the nutritive capillary circulation thus leading to ischaemia and to impaired wound healing.

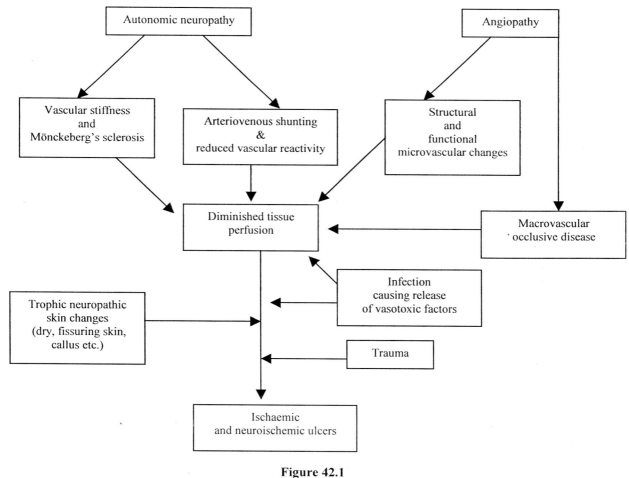

Figure 42.1
The pathway to ischaemia and ulceration.

– Directly, *via* vascular pathology. Macrovascular disease results in atherosclerosis as well as stenosis and therefore a limitation of the blood flow to the affected limb. The incidence of peripheral vascular disease is substantially increased in patients with foot ulcers. In areas lacking adequate collateral circulation such as the toes, the risk of ischaemia is increased. This risk is aggravated in patients with neuropathy because of their greater predisposition to trauma. Most foot ulcers occur at the level of the toes. Microvascular dysfunction is also affected in diabetes mellitus. This manifests as increased membrane thickness and permeability as well as diminished vessel reactivity. Sympathetic nerve activity may also contribute to microvascular function by diminishing endothelial reactivity. Thus, although there is no microvascular occlusive disease as a number of authors aver, there is a functional disorder that results in diminished tissue blood supply.

– Trauma, infection and trophic changes can compound the ischaemic process thus resulting in necrosis and ulcers.

The pathogenesis of ischaemic foot ulcers is summarized in Figure 42.1.

CONCLUSIONS

Foot ulcers are a dreaded complication of diabetes mellitus since they frequently lead to amputation, sepsis and increased mortality. In the United States of America, the costs of care for patients with diabetic foot ulcers have been found to be three times greater ($15,309 *vs.* $5,226) than for the general population of patients [32]. The total cost of care for patients with foot ulcers was found to be about $1.5 billion. The figures for Romania are not known but it is clear from the foregoing that foot ulcers are a source of major economic burden.

The majority of foot ulcers in our study are neuropathic and experience shows that, excluding aggravating factors such as infection, these ulcers will heal. However, when complicated by ischaemia or infection, the prognosis becomes graver.

Our experience also shows that 30.4% of foot ulcers are ischaemic and neuroischaemic. The pathogenesis of ischaemia is indirect and direct.

The indirect pathway is *via* sympathetic damage that increases vessel stiffness and leads to sclerosis. This rigidity diminishes the capacity of the circulation to expand to accommodate increased blood flow requirements in times of greater demand. Sympathetic damage also causes increased arteriovenous shunting which, although resulting in increased total foot blood flow, may cause reduction in capillary flow and hence tissue ischemia. The ischaemia is aggravated by the oedema that occurs as a result of the increased foot blood flow, capillary pressure and basement membrane dysfunction.

Direct factors include atherosclerosis and large vessel stenosis that cause reduction in blood flow and microvascular dysfunction in the form of decreased microvascular reactivity especially when there is poor glycemic control. Sympathetic nerve dysfunction may also reduce microvascular reactivity.

Trauma is an associated factor that aggravates foot ulcers and adversely affects prognosis. Our study showed that 76% of foot ulcers are present at the level of the toes, which are highly prone to trauma. Also, 85.7% of multiple ulcers were located at the level of the toes. These ulcers are frequently located at the lateral aspects of the toes where the neurovascular bundle is to be found. The toes are lacking in collateral circulation therefore, the increased risk of trauma, together with the compromise of the circulation against the background of ischemic change already elucidated above, predispose these ulcers to the development of gangrene.

In our study, we found that 15.2% of foot ulcers were associated with infection. Infection may compromise the blood circulation by the release of vasotoxic factors that lead to intravascular coagulation and tissue necrosis.

All foot ulcers must be treated aggressively as they can very easily lead to gangrene and therefore to amputation. The management of every ulcer must take into consideration the state of the peripheral circulation as this is vital to the promotion of healing and to the avoidance of gangrene. Every effort must therefore be made to eliminate or to treat the factors discussed above, which contribute to ischemia.

Bearing in mind the high cost of foot ulcer care as well as the risk of amputation, prevention is a much better option. Thus, education is important in foot care. In Bucharest, we have begun the first comprehensive programme in Romania specially designed for the education of patients with diabetes with regard to foot disorders. In this programme, patients are taught basic foot care, the recognition of signs and symptoms of neuropathy, arteriopathy, infection and trauma as well as how to cater for their feet. At the same time, regular education is carried out as part of every patient consultation. It is hoped that this will diminish the frequency of foot ulcers as well as impact positively on the morbidity, mortality and quality of life of diabetic patients. The consequence of this would be to reduce the costs of diabetes care as well as to improve the quality of life of these patients.

REFERENCES

1. Nwabudike LC, Ionescu-Tîrgoviște C, Forsea D, Anghel V. Dermatoses encountered in diabetes. *Acta Diabetologica Romana*, **25**: 136–137, 1999.

2. Nwabudike LC, Ionescu-Tîrgoviște C, Coravu D, Văcaru G. The cutaneous manifestations of diabetic neuropathy. *Jurnalul Român de Diabet, Nutriție și Boli Metabolice*, **8**: 27–30, 2001.

3. Faglia E, Faales F, Morabito A. New ulceration, new major amputation and survival rates in diabetic subjects hospitalized for foot ulceration from 1990–1993. A 6.5-year follow-up. *Diabetes Care*, **24**: 78–83, 2001.

4. Vereanu I, Pătrașcu T. The diabetic foot. Vasculopathy *vs.* Neuropathy. In Cheța: D (ed). *Vascular Involvement in Diabetes: Clinical, Experimental and Beyond.* Ed. Academiei Române.

5. Nwabudike LC, Ionescu-Tîrgoviște C. Clinical characteristics of patients with foot ulcers and diabetes mellitus. *Diabetes Metab*, **29**: 4S289, 2003.

6. Boulton AJM. The diabetic foot: Neuropathic in aetiology? *Diabetic Med*, **7**: 852–858, 1990.

7. Goebel F-D, Füessl HS. Mönckeberg's sclerosis after sympathetic nerve denervation in diabetic and nondiabetic subjects. *Diabetologia*, **24**: 347–350, 1983.

8. Chantelau E, Ma XY, Herrnberger S, Dohmen C, Trappe P, Baba T. Effect of medial arterial calcification on O_2 supply to exercising diabetic feet. *Diabetes*, **39**: 938–941, 1990.

9. Suzuki E, Kashiwagi A, Yoshihiko N, Egawa K, Shimizu S, Maegawa H, Haneda M, Yasuda H, Morikawa S, Inubushi T, Kikkawa R. Increased arterial wall stiffness limits flow volume in the lower extremities in type 2 diabetic patients. *Diabetes Care*, **24**: 2107–2114, 2001.

10. Edmonds ME. The neuropathic foot in diabetes. Part 1: Blood flow. *Diabetic Med*, **3**: 111–115, 1986.

11. Watkins PJ, Edmonds ME. Sympathetic nerve failure in diabetes. *Diabetologia*, **25**: 73–77, 1983.

12. Netten PM, Wollersheim H, Gielen MJ, Den Arend JA, Lutterman JA, Thien T. The influence of ulnar nerve blockade on skin microvascular blood flow. *Eur J Clin Invest*, **25**: 515–522, 1995.

13. Uccioli L, Mancini L, Giordano A, Solini A, Magnani P, Manto A, Cotroneo P, Greco AV, Ghirlanda G. Lower limb arterio-venous shunts, autonomic neuropathy and diabetic foot. *Diabetes Res Clin Pract*, **16**: 123–130, 1992.

14. Nabuurs-Franssen MH, Houben AJHM, Tooke JE, Schaper NC. The effect of polyneuropathy on foot microcirculation in type 2 diabetes. *Diabetologia*, **45**: 1164–1171, 2002.

15. Colberg SR, Parson HK, Holton RD, Nunnold T, Vinick AI. Cutaneous blood flow in type 2 diabetic individuals after an acute bout of maximal exercise. *Diabetes Care*, **26**: 1883–1888, 2003.

16. Rendel M, Bamisedun O. Diabetic cutaneous microangiopathy. *Am J Med*, **93**: 611–618, 1992.

17. Melton LJ, Macken KM, Palumbo PJ, Elveback LR. Incidence and prevalence of peripheral vascular disease in a population based cohort of diabetic patients. *Diabetes Care*, **3**: 650–654, 1980.

18. Ramsey SD, Newton K, Blough D, McCulloch DK, Sandhu N, Reiber GE, Wagner EH. Incidence, outcomes and cost of foot ulcers in patients with diabetes. *Diabetes Care*, **22**: 382–387, 1999.

19. Kalani M, Brismar K, Fagrell B, Östergren J, Jörneskog G. Transcutaneous oxygen tension and toe blood pressure as predictors for outcome of diabetic foot ulcers. *Diabetes Care*, **22**: 147–151, 1999.

20. Kessler L, Bilbault P, Ortega F, Grasso C, Passemard R, Stephan D, Pinget Michel, Schneider F. Hyperbaric oxygenation accelerates the healing rate of nonischemic chronic diabetic foot ulcers: a prospective randomized study. *Diabetes Care*, **26**: 2378–2382, 2003.

21. Apelqvist J, Castenfors J, Larsson J, Stenstrom A, Agardh CD. Prognostic value of ankle and toe blood pressure levels in outcome of diabetic foot ulcers. *Diabetes Care*, **12**: 373–378, 1989.

22. Faglia E, Favales F, Quarantiello A, Calia P, Clelia P, Brambilla G, Rampoldi A, Morabito A. Angiographic evaluation of peripheral arterial occlusive disease and its role as a prognostic determinant for major amputation in diabetic subjects with foot ulcers. *Diabetes Care*, **21**: 625–630, 1998.

23. Malik RA, Metcalfe J, Sharma AK, Day JL, Rayman G. Skin epidermal thickness and vascular density in type 1 diabetes. *Diabetes Med,* **9:** 263–267, 1992.

24. Yue DK, Mclennan SV, Turtle JR. Pathogenesis of diabetic microangiopathy: The roles of endothelial cell and basement membrane abnormalities. *Diabetic Med,* **9:** 218–220, 1992.

25. Boulton AJM, Roberts VC, Watkins PJ. Blood flow patterns in painful diabetic neuropathy. *Diabetologia,* **27:** 563–567, 1984.

26. Hamdy O, Abou-Elenin K, LoGerfo FW, Horton ES, Veves A. Contribution of nerve-axon reflex-related vasodilation to the total skin vasodilation in diabetic patients with and without neuropathy. *Diabetes Care,* **24:** 344–349, 2001.

27. Kilo S, Berghoff M, Hilz M, Freeman R. Neural and endothelial control of the microcirculation in diabetic peripheral neuropathy. *Neurology,* **54:** 1246–1256, 2000.

28. Caballero AE, Arora S, Saouaf R, Lim SC, Smakowski P, Park YJ, King GL, LoGerfo FW, Horton ES, Veves A. Microvascular and macrovascular reactivity is reduced in subjects at risk for type 2 diabetes. *Diabetes,* **48:** 1856–1862, 1999.

29. Kingwell BA, Formosa M, Muhlmann M, Bradley JS, McConell GK. Type 2 diabetic individuals have impaired leg blood flow responses to exercise. Role of endothelium-dependent vasodilation. *Diabetes Care,* **26:** 899–904, 2003.

30. Jorneskog G, Brismar K, Fagrell B. Pronounced skin capillary ischemia in the feet of diabetic patients with bad metabolic control. *Diabetologia,* **41**: 410–415, 1998.

31. Arora S, Smakowski P, Frykberg RG, Simeone LR, Freeman R, LoGerfo FW, Veves A. Differences in foot and forearm skin microcirculation in diabetic patients with and without neuropathy. *Diabetes Care,* **21:** 1393–1344, 1998.

32. Harrington C, Zagary MJ, Corea J, Klitenic J. A cost analysis of diabetic lower-extremity ulcers. *Diabetes Care,* **23:** 1333–1338, 2000.

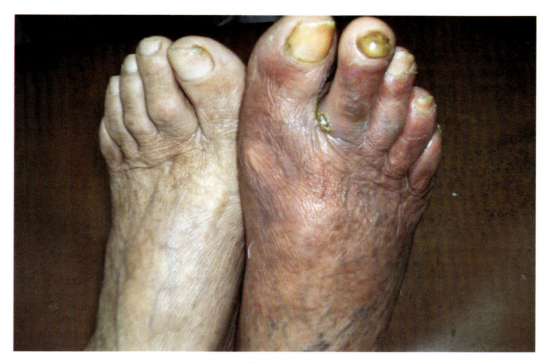

Plate 42.1

Ischaemic foot.

Note the small ulcer with necrotic base at the base of the right second toe. The ischaemia of that foot is a marked contrast to the left foot. This is not an uncommon sight in diabetes foot care.

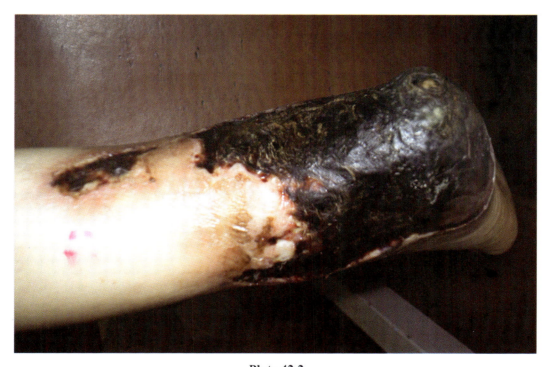

Plate 42.2

Necrotic heel ulcer.

Extensive heel and lower leg gangrene. This often begins as a minor fissure in the heel that becomes infected and, in this case compounded by inadequate care.

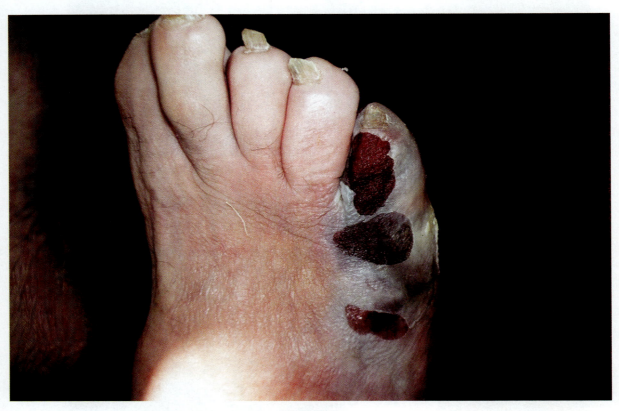

Plate 42.3
Gangrene of the toe and lateral foot.
Toe and lateral foot gangrene resulting, in this case, from an ulcer on the plantar surface of the foot that became infected leading to thrombosis and gangrene.

43

THE DIABETIC FOOT –
VASCULOPATHY *VERSUS* NEUROPATHY

Ion VEREANU, Traian PĂTRAȘCU

The diabetic foot is a severe complication of diabetes mellitus usually invalidating and relatively frequent in occurrence (15%). The complex pathogenesis of this complication explains the extremely varied character of this disorder, bringing about a wide range of surgical interventions. This material is a comparative analysis of the lesions resulting from diabetic vasculopathy and neuropathy with its implications for the definition of their clinical features and for the choice of adequate surgical treatment.

The study comprises a group of 200 patients with surgical complications of the diabetic foot admitted into the department of surgery of the Cantacuzino Hospital in the year 2001. The assessment of the pathogenic factors in causation was made on the basis of clinical examination and of clinical studies such as Doppler echography and oscillometry. The ischaemic component is present in quite many cases (over 60% predominantly arteriopathic or mixed). In the context of the clinical picture it is obvious that gangrene is more common in the ischaemic foot (71%) compared to the neuropathic foot (14%). The analysis of the lesions operated upon indicates a wide range of interventions in both pathogenic lesions but the prevalence of major amputations is more obvious in the ischaemic foot.

The post-operative course was favourable in 80–90% of cases in all-pathogenic types; treatment failures (successive amputations) predominated in cases with vasculopathy. Long term specialized supervision of all patients operated upon for diabetic foot lesions is necessary in order to achieve early diagnosis of possible postoperative complications requiring a sub-segment operation.

The diabetic foot is defined as the totality of the morphologic and functional changes occurring at the level of the foot in diabetes mellitus. It is a frequently encountered complication of this disease and its incidence has been clearly on the rise in the past decades.

It is thought that about 15% of patients develop lesions at the level of the foot and these are a frequent cause of hospital admissions for the diabetic patient. The raised costs of treatment are compounded by the invalidating character of this complication. The hazzard of amputation is thought to be 15 times greater in diabetic patients than the rest of the population and 50% of all nontraumatic amputations are due to the diabetic foot [1, 2].

The large number of cases seen in the Surgical Clinic of the Dr. I. Cantacuzino Hospital (350–450/year) is for the most part due to the close collaboration between this department and the specialised centers in Bucharest, namely "N. Paulescu" Institute of Diabetes, Nutrition and Metabolic Diseases and The Clinic of Diabetes, Nutrition and Metabolic Diseases at the Malaxa Hospital. The high frequency of diabetic foot cases that have become surgical, and particularly the high proportion of cases that require amputation leading thus to physical and social impairment, suggests the existence in the countryside of significant deficiencies in prevention as well as treatment of early lesions of the diabetic foot.

The great variety of surgical lesions of the diabetic foot is responsible for a wide range of surgical interventions ranging from simple drainage incisions of purulent collections to major amputations (leg and thigh). This fact is due to the complex pathogenesis of this disease, the predominance or the association, to different degrees, of the essential pathogenic factors of vasculopathy and neuropathy, combined with sepsis. For this reason, we thought it useful in this study to achieve a comparative analysis of lesions of vasculopathy and diabetic neuropathy and the implications for the definition of the clinical picture as well as for the choice of the adequate and optimum approach to treatment.

METHOD AND CLINICAL MATERIAL

We carried out a retrospective study of 200 patients with surgical complications of the diabetic foot admitted to the surgical department of Dr. I. Cantacuzino Hospital during the year 2001. The cases were recorded in the order in which the surgical interventions were carried out.

The assessment of the roles of the pathogenic factors in each case was carried out on the basis of clinical examination (very suggestive in the advanced stage of the lesions), of oscillometry (segmental measurement of the degree of pulsation of lower limb arteries), of Doppler echography and rarely of arteriography.

In the group under study, most cases were the result of the predominantly ischaemic diabetic foot – vasculopathy/arteriopathy (41%) – followed by the diabetic foot predominated by neuropathy (36%) and the mixed diabetic foot (23%). We use the terms predominantly ischaemic and predominantly neuropathic because, on the one hand, the methods available to us do not permit an exact delineation of the involvement of these factors and, on the other hand, there is a close association even if one of them participates to a smaller extent.

The gender distribution of predominantly ischaemic and mixed type of the diabetic foot was relatively equal as opposed to the neuropathic foot that showed a high male predominance (73%) (Figure 43.1).

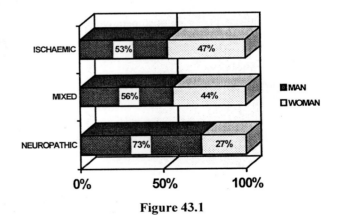

Figure 43.1

Sex distribution.

The age distribution shows major differences between the different pathogenic types. Most patients (86%) with ischaemic diabetic foot were over 60 years of age while most with predominantly neuropathic foot (75.5%), were below 60 years (Table 43.1).

Table 43.1

Age distribution

	Neuropathic	Mixed	Ischaemic
Below 40 yrs.	5.5%	2%	1.2%
41–60 yrs.	73%	39%	17%
61–70 yrs.	26%	41%	53%
Above 70 yrs.	4.4%	18%	47%

With regard to the type of diabetes, we noted a predominance of type II, representing approximately 3/4 of cases; this was the case for all the pathogenic types of diabetic foot (Figure 43.2).

The patients in the study group generally have a long history of diabetes (for all pathogenic categories): over half of them have a history of diabetes stretching beyond 10 years (Table 43.2). However, the predominantly ischaemic patient group, shows a slight superiority (22% compared to 15%) of recently diagnosed diabetes < 1 year.

At the time of admission, the majority of patients had already undergone surgery for complications at the level of their feet especially

in the neuropathic group (52.7% / 39%) (see Figure 43.3).

Table 43.2

Duration of diabetes

	Neuropathy	Mixed	Ischaemic
Below 1 yr.	15.2%	8.6%	22%
2–10 yrs	33.3%	34.7%	22%
Above 10 yrs	51.5%	56.7%	56%

Although various types of surgical lesions may be encountered in all pathologic forms of the diabetic foot, it is evident that gangrene of ischaemic origin (71%) predominates over neuropathic gangrene (14%) (Table 43.3).

A wide range of surgical interventions were carried out in both pathogenic forms but with significant differences in the sense of an obvious prevalence of major amputations in the ischaemic foot where their frequency was 10 times greater than in the neuropathic foot (Table 43.4). Surgical treatment has been accompanied by antibiotic treatment and metabolic control in all cases.

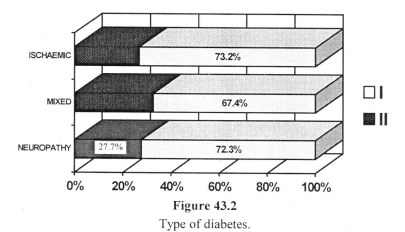

Figure 43.2

Type of diabetes.

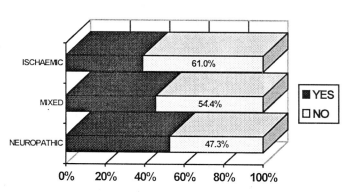

Figure 43.3

Previous surgery.

Table 43.3

Lesions of the diabetic foot

			Neuropathic	Mixed	Ischaemic
Gangrene	*Localised*	Dry	–	6%	14%
		Wet	3%	39%	30%
	Extensive		11%	9%	35%
Suppuration	*Abscess*		23%	10%	8%
	Inflammatory swellings		–	–	–
	Fasceitis		–	–	–
Mal perforans			14%	9%	–
Osteitis, osteoarthritis, suppuration			21%	24%	8%
Other lesions			6%	3%	5%

Table 43.4

Types of surgical intervention

	Neuropathic	Mixed	Ischaemia
Amputation of phalanges	3%	5%	7%
Wedge amputation	46%	62%	25%
Transmetatarsian amputation	20%	12%	8%
Tarsometatarsian amputation	0	0	0
Resection of metatarsophalangean joints	5%	0	0
Incisions, necrectomies etc.	20%	21%	7%
Leg amputation	5%	0	11%
Thigh amputation	1%	0	42%

RESULTS

The immediate post-operative course was favourable in 80–90% of the cases in all pathogenic groups (Figure 43.4). Cases that required a follow-up operation were considered treatment failures and required frequently successive amputations at higher levels than the first operation; in this category there is a predominance of cases with vascular specificity.

Two deaths were recorded (1%) inpatients over 65% years, with organic complications and organic failure generally associated with advanced septic lesions.

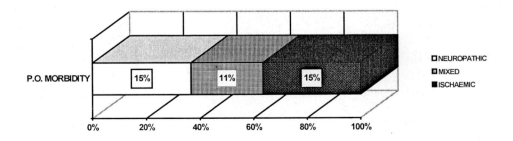

Figure 43.4

Results of surgical treatment.

DISCUSSION

Knowledge of the pathogenesis of the diabetic foot is essential for understanding the variety of its clinical forms as well as the adequate therapy, which may be different for choosing in individual cases.

Long-term hyperglycaemia is thought to be the principal pathogenic factor in all-specific complications of diabetes mellitus. The effects of this disorder occur through several abnormal metabolic pathways whose products are the essential causes of the vascular and neurologic lesions [3, 4].

According to data from the literature, ischaemia is a determining factor in 15% and an associated factor in 20–40% of cases [2, 5]. Our own statistical data are obviously much more substantial: 41% as a determining, and 21% as an associated factor thus emphasising the pathogenic importance of the ischaemic element. The high incidence of vascular involvement in our series could be explained by the large number of patients of advanced age in which there is a significant increase in the incidence of vascular disorders.

Diabetic macroangiopathy is an atherosclerotic angiopathy morphologically similar to that of normoglycaemic individuals thus differing, however, in the raised incidence, younger age of occurrence and higher rate of complications.

A distinctive element is also the preferential location of aterosclerosis in diabetic patients at the level of the leg arteries, *i.e.* the tibial and peroneal arteries. Not infrequently the proximal arteries (ilio-femoral) and the distal ones (leg arteries at the level of the ankle and the dorsal foot arteries) are free of disease or affected to a much smaller degree by the process of aterosclerosis and this fact is frequently used in vascular reconstruction. The development of aterosclerosis distal to the knee favours the development of collateral vessels around it. These peculiarities explain the frequent absence of intermittent claudication in these patients as the thigh muscles are more affected by obstruction of thigh vessels in comparison with those at the level of the leg. Co-existing peripheral neuropathy with diminished pain sensitivity compounds this.

Aside from the process of aterosclerosis affecting the vascular intima, which is frequent in diabetic patients, there is also involvement of the tunica media, which though not an obstructive phenomenon, interferes with the oxygenation of tissues through the limitation of the elasticity of the vessel walls.

Although macroangiopathy is the dominant ischaemic element in the diabetic foot, microangiopathy, which has capillary basement membrane thickening as a morphologic change (non-obstructive lesion) influencing the functions of transfer through the capillary wall, is significant.

In addition to these circulatory changes, the diabetic patient is frequently subjected to hypercoagulability and increased blood viscosity secondary to many factors such as increased levels of fibrinogen, platelet hyperactivity, diminished fibrinolysis, increase in von Willebrand factor levels and increased erythrocyte membrane rigidity (hyperglycaemic glycosylation).

The presence of any factors mentioned above could determine the diminution of the blood flow to the tissues [6, 7].

Diabetic neuropathy in the lower limbs is usually bilateral and symmetrical. This form of lesion, also known as diffuse neuropathy, is due to vascular structural and metabolic changes. In contrast to this kind of neuropathy, which is diffuse, symmetric and progressive, there also exists a focal neuropathy that occurs in clearly defined areas (asymmetric and localised) secondary to an acute ischaemic episode or a localised phenomenon due to neural compression.

Diabetic neuropathy (diffuse form) is thought to be present in generally 60–65% of the diabetic population and responsible for lesions of the diabetic foot in 60% of cases [3, 8]. In our statistics, the neuropathic factor was present in almost 60% of cases. Somatic, motor and sensory fibres as well as those of the autonomic nervous system are affected.

Motor neuropathy results in muscle atrophy and thus affects the intrinsic muscles of the leg (lumbricals and others) especially. The direct effects of these changes are an imbalance between muscle groups of the leg with the occurrence of hammer toes (medial flexion of the toes), and sole deformities leading to changes in the plantar pressure points. The striking result of this process is the development of a severe degenerative neuropathy with a complete change of the architecture of the foot designated as the Charcot foot (disintegration of the tarso-metatarsian joints, inversion of the arch of the foot and plantar pressure ulcers).

Sensory neuropathy involving the fibres responsible for the perception of pain, temperature, and pressure stimuli, could paradoxically produce the sensation of pain and paraesthesia. This hampers the correct diagnosis of the origin of the pain in the diabetic foot. It is also felt that sensory neuropathy is responsible for the diminution of the neuroinflammatory reaction as an important mechanism of protection against infections.

Autonomic neuropathy has as consequences a diminished sole blood flow *via* increase in arterio-venous shunts and diminished sweat function with hypohidrosis. It results a hypovascular foot with dry skin that is sensitive to microtrauma and infection as a consequence.

To these two essential pathogenic factors of the diabetic foot is added *infection* associated with significant long-term morbidity necessitating, not infrequently, surgical intervention, which is frequently mutilating.

The frequency of infections in the context of the diabetic foot is high. It is thought that 25% of patients with diabetes mellitus will develop a foot ulcer that is infected in 40–80% of cases, being the most frequent cause of hospitalisation in diabetic patients in the USA [9]. The infection must be approached with the utmost seriousness because its prognosis is reserved – a proportion ranging from 25–50% undergo distal amputation while a proportion of 10–40% undergo proximal amputations [10].

The increased frequency of these infections in the context of the diabetic foot has a series of causes amongst which are: skin changes secondary to vasculopathy and neuropathy, the compartmented anatomic structure of the foot contributing to rapid compression and ischaemia following infection, the presence of some immunologic deficits as well as a reduced capacity to heal.

The determination of the microbial population in a wound developed in the diabetic foot is usually difficult to interpret in the sense of the real pathogenic cause as these wounds could be contaminated by normal cutaneous flora that has no significant relationship to the disease. Generally, it is thought those monomicrobial infections, especially with gram-positive microbes characterise acute lesions of recent onset while chronic wounds have a complex aerobic and anaerobic gram-positive and gram-negative flora [11].

The obtaining of samples for bacteriologic examination must be done from the depths of the wounds under strict aseptic conditions in order to avoid false-positive cultures resulting from skin contamination (insignificant organisms).

Not infrequently, infections affect bony structures as a result of contiguity. In severe infections, profound osteomyelitis is present in 50–60% of cases and, in the milder cases, 10–20%. It is thought that ulcers 2 cm in diameter or greater and 3–5 mm deep or more are associated with contiguous osteomyelitis. Bacteriologic examination by bone biopsy shows, in these cases, a multibacterial infection in which *Staphylococcus aureus* can be found in about 40% of cases, *Staphylococcus epidermidis* in 25%, *streptococcus* 30% and *enterobacteria* 40% [11, 12].

Clinical diagnosis suggests which pathogenic element participates in the pathogenesis of each case. The diminution or absence of the pulse, cutaneous changes (stretched, shiny skin, modification of colour with change of position) the frequent presence of onychomycosis, muscle atrophy and pain indicate ischaemia while changes in sensitivity are major clinical elements in favour of the neuropathic foot. The fact that pathogenic factors are associated in variable proportions explains the large range of clinical forms as well as the lack of absolute specificity connected with these forms.

Gangrene in its different forms, localised or extensive, "dry" or "wet", constitutes, as is to be expected, the dominant lesion for the predominantly ischaemic (79%) and mixed (54%) diabetic foot.

It also occurs in the predominantly neuropathic foot. This is due to a participation of the vasculature and these results, mainly, from thrombosis in the proximity of some septic foci, while the compartment of anatomy of the foot favours this mechanism through compression.

Suppuration is thrice as frequent in the predominantly neuropathic foot (23% compared to 8%). It can affect the toes or the foot involving the plantar spaces or the dorsum of the foot. The triggering factor passes usually unnoticed, just as the onset of the infection due to the underlying neuropathy; fever and chills dominate, especially in infections of the mid-plantar space associated with metabolic imbalance (hyperglycaemia) that fails to respond to the usual medication. Local signs of infection (swelling, oedema, redness and pain) could be present but most times they are attenuated and not very suggestive for the unexperienced observer. The opening of such suppuration frequently exposes underlying extensive necrosis of the plantar fascia.

Aside from these forms of plantar infection associated with suppuration, inflammatory swellings of the dorsum of the foot may be encountered. These are true nonsuppurating cellulitis with an unfavourable course on the background of diabetes, resulting from cutaneous necrosis secondary to thrombosis of the skin vessels involved in inflammation.

Mal perforans is a chronic foot ulcer surrounded by hyperkeratosis. It is painless and appears in an area of maximum pressure, usually corresponding to the distal extremities of the metatarsal bones. This is a lesion encountered in the neuropathic foot (14%) or in the mixed foot (9%). It must be differentiated from ischaemic ulcers with varying locations but especially over bony prominences that are usually in contact with the footwear and it is superficial and painful. The lesions affect the soft tissues producing hyperkeratosis and ulcers, but could also affect the bone leading to osteoporosis, osteolysis and osteoarthritis. All the components of diabetic neuropathy contribute to the occurrence of this lesion (Figure 43.5).

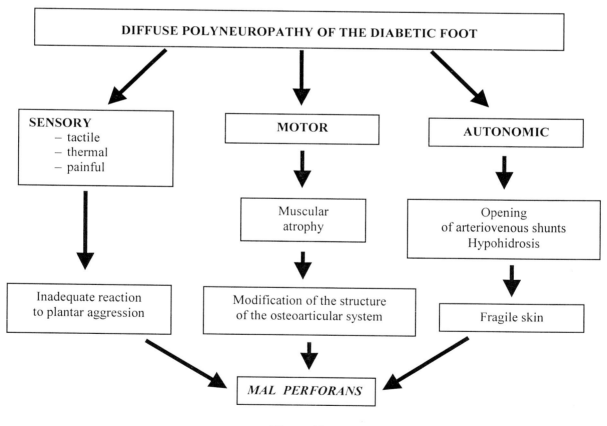

Figure 43.5
The pathogenesis of *mal perforans*.

Cases characterised by *involvement of the osteoarticular system* of the foot are not rare. The degree of involvement is variable and can sometimes lead to true destruction and disorganisation of the skeleton of the foot. Without doubt, bony lesions are caused by extension from a suppuration of the soft tissues but there are frequently cases when this method of propagation is not obvious. These bony lesions are almost thrice as frequent in the predominantly neuropathic diabetic foot.

The nonclinical tests are essential for the pathogenic diagnosis of the diabetic foot. It must include objective methods for the documentation of diabetic neuropathy as well as a series of noninvasive tests of the circulation of the lower limbs such as segmental blood pressure measurements taken at different levels including at the hallux with the use of a pulsatile Doppler listening device (when the pulse is not perceptible), digital photoplethysmography, B-mode ultrasound for the study of the morphology of the vessels as well as Doppler (Duplex) studies for blood vessel flow to which have been added, in recent times, techniques perfected by computerised tomography (spinal CT) or angiography using magnetic resonance. Angiography using contrast is considered the "gold standard", but is reserved for cases that must undergo vascular intervention because of the risks connected with its utilisation. The current level of equipment of general surgical services does not permit the frequent use of these procedures. Vascular evaluation is carried out most frequently by clinical examination, oscillometry and, in recent times, by Doppler ultrasound.

The distribution by sex and age-group shows the significant differences between categories of patients with lesions of the diabetic foot; the predominantly neuropathic foot appears usually in men before the age of 60 while the predominantly ischaemic foot occurs in equal proportions in both sexes and is characterised by an average age of over 70 years.

In most cases, the diabetic foot is a late complication in the course of diabetes mellitus. From our statistics, it can be seen that an appreciable number of cases (15–20%), sometimes presenting with severe lesions requiring mutilating surgery, occur within the first year of the development of the disease. The lack of thorough control of the disease and lack of sanitary education are also significant in explaining the fact that the overwhelming majority of cases of the diabetic foot with complications of a surgical nature (> 70%) occur in patients with type 2 diabetes. More frequent contact of type 1 diabetic patients with specialised centres probably allow for the timely and useful observation of the appearance of complications.

The frequency of preceding operations in the study group, greater in the neuropathic (53%) than in the ischaemic (39%) foot, demonstrates the progressive nature of the underlying disease; surgery in the context of the diabetic foot is nothing more than a consequence of the stage of progression.

The treatment of complications brought on by the diabetic foot is complex and presupposes a multidisciplinary approach in order to obtain good and lasting results with the reduction of the rate of lesion recurrence. This work, in the main part, concerns the contribution of the general surgeon regarding this pathology and also recalls the intervention of other therapeutic factors.

The statistics presented show that in the survey group the majority of surgical interventions are amputations and only a small number of cases benefit from conservative treatment (drainage incisions and limited excision of necrotic tissue). This fact is due to the advanced stage of lesions as a result of late presentation to the specialist. The major objective of surgery is to excise the lesions (or amputation) in order to obtain, by surgery, as little mutilation as possible. This is why the establishment of the level of amputation is essential and there are, at present, numerous attempts estimating the chances of success of every level of amputation. In the surgical clinic of the Dr. I. Cantacuzino Hospital, a prognostic index has been realised (T. Pătrașcu) that constitutes a valid guide for the assessment of chances of success that a distal amputation might have in a given situation [13]. Thus, repeated, serial amputations that are traumatic for the patient and also increase the cost of hospitalisation are avoided. The validity index of this score is 93%. A critical look at the factors included in this score leads us to believe that the replacement of oscillometry with more modern methods of evaluating the blood flow could greatly improve the validity of the score.

Irrespective of the level, the amputation technique must respect the classic principles accepted of the best possible functionality of the stump. This is unfortunately not always possible because, in the case of the diabetic foot, the major factors that must be borne in mind are the circulatory, septic and tissue factors. For these reasons, in the places of election for different levels of amputation, some amputation techniques, such as the flap, are inadequate for the diabetic foot. Thus, aside from ischaemic factors that "raise" the level of amputation, septic factors may oblige, in the first instance to a distal amputation with an open stump (as non-mutilating as possible), followed by the elimination of the pus and after that the covering of the stump.

As can be seen from Figure 43.7, especially in the predominantly neuropathic foot, distal amputations are most frequently practiced. In this context, our most frequent option is for "wedge" amputations that take the digit together with a part of the metatarsal bone. In order to modify the dynamics of the foot as little as possible, the site of transmetatarsal sectioning should be as distal as possible especially for the first toe (thus preserving the medial arch of the foot). In the case of resection of multiple digits, the preservation of the length and form of the foot are indicated, thus the successive resection of metatarsal bones is done as distally as possible. We do not recommend the preservation of the outermost digits (I&V) because of the very poor functional outcome. In these cases, the fifth metatarsal is not conserved but the first can be (with easier prosthesis).

We utilised toe amputations less frequently (37%). These amputations are always transdiaphysean and do not preserve the heads of the joints for good healing. When amputation of the second digit is necessary, a wedge amputation that brings together metatarsals I and II are carried out preventing this deformity.

Of the amputations leading to a shortening of the length of the foot, we used transmetatarsial amputations in 8–20% of cases. For good postoperative function, the orientation of the amputation must respect an oblique line (15°)

increasing progressively towards the hallux and the coverage of the stump must be carried out mainly with the plantar skin that is much thicker and better vascularised.

We lay special emphasis on interventions on the osteoarticular system of the metatarso-phalangeal joints in the presence of *mal perforans*, a lesion characteristic of a neuropathic pathogenesis. These operations are related to cases of *mal perforans* resistant to known methods of medical treatment and consist in either resection of the head of the corresponding metatarsal bones or in the resection of the metatarsophalangeal joints in the presence of supurative osteoarthritis. In order to suppress the maximum point of pressure corresponding to the metatarsal head, where there is no bone lesion, it is possible to carry out a simple diaphyseal osteotomy at the level of the corresponding metatarsal bone. The results obtained in these cases are very good with rapid healing of the *mal perforans*. Recurrence of these lesions is prevented by recommending the patient to a specialised service for shoe soles as well as for orthopaedic boots to accommodate the change in plantar pressure points.

As can be seen from our experience, the majority of major or proximal amputations have been carried out in the presence of the diabetic foot with a strong vascular component (53% compared to 6%). The very occasional case where thigh amputation is practised in the context of the predominantly neuropathic foot is due to the widespread nature of the septic factor.

Every time there is a possibility of choice, we prefer leg amputations to thigh amputations, as prosthesis is easier to achieve. Even with 0 oscillometry below the knee we prefer this level because there is a network of communicating vessels around the knee, that ensures blood circulation proximal to the leg and this is not detected by oscillometry. Bearing in mind the existence of the vascular factors, we opt, in leg amputation, for the technique of circular amputation without flaps and in this manner obtain satisfactory results. With regard to the level of amputation, this is higher in comparison with "elective amputation" as the principal objective is the preservation of the insertion for the quadriceps on the anterior tubercle of the tibia for extension and those of the biceps femoralis and semimembranosus for flexion. These conditions are met when the section passes at 8–10 cm distal to the tibial tubercle.

Thigh amputation, an intervention practised almost exclusively for the predominantly ischaemic diabetic foot, presents difficulties with regard to prosthesis, requiring a great deal of physical effort on the part of the patient with multiple disorders and advanced age. It is thought that only 1/4 of patients with thigh amputations will be capable of utilising the corresponding prosthesis [14].

The septic factor is another element that must be borne in mind in the treatment of lesions of the diabetic foot. Timely surgical intervention, wide opening and excision of the compromised tissues, leaving the wound open, at least in the first instance, are the basic principles of treatment of this type of lesion. Special attention must be accorded to the correct diagnosis of the suppuration in order to seek the sources of the expansion that may be less noisy and that may progress on their own if not treated. We have sometimes found in suppurative lesions of the foot with significant destruction of the leg that during the amputation procedure there are high tracts that oblige that the stump be left open.

The presence in the context of these suppurations of necrotising fasciitis obliges dissection to the point of finding healthy tissue no matter at what level the suppuration is found. Failure to observe this rule prolongs and sometimes compromises the healing that could be obtained at the cost of a more ample operation.

Progress in the treatment of open wounds that are a result of suppuration is the use of diverse types of dressings that have moist agents as their basis. These encourage the absorption of detritus and of germs, stimulating, at the same time, as a result of the ions that they offer, the granulation of these wounds, thus clearly shortening the healing time.

Antibiotic treatment is an essential component associated with surgery in the treatment of infectious complications of the diabetic foot. In mild infections most frequently caused by gram-positive organisms (especially *Staphylococcus* and *Streptococcus*), specific antibiotic therapy may be utilised such as semisynthetic penicillins, 1st generation cephalosporins and fluoroquinolones.

In severe infections that are usually long-standing with a history of prior antibiotic therapy, the microbial flora is mixed (aerobes and anaerobes) and therapy should be broad spectrum. In polymicrobial infections, 2nd, 3rd and 4th generation cephalosporins, fluoroquinolones with clindamycin, metronidazole or carbapenem may be used.

The antibiotic therapy can be maintained or modified on the basis of the results of the culture as well as response to treatment.

The duration of treatment is variable and related to the gravity of the infection (usually 7–14 days in mild cases and 2–4 weeks in severe ones).

The route of administration is parenteral for severe infections and oral for milder infections without systemic effects.

In the presence of osteomyelitis the parenteral route is mandatory for a long period of time (4–6 weeks). Treatment is carried out on the basis of cultures obtained by biopsies of bone fragments from the osteomyelitic focus. Chronic osteomyelitis obliges the excision of the infected bone. *Staphylococcus aureus* is very frequently found in bone cultures from these infections. Fluoroquinolones and clindamycin are very active in the treatment of osteomyelitis and are considered the latest therapies.

Aside from surgical and antibiotic treatment, proper management of the underlying diabetes is essential. The significant number of cases that are admitted with metabolic imbalance is great even though the patients come from a specialised centre [15]. This can be explained by the lack of response to hypoglycaemic medication due to the presence of sepsis. This resistance to treatment disappears after correct surgical drainage. The drainage may comprise the first step in the surgical treatment and allows the assessment of the lesions as well as the limitation of the tissue-destroying factors and it is then followed by adequate surgical therapy of the remaining lesions.

Vascular factors, with their implications, are a frequently encountered element of the patient with diabetes. Thus, the incidence of vascular disease is 15% at 10 years and 45% at 20 years from the diagnosis of the disease [16]. Research carried out in specialised centres shows that diabetic patients have obstructive arterial disease situated distal to the popliteal arteries and this is the cause of the majority of cases of peripheral ischaemic phenomena. Increasingly, vascular surgery centres emphasise *the good results obtained from the procedure of peripheral vascular reconstruction in diabetic patients at the level of the distal arteries of the leg or at the level of the dorsal arteries of the foot.* The preference for reconstruction utilising the patient's veins usually from the area of the greater or lesser saphenous vein and even of the veins at the level of the arms [17, 18] are worthy of mention (minimal, nonischaemic trauma for the graft). Our experience in this field is small, limited to only a few cases presenting with ischaemic lesions following reconstructive surgery. These have benefited from distal, peripheral amputation, which is an obvious advantage. In the future, vascular monitoring of the diabetic patient will permit the use of repermeabilisation or of timely reconstruction which certainly contributes to the diminution of the frequency of ischaemic gangrene and hence of amputations.

For reasons easy to understand, different procedures utilised in plastic surgery such as free tissue transfer, various types of flaps, etc.) are more difficult to apply in lesions of the diabetic foot. For this kind of procedure, it is first of all necessary to have a satisfactory circulation, as a condition for the healing of wounds and a good metabolic balance is necessary. The use of this procedure is problematic in the ischaemic diabetic foot where it can only be taken into consideration after a repermeabilisation or vascular reconstruction procedure. In the neuropathic diabetic foot, these procedures could be utilised after the elimination of the infection and the achievement of good metabolic balance. In the Cantacuzino surgical clinic, we have frequently followed a simpler procedure, *i.e.* the use of dermoepidermal grafts in order to cover some cutaneous defects in the case of the predominantly neuropathic foot; cases with larger defects in this category were referred to the plastic surgery clinics.

Good early results were obtained following surgical treatment for 84–89% of patients in the Cantacuzino Hospital. The majority of failures followed distal operations (26–28% of cases) especially on a clearly vascular background (17 of 28 cases).

All patients operated on for lesions of the diabetic foot must remain under the care of specialised services that are versed in the pathology of the diabetic foot in order to prevent and diagnose the possible reappearance of some complications in a timely manner.

CONCLUSIONS

1. The diabetic foot is a major complication of diabetes mellitus.

2. The education of the diabetic patient associated with follow-up monitoring by a diabetologist or a general practitioner properly trained for this is a basic condition for the improvement of clinical results.

3. The ischaemic factor is a major element in the course and prognosis of the diabetic foot. The timely monitoring of the diabetic patient in relation to the circulatory deficit of the lower limbs allows for timely reconstructive and revascularisation surgery.

4. Surgical complications of the diabetic foot require early intervention such as debridement with wide excision associated with adequate antibiotic treatment and proper metabolic balance.

5. The multitude of pathogenic factors as well as the complexity of lesions in the diabetic foot requires a multidisciplinary approach to this disorder.

REFERENCES

1. Reiber GE. Epidemiology of foot ulcers and amputations in the diabetic foot. In: Bowker JH and Pheifer M. (ed) *The diabetic foot*, 6th ed. Mosby, 2001, 3–12.
2. van Damme H, Paquet PH, Maertens B, Damas P, Scheen A.J. – Le pied diabetique: etiopatogenie, prevention et traitement – *Revue medicale de Liege*, **XLIX**: 1–1994, 1–11.
3. Tanenberg RJ, Schumer MP, Douglas AG, Pfeifer AM. – Neuropathic problems of the lower extremities in diabetic patients. In: Bowker JH and Pheifer M (ed.). *The Diabetic Foot*, 6th ed. Mosby, 2001, 33–64.
4. Caputo GM, Covanagh PR, Ulbrecht JJ, Gibbons GW. Assessment and management of foot disease in patients with diabetes. *N Engl J Med*, **331**: 854–860, 1994.
5. Elkeles RJ, Wolf I. The diabetic foot. *Bul M Journal*. **303**: 1053–1055, 1991.
6. Colwell JA, Lyons LT, Klein RL, Joke JR. Atherosclerosis and thrombosis in diabetes mellitus: new aspects of pathogenesis. In: Bowker

JH, and Pheifer M (ed.) *The diabetic foot*, 6th ed. Mosby, 2001, 65–106.

7. Mc Millan ED. Hemorheology Principles and Concepts, In: Bowker JH, and Pheifer M. *The diabetic foot* 6th ed. Mosby, 2001, 107–124.

8. Boulton A. Peripheral neuropathy and the diabetic foot. – *Foot*, **2**: 67–72, 1992.

9. Lipsky AB. Infectious problems of the foot in diabetic patients. In: Bowker JH and Pheifer M. *The diabetic foot*. 6th ed. Mosby, 2001, 467–482.

10. International Working Group on the Diabetic Foot. *International Consensus on the Diabetic Foot*, 2003 (in press).

11. Lipsky BA, Pecorano RE, Wheat JL. The diabetic foot: soft tissue and bone infection. *Infect Dis Clin North Am*. **4**: 409–432, 1990.

12. Lipsky BA. – Osteomyelitis of the foot in diabetic patients. *Clin Infect Dis*, **25**: 1318–1326, 1997.

13. Pătraşcu T, Dorah H, Păcescu E, Vereanu I – Gangrena diabetică – Indicele de prognostic terapeutic – studiu prospectiv. *Revista Chirurgia*, **6**: 2002.

14. Bowker JH, Giovanni TP. Minor and major limb amputation in persons with diabetes mellitus. In: Bowker JH, and Pheifer M. *The diabetic foot*, 6th ed, Mosby, 2001, 603–638.

15. Vereanu I. Amputaţiile distale în tratamentul piciorului diabetic. *Rev. Chirurgia (Bucureşti)*, **94**: 2, 103–111, 1999.

16. Hu MY, Allen BT. The role of vascular surgery in the diabetic patient. In: *The Diabetic Foot*. 6th ed, Mosby, 2001, 524–564.

17. Rosenblatt MS, Quist WC, Sidawy AM. Results of vein graft reconstruction of the lower extremity in diabetic and nondiabetic patients. *Surg Gynec Obstetr*, **71**: 331–335, 1990.

18. Shah DM, Darling RCR, Chang B. Long-term results of in situ saphenous vein bypass. Analysis of 2058 cases. *Am Surg*, **222**: 438–448, 1995.

44

MODIFIABLE RISK FACTORS AND RECONSTRUCTIVE SURGERY IN LOWER LIMB ATHEROSCLEROSIS IN DIABETIC PATIENTS

Viorel ŞERBAN, Mihai IONAC*, Adrian VLAD*, Mihaela ROŞU, Alexandra SIMA*

> *"Any fool can cut off a leg, it takes a surgeon to save one."*
> **George C. Ross**
> *1854*

The known risk factors for coronary artery disease also contribute to the development of peripheral arterial disease. Some of them (dyslipidemia, cigarette smoking, hypertension, diabetes mellitus, "atherogenic" diet, physical inactivity, obesity, hyperhomocysteinemia, inflammation, microalbuminuria) may be modified by lifestyle changes and/or pharmacological methods, and the clinical manifestations of atherosclerosis may thus be delayed.

A common pattern encountered in higher risk populations is the aggregation of multiple major risk factors (the metabolic syndrome).

With an aging population and often an unhealthy lifestyle, the incidence of peripheral arterial disease increases. Sometimes, this disease raises major therapeutical problems and may lead to high-level amputations, with an important decrease of patients' quality of life and major social implications.

The diabetic foot represents an entity that is distinct from the peripheral arterial disease in the diabetic patient. The main pathogenic mechanisms involved in its genesis are neuropathy, infection, microvascular dysfunction, and ischemia.

The improved technical possibilities allow for early diagnosis and surgical correction of the vascular lesions, resulting in a reduction in the number and extent of amputations.

Reconstructive arterial surgery is the "golden standard" for restoring the arterial blood flow in the ischemic leg.

Three vascular reconstruction techniques are commonly used:
1. Standard distal (infrageniculate) bypass;
2. Sequential bypass for multilevel arterial occlusive disease of the lower limbs;
3. Proximal percutaneous transluminal angioplasty combined with distal bypass.

These procedures are completed by an aggressive therapy of the concomitant infections, debridements, flap coverage and correction of underlying bony structural abnormalities. Sometimes, limited amputations may be required.

---

*Viorel Şerban, Mihai Ionac and Adrian Vlad contributed equally to this work and should be regarded as first authors.

MODIFIABLE RISK FACTORS FOR PERIPHERAL ARTERIAL DISEASE

From an epidemiological perspective, a "risk factor" is a characteristic or feature of an individual or population that is present early in life and is associated with an increased risk of developing future disease. For a risk factor to be considered causal, it must pre-date the onset of disease and must have biological credibility. Several risk factors are modifiable, and trials have demonstrated that lowering these factors reduces vascular risk [1].

Given our current understanding of the pathophysiology of atherothrombosis, it is surprising that the conceptual basis for considering specific "cardiovascular risk factors" did not formally exist until the initial findings of the Framingham Heart Study began to appear in the early 1960s.

The well-known modifiable risk factors associated with coronary atherosclerosis also contribute to the occurrence of peripheral arterial disease (PAD) (Table 44.1).

Table 44.1

Risk of peripheral arterial disease in persons with modifiable risk factors [2, modified]

Risk factor	Relative risk
Dyslipidemia (*per* 40 to 50 mg/dl increase in total cholesterol)	1.2–1.35
Cigarette smoking	2.0–5.0
Hypertension	2.5–4.0
Insulin resistance and diabetes	3.0–4.0
Atherogenic diet	
Physical inactivity and obesity	
Estrogen status	
Hyperhomocysteinemia	6.8
Lipoprotein(a)	2
Fibrinogen (*per* 0.7 g/l increase in fibrinogen)	1.35
Markers of fibrinolytic function	
Markers of inflammation	2.1
Microalbuminuria	
Intimal-media thickness	

AGGREGATION OF RISK FACTORS

Multiple major risk factors

A common pattern encountered in higher risk populations is the aggregation of multiple major risk factors. Multiple major risk factors are especially common in middle-aged and older persons, in whom age also counts as a risk factor. The risk for atherosclerosis has been evaluated in large prospective studies such as the Framingham Heart Study [3], the PROCAM Study [4], the MONICA study [5], the ARIC study [6], the Cardiovascular Health Study [7], and many others. Estimations of risk accompanying multiple major risk factors have been the basis of "global risk assessment" used in many cardiovascular prevention guidelines.

Metabolic syndrome: multiple metabolic risk factors

With the worldwide increase in overweight/obesity and sedentary life habits, an alternate pattern of risk factors is emerging. This pattern consists of several metabolic risk factors occurring in individuals; this aggregation of risk factors is known by several names: syndrome X, insulin resistance syndrome, the deadly quartet, and the metabolic syndrome. According to ATP III [8], the risk factors that make up the metabolic syndrome are the following:
- Atherogenic dyslipidemia
  - elevated small, dense lipoproteins
  - low HDL cholesterol
  - elevated triglycerides
- Elevated blood pressure
- Insulin resistance ± glucose intolerance
- Prothrombotic state
- Proinflammatory state

ATP III cholesterol guidelines [8] proposed a clinical diagnosis for the metabolic syndrome. This syndrome is based on risk factors that can be readily identified in clinical practice. According to ATP III, the diagnosis of the metabolic syndrome can be made if three out of the following five risk factors are present:
- Increased waist circumference (Table 44.2)
- Elevated triglycerides ≥ 150 mg/dl
- Reduced HDL cholesterol
  - men < 40 mg/dl
  - women < 50 mg/dl

- Elevated blood pressure
  - systolic blood pressure ≥ 130 mmHg
  - or diastolic blood pressure ≥ 85 mmHg
- Elevated fasting glucose ≥ 110 mg/dl

Table 44.2

The definition of increased waist circumference [8]

	Europe and United States	Asian Pacific Region	Japan
Men	≥ 102 cm	≥ 90 cm	≥ 90 cm
Women	≥ 88 cm	≥ 80 cm	≥ 85 cm

An alternate approach to the diagnosis of the metabolic syndrome has been proposed by the World Health Organization [9]. This approach begins with the assumption that insulin resistance is the underlying component of the metabolic syndrome and it requires evidence of insulin resistance for diagnosis, *i.e.*, impaired fasting glucose, impaired glucose tolerance, categorical hyperglycemia, or hyperinsulinemia. Other components that confirm the diagnosis are those listed by ATP III. In contrast, the ATP III diagnosis places more emphasis on obesity being the primary underlying cause of the metabolic syndrome as it views insulin resistance as one of several risk factors for atherosclerosis.

The risk of peripheral artery disease (PAD) and intermittent claudication increases progressively with the burden of contributing factors [10]. In the Framingham Heart Study, the occurrence of claudication in men whose risk factor was smoking *versus* nonsmoking was 2.6 *versus* 0.8 *per* 8 years *per* 1000 population. In male smokers who were also hypertensive, hypercholesterolemic, and diabetic, the risk was 44.3 *per* 8 years *per* 1000 [11]. Similar observations have been made in women.

DYSLIPIDEMIA

Until recently, the role of cholesterol in the pathogenesis of atherosclerosis remained controversial. The importance of serum (or plasma) cholesterol emerged from a series of large epidemiological studies. Further refinements in analytical methodologies, especially the use of the ultracentrifugation (which allows separation of plasma lipoproteins), provided important data on the relationship between low-density lipoproteins (LDL) and possibly very low-density lipoproteins (VLDL) and atherosclerosis. The role of high-density lipoproteins (HDL) as a protective fraction also resulted. Total cholesterol and HDL cholesterol are often paired. This has led to wide use of the total cholesterol to HDL cholesterol ratio. In prospective studies, the risk of coronary artery disease increases in a log-linear fashion with the increase of the ratio; risk has been noted to rise more sharply at values >5.0. One reason for the powerful prediction of this ratio is the fact that elevated cholesterol concentrations are an indicator of elevated atherogenic lipoproteins, whereas a low HDL cholesterol is a marker for the metabolic syndrome.

Abnormalities in lipid metabolism are associated with an increased prevalence of PAD. Elevations in total or LDL cholesterol increased the risk of PAD and claudication in some studies but not in others [12]. In a large Israeli study involving 10,059 men aged 40 to 65 years [cited by 2], the odds ratio for development of claudication was 1.35 for each increase in serum cholesterol of 50 mg/dl. Similar observations were made in the Framingham Heart Study, in which the odds ratio for claudication was 1.2 for each 40 mg/dl increase in total cholesterol [12]. In a cohort of patients participating in a lipid research clinic protocol, however, LDL cholesterol was not associated with PAD based on a multiple logistic regression analysis that included cigarette smoking, blood pressure, glucose and obesity. Hypertriglyceridemia independently predicts risk for PAD [1, 2].

Despite these results, until recently, enthusiasm for treating patients with drugs to lower cholesterol lagged for two reasons: (1) the drugs themselves had undesired effects, and (2) little direct evidence actually demonstrated reduced morbidity and mortality. However, recent trials, notably those using hydroxymethylglutaryl coenzyme A reductase inhibitors, have established beyond any doubt that lipid-lowering therapy in high-risk or even moderate-risk subjects reduces cardiovascular morbidity and mortality [13–18].

Physicians must therefore consider evaluation and management of dyslipidemia an integral part of their practice.

CIGARETTE SMOKING

Cigarette consumption constitutes the most important modifiable risk factor for atherosclerosis. Studies in the early 1950s first reported strong positive associations between cigarette exposure and coronary heart disease. Over the next 40 years, a large number of prospective studies have clearly documented the effects of smoking on coronary risk. Moreover, these effects are dose-dependent; consumption of as few as one to four cigarettes daily increases coronary artery disease risk. Besides myocardial infarction, cigarette consumption directly relates to increased rates of sudden death, aortic aneurysm formation, symptomatic PAD and ischemic stroke [1].

Smoking affects atherothrombosis by several mechanisms. In addition to accelerating athero-sclerotic progression, long-term smoking may enhance oxidation of LDL cholesterol and reduce levels of HDL cholesterol. Smoking also impairs endothelium-dependent artery vasodilation; has multiple adverse hemostatic effects; increases inflammatory markers such as C reactive protein (CRP), soluble intercellular adhesion molecule-1 (ICAM-1), and fibrinogen; causes spontaneous platelet aggregation; and increases monocyte adhesion to endothelial cells. Compared with nonsmokers, smokers have an increased prevalence of arterial spasm and may have reduced thresholds for ventricular arrhythmia [1].

Data derived from several observational studies (including the Edinburgh Artery Study, the Framingham Heart Study, and the Cardiovascular Health Study, among others) indicate a 2-fold to 5-fold increased risk of PAD in smokers [2, 12]. In the Whitehall Study [cited by 2], approximately 84% of patients with claudication were current smokers or ex-smokers, and in another large recent study [cited by 2], 90 percent of patients with PAD were current or former smokers. Progression of disease to critical limb ischemia and limb loss is more likely to occur in patients who continue to smoke than in those who stop. Smoking may even increase the risk of development of PAD more than it does for coronary artery disease [1, 2].

Cessation of cigarette consumption constitutes the most important intervention in preventive cardiology. Trials of nicotine replacement therapy using either transdermal nicotine or nicotine chewing gum have both proven to greatly increase abstinence rates after cessation. Such pharmacological programs, as well as physician-guided counseling, are cost-effective and should be provided as a standard prevention service. Unfortunately, although the elevated cardiovascular risks associated with smoking decrease significantly after cessation, the risks of cancer of the lungs, pancreas, and stomach persist for more than a decade, as do the risks of developing chronic obstructive pulmonary disease. Thus, primary prevention remains the most important population-based component of any smoking reduction strategy.

HYPERTENSION

Elevated levels of blood pressure consistently correlate with elevated risks of stroke and myocardial infarction. Although hypertension often clusters with insulin resistance and obesity, the risk imposed by hypertension increases in the presence of other cardiovascular risk factors.

Even among individuals without diastolic hypertension, isolated increases in systolic pressure are a risk factor. Pulse pressure, a potential surrogate for vascular wall stiffness, also potently predicts both first and recurrent myocardial infarction [1].

Hypertension increased the risk of claudication 2.5-fold in men and 4-fold in women in the Framingham Heart Study [11], and the risk increased proportionally with the severity of hypertension [11, 12]. Similarly, in the Edinburgh Artery Study, elevations in systolic blood pressure correlated with PAD. However, this finding has not been consistently shown in all epidemiological studies. In the British Whitehall Study and a large Finnish study [cited by 2], hypertension was not found to be associated with claudication.

In regard to treatment, blood pressure reduction greatly decreases risk, even among individuals with mild to moderate hypertension. In the elderly, randomized trial data have also indicated the efficacy of treating isolated systolic hypertension [19].

INSULIN RESISTANCE AND DIABETES

Compared to unaffected individuals, diabetic patients have a greater atherosclerotic burden both in the major arteries and in the microvascular circulation. Thus, insulin resistance and diabetes rank among the major cardiovascular risk factors.

However, although hyperglycemia is associated closely with microvascular disease, insulin resistance itself promotes atherosclerosis even before it produces frank diabetes.

In patients with diabetes mellitus (DM), PAD is often extensive and severe, and these patients have a greater propensity for vascular calcification. Involvement of the femoral and popliteal arteries is similar to that of nondiabetic persons, but distal disease affecting the tibial and peroneal arteries occurs more frequently. The risk of development of PAD increases 3-fold to 4-fold in patients with DM [2, 11, 12]. In the Framingham cohort, glucose intolerance contributed more as a risk factor for claudication than it did for coronary artery disease or stroke.

Despite evidence concerning pathophysiological abnormalities associated with DM and epidemiological data describing increased hazards associated with hyperglycemia, clinical trials have failed to demonstrate that improved glycemic control significantly reduces cardiovascular risk [20, 21].

ATHEROGENIC DIET

The nutrient composition of the diet contributes to the development of atherosclerotic disease in several ways. Among these, high intakes of saturated fatty acids and cholesterol promote atherogenesis by raising the serum cholesterol level. This was proved by epidemiological studies [22]. However, no large, heart-diet clinical trials have been conducted to test whether reducing intakes of saturated fats and cholesterol in the diet will reduce risk for coronary artery disease. Meta-analyses of several smaller clinical trials strongly suggest that replacing saturated fatty acids with unsaturated fatty acids in the diet will lower serum cholesterol levels and reduce incidence of coronary artery disease. Other dietary factors also associate with risk of atherosclerosis, either in a positive or negative way. Factors that seemingly increase the risk for coronary artery disease are transfatty acids, whereas putative protective factors include unsaturated fatty acids (N-9, N-6, and N-3), folic acid, fruits and vegetables, anti-oxidant vitamins, alcohol, and higher intakes of plant sterols and viscous fiber [8]. In addition, the risk of atherosclerosis may be increased by high intakes of sodium and low intakes of potassium, magnesium, and calcium, all of which may raise the blood pressure. Support for the beneficial effects of N-9 fatty acids comes from the Seven Country Study [cited by 1] in which high intakes of N-9 fatty acids were associated with lower rates of coronary artery disease. Higher intakes of N-9 and low consumption of saturated fatty acids are characteristic of the "Mediterranean diet". A large body of epidemiological data supports a coronary artery disease reducing action of moderate alcohol consumption [23]. Limited clinical trial data support benefit from higher intakes of N-3 fatty acids. In spite of several lines of evidence that oxidative stress contributes to the risk of coronary artery disease, clinical trials of anti-oxidant vitamins have failed to confirm a protective action [24]. It should be noted, however, that these studies were limited to high-risk patients and vitamins were given as a supplement. Several epidemiological studies suggest that diets rich in anti-oxidants are accompanied by reduced risk for coronary artery disease. Finally, numerous recent studies document that high intake of plant stanol/sterols or viscous fiber lower serum cholesterol levels beyond what can be achieved by reducing intake of saturated fatty acids and cholesterol [25].

PHYSICAL INACTIVITY AND OBESITY

The mechanisms by which exercise lowers cardiovascular risk remain uncertain, but likely include favorable effects on blood pressure, weight control, lipid profiles, and improved glucose tolerance. Exercise also improves endothelial function, enhances fibrinolysis, reduces platelet reactivity, and reduces propensity for in-situ thrombosis.

Controversy remains as to whether obesity itself is a true risk factor for cardiovascular disease or whether its impact on vascular risk is mediated solely through interrelations with glucose intolerance, insulin resistance, hypertension, physical inactivity, and dyslipidemia. Nonetheless, obesity is epidemic and weight control must play a fundamental role in all preventive cardiology practices, preferably in conjunction with advice regarding diet and exercise [1].

ESTROGEN STATUS

Before menopause, women have lower age-adjusted incidence and mortality rates for coronary heart disease than men do. Gender-specific incidence rates converge after menopause, suggesting a major role for estrogen in delaying progression of atherosclerosis. However, Women's Health Initiative randomized trial demonstrated an increase in cardiovascular mortality in post-menopausal women receiving hormone replacement therapy [26].

HYPERHOMOCYSTEINEMIA

Homocysteine is an amino acid derived from the demethylation of dietary methionine. Patients with rare inherited defects of methionine metabolism can develop severe hyperhomo-cysteinemia (plasma levels >100 μmol/l) and can have premature atherothrombosis. The mechanisms that account for these effects remain uncertain, but may include endothelial toxicity, accelerated oxidation of LDL cholesterol, impairment of endothelial-derived relaxing factor, and reduced flow-mediated arterial vasodilation.

In contrast to severe hyperhomocysteinemia, mild to moderate elevations of homocysteine (plasma levels >15 μmol/l) are common in general populations, primarily due to insufficient dietary intake of folic acid.

Although a nonfasting evaluation of total plasma homocysteine suffices for most clinical purposes, measurement of homocysteine levels 2 to 6 hours after ingestion of an oral methionine load (0.1 g/kg body mass) can identify individuals with impaired homocysteine metabolism despite normal fasting levels.

By contrast, prospective epidemiological studies (where homocysteine levels are ascertained before the onset of cardiovascular events) have provided mixed data.

In a meta-analysis of studies relating homocysteine to atherosclerotic disease [cited by 2], the odds ratio for PAD in patients with increased homocysteine levels was 6.8. High levels of homocysteine have been detected in 30 to 40 percent of patients with PAD. Plasma levels of B complex vitamins, including folate, cobalamin, and pyridoxal 5′-phosphate, all inversely relate to the plasma homocysteine concentration [2, 27].

Folic acid, given in doses of up to 400 μg/day, can be expected to reduce homocysteine levels approximately 25 percent, whereas the addition of vitamin B_{12} will likely reduce levels another 7 percent. Because this therapy is inexpensive and has low toxicity, vitamin supplementation may be a more cost-effective approach for high-risk groups than screening [28].

LIPOPROTEIN (a)

Although the normal function of lipoprotein(a) [Lp(a)] is unknown, the close homology between Lp(a) and plasminogen has raised the possibility that this unusual lipoprotein may inhibit endogenous fibrinolysis by competing with plasminogen for binding on the endothelial surface. More recent data demonstrate accumulation of Lp(a) and co-localization with fibrin within atherosclerotic lesions, both in stable patients and among those with unstable angina pectoris [29]. Apoprotein(a) [apo(a)] may also induce monocyte chemotactic activity in the vascular endothelium, whereas Lp(a) may increase release of plasminogen activator inhibitor (PAI). Thus, several mechanisms may contribute to a role for Lp(a) in atherothrombosis [1].

Many retrospective and cross-sectional studies suggest a positive association between Lp(a) and vascular risk. Increased levels of Lp(a) impart a 2-fold increased risk of PAD, with higher levels associated with a greater risk for critical limb ischemia [2].

Prospective studies of Lp(a) have not always found consistent evidence of association. The predictive value of Lp(a) in women is controversial.

Even in the positive studies of Lp(a), it is unclear whether evaluation of this lipoprotein adds to the predictive value of total and HDL cholesterol. Indeed, LDL reduction markedly reduces any adverse hazard associated with Lp(a).

Whereas niacin can modestly reduce Lp(a) levels, specific Lp(a)-lowering therapies are not available. For all of these reasons, most authors do not recommend general Lp(a) screening [1].

FIBRINOGEN

Plasma fibrinogen critically influences platelet aggregation and blood viscosity, interacts with plasminogen binding, and in combination with thrombin mediates the final step in clot formation. In addition, fibrinogen associates positively with age, obesity, smoking, DM, and LDL cholesterol and inversely with HDL cholesterol, alcohol use, physical activity, and exercise level [30].

Given these relationships, it is not surprising that fibrinogen was among the first "novel" risk factors to be evaluated in epidemiological studies. Reports from the Gothenburg, Northwick Park, and Framingham heart studies [cited by 1] found significant positive associations between fibrinogen and future risk of cardiovascular events. A series of prospective studies have since confirmed these results, and a recent meta-analysis indicates that the relative risk of future cardiovascular events is 1.8 times higher for individuals in the top tertile as compared with those in the bottom tertile of baseline fibrinogen concentration [31]. Women may have higher risks than men, at the same level of fibrinogen.

An increase in fibrinogen is also associated with an increased risk of PAD [2]. The Edinburgh Artery Study noted a 35 percent increased risk for PAD over 5 years for each 0.7 g/l increase in fibrinogen [32].

Due to the consistency of these data, many consider fibrinogen an independent marker of risk for atherosclerosis. However, two issues have limited clinical screening for fibrinogen to improve risk prediction: (1) inadequate standardization between competing laboratory techniques, and (2) wide intraindividual variation in plasma levels over time.

Fibrinogen elevation occurs as part of the acute-phase response and may thus be associated with risk owing to its role as a marker of systemic inflammation.

MARKERS OF FIBRINOLYTIC FUNCTION

Impaired fibrinolysis can result from an imbalance between the clot-dissolving enzymes – tissue-type plasminogen activator (t-PA) or urokinase-type plasminogen activator (u-PA) – and their endogenous inhibitors, primarily PAI-1. Plasma levels of PAI-1 peak in the morning whereas concentrations of t-PA demonstrate a less prominent circadian variation. On this basis, a relative hypofibrinolytic state may prevail in the morning that, along with increased platelet reactivity, may contribute to the increased risk of acute arterial events seen in this time period.

A highly consistent series of prospective studies have linked abnormalities of fibrinolysis to increased risk of arterial thrombosis. For example, prospective associations exist between *PAI-1* antigen and activity levels and the risk of first and recurrent myocardial infarction [30]. Perhaps paradoxically, individuals at risk for future coronary as well as cerebral thrombosis consistently have elevated levels of circulating *t-PA* antigen. These latter effects may represent evidence of underlying endothelial dysfunction among individuals at risk or of direct relationships between t-PA and PAI-1, or they may represent a biological response to impaired fibrinolysis. In this regard, reduced *clot lysis time*, an overall indicator of net fibrinolytic function, also predicts coronary risk. Finally, several studies indicate that levels of *D-dimer*, a peptide released by plasmin action on fibrin, also predict myocardial infarction, peripheral atherothrombosis, and recurrent coronary events [33].

Despite these data, the clinical use of fibrinolytic markers to determine vascular risk may offer little marginal value.

MARKERS OF INFLAMMATION

Inflammation characterizes all phases of atherosclerosis. Formation of the fatty streak, the earliest phase of atherogenesis, involves recruitment of leukocytes due to expression of leukocyte adhesion molecules on endothelial cells, in turn triggered by primary proinflammatory cytokines such as interleukin (IL)-1 or tumor necrosis factor (TNF) alpha. Subsequent migration of inflammatory cells into the subendothelial space requires chemotaxis controlled by chemokines induced by the primary cytokines. Mononuclear cells within this initial infiltrate as well as intrinsic vascular cells subsequently release growth factors that stimulate proliferation of the smooth muscle cells and hence the progression of plaques. Finally, the thrombotic complications of plaques often involve physical disruption, usually associated with signs of inflammation [34]. Other proinflammatory cytokines such as CD154 (CD40 ligand) can induce tissue factor procoagulant expression and promote thrombus formation [1].

The primary proinflammatory cytokines IL-1 and TNF-α induce, in turn, the expression of another cytokine, IL-6. This is a "messenger" cytokine that can determine the synthesis in the liver of acute-phase reactants. In this manner, local inflammation (in this case, the artery wall) can produce a reflection in the peripheral blood. This cytokine cascade orchestrates the expression of effector molecules (*e.g.*, the adhesion molecules).

Given this underlying pathophysiology, it is not surprising that several markers of low-grade systemic inflammation have also proved useful for cardiovascular risk prediction [35]. These markers include nonspecific acute-phase reactants such as high sensitivity C reactive protein (*hs-CRP*), adhesion molecules such as *ICAM-1*, which are involved in mononuclear cell attachment to the vascular endothelium, and cytokines such as *IL-6* and *TNF*. Each of these inflammatory markers can be measured in the plasma and may thus provide a window on the inflammatory processes at the level of the arterial wall.

Among the inflammatory markers, hs-CRP will likely prove the most clinically useful because it is easy and inexpensive to measure with commercial assays. CRP has proved to have strong predictive value both among currently healthy men and women as well as among the elderly, high-risk smokers, those with stable and unstable angina pectoris, and those with prior myocardial infarction [36–38]. In these studies, individuals with hs-CRP levels in the upper quartile had relative risks of future vascular events three to four times higher than individuals with

lower levels, effects that were independent of all other traditional cardiovascular risk factors. Moreover, plasma levels of hs-CRP appear to add to the predictive value of plasma lipid measurements, and thus may provide an improved method to determine future vascular risk [1].

Patients with PAD have elevated levels of hs-CRP. In the Physicians' Health Study [cited by 2], the relative risk of development of PAD among men in the highest quartile for hs-CRP concentration was 2.1.

Evidence also suggests that hs-CRP may represent a modifiable risk marker. In a randomized trial of low-dose aspirin, the relative efficacy of this agent in decreasing coronary risk was the greatest among those with evidence of low–grade inflammation as determined by hs-CRP but it was sequentially smaller as levels of hs-CRP declined, data that suggest potentially important antiinflammatory effects for aspirin. Similarly, in the Cholesterol and Recurrent Events (CARE) trial, the risk reduction associated with pravastatin was greater among individuals with a persistent inflammatory response as determined by hs-CRP, such that statin therapy attenuated almost completely the elevated risk associated with inflammation [38]. Moreover, therapy with pravastatin in the CARE trial significantly reduced levels of hs-CRP over a 5-year period [39]. This finding corroborates human experimental studies that suggest that lipid lowering attenuates inflammation [40] and that the use of statins reduces macrophage content and activity within atheromatous plaque [41]. Thus, lipid lowering by statins appears to mitigate the inflammatory processes that undermine plaque stability.

The observation that elevated levels of CRP, IL-6, TNF, IL-1 and soluble ICAM-1 all associate with future vascular events provides a potent stimulus to consider targeted antiinflammatory therapies as a novel method to both treat and prevent vascular thrombosis.

MICROALBUMINURIA

Microalbuminuria (defined as an albumin-creatinine ratio of 10–25 mg/mmol on the first-morning urine sample, or an albumin excretion rate of 20–200 μg/min on a timed collection) is present in 20–30% of all patients with type 2 DM, and is especially common in those with hypertension, endothelial dysfunction and other features of insulin resistance. Although microalbuminuria is predictive of worsening microvascular disease in the kidney (5–10% *per* year progress to overt diabetic nephropathy), an increased albumin excretion rate (AER) reflects a generalized abnormality of vascular function and is associated with 2–4 fold increases in cardiovascular and all-cause mortality. The extent to which microalbuminuria is a risk factor independent of other variables in type 2 DM, *e.g.* blood pressure and smoking, has been highlighted by recent cohort studies, *e.g.* the Heart Outcome Prevention Evaluation study [24]. The presence of microalbuminuria at baseline increased the adjusted relative risks (RR) of a major cardiovascular event (RR 1.83), all-cause death (RR 2.09) and hospitalization for heart failure (RR 3.23) in both diabetic and non-diabetic subjects. This study also highlighted that AER is a continuous risk factor, and that levels of AER below the arbitrary threshold for defining microalbuminuria are associated with a relatively increased cardiovascular risk. Similarly, microalbuminuria affects 10–15% of middle-aged non-diabetics and is associated with coronary, peripheral and cerebral vascular complications. Detection of microalbuminuria, especially in type 2 DM, signifies the need to intensify blood pressure control as part of a multiple risk factor intervention strategy in a high-risk group. As hypertensive patients with type 2 DM are frequently treated by more than one antihypertensive agent, ACE inhibitors and low-dose diuretics are preferably recommended in order to provide sufficient blood pressure control and target organ protection [42].

INTIMAL-MEDIA THICKNESS

Carotid wall thickness is measured by B-mode ultrasound, as the mean of the maximum intimal-media thickness (IMT) in 12 or 16 carotid segments.

Higher IMT in young and middle-aged adults is associated with childhood and current cardiovascular risk factors, as well as risk factor load [43].

An increased thickness of the carotid artery wall is thought to be a sign of early atherosclerosis. Carotid ultrasonography is useful as a non-invasive and easy screening method for coronary artery

disease and PAD [44, 45], and subsequently for following up the progression of atherosclerosis.

RECONSTRUCTIVE VASCULAR SURGERY IN CRITICAL ISCHEMIA OF THE LOWER LIMBS

With an aging population and improved treatment possibilities for many of the other atherosclerotic manifestations, the estimated incidence of critical limb ischemia (CLI) has increased to ca. 1 000/million inhabitants/year. CLI is defined as persistent pain requiring analgesia for more than 2 weeks, or ulceration, or gangrene of the foot, plus an ankle systolic pressure below 50 mmHg [46]. In diabetic patients the ankle pressure can be seldom recorded due to vascular calcification, therefore the pressure criterion is replaced by absence of ankle pulses.

CLI represents the end result of PAD and may lead to the loss of the patient's leg or life, unless proper therapeutical measures are taken. Leg loss carries a significant morbidity and mortality, and one third of the patients who survive will never ambulate again [47].

In contrast, improved diagnostic methods and reconstructive arterial surgery have made it possible to identify and to correct the atherosclerotic lesions causing ischemia, thus achieving long term salvage of the lower extremities. This had the greatest impact on improving quality of life in patients with CLI. Thirty years ago (and tragically in many Romanian hospitals today too!), major amputation was the method of choice in this situation. Today, a reconstructive procedure is the primary option for the vast majority of the patients. Therefore, an amputation has to be regarded either as the last choice, or as an indication of failed therapy.

ETIOLOGY, PATHOPHYSIOLOGY, EPIDEMIOLOGY

Atherosclerosis in the large arteries is the fundamental process in the pathogenesis of CLI. It occludes or severely narrows the arteries, reducing the blood flow and perfusion pressure in the peripheral tissue [48]. Even if the arterial occlusion may affect any level, patients with DM are more likely to have atherosclerotic disease affecting the territories of profunda femoris and infrageniculate arteries, with sparing of the foot arteries, which allows for successful arterial reconstruction to these distal vessels [49].

DM is an important factor in the development of CLI [11, 50]. The specific feature of DM is the localization of the atherosclerotic process in arteries in the crural region compared to more proximal localizations in most non-diabetic atherosclerotic disease, and the high frequency of mediasclerosis in the arterial wall leading to incompressibility of the arteries [46]. Diabetic neuropathy further complicates the situation by affecting sensory, proprioceptive and autonomic nerves. Loss of muscle function results in deformities and sensory loss predisposes the foot to pressure lesions with or without ischemia.

One of the most serious impediments in approaching vascular disease in patients with DM is the misconception that they suffer an untreatable occlusion of the microcirculation [51]. This idea originated from a retrospective histological study that showed the presence of periodic-acid-Schiff-positive material occluding the arterioles in amputated limb specimens from patients with DM. However, subsequent prospective staining and arterial casting studies and physiological studies have shown the absence of an arteriolar occlusive lesion. Eliminating the notion of "small vessel disease" or "microangiopathy" is fundamental to the principles of limb salvage in patients with DM, because arterial reconstruction is almost always possible in these patients.

Despite the fact that there is no occlusive lesion in the diabetic microcirculation, other structural changes do exist, most notably, a thickening of the capillary basement membrane. However, this does not induce the narrowing of the capillary lumen and arteriolar blood flow may be normal or even increased despite these changes. It seems, therefore, that a nonocclusive microcirculatory (capillary and arteriolar) dysfunction exists in DM and contributes probably to the development of neuropathy.

It is very clear that the prevalence of DM influences the incidence of CLI. In the western world the prevalence of DM varies between 2 and 5%. The total prevalence of DM in the population has been estimated to increase from 5,700/million inhabitants in the age group under 45 years to 79,700 in those over 65 years [52]. The corresponding amputation incidence increases from 1,200–1,400 to 9,500–12,000/million diabetics/year [53]. DM is an independent risk factor for PAD, but is also associated with other manifestations of atherosclerosis [50, 54]. Up to 10% of elderly diabetics develop ischemic ulcers and gangrene. In a 10-year follow-up of non-diabetic and diabetic claudicants, the amputation incidence was 8% and 34% respectively [55]. The CLI incidence in diabetics is at least five-fold greater compared to nondiabetics and amputation rates are 10–15 times those of nondiabetics [46].

THE DIABETIC FOOT

The diabetic foot represents an entity that is distinct to the PAD in the diabetic patient. Problems of the diabetic foot are the most common cause for hospitalization in patients with DM, with huge annual health care costs (*e.g.,* more than $1 billion in the USA) [56]. Diabetic foot ulceration will affect 15% of all individuals with DM during their lifetime and is clearly a significant risk factor in the pathway to limb loss [57]. The main pathogenetic mechanisms in diabetic foot disease are neuropathy, infection, microvascular dysfunction, and ischemia [58]. Acting together, they contribute to the sequence of tissue necrosis, ulceration, and gangrene.

Infection

The spectrum of infection in diabetic foot disease ranges from superficial ulceration to extensive gangrene with fulminant sepsis. Classical signs of infection may not always be present in the infected diabetic foot, due to the consequences of neuropathy, alterations in the foot microcirculation, and leukocyte abnormalities. Fever, chills, and leukocytosis may be absent in up to two thirds of patients with DM with extensive foot infections, and hyperglycemia is often the sole presenting sign. Therefore, a complete examination of the infected areas is mandatory and the wound should be thoroughly inspected, including unroofing of all encrusted areas, to determine the extent of involvement.

Most infections are polybacterial, the most common pathogens being *staphylococci, streptococci,* and *enterococci;* anaerobes and gram-negative bacilli are also commonly cultured.

Cultures should be obtained from the base of an ulcer or abscess cavity after debridement. Osteomyelitis is common in diabetic foot ulceration, appearing in almost 70% of benign-appearing ulcers and should be presumed if the bone is palpated on probing in an open ulcer [59].

Ischemia

Ischemia is a fundamental consideration to the reconstructive surgeon faced with the diabetic foot. Even moderate ischemia may lead to ulceration, therefore the biologically compromised foot necessitates maximum circulation to heal an ulcer.

This leads to three fundamental principles:

1. all diabetic foot ulcers should be evaluated for an ischemic component;

2. correction of a moderate degree of ischemia will improve healing in the biologically compromised diabetic foot;

3. whenever possible, the arterial reconstruction should be designed to restore normal arterial pressure to the target area.

Neuropathy

Despite important advances in DM care, neuropathy is a common complication, afflicting 50% to 60% of all patients [60, 61]. A direct causal relation between diabetic neuropathy and foot ulceration has been documented; peripheral neuropathy is present in more than 80% of the diabetics who have foot lesions [62]. The combination of motor and sensory neuropathy along with loss of the neurogenic inflammatory response, microcirculatory dysfunction and peripheral vascular disease results in a biologically compromised foot.

The causes of diabetic neuropathy are not exactly known and may be due to a combination of metabolic and vascular defects including hyperglycemia, nerve hypoxia and nerve compression [63–65]. Traditionally this diffuse symmetrical sensorimotor polyneuropathy of DM is considered progressive and irreversible, and patients are not referred to surgical treatment until ulceration, infection or the need for amputation occurs.

Alternatives to this generally accepted view are offered by clinical trials that have shown improvements of the nerve function after the revascularization of the extremity or after nerve decompression procedures.

The role of peripheral vascular disease remains considerable, because it seems likely that a decrease in total limb blood flow would intensify nerve ischemia. Although neuropathy itself is not an indication for arterial reconstruction, it seems that the long-term reversal of hypoxia in the ischemic limbs halts the normally expected progression of this diabetic complication [65]. On the other hand, it has been demonstrated that at least one of the factors involved in the diabetic neuropathy is the result of endoneurial edema caused by various biochemical reactions triggered by hyperglycemia. Over time, these biochemical alterations render the nerve susceptible to compression and clinical symptoms become manifest. Internal and external limiting structures create a double crush phenomenon to the nerve structure. Decompression of the nerve trunk at normal anatomical areas of narrowing, such as the carpal, cubital, and tarsal tunnels is one of the adjuncts to the overall treatment plan for diabetic neuropathy. Although surgeons cannot operate on the metabolic neuropathy itself, they can release superimposed compression neuropathies. Because nerve compression can be treated, there is cause for optimism in treating diabetic neuropathy [66]. Indications for nerve decompression at the level of the tarsal tunnel include painful paresthesias, decreased sensation, and foot ulcers. The results were consistent, with return of protective sensation, no new ulcer formation and significant decrease of the burning pain in 50% to 70% of the cases [64, 67–69].

In conclusion

Treatment of the diabetic foot should be directed towards the pathogenic factors outlined previously. In general, this can be broken down into a few simple guidelines:

1. prompt control of infection; this assumes first priority in the management of any diabetic foot problem;

2. evaluation for ischemia;

3. prompt arterial reconstruction once active infection has resolved;

4. secondary procedures, such as further debridement, toe amputations, local flaps, and even free flaps, may then be carried out separately in the fully vascularized foot;

5. Surgical decompression of peripheral nerves in symptomatic neuropathy.

PRINCIPLES OF ARTERIAL RECONSTRUCTION IN THE DIABETIC LOWER EXTREMITY

The aim of the treatment of CLI is lower limb salvage. To obtain this it is necessary to substantially improve the arterial blood flow. Reconstructive arterial surgery is the "golden standard" in improving arterial blood flow in the ischemic leg and it is the preferred option for most of the patients.

When to operate?

The most important observation is the presence or absence of a palpable foot pulse; in simplest terms, if the foot pulses are not palpable, it can be assumed that occlusive disease is present. A variety of noninvasive arterial tests may be ordered. However, in the presence of DM, all of these tests have significant limitations. Medial arterial calcinosis occurs frequently and unpredictably in patients with DM, and its presence can result in noncompressible arteries with artifactually high segmental systolic pressures and ankle-brachial indices.

Because the foot vessels are often patent in the patient with DM and because of the success of bypass grafting to these vessels, an appropriate evaluation for ischemia is essential in patients with DM. unless recognized and corrected, limb salvage efforts will fail even if infection and neuropathy have been appropriately treated.

Other tests as segmental doppler wave forms and pulsed volume recordings, and regional transcutaneous oximetry measurements, have important limitations [70] and they emphasize the continued importance of a thorough bedside evaluation and clinical judgment. The status of the foot pulse is the most important aspect of the physical examination. An absent foot pulse is an indication for contrast arteriography in the clinical setting of tissue loss, poor healing, or gangrene, even if neuropathy may have been the antecedent cause of skin breakdown or ulceration. Importantly, even when the tibial arteries are occluded, it is absolutely essential that arteriograms do not stop at the midtibial level,

because the foot vessels are often spared by the atherosclerotic occlusive process. Therefore, the complete infrapopliteal circulation should be incorporated, including the foot vessels. The advent of digital subtraction angiography has greatly helped in the visualization of these distal vessels. Both anteroposterior and lateral foot views should be included. Excessive plantar flexion should be avoided because this may impede flow in the dorsalis pedis artery. Inadequate arteriography may fail to visualize the vessel at malleolar level favorable for limb salvage and mistakenly deem the extremity as "un-reconstructible". Therefore, the liberal employment of intraoperative angiography is recommended in case of any concerns regarding the accuracy of the initial diagnostic arteriogram. A complete arteriogram will facilitate choosing an outflow artery that will restore a palpable foot pulse.

Which techniques to use?

Restoration of the foot pulse is a fundamental goal of revascularization in the diabetic foot. This goal has been achieved in our institution by using three types of vascular reconstruction:

1. Standard distal (infrageniculate) bypass;

2. Sequential bypass for multilevel arterial occlusive disease (MLAOD) of the lower limbs;

3. Proximal percutaneous transluminal angioplasty (PTA) combined with distal bypass.

1. Distal bypass

The common femoral or popliteal vessels are usually used as inflow sites of the proximal anastomoses. The outflow vessels include posterior tibial artery that has continuity with the plantar arch in most than half of the cases [71]. Anterior tibial and pedal arteries have been proved in our and others' hands to be equally efficient and with long-term patency rates (Plate 44.1). Although peroneal artery is not in continuity with the foot vessels and may not achieve maximal flow, particularly to the forefoot, excellent results have been reported with peroneal artery bypass grafting [72]. Minor atheromatous lesions (less than 30% reduction of luminal diameter) in the inflow vessels may be tolerated. Autologous vein was used throughout. The saphena magna is usually implanted reversed in all cases except where it is not available, when an upper limb vein or a

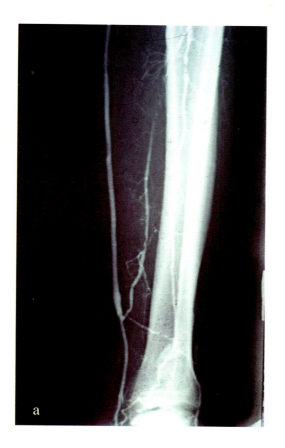

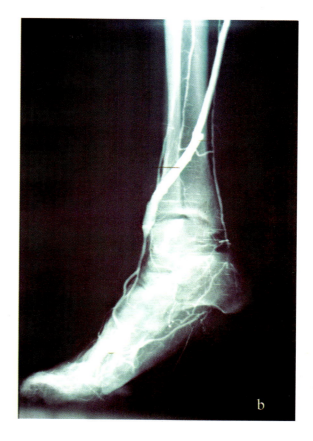

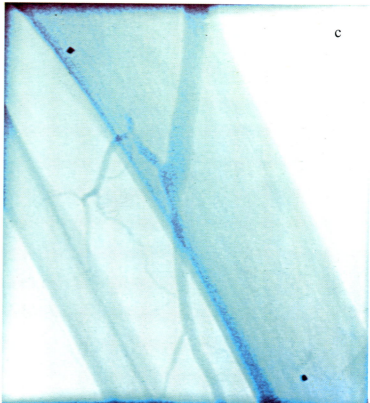

Plate 44.1

a – Popliteal to tibial posterior bypass, 18 months follow-up; b – Popliteal to pedal bypass, 12 months follow-up; c – Femoral to peroneal bypass, 12 months follow-up.

polytetrafluoroethylene (PTFE) graft may serve as an option (Figure 44.1).

2. Sequential bypass

Lower extremity ischemia resulting from multilevel arterial occlusive disease (MLAOD) poses a challenging problem. Both inflow and outflow revascularization procedures are required for successful surgical treatment and there is considerable debate regarding the timing of the multiple revascularization procedures [73]. Some authors advocated a staged approach in which inflow reconstruction is performed initially with the outflow procedure being delayed and reserved for those patients whose ischemic symptoms persist after inflow bypass [74]. This approach would offer the advantage of decreased time under anesthesia and reduced operative time and stress, also reporting an overall reduction in morbidity and mortality for inflow bypass alone as compared with simultaneous inflow and outflow procedures.

We and other authors routinely perform simultaneous inflow and outflow reconstructions as the preferred procedure [72, 75, 76]. We feel that in instances where both procedures are ultimately necessary, simultaneous performance avoids the need for two distinct operative procedures and thereby avoids the increased morbidity and mortality associated to multiple interventions. Additionally, some patients have a critical level of ischemia that mandates simultaneous reconstructions. In these instances staging the procedures may result in delay in achieving optimal revascularization and could therefore place the patient at risk for suboptimal outcome. The presence of DM has been proposed as a factor that may necessitate the performance of simultaneous rather than staged inflow and outflow revascularization procedures [74]. Because patients with DM are particularly predisposed to the development of infrageniculate arterial occlusive disease [49], and because they may exhibit decreased immune function [52], they would be more likely to require a combined procedure to relieve their ischemic symptoms.

The inflow artery was in all cases the common femoral. The popliteal artery was used as an intermediate outflow site, the anastomosis being performed either side-to-side or end-to-side. The distal outflow procedure was a popliteal- or previous graft-to-posterior tibial/peroneal or anterior tibial arteries bypass (Figure 44.1). Autogenous reversed ipsilateral saphena magna is used routinely. When the vein is short or narrow, composite conduits including cephalic vein or PTFE grafts may be used (Figure 44.1).

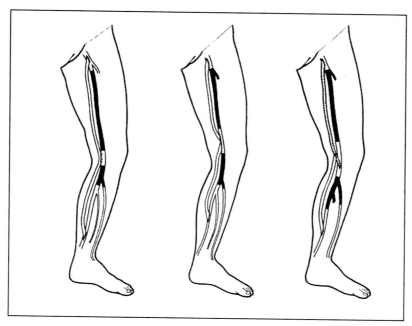

Figure 44.1
Possible configurations for sequential bypass.

3. PTA combined with distal bypass

Before the era of the interventional cardiology, the "golden standard" for the multilevel vascular obstructions was the sequential bypass. With the advent of the endovascular techniques that allow percutaneous arterial dilation and stenting, the patients benefit of new alternatives for the treatment of multilevel obstructions, lowering the complications rate with excellent immediate and long-term results [77]. However, using only endovascular techniques in the lower extremities the patency at one year is estimated around 70% [78]. The zone of dilation, severity of the stenosis and the presence of a good run-off influence the results of PTA. A good run-off can be obtained by associating PTA & stenting to distal bypass surgery [79, 80]. This combined approach may be applied at the following levels: iliac PTA & stenting – infrainguinal bypass, superficial femoral PTA & stenting – infrapopliteal bypass (Figure 44.2), being less invasive than a sequential bypass, significantly decreasing patient's stress and the operative time. It has been demonstrated that the distal bypass consecutive to proximal dilation and stenting has increased the patency of the percutaneous procedure. The presence of DM seems not to alter the long-term results [79] (Figure 44.2).

Because of the presence of medial arterial calcification in patients with DM, severe calcification of the outflow artery may be encountered, but this should not preclude attempts at arterial reconstruction. Moreover, active infection in the foot is not a contraindication to distal bypass grafting, as long as the infectious process is controlled and is located away from the proposed incision area.

Bypasses to tibial and pedal arteries demand meticulous attention and a fine, atraumatic technique. The relatively small caliber of these vessels allows little margin for iatrogenic intimal flaps or tears at the anastomotic site that invariably cause early graft failure.

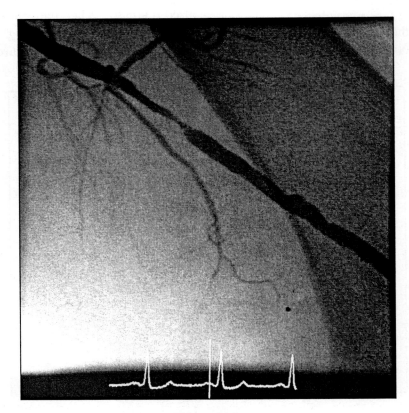

Figure 44.2a

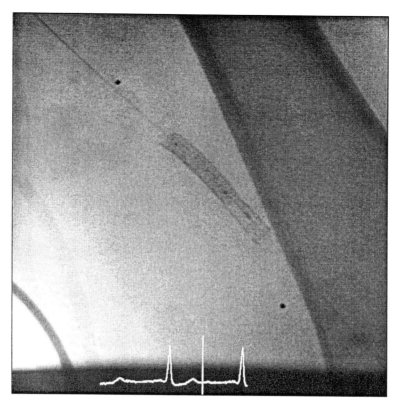

Figure 44.2b

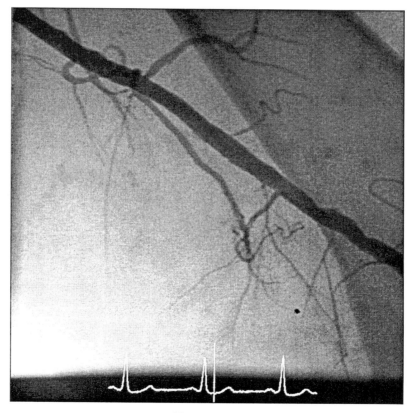

Figure 44.2c

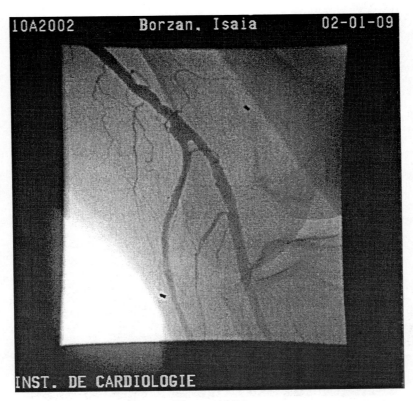

Figure 44.2d

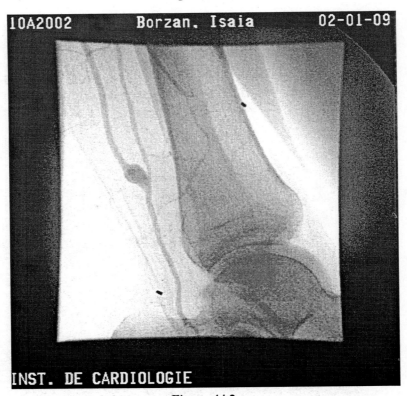

Figure 44.2e

(a) – (c) Femoral percutaneous transluminal angioplasty (PTA),
combined with (d) – (e) Popliteal to tibial posterior bypass, 30 months follow-up.

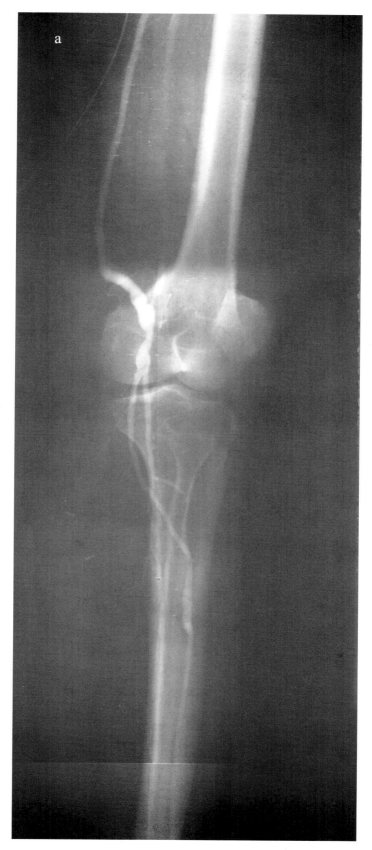

Plate 44.2

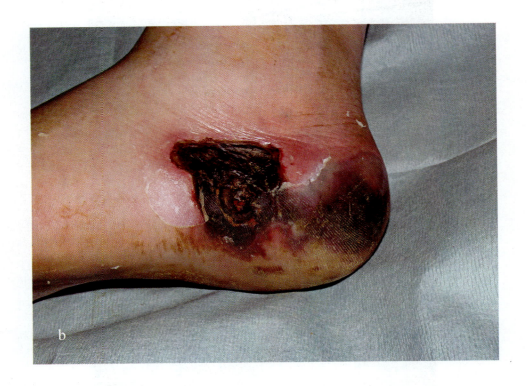

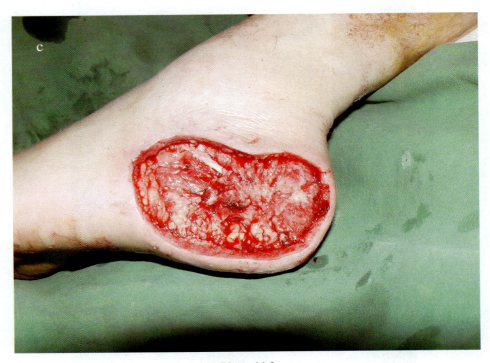

Plate 44.2

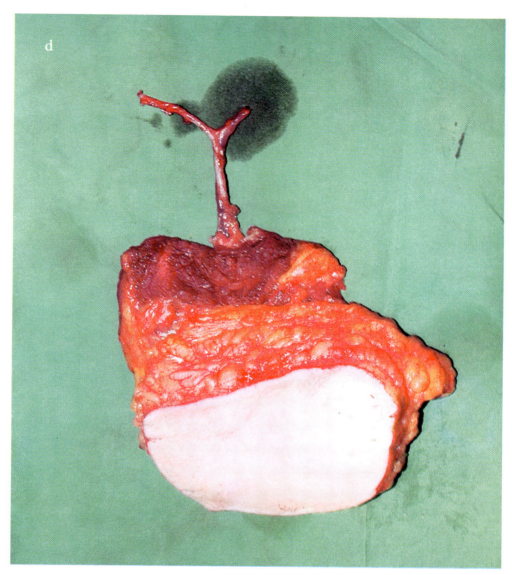

Plate 44.2

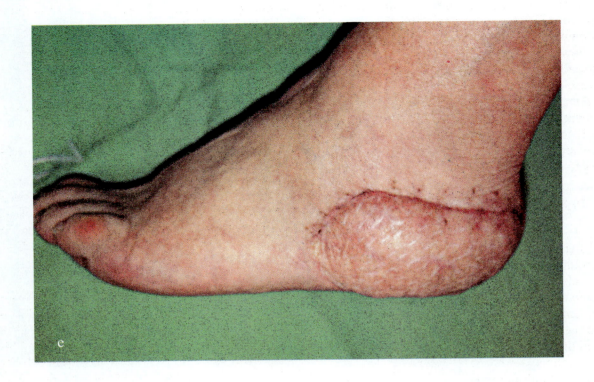

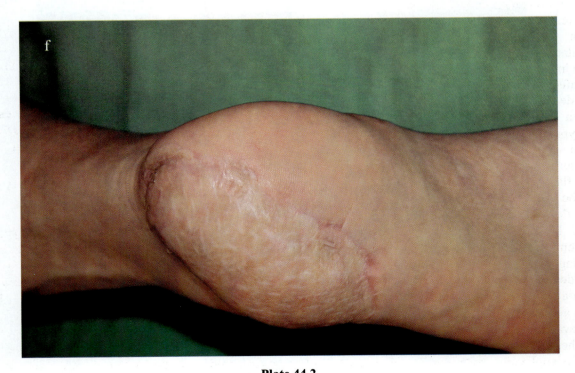

Plate 44.2

a – Sequential femoral-popliteal to tibial anterior bypass combined with (b – f) – Latissimus dorsi free flap for reconstruction of the calcaneum, 36 months follow-up. The free flap was revascularized to the patent pedal artery.

Therefore, the routine use of an operating microscope when performing the distal anastomosis has several advantages. It provides high-power and variable magnification to create technically perfect anastomoses on diseased atherosclerotic vessel walls. In addition the operating microscope insures excellent illumination and fixed visual field. The perfect visual control also reinforces the use of microsurgical atraumatic technique, avoiding any injury to the vessel intima.

Is revascularization successful enough?

After successful revascularization, secondary procedures may be performed for both limb and foot salvage. Once the gangrenous tissue has become demarcated after revascularization, debridements or minor digital amputations are performed. As soon as clean granulation tissue covers the wounds these are skin-grafted. Because of the architecture of the diabetic foot, underlying bony structural abnormalities are often the cause of ulceration and may be corrected with metatarsal head resection or osteotomy.

In the septic neuroischemic foot, major amputation may be considered as unavoidable, but if the infection is not immediately life-threatening, the infected part of the foot should be drained and debrided properly and left wide open, sometimes with a guillotine amputation in order not to risk the bypass graft.

In patients with extensive tissue loss and exposure of the underlying bone, tendons, both local flaps and free flaps may be used. Heel ulcers may be treated with partial calcanectomy and local (*e.g.*, flexor tendon) or even free flap coverage.

It has been demonstrated that combining revascularization techniques with free flap coverage has many advantages [81]: (1) it provides immediate soft tissue coverage, limiting amputation level and healing time, resulting in early ambulation; (2) it provides extra run-off to the revascularization, illustrated by a decrease in peripheral resistance, contributing to its patency; (3) the application of healthy, well vascularized tissue limits infection and enhances neovascularization; (4) a full-length limb is preserved. We believe this combined approach offers a valuable alternative to primary amputation

in this group of patients with extensive ischemic defects (Plate 44.2).

What can be expected in the immediate and late postoperative period?

Postoperative pharmacotherapy consists of aspirin 250 mg daily and low molecular weight heparin for prophylaxis of venous thromboembolism. After discharge, patients should be recalled every three months during the first postoperative year. Later, follow-ups are scheduled at 6-months intervals. At the follow-up visits pulses are palpated and ankle pressures evaluated by hand-held Doppler.

Early mortality and complications

Despite the high incidence of coexisting coronary disease and congestive heart failure, the in-hospital mortality is less than 1% in DM group of patients [52, 72–74]. Therefore, a more aggressive approach toward invasive perioperative cardiac monitoring and treatment should be adopted. Early complications develop in approximately 10% of the patients and are controlled either by reinterventions or by standard wound care. The morbidity and mortality rates seem not to differ significantly between diabetic and nondiabetic patients [76].

Foot salvage and clinical outcome

Cumulative patency and limb salvage rates do not vary significantly between diabetic and nondiabetic patients, and they vary between 80% and 100% at 5 years [71–74, 76].

SUMMARY

This aggressive and systematic approach to diabetic foot disease has resulted in improved limb salvage among patients with DM. At the authors' institution, there has been a significant reduction in every category of lower limb amputation since 1997 [72]. Concomitant with this decrease, the number of patients who undergo arterial reconstruction has increased, and distal bypass procedures are more often utilized.

The presented data confirm that distal bypass is an effective and durable procedure that can be performed safely even for high-risk patients, including diabetics with multiple comorbidities, requiring revascularization for limb salvage. The use of an operating microscope during performance of distal anastomoses is highly recommended. Infrapopliteal bypass should be considered for all patients with critical limb ischemia before major amputation is contemplated.

Better awareness and understanding of the complex pathophysiology of diabetic vascular disease will lead to further decreases in lower limb amputation and will reduce the overall morbidity and mortality of DM.

REFERENCES

1. Ridker PM, Genest J, Libby P. Risk Factors for Atherosclerotic Disease. In: Braunwald E, Zipes DP, Libby P (eds). *Heart Disease. A Textbook of Cardiovascular Medicine.* 6th Edition, W. B. Saunders Company, 2001, 1010–1039.

2. Creager MA, Libby P. Peripheral Arterial Diseases. In: Braunwald E, Zipes DP, Libby P (eds). *Heart Disease. A Textbook of Cardiovascular Medicine.* 6th Edition, W. B. Saunders Company, 2001, 1457–1484.

3. Wilson PWF, D'Agostino RB, Levy D, *et al.* Prediction of coronary heart disease using risk factor categories. *Circulation,* **97:** 1837–1847, 1998.

4. Assman G, Cullen P, Schulte H. Simple scoring scheme for calculating the risk of acute coronary events based on the 10-year follow-up of the prospective cardiovascular Munster (PROCAM) study. *Circulation,* **105:** 310–315, 2002.

5. Kuulasmaa K, Tunstall-Pedoe H, Dobson A, *et al.* Estimation of contribution of changes in classic risk factors to trends in coronary-event rates across the WHO MONICA Project populations. *Lancet,* **355:** 675–687, 2000.

6. Sharrett AR, Ballantyne CM, Coady SA, *et al.* Atherosclerosis Risk in Communities Study Group: Coronary heart disease prediction from lipoprotein cholesterol levels, triglycerides, lipoprotein(a), apolipoproteins A-1 and B, and HDL density subfractions: The Atherosclerosis Risk in Communities (ARIC) Study. *Circulation,* **104:** 1108–1113, 2001.

7. Kuller L, Fisher L, McClelland R, *et al.* Differences in prevalence of and risk factors for subclinical vascular disease among black and white participants in the Cardiovascular Health Study. *Arterioscler Thromb Vasc Biol,* **18:** 283–293, 1998.

8. Third report of the National Cholesterol Education Program (NCEP) expert panel on detection, evaluation, and treatment of high blood cholesterol in adults (Adult Treatment Panel III). Final Report. *Circulation,* **106:** 3143–3421, 2002.

9. World Health Organization Dept. of Non-communicable Disease Surveillance. Definition, diagnosis and classification of diabetes mellitus and its complications: Report of a WHO consultation. *Geneva World Health Organization,* 1999.

10. Gaede P, Vedel P, Larsen N, *et al.* Multifactorial intervention and cardiovascular disease in patients with type 2 diabetes. *N Engl J Med,* **348:** 383–393, 2003.

11. Kannel WB, McGee DL. Update on some epidemiologic features of intermittent claudication: The Framingham Study. *J Am Geriatr Soc,* **33:** 13–18, 1985.

12. Murabito JM, D'Agostino RB, Silbershatz H, *et al.* Intermittent claudication. A risk profile from the Framingham Heart Study. *Circulation,* **96:** 44–49, 1997.

13. Shepherd J, Cobbe SM, Ford I, *et al.* for the West of Scotland Coronary Prevention Study Group. Prevention of coronary heart disease with pravastatin in men with hypercholesterolemia. *N Engl J Med,* **333:** 1301–1307, 1995.

14. Sacks FM, Pfeffer MA, Moye LA, *et al.* for the Cholesterol and Recurrent Events Trial Investigators. The effect of pravastatin on coronary events after myocardial infarction in patients with average cholesterol levels. *N Engl J Med,* **335:** 1001–1009, 1996.

15. The Long-Term Intervention with Pravastatin in Ischaemic Disease (LIPID) Study Group. Prevention of cardiovascular events and death with pravastatin in patients with coronary heart disease and a broad range of initial cholesterol levels. *N Engl J Med,* **339:** 1349–1357, 1998.

16. Scandinavian Simvastatin Survival Study Group. Randomised trial of cholesterol lowering in 4444 patients with coronary heart disease: The Scandinavian Simvastatin Survival Study (4S). *Lancet,* **344:** 1383–1389, 1994.

17. Heart Protection Study Collaborative Group. MRC/BHF Heart Protection Study of cholesterol lowering with simvastatin in 20, 536 high-risk individuals: a randomised placebo-controlled study. *Lancet,* **360:** 7–22, 2002.

18. Sever PS, Dahlöf B, Poulter NR, *et al.* for the ASCOT investigators. Prevention of coronary and stroke events with atorvastatin in hypertensive patients who have average or lower-than-average cholesterol concentrations, in the Anglo-Scandinavian Cardiac Outcomes Trial–Lipid Lowering Arm (ASCOT-LLA): a multicentre randomised controlled trial. *Lancet,* **361:** 1149–1158, 2003.

19. Staessen JA, Fagard R, Thijs L, *et al.* Randomised double-blind comparison of placebo and active treatment for older patients with isolated systolic hypertension. The Systolic Hypertension in Europe (Syst-Eur) Trial Investigators. *Lancet*, **350**: 757–764, 1997.

20. UK Prospective Diabetes Study Group. Intensive blood-glucose control with sulphonylureas or insulin compared with conventional treatment and risk of complications in patients with type 2 diabetes (UKPDS 33). *Lancet*, **352**: 837–853, 1998.

21. Sichiri M, Ohkubo Y, Kishikawa H, *et al.* Long-term results of the Kumamoto study on optimal diabetes control in type 2 diabetic patients. *Diabetes Care*, **23**(Suppl 2): B21–B29, 2000.

22. Stamler J, Greenland P, Van Horn L, *et al.* Dietary cholesterol, serum cholesterol, and risks of cardiovascular and noncardiovascular diseases. *Am J Clin Nutr*, **67**: 488–492, 1998.

23. Mukamal KJ, Rimm EB. Alcohol's effects on the risk for coronary heart disease. *Alcohol Res Health*, **25**: 255–261, 2001.

24. Yusuf S, Sleight P, Pogue J, *et al.* Effects of an angiotensin-converting-enzyme inhibitor, ramipril, on cardiovascular events in high-risk patients. The Heart Outcomes Prevention Evaluation Study Investigators. *N Engl J Med*, **342**: 145–153, 2000.

25. Law M. Plant Sterol and stanol margarines and health. *Br Med J*, **320**: 861–864, 2000.

26. Rossouw JE, Anderson GL, Prentice RL, *et al.* Writing Group for the Women's Health Initiative Investigators. Risks and benefits of estrogen plus progestin in healthy postmenopausal women: principal results from the Women's Health Initiative randomized controlled trial. *JAMA*, **288**: 321–333, 2002.

27. Şerban V. Homocisteina şi diabetul zaharat. In: Şerban V (ed). *Actualităţi în diabetul zaharat*, Editura Brumar, Timişoara, 2002, 263–279.

28. Homocysteine Lowering Trialists' Collaboration. Lowering blood homocysteine with folic acid based supplements: Meta-analysis of randomised trials. *BMJ*, **316**: 894–898, 1998.

29. Dangas G, Mehran R, Harpel PC, *et al.* Lipoprotein(a) and inflammation in human coronary atheroma: Association with the severity of clinical presentation. *J Am Coll Cardiol*, **32**: 2035–2042, 1998.

30. Scarabin PY, Aillaud MF, Amouyel P, *et al.* Associations of fibrinogen, factor VII and PAI-1 with baseline findings among 10,500 male participants in a prospective study of myocardial infarction – the PRIME Study. Prospective Epidemiological Study of Myocardial Infarction. *Thromb Haemost*, **80**: 749–756, 1998.

31. Danesh J, Collins R, Appleby P, *et al.* Association of fibrinogen, C-reactive protein, albumin, or leukocyte count with coronary heart disease: Meta-analyses of prospective studies. *JAMA*, **279**: 1477–1482, 1998.

32. Smith FB, Lee AJ, Hau, CM, *et al.* Plasma fibrinogen, haemostatic factors and prediction of peripheral arterial disease in the Edinburgh Artery Study. *Blood Coagul Fibrinolysis*, **11**: 43–50, 2000.

33. Moss AJ, Goldstein RE, Marder VJ, *et al.* Thrombogenic factors and recurrent coronary events. *Circulation*, **99**: 2517–2522, 1999.

34. Ross R. Atherosclerosis – an inflammatory disease. *N Engl J Med*, **340**: 115–126, 1999.

35. Libby P, Ridker PM. Novel inflammatory markers of coronary risk: Theory *versus* practice. *Circulation*, **100**: 1148–1150, 1999.

36. Koenig W, Sund M, Froelich M, *et al.* C-reactive protein, a sensitive marker of inflammation, predicts future risk of coronary heart disease in initially healthy middle-aged men: Results from the MONICA (Monitoring Trends and Determinants in Cardiovascular Disease) Augsberg Cohort Study, 1984 to 1992. *Circulation*, **99**: 237–242, 1999.

37. Roivainen M, Viik-Kajander M, Palosuo T, *et al.* Infections, inflammation, and the risk of coronary heart disease. *Circulation*, **101**: 252–257, 2000.

38. Ridker PM, Rifai N, Pfeffer MA, *et al.* Inflammation, pravastatin, and the risk of coronary events after myocardial infarction in patients with average cholesterol levels. Cholesterol and Recurrent Events (CARE) Investigators. *Circulation*, **98**: 839–844, 1998.

39. Ridker PM, Rifai N, Pfeffer MA, *et al.* Long-term effects of pravastatin on plasma concentration of C-reactive protein. The Cholesterol and Recurrent Events (CARE) Investigators. *Circulation*, **100**: 230–235, 1999.

40. Aikawa M, Voglic SJ, Sugiyama S, *et al.* Dietary lipid lowering reduces tissue factor expression in rabbit atheroma. *Circulation*, **100**: 1215–1222, 1999.

41. Williams JK, Sukhova GK, Herrington DM, *et al.* Pravastatin has cholesterol-lowering independent effects on the artery wall of atherosclerotic monkeys. *J Am Coll Cardiol*, **31**: 684–691, 1998.

42. Donnelly R, Yeung JM, Manning G. Microalbuminuria: a common, independent cardiovascular risk factor, especially but not exclusively in type 2 diabetes. *J Hypertens Suppl 2003*, **21**(Suppl 1): S7–S12, 2003.

43. Davis PH, Dawson JD, Riley WA, *et al.* Carotid intimal-medial thickness is related to cardiovascular risk factors measured from childhood through

middle age: The Muscatine Study. *Circulation*, **104**: 2815–2819, 2001.

44. Gerstein HC, Anand S, Yi QL, *et al.* The Relationship Between Dysglycemia and Atherosclerosis in South Asian, Chinese, and European Individuals in Canada. A randomly sampled cross-sectional study. *Diabetes Care*, **26**: 144–149, 2003.

45. Mattace Raso F, Rosato M, Talerico A, *et al.* Intimal-medial thickness of the common carotid arteries and lower limbs atherosclerosis in the elderly. *Minerva Cardioangiol*, **47**: 321–327, 1999.

46. Second European consensus document on chronic critical leg ischemia. *Eur J Vasc Surg*, **6**(Suppl A), 1992.

47. De Frang RD, Taylor LM Jr, Porter JM. Basic data related to amputations. *Ann Vasc Surg*, **5**: 202–207, 1991.

48. Taylor LM, Porter JM. Natural history and nonoperative treatment of chronic lower extremity ischemia. In: Rutherford RB (ed). *Vascular surgery*, W. B. Saunders Company, 1995, 751–765.

49. Veith FJ, Gupta SK, Wengerter KR, *et al.* Changing atherosclerotic disease patterns and management strategies in lower limb threatening ischemia. *Ann Surg*, **212**: 402–414, 1990.

50. Adler AI, Boyko EJ, Ahroni JH, *et al.* Lower extremity amputation in diabetes: The independent effects of peripheral vascular disease, sensory neuropathy and foot ulcers. *Diabetes Care*, **22**: 1029–1035, 1999.

51. LoGerfo FW, Coffman JD. Vascular and microvascular disease of the foot in diabetes. *N Engl J Med*, **311**: 1615–1619, 1984.

52. Akbari CM, LoGerfo F. Diabetes and peripheral vascular disease. *J Vasc Surg*, **30**: 373–384, 1999.

53. van Houtum WH, Lavery LA. Outcomes associated with diabetes-related amputations in the Netherlands and in the state of California, USA. *J Int Med*, **240**: 227–231, 1996.

54. Lehto S, Pyörälä K, Rönnemaa T, *et al.* Risk factors predicting lower extremity amputations in patients with NIDDM. *Diabetes Care*, **19**: 607–612, 1996.

55. Siitonen OI, Niskanen LK, Laakso M, *et al.* Lower-extremity amputations in diabetic and nondiabetic patients. *Diabetes Care*, **16**: 16–20, 1993.

56. Grunfeld C. Diabetic foot ulcers: etiology, treatment, and prevention. *Adv Intern Med*, **37**: 103–132, 1991.

57. Reiber GE. The epidemiology of diabetic foot problems. *Diabet Med*, **13**: S6–S11, 1996.

58. Vereşiu IA. Piciorul diabetic. In: Şerban V, Vlad A, Sima A (eds). *Diabetul zaharat al vârstnicului*, Editura Brumar, Timişoara, 2003, 241–282.

59. Grayson ML, Gibbons GW, Balogh K. Probing to bone in infected pedal ulcers: a clinical sign of underlying osteomyelitis in diabetic patients. *JAMA*, **273**: 721–723, 1995.

60. The DCCT Research Group. Factors in the development of diabetic neuropathy: baseline analysis of neuropathy in the feasibility phase of the Diabetes Control and Complications Trial (DCCT). *Diabetes*, **37**: 476–481, 1988.

61. Dyck PJ, Kratz KM, Karnes JL. The prevalence by staged severity of various types of diabetic neuropathy, retinopathy, and nephropathy in a population-based cohort: The Rochester Diabetic Neuropathy Study. *Neurology*, **43**: 817–824, 1993.

62. Caputo GM, Cavanagh PR, Ulbrecht JS, *et al.* Assessment and management of foot disease in patients with diabetes. *N Engl J Med*, **331**: 854–860, 1994.

63. Stevens MJ, Feldman EL, Greene DA. The aetiology of diabetic neuropathy: the combined roles of metabolic and vascular defects. *Diabet Med*, **12**: 566–579, 1995.

64. Aszmann OC, Kress KM, Dellon AL. Results of decompression of peripheral nerves in diabetics: a prospective, blinded study. *Plast Reconstr Surg*, **106**: 816–822, 2000.

65. Akbari CM, Gibbons GW, Habershaw GM, *et al.* The effect of arterial reconstruction on the natural history of diabetic neuropathy. *Arch Surg*, **132**: 148–152, 1997.

66. Dellon AL. A cause for optimism in diabetic neuropathy. *Ann Plast Surg*, **20**: 103–105, 1988.

67. Caffee HH. Treatment of diabetic neuropathy by decompression of the posterior tibial nerve. *Plast Reconstr Surg*, **106**: 813–815, 2000.

68. Dellon AL. Treatment of symptomatic diabetic neuropathy by surgical decompression of multiple peripheral nerves. *Plast Reconstr Surg*, **89**: 689–697, 1992.

69. Wieman TJ, Patel VG. Treatment of hyperesthetic neuropathic pain in diabetics: Decompression of the tarsal tunnel. *Ann Surg*, **221**: 660–664, 1995.

70. Ubbink DT, Tulevski II, de Graaf JC, *et al.* Optimisation of the non-invasive assessment of critical limb ischemia requiring invasive treatment. *Eur J Endovasc Surg*, **19**: 131–137, 2000.

71. Sugawara Y, Sato O. Tibioperoneal bypass for popliteal arterial occlusion. *J Cardiovasc Surg*, **39**: 19–23, 1998.

72. Ionac M, Păscuţ M, Slovenski M, *et al.* Microscope-aided femoral- or popliteal-to-distal

bypass for salvage of limbs with critical ischemia. *Rom J Hand Reconstr Microsurg*, **4:** 35–38, 1999.

73. Nypaver TJ, Ellenby MI, Mendoza O, *et al.* A comparison of operative approaches and parameters predictive of success in multilevel arterial occlusive disease. *J Am Coll Surg*, **179:** 449–456, 1994.

74. Scher KS, McFall T, Steele FJ. Multilevel occlusive vascular disease presenting with gangrene. *Am Surg*, **57:** 96–100, 1991.

75. Harward TR, Ingegno MD, Carlton L, *et al.* Limb-threatening ischemia due to multilevel arterial occlusive disease. Simultaneous or staged inflow/outflow revascularization. *Ann Surg*, **221:** 498–503, 1995.

76. Faries PL, LoGerfo FW, Hook SC, *et al.* The impact of diabetes on arterial reconstructions for multilevel arterial occlusive disease. *Am J Surg*, **181:** 251–255, 2001.

77. de Sanctis JT. Percutaneous interventions for lower extremity peripheral vascular disease. *Am Fam Physician*, **64:** 1965–1972, 2001.

78. Rodriguez-Lopez JA, Soler L, Werner A, *et al.* Long-term follow-up of endoluminal grafting for aneurysmal and occlusive disease in the superficial femoral artery. *J Endovasc Surg*, **6:** 270–277, 1999.

79. Cheng SW, Ting AC, Lau H. Combined long-segment angioplasty and stenting of the superficial femoral artery and popliteal-distal bypass for limb salvage. *J Cardiovasc Surg*, **41:** 109–112, 2000.

80. Ionac M, Mut B, Dorobanţu C, *et al.* Percutaneous and microsurgical procedures for ischemic limb salvage in a diabetic patient. One year follow up. *Timişoara Med J*, **52:** 64–68, 2002.

81. Vermassen FE, van Landuyt K. Combined vascular reconstruction and free flap transfer in diabetic arterial disease. *Diabetes Metab Res Rev*, **16:** S33–S36, 2000.

45

OPHTHALMOLOGICAL ASPECTS OF DIABETES MELLITUS

Benone CÂRSTOCEA, Luiza Otilia GAFENCU

Diabetic retinopathy and senile macular degenerescence represent the two major causes for permanent loss of sight. An early diagnosis, regular check-ups and a good cooperation among diabetologist, family physician and ophthalmologist, can ensure delayed evolution and complication prevention (*e.g.*, the gradual loss of sight).

The risk of developing diabetic retinopathy is about 50% for patients with diabetes for more than 15 years. Only 30% of them reach severe forms of diabetic retinopathy. This risk is greater in patients with type 1 diabetes, compared to those with type 2.

It is worth mentioning that all the eye structures suffer in the presence of diabetes mellitus. Often precocious signs of the disease are ignored or given no importance.

In time, a series of etiologic hypotheses for diabetic retinopathy were brought forward. Today, Aldose reductase altered activity and the release of angiogenetic factors are considered to be the main mechanisms responsible for the pathological alteration of the retina.

Treatment differs according to the stage of the disease. The therapeutic choices are pharmacological, physical or surgical. While in the initial phases therapy consists mainly in normalizing glycemia, in the later stages laser photocoagulation or surgery is recommended. Laser treatment allows for stopping the disease and preventing further complications. Surgery is reserved for proliferative diabetic retinopathy with major complications.

Another important ocular complication of diabetes mellitus is cataract. Treatment is exclusively surgical.

The neovascular secondary glaucoma represents in many cases a difficult condition to manage, evolving despite of every preventive procedure, finally leading to blindness. A particular observation is the occurrence of pseudoexfoliative glaucoma in patients who have undergone previous retinal photocoagulation.

In ophthalmology, few diseases have such a large and/or severe resounding as diabetes mellitus has. According to statistics, in Europe as well as in America, diabetic retinopathy and the age related macular degenerescence, are the most frequent causes of blindness. Hence, the importance and weight the diabetic retinopathy should get in this chapter.

We should also take into account from the very beginning that all the eye structures and annexes, except the sclera, can be altered by diabetes mellitus (Table 45.1).

The first conclusion coming out of the above chart would be to split the ocular complications of diabetes into ocular complications and extraocular complications.

Such a separation does not point out the clinical values; frequently, these complications coexist.

A second conclusion stands that at least the extraocular alterations are definitely a local manifestation of the diabetic angiopathy.

The third conclusion stands that even signs and symptoms apparently without any importance – xanthelasma, vascular alterations of the conjunctiva or diplopia (as a consequence of paresis of an ocular muscle) could lead to finding out a serious ocular disease, such as diabetic retinopathy. They are, sometimes, signs of an ignored or neglected diabetes mellitus [1, 2, 3].

In addition, a subjective category of symptoms, as for example the chromatic discrimination, visual acuity alterations, or transitory refraction changes related to the time of the main meals, can also be considered as the first sign in a neglected diabetes mellitus [1, 3].

Table 45.1

Ocular complications of diabetes mellitus

Tissue	Complications Determined by Diabetes Mellitus
Eyelids	Xanthelasma
Conjunctiva	Microaneurysms
Extraocular muscles	Paresis of the oculomotorial nerves
Lacrimal system	Mucormycosis
Cornea	Descemetic folds
Iris	Rubeosis iridis Uveal ectropion Vacuolisation of the pigmented epithelium
Crystalline lens	Refractive changes Cataract
Ciliary body	Pigmented epithelium basal membrane thickening
Vitreous	Asteroid hyalosis Posterior detachment
Retina	Diabetic retinopathy

DIABETIC RETINOPATHY

ETIOLOGIC MECHANISMS IN DIABETIC RETINOPATHY

Diabetic retinopathy was unknown until 1921, the year when insulin was discovered. The new treatment of diabetes gave the possibility to observe and describe the ocular involvement of this systemic disease. The risk for diabetic retinopathy appearance is almost constant for the majority of diabetic patients, suffering from the illness for more than 15 years. The prevalence of proliferative retinopathy is about 50% in subjects with type 1 diabetes and is lower in those with type 2 diabetes, after a duration of 20 years or longer. About 30% diabetic patients reach cecity in 20 years [2, 4, 5, 6].

Today there are large possibilities for precocious diagnosis and treatment of diabetic retinopathy. The collaboration among family physician, diabetologist and ophthalmologist needs to be consolidated for the proportion of blind people due to diabetic retinopathy to decrease. Heightened emphasis on identifying patients at risk and the new methods of screening can reduce the number of patients that do not have regular eye examination. A very important issue is also the access to educational materials and facilities to control their disease. Unfortunately, it seems that only 50% of patients with diabetes receive regular ophthalmologic examinations and many become blind because of no treatment [4].

The physiopathology of diabetic retinopathy starts with its unique biochemical anomaly – the increase of glycemia. Hyperglycemia is the major etiologic agent in all of the microvascular complications of diabetes [1, 2, 7].

From the pathogenetic point of view, many theories have been put forward so far, each of them being still valid:

1. the theory of Aldose reductase;
2. the theory of the angiogenic factors;
3. the theory of the growth hormone;
4. the theory of the hemorheologic alterations;
5. the theory of the A_1 glycosylated hemoglobin.

1. The Aldose reductase is the enzyme that catalyses the transformation of carbohydrates into alcohol: glucose into sorbitol, the galactose into dulcitol. Both sorbitol and dulcitol hardly diffuse through the cellular membrane. Their intracellular concentration increases and the newly created osmotic forces will determine an intracellular infusion of water, unbalancing in this way the electrolytic scales. The latest researches have pointed out high concentrations of Aldose reductase at pericyte level in the retina. This may be the trigger element of diabetic retinopathy. The cellular edema that appears due to the intracellular accumulation of sorbitol may cause the early destruction of the pericytes and the weakening of the capillary wall [2, 8, 9].

2. The angiogenic factors theory was suggested by Michaelson. He was the first scientist who stated that hypoxic retina produces an angioproliferative factor that diffuses in the ischemic area inducing neovascularization. There are many clinical studies sustaining the theory [2, 10]. Thus, at the level of the neoplasm, an angiogenic factor has been discovered that stimulates new vessels to appear [11]. A second proof is given by the neovascularization of the optic nerve and especially of the iris in diabetes; this can be remitted by using laser panphotocoagulation of the ischemic retina [12, 13].

The most investigated angiogenic factor with reference to retinal and choroidal neovascularizing diseases is the vascular endothelial growth factor (VEGF). There are also other factors such as acidic fibroblast growth factor (FGF-1) or basic fibroblast growth factor (FGF-2). This fact indicates that a mixture of these factors can be involved in this complex mechanism of neovascularization. VEGF expression is substantial up-regulated by hypoxia. VEGF levels in the vitreous of patients undergoing vitrectomy for proliferative diabetic retinopathy are substantially increased in comparison with individuals undergoing the same surgery for other non-vasoproliferative diseases [1, 2, 14, 15, 16, 17].

VEGF is determined by immunocytochemistry in retinal glial cells, in particular Muller cells, and in glial cells of the optic nerves of the patients suffering from diabetes.

The nonperfused retinal area is responsible also of forming microaneurysms and vascular shunts. The formation mechanisms of microaneurysms include a proliferation of the endothelial capillary cells, weakness of the capillary wall due to the loss of pericytes, abnormalities of the adjacent retina and increased intraluminal pressure. With the increasing formation of microaneurysms excessive vascular permeability can occur. As a result, retinal edema develops, especially in the macular area. It is accompanied by retinal hard exudates, which consist of lipid deposits. Adjacent to these areas of nonperfusion, clusters of microaneurysms and hypercellular vessels develop. They are referred as intraretinal microvascular abnormalities (IRMA) [1, 2, 3, 18].

3. The growth hormone theory. Growth hormone seems to have a causative role in the development and progression of diabetic vascular complications. Poulson was the first who described the regression of the proliferative diabetic retinopathy at a woman suffering from a postpartum hemorrhagic necrosis of the pituitary gland (Sheehan syndrome). Surgical ablation of the pituitary gland was debated steadily between the years 1950–1960 and nowadays it is no longer used, both due to important postoperative complications (the necessity to replace the thyroid hormone deficit, as well as important glycemia variations) and due to the development of the laser therapy [19].

4. The hemorheologic alterations are just as well responsible for the increasing hypoxia in the retina. The liver synthesizes increased quantities of fibrinogen and α_2 plasmatic globulin under the growth hormone influence. The former high sanguineous levels, but also the other plasmatic proteins, may reduce the rejection forces among red cells, increasing their agglutination capacity. At the same time, diabetes may be also associated with a decrease in plasminogen activating factor release at endothelial cell level and an increased concentration of the VIII Willebrand factor, also as an answer from the injuries suffered by the endothelial cells. The result consists in increasing the platelets ability to aggregate that, once fixed on the vascular walls, will turn the arachidonic acid that still exists in their own membranes into A_2 thromboxane, the most powerful vessel constrictor and well-known factor of aggregating the platelets. These aggregated platelets and blood red cells will finally cause capillary occlusion and areas of ischemic retina [1, 2, 8].

5. The increased concentration of the A_1 glycosylated hemoglobin seems to be another mechanism in the pathogenesis of diabetic retinopathy. Ordinarily, the concentration of A_1 glycosylated hemoglobin represents 3–6% of the total hemoglobin. In diabetic patients, this level is up to 10–20%. When glycemia is increased, the glucose bounds to the amino groups of the proteins. The process is called glycation. Glycosylated hemoglobin can be easily quantified and compared with the help of the chromatography techniques. In A_1 glycosylated hemoglobin, the glucose stops the activity of the 2,3-diphosphoglycerate by releasing the oxygen out of the red blood cells. In spite of the natural transport of oxygen, retina gets hypoxic. In early diabetic retinopathy, the reduced capacity of the blood cells to deliver oxygen stimulates the self-regulated mechanisms that increase the blood flow. Later these mechanisms become insufficient [1, 2, 3, 20].

All these metabolic diabetic deviations eventually interfere in the alteration of the three capillary walls constituents. Thus, the capillary basal membrane thickens by depositing collagen and glycoproteins. The thickening degree of the basal membrane is strongly connected with long-standing disease, evolution and the level of glycemia. This hyalinization, especially at meta-arteriole level, will unavoidably and gradually obliterate the vascular lumen, thus slowing the blood flow and consecutively accentuating retinal hypoxia. The first vascular occlusions appear in the arteriolar sector followed later by capillary bed atrophy. The endothelial cells suffering from metabolic stress loose their role of blood-retinal barrier. Hyperglycemia causes a selective degenerescence of the microvascular intramural pericytes. The pericytes/endothelial cells ratio (usually 1) decreases. Therefore, the vascular tonus is altered.

All these alterations of the capillary wall determine chronic hypoxia and ischemia and together with microaneurysms, edema, hard and soft exudates and, finally, neovascular proliferation [1, 2, 3, 8].

The conclusion of the latest physiopathologic studies is that any of the earlier mentioned pathogenic mechanisms, and perhaps other still unknown processes, might initiate or accelerate diabetic retinopathy.

The diabetic retinopathy incidence depends on a range of risk factors:

– time of onset and duration;

– age;
– type of the diabetes mellitus;
– glycemic profile;
– renal diseases;
– arterial hypertension;
– pregnancy.

Referring to glycemia level, the authors' own remark, in over the 20 years long run steadily study, is that variations in glycemia play a tremendous role in the occurrence and especially the evolution of diabetic retinopathy. The day-timed curve of the glycemia that concentrates between +/–20mg seems to be an element of good prognostic of the disease [5].

CLINICAL ASPECTS OF DIABETIC RETINOPATHY

The main clinical signs of diabetic retinopathy are:
– decrease of the visual acuity. It varies depending on the degree of macular alteration. Visual acuity decreases or is lost in case of severe macular edema, macular hemorrhages, foveal neovascularization or macular detachment;
– pathological values of the contrast sensitivity, even when visual acuity is good and there are no ophthalmologic alterations;
– altered darkness adaptation that appears in the stage of nonproliferative retinopathy and gets more and more evident as soon as the retinopathy advances;
– the presence of the relative scotoma on visual field investigation is explained through the existence of non-perfusion areas. The morphological substratum of the perimetry alterations is represented by the retinal injuries by microangiopathy: hemorrhages, exudates, macular edema;
– chromatic sense disturbances are precocious in 40–50 % of the cases even before the retinopathy is evident and while the retinopathy is present, in 80% of the cases. The chromatic alterations correspond to the retinal injuries. Dyschromatopsia in blue-yellow axis is due to some selective decrease of the spectral sensitiveness to the blue light. In diabetes, the sensitivity of the blue color perceptive cones is affected. Red or green perceptive cones are not affected. Dyschromatopsia may become an obstacle for the suffering person when appreciating the level of the glycemia, at the colorimetric tests;
– the most important electrophysiological alterations are those noticed on electroretinogram. Even the diabetic patients without discernible retinopathy on ophthalmoscopy show a decrease in the amplitude of the oscillatory potentials. The a and b waves have a normal aspect. This can be explained starting from minimum ischemic phenomena at internal glandular layer level. The oscillatory potentials may be therefore a useful mark in the progression of retinopathy. As soon as retinopathy evolves the amplitude of the b wave decreases as well [1, 2, 8, 18].

From the clinical and histopathological point of view, the alteration of retinal capillaries in the diabetic microangiopathy covers a large range of aspects: microaneurysms, hemorrhages, edema, etc.

Microaneurysms are saccular dilatations of the capillary wall. They produce a red dot globe aspect on ophthalmoscopy. Usually they are close to the area of ischemic retina and have 15–50 microns in diameter; when associated with the initial dilatation of the capillary vessel their dimensions multiply by 2 or 3. They are more often situated on the venous side of the capillary web than on the arterial one. The majority of microaneurysms are encircled by a thin wall with a thin basal membrane and, sometimes, important hyaline PAS-positive deposits can be visible. Their occurrence is in close connection with the disappearance of pericytes. On fluorescein angiography, microaneurysms show a limited fluorescence with maximum intensity during arteriovenous time and disappearance during the tardive venous time. Their number is greater than what is visible on ophthalmoscopy. Microaneurysms may be difficult to differentiate from small, punctate hemorrhages also seen in early stages of diabetic retinopathy. On the early frames of the angiography, they are easily distinguished from intraretinal hemorrhages by their bright hyperfluorescence, whereas hemorrhages block fluorescence. An increased number of micro-aneurysms are associated with the progression of diabetic retinopathy [1, 2, 3] (Figures 45.1, 45.2, Plate 45.1).

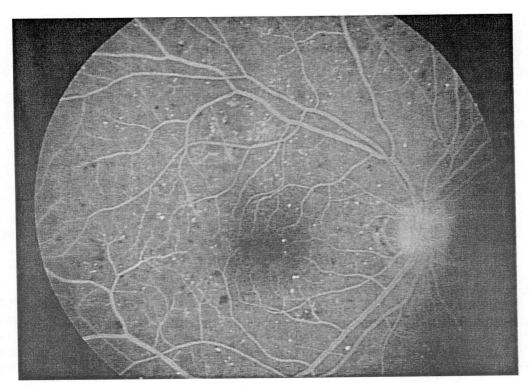

Figure 45.1
Non proliferative diabetic retinopathy FA (fluorescein angiography).

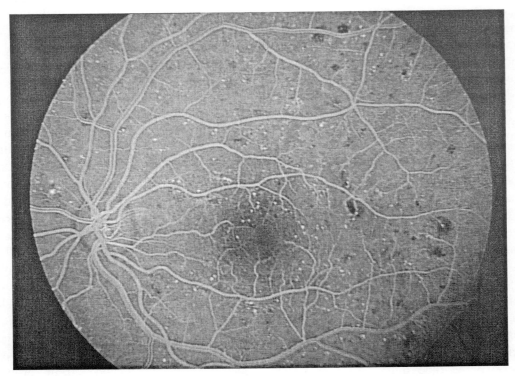

Figure 45.2
Non proliferative diabetic retinopathy FA (fluorescein angiography).

Hemorrhages are red cells conglomerates situated inside the granular layer that usually diffuse to the external plexiform layer and appear, when examined by ophthalmoscopy, as small round well shaped hemorrhages. In advanced stages of diabetic retinopathy, they may become confluent. The flame shaped hemorrhages, located in the nerve fibers layer, are present in advanced stages of the disease. Irrespective of the hemorrhage type, they induce an important macrophagic reaction, and their resorption may last for several weeks. The extensive hemorrhages result in alteration or tearing of the new vessels and develop preretinal or in the vitreous cavity. When examined by fluorescein angiography their aspect is as black spots and they hinder the fluorescence of the retina [2, 21].

The retinal edema has a starting point the disturbances of permeability of the retinal capillary vessels and in other types of injuries: microaneurysms or neo-formation vessels. The edema is a transudate accumulation in the outer plexiform layer. The accumulation of liquid extends the nervous fibers, tears the processes of Muller cells and progresses closer and closer. In the early stages, the macular edema is not ophthalmoscopically noticed. Later, the liquid accumulation goes to increasing the space between the anterior profile line and the posterior one. The thickening of the retina can be examined especially by biomicroscopy of posterior pole. The edema becomes evident on fluorescein angiography, in its debut stage, under the shape of a homogeneous fluorescein diffusion. On ophthalmoscopy, macular microcystic edema has a grey-whitish or yellow color and its angiofluorographic picture resembles "flower petals" around the macula, as a consequence of fluorescein accumulation in the perifoveal retinal cystic spaces [2, 21].

The transudate can be reabsorbed in several weeks, but once the chronic stage has set in, the transudate will be replaced together with the degeneration of retinal tissue, by an exudate.

From the histopathologic point of view, there are two types of exudates:

– Hard, dry exudates are localized in the outside layers, especially in the outside plexiform layer, where they dislocate nervous fibers. They are amorphous, rich in lipoproteins and glycolipids. On ophthalmoscopy, they look like white-yellowish shining, well marked spots with irregular margins. They are of small size and isolated, in the incipient stages of retinopathy; their tendency is to cluster around the capillary vessels or microaneurysms whose wall they have passed through. When the exudates are distributed around the fovea, they may form the aspect of a "macular star". The large size exudates may look hypofluorescent when examined by angiography while the small ones cannot be visualized [21]. The hard exudates may persist for months or even years, before they are gradually removed by the macrophages.

– The soft, "cotton wool", superficial exudates are larger than the hard ones and are not specific for diabetic retinopathy. They may also appear in the hypertensive retinopathy, venous occlusion, nephropathies. On ophthalmoscopy, they look like white-grayish nodules, with blurred margins, placed in the nerve fibers layer. The soft exudates are considered to be cytoplasmatic debris, located in the nerve fiber layer because of the blocked axoplasmatic flux, due to the micro-infarcts, situated at this level. They are more often found in the first stages of proliferative retinopathy, especially in the proximity of the optic nerve head, where the axons are larger and in greater number.

On fluorescein angiography, they cannot be noticed. These exudates usually disappear in weeks or months [1, 2, 3, 8, 21, 22].

The arterial and the arteriolar occlusions are not always visualized on ophthalmoscopy. They are visualized on fluorescein angiography when, beside the occlusion, appear large areas of capillary nonperfusion as well as narrowing or segmentary dilatations of the distal arterioles. The vascular modifications are more characteristic at the venous level, where even simple diffuse dilatations might be considered as a first sign of diabetic retinopathy [2, 21].

The veins dilatation is a sign of the increased blood flow need of a hypoxic retina. Later, the veins become tortuous, present constrictions and typical segmentary dilatations. At this moment, the fluorescein angiography points out large areas of ischemia in the retina. First, hypoxia determines capillary dilatation encircling the nonperfused areas. Later, a tearing of the blood retinal barrier appears and the exudates and hemorrhages become visible.

From the clinical point of view, the appearance of the neovascularization marks the entry in the proliferative stage of diabetic retinopathy. The new vessels, which are very fragile, have venous origin, though they might also form at the arteriolar level. Histologically, the new vessels are formed by the endothelial fenestrated cells and pericytes. In some areas, the vessels may have endothelial cells with a normal aspect or, some of them may have areas of necrosis. When diabetic retinopathy progresses, a fibrous membrane adds to the vascular component. Initially, the fibrovascular membrane is located intraretinally. Later it insinuates between the internal limiting membrane and the posterior hyaloid membrane, thus settling firm vitreoretinal adherences. Further on, the new vessels may get oriented from the retina to the vitreous, perpendicularly to the retinal plane, especially if posterior vitreous detachment appears. In addition, a preretinal hemorrhage may be present. The fibrous component plays the holder part for other new vessels to develop and it is responsible for the retinal tractions that appear in the stage of proliferative diabetic retinopathy.

Although new vessels may arise anywhere in the retina, they are most frequently seen posteriorly, within about 45 degrees of the optic disc.

The new vessels do not develop from the very beginning into the vitreous cavity; they are attracted into it, once the hinder detachment of the vitreous appears. Thus, the importance of the vitreous in the progression of the proliferative retinopathy is confirmed. The hinder detachment may determine as well some traction on the optic nerve or on the macula, both of them being important causes for visual acuity depreciation. The majority of the retinal detachments as part of the proliferative diabetic retinopathy is secondary and has the following characteristics:

– the presence of the newly formed fibrovascular membranes, located prior to the detached retina, adherent to it;

– the detached surface is situated with the concavity ahead;

– the progressive detachment might stand for months or even years and it does not suffer modifications at rest.

When a rhegmatogenous detachment appears, the ophthalmoscopic aspect is typical:

– the retinal prominence, colored grey-blue which becomes slightly wavy when the eye moves;

– the vessels have a dark color and the arteries cannot be differentiated from veins;

– the prominence of the detached retina changes depending on the age and the topography of the detachment or on the vitreous state of liquefaction and the extension of its posterior detachment (Plate 45.2).

The retinal tear is usually located at the posterior pole, near the areas presenting fibrovascular modifications.

The papillary new vessels originate at the level of the peripapillary arteriolar system. They develop both in parallel with the retina and ante-posterior to the vitreous and seem to be independent from other vessels of neoretinal formation. This neovascularization associated with large areas of non-perfusion around the optic nerve contains large vascular curls, well differentiated into afferent arteriolar and efferent venous trees. They divert a part of the sanguineous mass, which is intended to the retina, thus aggravating the hypoxia and creating a vicious circle. Irrespective of location, the new vessels are pointed out with the help of fluorescein angiography [1, 2, 3, 8, 21].

In conclusion, diabetic retinopathy can be classified into a preclinical stage without distinguishable modifications on ophthalmoscopy and a clinical stage when its symptoms are noticeable. The preclinical stage refers to the increase of the blood flow and to the alteration of the retinal capillary basal membrane. The clinical stage must be subdivided in nonproliferative diabetic retinopathy or background, preproliferative diabetic retinopathy and proliferative diabetic retinopathy.

The first pathological modifications that must be searched for during an ophthalmologic examination are within the nonproliferative diabetic retinopathy. The featured injuries comprise: microaneurysms, profound and superficial hemorrhages, hard profound exudates, outstanding modifications of the vascular lumen especially of the capillaries and veins, retinal or macular edema. The maculopathy, frequently found in non-insulin dependent patients, determine a decrease in visual acuity. It is the consequence of edema, hemorrhages or hard exudates located in the macular area. Although, usually it associates with severe cases of

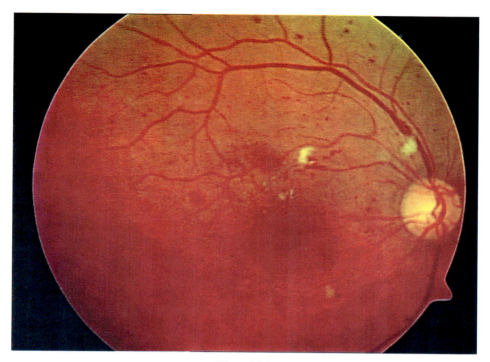

Plate 45.1
Nonproliferative diabetic retinopathy – Ophtalmoscopy.

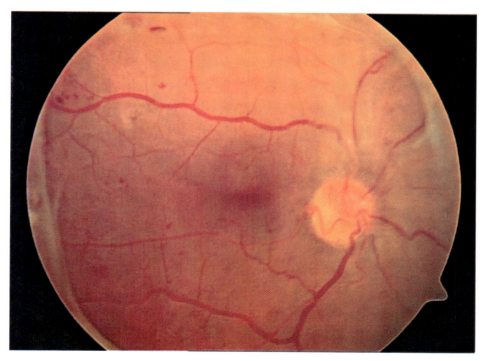

Plate 45.2
Proliferative diabetic retinopathy.

nonproliferative retinopathy, incidentally it may appear in diabetic patients suffering from minor microaneurysms or hemorrhages. Sometimes, the decrease in the visual acuity is due to a non-vascular fibrous epiretinal membrane that insinuates in the macular area between the internal limiting membrane and posterior hyaloid [1, 2, 3, 8].

The prognostic for the patients diagnosed with nonproliferative diabetic retinopathy is relatively good, only 3% of the patients suffering a severe decrease of their visual acuity [1, 2, 5].

The preproliferative diabetic retinopathy is mainly characterized by the accentuation of the retinal hypoxic and ischemic signs. The hemorrhages and hard exudates increase numerically. Exudates having a cotton-like aspect appear and they are a sign of altered nervous fibers; the arteries have increased reflex, the veins get swollen and of irregular caliber. Large nonperfused retinal areas are visualized on fluorescein angiography. In this stage the inner retinal microvascular anomalies, represented by the capillary shunts, are difficult to be differentiated from the possible neovessel shunts. Usually fluorescein does not diffuse, as is the case with new vessels. According to ETDRS (Early Treatment Diabetic Retinopathy Study), these alterations at the retinal level stand as an important risk factor for proliferative diabetic retinopathy development. About 50% of patients progress from preproliferative to proliferative disease in 12 to 24 months. That is why they should be under strict surveillance [1, 2, 5, 8].

The diagnosis of proliferative diabetic retinopathy is based on the presence of the new vessels as a sign of an important hypoxia. This neovascularization has a chronological progression and it may be from ophthalmologic and didactic point of view linked to three colors: red, pink and white.

Initially the red new vessels, characterized by a few fibrous tissues, are displayed on the inner surface of the retina. In the second stage both the neo-vessels and the fibrous tissue speedily develop. This fibro-vascular shape becomes pink. While the fibrous conjunctive tissue continues to develop, the vascular component gradually suffers a regression. The fibrous tissue condenses, contracts and gives a whitish aspect to the injury. There are cases when the proliferative retinopathy

is asymptomatic until a preretinal or intravitreal hemorrhage appears. In itself, the neovascularization rarely leads to a sudden and profound decrease of visual acuity if the vitreous stays attached [1, 2, 3, 5, 8].

CLASSIFICATION OF DIABETIC RETINOPATHY

The classification of diabetic retinopathy is generally based on the severity of intraretinal microvascular changes and the presence or absence of the retinal neovascularization.

In our opinion, three classifications are worth mentioning:
- **VAHEX** (L'Esperance and James);
- **ALFEDIAM** (French Association for Studying the Diabetes and Metabolic Diseases);
- **ETDRS** (Early Treatment Diabetic Retinopathy Study).

The **VAHEX** classification (V – venous dilatation, A – aneurisms, H – hemorrhages, E – edema, X – exudates) was proposed by L'Esperance and James and includes two important stages and an intermediary one. [1, 22] (Figure 45.3).

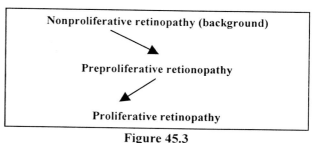

Figure 45.3
Stages of diabetic retinopathy.

Preproliferative retinopathy

Even today, after more than 20 years, the classification is still valid essentially for the diagnosis and therapeutic implications of the intermediary stage of preproliferative retinopathy as a progression stage from the background to the proliferative retinopathy.

This moment can be visualized on fluorescein angiography, when large ischemic areas and perivascular diffusion are present. At this time retinal panphotocoagulation is of utmost importance and really effective.

The **VAHEX** classification pays less importance to diabetic macular edema responsible for the important decrease of visual acuity.

It is worth remembering that, at that time, photocoagulation in the area within the inner temporal arcades was less considered.

The **ALFEDIAM** classification is used in France and other areas under French language influence. It includes two important categories of retinal interest in diabetes mellitus [1, 22].

A. the diabetic retinopathy

B. the diabetic maculopathy.

A. Diabetic retinopathy

According to **ALFEDIAM**, it reaches the following stages:

1. Minimum non proliferative diabetic retinopathy:

– clinical: limited number of microaneurysms and spotted retinal hemorrhages;

– fluorescein angiography: capillary micro-occlusions, localized intraretinal diffusion.

2. Moderate diabetic nonproliferative retinopathy:

– clinical: microaneurysms and spotted hemorrhages, a "flame" pattern, numerous venous anomalies (minimum in two quadrants), retinal "spotted" hemorrhages within the four quadrants;

– fluorescein angiography: localized ischemic retinal areas.

3. Severe diabetic non proliferative retinopathy (preproliferative):

– clinical: severe retinal hemorrhages within the four quadrants, venous anomalies in minimum two quadrants, numerous microaneurysms;

– fluorescein angiography: extended territories of retinal ischemia, diffusion

4. Proliferative diabetic retinopathy in debut:

– clinical: retinal new vessels of small size in one or more quadrants of the peripheral retina.

5. Moderate diabetic proliferative retinopathy:

– clinical: extended areas of neovascularization, measuring more than one half of the papillary diameter, extending in one or more quadrants, minimum papillary neovascularization.

6. Severe diabetic proliferative retinopathy:

– clinical: prepapillary important vascularization in addition to the signs from the previous stage.

7. Complicated proliferative diabetic retinopathy:

– preretinal and intraretinal hemorrhages;

– tractional retinal detachment (sometimes rhegmatogenous);

– rubeosis iridis, secondary neovascular glaucoma.

B. Diabetic Maculopathy

1. Edematous:

– focal macular edema with or without exudates;

– diffused macular edema – cystoid,
                              – noncystoid;

2. Ischemic.

The ALFEDIAM classification allows a precocious diabetic retinopathy diagnosis. A long subsequent follow up comprising of thorough examination, fluorescein angiography, retinal photographs, modification of the surveillance rhythm and indications of therapeutic intervention is recommended.

More complicated than ALFEDIAM, the ETDRS classification is pre-eminently used by the American or by the Anglo-Saxon School of Ophthalmology.

ETDRS Classification (Early Treatment Diabetic Retinopathy Study) starts with comparing the color stereo-pictures of the fundus seven areas [23, 24].

Retinal-photographs are taken under 30 degrees angle and are centered as follows:

– negative 1 – papilla;

– negative 2 – macula;

– negative 3 – temporal area of the macula;

– negative 4–7–tangents to a line situated at the superior and inferior margins of the papilla and a vertical line passing through the centre of the papilla (Figure 45.4 a, b).

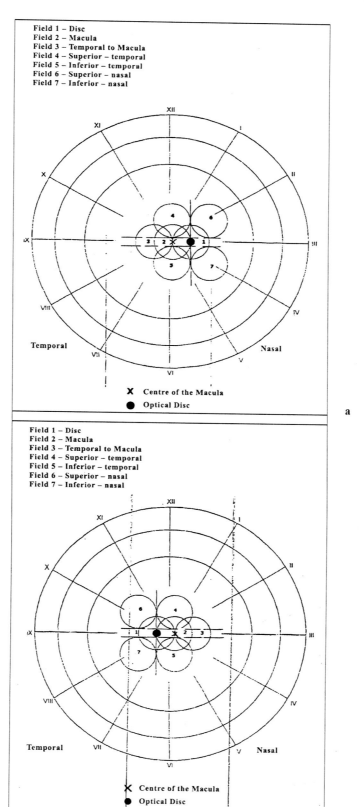

Figure 45.4
Retinal field.

The **EDTRS** classification:
– the absence of diabetic retinopathy;
– isolated microaneurysms;
– minimum nonproliferative diabetic retinopathy;
– moderate nonproliferative diabetic retinopathy;
– severe nonproliferative diabetic retinopathy;
– proliferative diabetic retinopathy in debut;
– moderate proliferative diabetic retinopathy;
– high-risked proliferative diabetic retinopathy;
– evolved proliferative diabetic retinopathy – partially visible fundus, undetached macula;
– evolved proliferative diabetic retinopathy, invisible fundus, detached macula;
– non-gradual diabetic retinopathy.

The authors used the **VAHEX** classification for a long period but the need to work according to the standards of the European States has determined to start using the **ETDRS** classification in the last 5 years, matching the rhythm of follow-up and of treatment with our own possibilities, as we further point out. In 1994, A. Barar suggested his personal approach inspired by **ETDRS**'s principles on diabetic retinopathy of follow-up and treatment [25]. It is simple and useful but, unfortunately, it has not been put into the Romanian ophthalmologic practical applications.

According to EDTRS, diabetic maculopathy is actually reduced to two stages:
– extrafoveal macular edema (ME)
– clinically significant macular edema (CSME) (Plates 45.3; 45.4).

The implications of the various diabetic retinopathy classifications are practically directed towards precocious diagnosis, treatment and follow-up.

Precocious diagnosis is linked on the compulsory ophthalmologic examination once a year for each diabetic or nondiabetic patient 40 or older (diabetes mellitus cases were diagnosed for the first time this way), yearly ophthalmoscopic or biomicroscopic fundus examination for each type 2 diabetic person registered and every 6 months examination for each registered type 1 diabetic patient. Newly diagnosed nonproliferative diabetic retinopathy intensifies the rhythm of examination with retina pictures every 6 months and fluorescein angiography once a year. Nonproliferative diabetic retinopathy does not require any special ophthalmologic treatment. Preproliferative diabetic retinopathy (ALFEDIAM's

severe nonproliferative diabetic retinopathy and EDTRS's severe nonproliferative diabetic retinopathy) and subsequent stages enforce ophthalmologic treatment together with a good metabolic control of diabetes and of the associated risk factors.

MANAGEMENT OF THE DIABETIC RETINOPATHY

The diabetic retinopathy treatment has as main purposes stopping the progression of the diabetic retinopathy and preserving visual acuity. Focusing on the purpose, the followings are necessary:
– combating the risk factors;
– precocious diagnosis;
– careful follow-up;
– a good metabolic control;
– other medical treatments (aspirin and antiplatelet treatments, lipid-lowering treatments, aldose reductase inhibitors, growth hormone inhibitors);
– panretinal laser photocoagulation;
– macular edema treatment;
– posterior vitrectomy;
– surgical treatment of cataract;
– neovascular secondary glaucoma treatment.

It is the ophthalmologist's task to precocious diagnose diabetic retinopathy (which may be done in any ophthalmologic unit provided with a minimal equipment), to follow up (the equipment is to be completed with fundus camera for retin photography and angiography) and finally, to perform laser treatment (blue-green ionized Argon, Krypton lasers for photocoagulation, frequency-doubled Neodymium: Yttrium-Aluminium-garnet, organic dye lasers). Surgical interventions require a special training and complete surgical equipment for vitreoretinal surgery [4, 26, 27].

Retinal panphotocoagulation is the best treatment for preproliferative retinopathy (severe nonproliferative) and of the proliferative retinopathy. At the beginning of the 80's photocoagulation was considered to destroy the hypoxic retina engendering angiogenic factors. Panphotocoagulation seems to achieve also a total posterior detachment of the vitreous, which stops the fibrovascular proliferation. A third assumption justifying panphotocoagulation is a better retina oxygenation with the oxygen normally diffusing from the choriocapillaris *via* the destroyed pigmented epithelium. Finally, the fourth theory assumes that pigmented retinal epithelium cells may produce growth-stimulating and/or growth-inhibiting factors and that the response to these cells to photocoagulation injury may change the balance of these factors. The four assumptions on panphotocoagulation – apparently all of them valid – lead to two ways of proceeding with panphotocoagulation:

a) Higher parameters, more aggressive, with laser impacts capable to destroy the retina until the VIII layer, destruction of the ischemic retinal territories and contraction of the internal limiting membrane in order to proceed to the detachment of the vitreous.

b) Less aggressive photocoagulation, sufficient to destroy the pigment epithelium, answering in this way the latter mentioned theories.

In practice, retinal panphotocoagulation is accomplished by the coagulation of the whole peripheral retina, except the area within the arch described by the large temporal vessels. The procedure is done in successive sessions, with laser impacts to permit a space among them not larger than the impact diameter; the number of the sessions is 4–6 or 8 within a 2–5 weeks period. Depending on the used parameters, between 250–800 impacts/session can be applied. The photocoagulation is best achieved when starting in inferior quadrants because of impaired visibility in these regions. The photocoagulated areas extend from the extreme periphery giving free access to the temporal vessels, respectively to the nasal margin of the papilla. A total number of 1 200–2 500 laser impacts may grant panphotocoagulation that is done in policlinics, in the obscure room, under the topic anesthesia rarely under retro-bulbar anesthesia; the laser treatment preparation includes, beside the consent of the patient who should be well informed, the maximum medical mydriasis. The used lasers are: (488–514 nm) blue-green Argon laser, (532 nm), Nd:YAG frequency doubled laser or 810 nm laser diodes. Rarely, may be used the dye laser (yellow-red) or (648 nm) the Krypton laser, especially when a vitreous hemorrhage is present or there are extended retinal hemorrhages. The way of the radiation delivery is done by adapting the laser to a biomicroscope with the help of a contact lens

(three mirrors Goldmann, Volk, panfunduscope Rodenstock, Mainster-Wide Field) or rarely by choosing an indirect ophthalmoscope. The choice of the contact lens directly influences in choosing the diameter of the laser beams; the diameter of the laser beam at the level of the retina is double the one displayed on panfundoscope or quadrisphere. In the concavity of the contact lens, a drop of methylcellulose will be instilled, before applying it to the eye not to permit the appearance of the air bubble that may spoil the visibility of the retina and also deform, diverge or alter the laser radiation [12, 13, 28, 29].

The parameters of the laser are:

– the dimension of the laser beam – as a rule, 500 μ is used for the periphery and 200 μ for the posterior pole. The type of lenses used will also be carefully considered;

– the time (the duration of the impact) – between 0.1 and 0.5 seconds, usually 0.2 sec;

– the intensity of the beam will be chosen so that from the three elements combination (diameter, time, intensity) to get a whitish well shaped spot on the retina. Anyway, the intensities will be between 100–500 milliwatt, more power being dangerous for the transparent mediums and for the retina.

– working organization: the modern lasers make possible that trains of impulses be applied or automatically released. The attention of the ophthalmologist should be special to avoid the sudden coagulation of the retinal vessels (Plate 45.5; 45.6).

A well-done photocoagulation will not generate negative secondary effects; the patient will only complain of a simple temporary immediate post-treatment impaired visual acuity. However, several secondary iatrogenic effects have to be noticed:

– increased intraocular pressure: due to the excessive pressure on the globe, especially when a session lasts excessively long;

– corneal epithelial defects by excessive manipulation of the lens on the surface of the cornea during photocoagulation;

– "spotted" or diffused crystalline lens opacity when using the laser at high energy;

– retinal hemorrhages or retinal vessels obstructions if sudden laser impacts are applied on retinal vessels;

– fibrous proliferation starting with the areas in which using high energies the tearing of the internal limiting membrane took place;
– alteration of scotopic visual field;
– altered dark adaptability;
– progression of lens opacities.

The above secondary effects are less important than letting diabetic retinopathy evolve. A correct photocoagulation leads to adequate control of the progressive diabetic retinopathy, by preserving and rarely by improving the visual acuity. Still, the patients should be warned about possible persistent secondary effects.

The failure in retinal neovascularization regression and the fibrous proliferation accentuation, as well as the occurrence of hemorrhages, implies a reevaluation of the case and a possible repetition of photocoagulation [2, 8].

A strange observation of ours, on patients subject to panphotocoagulation, who have had a good evolution in the latest 10 years, consists in the appearance of the pseudoexfoliation syndrome, four times more frequent than at the normal subjects. These eyes evolve similarly to those having normal pressure glaucoma.

In diabetic macular edema, laser photo-coagulation is one of the few available methods to determine functional and anatomic improvements. The optical coherence tomography, retin photography and fluorescein angiography prove together the importance of photocoagulation. Focal photocoagulation consists of multiple impacts over the entire macular edema area, with 100μ diameter, 0.10 seconds exposing time and the minimum energy necessary to get to a white spot [2, 30, 31, 32, 33].

Association of the macular edema with proliferative diabetic retinopathy represents a debatable problem. According to our experience in this case, the beginning should be with macular photocoagulation "grid" pattern and then, 4 to 8 laser sessions to cover the retinal periphery, as proceeding with any retinal panphotocoagulation. After the laser treatment, the patient is clinically and on fluorescein angiography examined, every three months in the first year and then every six months [2, 30, 31, 32, 33, 34].

Other treatment possibilities of chronic diabetic macular edema are:
– triamcinolone intravitreal injection;
– posterior vitrectomy and peeling of the internal limiting membrane.

The posterior vitrectomy or, in other words, vitreoretinal surgery for the diabetic retinopathy is currently recommended in:
– massive vitreous hemorrhages: vitrectomy is performed if it is not reabsorbed after 2–3 months, and the fundus cannot be examined or treated by laser;
– the tractional retinal detachment: when the macula is detached or just tracted;
– the mixed rhegmatogenous and tractional detachment of the retina: even when there is no macular detachment.

Other indications of the vitreoretinal surgery for diabetic retinopathy are:
– chronic non-responsive macular edema: internal limiting membrane peeling;
– preretinal fibrosis covering and tractioning the macula [35];
– persistent premacular hemorrhages;
– macular edema with hard and huge exudates intraretinal or beneath the retina;
– red blood cell-induced (erythroclastic) glaucoma;
– cataract and vitreous hemorrhage precluding a view of posterior segment complications [2, 36, 37, 38, 39].

The purpose of the vitrectomy is:
– Replacement of the opaque vitreous;
– Eliminating the antero-posterior vitreoretinal and tangential tractions;
– Detached retina reapplication;
– Control upon the bleeding sources by using the endophotocoagulation, endodiathermy or simply by internal tamponade;
– Completing the pre-surgery retinal pan-photocoagulation;
– Cryocoagulation of the retinal extreme periphery, which is inaccessible to the photocoagulation.

The choice for vitreoretinal surgery should seriously take into account the risks to benefits ratio, considering on the one hand the difficulties of the vitreoretinal surgery, and on the other hand le mot d'esprit: "an inadequate surgery can cause a greater disaster than the disease itself" [1, 2, 22].

CATARACT AND DIABETES MELLITUS

Refraction alterations and diabetic cataract represent the two most important alterations of the

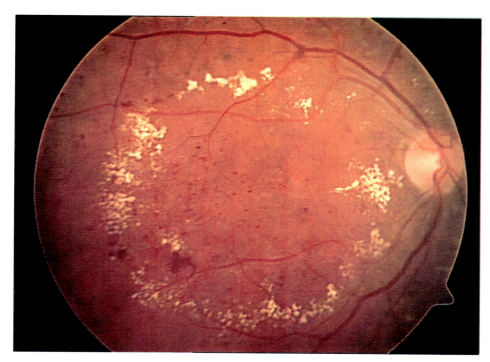

Plate 45.3
Extrafoveal macular edema.

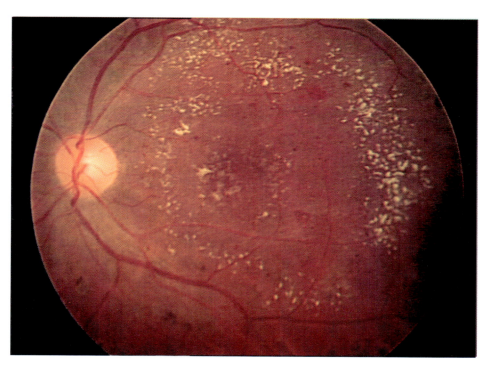

Plate 45.4
Clinically significant macular edema.

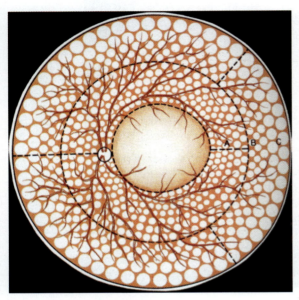

Plate 45.5

Principles of panretinal photocoagulation.

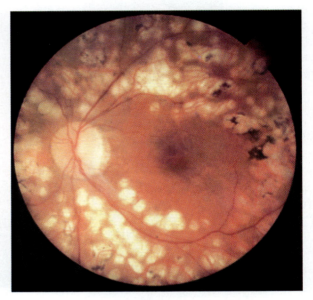

Plate 45.6

Panretinal photocoagulation.

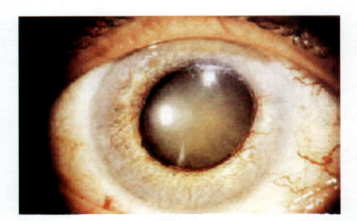

Plate 45.7

Severe *rubeosis iridis*.

lens in diabetes mellitus. Refraction changes are often quickly reversible in diabetic patients. A long running hyperglycemia can be the explanation for transitory myopia or, conversely, excessive reduction of the blood glucose level can cause hypermetropia.

The diabetic cataract was probably the most elaborately studied experimental cataract. The reason is the aldose reductase, the enzyme suspected of initiating the cataractogenic process [1, 2, 8]. The concept assuming as a basis aldose reductase developed 25 years ago when Van Heyningen put into evidence the presence of sorbitol in the lens of diabetic rats. Later, also experimentally, it was demonstrated how the aldose reductase enzyme initiates the disorders at the lens level leading to the occurrence of diabetic cataract. The first noticed alteration is represented by the appearance of some vacuoles at the periphery of the lens that later tend to agglomerate at the level of the anterior cortical. Successively, a dense nuclear opacity may appear. The vacuoles are actually altered fibers of the lens. Under aldose reductase action, the glucose is crystallized into sorbitol accumulating at the level of the lens fibers. Usually, polyols do not easily penetrate biological membranes; that is why if they are not quickly metabolized, they might accumulate, causing an increase in cellular osmosis. Such a created hypertonicity is corrected by a corresponding influx of water determining the vacuolization of the fibers. Successively, other important alterations on the permeability of the membrane lacking its amino acids, potassium ions and myoinositol happen; usually they have a greater concentration in the lens than in the aqueous humor. The accumulation in sodium and chlorine and the other main electrolytic alterations will cause finally opacification of the lens. To conclude, we remark that the biochemical alterations noticed at the begining stage of the diabetic cataract are caused by the osmotic modifications following the sorbitol accumulation.

From the clinical viewpoint, three forms of cataract might be individualized:

– the "real" diabetic cataract appearing rarely on young patients under the form of some posterior subcapsular opacity because of a serious diabetes with a rapid evolution. The distinctive character of the cataract consists of a rapid bilateral involvement, sometimes in hours or days, being more extended on the surface than in the deeper layers. The most typical shape of the opacities is compared to a "snow storm" consisting in white and grey snowflakes, which are located subcapsular, posteriorly or anteriorly. The most frequent shape is in "the posterior plate" causing an important decrease of visual acuity. Sometimes the whole process may have the aspect of a "juicy milk" cataract. At children, the first sign is frequently a white pupil (leukocoria);

– the senile cataract occurring in diabetic patients is hard to differentiate from both the clinical and the histopathological point of view, from the senile forms, which are encountered in the nondiabetic population. If brown nuclear compact forms or a posterior subcapsular opacity are present, we might think about a possible diabetic factor. The senile cataract appears precociously at diabetic patients and evolves more rapidly. It is the most frequent form of diabetic cataract. Sometimes, the opaqueness of the lens may partially disappear due to an adequate correction of glycemia;

– the cataract which may appear in dormant diabetes has a bilateral evolution and is present in middle-aged patients, 40–60 years old. The patient generally feels well but there is usually a slight tendency to develop obesity. The glycemia may seem to be in the normal standard but facing a patient with diabetic heredity, the test of the induced hyperglycemia is highly recommended.

Besides these three forms of cataract, diabetic patients may present also a type of cataract with the iatrogenic elements. This is due to the accelerated evolution of an incipient cataract in a patient after panphotocoagulation, as well as the cataract consecutive to posterior vitrectomy.

The attitude towards diabetic cataract does not differ from the attitude towards other types of cataract: the extraction of the lens by phacoemulsification with the posterior chamber implant of an intraocular artificial lens. It is preferable to use lenses with large diameter (6mm or more) and to avoid, as much as possible, intraoperative tearing of the posterior capsule. Cataract surgery does not influence the evolution of diabetic retinopathy; on the contrary, the intraoperative complications happening during the cataract surgery (tearing of the capsule, posterior luxation of lens material, injury of the iris) might accelerate the evolution of diabetic retinopathy.

The impossibility to finish with retinal panphotocoagulation, due to lens opacities, calls for crystalline lens extraction with IOL intrasaccular implant followed complete retinal photocoagulation. The cataract and posterior vitrectomy represented for a long time a problem with several disputed solutions:

– surgery in sequence: cataract surgery and then posterior vitrectomy;

– surgery in sequences: posterior vitrectomy followed by cataract surgery some time later;

– simultaneous surgery (the combination cataract extraction – vitrectomy). This third choice is in our opinion better: moving away the lens even if it is partially opaque is a necessary solution to have a good intraoperative control of the fundus during the vitreoretinal surgery. On the other hand, the cataractogenous effect of the vitrectomy – even it is well performed – pleads for mixed surgery [2, 8, 40, 41, 42].

GLAUCOMA AND DIABETES

Traditionally, diabetes mellitus was not registered among the risk factors of the primary glaucoma; however, today when the role of ocular blood flow in the pathogenesis of the glaucoma became very important, the possible glaucoma-diabetes mellitus correlations should be reevaluated.

Diabetes mellitus is one of the main causes of secondary neovascular glaucoma. The angiogenic factors generated by the ischemic retina play the essential role. They are capable to diffuse to the anterior segment and generate iris neovascularization. The iris rubeosis represents the initial stage of secondary neovascular glaucoma; yet some cases of rubeosis iridis are not progressive. That is why an identification of the two entities should be avoided. The iris neovascularization starts from the iris venula, without any rule – from the level of the pupil, from the level of the angle or simultaneously. A fine preirian fibrous membrane appears later, invading the angle. The rubeosis iridis frequency is 5% in patients without diabetic proliferative retinopathy, and 43–65% in patients suffering from proliferative retinopathy [1, 2, 3, 8] (Plate 45.7).

Rubeosis iridis treatment includes retinal panphotocoagulation and possible vitreo-retinal surgery. The photocoagulation attempts on the iris vessels proved inefficient. A viable alternative used by the authors, represents the microdissection of the preirian fibrous membrane during vitreoretinal surgery. The evolution of the rubeosis iridis towards invading the angle leads to secondary neovascular glaucoma, characterized by the painful red eye, a severe decrease of the visual acuity, increased intraocular pressure, corneal edema, florid rubeosis iridis and pupil distortion [41, 43].

The treatment outcome in these cases is limited; if retinal panphotocoagulation is not possible retinal transcleral pancryocoagulation should be performed. The medical treatment is not efficient, yet, it is important to note that pilocarpine is counter indicated. In addition, the topic administration of acetazolamide inhibitors, beta-blockers, mydriatics is also avoided. The surgical treatment – filtering procedures using antimetabolites or artificial drainage shunts gives a limited and transient efficiency. In our opinion, more efficient are the cyclodestructive – cryo or laser proceedings. Anyhow, these eyes are often not functional anymore, and for calming pains generated by high intraocular pressure, retrobulbar alcohol injection or enucleation, are necessary [8, 43, 44, 45, 46].

In this subchapter, we come back to our remark on the occurrence of the pseudoexfoliation syndrome of which 80% of the laser treated patients suffer from. With a good evolution after more than ten years since they have been subjected to panphotocoagulation, in spite of a normal eye tension, a good visual acuity and normal ophthalmoscopic aspect and fluorescein angiography result on retina, the above patients developed obvious ischemia of the optic nerve and approached the evolution towards normal tension glaucoma.

Further studies are needed to clarify these remarks, especially if confirmed by other authors.

We have insisted on three of the most important ocular symptoms of diabetes mellitus, mainly due to their dramatic implications on the visual functions. We think that other symptoms (mentioned in Table 45.1) are also products of diabetic microangiopathy.

To conclude, diabetes mellitus is one of the most important diseases among the ophthalmologic illnesses, and it might generate a new branch of ophthalmologic science – ophtalmo-diabetology.

REFERENCES

1. Massin P, Erginay A, Gaudric, A. *Retinopathie diabetique*, Elsevier, 2000.
2. Ryan JS. *Retina*, Mosby, 2001
3. Bălă R. *Manifestări oculare în diabetul zaharat*, Referat teză doctorat, UMF, Bucureşti, 2002.
4. Klein R. Barriers to prevention of vision loss caused by diabetic retinopathy. *Arch Ophthalmol*, 115: 1073–1075, 1997.
5. Cârstocea B, Gafencu LO, Lazanu R. 12 ani de experienţă clinică în tratamentul retinopatiei diabetice. *Revista de Medicină Militară*, 4: 23–32,1994.
6. Cârstocea B. Afecţiuni vasculare ale ochiului şi anexelor. In: Olteanu M (ed). *Tratat de Oftalmologie*, Ed. Medicală, Bucureşti, 1988.
7. Cârstocea B, Apostol S. Noi aspecte în patologia şi tratamentul retinopatiei diabetice. *Jurnalul Medicinii Româneşti*, 5: 48–60,1994.
8. Kanski J J. *Clinical Ophthalmology, a Systematic Approach*, Butterworth-Heinemann, 2000, 466.
9. Van den Enden MK, Nyengaard JR, Ostrow E, Burgan JH, Williamson JR. Elevated glucose levels increase retinal glycolysis and sorbitol pathway metabolism: implications for diabetic retinopathy. *Invest Ophthalmol Vis Sci*, 36: 1675–1685, 1995.
10. Williamson JR, Chang K, Franzos M, Hasan ES, Ido Y, Kawamura T, Ntengaard JR, van den Enden M, Kilo C, Tilton RG. Hyperglycemic pseudohypoxia and diabetic complications. *Diabetes,* 42: 801–813, 1993.
11. Vinores SA, Kuchle M, Mahlow J, Chiu C, Green WR, Campochiaro PA. Blood-ocular barrier breakdown in eyes with ocular melanoma: a potential role for vascular endothelial factor/vascular permeability factor. *Am J Pathol*, 147: 1289–1297, 1995.
12. Cârstocea B. Laseri româneşti în Oftalmologie. Teză de doctorat. UMF. Bucureşti, 1991.
13. Dumitra CD. *Biofotonica. Bazele fizice ale aplicaţiilor laserilor în medicină şi biologie*, Ed. All Media, Bucuresti, 1999.
14. Aiello LP, Avery RL, Thieme HH, Iwamoto MA, Park JE, Nguen HV, Arrigg PG, Keyt BA, Jampel HD, Shah ST, Pasquale RL, Aiello LM, Ferrara N, King GL. Vascular endothelial growth factor in ocular fluid of the patients with diabetic retinopathy and other retinal disorders. *N Engl J Med*, 331: 1480–1487, 1994.
15. Aiello LP, Northrup JM, Keyt BA, Takagi H, Iwamoto MA. Hypoxic regulation of vascular endothelial growth factor in retinal cells. *Arch Ophthalmol*, 113: 1538–1544, 1995.
16. Lutty GA, McLeod DS, Merges C, Diggs A, Plouet J. Localization of vascular endothelial growth factor in human retina and choroids. *Arch Ophthalmol*, 114: 971–977, 1996.
17. Hanneken A, de Juan E Jr, Lutty GA, Fox GM, Schiffer S, Hjelmeland LM. Altered distribution of basic fibroblast growth factor in diabetic retinopathy. *Arch Ophthalmol* 109: 1005–1911, 1991.
18. Olteanu M, Cârstocea B Dordea S. Retinopatia diabetică-clasificare, etiopatogenie, tratament. *Oftalmologia*, 3: 34–39, 1982.
19. Smith LEH, Kopchick JJ, Chen W, Knapp J, Kinose F, Daley D, Foley E, Smith RG, Shaeffer JM. Essential role of growth hormone in ischemia-induced retinal neovascularization. *Science,* 276: 1706–1709, 1997.
20. Diabetes Control and Complications Trial Research Group. The relationship of glycemic exposures (HbA$_1$C) to the risk of development and progression of retinopathy in Diabetes Control and Complications Trial. *Diabetes,* 44: 968–983, 1995.
21. Cohen YH, Quentel G. *Diagnostic angiographique des maladies retiniennes*, Elsevier, Paris, 1997.
22. Massin P, Angioi-Duprez K, Bacin F, *et al.* Recomandations de L'Alfediam. Depistage, surveillance et traitement de la retinopathie diabetique. *Diab Metab*, 22: 203–209, 1996.
23. Early Treatment Diabetic Retinopathy Study Research Group: Early Treatment Diabetic Retinopathy Study design and baseline patient characteristics, EDTRS report no. 7. *Ophthalmology,* 98: 741–756, 1991.
24. Early Treatment Diabetic Retinopathy Study Research Group. Fundus photographic risk factors for progression of diabetic retinopathy, EDTRS report no.12. *Ophthalmology,* 98: 822–823, 1991.
25. Barar A. Model de fişă de urmărire a retinopatiei diabetice în vederea tratamentului. *Soc Rom De Oftalmologie*, Craiova, 1994.
26. UK Prospective Diabetes Study (UKPDS) Group. Intensive blood-glucose control with sulphonylureas or insulin compared with conventional treatment and risk of complications in patients with type 2 diabetes (UKPDS 33). *Lancet,* 352: 837–853, 1998.
27. UK Prospective Diabetes Study Group. Tight blood pressure control and risk of macrovascular and microvascular complications in type 2 diabetes: UKPDS 38. *BMJ,* 317: 703–713, 1998.
28. Early Treatment Diabetic Retinopathy Study Research Group. Early photocoagulation for diabetic retinopathy, EDTRS report no. 9. *Ophthalmology,* 98: 767–785, 1991.

29. Ferris F. Early photocoagulation in patients with either type I or type II diabetes. *Trans Am Ophthalmol Soc*, **94**: 505–537, 1996.

30. Early Treatment Diabetic Retinopathy Study Research Group. Photocoagulation for diabetic macular edema, EDTRS report no. 4. *Int Ophthalmol Clin*, **27**: 265–272, 1987.

31. Early treatment Diabetic Retinopathy Study Research Group. Techniques for scatter and local photocoagulation treatment of diabetic retinopathy, EDTRS report no. 3. *Int Ophthalmol Clin*, **27**: 254–264, 1987.

32. Early Treatment Diabetic Retinopathy Study Research Group. Treatment techniques and clinical guidelines for photocoagulation of diabetic macular edema, EDTRS report no 2. *Ophthalmology*, **94**: 761–774, 1987.

33. Early Treatment Diabetic Retinopathy Study Research Group. Photocoagulation for diabetic macular edema: relationship of treatment effect to fluorescein angiographic and other retinal characteristics at baseline, EDTRS report no. 19. *Arch Ophthalmol*, **113**: 1114–1115, 1995.

34. Vender JF, Ducker JS, Benson WE, Brown GC, McNamara JA, Rosenstein RB. Long –term stability and visual outcome after favorable initial response of proliferative diabetic retinopathy to panretinal photocoagulation. *Ophthalmology*, **98**: 1575–1579, 1991.

35. Lewis H, Abrams GW, Blumenkranz MS, Campo RV. Vitrectomy for diabetic macular edema associated with posterior hyaloidal traction. *Ophthalmology*, **99**: 753–759, 1992.

36. Diabetic Retinopathy Vitrectomy Study Research Group. Early vitrectomy for severe vitreous hemorrhage in diabetic retinopathy: two-year results of a randomized clinical trial. Diabetic Retinopathy Vitrectomy Study report no. 2. *Arch Ophthalmol*, **103**: 1644–1652, 1985.

37. Diabetic Retinopathy Vitrectomy Study Research Group. Early vitrectomy for severe proliferative diabetic retinopathy in eyes with useful vision: clinical application of results of a randomized trial. Diabetic Retinopathy Study report no. 4. *Ophthalmology*, **95**: 1321–1334, 1988.

38. Diabetic Retinopathy Vitrectomy Study Research Group. Early vitrectomy for severe proliferative diabetic retinopathy in eyes with useful vision: results of a randomized trial. Diabetic Retinopathy Vitrectomy Study report no.3. *Ophthalmology*, **95**: 1307–1320, 1988.

39. Diabetic Retinopathy Vitrectomy Study Research Study Group. Early vitrectomy for severe vitreous hemorrhage in diabetic retinopathy: four-year results of a randomized trial. Diabetic Retinopathy Study report no. 5. *Arch Ophthalmol*, **108**: 958–964, 1990.

40. Foster RE, Lowder C, Meisler DM, Zakov ZN, Meyers SM, Ambler JS. Combined extracapsular cataract extraction, posterior chamber intraocular lens implantation and pars plana vitrectomy. *Ophthalmic Surg*, **24**: 446–452, 1993.

41. Abrams GW. *En bloc* dissection techniques in vitrectomy for diabetic retinopathy. In Lewis H, Ryan SJ (eds). *Medical and surgical retina: advances, controversies and management*, St. Louis, Mosby, 1994.

42. Kokame GT, Flynn HW Jr, Blankership GW. Posterior chamber intraocular lens implantation during diabetic par splana vitrectomy. *Ophthalmology*, **96**: 603–610, 1989.

43. Olteanu M, Cârstocea B, Bărăcan C. Locul criocoagulării în tratamentul retinopatiei diabetice. *Oftalmologia*, **3**: 47–56, 1983.

44. Tsai JC, Bloom PA, Franks WA, Khaw PT. Combined transscleral diode laser cyclophoto-coagulation and transscleral retinal photo-coagulation for refractory neovascular glaucoma. *Retina*, **16**: 164–166, 1996.

45. Chew EY, Ferris FL 3rd, Csaky KG, Murphy RP, Agron E, Thompson DJ, Reed GF, Schachat AP. The long-term effects of laser photocoagulation treatment in patients with diabetic retinopathy: the early treatment diabetic retinopathy follow-up study. *Ophthalmology*, **110**: 1683–9, 2003.

46. Browning DJ. Positioning the obese or large-breasted patient for macular laser photo-coagulation. *Am J Ophthalmol*, **137**: 178–9, 2004.

46

CUTANEOUS VASCULAR INVOLVEMENT IN DIABETES MELLITUS

Ioan NEDELCU, Irina MĂRGĂRITESCU, Laura-Elena NEDELCU

The incidence of cutaneous-mucosal manifestations in diabetes mellitus patients was differently appreciated. The physiopathologic mechanisms responsible for the cutaneous-mucosal manifestations in diabetes mellitus patients are similar to those involved in the diabetes mellitus general physiopathology.

Diabetic dermopathy

The existence of a correlation between the presence of diabetic dermopathy and the severity of diabetes, as well as between the antidiabetic therapy and diabetic dermopathy evolution was noticed.

Peri-vascular inflammatory infiltrates, with the accumulation of lymphocytes, are described in older lesions of diabetic dermopathy. Diabetic dermopathy lesions, especially when localized at the lower legs, impose the differential diagnosis with necrobiosis lipoidica.

Facial erythrosis

This clinical aspect defines the situation of a patient with long term evolution of overt diabetes mellitus. Initially considered as the exclusive appendage of overt diabetes mellitus, the involvement of latent diabetes, and even the predilection for juvenile-onset diabetes, were both demonstrated.

Purpuric dermatitis of the lower legs

Purpuric lesions and hemosiderin pigmentation intermingle with clinical manifestations of diabetic dermopathy, displaying a polymorphous clinical aspect, which is highly evocative for the diagnosis.

Diabetic necrosis

Diabetic gangrene is a frequent clinical feature in diabetic patients with advanced angiopathy.

Nail folds telangiectasia of the diabetic patient

The nail bed is used for *in vivo* investigation, through capillaroscopy, of cutaneous micro-vascularization. Capillaroscopy studies confirmed that venous dilatation of the periungual microcirculation may be a valuable indicator in the study of functional microangiopathy, while venular tortuosity offers extremely valuable information on the diabetic structural microangiopathy. Venous dilatation of the periungual microcirculation represents a good indicator of diabetic microangiopathy, but needs to be differentiated from nails folds venular dilatations in connective tissue diseases.

Erysipelas-like erythema of diabetics

Prognostic and evolution significance of diabetic erysipelas-like erythema may be severe, with possible appearance of more or less extensive diabetic gangrenes.

Necrobiosis lipoidica diabeticorum

Usually, lesions of necrobiosis lipoidica diabeticorum are asymptomatic plaques, but in rare cases patients may claim pruritus, burning , tenderness, hypohidrosis, etc.

Necrobiosis lipoidica plaques' evolution is slightly progressive, covering large, extensive surfaces, generating an impressive clinical aspect. Even if the evolution of necrobiosis lipoidica diabeticorum seems to be independent of glycemia level and antidiabetic treatment, recent studies show that a good treatment of diabetes mellitus can reduce the appearance of necrobiosis lipoidica lesions.

The relationship between necrobiosis lipoidica and overt diabetes mellitus may be proved in 60-65% of cases. 90% of the patients with necrobiosis lipoidica but without overt diabetes mellitus have a modified response to glucose tolerance test, either enhanced with cortisone or not, or possess significant familial antecedents for diabetes. Based on arguments such as the relatively low incidence of necrobiosis lipoidica in diabetes mellitus patients, the existence of good clinical response to different therapies without effect in diabetes mellitus, the association of necrobiosis lipoidica with other diseases, and the lack of any correlation between the extension and the clinical expression of necrobiosis lipoidica and the severity of diabetes mellitus, we consider that the direct linkage between necrobiosis lipoidica lesions and diabetes mellitus is at least debatable.

The skin suffering in diabetes mellitus is a polymorphous one, both in what concerns clinical manifestations, and the physiopathologic significance [1, 2]. Cutaneous lesions may constitute, rather frequently, the first sign of disease and their recognition, by the informed physician, plays a significant role in early diagnosis of a clinically unrecognized diabetes mellitus [2, 3, 4].

Long-term diabetic metabolic sufferance may induce cutaneous manifestations, often with severe significance, sometimes with vital risk, and their identification allows a right prognostic and therapeutic evaluation in the proper case.

Statistic-oriented studies reported various percents, sometimes important, of cases in which the identification of some cutaneous manifestations allowed the diagnosis of a clinically ignored diabetes mellitus [2, 4, 5, 6, 8], but the link between those and diabetes seems to be more or less specific. These affections might be regarded as complications of diabetes, or as proofs of existence of glycoregulation disturbance [5, 7, 8, 9].

The incidence of cutaneous-mucosal manifesttations in diabetic patients was differently appreciated. Recent studies [10] imposed the idea that the cutaneous manifestations are present in at least 2/3 of the diabetes mellitus patients, both in type 1 and in type 2 diabetes.

Regarding the report between the precocity of cutaneous-mucosal lesions appearance and the moment of diabetes onset, it is considered that 80% of lesions are present in the first 5 years of evolution [8, 11].

The physiopathologic mechanisms responsible for the cutaneous-mucosal manifestations appearance in diabetes are similar to those involved in the diabetes mellitus general physiopathology and discussed in the physiopathology chapter.

It is difficult to classify the diabetes mellitus-related cutaneous-mucosal lesions, mainly because of their clinical and physiopathologic polymorphism [12, 13, 14], but also because of very numerous criteria possible to be elected for classification. A didactical and nosologic satisfactory classification is the one proposed next [2, 9, 15] (Table 46.1).

Analyzing this classification from the point of view of involved pathophysiology, we consider the opportunity of a detailed description of cutaneous manifestations induced by the vascular mechanism.

DIABETIC DERMOPATHY
(syn. "shin spots" dermopathy, spotted legs syndrome, pretibial pigmented spots)

Diabetic dermopathy is a rather frequently encountered clinical manifestation, as shown by its numerous synonyms. It is most often present at the lower legs skin level, but it is possible to be present in other cutaneous territories, such as forearms, thighs, and, generally, the skin that covers bony prominences [6].

Because of its high frequency, diabetic dermopathy is considered to be the most common and the most frequently encountered cutaneous manifestation in diabetes mellitus [3, 16], in many cases representing, in fact, the first clinical manifestation of diabetes mellitus.

Clinically, diabetic dermopathy is characterized by the presence of hyper-pigmented, atrophic round-oval or slightly polygonal shaped, with relatively clear borders maculae, having the diameter between a few millimeters and a few centimeters, and electively distributed on the anterior side of the lower leg, but being possible to appear in other skin areas, such as thighs, or the skin that covers the bony prominences such as that of forearms (Plate 46.1).

The aspect of primitive cutaneous lesion in diabetic dermopathy is at the beginning that of a round-oval shaped papule, dark-red colored, which slowly grows in surface as it is getting older, until it becomes a 1–2 centimeters erythematous or erythemato-vesiculous plaque (Plate 46.2).

At maturity, those plaques develop a light brown colour, with relatively irregular borders and become superficial, frequently with a bilateral, asymmetric distribution on the affected extremities. In some patients, a linear distribution of plaques was described. The surface is depressible; the plaques are not painful and not itchy [17, 18].

The final brown colour of cutaneous lesions in diabetic dermopathy was attributed to the presence of hemosiderin in the perivascular histiocytes [3, 6, 19].

The natural evolution of diabetic dermopathy's cutaneous lesions is to progressive healing in 12 to 18 months, without ulceration, but because the slow healing process is associated with the appearance of new lesions, an overall quasi-stationary clinical picture is established, the so-called "permanently spotted shin" [17, 18, 20].

Table 46.1

The didactical classification of diabetes mellitus-related cutaneous-mucosal lesions

1. Cutaneous infections in diabetic patients;
2. Cutaneous lesions induced by vascular disturbances:
a) Diabetic microangiopathy:
– Diabetic dermopathy;
– Facial erythrosis (rubeosis);
– Purpuric dermatitis of the lower limbs;
– Periungual telangiectasia;
– Erysipelas-like erythema;
– Necrobiosis lipoidica diabeticorum.
b) Diabetic macroangiopathy:
– Lower limbs ischemic gangrene.
c) Diabetic micro- and microangiopathy:
– Diabetic ischemic acral complex.
3. Diabetes mellitus dermal manifestations:
a) Diabetic thick skin;
b) Diabetic yellow skin.
4. Lesions induced by neurological disturbances (diabetic neuropathy):
a) Diabetic neuropathic acral complex;
b) Diabetic bullous dermatosis.
5. Cutaneous manifestations induced by diabetic metabolic disturbances:
a) Fatty metabolism disturbances:
– Xanthomas;
– Xanthelasma.
b) Carotene metabolism disturbances:
– Cutaneous carotenemia (xanthosis diabetica, carotenosis).
6. Anti-diabetic treatment complications:
a) Insulin lipodystrophy:
– Insulin lipoatrophy;
– Insulin lipohypertrophy.
b) Diabetic keloid;
c) Allergic cutaneous reactions induced by anti-diabetic medications (anti-diabetic sulphamides, insulin);
d) Hematologic alterations (thrombocytopenia);
e) Alcohol ingestion vascular syndrome;
f) Other local reactions to insulin injection:
– Erythema;
– Hemorrhagic necrosis.
g) Insulin induced edema.
7. Diabetes mellitus associated lipodystrophy syndromes:
a) Lawrence- Seip syndrome (lipoatrophic diabetes, total lipoatrophy);
b) Partial lipoatrophy (progressive lipodystrophy).
8. Significant morbid associations:
– *Granuloma annulare*;
– *Acanthosis nigricans*;
– Hemochromatosis;
– *Porphyria cutanea tarda*;
– Werner's syndrome;
– Acromegaly;
– Mauriac's syndrome;
– Achard-Thiers syndrome;
– Migrating necrolytic erythema;
– Skin tags (acrochordons);
– Kyrle's disease.
9. Occasional associations:
– Vitiligo;
– Urbach-White lipoproteinosis;
– Scleredema of Buschke;
– Dupuytren disease;
– Peyronie disease;
– *Pseudoxanthoma elasticum*;
– Calciphylaxis;
– *Lichen planus*.
10. Diabetes mellitus and pruritus.

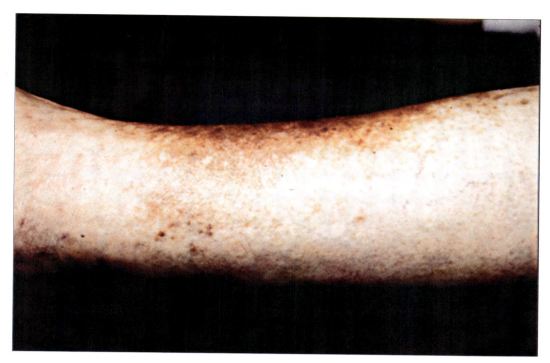

Plate 46.1
Diabetic dermopathy – "shin spots".

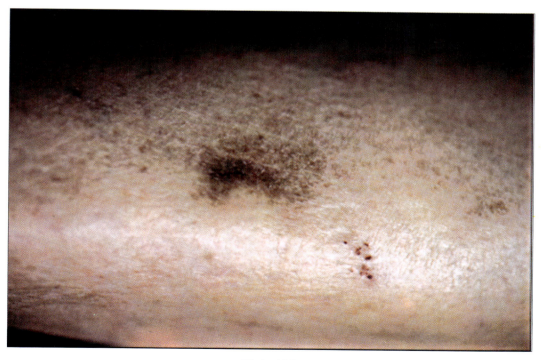

Plate 46.2
Diabetic dermopathy – "shin spots" – early lesion.

Diabetic dermopathy is noticed in almost 50% of diabetes patients, after the age of 30, and most often in male (male/female – 2/1) [3].

Regarding the genesis of diabetic dermopathy, according to data in literature, one may appreciate that cutaneous lesions are more frequent as the history of diabetes is longer [21, 22], without being able to formulate a diabetes-specific cause-effect relationship. The existence of a correlation between the presence of diabetic dermopathy and the severity of diabetes, or between the anti-diabetic therapy and diabetic dermopathy evolution was not noticed [8, 15].

The initial description of diabetic dermopathy lesions, done by Melin, in 1964 [23], did not mention the existence of pre-existent cutaneous disturbances in the distribution area (trauma, piodermitis, etc.) [21, 23].

Recent studies describe the onset of diabetic dermopathy with eruptions consisting of distinct papulous erythematous elements, or erythematous plaques, sometimes squamous and erosive, correlated or not with a local trauma [6]. Some investigators observed reproduction of the lesions after local thermal trauma [24]. It can be appreciated that in diabetic dermopathy it is possible to define, in fact, a post-traumatic atrophy and a post-inflammatory hyper-pigmentation on a skin with vascular deficit [4, 17], context in which diabetic microangiopathy plays an important role, such as the diabetic neuropathy [3, 17]. This hypothesis is supported by the fact that diabetic dermopathy is encountered in patients that also present other signs of diabetic angiopathy (retinopathy, nephropathy, neuropathy), [3, 20, 21, 23, 25] and a consecutive angiopathic capillary fragility [8].

In optic microscopy, with hematoxylin-eosine standard staining, in early stages, the diabetic dermopathy lesions consist of epidermal and papillary dermal edema, with numerous extravasated erythrocytes and a mild lymphohistiocytic infiltrate [3, 20, 21, 25]. In older lesions, one can notice an arteriolar and superficial dermal capillaries wall-thickening, with PAS positive fibrillar deposits, rare extravasated erythrocytes and hemosiderin deposition in peri-vascular histiocytes (positive Pearl stain for iron). Peri-vascular inflammatory infiltrates, mainly with the accumulation of lymphocytes, are described in older lesions of diabetic dermopathy [20, 21, 25]. In electron microscopy, the basal lamina thickening was noticed only in few cases [19].

The number of cutaneous lesions allows the appreciation of the specific correlation between dermopathy and diabetes mellitus. It is appreciated that the presence of only one or two cutaneous lesions would reflect a low specificity (those lesions may appear in 20% of control group patients, with glucose tolerance test in normal range) [22], while the presence of more than four dermopathy lesions is encountered only in the diabetic population [18] on which diabetic retinopathy is also present.

Diabetic dermopathy lesions, especially when localized at lower legs, impose the differential diagnosis with necrobiosis lipoidica.

FACIAL ERYTHROSIS/RUBEOSIS
(syn. von Noorden rubeosis diabetica)

Facial erythrosis defines the situation of a patient with overt diabetes mellitus with long-term evolution [3, 25]. Particular red colour of the face, and sometimes hands and feet, that appears in patients with photo-type II-III (frequently light – red or yellow – colored hair), on which diabetes evolves for many years is what characterizes the ailment. Diabetic's facial erythema was initially described as having a peculiar topography, on the forehead and zygomatic region. Initially it was considered the exclusive appendage of overt diabetes mellitus. Lately, it was demonstrated the involvement of latent diabetes mellitus and even the predilection for juvenile-onset diabetes. Further studies have shown that diabetic facial erythrosis' topography is not exclusively facial, as initially supposed, being able to involve the hands and feet of diabetics, following the decrease of vascular tonus or diabetic microangiopathy [3, 26].

Initially regarded as a simple capillary congestion, diabetic erythrosis was proved to be the expression of the pathological visualization of some very fine venous plexuses in the capillaries depleted chorion [8, 11]. Capillaroscopy studies demonstrated that those venous plexuses possess a lowered vascular tonus, and dilate consecutive to diabetic metabolic imbalance. The clinical reality that rubeosis improves with the diabetes metabolic balancing (correction of acidosis, but not only), is the major clinical proof in favor of this interpretation of diabetic erythrosis, joining the paraclinical data (capillaroscopy).

From the physiopathologic aspect, the hypothesis is that hyperglycemia would determine, through specific mechanisms, a sluggish microcirculation, so that diabetic patients develop a functional microangiopathy, with chorionic venous plexus dilatation, associated with other territories veins dilatation (such as the retinal ones, noticed on eye ground examination) [27]. This venous dilatation associated with imbalanced diabetes mellitus may return to normal state with glycemic control. This may represent a major argument in favor of the functional character, at least at the beginning of microangiopathy, and on the other side, it may be considered a good prognostic sign in appreciation of diabetes mellitus evolution under treatment.

PURPURIC DERMATITIS OF THE LOWER LEGS
(syn. pigmented purpura, chronic purpura)

Chronic pigmented purpura (pigmented purpuric dermatosis), condition described in older diabetic patients, usually occurs on the anterior and lateral aspects of the lower legs, often on the same territories where the patient also has diabetic dermopathy lesions [28]. The presence of purpuric lesions shaped as small, round-oval, sometimes polygonal maculas, a few millimeters or even centimeters in diameter, with typical brick-red colour, uniformly distributed or intermingled with older lesions (in which the hemoglobin was already degraded and the hemosiderin was ingested by the histiocytes), with skin developing a yellow-tan hyperpigmentation, conferring the lower legs the typical "salt and pepper" configuration, characterizes the clinical aspect [28] (Plate 46.3).

Purpuric lesions and hemosiderin pigmentation intermingle with clinical manifestations of diabetic dermopathy, displaying a polymorphous clinical aspect, which is highly evocative for the diagnosis.

The capillary hyper-permeability with erythrocytes extravasation in diabetic purpura recognizes at least two pathogenic mechanisms: on the one side the involvement of diabetic microangiopathy, and on the other side, the aggravation of capillaries situation following the cardiac failure and lower extremities edema with erythrodiapedesis at the superficial vascular plexus level [2, 3, 25].

Diabetic purpuric and pigmented dermatitis of the lower legs, by itself, does not represent a gravity factor, but it can constitute a prognosis indicator, showing the aggravation of diabetes

complications on the vital internal organs level, suggesting the necessity of fast, sustained therapeutic intervention.

DIABETIC CUTANEOUS NECROSIS
(syn. diabetic wet gangrene)

Diabetic cutaneous gangrene is a clinical frequent eventuality in diabetic patients with advanced angiopathy. Diabetic necrosis may be strictly cutaneous, situation in which the evolution is less severe, or may involve totally the cutaneous and subcutaneous structures, with severe evolution and reserved prognosis, sometimes being necessary a high level amputation, far from the gangrenous area [3, 7, 25] (Plate 46.4).

The vascular factor, through macro- and microangiopathy, is essential, being involved in diabetic gangrene pathogenesis. Once installed, the total obstruction of blood circulation in a cutaneous sector or extremity segment (such as fingers, distal leg), induces prolonged ischemic sufferance, with either partial cutaneous necrosis, or total necrosis of the affected limb segment, clinical context in which atrocious pain represents the most dominant symptom. In the following moments, the cutaneous necrosis suffers bacterial and/or fungal superinfection, with exudation (wet gangrene). The overlying infectious factor aggravates the clinical picture and darkens the prognosis [7, 15].

On this compromised vascular field, through both diabetic macro and microangiopathy, an important aggravating role is played by the apparently promoting and/or favoring factors of mal-evolution, among which the most important are microtraumas and bad hygiene [24].

The sufferance onset is apparently following a minor trauma, after which appears a red-violaceous lesion, with relatively clear contour, having the tendency of progressive evolution. From red-violaceous, the colour will become black (Plate 46.5; 46.6).

Concomitant with necrosis maturation, in self-limited evolution cases, the gangrene isolates itself from the healthy surrounding tissue, creating a slightly depressed groove. In the unfavorable evolution cases, the gangrene area extends step by step, from a day to another, with an excruciating painful phenomenon and metabolic intoxication state, gets superinfected, exudates and develops a fetid smell (Plate 46.7).

This clinical picture imposes frequently the high-level amputation, at enough distance from necrosis area, in an area with good enough vasculature, in order to assure the success of operation [7]. Patient's young age is a good prognosis factor, presuming the existence of some functional reserve that will offer the body a better management of the disease, while long history of diabetes and the gravity of clinical manifestations of diabetes often constitute poor factors of prognosis. Regardless the favorable and/or aggravating factors situation, it is considered that the occurrence of diabetic gangrene is an indicator of great gravity in the evolution and prognosis of a diabetes mellitus patient [3, 29].

NAILS FOLDS TELANGIECTASIAS OF THE DIABETIC PATIENT

The nail bed is used for *in vivo* investigation, through capillaroscopy [30], of cutaneous micro-vascularization. Capillaroscopy studies confirmed that venous dilatation of the periungual microcirculation might be of great value indicating functional microangiopathy [27], while venular tortuosity offers extremely valuable information upon diabetic structural microangiopathy. It was observed that nail folds venous dilatation is detectable in 49% of diabetic patients, compared with only 10% in control group [31]. Nail folds venous dilatation constitutes a good indicator of diabetic microangiopathy [30], but needs to be differentiated from periungual microcirculation changes seen in connective tissue diseases. In the latter, periungual vessel changes are typical, displaying mega-capillaries with wide, irregularly shaped curves [30].

ERYSIPELAS-LIKE ERYTHEMA OF DIABETICS

The occurrence, on the lower legs or dorsum of the feet, in long term-standing diabetic patients with severe angiopathy [26], of erythematous plaques with sharp margins, local edema and radiological signs of underlying bone rarefaction/destruction, defines the clinical picture of erysipelas-like erythema in diabetes mellitus [32].

The clinical aspect that is visually similar to that of erysipelas, because adds painful symptoms, is not in reality an erysipelas, because lacks systemic and local hyperpyrexia and altered hematologic values (absence of leukocytosis and elevated erythrocyte sedimentation rate).

Diabetic erysipelas-like erythema clinical manifestations are edema and erythema representing functional microangiopathy superimposed on a compromised macrocirculation, similar to that seen in the diabetic arterial gangrene.

Prognostic and evolution significance of diabetic erysipelas-like erythema is severe for patient evolution in the near future more or less extensive diabetic gangrenes being possible to appear [26, 32].

NECROBIOSIS LIPOIDICA
(syn. necrobiosis lipoidica diabeticorum)

Necrobiosis lipoidica diabeticorum, in its full clinical maturity phase, consists of atrophic, round-oval or polycyclic, very well defined plaques, with a diameter varying from few to several tens of centimeters, with characteristic waxy-yellow appearance, electively located on the anterior and lateral sides of the lower legs (Plate 46.8).

The dermatosis onset is by small size lesions, with papular or small plaques aspect, well-circumscribed, round-oval shaped, dusky-red colored, with firm consistency, covered by fine, adherent scales. The lesions multiply and join by the periphery, building larger, indurated, oval or serpiginous, with centre yellow colored, slightly depressed (evocative of lipid deposits), atrophic plaques, with slightly elevated borders, and the surrounding skin red-bluish colored [3, 25, 29, 33].

In a chronic stage, peri-lesional inflammation signs disappear and the plaques gain the characteristic aspect, well delineated, sclerotic, round-oval or polycyclic, with atrophic, shiny surface, yellow-brown characteristic colored, less indurated than in the previous stages (Plate 46.9).

On the surface of mature lesions one can notice numerous telangiectasias, and through its transparency the subjacent vessels.

Sometimes, those plaques may develop a sclerodermiform pattern [3, 17, 33]. The scales on the plaques surface are usually fine, but in the pre-ulceration moments they become thick, with ichthyosis-like aspects. In natural evolution, in

30% of patients, necrobiosis lipoidica plaques, and especially those with greater dimensions, ulcerate, frequently as a result of minor trauma. Ulcerated lesions are painful, even worse when they become infected, and may heal spontaneously or under treatment, with unaesthetic scars.

Diabetic necrobiosis lipoidica plaques election sites are, as for the non-diabetic necrobiosis lipoidica, the internal perimalleolar and pretibial lower legs areas (Plate 46.10).

There have been described diabetic necrobiosis lipoidica lesions in other cutaneous areas, such as: thighs, feet, abdomen, hands, forearms, face, penis, eyelids and so on [3, 34, 35].

Usually, diabetic necrobiosis lipoidica plaques are asymptomatic, but in rare cases patients may claim pruritus, burning sensations, hypo- or hypersensitivity on touch, hypohidrosis, etc. [35, 36, 37].

In exceptionally rare situations, necrobiosis lipoidica plaques display, at the periphery, a comedon-like lesion covered surface, that histologically represents areas of transepidermal evacuation of necrotic material at the follicular opening area [38, 39].

The evolution of necrobiosis lipoidica plaques is slightly progressive, with the covering of large, extensive surfaces, generating an impressive clinical aspect. In 3 to 4 years, one of five necrobiosis lesions will spontaneously heal, with various degrees of unaesthetic scars. Typically, the evolution of diabetic necrobiosis lipoidica seems to be independent of glycemia level and antidiabetic treatment choice [3, 25], but recent studies showed that a good treatment of diabetes mellitus can reduce the necrobiosis lipoidica lesions appearance [40, 41].

From nosologic point of view, necrobiosis lipoidica is a degenerative sufferance of collagen fibers that, in microscopy, shows necrobiotic aspects [3, 25].

The incidence of necrobiosis lipoidica among diabetes mellitus patients is only 0.3% [3, 25]. The ailment was described as being characteristic to Caucasians and female patients, with sex ratio female/male: 3/1. Elective age for necrobiosis lipoidica's onset is decades 3 and 5, but exceptionally it was diagnosed in newborns. A study concerning the aspects of HLA antigens and necrobiosis lipoidica diabeticorum showed an increase of HLA A2 in patients free of necrobiosis lipoidica [42].

The necrobiosis lipoidica – clinically manifest diabetes mellitus relationship may be proved in 60–65% of cases, and 90% of the necrobiosis lipoidica patients without clinically manifest diabetes mellitus present a modified response to glucose tolerance test, either enhanced with cortisone or not, or possess significant familial antecedents for diabetes [3, 25]. The onset of diabetic necrobiosis lipoidica usually occurs after the onset of diabetes mellitus, but sometimes the two ailments may evolve simultaneously from the beginning. In rare cases, the onset of necrobiosis lipoidica may precede, sometimes even with years, the onset of diabetes mellitus. It is considered that there are no correlations between the gravity of necrobiosis lipoidica and the severity of diabetes mellitus [3, 8, 25], but other studies showed a linkage between the necrobiosis lipoidica appearance and the gravity of diabetes mellitus (presence of nephropathy, neuropathy and/or retinopathy) [41, 43, 44].

Typical alterations of necrotizing neutrophilic vasculitis are present on the histopathology examination on biopsies taken from early lesions of necrobiosis lipoidica, with hematoxylin-eosine stain [35]. In advanced lesions, in the superficial dermis one may find squamous cells and collagen necrobiotic degeneration, associated with the destruction of annexial structures: glands, pilous follicles, etc. (Plate 46.11)

In deep dermis, there is a granulomatous infiltrate rich in epithelioid cells, histiocytes, and gigantic multinucleate cells, sometimes with asteroid bodies [3, 25, 35, 36] (Plate 46.12).

Dermal vessels present endothelial proliferation, with intraluminal inclusions and thick capillaries walls, with PAS-positive deposits that proved to be IgM, C3, C4 and fibrin in immunofluorescence [45] (Plate 46.13).

In electron microscopy, there is focal degeneration of endothelial cells in dermal vessels [46]. Sometimes, the collagen necrobiotic degeneration can be associated with epithelial degeneration, such as squamous cell carcinoma [47, 48].

Physiopathologically, the granulomatous reaction is the consequence of dermal collagen alteration [25] subsequent to microangiopathy, as suggested by Doppler laser flowmetry studies [3], and complicated with coagulability disturbances (increased platelet adherence through increased blood F VIII-related antigen, alpha$_2$-macroglobulin and fibronectin levels) [3, 49, 50].

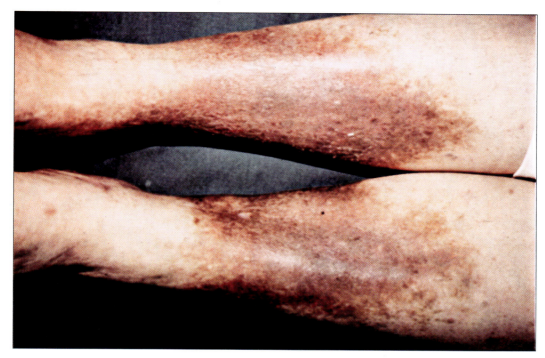

Plate 46.3
Purpuric and pigmentary dermatitis of diabetic patients' lower extremities.

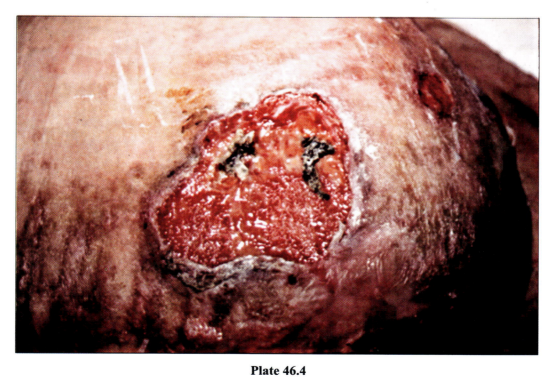

Plate 46.4
Extensive cutaneous necrosis of the abdominal wall developed after surgery for giant eventration in a 68 year old patient with a long-standing (over 40 years) diabetes mellitus.

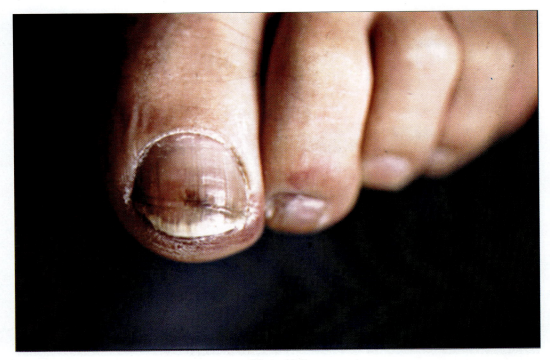

Plate 46.5
Subungual and periungual patch necrosis of the great toe in a 45 year patient with long-standing (over 20 years) diabetes mellitus.

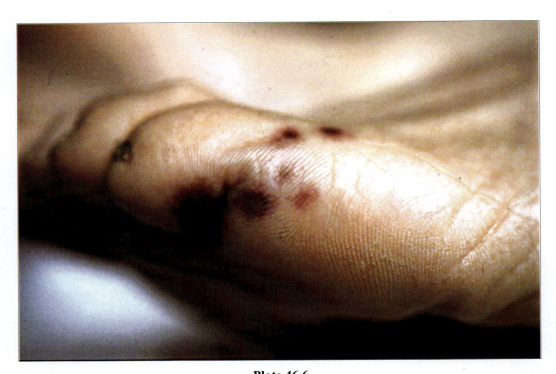

Plate 46.6
Patch necrosis of the fifth right toe in a 45 year old patient with long-standing (over 20 years) diabetes mellitus.

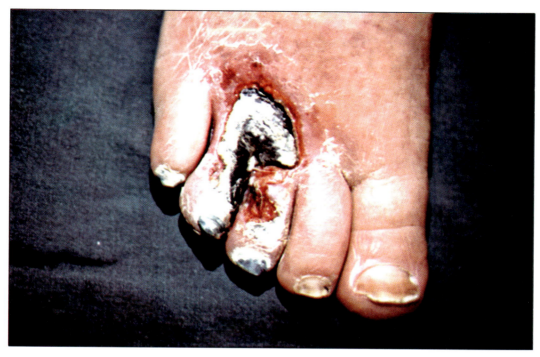

Plate 46.7
Patch gangrene on the dorsum of the third and fourth right toes in a 64 year old patient with long-standing (over 25 years) diabetes mellitus.

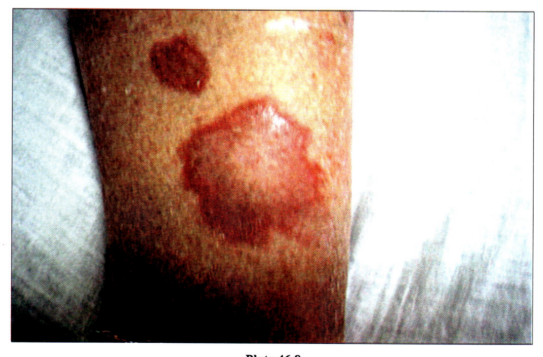

Plate 46.8
Necrobiosis lipoidica on the anterior aspect of the left shin in a 42 year old patient with long-standing (over 10 years) diabetes mellitus.

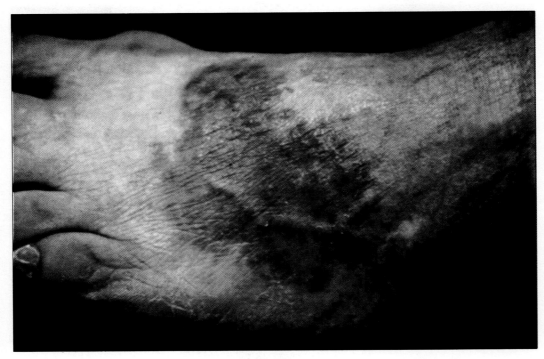

Plate 46.9
Necrobiosis lipoidica on the dorsum of the left leg in a 42 year old patient with long-standing
(over 10 years) diabetes mellitus.

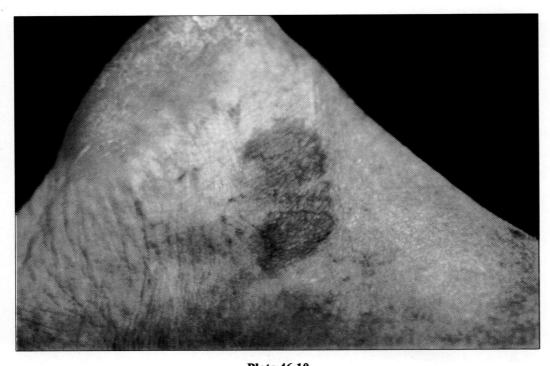

Plate 46.10
Necrobiosis lipoidica behind the left external malleolus in a 42 year old patient with long-standing
(over 10 years) diabetes mellitus.

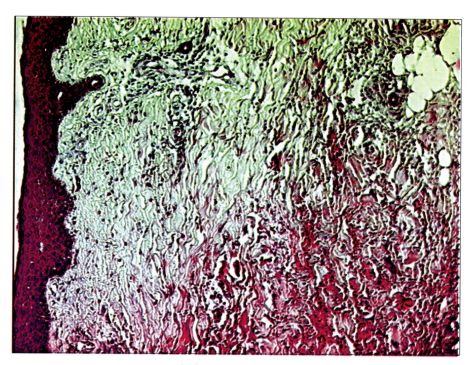

Plate 46.11
Necrobiosis lipoidica hematoxylin and eosin (×20) – general view image showing atrophic epidermis, thick dermis with irregular collagen fibers, diffuse cellular inflammatory infiltrate in the lower dermis and destruction of the annexial structures.

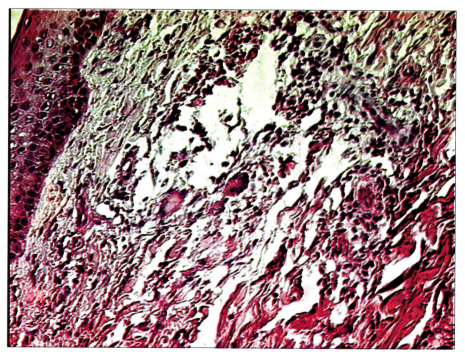

Plate 46.12
Necrobiosis lipoidica hematoxylin and eosin (×40) – details showing components of the granulomatous infiltrate with lymphocytes, epithelioid and multinucleate giant cells and thick wall vessels with perivascular inflammatory infiltrate.

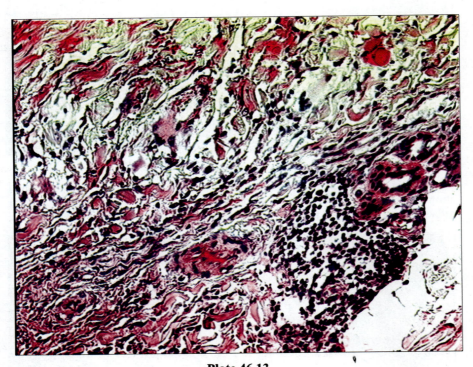

Plate 46.13

Necrobiosis lipoidica hematoxylin and eosin (×40) – details showing thick dermal vessels with endothelium proliferation and intraluminal occlusion.

Based on arguments such as the relatively low incidence of necrobiosis lipoidica in diabetes mellitus patients (only 0.3%) [3, 25], the existence of good clinical response to different therapies (topical tretinoin or retinoids) [51, 52], chloroquine [53], PUVA - therapy [54, 55], pulsed dye laser [56], Promogran [57]), GM-CSF (granulocyte - macrophage colony stimulating factor) [58], without effect in diabetes mellitus, the association of necrobiosis lipoidica with other diseases (such as ataxia-telangiectasia without diabetes cases) [3, 59], and because of the lack of any correlation between extension and the clinical expression and gravity of diabetes mellitus, we consider that the notion of direct linkage between necrobiosis lipoidica lesions and diabetes mellitus is at least debatable.

REFERENCES

1. Krall L.P., *et al.* Disorders of the skin in diabetes. In: Marble A *et al* (ed): *Joslin's diabetes mellitus*, 11th edition, Lea & Febiger, Philadelphia, 1973, p 653

2. Bucur G, *et al. Boli dermatovenerice*, ed. a II-a. Editura Medicală Națională, București, 2002.

3. Weissman K. Skin disorders in diabetes mellitus. In: Chapter 56, Metabolic and Nutritional Disorders. In: Rook, Wilkinson, Ebling (ed):*Textbook of Dermatology*, Champion R.H. *et al*, 6th edition, Blackwell Scientific Ed, Oxford, England, 1998, p. 2. 673–77.

4. Huntley AC. Cutaneous manifestations of diabetes – general considerations. The Skin in Diabetes, Jelinek JE, Ed. Philadelphia, Lea & Febiger, 1986, p. 23–30.

5. Schirren C, *et al.* Die Beteiligung der Haut beim Diabetes mellitus, Mat Med Nordmark, **22(3)**: 145, 1970.

6. Bauer M, *et al.* Diabetic Dermangiopathy – a spectrum including pigmented pretibial patches and necrobiosis lipoidica diabeticorum. *Br J Derm*, **83**: 528–535, 1970.

7. Brownlee M. Complications of diabetes mellitus.In section VIII: Disorders of Carbohydrate and Lipid Metabolism. In: *Williams Textbook of Endocrinology*, Larsen P.R., 10th edition, WB Saunders, Philadelphia, 2003, p. 1510–65.

8. Mincu I. *Diabetul zaharat*. Editura Medicală, București, 1977.

9. Diaconu DJ, *et al. Dermato-venerologie*. Editura Didactică și Pedagogică, București, 1999.

10. Nern K. Dermatologic conditions associated with diabetes. *Curr Diab Rep*, **2(1)**: 53–59, 2002.

11. Schirren C, *et al. Die Beteiligung der Haut beim Diabetes mellitus, Handbuch der Diabetes mellitus.* Lehman Verlag, München, 1971.

12. Yosipovitch G, *et al.* The prevalence of cutaneous manifestations in IDDM patients and their association with diabetes risk factors and microvascular complications. *Diabetes Care*, 21: 506–509, 1998.

13. Jelinek JE. The skin in diabetes. *Diabet Med*, **10**: 201–213, 1993.

14. Hanna W, *et al.* Pathologic features of diabetic thin skin. *J Am Acad Dermatol*, **16**: 546–553, 1987.

15. Grosshans E *et al. Diabète et affections cutanées, Précis de Diabétologie*, Ed. Masson, Paris, 1977.

16. Bernstein JE. Cutaneous manifestations of diabetes mellitus. *Curr Concepts Skin Disord*, 1: 3, 1980.

17. Huntley AC. The cutaneous manifestations of diabetes mellitus. *J Am Acad Dermatol*, **7**: 427–55, 1982.

18. Murphy RA. Skin lesions in diabetic patients: The "spotted leg" syndrome. *Lahey Clin Found Bull*, **14**: 10–14, 1965.

19. Fisher ER, *et al.* Histologic, histochemical, and electron microscopic features of the shin spots of diabetes mellitus. *Am J Clin Path*, **50**: 547–554, 1968.

20. Binkley GW, *et al.* Diabetic dermopathy – a clinical study. *Cutis*, **3**: 955–958, 1967.

21. Binkley GW. Dermopathy in diabetes mellitus. *Arch Dermatol*, **92**: 625, 1965.

22. Danowski TX *et al.* Shin spots and diabetes mellitus. *Am J Med Sci*, **251**: 570–5, 1966.

23. Melin H. An atrophic circumscribed skin lesion in the lower extremities of diabetic. *Acta Med Scand*, **176 (Suppl. 423)**: 1–75, 1964.

24. Lithner F. Cutaneous reactions of the extremities of diabetics to local thermal trauma. *Acta Med Scand*, **198**: 319–325, 1975.

25. Freinkel RK. Diabetes Mellitus, Alterations and Disorders of the Endocrine System. In: Fitzpatrick's *Dermatology in Internal Medicine*, Freedberg I.M. *et al*, V-th Edition, McGraw-Hill Ed, New York, 1999, p. 1969 – 75.

26. Lithner F. Cutaneous erythema, with or without necrosis. Localized to the legs and feet – a lesion in elderly diabetics. *Acta Med Scand*, **196**: 333–42, 1974.

27. Ditzel J. Functional microangiopathy in diabetes mellitus. *Diabetes*, **17**: 388–397, 1968.

28. Lithner F. Purpura, pigmentation and yellow nails of the lower extremities in diabetes. *Acta Med Scand*, **199**: 203–208, 1976.

29. Perez MI *et al.* Cutaneous manifestations of diabetes mellitus. *J Am Acad Dermatol*, **30**: 519–531, 1994.

30. Grassi W *et al.* Nailfold computed videomicroscopy in morpho-functional assessment of diabetic microangiopathy. Acta *Diabetol Lat*, **22**: 223–228, 1985.

31. Landau J, *et al.* The small blood-vessels of the conjunctiva and nailbed in diabetes mellitus. *Lancet* 2:731–734, 1960.

32. Lithner F *et al.* Skeletal lesions of the feet in diabetics and their relationship to cutaneous erythema with or without necrosis of the feet. *Acta Med Scand,* 200:155–161, 1976.

33. Huntley AC. Cutaneous manifestations of diabetes mellitus. *Dermatol Clin,* 7: 531–546, 1989.

34. Wilson Jones E. Necrobiosis lipoidica presenting on the face and scalp. *Trans St Johns Hosp Dermatol Soc,* 57: 202, 1971.

35. Boulton AJ *et al.* Necrobiosis lipoidica diabeticorum: a clinicopathologic study. *J Am Acad Dermatol,* 18: 530–537, 1988.

36. Hatzis J, Varelzidis A, Tosca A *et al.* Sweat gland disturbances in granuloma annulare and necrobiosis lipoidica. *Br J Dermatol,* 108: 705–9, 1983.

37. Mann RJ, Harman RRM. Cutaneous anaesthesia in necrobiosis lipoidica. *Br J Dermatol,* 110: 323–5, 1984.

38. Parra AC. Transepithelial elimination in necrobiosis lipoidica. *Br J Dermatol,* 96: 83–6, 1977.

39. McDonald L *et al.* Perforating elastosis in necrobiosis lipoidica diabeticorum. *Cutis,* 57(5): 336–8, 1996.

40. Imakado S, *et al.* Diffuse necrobiosis lipoidica diabeticorum associated with non-insulin dependent diabetes mellitus. *Clin Exp Dermatol,* 23(6): 271–3, 1998.

41. Cohen O, *et al.* Necrobiosis lipoidica and diabetic control revisited. *Med Hypotheses,* 46(4): 348–50, 1996.

42. Soler NG, *et al.* HLA antigens and necrobiosis lipoidica diabeticorum – a comparison between insulin-dependent diabetics with and without necrobiosis. *Postgrad Med J,* 59(698): 759–62, 1983.

43. Demis: Clinical Dermatology; Volume 1, unit 4–8:1–7, revision CD–94. Lippincott-Raven, Philadelphia, 1997.

44. Kelly WF, *et al.* Necrobiosis lipoidica diabeticorum: association with background retinopathy, smoking and proteinuria. A case controlled study. *Diabet Med,* 10(8): 725–8, 1993.

45. Quimby SR, *et al.* The cutaneous immunopathology of necrobiosis lipoidica diabeticorum. *Arch Dermatol* 124(9):1364–71, 1998.

46. Heng MCY, *et al.* Focal endothelial cell degeneration and proliferative endarteritis in trauma-induced early lesions of necrobiosis lipoidica diabeticorum. *Am J Dermatopath,* 13: 108–114, 1991.

47. Clement M, Guy R, Pembroke AC. Squamous cell carcinoma arising in long-standing necrobiosis lipoidica. *Arch Dermatol,* 121: 24–25, 1998.

48. Gudi VS, *et al.* Squamous cell carcinoma in an area of necrobiosis lipoidica diabeticorum: a case report. *Clin Exp Dermatol,* 25(8): 597–9, 2000.

49. Majewski BBJ *et al.* Serum alpha2 globulin levels in granuloma annulare and necrobiosis lipoidica. *Br J Dermatol,* 105: 557–62, 1981.

50. Majewski BBJ, *et al.* Increased factor VIII-related antigen in necrobiosis lipoidica and widespread granuloma annulare without associated diabetes. *Br J Dermatol,* 107: 641–5, 1982.

51. Boyd AS. Tretinoin treatment of necrobiosis lipoidica diabeticorum. *Diabetes Care,* 10(22): 1753–1754, 1999.

52. Elson ML. The role of retinoids in wound healing. *J Am Acad Dermatol,* 38: S79–S81, 1998.

53. Nguyen K, *et al.* Necrobiosis lipoidica diabeticorum treated with chloroquine. *J Am Acad Dermatol,* 46(2): S34–6, 2002.

54. Ling TC *et al.* PUVA therapy in necrobiosis lipoidica diabeticorum. *British Journal of Dermatology,* 143(suppl 57): 42–85, 2000.

55. Ling TC, *et al.* PUVA therapy in necrobiosis lipoidica diabeticorum. *J Am Acad Dermatol,* 46(2): 319–20, 2002.

56. Moreno-Arias GA, *et al.* Necrobiosis lipoidica diabeticorum treated with the pulsed dye laser. *J Cosmet Laser Ther,* 3(3): 143–6, 2001.

57. Omugha N, *et al.* The management of hard-to-heal necrobiosis with Promogran. *Br J Nurs,* 12(Suppl 15): S14–S20, 2003.

58. Remes K, *et al.* Healing of chronic leg ulcers in diabetic necrobiosis lipoidica with local granulocyte-macrophage colony stimulating factor treatment. *J Diabetes Complications,* 13(2): 115–8, 1999.

59. Thibaut S, *et al.* Ataxia-telangiectasia and necrobiosis lipoidica: an explainable association. *Europ J Derm,* 4: 509–513, 1994.

ABSTRACTS
(in Romanian)

1. COMPLICAȚIILE CARDIOVASCULARE ALE DIABETULUI ZAHARAT: AMPLOAREA FENOMENULUI

Dan CHEȚA, Cristian PANAITE, Bogdan BALAȘ, Gabriela RADULIAN

Complicațiile cardiovasculare ale diabetului zaharat au devenit o problemă majoră atât pentru cercetători, cât și pentru clinicieni. Impactul din ce în ce mai mare asupra societății nu este câtuși de puțin surprinzător, dacă ținem cont de creșterea pe care atât bolile cardiovasculare cât și diabetul *per se* o înregistrează.

În acest capitol introductiv sunt trecute în revistă manifestările diverse pe care le poate îmbrăca boala cardiovasculară în diabet, aducând argumente puternice de epidemiologie. Au fost investigate trăsăturile caracteristice ale complicațiilor macrovasculare (boala coronariană, periferică și boala cerebrovasculară) cât și ale complicațiilor microvasculare (nefropatia și retinopatia).

Aspectele sociale și financiare studiate au relevat adevăratele dimensiuni ale problemei. Resurse financiare uriașe sunt alocate în fiecare an pentru tratamentul diabetului, complicațiile vasculare aflându-se pe primul loc.

În ce privește România, datele privind epidemia de diabet și complicațiile vasculare sunt puține și uneori contradictorii. Cele mai importante informații sunt cele oferite de studiul EPIDIAB, pe scurt prezentat.

În lumina noilor studii, se desprind câteva principii ce trebuie urmate pentru a diminua riscul cardiovascular asociat diabetului. În opinia noastră, o abordare multifactorială a acestui risc este cea mai benefică. Cu toate acestea, dificultăți de ordin practic încă trebuiesc depășite în implementarea strategiilor de prevenție, înainte de a reuși în această încercare ambițioasă, dar foarte necesară.

2. DISFUNCȚIA ENDOTELIALĂ ÎN DIABET

Maya SIMIONESCU, Doina POPOV, Anca SIMA

Prin poziția strategică între sânge și țesuturi, endoteliul vascular îndeplinește funcții vitale care asigură homeostazia mediului intern; totodată, endoteliul poate fi afectat de orice modificări care pot apărea în sânge sau țesuturi, unele dintre ele reprezentând „agresori" pentru celula endotelială (CE). În funcție de intensitatea sau de durata factorilor agresori (hiperglicemie, hipercolesterolemie, inflamație, hipertensiune etc.), răspunsul CE este de modulare a funcțiilor constitutive, urmată de instalarea disfuncției endoteliale și, în cele din urmă, de lezare și moarte celulară.

Disfuncția endotelială poate fi definită ca o modificare funcțională (adesea reversibilă) însoțită de o schimbare a fenotipului celular. În hiperglicemie, disfuncția celulei endoteliale se manifestă prin modificări de permeabilitate, scăderea densității sarcinilor anionice ale plasmalemei luminale, sinteza crescută de componente ale laminei bazale și ale matricei extracelulare perivasculare, expresia de noi molecule de adeziune și o producție perturbată de vasodilatatori/vasoconstrictori, de factori de coagulare și de fibrinoliză etc.

Date recente au evidențiat markeri specifici care definesc disfuncția CE în diabet: acumularea excesivă a compușilor de glicare avansată (AGE) și de lipoxidare avansată (ALE), stresul oxidativ crescut, exprimarea de noi molecule de adeziune la suprafața plasmalemei, alterări ale reactivității vasculare și scăderea biodisponibilității oxidului nitric (NO). La nivel molecular au fost identificate căile biochimice majore care induc disfuncția vasculară în hiperglicemie: creșterea fluxului de glucoză prin calea poliolilor, formarea de produși AGE și activarea protein kinazei C, molecule implicate în transmiterea intracelulară a semnalelor.

O caracteristică definitorie a disfuncției endoteliale este scăderea biodisponibilității NO. Factorii care contribuie la acest proces sunt reducerea expresiei sintetazei endoteliale a NO (eNOS), lipsa substratului și a cofactorilor pentru eNOS, o activare deficientă a eNOS datorată alterării semnalizării celulare sau accelerarea inactivării NO de către speciile reactive ale oxigenului. În același timp, producția crescută de endoteline (în special endotelina-1) are ca rezultat scăderea capacității de vasorelaxare dependentă de endoteliu. În plus, stresul de curgere poate activa factori de transcripție care, la rândul lor, pot regla gene responsabile de remodelarea peretelui vascular, crescându-i rezistența mecanică și conducând în final la blocarea vasorelaxării.

Datele acumulate până în prezent probează că endoteliul vascular este o țintă terapeutică în diabet. În restabilirea funcției endoteliale și-au dovedit eficiența utilizarea inhibitorilor glicării ireversibile, a anti-oxidanților, a inhibitorilor sistemului renină-angiotensină, precum și L-arginina.

O nouă familie de receptori nucleari, receptorii de activare a proliferării peroxizomilor (PPAR) reglează expresia unor gene care controlează metabolismul lipidic şi al glucozei (PPAR-α, PPAR-(β)δ, PPAR-γ). Studii farmacologice şi genetice au arătat că PPAR-α reglează calea oxidării acizilor graşi şi PPAR-γ modifică sinteza acizilor graşi şi stocarea lor în ţesutul adipos. În prezent, agoniştii sintetici ai PPAR sunt folosiţi cu succes în tratamentul diabetului de tipul 2 şi al dislipidemiei: glitazonele, medicamente cu potenţial antidiabetic, sunt liganzi sintetici de mare afinitate pentru PPAR-γ, iar fibraţii (agenţi hipolipidemici) sunt liganzi cu mare afinitate pentru PPAR-α.

În restabilirea funcţiei endoteliale, eficacitatea tratamentului poate diferi în raport cu cauza disfuncţiei celulei endoteliale sau cu patul vascular afectat (artere, arteriole, capilare etc.). Testări clinice ulterioare vor proba dacă reversia disfuncţiei endoteliale conduce la scăderea morbidităţii şi mortalităţii cauzate de diabet.

3. *PEROXISOME PROLIFERATOR-ACTIVATED RECEPTORS* (PPARs) – POTENŢIALE ŢINTE PENTRU ATEROSCLEROZA DIABETICĂ

Gabriela ORĂŞANU, Ouliana ZIOUZENKOVA, Jorge PLUTZKY

Cercetările recente au evidenţiat existenţa unor conexiuni extrem de importante între patologia cardiovasculară şi cea diabetică, ateroscleroza şi diabetul zaharat fiind condiţii cronice întâlnite frecvent în cadrul aceluiaşi pacient. Oamenii de ştiinţă au demonstrat că, pe lângă binecunoscuta relaţie de cauzalitate (diabetul zaharat fiind una dintre cele mai frecvente cauze de ateroscleroză), factori comuni, genetici şi de mediu pot determina apariţia concomitentă a celor două patologii. Studiile clinice, dar şi cele de cercetare fundamentală din biologia vasculară, au arătat că procesele inflamatorii vasculare sunt implicate în etiopatogenia, progresia şi apariţia complicaţiilor celor două boli.

Înţelegerea mecanismelor biologice care determină ateroscleroza diabetică a stârnit un considerabil interes. Receptorii de proliferare a peroxizomilor (*peroxisome proliferator-activated receptors* – PPARs) au fost implicaţi în mecanismele moleculare complexe care stau la baza aterosclerozei şi diabetului zaharat. Aceşti receptori sunt factori de transcripţie nucleari, activaţi de către liganzi specifici, care joacă un rol important în reglarea metabolismului glucidic şi lipidic. Mai mult, PPARs modulează răspunsul inflamator nu numai prin efectele lor metabolice, cât şi prin acţiunea directă asupra celulelor vasculare şi inflamatorii. Aceste date au importante implicaţii clinice. Tiazolidindionele (TZDs), activatoare ai PPARγ, sunt frecvent utilizate la pacienţii diabetici cu risc crescut de apariţie a complicaţiilor aterosclerotice.

În prezent, prin identificarea genelor ţintă, se încearcă clarificarea mecanismelor prin care aceşti receptori îşi exercită acţiunea la nivel molecular. Noii modulatori ai PPARs ar putea fi utilizaţi în mod specific în tratarea pacienţilor cu prediabet, care prezintă factori de risc pentru apariţia bolilor cardiovasculare.

4. LIPOPROTEINELE ŞI SEMNALIZAREA PPAR ÎN DIABET

Ouliana ZIOUZENKOVA, Gabriela ORĂŞANU

Lipoproteinele bogate in trigliceride (LBT) pot induce apariţia diabetului zaharat de tip 2. Mecanismele moleculare responsabile de acţiunea acestora implică activarea factorilor de transcripţie, care pot stimula sau inhiba procesele inflamatorii. Acest capitol descrie principalele căi de activare a factorului de transcripţie PPARα. Acţiunea sa antiinflamatorie contracarează efectele proinflamatorii ale factorilor de transcripţie NFκB şi AP-1. Complexitatea compoziţiei, precum şi diferitele căi de absorbţie ale LBT explică multitudinea efectelor pe care acestea le exercită. Înţelegerea mecanismelor prin care LBT activează anumiţi factori de transcripţie deschide noi perspective în prevenţia şi tratamentul dislipidemiilor la pacienţii cu diabet zaharat de tip 2.

5. IMPLICAREA METABOLISMULUI ICOSANOIZILOR ÎN COMPLICAŢIILE VASCULARE ALE DIABETULUI ZAHARAT

Mihai NECHIFOR

Icosanoizii (prostaglandine, tromboxani, prostacicline, lipoxine, hepoxiline, izoprostani, hidroperoxizi intermediari etc.) şi acizii graşi precursori (acidul arahidonic, linoleic, eicosapentaenoic şi docosahexaenoic) se sintetizează la nivelul vaselor de sânge şi a elementelor figurate ale sângelui şi au acţiuni importante pentru funcţionarea normală a sistemului circulator.

Modificări în sinteza componentelor sistemului icosanoizilor sunt implicate în numeroase procese patologice cu impact major asupra organismului uman, între care angiopatia diabetică.

PGI$_2$(prostaciclina) este unul dintre principalii factori protectori ai endoteliului vascular față de acțiunea aterogenă a hiperglicemiei și față de efectul citotoxic al radicalilor peroxidici.

Alți icosanoizi cum sunt TxA$_2$, izoprostanii, leucotrienele au un efect proaterogen.

În condiții de hiperglicemie și dislipidemie icosanoizii proaterogeni (ex. TxA$_2$ cu acțiune proagregantă plachetară) se sintetizează în exces.

Noi am testat, în condiții de hiperglicemie la șobolanii Wistar la care s-a produs experimental diabet aloxanic (aloxan 175mg/kg subcutanat) și în condiții de hipervitaminoză D$_2$ (30 000 UI/kg/zi, 42 zile), un analog prostaglandinic de sinteză al PGF$_{2\alpha}$, produs la ICCF București, cloprostenol optic activ (ClPGOA, 50 µg/kg/zi).

Examinările macroscopice și optic microscopice ale leziunilor vasculare, după șase săptămâni la șobolanii Wistar ce au avut valori ale glicemiei mai mult decât duble față de valorile anterioare inducerii diabetului zaharat, au arătat că acest analog de PGF$_{2\alpha}$, fără acțiune vasoconstrictoare, dar cu acțiune luteolitică, reduce semnificativ suprafața lezională arterială determinată planimetric.

Considerăm că unii analogi prostaglandinici (alții decât cei ai PGI$_2$) pot avea un efect parțial protector vascular în angiopatia diabetică.

6. BAZELE GENETICE ALE COMPLICAȚIILOR VASCULARE DIN DIABETUL ZAHARAT

Dănuț CIMPONERIU, Pompilia APOSTOL, Irina RADU, Dan CHEȚA, Cristian PANAITE, Bogdan BALAȘ

Diabetul zaharat și complicațiile sale au fost asociate cu reducerea calității și speranței de viață. Afectarea micro- (nefropatia, retinopatia și neuropatia diabetică) și macrovasculară reprezintă o complicație redutabilă a acestor pacienți.

Nefropatia diabetică este o boală la care contribuie factori hemodinamici, metabolici, citokine, factori de creștere și parametrii antropometrici. În plus, s-a observat existența unei componente genetice care contribuie suplimentar la apariția bolii, independent de controlul glicemic. Pe lângă investigarea genelor candidate, studiile *in vivo, in vitro* și *in silico* au adus informații suplimentare referitoare la componenta genetică a nefropatiei diabetice. Rezultatele numeroaselor studii realizate rămân în continuare contradictorii. Așadar, putem spune că nefropatia diabetică este o boală multifactorială și poligenică care apare ca urmare a acțiunii factorilor de mediu, pe un fond genetic de susceptibilitate. Acest fond este rezultatul balanței dintre alelele de risc și cele protective. În momentul de față nu se cunoaște nici un polimorfism sau test genetic cu valoare predictivă pentru apariția sau evoluția nefropatiei diabetice.

Retinopatia diabetică reprezintă cauza principală a orbirii la adulții diabetici. Numeroși factori au fost asociați retinopatiei diabetice, printre care: factorul de creștere al endoteliului vascular, aldozo-reductaza, paraoxonaza, $\alpha 2\beta 1$ integrina, IGF-1, enzima de conversie a angiotensinei, receptorul pentru produșii finali de glicozilare, sistemul renină-angiotensină, genele TNF, familia enzimelor NOS, LDL, endotelina, poli (ADP-riboza) polimeraza-1 și GLP-1. Sunt prezentate efectele tuturor acestor factori în retinopatia diabetică. Este dificil de definit rolul influențelor genetice asupra RD datorită diferențelor în metodele de alegere a pacienților, criteriilor de selecție ale acestora, factorilor de risc, variației etnicității și diferențelor clinice în evaluarea stadiului retinopatiei.

Neuropatia diabetică, cu cele două forme majore ale sale, autonomică și periferică, constituie una din complicațiile redutabile ale sistemul nervos la pacienții cu diabet zaharat. Neuropatia este o boală multistadială, consecință a acțiunii factorilor de risc la persoanele cu susceptibilitate genetică. Cascada de evenimente este inițiată de perturbarea cronică a glicemiei care determină în principal formarea produșilor de glicozilare avansată, activarea căii poliol și creșterea stresului oxidativ, având drept rezultat alterarea proprietăților structurale și funcționale ale neuronilor. Genele care codifică pentru proteine implicate în aceste procese, în special cele pentru aldozo-reductază și superoxid dismutaza, au fost considerate gene de risc pentru neuropatie. Studiile realizate până în prezent nu au reușit să identifice markeri cu valoare predictivă certă.

Complicațiile macrovasculare. Principalele complicații macrovasculare întâlnite la pacienții diabetici sunt: boala coronariană, afectarea arterială periferică și boala cerebrovasculară. Alterarea endoteliului vascular la pacienții diabetici, cauzată de perturbarea generală a metabolismului, reprezintă cauza majoră a declanșării complicațiilor macrovasculare. Numeroase studii au demonstrat implicarea componentei genetice în apariția acestor complicații. S-a stabilit că predispoziția genetică este poligenică, principalele gene candidate fiind cele implicate în metabolismul lipidic.

7. ROLUL HIPERGLICEMIEI ÎN DEZVOLTAREA COMPLICAȚIILOR DIABETULUI, INVESTIGAT CU AJUTORUL MODELULUI ȘOARECILOR TRANSGENICI

Doina POPOV, Dorel Lucian RADU

Recent, a fost introdus un nou model experimental pentru diabetul de tip 1, cu ajutorul șoarecilor dublu transgenici (dTg), obținuți prin încrucișarea șoarecilor transgenici care exprimă hemaglutinina virusului gripal murin PR8 pe suprafața celulelor β-pancreatice, sub controlul promotorului genei pentru insulină al șobolanului, cu șoareci transgenici care exprimă receptorul pentru hemaglutinina aceluiași virus, pe limfocitele T (Radu și colab., 1999 și 2000). În studiul de față, am urmărit modificările structurii fine ale organelor predilect afectate de diabet: miocardul ventricular, glomerulii renali și aorta la șoarecii dTg diabetici, comparativ cu animale non-diabetice de aceeași vârstă (control). Rezultatele obținute au arătat că șoarecii diabetici dTg prezintă: hipertrofie a ventriculului stâng (la glicemie 365–475 mg/dl), urmată de cardiomiopatie dilatativă (la glicemie peste 600 mg/dl), fibroză interstițială a miocardului, îngustarea capilarelor miocardului sub presiunea matricei pericapilare hiperplazice, încărcarea cu lipide a epicardului (proces care nu a fost descris încă în diabet), hipertrofie renală, glomerulopatie, precum și activarea endoteliului și celulelor musculare netede din peretele aortei. Etapa următoare de parcurs o constituie înțelegerea mecanismelor biochimice afectate de hiperglicemia circulantă, ce conduc la modificările morfologice specifice observate la șoarecii diabetici dTg.

8. EXCITABILITATEA NERVULUI UMAN: MECANISME ȘI EFECTE FUNDAMENTALE ALE HIPERGLICEMIEI, HIPOXIEI ȘI ISCHEMIEI

Gordon REID

Etiologia neuropatiei diabetice este încă foarte puțin cunoscută, deși este clar că hipoxia și hiperglicemia joacă un rol important. Acest capitol va descrie câteva din efectele directe ale hipoxiei și hiperglicemiei asupra conducției și excitabilității nervului și va începe cu explicarea cunoștințelor existente despre excitabilitatea axonului, atât în sensul canalelor ionice „clasice" dependente de voltaj, cât și în sensul canalelor mai recent descoperite, ale căror activitate depinde de starea metabolică a axonului. Până acum cunoștințele despre aceste canale au provenit din studierea altor specii, dar în ultimul deceniu acestea au fost studiate și în axonii umani. Voi descrie un model *in vitro* de diabet prin aplicarea soluțiilor hipoxice și hiperglicemice nervului extras, arătând că acidoza intracelulară este un factor major în inducerea depolarizării axonului, depolarizare care ar putea duce la moartea acestuia. Voi descrie încercările de înțelegere a activității spontane în timpul și după ischemie, prin înregistrări directe din nervii umani; probabil că activitatea spontană în axoni duce la durerea neuropatică. Deși este prea devreme să putem spune cât de mult aceste experimente clarifică cauzele neuropatiei diabetice, ele au arătat totuși un număr de mecanisme candidate, care sugerează direcțiile de urmat pentru viitorii ani de cercetare.

9. GLICAREA INSULINEI ȘI ROLUL SĂU POSIBIL ÎN PATOGENIA DIABETULUI

Elena GANEA

Este unanim acceptat faptul că, hiperglicemia joacă un rol important în producerea complicațiilor diabetului zaharat. Hiperglicemia prelungită induce acumularea continuă a produșilor de glicozilare neenzimatică (glicare) în diferite țesuturi din organism, inclusiv în pereții vaselor de sânge, fiind asociată cu complicațiile micro- și macrovasculare. Efectele negative, cumulative ale acestor produși de glicare avansată (AGEs) se manifestă după un timp îndelungat, de luni sau chiar ani; de aceea, multă vreme s-a considerat că insulina plasmatică, având un timp de înjumătățire de numai 4–5 min, nu poate fi supusă procesului de glicare.

Datorită progresului continuu al tehnicilor moderne de laborator, prezența insulinei glicate s-a demonstrat: a) în experimente efectuate *in vitro* în condiții hiperglicemice; b) în extracte și insule pancreatice izolate de la diferite modele animale cu diabet tip 2; c) în celule β-pancreatice menținute în cultură în condiții hiperglicemice și recent d) în plasma umană.

Datele experimentale sugerează că glicarea *in vivo,* atât a insulinei, cât şi a proinsulinei, la animale diabetice are loc în insulele β-pancreatice, în timpul sintezei şi stocării insulinei, înainte ca granulele mature să fuzioneze cu membrana plasmatică şi să-şi golească conţinutul în lichidul extracelular. În diabet, mediul hiperglicemic extracelular poate induce o creştere a concentraţiei intracelulare de glucoză, transportată în celulele β de către transportorul GLUT2. Insulina poate fi glicată intracelular de către glucoză, dar şi de metabolitul acesteia, glucozo-6-fosfat, care este un agent de glicare mult mai activ decât glucoza.

Principalul loc de glicare al insulinei umane, *in vitro,* a fost identificat la fenilalanina aminoterminală a lanţului β şi, detectându-se ulterior şi un al doilea loc, la glicina aminoterminală a lanţului α. Monomerul de insulină, este stabilizat, pe lângă cele trei punţi disulfurice, de o reţea de interacţii intra şi intermoleculare, legături van der Waals, punţi de hidrogen, ionice. Modificarea încărcării electrice de la suprafaţa moleculei, indusă de glicare, poate influenţa formarea unora din aceste legături, ca şi interacţiile proteină-proteină sau proteină-apă, contribuind la destabilizarea conformaţiei native.

Glicarea insulinei produce scăderea activităţii ei biologice. S-a constatat că insulina glicată, comparativ cu insulina nativă, are o capacitate scăzută de reglare a metabolismului glucozei plasmatice, de stimulare a captării intracelulare a glucozei, a oxidării glucozei şi a sintezei glicogenului. Deşi numeroase studii au arătat că funcţiile biologice ale insulinei (transportul şi metabolismul glucozei, creşterea celulară şi mitogeneza) sunt legate de interacţia cu receptorul pentru insulină, date recente sugerează şi implicarea unor procese post-receptor.

În concluzie, insulina glicată a fost detectată şi caracterizată în plasma umană, activitatea ei biologică scăzută faţă de normal sugerând contribuţia acesteia la intoleranţa la glucoză şi rezistenţa la insulină, întâlnite în diabetul zaharat de tip 2.

10. MECANISME MOLECULARE ALE TRANSDUCŢIEI INSULINEI ŞI ROLUL METFORMINULUI ÎN REZISTENŢA LA INSULINĂ

Florin GRIGORESCU

Acţiunea insulinei la nivel celular este iniţiată de fixarea pe un receptor membranar specific pentru insulina (IR), urmată de activarea tirozin-kinazei receptorului şi fosforilarea specifică a substratelor receptorului insulinei (IRS). Asocierea proteinelor de semnalizare intracelulare duce, în cele din urmă, la stimularea funcţiilor mitogenice sau metabolice ale insulinei. Alterările fiecărei etape ale acestei cascade de evenimente pot să producă rezistenţă la insulină (mecanism primar), deşi rezistenţa la insulină întâlnită în variate condiţii clinice (ex. obezitate, diabet de tip 2, sindromul ovarului polichistic) poate implica alte mecanisme reglatorii cu specificitate de ţesut (mecanisme secundare). Această distincţie este importantă în ameliorarea rezistenţei la insulină prin agenţi farmacologici. Metforminul (N_1N_1- dimetilbiguanid), medicament utilizat curent în tratamentul diabetului, are efecte benefice prin scăderea glicemiei, ameliorarea metabolismului lipidic şi acţiunea cardio-protectivă, deşi mecanismul molecular rămâne necunoscut. Pentru înţelegerea mecanismelor moleculare ale metforminului, am dezvoltat un model experimental la şobolani care permite studierea evenimentelor transducţionale hepatice, după injectarea unui bolus de insulină în vena portă şi după administrarea acută sau cronică *per os* a metforminului. Rezultatele diverselor protocoale experimentale, incluzând studiul fosforilării şi activarea PtdIns 3' kinazei, sugerează că metforminul acţionează la nivel transducţional prin modificarea cineticii de asociere IR/IRS şi utilizarea în particular a substratului IRS-2 în ficat. Aceste date reiterează cunoştinţele asupra rolului particular al IRS-2 în homeostazia glucidică şi oferă o nouă viziune asupra mecanismelor implicând IRS-2 în alte ţesuturi, ca de exemplu în efectul leptinei la nivel hipotalamic sau efectele insulinei la nivel vascular.

11. RELAŢIA DINTRE DIABET ŞI ATEROSCLEROZĂ – ROLUL INFLAMAŢIEI

Eduard APETREI, Ruxandra CIOBANU-JURCUŢ

Bolile cardiovasculare reprezintă principala cauză de deces la pacienţii cu diabet zaharat. Ateroscleroza este responsabilă pentru aproximativ 80% din mortalitatea pacienţilor cu diabet, şi mai mult de 75% dintre spitalizările pentru complicaţii ale diabetului sunt atribuibile bolilor cardiovasculare.

În ultimii ani, au apărut dovezi că inflamația joacă nu numai un rol în dezvoltarea sindroamelor coronariene acute, dar este și un factor cheie în inițierea, progresia și pașii finali ai dezvoltării aterosclerozei – respectiv fisura și ruptura plăcii. Dovezi importante au fost aduse de studiile prospective care au identificat mai mulți markeri ai inflamației sistemice ca factori predictivi pentru morbiditatea cardiovasculară, nu numai la indivizii sănătoși, ci mai ales la pacienții cu boală coronariană stabilă sau instabilă.

În timp ce, în ceea ce privește ateroscleroza, s-au acumulat dovezi impresionante asupra existenței unei componente inflamatorii, în ultimii ani s-a recunoscut și în cazul insulinorezistenței o componentă inflamatorie importantă. S-a propus o ipoteză prin care defectele de acțiune ale insulinei asupra principalelor țesuturi (adipos, muscular și hepatic) ar conduce la o înrăutățire a statusului inflamator subclinic latent. Independent de agentul primar și de evenimentele inițiale, relația dintre insulinorezistență și inflamație este bidirecțională; orice proces în care apare inflamație cronică poate conduce la scăderea acțiunii periferice a insulinei, iar insulinorezistența va conduce la accentuarea statusului inflamator, cu crearea unui cerc vicios.

În consecință, reducerea inflamației ar putea avea efecte benefice asupra dezvoltării diabetului și altor dezordini metabolice, precum și în prevenirea aterogenezei accelerate a pacientului diabetic. Sunt necesare investigații suplimentare pentru studierea acestei posibilități și eventual, pentru aducerea de progrese spectaculoase în ceea ce privește prevenirea și tratamentul diabetului zaharat.

12. REZISTENȚA LA INSULINĂ ȘI DISFUNCȚIA ENDOTELIALĂ

Amorin-Remus POPA, Katalin BABEȘ, Petru Aurel BABEȘ

Capitolul discută dovezile și implicațiile funcționale ale endoteliului ca țesut țintă pentru insulină, în strânsă relație cu sindromul de rezistență la insulină. Endoteliul vascular răspunde la acțiunea insulinei printr-o creștere a eliberării de oxid nitric, dar acest mecanism este afectat în condițiile rezistenței la insulină.

În capitol se discută, de asemenea, și implicațiile fizio-patologice ale acestor anomalii, în creșterea riscului cardiovascular la subiecții cu rezistență la insulină. Insulina are un efect dependent de doză în ceea ce privește dilatarea vaselor mușchiului scheletic. Rezistența la acțiunea insulinei de a stimula metabolismul glucozei, aspect care caracterizează clinica obezității, diabetului zaharat tip 2 și a hipertensiunii arteriale este asociată cu o alterare a vasodilatației mediate de insulină. Datele sugerează că insulina dilată vasele mușchiului scheletic prin eliberarea de NO din endoteliu. Vasodilatația mediată de insulină pare a crește acțiunea insulinei de stimulare a captării glucozei la nivelul mușchiului scheletic. Vasodilatația intermediată de insulină este dependentă de NO, ea fiind alterată în stările de rezistență la insulină.

Rezistența la insulină este însoțită de creșteri cronice ale acizilor grași liberi care pot fi cauza disfuncției endoteliale din stările de rezistență la insulină. Există dovezi privind prezența unui mecanism care leagă rezistența la insulină din diabet sau obezitate cu defecte în acțiunea vasodilatatoare a insulinei și cu disfuncția endotelială, aspecte care favorizează boala macrovasculară și hipertensiunea.

A fost demonstrată importanța eNOS în reglarea tonusului vascular și a hemodinamicii. Disfuncția endotelială reprezintă un eveniment precoce și central care va conduce la boala macrovasculară la pacienți cu rezistență la insulină.

13. DISFUNCȚIA ENDOTELIALĂ ȘI DIABETUL ZAHARAT DE TIP 2

Cristian GUJA, Constantin IONESCU-TÎRGOVIȘTE

În ultimii ani s-au acumulat foarte multe date care vin să susțină rolul major pe care îl are afectarea endoteliului vascular în patogenia complicațiilor macro- și microvasculare ale diabetului zaharat (DZ). Endoteliul vascular este metabolic un țesut foarte activ, el secretând un număr mare de substanțe bioactive ce au rolul de a menține un echilibru între forțe opuse cum ar fi: vasodilatația (oxidul nitric, prostaciclina, bradikinina etc.) și vasoconstricția (endotelina-1, angiotensina II, tromboxan A2 etc.), tromboza și fibrinoliza, proliferarea celulară și inhibarea acesteia etc.

Disfuncția endotelială (DE) constă în scăderea/pierderea activității endoteliale fiziologice și reprezintă un marker precoce al riscului cardiovascular. Deoarece reglarea tonusului vascular reprezintă cea mai studiată funcție a endoteliului, DE este mai frecvent definită ca fiind pierderea capacității vasodilatatorii mediată de endoteliu (prin secreția de NO). La apariția DE contribuie un mare număr de factori dintre care mai studiați sunt: scăderea biodisponibilității NO (reducerea producției endoteliale prin scăderea expresiei Nitric Oxid Sintetazei endoteliale și creșterea degradării NO, în special prin producție crescută de anion superoxid), creșterea producției de Endotelină-1 și de Angiotensină II.

Mecanismele apariţiei DE în DZ tip 2 sunt multiple, principala cauză fiind reprezentată de hiperglicemia cronică. Aceasta acţionează prin intermediul creşterii semnalizării mediate de diacilglicerol – protein kinaza C, prin creşterea activităţii aldozo reductazei cu acumularea de produşi ai căii poliol şi prin acumularea produşilor finali de glicozilare avansată (AGE). Precursorul comun al tuturor acestor mecanisme pare a fi stresul oxidativ crescut, caracteristic „mediului intern diabetic". Alţi mediatori ai DE din DZ sunt reprezentaţi de insulinorezistenţa *per se*, stresul oxidativ, dislipidemie, starea protrombotică, hiperexpresia factorilor de creştere etc.

Dat fiind rolul major al DE în apariţia complicaţiilor vasculare ale DZ, intervenţia terapeutică cu scopul de a ameliora funcţia endotelială este esenţială. Este evidentă importanţa unui bun control metabolic, a tratării dislipidemiei diabetice şi a HTA. În plus, dată fiind asocierea dintre DE şi insulinorezistenţă, ameliorarea sensibilităţii la insulină (optimizarea stilului de viaţă, Metformin, Tiazolidindione etc.) pare a fi la fel de importantă. În sfârşit, există dovezi privind efectul benefic direct asupra DE al gliclazidului, statinelor, fibraţilor, inhibitorilor enzimei de conversie şi al vitaminelor antioxidante.

14. HEMODINAMICA RENALĂ ÎN DIABET

Tudor NICOLAIE, Dana M. NEDELCU

Nefropatia diabetică, cauză majoră de morbiditate şi mortalitate în diabetul zaharat, reprezintă una din frecventele etiologii ale insuficienţei renale cronice, în multe ţări ea constituind principalul motiv al necesităţii de suplinire a funcţiei renale.

Dintre multiplii factori identificaţi în iniţierea, întreţinerea şi progresia nefropatiei diabetice este analizată contribuţia hemodinamicii renale în afectarea rinichiului specifică diabetului zaharat.

În cursul diabetului zaharat, indiferent de tipul său, 1 sau 2, chiar de la debutul bolii s-au identificat modificări ale hemodinamicii renale. La modelele animale de diabet zaharat şi la loturile de pacienţi diabetici s-a semnalat instalarea hiperperfuziei glomerulare, creşterea presiunii în capilarele glomerulare şi hiperfiltrarea. Aceste fenomene induc creşterea producţiei de matrice în celulele mezangiale, îngroşarea membranei bazale glomerulare şi exprimarea unor factori care contribuie la scleroză, precum TGF-β şi colagenul de tip IV. Sunt analizaţi factorii metabolici şi hormonali, care acţionând asupra hemodinamicii sistemice sau locale, la nivelul rinichiului diabetic, iniţiază şi întreţin nefropatia diabetică. Este prezentată influenţa hiperglicemiei, a corpilor cetonici, a tipului de dietă, a insulinei, glucagonului, hormonului de creştere, peptidului natriuretic atrial şi a omologului de somatostatină -octreotid-, directă sau prin mediatori cu efect hemodinamic, asupra filtrării glomerulare şi fluxului plasmatic renal. Intervenţia prostaglandinelor şi a hormonilor presori, ca angiotensina II, este subliniată în dezechilibrarea sistemelor vasodilatatoare şi vasoconstrictoare care reglează rezistenţa vasculară în diabet. Participarea importantă a angiotensinei II în instalarea şi dezvoltarea nefropatiei diabetice este demonstrată prin prezentarea rezultatelor studiilor UKPDS, MICRO-HOPE, AIPRI, RENAAL, care demonstrează efectul renoprotector în diabetul zaharat al inhibitorilor enzimei de conversie şi al antagoniştilor receptorului 1 al angiotensinei II, administraţi individual sau asociaţi. Disfuncţia endotelială şi nivelul crescut al endotelinei 1, elemente care au fost mult studiate în diabetul zaharat, intervin şi prin verigă hemodinamică în iniţierea şi dezvoltarea nefropatiei diabetice.

Sunt prezentate studiile personale având ca scop evaluarea sensitivităţii şi gradului de predictibilitate pe care ultrasonografia Doppler o prezintă în detectarea afectării premature a hemodinamicii renale la pacienţii cu diabet zaharat.

Datele prezentate argumentează posibilitatea de lansare a ipotezei că hemodinamica renală reprezintă placa turnantă a vectorilor patogenici care acţionează în diabetul zaharat în iniţierea, întreţinerea şi progresia nefropatiei diabetice.

15. MICROALBUMINURIA ŞI BOALA CARDIOVASCULARĂ

Cristian SERAFINCEANU

Microalbuminuria (MA), definită ca prezenţa persistentă în urina pacienţilor diabetici a unei cantităţi de albumină de 30–300 mg/24h (20–200μg/min), a fost descrisă iniţial ca fiind strâns legată de stadiul incipient al bolii renale diabetice. Deşi această presupunere iniţială este aproape complet valabilă şi în prezent pentru pacienţii cu diabet zaharat tip 1, cercetările ulterioare au demonstrat că la pacienţii cu diabet zaharat tip 2, ca şi la nediabetici, MA este asociată independent atât cu hipertensiunea arterială cât şi cu riscul apariţiei de evenimente cardiovasculare. De fapt, prezenţa MA pare să dubleze riscul cardiovascular la aceşti pacienţi, deci MA trebuie considerată ca un semn precoce de afectare nu numai renală, ci şi cardiovasculară. Studiile epidemiologice au oferit date noi despre agregarea familială a MA, asocierea sa cu hipertensiunea arterială şi posibilii markeri genetici cu semnificaţie predictivă. Prezenţa MA s-a dovedit predictivă pentru apariţia în viitor a evenimentelor cardiovasculare, la pacienţii cu diabet zaharat tip 2, dar şi la subiecţi non-diabetici.

Mecanismele posibile prin care MA poate produce leziune cardiovasculară sunt complexe şi nu pe deplin înţelese încă. MA pare să reflecte o modalitate „dezavantajoasă" de alterare a factorilor de risc cardiovascular „clasici": dislipidemia şi hipertensiunea arterială. Pe de altă parte, a fost dovedită existenţa unei relaţii intrinseci puternice între MA şi factorii de risc cardiovascular „non-convenţionali": markerii de disfuncţie endotelială, insulinorezistenţa şi starea de inflamaţie subclinică. Din acest punct de vedere, MA poate fi considerată ca un marker de leziune microvasculară generalizată sau ca o manifestare directă a disfuncţiei endoteliale. Asocierea MA cu markerii de inflamaţie cronică pare să îi confere acesteia semnificaţia de marker de risc cardiovascular.

În lumina acestor date recente, este deosebit de importantă definirea unei abordări terapeutice multifactoriale pentru prevenirea bolii cardiovasculare la pacienţii care prezintă MA, diabetici ca şi non-diabetici. Noile strategii terapeutice în această direcţie vor trebui să includă printre componentele lor esenţiale sensibilizantele la insulină (thiazolidindionele), blocantele sistemului renină-angiotensină şi statinele.

16. FACTORII DE RISC CARDIOVASCULAR ÎN DIABETUL DE TIP 1 ŞI DE TIP 2: FACTORI DE RISC CONVENŢIONALI ŞI FACTORI LEGAŢI DE DIABET?

Eckhard ZANDER, Wolfgang KERNER

Atât în tipul 1, cât şi în tipul 2 de diabet, complicaţiile macrovasculare ameninţă sănătatea şi micşorează speranţa de viaţă. Complicaţiile cardiovasculare apar mai devreme decât la populaţia nediabetică şi progresează mai rapid. Spre deosebire de populaţia nediabetică, pacienţii cu diabet nu au beneficiat la fel de mult de progresele făcute în reducerea mortalităţii cardiovasculare. În afara factorilor de risc clasici, alţi factori neconvenţionali par să explice acest exces de mortalitate. În lucrarea de faţă am trecut în revistă factorii de risc convenţionali şi neconvenţionali pentru morbiditatea şi mortalitatea în ambele tipuri de diabet. Trebuie luat în considerare şi faptul că cele două tipuri de diabet au o etiologie şi manifestări clinice diferite.

Hiperglicemia este cel mai probabil candidat ca factor de risc. HbA1c trebuie să fie sub valoarea de 7%. Încă nu s-a stabilit dacă hiperinsulinemia asociată cu insulinorezistenţa este aterogenă. Rolul nivelelor crescute de colesterol pentru boala cardiovasculară în diabet a fost arătat în studiul MRFIT. Cele mai multe ghiduri stabilesc pentru LDL-colesterol o valoare ideală mai mică de 2.6 mmol/l (<100 mg/dl). Hipertensiunea este un alt factor important ce reduce speranţa de viaţă în ambele tipuri de diabet şi accelerează micro- şi macroangiopatia. Valorile ţintă se situează sub 130/80 mmHg. Fumatul înrăutăţeşte de asemenea angiopatia diabetică. Tromboza datorată stării de hipercoagulabilitate în vasele aterosclerotice creşte morbiditatea cardiovasculară. În ambele tipuri de diabet există date despre creşterea morbidităţii cardiovasculare de către hipertensiune, hiperlipoproteinemie şi proteinuria asociată.

17. GLICEMIA BAZALĂ MODIFICATĂ ŞI SCĂDEREA TOLERANŢEI LA GLUCOZĂ: DIFERENŢE PRIVIND PREVALENŢA, CARACTERISTICILE METABOLICE ŞI RISCURILE ASOCIATE

Radu LICHIARDOPOL

În 1997, Asociaţia Americană de Diabet a recomandat scăderea nivelului glicemiei pentru diagnosticul diabetului zaharat la 7.0 mmol/l (126 mg/dl) şi a propus o nouă categorie a intoleranţei la glucoză: glicemia *à jeun* modificată (IFG: *Impaired Fasting Glucose*), considerând-o echivalentă cu scăderea toleranţei la glucoză (IGT: *Impaired Glucose Tolerance*).

Până în prezent s-au acumulat numeroase dovezi care atestă că între IFG şi IGT există diferenţe substanţiale privind prevalenţa, fenotipul, riscul cardiovascular şi riscul progresiei spre diabet.

Marile studii epidemiologice (DECODE, DECODA) au evidenţiat că aceste categorii ale intoleranţei la glucoză se manifestă cel mai frecvent sub forma creşterii izolate a glicemiei: fie numai *à jeun* (IFG), ori numai după încărcare orală cu glucoză (IGT cu glicemie *à jeun* normală). Aceste *pattern*-uri distincte ale intoleranţei la glucoză se menţin de-a lungul istoriei naturale a bolii în cursul progresiei spre diabet, sugerând expresia unor mecanisme fiziopatologice diferite, care, probabil, reclamă intervenţii profilactice şi terapeutice diferite.

În consecință, clasificarea intoleranței la glucoză ar trebui să considere, în cadrul spectrului intoleranței la glucoză, stările manifestate prin hiperglicemie izolată *à jeun*, stările manifestate prin hiperglicemie izolată după încărcarea orală cu glucoză și stările intermediare aflate între aceste două extreme.

18. DISFUNCȚIA ENDOTELIALĂ, ATEROSCLEROZA ȘI ARTERIOSCLEROZA LA PACIENȚII DIABETICI CU ȘI FĂRĂ AFECTARE RENALĂ

David J.A. GOLDSMITH, Andy SMITH, Karim BAKRI, Rashed BAKRI, Adrian COVIC

Complicațiile micro- și macrovasculare ale diabetului zaharat reprezintă principalele cauze de mortalitate la această categorie de pacienți. Atât în țările industrializate, cât și în cele în curs de dezvoltare se constată o creștere impresionantă a prevalenței diabetului zaharat de tip 2, cu consecințe nefaste previzibile. La fel de importantă ca și combaterea obezității și a sedentarismului la nivelul întregii societăți, identificarea unor markeri ai bolilor cardiovasculare (sau a susceptibilității pentru acestea), în vederea unor acțiuni țintite de prevenție, reprezintă o prioritate a cercetării medicale.

Funcția endotelială joacă un rol esențial în patogeneza afectării cardiovasculare la pacienții diabetici. În rândurile de mai jos va fi discutat rolul controlului endotelial asupra tonusului musculaturii netede vasculare și modul în care pierderea integrității funcției endoteliale este generată de către alterarea transducției, de către reducerea eliberării sau distrucția accelerată a factorilor de relaxare endoteliali sau, în fine, de către sensibilitatea redusă a celulei musculare netede față de aceștia.

Rigiditatea arterială (măsurată, în mod direct, prin viteza undei de puls sau, indirect, prin evidențierea unei presiuni a pulsului lărgită), s-a dovedit a fi un marker înalt semnificativ al hipertensiunii arteriale sistolice izolate, cel mai frecvent la pacienți vârstnici, dar evidențiată de asemenea la diabetici, în special la aceia cu afectare renală. Pacienții cu artere mai rigide prezintă mai frecvent hipertrofie ventriculară stângă și un prognostic mai rezervat. Creșterea rigidității arteriale la pacientul diabetic (și renal) se datorează atât fenomenelor de atero-, cât și de arterioscleroză (prin îngroșarea mediei arteriale și calcificări). Măsurile terapeutice de reducere a amplitudinii atero- și arteriosclerozei sunt subiectul a numeroase studii clinice și experimentale. Există speranțe îndreptățite că rezultatele acestor studii vor putea fi transmise în activitatea practică de prevenție a vasculopatiei diabetice, ceea ce ar îmbunătăți considerabil supraviețuirea pacienților diabetici.

19. SISTEMUL RENINĂ-ANGIOTENSINĂ-ALDOSTERON ȘI DIABETUL ZAHARAT

Marius Marcian VINTILĂ, Monica Mariana BĂLUȚĂ, Vlad Damian VINTILĂ

Sistemul renină-angiotensină-aldosteron (SRAA) reprezintă un mecanism important în patologia hipertensiunii, în inițierea și progresia aterosclerozei, ducând în final la producerea de evenimente cardiovasculare. Noi dovezi sugerează că inhibiția SRAA ar putea duce la prevenirea diabetului.

Diabetul crește riscul pentru boala cardiovasculară aterosclerotică. Atât diabetul de tip 1, cât și cel de tip 2, sunt factori de risc independenți pentru boala cardiacă ischemică și cardiomiopatia diabetică, ambele afecțiuni ducând la insuficiență cardiacă indiferent de cauza inițială. Boala macrovasculară, în special boala coronariană, este prima cauză de deces la pacienții diabetici.

Fără legătură cu prezența diabetului, disfuncția endotelială este una din manifestările precoce ale bolii vasculare, cu mult înainte de dezvoltarea aterosclerozei. Dovezi oferite de studiile clinice sugerează că întreruperea unei verigi patologice prin blocarea enzimei de conversie poate duce la îmbunătățirea disfuncției endoteliale.

Date sigure indică faptul că insulinorezistența joacă un rol major în dezvoltarea intoleranței la glucoză și consecutiv a diabetului. Angiotensina II are un rol negativ în modularea cascadei postreceptor pentru insulină, crescând astfel insulinorezistența.

Expresia enzimei de conversie în țesutul adipos este direct corelată cu insulinorezistența. Există ipoteza că blocarea SRAA previne diabetul prin activarea recrutării și diferențierii adipocitelor. Formarea mai multor adipocite contracarează depunerea de lipide în alte țesuturi (mușchi, ficat, pancreas) crescând astfel sensibilitatea la insulină și prevenind diabetul de tip 2.

Hipertensiunea contribuie la geneza și progresia complicațiilor cronice ale diabetului. La diabetici, hipertensiunea e caracterizată prin activarea SRAA și se asociază cu anomalii în funcționarea sistemului nervos autonom, cu dispariția fenomenelor de scădere tensională nocturnă și/sau de diminuare a ritmului cardiac, precum și cu disfuncție endotelială. Aceste elemente par să joace un rol în apoptoza miocitelor, care împreună cu afectarea micro- și macrovasculară stau la baza producerii cardiomiopatiei diabetice.

Administrarea inhibitorilor enzimei de conversie poate încetini progresia distrugerii renale, atât la diabetici, cât și în alte boli parenchimale renale. Acest efect pare a fi unul suplimentar, indiferent de efectul asupra scăderii tensiunii arteriale și se presupune a fi rezultatul diminuării selective a presiunii intraglomerulare.

În cazul sindromului metabolic, modularea SRAA prin inhibiția enzimei de conversie sau prin blocarea receptorilor angiotensinei reprezintă o primă linie de intervenție. Efectul este și acela al reducerii stimulării simpatice centrale și periferice, întotdeauna prezentă la acest grup de pacienți.

Aldosteronul inițiază fenomenele inflamatorii și de fibroză perivasculară, are efect cumulativ cu angiotensina II în inducerea expresiei PAI-1 și are un rol prooxidativ, important în geneza aterosclerozei. Este implicat în procesul de remodelare cardiacă producând hipertrofie miocitară și fibroză interstițială și perivasculară. Studii recente au dovedit efectele pozitive ale blocadei efectelor aldosteronului în prevenirea recăderii episoadelor de insuficiență cardiacă și supraviețuirea pacienților cu insuficiență cardiacă severă (spironolactonă-RALES) sau la supraviețuirea pacienților cu insuficiență cardiacă post infarct miocardic (eplerenone-EPHESUS).

20. IMPLICAREA NEUROPATIEI AUTONOME ÎN COMPLICAȚIILE CARDIOVASCULARE DIN DIABETUL ZAHARAT

Ioana Maria BRUCKNER, Mihaela Victoria VLĂICULESCU, Anca Maria NEGRILĂ

Neuropatia diabetică reprezintă o entitate clinică bine definită în patologia pacientului cu diabet zaharat. Deși în trecut atenția clinicienilor a fost îndreptată preponderent către neuropatia diabetică periferică senzitivo-motorie, în ultimii ani neuropatia autonomă reprezintă un subiect tot mai des abordat în literatura de specialitate ca o complicație frecventă și severă a diabetului zaharat.

Alterarea balanței vegetative simpatic/parasimpatic în cadrul neuropatiei autonome cardiovasculare se însoțește de o morbiditate considerabilă și un prognostic cardiovascular nefavorabil, diagnosticul cât mai precoce și influențarea terapeutică adecvată fiind obligatorii în abordarea acestor pacienți.

Deoarece simptomatologia asociată neuropatiei autonome cardiovasculare poate fi proteiformă și uneori nespecifică și date fiind implicațiile prognostice ale acestei complicații, sunt necesare metode de diagnostic cu specificitate și sensibilitate înalte.

Introducerea în practica clinică curentă a setului de teste cardiovasculare reflexe Ewing a permis decelarea precoce a neuropatiei vegetative, în stadii asimptomatice. La acestea se pot asocia explorări precum ecocardiografia, monitorizarea electrocardiografică Holter și ambulatorie a tensiunii arteriale, eventual explorări imagistice ale circulației coronariene, al căror aport în diagnostic este deocamdată controversat.

Numeroase studii prospective au demonstrat creșterea mortalității în rândul pacienților diabetici cu neuropatie autonomă cardiovasculară, cei mai importanți factori predictivi fiind reducerea variabilității ratei cardiace și influențarea repolarizării ventriculare, apreciată prin prelungirea intervalului QT și modificarea dispersiei sale. Totodată, trebuie avut în vedere și faptul că disfuncția autonomă poate fi și consecința unei afectări ischemice miocardice sau a prezenței insuficienței cardiace, elemente ce pot contribui suplimentar la creșterea mortalității.

Obținerea unui echilibru metabolic pare sa fie modalitatea cea mai eficientă de prevenire și încetinire a evoluției neuropatiei autonome cardiovasculare. La acest deziderat se adaugă mijloace terapeutice specifice manifestărilor particulare ale neuropatiei autonome cardiovasculare.

21. *SCREENING*-UL COMPLICAȚIILOR SUBCLINICE CE APAR LA TINERI CU DIABET ZAHARAT TIP 1: EXPERIENȚĂ ACUMULATĂ LA BRUXELLES

Harry DORCHY

Studii clinice efectuate începând cu 1970 de către grupul de diabetologie pediatrică de la Universitatea Liberă din Bruxelles au demonstrat că *screening*-ul pentru stadii subclinice de retinopatie, neuropatie și nefropatie ar trebui efectuat la pubertate și la cel puțin 3 ani după diagnosticarea diabetului. Astfel, s-ar putea preveni apariția unor leziuni potențial invalidante prin detectarea acestor afecțiuni în stadii subclinice, reversibile prin îmbunătățirea controlului metabolic. Un studiu de angiografie retiniană cu fluoresceină din 1974 a arătat că dezvoltarea microanevrismelor, leziuni ireversibile, ar putea fi precedată de scurgeri de fluoresceină datorate dezorganizării barierei hemato-retiniene. Factorii de risc pentru dezvoltarea precoce a retinopatiei includ: durata diabetului, vârsta la diagnosticare (copiii mai tineri ajung mai târziu la retinopatie), pubertatea și sexul (debutul este mai precoce cu un an la fete comparativ cu băieții), control metabolic deficitar pe durata a câțiva ani, nivele mari ale colesterolului și indexul de masă corporală (IMC) crescut. Pe de altă parte, îmbunătățirea rapidă a controlului glicemic poate agrava retinopatia diabetică (1985). S-a putut stabili o relație între anomalii minime EEG, frecvența comelor hipoglicemice severe (cu sau fără convulsii) și retinopatie (1979). Desincronizarea potențialelor de acțiune în neuronii din nervii distali precede încetinirea vitezei de conducere (1981). O singură valoare ridicată a hemoglobinei glicozilate a fost asociată cu scăderea conducerii în nervul motor peronier (1985), fapt neobservat și la nervul femural. Răspunsul dependent de simpatic al pielii (1996) și analiza statistică a variabilității frecvenței cardiace (2001) ar putea prezenta interes pentru diagnosticarea precoce a neuropatiei autonome. Microproteinuria precoce are etiologie multiplă, atât glomerulară (microalbumina), cât și tubulară (β2-microglobulina). Testarea la efort până la epuizare nu a furnizat informații în plus față de excreția bazală (1976). Microtransferinuria și pierderile urinare de glicozaminoglicani (2001) ar putea de asemenea să fie markeri de predicție ai disfuncției glomerulare. Antrenamentul fizic a redus proteinuria de efort la jumătate (1988). Nivele serice crescute de lipoproteină (a) nu au fost asociate cu prezența complicațiilor subclinice (1996). Pe de altă parte, testarea ultrasensibilă a proteinei C reactive ar putea fi un indicator interesant al riscului de a dezvolta complicații precoce (2002). Controlul metabolic deficitar a fost asociat cu nivele crescute de trigliceride, colesterol total, LDL colesterol și apolipoproteină B (1990). Au fost decelate scăderi ale nivelelor de glutation peroxidază, glutation reductază și vitamina C, denotând un stres oxidativ moderat, cu toate că nu s-au depistat creșteri ale peroxidării LDL colesterolului (1998). Eritrocitele au manifestat o activitate glicolitică crescută, iar neutrofilele o migrare scăzută, raportat la gradul de control metabolic (1992). De asemenea, controlul metabolic a influențat nivelele serice de triiodotironină (1985), concentrațiile magneziului (1999) și infecția cu *Helicobacter pylori* (1997). Terapia cu insulină ar putea activa calea complementului dacă se folosesc preparate intermediare sau retard fără protaminsulfat (1992), și provoacă creșteri ale IMC la adolescenții cu regim de 4 injecții pe zi (1988). Bunăstarea pacienților a fost invers proporțională cu nivelele hemoglobinei glicozilate (1997).

22. COMPLICAȚIILE DIABETULUI ZAHARAT TIP 1 LA COPII ȘI ADOLESCENȚI

Stuart J. BRINK

În general, la majoritatea copiilor și adolescenților, complicațiile diabetului zaharat de tip 1 sunt subclinice, dar încep să se manifeste după o perioadă mai lungă de timp și un control metabolic mai precar. Nu există o perioadă de grație pentru instalarea acestor complicații deși se pare că există o fază accelerată de apariție în jurul pubertății. Durata diabetului și controlul glicemic pe termen lung, vârsta și pubertatea sunt factori critici asociați cu dezvoltarea complicațiilor microvasculare și eventual macrovasculare ale diabetului. Factorii genetici accesibili prin analiza antecedentelor familiale, precum și statusul lipidic, tensiunea arterială și fumatul sunt de asemenea factori importanți în apariția și severitatea acestor complicații. DCCT a demonstrat importanța îmbunătățirii controlului glicemic și în special menținerea acestor efecte benefice pe o perioadă lungă de timp, chiar în cazul în care controlul nu este susținut, pentru cel puțin 6 ani după terminarea studiului. Evenimentele principale urmărite în DCCT, retinopatia, nefropatia și neuropatia, s-au regăsit în proporții mult scăzute la pacienții la care s-a urmărit menținerea de valori scăzute ale glicemiei și HbA1c. Mecanismul principal prin care s-a obținut această scădere a riscului a implicat utilizarea aceloraşi principii de tratament în cadrul unei echipe multidisciplinare de asistente, nutriţionişti, psihologi, fizioterapeuţi, precum şi medici, toţi conlucrând pentru obţinerea unor valori glicemice specifice. Alte studii intervenţionale sau de cohortă efectuate la copii sau adolescenţi în Paris, Franţa, Bruxelles, Belgia, Oslo, Norvegia, Sydney, Australia şi Leicester, Anglia au susţinut concluziile DCCT cu privire la tinerii cu diabet zaharat de tip 1. Cu ajutorul educaţiei medicale şi a terapiei suportive incidenţa complicaţiilor microangiopatice poate fi redusă. Controlul metabolic este esenţial.

23. O ABORDARE ŞTIINŢIFICĂ A MANAGEMENTULUI BOLILOR CARDIOVASCULARE DIN DIABETUL ZAHARAT

Umair MALLICK, Maria DOROBANŢU, Billy IQBAL, Dan CHEŢA

Diabetul zaharat şi complicaţiile sale cardiovasculare sunt o cauză importantă de morbiditate şi mortalitate în lumea întreagă. Bazându-se pe tehnici noi de diagnostic şi tratament, în lumina unor dovezi clinice şi epidemiologice, mulţi experţi au imaginat scheme complexe pentru managementul pacienţilor cu boli cardiovasculare. Relaţia dintre numeroşii factori de risc, în diferite grupe populaţionale din ţările industrializate sau în curs de dezvoltare, trebuie înţeleasă mai bine pentru a putea defini strategiile de prevenire şi diminuare a poverii clinice şi economice dată de diabetul zaharat şi bolile cardiovasculare.

Acest capitol se adresează cititorilor care au cunoştinţe medicale de bază, sperând să le oferim un sumar de concepte fundamentale referitoare la epidemiologia şi fiziopatologia diabetului zaharat şi bolilor cardiovasculare. Deşi multe din aceste probleme sunt discutate în alte capitole ale cărţii, noi încercăm să le prezentăm utilizând o abordare care integrează principii ale medicinii bazate pe dovezi. Pentru mai multe informaţii recomandăm consultarea literaturii de specialitate.

24. O ABORDARE PRACTICĂ A RISCULUI MULTIFACTORIAL DIN DIABETUL ZAHARAT TIP 2

Nicolae HÂNCU, Anca CERGHIZAN, Cornelia BALA

Diabetul zaharat tip 2 este asociat cu o creştere a riscului de mortalitate şi morbiditate prin boli cardiovasculare. Riscul este multifactorial, incluzând cel puţin un cvintet de factori: hiperglicemia, hipertensiunea arterială, dislipidemia, obezitatea şi fumatul. La aceştia se poate adăuga şi starea protrombotică. Reducerea mortalităţii şi morbidităţii cardiovasculare se poate obţine doar printr-o abordare multifactorială, prin care să se obţină un control al celor cinci factori de risc. Abordarea multifactorială presupune următoarele etape: 1) identificarea şi evaluarea fiecărui factor de risc, 2) evaluarea riscului cardiovascular global, 3) intervenţia asupra fiecărui factor de risc. Implementarea managementului multifactorial al riscului cardiovascular în diabetul zaharat tip 2 implică un mare efort din partea practicienilor, dar acesta merită făcut deoarece există dovezi clare asupra beneficiilor ce pot fi obţinute.

25. HIPERTENSIUNEA ÎN DIABETUL ZAHARAT

Gheorghe S. BĂCANU, Viorel ŞERBAN, Romulus TIMAR, Adrian VLAD, Laura DIACONU

Prevalenţa hipertensiunii arteriale la pacienţii cu diabet zaharat este de 1,5–3 ori mai mare decât în populaţia generală. Prevalenţa crescută, de până la 60–80%, a hipertensiunii arteriale în diabetul zaharat de tip 2, este explicabilă prin existenţa unor factori etiopatogenici comuni pentru aceste două afecţiuni, insulinorezistenţa şi obezitatea androidă. În diabetul zaharat de tip 1, prevalenţa hipertensiunii arteriale este mai scăzută, de 10–30%, asocierea ei sugerând prezenţa nefropatiei diabetice. Din punct de vedere al riscului cardiovascular, diabetul zaharat este considerat un echivalent al prezenţei cardiopatiei ischemice, iar asocierea HTA agravează acest risc. Studiul MRFIT a arătat că prezenţa HTA s-a asociat cu o creştere a riscului pentru mortalitatea cardiovasculară de 3 ori mai mare la pacienţii cu diabet zaharat comparativ cu persoanele nediabetice. De asemenea, HTA, alături de hiperglicemie, favorizează apariţia şi progresia nefropatiei şi retinopatiei diabetice. Din aceste motive în diabetul zaharat se impune acordarea unei importanţe egale, atât asigurării unui bun echilibru glicemic, cât şi a unor valori normale ale tensiunii arteriale. Dislipidemiile şi obezitatea sunt frecvent asociate DZ şi necesită a fi tratate pentru a reduce riscul cardiovascular.

Numeroase studii clinice au demonstrat eficiența tratamentului agresiv al hipertensiunii arteriale de a reduce incidența complicațiilor macro- și microvasculare ale diabetului zaharat, însă strategia ideală de tratament nu a fost clar definită.

Acest capitol prezintă particularitățile hipertensiunii arteriale la pacientul cu diabet zaharat și își propune să ofere clinicienilor un ghid de tratament al hipertensiunii arteriale în diabetul zaharat alcătuit pe baza concluziilor studiilor efectuate în acest domeniu, până la ora actuală.

26. MONITORIZAREA AMBULATORIE A TENSIUNII ARTERIALE ÎN DIABET – STUDIU ASUPRA NEFROPATIEI DIABETICE

Adrian COVIC, Paul GUSBETH-TATOMIR, David J.A. GOLDSMITH

Prevalența diabetului zaharat este în creștere în întreaga lume. Odată cu creșterea speranței de viață, incidența diabetului zaharat tip 2 este în continuă ascensiune, iar cu aceasta și incidența complicațiilor micro- și macrovasculare. Nefropatia diabetică reprezintă o complicație majoră a diabetului zaharat de tip 1 și 2, care, în majoritatea cazurilor, progresează spre insuficiență renală cronică terminală (IRCT). Există de asemenea o creștere impresionantă a prevalenței IRCT datorată nefropatiei diabetice, determinând o presiune importantă asupra programelor naționale de substituție a funcției renale în majoritatea țărilor de pe glob. Morbiditatea și mortalitatea pacienților diabetici dializați (în special de cauze cardiovasculare) este mult mai ridicată comparativ cu a celor nediabetici.

Un determinant major al morbimortalității cardiovasculare (dar și al progresiei nefropatiei diabetice) este reprezentat de către hipertensiunea arterială. Măsurarea clinică a tensiunii arteriale, după cum au dovedit-o studiile ultimilor ani, prezintă mai puțină acuratețe în predicția lezării organelor-țintă în comparație cu monitorizarea continuă ambulatorie a tensiunii arteriale.

Monitorizarea continuă ambulatorie s-a dovedit a fi un instrument deosebit de util în evaluarea tensiunii arteriale în scop diagnostic și terapeutic. Un profil tensional zi-noapte anormal, determinat prin monitorizarea continuă ambulatorie, este predictiv pentru dezvoltarea ulterioară a nefropatiei diabetice și se asociază cu progresie mai rapidă către stadiul proteinuric și apoi către insuficiență renală cronică. Concomitent, riscul cardiovascular al pacienților diabetici cu ritm circadian anormal al tensiunii arteriale este mult crescut. Conform unor studii recente, pe care autorii le discută pe larg, pacienții diabetici și non-diabetici, la care reducerea fiziologică a TA în cursul nopții este absentă (în principal datorită neuropatiei autonome), prezintă un risc augmentat de deces prin evenimente cardiovasculare majore. Un tratament antihipertensiv individualizat, care să se adreseze ritmului circadian anormal, în intenția de a-l corecta, ar putea îmbunătăți semnificativ prognosticul cardiovascular și general la pacienții cu diabet zaharat.

27. INFARCTUL MIOCARDIC LA PACIENȚII CU DIABET ZAHARAT

Carmen GINGHINĂ, Dinu DRAGOMIR, Mirela MARINESCU

Se consideră că riscul coronarian al unui pacient diabetic este similar cu cel al unui pacient non-diabetic de aceeași vârstă cu un infarct miocardic în antecedente. Ca și în rândul populației generale, la diabetici infarctul miocardic rămâne apanajul vârstei de peste 40 de ani. În grupa diabeticilor de vârstă tânără, incidența IMA este mai mare comparativ cu non-diabeticii.

Incidența infarctului miocardic la diabetici nu depinde de tipul tratamentului antidiabetic, ci mai degrabă de dezechilibrul metabolic și de vechimea diabetului zaharat.

Producerea infarctului miocardic la diabetici are implicații metabolice importante: stimulare simpatică excesivă, scăderea secreției de insulină, hiperproducție de cortizol și glucagon, creșterea producției de acizi grași liberi, și frecvent cetoacidoza diabetică. Complicațiile metabolice acute ale diabetului zaharat au efecte adverse importante asupra evoluției și tratamentului infarctului miocardic la acest segment de pacienți.

„Statusul diabetic" al unui bolnav cu infarct miocardic se caracterizează prin anomalii mai marcate ale coagulării, trombolizei spontane și funcției plachetare.

IMA la pacienții diabetici este mai frecvent silențios sau se poate manifesta prin insuficiența acută de pompă, decompensare metabolică sau ambele. Asocierea IMA la debut cu cetoacidoză (sau comă cetoacidozică) este o combinație mai rară, dar foarte gravă. IMA la pacienții diabetici evoluează frecvent în perioada acută cu multiple complicații, ceea ce face ca rata mortalității intraspitalicești să fie aproape dublă fața de persoanele non-diabetice cu IMA.

O atenție deosebită trebuie acordată diagnosticului formelor de IMA fără supradenivelare de segment ST, mai ales în situațiile în care durerea este absentă și în care criteriul enzimatic are o mare importanța diagnostică.

Tratamentul IMA la diabetici presupune aceleași linii generale cu non-diabeticii: utilizarea pe scară largă a agenților trombolitici, a antiagregantelor plachetare și a inhibitorilor de enzimă de conversie a angiotensinei (IEC). Nu trebuie evitate β-blocantele, dar se impune respectarea contraindicațiilor specifice. În plus, strategia terapeutică impune echilibrarea metabolică riguroasă. Îmbunătățirea controlului metabolic cu insulină este asociată cu o evoluție mai bună a pacienților diabetici după o angioplastie coronariană percutană.

Diabeticii beneficiază în mod special de terapia cu receptori GP-IIb/IIIa cu efect în reducerea complicațiilor post-procedurale.

S-a constatat că diabeticii cu infarct miocardic prezintă adesea o afectare multicoronariană cu leziuni aterosclerotice difuze, mai ales la nivelul patului distal. Datele studiilor arată ca la pacienții diabetici se preferă revascularizarea chirurgicală deoarece folosirea procedurilor intervenționale se asociază cu o rată crescută de restenoză și de complicații post-procedurale. În ultimul timp, folosirea stenturilor coronariene asociată angioplastiei scade rata de restenoză.

În mod frecvent normalizarea profilului lipidic la pacientul diabetic cu infarct miocardic nu se poate realiza cu o singură clasă de medicamente, de aceea se recomandă terapia asociată statină-fibrați.

Evoluția și prognosticul diabeticului cu infarct miocardic trebuie considerate în raport cu coexistența celorlalte complicații ale DZ, și în primul rând a microangiopatiei diabetice și neuropatiei autonome cardiace. La diabetici sunt considerați factori de prognostic nefavorabil pe termen lung: vârsta bolnavului, sexul feminin, asocierea HTA, profilul aterogen al lipoproteinelor (particule mici și dense de LDL-colesterol), tulburări de ritm ventriculare, afectarea coronariană multivasculară difuză și distală, reducerea rezervei de flux coronarian, insuficiența cardiacă congestivă.

28. CALCIFICĂRI ALE ARTEREI CORONARE ÎN DIABET

Dana DABELEA

Calcificarea Arterială Coronariană reprezintă unul din noii markeri sub-clinici ai bolii vasculare coronariene, intens studiat în prezent. Prezența calciului în intima arterelor coronare, la nivelul plăcii de aterom, poate fi vizualizată radiologic prin tomografie computerizată de mare rezoluție și viteză (*Electron-Beam Computed Tomography*). Calcificarea coronariană se corelează semnificativ cu manifestările clinice ale cardiopatiei ischemice, cu severitatea stenozei coronariene și cu evenimentele coronariene acute. În plus, ea poate fi detectată cu mult timp înainte ca boala coronariană să devină clinic manifestă, ceea ce o face utilă în predicția riscului cardiovascular și, posibil, în prevenirea cardiopatiei ischemice în populațiile sau la pacienții cu risc crescut. Un asemenea grup este cel al pacienților cu diabet zaharat, a căror morbiditate și mortalitate coronariană sunt semnificativ mai mari decât cele întâlnite în populația nediabetică. Cunoștințele actuale privitoare la rolul și importanța calcificării coronariene în diabetul zaharat sunt date pe scurt în acest articol.

29. INSUFICIENȚA CARDIACĂ ÎN DIABETUL ZAHARAT

Katalin BABEȘ, Amorin-Remus POPA, Petru Aurel BABEȘ

Supramorbiditatea cardiacă din diabetul zaharat se datorează în mare parte insuficienței cardiace. Populația europeană prezintă insuficiență cardiacă într-o proporție de 0,4–2 %, prevalența crescând cu vârsta, afectând 6–10 % din cei peste 65 de ani. Reducerea activității fizice asociată cu supraalimentarea cu o dietă nesănătoasă, creșterea mediei de vârstă, sunt factorii care determină creșterea explozivă a numărului de diabetici; acesta se preconizează să ajungă la aproximativ 300 de milioane în 2025, reprezentând 5,4% din populația globului.

Interrelația dintre diabetul zaharat și bolile cardiovasculare este în atenția multor studii recente. Conform acestora, 28 % din bolnavii cu cardiopatie ischemică au diabet și aproximativ 70 % din cei cu sindrom coronarian acut au tulburări ale metabolismului glucidic; dintre bolnavii spitalizați pentru insuficiență cardiacă, 35% beneficiază și de tratament antidiabetic. Insuficiența cardiacă a diabeticului are la bază, în afara patologiei aterosclerotice, asocierea frecventă a hipertensiunii arteriale (la peste 1/3 din diabetici) și o afectare specifică miocardică: cardiomiopatia diabetică.

Hiperglicemia induce mecanisme maladaptative care pot interfera cu metabolismul energetic miocardic, cu funcția contractilă a miofibrelor, cu cuplarea excitație-contracție, rezultând modificări citoscheletale și creșterea activității neuro-hormonale. Aceste modificări metabolice pot induce remodelarea cardiacă și mecanisme care activează un cerc vicios, insuficiența cardiacă și insulinorezistența influențându-se negativ reciproc. Prima manifestare a bolii cardiace este insuficiența diastolică, prezentă la diabeticii tineri, aparent sănătoși, fără alți factori cardiovasculari adiționali.

Tratamentul insuficienței cardiace urmează principiile ghidului Societății Europene de Cardiologie. Conform acestuia, principalele clase de medicamente folosite sunt: diureticele, inhibitorii enzimei de conversie, beta-blocantele, antioxidantele precum și controlul metabolic riguros al diabetului.

În prezent, efortul terapeutic este tardiv, tratamentul fiind inițiat în stadiile avansate ale bolii, când se poate obține cel mult o modestă ameliorare a simptomatologiei. Pentru a îmbunătăți prognosticul acestor bolnavi este necesar efortul comun al cardiologilor și al diabetologilor de a iniția tratamentul în stadiile incipiente.

30. EVOLUȚIA CLINICĂ ȘI PARTICULARITĂȚILE DE TRATAMENT ALE PACIENTULUI DIABETIC CU INSUFICIENȚĂ CARDIACĂ

Dinu DRAGOMIR, Carmen GINGHINĂ, Mirela MARINESCU

În ultimul timp se remarcă tendința de creștere a numărului de pacienți diabetici cu insuficiență cardiacă și implicit a costurilor legate de asistența ambulatorie și mai ales de necesitatea spitalizărilor repetate.

Insuficiența cardiacă (IC) a diabeticului are la bază, în afara cunoscutei patologii aterosclerotice cardiace (macroangiopatia coronariană), asocierea frecventă cu hipertensiunea arterială (la peste jumătate din pacienții cu diabet zaharat) și, nu în ultimul rând, o afectare specifică miocardică, așa-numita cardiomiopatie diabetică. Diabeticii cu insuficiență cardiacă și macroangiopatie coronariană au frecvent o afectare multicoronariană, cu leziuni aterosclerotice difuze. Prezența ischemiei miocardice la pacienții diabetici poate fi explicată și prin insuficiența microcirculației coronariene, în condiții de artere coronare epicardice permeabile. Hipertensiunea arterială și diabetul zaharat coexistă frecvent la același pacient, crescând riscul semnificativ pentru insuficiență cardiacă. Conceptul de cardiomiopatie diabetică presupune o afectare miocardică specifică, difuză, în lipsa leziunilor coronarelor epicardice, dar majoritatea autorilor includ în această noțiune și leziunile microangiopatice coronariene care, așa cum se știe, sunt generalizate în diabetul zaharat și pot fi evidențiate relativ ușor în faza precoce, având diferite alte localizări (retiniană, renală etc.). Explorarea non-invazivă (ecocardiografică și radioizotopică) aduce elemente valoroase de diagnostic, evidențiind disfuncție ventriculară inițial diastolică și evolutiv se asociază disfuncția sistolică de efort și ulterior de repaus.

Severitatea disfuncției ventriculare la pacienții diabetici cu insuficiență cardiacă este corelată cu gradul controlului metabolic și cu prezența unei disfuncții autonome cardiace – neuropatia autonomă cardiacă a diabeticului (NAC) – chiar și atunci când nu există o microangiopatie coronariană evidentă. Tratamentul farmacologic al pacienților diabetici cu IC este în linii mari similar cu al pacienților non-diabetici cu IC. Diabeticii prezintă câteva particularități de tratament al IC legate de frecvența disfuncției renale și a tulburărilor hidroelectrolitice, asocierea frecventă a HTA și natura obscură a aterosclerozei coronariene ± cardiomiopatia diabetică. IEC și beta-blocantele au un beneficiu terapeutic particular la pacienții diabetici. Tratamentul diuretic presupune precauții speciale la diabetici; un loc important au câștigat diureticele de tip *tiazid-like* (indapamida).

La pacienții diabetici este dovedită eficiența terapiei metabolice și antioxidante asociate tratamentului convențional al insuficienței cardiace pentru îmbunătățirea prognosticului acestei categorii de pacienți. Folosirea combinată a unor strategii de tratament alternativ (nonfarmacologic) aduce beneficii din punct de vedere al mortalității și morbidității cardiovasculare și poate constitui o punte pentru transplant cardiac la diabeticul cu insuficiență cardiacă refractară la tratament.

31. CARDIOMIOPATIA DIABETICĂ

Viorel MIHAI

Diabetul zaharat, atât tipul 1 cât şi tipul 2, este asociat cu un exces de morbiditate şi mortalitate cardio-vasculară, fiind implicaţi factori precum: hipertensiunea arterială, boala cardiacă ischemică, disfuncţia microvasculară. În ultimii 30 de ani, multiple argumente (epidemiologice, studii *post-mortem*, studii experimentale pe animale şi non-invazive umane) indică existenţa unei cardiomiopatii diabetice specifice.

Într-un prim stadiu, cardiomiopatia diabetică se caracterizează prin disfuncţie diastolică a ventriculului stâng, adesea asimptomatică. În patogeneza disfuncţiei diastolice sunt implicate defecte in structura proteinelor contractile cardiace, anomalii ale Ca^{2+}, lipo- şi gluco-toxicitatea, neuropatia autonomă, precum şi anomalii genetice. Această formă uşoară de cardiomiopatie poate deveni severă, în prezenţa hipertensiunii arteriale şi/sau bolii cardiace ischemice. Prin urmare, diagnosticul precoce al disfuncţiei cardiace se impune pentru ameliorarea prognosticului cardiovascular al pacienţilor diabetici.

Studiul ecocardiografic al unui lot de bolnavi tineri cu diabet tip 1, fără hipertensiune arterială, boală cardiacă ischemică, fără simptome de insuficienţă cardiacă şi fără complicaţii cronice diabetice, demonstrează o incidenţă mare a disfuncţiei diastolice asimptomatice (34%). Disfuncţia diastolică se corelează cu controlul metabolic al diabetului zaharat şi este însoţită de o scădere a performanţei cardiace la efort.

Având în vedere potenţialul evolutiv al disfuncţiei cardiace diastolice spre forme clasice, severe de cardiomiopatie congestivă, evaluarea ecocardiografică de rutină este necesară, în condiţiile unei prevalenţe crescute a afectării cardiace asimptomatice evidenţiată de studiul nostru.

32. INFLAMAŢIA ŞI INSUFICIENŢA CARDIACĂ LA PACIENŢII DIABETICI

Ioana Maria BRUCKNER, Ilinca SĂVULESCU-FIEDLER, Ion Victor BRUCKNER

Prevalenţa diabetului zaharat în rândul pacienţilor cu insuficienţă cardică este crescută, fapt dovedit de numeroase studii clinice (SOLVD, NETWORK, V-HeFT etc.). Pe de altă parte, studiul Framingham demonstrează creşterea incidenţei insuficienţei cardiace la pacienţii diabetici, independent de coasocierea cu hipertensiunea arterială sau boala cardiacă ischemică. De altfel, cea mai frecventă cauză de deces a pacienţilor diabetici o reprezintă suferinţa cardiacă. Concordant celor spuse, studiul UKPDS conchide că fiecărei creşteri cu 1% a hemoglobinei glicozilate îi corespunde o creştere de 16% a riscului de spitalizare şi/sau deces prin insuficienţă cardiacă.

Legăturile dintre cele două condiţii morbide se realizează prin variate mecanisme, printre care apariţia mai frecventă, la pacienţii diabetici, a ischemiei miocardice explicată, atât prin microangiopatie şi disfuncţie endotelială, cât şi prin macroangiopatie agravată şi mai precoce prin coasocierea hipertensiunii, obezităţii, dislipidemiei, hiperinsulinismului şi stării procoagulante.

De asemenea, în absenţa leziunilor coronariene la persoanele cu diabet apare o afectare miocardică difuză, autonomizată, sub denumirea de cardiomiopatie diabetică. Modificările de la nivel celular din această suferinţă, necroza miocitară şi apoptoza, sunt legate de stresul oxidativ, rezultat deopotrivă al tulburării metabolice, al producţiei crescute de angiotensină II, inclusiv la nivel local, cardiac, dar şi al acţiunii produşilor de glicare proteică. Fiziopatologia cardiomiopatiei diabetice include explicaţii legate de scăderea rezervei coronariene prin disfuncţie endotelială şi microangiopatie, de acumularea de produşi finali de glicozilare avansată, de creşterea stresului oxidativ şi, nu în ultimul rând, de modificări metabolice care afectează direct furnizarea de energie necesară funcţiei miocitare.

Legătura dintre insulinorezistenţă şi insuficienţa cardiacă este bidirecţională; nu numai că cea dintâi conduce la disfuncţie ventriculară stângă, dar şi aceasta din urmă determină, prin mai multe mecanisme, scăderea sensibilităţii la insulină, cu creşterea subsecventă a riscului apariţiei diabetului zaharat de tip 2. Căile prin care se realizează aceasta sunt: hiperactivitatea simpatică, scăderea masei musculare scheletale şi a fluxului sanguin muscular, eliberarea de citochine proinflamatorii (în special $TNF\alpha$ şi IL-6) şi, nu în ultimul rând, limitarea importantă a activităţii fizice. Apare astfel un lanţ fiziopatologic autoîntreţinut. Multiple studii clinice, dintre care vor fi citate doar câteva în cele ce urmează, subliniază legătura dintre sindromul de rezistenţă la insulină, diabetul zaharat şi mediatorii inflamaţiei.

Injuria cardiacă iniţială, ca şi creşterea stresului telediastolic ventricular determină eliberarea de citochine cu origine cardiacă, care ajunse în circulaţie amplifică răspunsul imun. Prin căi multiple, implicând activarea celulelor inflamaţiei (în primul rând macrofage), activarea endotelială, amplificarea stresului oxidativ se realizează, atât cercuri vicioase de agravare a insuficienţei cardiace, cât şi condiţii de creştere a rezistenţei la insulină.

Pe de altă parte țesutul adipos, în special cel visceral, este o sursă de citochine inflamatorii. Acțiunea acestora, asociată modificărilor metabolice din diabet, întreține și agravează reacția inflamatorie sistemică.

Astfel, inflamația poate reprezenta o verigă importantă în relația insuficiență cardiacă – diabet zaharat, relație de asociere descrisă clinic, dar încă incomplet înțeleasă.

33. FUNCȚIA CARDIACĂ ÎN DIABET – EVALUARE ECOGRAFICĂ

Ion Victor BRUCKNER, Adriana Luminița GURGHEAN, Ioana Maria BRUCKNER

Diabetul zaharat reprezintă un factor de risc major și independent pentru boala cardiovasculară, având o incidență și prevalență în continuă creștere.

Totodată, este responsabil pentru evoluția rapid nefavorabilă a afecțiunilor cardiovasculare. Studiile epidemiologice au arătat că prognosticul, atât pe termen scurt, cât și îndelungat al pacienților diabetici cu boală cardiacă cunoscută este mult mai prost comparativ cu al pacienților nediabetici.

În diabetul de tip 2, complicațiile macrovasculare cum sunt boala coronariană ischemică, accidentul vascular cerebral, boala vasculară periferică au o incidență mult crescută comparativ cu populația generală, aceasta datorându-se asocierii cu ateroscleroza precoce. Pe de altă parte, la pacienții cu diabet de tip 1, se descrie o afectare difuză miocardică, în afara unei boli cardiace evidente, care reprezintă substratul cardiomiopatiei diabetice, entitate frecvent întâlnită la acești pacienți alături de complicațiile microvasculare.

Indiferent de tipul de diabet sau de mecanismul de apariție al afectării cardiace, leziunile apărute devin rapid ireversibile conducând la insuficiență cardiacă – stadiul final de evoluție al tuturor bolilor cardiovasculare.

De aceea, evaluarea cât mai complexă a pacienților diabetici, cu sau fără boală cardiacă evidentă, devine obligatorie în ideea de a preveni apariția sau de a întârzia progresia insuficienței cardiace.

Ecocardiografia, între alte investigații noninvazive, ocupă un loc aparte în evaluarea acestor pacienți, fiind o metodă cu disponibilitate, acuratețe și reproductibilitate crescute. Valoarea examenului ecocardiografic constă în capacitatea sa de a detecta precoce modificările morfologice (geometria, dimensiunile ventriculare, hipertrofia miocardică) și funcționale miocardice (disfuncția diastolică, anomaliile de cinetică segmentară, disfuncția sistolică globală). Tehnicile noi ecografice – ecografia de contrast, Doppler tisular miocardic au îmbunătățit semnificativ acuratețea acestei metode permițând o mai bună evaluare a afectării cardiace la această categorie de pacienți.

34. ISCHEMIA MIOCARDICĂ SILENȚIOASĂ LA PACIENȚII DIABETICI

Igor TAUVERON, Françoise DESBIEZ, Laurence MARTEL-COUDERC, Philippe THIEBLOT

Coronaropatia reprezintă o cauză majoră de moarte la pacienții diabetici. Ischemia cardiacă silențioasă apare frecvent la acești pacienți și are un prognostic la fel de prost ca și cel al anginei dureroase. Rămâne de discutat dacă neuropatia autonomă este implicată în patologie.

Factorii de risc asociați ischemiei silențioase la diabetici sunt asemănători cu cei descriși pentru boala coronariană nediabetică: vârsta, sexul masculin, dislipidemia, hipertensiunea arterială, fumatul, antecedentele familiale cardiovasculare. La diabetici se adaugă și boala arterială periferică și proteinuria (într-o mai mică măsură– microalbuminuria) ca factori majori de risc. Sunt evocate de asemenea și tratamentul cu insulină în diabetul zaharat tip 2 și retinopatia.

Criteriile de *screening* pentru ischemia silențioasă la diabetici nu sunt bine stabilite, dar există o tendință de a monitoriza pacienții care au cel puțin doi factori de risc. Validarea unei scale de risc, bazată pe un scor care să țină cont de influența fiecărui factor de risc, pare esențială.

Există mai multe metode de *screening*. În absența unei modificări inițiale a EKG, sugerăm testul de efort ca prim pas în stabilirea diagnosticului. Un rezultat negativ în condiții de efort maximal exclude o boală cardiacă ischemică. Un al doilea test este necesar dacă nu se poate face testul de efort sau în condiții submaximale de efort.

Înregistrarea Holter nu este suficient de sigură. Valoarea diagnostică a scintigrafiei miocardice nu este la fel de utilă ca în populația generală, dar valoarea sa prognostică rămâne satisfăcătoare. Ecocardiografia de stres are o specificitate și senzitivitate similară scintigrafiei, dacă este realizată de personal experimentat. Tomografia computerizată și RMN cardiovasculară urmează să fie validate. În cazul unei anomalii semnificative este necesară angiografia coronariană, pentru stabilirea diagnosticului, prognosticului și metodei terapeutice.

35. STATINELE ŞI DISLIPIDEMIA ÎN DIABET

Ioan Mircea COMAN, Anca Ileana COMAN

Punctul de plecare în morbiditatea cardiovasculară a diabeticilor este ateroscleroza precoce, iar argumentele pentru asocierea diabet – ateroscleroză vin din studiile epidemiologice. Insulinorezistenţa preexistentă şi hiperinsulinismul ar putea fi evenimente primare într-o cascadă de modificări ulterioare care permit definirea diabetului ca factor de risc major independent.

Boala coronariană la diabetici este multifactorială; pe lângă diabet, alţi factori (în special cei ce definesc sindromul metabolic) rămân importanţi. Dislipidemia pare să fie cel mai important factor de risc modificabil în diabet (mai ales în diabetul de tip 2).

Dislipidemia tipică în diabet este caracterizată de creşterea colesterolului total, LDL colesterolului şi trigliceridelor şi scăderea HDL colesterolului.

Statinele sunt inhibitori competitivi de HMG-CoA reductază, enzimă cheie în calea de sinteză a colesterolului. Scăzându-i sinteza, statinele scad concentraţia intracelulară de colesterol, iar apoi prin mecanism de *feedback* apare o supraexpresie a receptorilor LDL şi creşte transferul lipoproteinelor plasmatice.

Studiile au demonstrat de asemenea un efect protector nonlipidic (acţiune pleiotropă) parţial legată de inhibarea mevalonatului. Rămâne de demonstrat dacă componenta pleiotropă a efectului statinelor ar putea fi mai mare la pacienţii cu diabet faţă de populaţia generală.

Studiile intervenţionale aduc argumente pentru terapia cu statine. În ciuda unui procent mic de diabetici, studiul 4S a demonstrat că terapia cu simvastatin îmbunătăţeşte prognosticul în acest subgrup. O metaanaliză recentă a studiilor cu pravastatin (incluzând CARE şi LIPID) a arătat că atunci când LDL colesterol este mai mic decât 3 mmol/l, beneficiul maxim al terapiei apare la acei pacienţi care sunt diabetici. Studiul HPS a adus argumente puternice, demonstrând reducerea importantă a riscului evenimentelor coronariene majore, accidente vasculare cerebrale şi nevoia de revascularizare la pacienţii cu diabet, chiar la aceia la care nu fusese diagnosticată încă boala coronariană sau altă boală ocluzivă arterială. Pornind de la rezultatele sale s-ar putea avea în vedere terapia de rutină cu statine la toţi pacienţii cu diabet zaharat cu risc crescut de evenimente majore vasculare, indiferent de nivelul iniţial al colesterolului. Studiul ASCOT utilizând atorvastatinul, stopat înainte de termen, a arătat un beneficiu net al pacienţilor din braţul tratat cu statine. Folosind acelaşi medicament, studiul GREACE a demonstrat că scăderea riscului cardiovascular a fost mai mare la diabetici decât la celelalte subgrupuri analizate.

Recomandările Asociaţiei Americane de Diabet şi ale celui de-al III-lea Raport al Experţilor Programului Naţional American de Educaţie privind colesterolul recomandă statine ca principala opţiune la pacienţii diabetici cu LDL mai mare de 130mg/dl sau non-HDL mai mare de 160 mg/dl (reprezentând marea majoritate a diabeticilor) şi ca posibilă terapie la aproape toţi ceilalţi pacienţi cu LDL cuprins între 100–130 mg/dl şi non-HDL colesterol între 130–160 mg/dl.

Pentru întregul impact clinic al statinelor la diabetici ar trebui amintită folosirea lor ca „stabilizatori de placă" în sindroamele coronariene acute.

36. GLICOZAMINOGLICANII ÎN VASCULOPATIA DIABETICĂ: IPOTEZE ŞI DOVEZI RECENTE

Gabriela NEGRIŞANU, Laura DIACONU

Numeroase dovezi au evidenţiat că metabolismul glicozaminoglicanilor (GAG) poate fi alterat la pacienţii cu diabet zaharat. Reducerea conţinutului de glicozaminoglicani (GAG), în special de heparan sulfat (HS), la nivelul peretelui vascular poate avea un rol important în patogeneza complicaţiilor vasculare ale diabetului. HS este o moleculă cu structură similară heparinei, dar cu grad mai redus de sulfatare şi epimerizare, cu o puternică încărcătură electronegativă. HS formează situsurile anionice de la nivelul matricei extracelulare şi determină permeabilitatea selectivă pentru macromolecule (ca albumină, fibrinogen, lipoproteine aterogene) a membranelor bazale endoteliale. De asemenea, HS este implicat în proprietatea antitrombogenică a vaselor şi inhibă sinteza şi acţiunea unor factori de creştere (inclusiv TGF β) activaţi de hiperglicemie care induc sinteza colagenului şi a altor proteine fibrozante la nivelul matricei şi intervin în reglarea proliferării celulelor netede vasculare. Cauza reducerii

HS la nivel vascular nu este cunoscută, dar ar putea fi disfuncția endotelială indusă de hiperglicemie; în consecință, scăderea HS ar contribui, prin multitudinea de efecte enunțate, la patogeneza complicațiilor micro- și macrovasculare ale diabetului. Numeroase studii efectuate pe modele experimentale și la oameni au dovedit eficacitatea GAG de a reduce factorii de risc vasculari prezenți în diabetul zaharat, în plus au ameliorat starea clinică a pacienților cu complicații vasculare și au prevenit evenimentele tromboembolice. GAG și-au dovedit eficiența, atât în prevenția, cât și în vindecarea nefropatiei diabetice experimentale. La oameni, studiile de amploare redusă au demonstrat efecte benefice asupra excreței urinare de albumină. Sunt necesare studii pe termen lung care să dovedească că GAG pot vindeca nefropatia diabetică la oameni și nu doar albuminuria. Sintetizarea unor compuși cu eficiență asupra nefropatiei și macroangiopatiei diabetice fără activitate anticoagulantă ar fi deosebit de utilă pentru prevenția sau tratamentul pe termen lung al complicațiilor vasculare ale diabetului.

În acest capitol am analizat ipotezele formulate și dovezile disponibile la ora actuală cu privire la rolul GAG în patogeneza complicațiilor vasculare ale diabetului.

37. PROTECȚIA ÎMPOTRIVA COMPLICAȚIILOR VASCULARE ALE DIABETULUI, INDEPENDENTĂ DE CONTROLUL GLICEMIC: ROLUL GLICLAZIDULUI

Paul JENNINGS

Angiopatia diabetică este o combinație între modificările microvasculare specifice diabetului și modificările macrovasculare, conducând la ateroscleroză accelerată și moarte prematură. Atât microangiopatia, cât și macroangiopatia, se caracterizează prin alterări ale structurii și funcției celulelor endoteliale, reactivitate crescută a trombocitelor și un stres oxidativ crescut. Toate aceste modificări pot fi urmarea activității radicalilor liberi. Peroxizii lipidici generați astfel modulează cascada acidului arahidonic, demonstrând o legătură între stresul oxidativ și predispoziția pentru tromboze a diabeticilor.

Gliclazidul este o sulfoniluree de a doua generație, cu o structură unică datorată inelului amino-AZA bicyclo[3.3.0] octan. Gliclazidul, pe lângă efectul hipoglicemiant, s-a dovedit *in vitro* a avea proprietăți antioxidante. El previne astfel și oxidarea LDL-colesterolului atât *in vitro*, cât și *in vivo*. De asemenea, gliclazidul îmbunătățește permeabilitatea vasculară și relaxarea dependentă de endoteliu. Toate aceste studii dovedesc prezența unor efecte vasculare, independent de influența asupra controlului glicemic. Astfel, s-ar putea explica efectele vizibile clinic, precum prevenirea relativă a retinopatiei diabetice. În concluzie, gliclazidul prezintă proprietăți vasculoprotective ce îl fac de preferat în fața altor sulfonilureice.

38. INSULINA ȘI BOALA CARDIOVASCULARĂ ÎN DIABETUL DE TIP 2

Rodica POP-BUȘUI, Martin STEVENS

Impactul și efectele cardiovasculare ale insulinei au suscitat un interes crescând în ultimii ani. Acesta s-a datorat, pe de o parte, numeroaselor studii epidemiologice care au demonstrat existența unei strânse legături între obezitate, insulinorezistență și hipertensiunea arterială, creând baza așa-numitei ipoteze a hipertensiunii insulin-induse. Pe de altă parte, acest interes a fost stimulat de o serie de date experimentale care au arătat că acțiunile vasculare ale insulinei joacă un rol important în una dintre funcțiile ei de bază, și anume preluarea și utilizarea glucozei la nivel muscular. Noi date experimentale au demonstrat că, de fapt, efectele vasculare ale insulinei sunt cu mult mai complexe, printre care modularea tonusului vascular, a proliferării și migrării celulelor musculare netede vasculare, *via* stimularea eliberării de oxid nitric sau a apoptozei.

Ca urmare întregul concept al tratamentului cu insulină este azi reevaluat în lumina evidențelor ce sugerează că efectele insulinei asupra sistemului vascular pot fi foarte importante în prevenirea sau atenuarea progresiei afecțiunilor cardiovasculare.

39. NOI ABORDĂRI ÎN TRATAMENTUL SINDROAMELOR CORONARIENE ACUTE LA PACIENȚII DIABETICI

Maria DOROBANȚU, Șerban BĂLĂNESCU

Toți pacienții cu diabet zaharat și mai ales cei non-insulinodependenți au prevalență mare a bolii coronariene și mai ales a sindroamelor coronariene acute. Ei au afectare coronară difuză cu leziuni aterosclerotice lungi pe vase de diametru redus, au o stare de hipercoagulabilitate sistemică cu creșterea factorilor procoagulanți și scăderea activității fibrinolitice spontane concomitent cu plachete disfuncționale. Acestea se asociază cu inflamația peretelui vascular, determinat în parte de hiperglicemie, cu scăderea răspunsului vasodilatator dependent de endoteliu și creșterea citokinelor proinflamatorii și a moleculelor de adeziune care accelerează progresia aterosclerozei și transformă plăcile stabile în plăci vulnerabile. Pe acest fond există un risc mai mare al evenimentelor adverse cardiovasculare și de mortalitate după un eveniment coronarian major la diabetici față de populația nediabetică.

Creșterea constantă a prevalenței diabetului de tip 2, prevalența mare a bolii coronare și a sindroamelor coronariene acute la acești bolnavi asociate cu prognostic rezervat pe termen lung reprezintă o mare provocare pentru medicina cardiovasculară. Evoluția pacientului diabetic cu un sindrom coronarian acut depinde de măsurile terapeutice instituite la internare.

Atitudinea terapeutică agresivă cu angiografie precoce și intervenție coronariană percutanată (PCI) pare justificată în ciuda incidenței mai mari a complicațiilor acute, a revascularizării miocardice incomplete și a prognosticului mai prost în comparație cu nediabeticii. Cel mai bun tratament de revascularizare de care dispunem în prezent este asocierea între implantarea de stent și administrarea unui inhibitor GP IIb/IIIa, mai ales a abciximabului. Există dovezi numeroase care susțin utilizarea tratamentului metabolic agresiv cu insulină-glucoză-potasiu pentru normalizarea rapidă a anomaliilor metabolice asociate diabetului într-un sindrom coronarian acut, ceea ce conferă avantaje majore pe supraviețuirea pe termen lung. Toate metodele de tratament dovedite eficace în sindroamele coronariene acute trebuie să fie administrate și pacientului diabetic, fără teama de reacții adverse în prezența indicațiilor precise și ținând cont de contraindicații ferme. Tratamentul trombolitic și cel beta-blocant pun probleme speciale în această situație. Bypass-ul aortocoronar (CABG) este superior PCI ca metodă de revascularizare la diabeticul stabil, dar noile metode de intervenție percutanată nu au fost încă studiate comparativ cu CABG. Stenturile acoperite cu medicamente antiproliferative reduc incidența restenozei și se pot dovedi eficace și la diabetici, anulând astfel principalul dezavantaj al PCI la acești pacienți care este incidența crescută a revascularizării vasului-țintă.

40. STRATEGII DE REVASCULARIZARE CORONARIANĂ ÎN DIABET

Claude HANET

Diabetul zaharat este un factor de risc bine cunoscut pentru boala cardiovasculară aterosclerotică care, atunci când e prezent, este asociat cu creșteri ale mortalității și morbidității, comparativ cu pacienții nediabetici cu boală coronariană. Riscul absolut al morții datorate bolii cardiovasculare a fost demonstrat a fi mult mai mare decât la pacienții nediabetici de orice grupă de vârstă, proveniență etnică sau nivel al factorilor de risc [1].

În comparație cu pacienții nediabetici, cei diabetici au de asemenea un prognostic pe termen lung mai rezervat după procedura de revascularizare, fie prin bypass aorto-coronarian, fie prin angioplastie coronariană percutană. Diabetul este un factor de risc independent pentru progresia leziunilor și mortalitatea cardiacă după bypass [2, 3]. După angioplastie, diabetul a fost identificat ca factor de risc în apariția restenozei. Mai mult, incidența restenozei ocluzive după angioplastie cu balon este dramatic mai mare la pacienții diabetici, și se asociază cu efecte negative asupra funcției ventriculului stâng [4].

Mai multe studii multicentrice au fost concepute cu scopul de a determina strategia optimă de revascularizare pentru pacienții cu boală coronariană. Luând în considerare frecvența mare a efectelor adverse după revascularizarea miocardică la pacienții diabetici, această subpopulație a fost studiată cu o atenție specială pentru factorii susceptibili să afecteze atât prognosticul pe termen scurt, cât și cel pe termen lung.

41. PROGRAME DE ÎNTRERUPERE A FUMATULUI LA PACIENȚII DIABETICI

Laurence GALANTI

Fumatul este în general o problemă de importanță majoră a sănătății publice, de asemenea reprezentând un factor de risc pentru multe boli grave, în special pentru diabet. Cea mai mare majoritate a fumătorilor sunt dependenți cronici de tutun. În încercarea de a ordona stagiile acestei dependențe a fost descrisă „cariera fumătorului". Potențialul tutunului de a produce dependență este strâns legat de prezența nicotinei. Dependența apare dintr-o varietate de ritualuri și asocieri senzoriale cu fumatul, întărite imediat de o doză de nicotină din țigară. Există ghiduri de recomandări utile clinicienilor pentru a putea să ajute fumătorul în încercarea de a se lăsa de fumat. Aceste strategii implică o varietate de acțiuni: întrebarea pacientului dacă fumează sau nu și sfătuirea să renunțe, stabilirea gradului de dorință al pacientului de a renunța, asistența în încercarea de a renunța și urmărirea ulterioară a pacientului. Intervențiile trebuie să fie adaptate conform stadiului în care se află pacientul. În prezent, sunt disponibili o serie de agenți farmacologici, folosiți în tratamentul dependenței de nicotină, incluzând tratamentul substitutiv cu nicotina și bupropionul, dovediți a crește procentul celor ce reușesc să renunțe la fumat, și să prelungească durata de abstinență. Eficiența tratamentului medicamentos crește când este dublat de consiliere și terapie comportamentală.

42. ROLUL VASCULATURII ÎN ULCERELE PICIORULUI DIABETIC

Lawrence Chukwudi NWABUDIKE

Ulcerele piciorului diabetic sunt o complicație de temut a diabetului zaharat, ele putând fi neuropate, ischemice sau neuroischemice. Factorii etiologici asociați sunt infecția și traumatismul. Ischemia este un factor etiologic în 30,4% din cazurile noastre. Părțile piciorului fără circulație colaterală, cum ar fi degetele, sunt cele mai frecvent afectate. 76,0% din cazurile cu ulcere unice și 85,7% din cazurile cu ulcere multiple au avut leziuni la acest nivel. Patogeneza ischemiei la nivelul membrelor inferioare include lezarea nervilor simpatici, care determină rigiditatea pereților vasculari, scleroza medială vasculară (SMV) și deschiderea șunturilor arteriovenoase cu ocolirea circulației capilare. Factorii direcți, cum ar fi ateroscleroza, stenoza și modificările microvasculare (scărerea presiunii sanguine la nivelul gleznelor și degetelor, diminuarea fluxului sanguin capilar și a presiunii parțiale a oxigenului) predispun la ischemie. Trauma, infecția și modificările trofice contribuie la producerea ulcerelor la nivelul picioarelor, în condiții de ischemie.

43. PICIORUL DIABETIC – VASCULOPATIE *VERSUS* NEUROPATIE

Ion VEREANU, Traian PĂTRAȘCU

Piciorul diabetic este o complicație severă, de multe ori invalidantă și relativ frecventă a diabetului (15%). Patogenia complexă a acestei complicații explică caracterul extrem de variat al afecțiunii, fapt care are drept consecință o paletă largă de intervenții chirurgicale. Materialul prezentat face, pe baza unui studiu clinic, analiza comparativă a leziunilor consecutive vasculopatiei și neuropatiei diabetice cu implicațiile pe care le au în definirea tabloului clinic și a alegerii metodei adecvate de tratament chirurgical.

Cercetarea cuprinde un lot de 200 de bolnavi cu complicații chirurgicale ale piciorului diabetic internați în servicul de chirurgie Cantacuzino în anul 2001. Aprecierea participării factorilor patogenici în determinismul cazurilor s-a făcut pe baza examenului clinic și al examenelor paraclinice, ecografie Doppler, oscilometrie, arteriografie. Componenta ischemică este prezentă în mare parte din cazuri (peste 60% sub formă dominantă sau mixtă). În cadrul tabloului lezional este evidentă predominența gangrenei în piciorul de tip ischemic (71%) față de cel neuropat (14%). Analiza leziunilor de operație practicate indică o gamă largă de intervenții în ambele leziuni patogenice, dar este evidentă prevalența amputațiilor majore pentru piciorul ischemic.

Evoluția postoperatorie a fost favorabilă în 80–90% din cazuri în toate tipurile patogenice; eșecurile (amputații succesive) au predominat în cazurile cu determinism vascular. Toți bolnavii operați pentru leziuni ale piciorului diabetic trebuie să rămână însă sub supravegherea cabinetelor specializate pentru a putea preveni și surprinde la timp posibila reapariție de complicații succesive.

44. FACTORII DE RISC MODIFICABILI ȘI RECONSTRUCȚIA CHIRURGICALĂ ÎN ATEROSCLEROZA MEMBRELOR INFERIOARE LA PACIENȚII DIABETICI

Viorel ȘERBAN, Mihai IONAC, Adrian VLAD, Mihaela ROȘU, Alexandra SIMA

Factorii de risc cunoscuți pentru boala coronariană contribuie, în egală măsură, și la apariția arteriopatiei aterosclerotice a membrelor inferioare. Unii dintre aceștia (dislipidemiile, fumatul, hipertensiunea arterială, diabetul zaharat, alimentația „aterogenă", sedentarismul, obezitatea, hiperhomocisteinemia, inflamația, microalbuminuria) pot fi influențați prin mijloace farmacologice și/sau modificarea stilului de viață, întârziind astfel instalarea manifestărilor clinice ale aterosclerozei.

În anumite situații, factorii de risc se pot cumula la o singură persoană, constituind așa-numitul „sindrom X metabolic", situație în care probabilitatea apariției aterosclerozei este crescută.

Odată cu procesul de îmbătrânire a populației, caracteristic zilelor noastre, în condițiile unui mod de viață de multe ori nesănătos, incidența arteriopatiei membrelor inferioare se situează pe o curbă ascendentă. În unele situații, această afecțiune ridică probleme terapeutice mari medicului practician, putând duce la amputații înalte, deosebit de traumatizante pentru pacient și cu implicații sociale majore.

Piciorul diabetic constituie o entitate clinică distinctă de arteriopatia aterosclerotică a membrelor inferioare. În producerea lui, pe lângă ischemia dată de ateroscleroză, intervin neuropatia, infecția și disfuncția microcirculatorie.

Progresele tehnice înregistrate permit diagnosticarea precoce și corectarea leziunilor vasculare cauzatoare de ischemie, limitându-se astfel numărul și dimensiunea amputațiilor.

Chirurgia de reconstrucție arterială reprezintă „standardul de aur" pentru îmbunătățirea fluxului sanguin la nivelul membrului ischemic. În mod curent se folosesc trei tehnici de revascularizare:

1. bypass-ul distal;
2. bypass-ul secvențial;
3. angioplastia transluminală percutană, combinată cu bypass-ul distal.

Este necesar ca la aceste proceduri să se adauge tratamentul agresiv al infecțiilor concomitente, debridări tisulare, plastii de tegument și corectarea eventualelor anomalii osoase. În anumite situații se impune și efectuarea unor amputații, care sunt de obicei limitate ca întindere.

45. ASPECTE OFTALMOLOGICE ALE DIABETULUI ZAHARAT

Benone CÂRSTOCEA, Luiza Otilia GAFENCU

Retinopatia diabetică, complicație majoră a diabetului zaharat, reprezintă, alături de degenerescența maculară senilă, una din primele cauze de pierdere definitivă a vederii. Diagnosticul precoce al diabetului zaharat, examenele de specialitate periodice, precum și colaborarea perfectă dintre diabetolog, medicul de familie și oftalmolog pot asigura atât o evoluție favorabilă a bolii pe o perioadă lungă de timp, precum și prevenirea complicațiilor invalidante cum este scăderea vederii.

Conform statisticilor, riscul de apariție a retinopatiei diabetice este de aproximativ 50% la bolnavii cu evoluție a bolii de 15 ani sau mai mult. Doar 30% dintre aceștia evoluează către forma severă a retinopatiei diabetice. Oricum, riscul este mai mare la pacienții suferind de diabet zaharat tip 1 comparativ cu cei de tip 2.

Este important de subliniat faptul că toate structurile oculare suferă în cazul diabetului zaharat, semnele precoce de boală fiind, de multe ori, ignorate sau considerate simptome minore.

De-a lungul anilor au fost emise o serie de ipoteze etiologice privitoare la retinopatia diabetică. În prezent, se consideră că alterarea activității aldozoreductazei și eliberarea factorilor angiogenetici reprezintă principalele mecanisme implicate în apariția modificărilor de tip patologic la nivel retinian.

Tratamentul retinopatiei diabetice este complex, medicamentos, fizic sau chirurgical, şi diferă în funcţie de stadiul bolii. Dacă în fazele precoce ale acesteia atitudinea terapeutică pune accent pe echilibrarea glicemiei, în stadiile mai avansate se indică fotocoagularea laser sau intervenţia chirurgicală. Tratamentul laser permite stabilizarea bolii şi previne apariţia complicaţiilor. Tratamentul chirurgical se pretează cazurilor de retinopatie diabetică proliferantă, cu complicaţii majore.

O complicaţie importantă a diabetului zaharat la nivel ocular o reprezintă opacifierea cristalinului.Tratamentul acesteia este exclusiv chirurgical.

Glaucomul secundar neovascular reprezintă una din dramele cu care se confruntă oftalmologul. De multe ori acesta se dezvoltă în ciuda tuturor manevrelor preventive sau terapeutice, fizice sau chirurgicale. Din nefericire, evoluţia sa duce inevitabil către orbire.

O observaţie aparte o constituie apariţia glaucomului de tip pseudoexfoliativ la bolnavii cu fotocoagulare retiniană în antecedente.

46. IMPLICAREA VASCULARĂ CUTANATĂ ÎN DIABETUL ZAHARAT

Ioan NEDELCU, Irina MĂRGĂRITESCU, Laura-Elena NEDELCU

Incidenţa manifestărilor cutaneo-mucoase în diabetul zaharat a fost apreciată în mod diferit. Mecanismele fiziopatologice responsabile de manifestările cutaneo-mucoase din diabetul zaharat sunt similare cu cele implicate în fiziopatologia generală a diabetului zaharat.

Dermopatia diabetică

A fost observată existenţa unei corelaţii între prezenţa dermopatiei diabetice şi severitatea diabetului, precum şi între tratamentul antidiabetic şi evoluţia dermopatiei diabetice.

În leziunile mai vechi de dermopatie diabetică sunt descrise infiltratele inflamatorii perivasculare, cu acumularea de limfocite. Se impune diagnosticul diferenţial cu necrobioza lipoidică, în special când leziunile sunt localizate la membrele inferioare.

Eritroza facială

Acest aspect clinic defineşte situaţia unui pacient cu diabet zaharat clinic manifest, cu evoluţie de lungă durată. Iniţial considerată apanajul exclusiv al diabetului zaharat clinic manifest, a fost demonstrată implicarea diabetului latent; este considerată o manifestare predilectă a diabetului juvenil.

Dermatita purpurică a membrelor inferioare

Leziunile purpurice şi pigmentarea hemosideremică se combină cu manifestările clinice ale dermopatiei diabetice, prezentând un tablou clinic polimorf, înalt evocator pentru diagnostic.

Necroze cutanate diabetice

Gangrena diabetică este o manifestare clinică frecventă la pacienţii diabetici cu angiopatie avansată.

Telangiectaziile repliului unghial

Patul unghial este folosit pentru investigaţiile *in vivo*, prin capilaroscopie, ale microcirculaţiei cutanate. Studiile capilaroscopice confirmă că dilataţiile venoase periunghiale pot fi un indicator de valoare în studierea microangiopatiei funcţionale, în timp ce sinuozităţile venulare oferă informaţii preţioase asupra microangiopatiei diabetice structurale. Dilatările venoase periunghiale constituie un bun indicator al microangiopatiei diabetice, dar este necesară diferenţierea de dilatările venoase periunghiale din bolile de colagen.

Eritemul erisipeloid al diabeticilor

Semnificaţia prognostică şi evolutivă a eritemului erisipeloid diabetic este severă pentru evoluţia pacientului în viitorul apropiat, fiind posibil să apară gangrene diabetice mai mult sau mai puţin extinse.

Necrobioza lipoidică a diabeticilor

Uzual, plăcile de necrobioză lipoidică diabetică sunt asimptomatice, dar în cazuri rare pacienţii pot acuza prurit, arsuri, hipo sau hipersensibilitate la atingere, hipohidroză etc.

Evoluţia plăcilor de necrobioză lipoidică este lent progresivă, cu acoperirea unor suprafeţe extensive, generând un aspect clinic impresionant. Chiar dacă evoluţia necrobiozei lipoidice diabetice pare să fie independentă de nivelurile glicemiei şi de tratamentul antidiabetic, studii recente au arătat că un tratament eficace al diabetului zaharat poate reduce aspectul lezional al necrobiozei lipoidice.

Relaţia dintre necrobioza lipoidică şi diabetul zaharat clinic manifest poate fi dovedită în 60–65% din cazuri. 90% din pacienţii cu necrobioză lipoidică fără diabet zaharat clinic manifest prezintă un răspuns modificat la testul de toleranţă la glucoză, cu sau fără sensibilizare cu cortizon, sau au antecedente familiale semnificative de diabet. Pe baza unor argumente, precum incidenţa relativ joasă a necrobiozei lipoidice la pacienţii cu diabet zaharat, existenţa unui răspuns clinic bun la diferite tratamente fără efect asupra diabetului, asocierea necrobiozei lipoidice cu alte afecţiuni şi absenţa unei corelaţii între extensia şi expresia clinică a necrobiozei lipoidice şi gravitatea diabetului zaharat, considerăm că legătura directă dintre necrobioza lipoidică şi diabetul zaharat este cel puţin discutabilă.

SELECTED INDEX

A

Abciximab, 672, 675–677

Acid glycosaminoglycan, 353

Acidosis, 141, 143

ACTH, 378

Action potential, 348

Action stage, 692, 697

Action to control cardiovascular risk in diabetes (ACCORD), 423

Acupuncture, 699

Acute coronary syndrome (ACS), 670–677

Acute myocardial infarction (AMI), 485, 488–490, 492–494, 496–499, 501–511, 535, 541, 544, 547, 670, 671, 673–677

Adaptor protein-1 (AP-1), 52–55

Adenosine triphosphate (ATP), 140, 141

Adhesion molecule, 52, 53, 57, 180, 181, 184, 187, 248, 249, 251

Adipocyte, 37, 42, 43

Adipocyte, 3T3-L1, 158

Adiponectin, 212, 213, 309, 314

Adipose tissue, 196, 198

Adrenal insufficiency (Addison's disease), 376, 377

Adult treatment panel III (ATP III), 421, 427

Advanced glycation end-product (AGE), 21–25, 28, 29, 41, 42, 88, 89, 93, 96, 97, 105, 123, 130, 152, 207, 209, 210, 212, 213, 308, 378, 557–559, 569, 571, 579, 580, 581, 626, 636, 646, 647, 671

Advanced glycation end-product receptor (RAGE), 21, 22, 88, 89, 93, 96, 97, 105, 123, 210, 671

Advanced glycosylation end-product, *see advanced glycation end-product*

Advanced lipoxidation end-product, 22

Akinesis, 590, 594, 596

Albumin, 351–354

Albumin excretion rate, 235, 237, 239, 247, 250, 251

Albuminuria, 223, 390, 398, 448, 449, 457–459, 473, 626, 627, 629, 634, 635, 637–638

Aldose reductase (AR), 89, 90, 93–95, 100, 209, 646, 751, 760, 763

Aldose reductase inhibitor, 384

Aldosterone, 304, 306, 307, 312, 314

Alloxan, 73–75

Alopecia, 378

Alpha-1 adrenergic blocker, 464

α_1-blocker, 434

$\alpha2\beta1$ integrin, 93, 95

Altered insulin signaling, 196

Amadori product (AP), 152

Ambulatory blood pressure monitoring (ABPM), 328, 333, 473–479

Amino peptidase, 306

Amputation, 5, 7, 716, 718, 720, 722–725, 735–737, 743, 744

Anastomosis, 739, 743

Angiography, 604

Angiopathy, 646

Angiotensin, 85, 86, 89, 96

Angiotensin
I, 304–306, 314
II, 24, 30, 208, 225, 226, 304–310, 312–314, 446, 447, 452, 458, 570, 574, 575, 577–579, 581
converting enzyme (ACE), 83, 85, 96, 208, 209, 213–215, 226, 238, 247, 252, 304–309, 314, 453, 454, 456
converting enzyme inhibitor (ACEI), 209, 213–215, 226, 228, 304, 306–314, 382, 383, 432, 434, 452, 454–456, 458–461, 465, 529, 530, 546–549, 551, 552
receptor, 85, 86, 90, 305, 311
receptor blocker (ARB), 213, 214, 226, 251–253, 304, 310, 311, 455, 458
type 1 receptor, 226, 456, 457
type 2 receptor, 226, 456, 457

Angiotensinogen (AGT), 85, 86, 96, 304–306

Anionic charge, 627, 635, 638

Antibiotic therapy, 724

Antihypertensive and lipid lowering treatment to prevent heart attack trial (ALLHAT), 434

Antioxidant, 646, 647, 649

Antioxidant status, 357, 358

Aortic stiffness, 297, 298

Apolipoprotein, 88, 100, 102, 105, 354–356, 361

Apolipoprotein
AI, 37, 41
AII, 37
CIII, 37, 42, 56, 57
E, 39, 41, 43

Apoptosis, 557, 558, 570, 574–580